Basic and Clinical Anatomy of the

SPINE, SPINAL CORD, AND ANS

Basic and Clinical Anatomy of the

SPINE, SPINAL CORD, AND ANS

SECOND EDITION

GREGORY D. CRAMER, D.C., Ph.D.
Professor, Department of Anatomy
Professor and Dean
Department of Research
National University of Health Sciences
Lombard, Illinois

SUSAN A. DARBY, Ph.D.
Professor
Department of Anatomy
National University of Health Sciences
Lombard, Illinois

Illustrators
Theodore G. Huff, B.A., M.F.A.
Sally A. Cummings, M.A., M.S.

Photographer
Ron Mensching, B.S.

With 475 illustrations

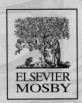

ELSEVIER
MOSBY

ELSEVIER
MOSBY
11830 Westline Industrial Drive
St. Louis, Missouri 63146

Basic and Clinical Anatomy of the Spine, Spinal Cord, and ANS, Second Edition
Copyright © 2005, 1995 by Mosby, Inc.

NOTICE

Knowledge and best practice in this field are constantly changing. As new research and experience broaden our knowledge, changes in practice, treatment and drug therapy may become necessary or appropriate. Readers are advised to check the most current information provided (i) on procedures featured or (ii) by the manufacturer of each product to be administered, to verify the recommended dose or formula, the method and duration of administration, and contraindications. It is the responsibility of the practitioner, relying on his or her own experience and knowledge of the patient, to make diagnoses, to determine dosages and the best treatment for each individual patient, and to take all appropriate safety precautions. To the fullest extent of the law, neither the Publisher nor the Authors assumes any liability for any injury and/or damage to persons or property arising out of or related to any use of the material contained in this book.

Library of Congress Cataloging-in-Publication Data

Cramer, Gregory D.
  Basic and clinical anatomy of the spine, spinal cord, and ANS/Gregory D. Cramer,
Susan A. Darby; illustrator, Sally A. Cummings; photographer, Ron Mensching – 2nd ed.
    p.; cm.
  Includes bibliographical references and index.
  ISBN-13: 978-0-323-02649-9 ISBN-10: 0-323-02649-4
  1. Spinal cord–Anatomy. 2. Spine–Anatomy. 3. Automatic nervous system–Anatomy.
  I. Title: Spine, spinal cord, and ANS. II. Darby, Susan A. III–Title.
    [DNLM: 1. Spinal Cord–anatomy & histology. 2. Autonomic Nervous System–anatomy
  & histology. WL 400 C889b 2005]
  QM465.C73 2005
  611′.82–dc22

                                                                2005047328

Publishing Director: Linda Duncan
Editor: Kathy Falk
Managing Editor: Christie Hart
Publishing Services Manager: Patricia Tannian
Project Manager: Sharon Corell
Designer: Jyotika Shroff

ISBN-13: 978-0-323-02649-9
ISBN-10: 0-323-02649-4

Printed in China
Last digit is the print number: 9 8 7 6 5 4

Contributors

WILLIAM E. BACHOP, PH.D.
Professor Emeritus
Department of Anatomy
National University of Health Sciences
Lombard, Illinois

BARCLAY W. BAKKUM, D.C., Ph.D.
Professor and Chairman
Department of Anatomy
National University of Health Sciences
Lombard, Illinois

ROBERT J. FRYSZTAK, Ph.D.
Associate Professor
Department of Physiology and Biochemistry
National University of Health Sciences
Lombard, Illinois

CHAE-SONG RO, M.D., Ph.D.
Associate Professor (Deceased)
Department of Anatomy
National University of Health Sciences
Lombard, Illinois

PETER C. STATHOPOULOS, M.Ed., M.S., D.C.
Professor (Retired)
Department of Anatomy
National University of Health Sciences
Lombard, Illinois

SHI-WEI YU, M.D.
Electron Microscopist
Pathology Department
Loyola University Medical Center
Maywood, Illinois

To

Chris and David
Dave, Katherine, and Jason

Thank you for your invaluable support, patience, and encouragement throughout the writing of the first and second editions of this text.

Forewords

In the decade since publication of the first edition of *Basic and Clinical Anatomy of the Spine, Spinal Cord, and ANS* (autonomic nervous system), this wonderful book by Cramer and Darby has remained the seminal text on the subject. With its extensive and meticulous referencing of original work and beautifully illustrative figures and photographs, it remains one of the most valuable and most used books on my shelf. Of course, as time passes, there is an evolution in concepts that mandates a revision. The second edition does this and more, comprehensively revisiting the topics addressed in the first edition while adding an important chapter on the pediatric spine and additional material on scoliosis and many other clinical conditions.

As I pointed out in the foreword to the first edition, this book fills a need for all practitioners involved in the care of patients with disorders of the spine. The book provides an exceptional basis for a course on spinal anatomy for students of physical medicine, chiropractic, and osteopathy. However, it is also detailed enough to fill a need for residents and provides an exceptional resource for the practicing spine specialist. I am unaware of any other text with the breadth and depth offered by this text, which, nevertheless, maintains a balance of readability and clinical relevance. The illustrations and photographs are a particular strength of the book. They have been useful to me on many occasions in explaining principles of clinical anatomy of the spine. The improvement in images resulting from technological advances since publication of the first edition can only serve to enhance the utility of the figures. I have no doubt that *Basic and Clinical Anatomy of the Spine, Spinal Cord, and ANS* will be the classic text on spinal and autonomic anatomy for the coming decade and into many future editions.

RAND S. SWENSON, D.C., M.D., Ph.D.
Associate Professor of Anatomy and Medicine
(Neurology)
Dartmouth Medical School
Hanover, New Hampshire

Drs. Cramer and Darby, with the able assistance of colleagues in Anatomy and Physiology at National University of Health Sciences, have updated and improved a remarkable resource for both clinicians and students.

The second edition of *Basic and Clinical Anatomy of the Spine, Spinal Cord, and ANS* is designed to facilitate a learner's understanding of important anatomic concepts and their relationship to clinical practice. The most important aspects of this book include comprehensive coverage of spinal anatomy and related neuroanatomy, with clear explanations of structural relationships; the extensive use of illustrations and photographs to enhance anatomic detail; and numerous well-referenced clinical pearls that relate anatomy to clinical care.

Several hundred pages of important new text and countless new MRI and CT scans, illustrations, and photographs have been added to the new edition. Of particular interest is the new chapter on the pediatric spine. The chapter on the mechanisms of pain of spinal origin has increased in size with the addition of new research, and the chapter on the biology of the intervertebral disc also contains significant new research.

Anatomy faculty and students will find that this book goes beyond a mere description of the structure of the spine and nervous system. It sets out to explain how a structure develops, to uncover patterns of distribution, and to foster an appreciation of the morphologic basis of variation. Anatomic facts are presented within the context of their mutual relationships and clinical relevance. This inevitably leads to comprehension of the underlying principles involved and facilitates anatomic reasoning and easier acquisition of additional morphologic facts and concepts.

For the clinician, this book provides essential background knowledge for the safe and appropriate care of patients with neuromusculoskeletal disorders of the spine. Valuable chapters have been included on the surface anatomy of the back, muscles that influence the spine, pain of spinal origin, and the microscopic anatomy of the zygapophyseal joints, intervertebral discs, and other tissues. Special emphasis is placed on structures that may be affected by manual spinal techniques. Each chapter is extensively referenced with new citations. I highly recommend this invaluable resource to all students and practitioners who regularly care for patients with spinal disorders.

ALAN H. ADAMS, M.S., D.C.
Vice President of
Academic Affairs and
Program Development
Texas Chiropractic College
Pasadena, Texas

Preface for the First Edition

Current anatomy texts that describe the spine, spinal cord, and autonomic nervous system frequently discuss this material in a rather general way. Often the pages devoted to these topics are scattered throughout the text, deemphasized, or relegated to later chapters. At the other end of the spectrum, several highly specialized texts on spinal anatomy describe a single region of the spine. In some instances even subregions of the vertebral column, such as the intervertebral discs or intervertebral foramina, become the sole topic of the text. These general and specialized texts both serve important purposes. However, we felt that a need existed for a cohesive, well-illustrated text covering spinal anatomy, which included the neuroanatomy of the spinal cord and the autonomic nervous system as well.

The purpose of this book is threefold:

- To provide an accurate and complete text for students studying the spine, spinal cord, and autonomic nervous system.
- To serve as a reliable reference to spinal anatomy and related neuroanatomy for clinicians and researchers.
- To help bridge the gap between the basic science of anatomy and the applied anatomy of clinical practice.

To accomplish the first purpose, the anatomy of the spine, spinal cord, and autonomic nervous system is organized with both the student and the clinician in mind. The first chapter on surface anatomy provides both the neophyte and the seasoned clinician with a valuable resource—a comprehensive view of surface landmarks and the vertebral levels of clinically relevant structures. General concepts also are emphasized throughout the book through many illustrations and photographs to help the reader establish a three-dimensional image of the spine, spinal cord, and autonomic nervous system.

The second purpose of the text was accomplished with a thorough search of the current literature in spinal anatomy, and the results of many of these clinically relevant studies are included in the text. Even though the science of anatomy is very old, a surprisingly large number of studies related to spinal anatomy continue to appear in the scientific literature. The past 25 years have also seen an explosion of new neuroanatomic information.

Including the results of recent investigative studies also provided a means by which the third objective of this book was attained. This objective was to serve as a bridge between the basic science of anatomy and the applied anatomy of clinical practice. Throughout the text the results of clinically relevant research have been presented with a red rule running beside them, thus providing a rapid reference to this clinically applicable information. In addition, a chapter on pain generators and pain pathways of the back has been included (Chapter 11). This chapter focuses on those structures that can be a source of back pain and details the manner by which the resulting nociceptive stimuli are transmitted and perceived by the patient.

Numerous magnetic resonance imaging scans have been included throughout this text. The purpose of these scans is not only to demonstrate clinically relevant anatomy, but also to aid the unfamiliar reader beginning the exciting process of learning cross-sectional spinal anatomy, which is often clearly demonstrated on these scans.

This book is designed to serve the needs and interests of many groups. The basic anatomy and concepts should be an aid to beginning students of spinal anatomy, whether they be allopathic, osteopathic, chiropractic, or physical therapy students. The text should also provide a ready source for those in clinical practice desiring a rapid reference on a specific topic related to the spine, since the book is arranged topically and exhaustively indexed. Finally, the inclusion of the results of recent research studies, as well as discussions on clinically related topics, will hopefully spark interest and highlight the importance of the spine for the new students, as well as the experienced individual.

GREGORY D. CRAMER

SUSAN A. DARBY

Preface for the Second Edition

We are very grateful for the warm reception given the first edition by professionals in many different disciplines. Those familiar with the first edition will find that this edition has kept the features that were well received. We are also grateful for the suggestions offered by those who read the first edition, and we have worked diligently to incorporate all of these suggestions into the second. This edition is significantly different from the first. The primary changes are related to the addition of new written material, photographs, and illustrations. More than 8,000 papers of interest were identified for this edition. Of these, more than 2,000 were retrieved. Summaries of the results of more than 700 of the retrieved papers that were identified as having relevant information appear in the second edition. The majority of these additions have significant clinical relevance. As a result, most of the chapters have been completely revamped and significantly updated. Important sections on the clinical anatomy of the vertebral artery (Chapter 5) and scoliosis (Chapter 6) have been added. Chapter 9 has an entirely new section on the motor control of movements, and Chapter 10 includes much new material on the autonomic innervation of the immune system, the role of the autonomic nervous system (ANS) in pain perception and specific pain syndromes, and neurotransmission. Chapter 11 has more than doubled in size, with a great deal of new, clinically relevant research on the mechanisms of pain of spinal origin being summarized for the reader. Chapter 12 was completely reorganized with many new x-rays and illustrations added to demonstrate the most common developmental anomalies. Chapter 13, which discusses the pediatric spine, is new and provides important and clinically relevant information. The photographs of anatomic material in this chapter that are provided by Dr. Shi-Wei Yu are unique and add significant value to the presentation of the anatomy of the pediatric spine. Chapter 14 has been dramatically changed by adding significant sections on the biology of the intervertebral disc and on the topic of intervertebral disc degeneration—the focus of a great deal of research over the past 10 years. In addition, sections on the microscopic anatomy of other spinal tissues (e.g., nerve, bone, muscle, ligaments, and other connective tissues) have been added to this chapter to allow the book to be used as a complete text of spinal anatomy (i.e., all topics needed to teach spinal anatomy are now covered in the text). The red-lining remains in the second edition, allowing doctors of chiropractic, medicine (orthopedic surgeons, neurologists, radiologists, neurosurgeons, head and neck surgeons, physiatrists, general practitioners treating back pain), physical therapists, and other health practitioners to quickly access detailed summaries of the literature on topics of particular clinical relevance.

Finally, more than 170 new photographs and illustrations have been added to the second edition. The vast majority of magnetic resonance imaging and computed tomography scans of the first edition have been replaced with similar images produced from new, higher resolution scanners. Some additional photographs and illustrations have been added to further clarify material presented in the first edition; however, most of the new photographs and illustrations are related to material that has been added to the second edition.

Our hope is that the result of this group effort is a text that effectively serves many important audiences (students of chiropractic, physical therapy, and occupational therapy; orthopedic residents; and practicing physicians and residents of the specialties listed)—audiences to which we are very grateful.

GREGORY D. CRAMER
SUSAN A. DARBY

Introduction

This book has been organized with two groups of readers in mind: those studying the spine for the first time, and those clinicians and researchers who have previously studied the spine in detail. Therefore we have accepted the daunting task of designing a book to act as a source of reference and as a book that is "readable." To this end an outline has been included at the beginning of each chapter. This format should help the reader organize his or her thoughts before beginning the chapter and also provide a quick reference to the material of interest. A complete subject index is also included at the end of the text for rapid referencing. In addition, items of particular clinical relevance and the results of clinically relevant research appear with a red rule beside the material throughout the book. This highlighting procedure is meant to aid students and clinicians alike in focusing on areas that are thought to be of particular current importance in the detection of pathologic conditions or in the treatment of disorders of the spine, spinal cord, and autonomic nervous system. Discussions of the clinical relevance of anatomic structures are included to relate anatomy to clinical practice as efficiently as possible.

Chapter 1 discusses surface anatomy. It contains information useful not only to the student who has yet to palpate his or her first patient, but also to the clinician who examines patients on a daily basis. Chapters 2 and 3 relate the general characteristics of the spine and spinal cord, using a basic approach. These chapters are directed primarily to the beginning student. A quick review of these chapters, with attention focused on the sections highlighted by a red rule, should also be of benefit to the more advanced student. Chapter 2 includes a section on advanced diagnostic imaging. This section is provided for the individual who does not routinely view computed tomography and magnetic resonance imaging scans. A brief description of the strengths and weaknesses of both imaging modalities and a concise overview of other less frequently used advanced imaging procedures are included. Chapters 3 and 4 relate soft tissues to the "bones" by describing the spinal cord and its meningeal coverings, and the muscles that surround and influence the spine. This material is followed by a detailed study of the regional anatomy of the spine in Chapters 5 through 8. These chapters also include information concerning the ligamentous tissues of the spine. A more thorough presentation of the anatomy of the spinal cord and autonomic nervous system is found in Chapters 9 and 10, and the development (from inception to adulthood) and histologic makeup of the spine and spinal cord are found in Chapters 12 through 14.

It should be noted that the first four chapters provide the groundwork for later chapters that are more detailed and contain additional information with specific clinical relevance. Therefore certain material is occasionally discussed more than once. For example, Chapters 2 and 3 are concerned with general characteristics of the spine and spinal cord, with a discussion of the various components of a typical vertebra, the vertebral canal, and the spinal cord within the canal. These structures are discussed again regionally (Chapters 5 through 8) to a much greater depth to explore their relative importance and clinical significance in each region of the spine and to appreciate the neuroanatomic connections within the spinal cord (Chapter 9).

Chapter 11 is devoted to pain producers (those structures that receive nociceptive innervation), the mechanisms and neuroanatomic pathways of nociception from spinal structures, and the peripheral, spinal, and supraspinal modulation of these impulses. This chapter is designed for readers who have already completed study in spinal anatomy and neuroanatomy. Chapter 12 discusses the development of the spine and is designed for use by students studying spinal anatomy and for clinicians who wish to refresh their knowledge of the development of the spine and spinal cord. Chapter 13 covers the pediatric spine and should be useful to all readers. Chapter 14 describes the microscopic anatomy of the zygapophyseal joints, intervertebral discs, and all other spine-related tissues. Since much of the current research on the spine is focused at the tissue, cellular, and subcellular levels, both students and clinicians should find this chapter useful at some point in their careers. Because of the rather specialized nature of the last four topics, they have been positioned at the end of the book.

CLARIFICATION OF ABBREVIATIONS AND TERMS

Vertebral levels are frequently abbreviated throughout this text. The initials C, T, and L are used to abbreviate cervical, thoracic, and lumbar, respectively. Vertebral levels can then be easily identified by placing the appropriate number after the abbreviated region. For example, "T7" is frequently used rather than "the seventh thoracic vertebra."

In addition, some potentially confusing terminology should be clarified. Throughout this text the term **kyphosis** is used when referring to a spinal curve that is concave anteriorly, and the term **lordosis** is used for a curve that is concave posteriorly. The term **hyperlordosis** refers to an accentuation of a lordosis beyond what is usually accepted as normal, and the term **hyperkyphosis** is used for an accentuation of a kyphosis beyond the range of normal. This is in contrast to the terminology of some texts that refer to normal spinal curves as being "concave anteriorly" or "concave posteriorly" and reserve the terms "kyphosis" and "lordosis" for curves that are deeper than normal. Although both sets of terminology are correct, the prior one was chosen for this text because we felt that this terminology would lend the most clarity to subsequent discussions.

Finally, we hope that you, the reader, believe as we do that the long-standing interest of clinicians in the anatomic sciences is not an accident. Greater awareness of structure leads to a keener perception of function, and an increased understanding of pathologic conditions is the natural consequence. This results in a better comprehension of current therapeutic approaches and the development of new treatment procedures based upon a scientific foundation. Therefore astute clinicians keep an eye toward developments in the structural sciences, being aware that their concepts of human mechanisms may be influenced by new discoveries in these disciplines. Whenever new information about the causes underlying dysfunction is available, new therapeutic approaches are sure to follow, and clinicians who have kept abreast of these recent discoveries will find themselves leaders in their field.

Acknowledgments

This project would not have been possible had it not been for the support of the members of the administration, faculty, students, and staff of the National University of Health Sciences, who allowed us the time and facilities necessary to review the literature, write several drafts of text, and work on the development of supporting figures. We greatly appreciate their support of, and in some instances commitment to, this work.

In addition, many people have helped with the production of this book. We would like to take this opportunity to thank those who helped with proofreading portions of various drafts of the first and second editions of this work and whose suggestions were extremely helpful in the development of the final manuscripts. These people include Robert Appleyard, Ph.D.; Joe Cantu, D.C.; Jim Christiansen, Ph.D.; John DeMatte, D.C.; Richard Dorsett, D.C.; Kris Gongaware, D.C.; James McKay, D.C.; Michael Kiely, Ph.D.; Allan Mathieu; Carol Muehleman, Ph.D.; Ken Nolson, D.C.; and Nancy Steinke, M.S. A special thanks to Lynn Zoufal who spent countless hours keying in editorial changes to the manuscripts.

We would also like to thank Patrick W. Frank for his beautiful dissections of the muscles of the back, which appear in Chapter 4. The work of Victoria Hyzny and Terese Black in the dissections that appear in Chapters 3, 5, 9, and 10 is greatly appreciated. The inexhaustible support of Joshua W. Little, who performed countless literature searches and monitored the files for the literature, was extremely valuable. Anna M. Rodecki, Kim Anderson, Terese Black, Michelle Steinys, D.C., and Gina Sirchio also assisted with searching the literature and compiling the reference lists, and we thank them. We thank Judy Pocius, Sheila Meadows, and Terese Black for organizational help with photographs and illustrations. We are also grateful for the computer graphics added by Dino Juarez to several of the magnetic resonance imaging scans found in Chapters 11 and 13.

The magnetic resonance imaging scans, computed tomograms, and x-ray films were graciously provided by Dennis Skogsbergh, D.C., DABCO, DACBR, of the Texas Back Institute. Many of the x-rays of spinal pathology and congenital anomalies were provided by Jeffery A. Rich, D.C., DACBR, Chairman of the Department of Diagnostic Imaging at the National University of Health Sciences. Dr. Rich also made significant contributions to the section on Advanced Diagnostic Imaging in Chapter 2. We would like to thank both of them for their contributions to this text. Where possible, diagnostic images are presented in a larger format than in the first edition (thank you for the suggestion, Dr. Barber).

We thank Michael L. Kiely, Ph.D., for his review of the entire manuscript for the first edition. We also appreciate the work and patience of the publishing staff at Elsevier Inc., particularly that of the executive editors: James Shanahan and Martha Sasser for the first edition, and Christie Hart for the second edition.

We would also like to gratefully acknowledge our parents, Dr. and Mrs. David Cramer and Mr. and Mrs. George Anderson, whose encouragement and early instruction gave us a strong desire to learn more and to help others.

The outstanding teaching of Drs. Joseph Janse, Delmas Allen, Liberato DiDio, William Potvin, Frank Saul, and Richard Yeasting will never be forgotten. Their example provided much of the motivation for beginning, and completing, this endeavor. Thank you all very much.

GREGORY D. CRAMER
SUSAN A. DARBY

Contents

PART III: SPINAL DEVELOPMENT, PEDIATRIC SPINE, AND MICROSCOPIC ANATOMY

PART I

CHARACTERISTICS OF THE SPINE AND SPINAL CORD

CHAPTER 1

Surface Anatomy of the Back and Vertebral Levels of Clinically Important Structures

Barclay W. Bakkum

Surface anatomy is defined as the configuration of the surface of the body, especially in relation to deeper parts. A thorough knowledge of surface anatomy is necessary for the proper performance of a physical examination. Information gathered by the eyes (inspection) and fingers (palpation) is often critical in the assessment of a patient. An understanding of the topography of the human body also allows the health care provider to locate the position of deep structures that may need further evaluation.

The locations of structures in reference to the surface of the body are always approximations, although it has been shown that reliability of locating spinal structures by palpation can be enhanced by training and experience (Byfield et al., 1992; Downey et al., 1999). Individual variations are common and are influenced by such factors as age, gender, posture, weight, and body type. Respiratory movements also can have marked effects on the locations of structures, especially those of the thorax. Determining the position of the contents of the abdomen can be particularly challenging, and the precise location of abdominal viscera can be established only by verification with appropriate diagnostic imaging procedures.

In keeping with the scope of this text, the surface anatomy included in this chapter is limited to the back.

Spinous processes and posterior bony landmarks are used as points of reference in the first part of the chapter. One reason for the use of these as landmarks is to help clinicians with examination and treatment of the back and spine when the patient is in the prone position. In addition, the vertebral levels of structures of the anterior neck and trunk, which are either visible by means of advanced imaging procedures (magnetic resonance imaging [MRI] or computed tomography [CT]) or palpable during physical examination, are included. Knowledge of the normal relationships between the viscera and the spine is becoming increasingly important in clinical practice, as clinicians are asked with greater frequency to interpret or review studies employing these advanced imaging procedures. On a more practical level, knowledge of these relationships helps the clinician quickly become oriented with the vertebral level of diagnostic images taken in the horizontal plane.

Because other texts discuss the location of organs with regard to abdominal regions or quadrants, that method of locating organs is not covered here.

THE BACK

The back, or dorsum, is the posterior part of the trunk and includes skin, muscles, vertebral column, spinal cord, and various nerves and blood vessels (Gardner, Gray, and O'Rahilly, 1975). The 24 movable vertebrae consist of, from superior to inferior, 7 cervical (C), 12 thoracic (or dorsal) (T), and 5 lumbar (L). Inferior to the lumbar vertebrae, five sacral vertebrae (S) fuse in the adult to form the sacrum. The lowermost three to five vertebrae fuse late in adult life to form the coccyx (Co).

Intervertebral discs are located between the anterior portions of the movable vertebrae and between L5 and the sacrum. There is no disc located between the occiput and C1 (atlas), or between C1 and C2 (axis). The discs are named for the vertebra located immediately above the disc; that is, the T6 disc is located between the T6 and T7 vertebrae.

Seven processes arise from the posterior portion of the typical vertebra. Several atypical vertebrae have variations in their anatomy and are discussed in Chapters 5, 6, and 7. The spinous process is a midline structure that is directed posteriorly and to a variable degree inferiorly. The transverse processes are a pair of lateral projections. The other four processes are articular, and each vertebra has a superior pair and an inferior pair. These processes are discussed in greater detail in Chapter 2.

The remainder of this chapter discusses visual landmarks of the back, palpatory landmarks of the back, spinal cord levels versus vertebral levels, and vertebral levels of structures in the anterior neck and trunk. This information enables the clinician to gain a thorough understanding of surface anatomy and serves as a reference for future patient assessment, both in the physical examination and through diagnostic imaging procedures, including x-ray examination, CT, and MRI.

Visual Landmarks of the Back

In the midline of the back is a longitudinal groove known as the median furrow (or sulcus) (Fig. 1-1). Superiorly it begins at the external occipital protuberance (EOP) (see the following discussion) and continues inferiorly as the gluteal (anal, natal, or cluneal) cleft (or crena ani) to the level of the S3 spinous tubercle, the remnants of the spinous process of S3. It is shallow in the lower cervical region and deepest in the lumbar region. The median furrow widens inferiorly to form an isosceles triangle with a line connecting the posterior superior iliac spines (PSISs) forming the base above, and the gluteal cleft forming the apex of the triangle below. The PSISs are often visible as a pair of dimples located 3 cm lateral to the midline at the level of the S2 spinous tubercle. The gluteal fold (or sulcus) is a horizontal skin fold extending laterally from the midline and roughly corresponds with the inferior border of the gluteus maximus muscle. This fold marks the lower extent of the buttock.

Several muscles are commonly visible in the back region. The trapezius is a large, flat, triangular muscle that originates in the midline from the EOP to the spinous process of T12 and inserts laterally onto the spine of the scapula. Its upper fibers form the "top of the shoulder," where the neck laterally blends into the thorax. The latissimus dorsi, extending from the region of the iliac crest to the posterior border of the axilla, forms the lateral border of the lower thoracic portion of the back. This muscle is especially noticeable when the upper

extremity is adducted against resistance. Between the trapezius medially and the latissimus dorsi laterally, the inferior angle of the scapula may be seen at approximately the level of the T7 spinous process. The erector spinae muscles form two large longitudinal masses in the lumbar region that extend approximately a handbreadth (10 cm) laterally from the midline. These muscle masses are responsible for the deepening of the median furrow in this region.

Besides these muscles, several bony landmarks usually are visible in the region of the back. The spinous process of C7 (the vertebra prominens) usually is visible in the lower cervical region. The spinous process of T1 often is visible also and actually is the most prominent spinous process in 30% to 40% of the population. When the patient's head is flexed, the spinous processes of C7 and T1, and often C6, usually are seen easily.

In the adult the vertebral column has several visible normal curves. In the cervical and lumbar regions the spine is anteriorly convex (lordotic), and in the thoracic and sacral areas it is posteriorly convex (kyphotic). Normally there is no lateral deviation of the spinal column, but such curvature is known as scoliosis when present. These curves are covered in more detail in Chapter 2.

Palpatory Landmarks of the Back

The following structures usually are not visible, but can be located on palpation. Some of the structures in this discussion of palpable landmarks cannot normally be felt, but their relation to landmarks that can be localized is given.

Cervical Region. The EOP (inion) is in the center of the occipital squama (Fig. 1-2). The superior nuchal line extends laterally from the EOP. The transverse process of the atlas may be found directly below and slightly anterior to the mastoid process of the temporal bone. Care must be taken when palpating this structure because of the relatively fragile styloid process of the temporal bone that lies just in front and the great auricular nerve that ascends in the fascia superficial to the C1 transverse process.

The spinous process of the axis is the first readily palpable bony structure in the posterior midline below the EOP (see Fig. 1-2), although according to Oliver and Middleditch (1991) the posterior tubercle of C1 may be palpable in some people between the EOP and the spinous process of C2. In the midline below the spinous process of the axis, the second prominent palpable structure is the spinous process of C7 or the vertebra prominens. In 60% to 70% of the population the vertebra prominens is the most prominent spinous process, whereas the spinous process of T1 is more evident in the

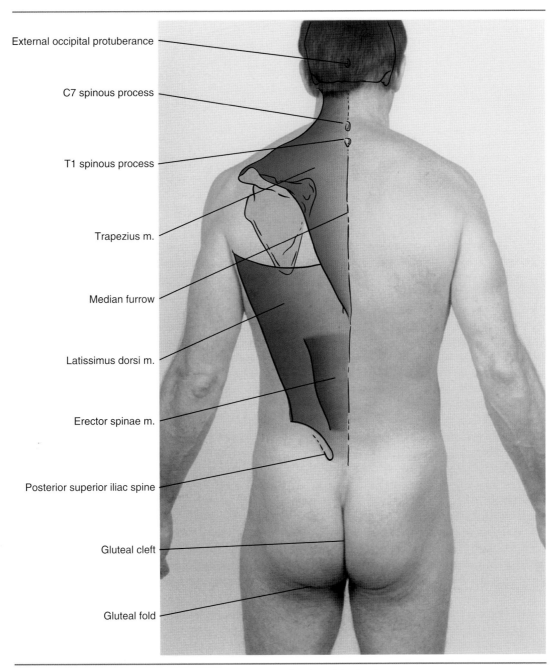

External occipital protuberance

C7 spinous process

T1 spinous process

Trapezius m.

Median furrow

Latissimus dorsi m.

Erector spinae m.

Posterior superior iliac spine

Gluteal cleft

Gluteal fold

FIG. 1-1   Visual landmarks of the back.

other 30% to 40%. The other cervical spinous processes are variably more difficult to palpate. The spinous process of C3 is the smallest and can be found at the same horizontal plane as the greater cornua of the hyoid bone. The spinous process of C6 is the last freely movable spinous process with flexion and extension of the neck. It is usually readily palpable with full flexion of the neck.

The zygapophysial joints between the articular processes of the cervical vertebrae (collectively known as the left and right articular pillars) can be found 1.5 cm lateral of the midline in the posterior neck. With the exception of C1, the tips of the transverse processes of the cervical vertebrae are not individually palpable, but the posterior tubercles of these processes form a bony resistance that may be palpated along a line from the tip of the mastoid process to the root of the neck, approximately a thumb breadth (2.5 cm) lateral of the midline. The anterior aspects of the transverse processes of the cervical vertebrae may be found in the groove

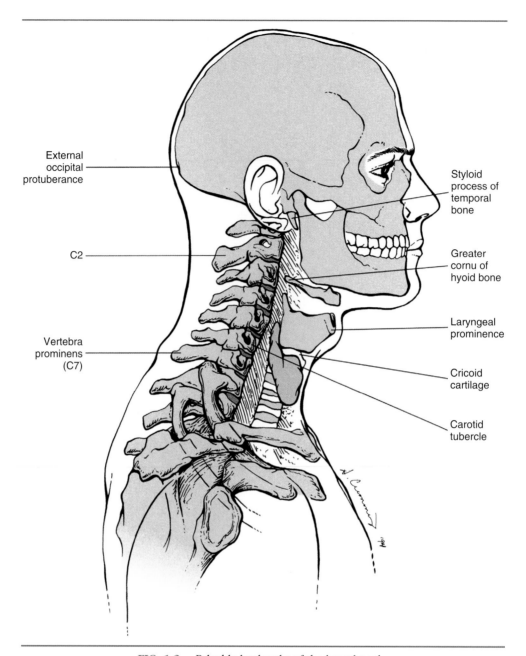

FIG. 1-2   Palpable landmarks of the lateral neck.

between the larynx and sternocleidomastoid muscle (SCM). It may be necessary to slightly retract the SCM laterally to palpate these structures. The anterior tubercles of the transverse processes of C6 are especially large and are known as the carotid tubercles (see Fig. 1-2). These may be palpated at the level of the cricoid cartilage. Care must be taken when locating the carotid tubercles (and the other cervical transverse processes), because they are in the proximity of the common carotid arteries, and they always should be palpated unilaterally.

Anteriorly, the superior border of the thyroid cartilage, forming the laryngeal prominence (Adam's apple)

in the midline, may be used to find the horizontal plane of the C4 disc. The body of C6 is located at the same horizontal level as the cricoid cartilage and the first tracheal ring.

Thoracic Region. The spinous process of T1 is the third prominent bony structure in the midline below the EOP; the spinous processes of C2 and C7 are the first and second, respectively (Fig. 1-3). The spinous process of T3 is located at the same horizontal plane as the root of the spine of the scapula. The spinous process of T4 is located at the extreme of the convexity of the thoracic kyphosis;

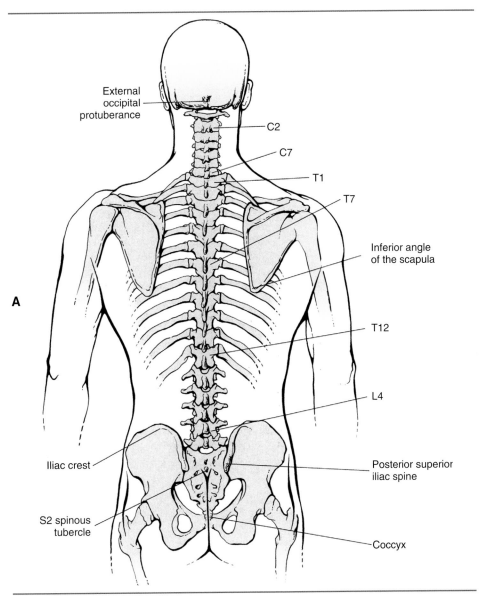

FIG. 1-3 Palpable landmarks of the back from, **A,** posterior view.

Continued

therefore it is usually the most prominent spinous process below the root of the neck.

When patients are standing or sitting with their upper extremities resting along the sides of their trunk, the inferior scapular angle usually is at the horizontal level of the spinous process of T7. This changes when the patient is lying prone with his or her upper extremities resting toward the floor in a flexed position (the most common posture of the patient when this region of the back is palpated). In this position the scapulae are rotated so that the T6 spinous process is more commonly found at the level of the inferior scapular angle.

The spinous processes of T9 and T10 often are palpably closer together than other thoracic spinous processes, but this is not a consistent finding. Located roughly halfway between the level of the inferior angle of the scapula and the superior margin of the iliac crests is the spinous process of T12.

Because the spinous processes of the thoracic vertebrae project in an inferior direction to different degrees, the remainder of the vertebrae are located variably superior to the spinous process of the same vertebral segment (Keogh and Ebbs, 1984). The tips of the transverse processes of T1-4 and T10-12 are located one spinous interspace superior to the tip of the spinous process of the same segment. The tips of the transverse processes of T5-9 are located two spinous interspaces superior to the tips of their respective spinous processes because these spinous processes project inferiorly to a greater degree. For example, the tips of the transverse

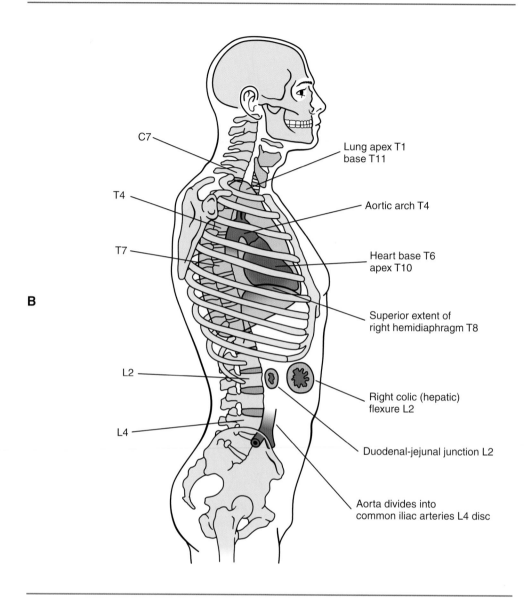

C7

Lung apex T1
base T11

T4

Aortic arch T4

T7

Heart base T6
apex T10

B

Superior extent of
right hemidiaphragm T8

L2

Right colic (hepatic)
flexure L2

L4

Duodenal-jejunal junction L2

Aorta divides into
common iliac arteries L4 disc

FIG. 1-3—cont'd   **B,** Lateral view.

processes of T3 are located in the same horizontal plane as the inferior tip of the spinous process of T2, whereas the tips of the transverse processes of T8 are at the same horizontal plane as the inferior tip of the spinous process of T6. The transverse processes of the thoracic vertebrae progressively get shorter from superior to inferior, so that the tips of the transverse processes of T1 are located 3 cm lateral to the midline, although those of T12 are 2 cm. Sometimes the transverse processes of T12 are small and not readily palpable. The angles of the ribs may be palpated 4 cm lateral to the midline at the horizontal levels of their respective transverse processes.

Lumbosacral Region. The posterior aspects of the spinous processes of the lumbar vertebrae differ from the thoracic vertebrae in that they present more of a flat surface. The spinous processes of L4 and L5 are shorter than the other lumbar spinous processes and are difficult to palpate, especially the L5 spinous process. The spinous process of L4 is the most inferior spinous process that has palpable movement with flexion and extension of the trunk. Usually it is in a horizontal plane with the superior margin of the iliac crests, although in approximately 20% of the population the iliac crests are even with the spinous process of L5 (Oliver and Middleditch, 1991).

The tips of the transverse processes of the lumbar vertebrae are located approximately 5 cm lateral to the midline and usually are not palpable. The mamillary processes are small tubercles on the posterior-superior aspect of the superior articular processes of the lumbar vertebrae. They are located approximately a finger breadth (2 cm) lateral to the midline at the level of the spinous process of the vertebra above and are not readily palpable.

The second spinous tubercle, the remnants of the spinous process of S2, is located at the extreme of the convexity of the sacral kyphosis and is the most prominent spinous tubercle on the sacrum. It is also on the same horizontal plane as the posterior superior iliac spines. The third spinous tubercle is located at the upper end of the gluteal cleft. The lowest palpable depression in the midline of the posterior aspect of the sacrum is the sacral hiatus. There are four pairs of posterior sacral foramina located 2.5 cm lateral to the midline and 2.5 cm apart, but usually these are not palpable. The tip of the coccyx is the last palpable bony structure of the spine and can be found in the gluteal cleft approximately 1 cm posterior to the anus.

SPINAL CORD LEVELS VERSUS VERTEBRAL LEVELS

The spinal cord is the extension of the central nervous system outside the cranium (Fig. 1-4). It is encased by the vertebral column and begins, on a gross anatomic level, at the foramen magnum, located halfway between the inion and the spinous process of C2. In the third fetal month the spinal cord, which is developing from the neural tube, extends the entire length of the embryo, and the spinal nerves exit the intervertebral foramina (IVFs) at their level of origin (Sadler, 2000). However, with increasing development the vertebral column and the dura mater lengthen more rapidly than does the neural tube, and the terminal end of the spinal cord gradually assumes a relatively higher level. At the time of birth the tip of the spinal cord, or conus medullaris, lies at the level of the L3 vertebral body. In the adult the conus medullaris usually is found at the L1-2 level (L1 body, 26%; L1 disc, 36%; L2 body, 20%), but may be found as high as the T12 disc (12%) or as low as the L2 disc (6%) (Fitzgerald, 1985). Chapter 3 and Table 3-1 provide further details on the inferior extent of the conus medullaris.

As a result of this unequal growth, the portion of the spinal cord from which the respective pairs of spinal nerve roots begin, known as the spinal cord level, is more superior than the level of the IVF from which the corresponding spinal nerve exits. Therefore the spinal nerve roots run obliquely inferior inside the vertebral (spinal) canal from their spinal cord level to their cor-

responding IVF. This obliquity is not equal throughout the length of the vertebral column. At the most superior levels of the vertebral column, the spinal nerve roots are nearly horizontal, and at more inferior levels they are progressively more oblique. In the lumbosacral region of the vertebral canal, the spinal nerve roots are nearly vertical and form a bundle known as the cauda equina.

A convenient method of locating various structures of the neck and trunk is to relate them to the vertebra, or portion of a vertebra, that lies at the same horizontal level as that structure. This plane is known as the vertebral level of a structure. *Unless otherwise noted, the vertebral body serves as the source of reference for the vertebral level.* Table 1-1 lists the vertebral levels of many of the clinically important visceral structures in the anterior neck and trunk. When locating structures within the vertebral canal, spinal cord levels must be distinguished from vertebral levels. The cervical spinal cord levels lie at even intervals between the foramen magnum and the spinous process of C6 (Keogh and Ebbs, 1984). The upper six thoracic spinal cord levels are between the spinous processes of C6 and T4, and the lower six thoracic spinal cord levels are between the spinous processes of T4 and T9. The lumbar, sacral, and coccygeal spinal cord levels are located between the spinous processes of T10 and L1, where the spinal cord ends as the conus medullaris.

The diameter of the spinal cord increases in two regions. These spinal cord enlargements are formed by the increased numbers of nerve cells necessary to innervate the limbs. The cervical enlargement includes the C4-T1 spinal cord levels and is at the level of the vertebral bodies of C4-7, or the spinous processes of C3-6 (Keogh and Ebbs, 1984). The lumbar enlargement is composed of the L2-S3 spinal cord levels and is found at the level of the T10-L1 vertebral bodies or the spinous processes of T9-12.

VERTEBRAL LEVELS OF STRUCTURES IN THE ANTERIOR NECK AND TRUNK

This section describes the vertebral levels of most of the clinically important structures found in the anterior neck and trunk. Knowledge of the surface locations for the deep structures of the anterior neck and trunk is essential for relating those structures to the whole person, especially during the physical examination. This information is summarized in Table 1-1.

Visual Landmarks

The most obvious visible structure in the anterior neck region is the laryngeal prominence (Fig. 1-5). It can be seen in the midline at the level of the C4 disc and is larger in adult men than in women. Moving inferiorly, the

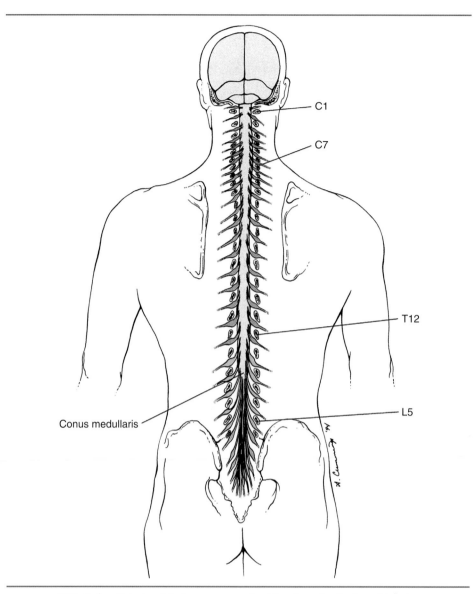

FIG. 1-4   Relationship between vertebral levels and spinal cord levels.

jugular notch (or incisure) of the sternum, or suprasternal notch, is at the superior margin of the manubrium and corresponds with the horizontal plane of the T2 disc or T1-2 interspinous space. The sternal angle (of Louis) at the inferior margin of the manubrium is at the level of the T4 disc. Near the inferior end of the sternum the xiphisternal junction is found. It corresponds not only with the body of T9 but also with the inferior margin of the pectoralis major muscle and the fifth costal cartilages. These relationships are quite variable depending on body type. Laterally the lowest portion of the costal margin is made up of the tenth costal cartilages. The horizontal plane at this level is termed the subcostal plane and goes through the body of L3 (Moore and Dalley, 1999).

The transpyloric plane is the horizontal plane at the halfway point between the upper border of the symphysis pubis and suprasternal notch. It corresponds with the L1 disc and usually is one handbreadth (10 cm) inferior to the xiphisternal junction. The vertebral level of the umbilicus is typically at the level of L3, but this varies depending on body type and weight. The pubic crest is identified with the level of the superior margin of the pubic symphysis. It extends 2.5 cm lateral to the midline and has a prominence on its lateral aspect known as the pubic tubercle. Typically the pubic crest is in the same plane as the coccyx, but again weight and body type can alter the tilt of the pelvis and therefore this relationship. The inguinal ligament extends from the anterior superior iliac spine at the level of the L5 disc to

Table 1-1   Vertebral Levels of Clinically Important Structures

Vertebral Level	Structure	Vertebral Level	Structure
C1	Transition of medulla oblongata into spinal cord		Superior extent of left hemidiaphragm
	Hard palate		Superior pole of spleen
	Anterior portion of soft palate		Left extent of inferior border of liver
C2	Inferior border of free edge of soft palate	T10	Apex of heart
	Nasopharynx and oropharynx join		Anteroinferior ends of oblique fissures of lungs
C2 disc	Superior cervical ganglion		Esophageal hiatus (diaphragm)
C3	Epiglottis	T11	Lowest extent of lungs (inferolateral angles of posterior aspects of lungs)
	Oropharynx becomes laryngopharynx		Inferior extent of esophagus
C3 disc	Common carotid arteries split into internal and external carotid arteries		Cardiac orifice of stomach
	Carotid sinus		Left suprarenal gland
C3 spinous	Greater cornua of hyoid bone	T12	Aortic hiatus (diaphragm)
C4 disc	Laryngeal prominence		Costodiaphragmatic recesses
C5	Vocal folds		Inferior pole of spleen
	Erb's point		Tail of pancreas
	Superior margin of lobes of thyroid gland		Orifice of gallbladder
C6	Middle cervical ganglion		Superior poles of kidneys (right slightly lower than left)
	Cricoid cartilage		Right suprarenal gland
	First tracheal ring	L1	Pyloric orifice of stomach
	Transition of larynx to trachea		Superior horizontal (first) part of duodenum
	Transition of laryngopharynx to esophagus		Left colic (splenic) flexure
C7	Inferior cervical ganglion	L1 disc	Transpyloric plane
T1	Stellate ganglion		Conus medullaris
	Inferior margin of thyroid gland		Hila of kidneys (right slightly below and left slightly above)
	Subclavian and internal jugular veins unite to form the brachiocephalic veins	L2	Duodenal-jejunal junction
	Apices of lungs		Right colic (hepatic) flexure
T2	Brachiocephalic veins unite to form superior vena cava		Head of pancreas
T2 disc	Suprasternal notch	L3	Subcostal plane (lowest portion of costal margin made up from the tenth costal cartilage)
T4	Aortic arch		
T4 disc	Sternal angle (of Louis)		
T5	Pulmonary trunk divides into right and left pulmonary arteries		Umbilicus (inconsistent)
	Pulmonary artery and primary bronchus enter right lung		Inferior horizontal (third) part of duodenum
	Trachea divides into primary bronchi		Right extent of lower border of liver
	Posterosuperior ends of oblique fissures of lungs		Inferior poles of kidneys (right slightly lower than left)
T6	Base of heart	L4	Beginning of sigmoid colon
	Pulmonary artery and primary bronchus enter left lung	L4 disc	Aorta divides into common iliac arteries
	Pulmonary veins exit right lung	L5	Common iliac veins unite to form inferior vena cava
	Superior vena cava enters right atrium		Ileocecal junction
T7	Pulmonary veins exit left lung		Vermiform appendix arises from cecum
	Inferior vena cava enters right atrium	L5 disc	Anterior superior iliac spine
	Horizontal fissure of right lung		Superolateral end of inguinal ligament
T8	Caval hiatus (diaphragm)	S3	Beginning of rectum
	Superior extent of right hemidiaphragm	Lower sacrum	Superior extent of uterus
	Superior border of liver	Coccyx	Pubic crest
T9	Xiphisternal junction		Ganglion impar
	Fifth costal cartilage		Superior margin of pubic symphysis
	Inferior border of pectoralis major muscle		Inferomedial end of inguinal ligament
	Inferomedial angles of posterior aspects of lungs		Bladder (empty)

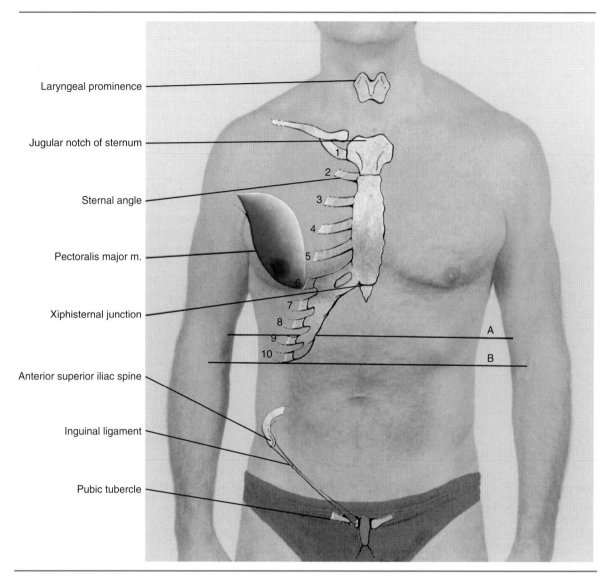

Laryngeal prominence

Jugular notch of sternum

Sternal angle

Pectoralis major m.

Xiphisternal junction

Anterior superior iliac spine

Inguinal ligament

Pubic tubercle

FIG. 1-5   Visual landmarks of the anterior trunk. *A*, The transpyloric plane. *B*, The subcostal plane. Note that the ribs have been numbered.

the pubic tubercle and demarcates the beginning of the thigh region.

Deeper Structures

Neural Structures. At the level of the atlas, the gross anatomic transition of the medulla oblongata into the spinal cord occurs as it exits the cranium via the foramen magnum. The conus medullaris, the inferior tip of the spinal cord, usually is found at the L1-2 level (see previous discussion).

The sympathetic trunks (Fig. 1-6) extend along the entire anterolateral aspect of the spinal column. In the cervical region the trunks are approximately 2.5 cm lateral to the midline. They are somewhat more laterally located in the thoracic and lumbar regions. Along the

anterior surface of the sacrum the trunks begin to converge until they meet as the ganglion impar on the anterior surface of the coccyx. Sympathetic ganglia are located at fairly regular intervals along these trunks. Typically there are three ganglia in the cervical region (see Fig. 1-6). The superior cervical ganglion can be found at the C2-3 interspace. The middle and inferior cervical ganglia typically are found at the C6 and C7 levels, respectively. Sometimes the inferior cervical ganglion and first thoracic ganglion unite to form the stellate (or cervicothoracic) ganglion, which is found at the T1 level. The sympathetic trunks are described in more detail in Chapter 10.

Several peripheral nerves become superficial approximately midway along the posterior border of the SCM (see Fig. 1-6). This area is sometimes called Erb's point

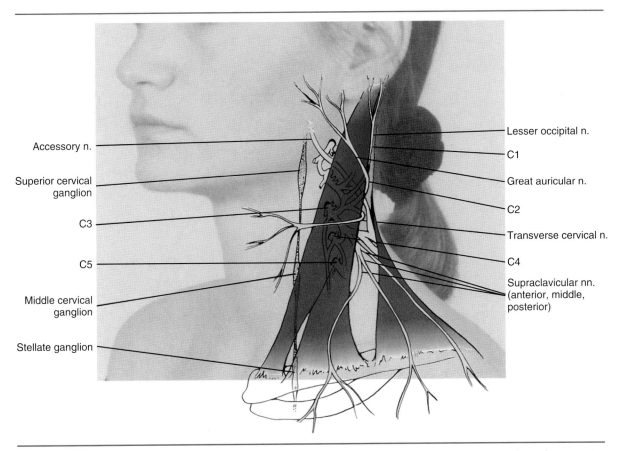

Accessory n.

Superior cervical ganglion

C3

C5

Middle cervical ganglion

Stellate ganglion

Lesser occipital n.

C1

Great auricular n.

C2

Transverse cervical n.

C4

Supraclavicular nn. (anterior, middle, posterior)

FIG. 1-6   Erb's point and the cervical sympathetic trunk. Note that Erb's point is located midway along the posterior border of the sternocleidomastoid muscle. Also note the sympathetic trunk connecting the cervical sympathetic ganglia.

and is roughly at the C5 level. These nerves include the transverse cervical nerve, which supplies the skin of the throat region; the lesser occipital nerve, which supplies the skin in the area of the mastoid process; and the great auricular nerve, which innervates the skin in the vicinity of the ear. In addition, the supraclavicular nerves arise by a common trunk that emerges from Erb's point. This trunk divides into three branches alternately called anterior, middle, and posterior *or* medial, intermediate, and lateral, which go to the skin of the upper chest region. Finally, the accessory nerve (cranial nerve XI) becomes relatively superficial in this region after sending motor branches into the deep surface of the SCM. It then courses in a posterolateral direction, across the posterior triangle of the neck, to reach the deep surface of the trapezius muscle, which it also supplies with motor innervation.

The roots of the brachial plexus, which arise from the ventral rami of the C5-T1 spinal nerves, are located just posterior to the lower one third of the SCM (Keogh and Ebbs, 1984). The upper (or lateral) margin of the plexus runs along a line from the junction of the middle and lower thirds of the SCM to the tip of the coracoid process of the scapula. The lower (or medial) border of the plexus extends from the junction of the posterior border of the SCM with the clavicle to one finger breadth (2 cm) inferior and medial to the tip of the coracoid process of the scapula.

Vascular Structures. The shape of the heart may be thought of as an isosceles triangle with a superior base and an inferior apex directed to the left of the midline (Fig. 1-7). The base of the heart usually can be found at the level of T6. The horizontal position of the apex of the heart typically is said to be at the level of T10, but this is variable depending on the patient's body type. It may be found as high as T9 (Moore and Dalley, 1999) or as low as T11 (Gardner, Gray, and O'Rahilly, 1975).

The ascending aorta emerges from the left ventricle of the heart roughly in the midline and runs superiorly. It then turns to the left and forms the aortic arch that can be found at the level of the T4 body. The thoracic portion of the descending aorta begins in the plane of the T4 disc and runs inferiorly slightly left of the midline along the anterior surface of the thoracic vertebrae. It becomes the

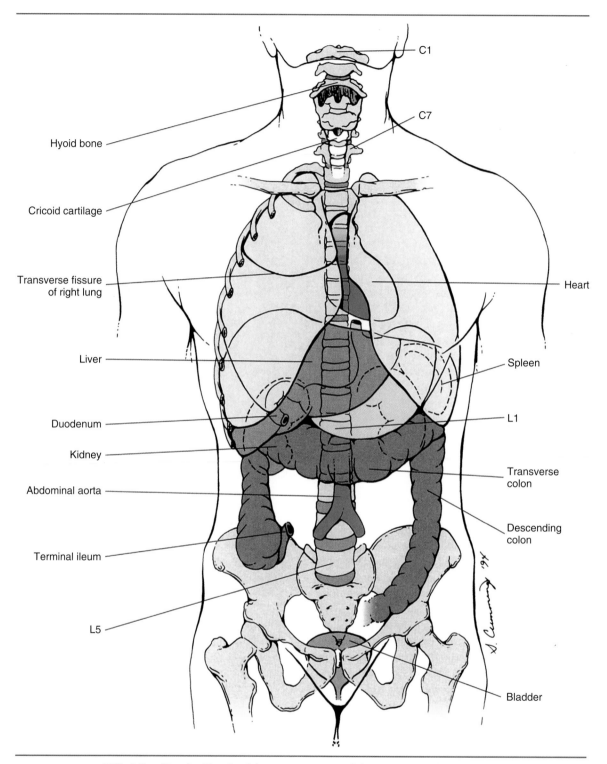

Hyoid bone

C1

C7

Cricoid cartilage

Transverse fissure
of right lung

Heart

Liver

Spleen

Duodenum

L1

Kidney

Abdominal aorta

Transverse
colon

Terminal ileum

Descending
colon

L5

Bladder

FIG. 1-7   Vertebral levels of deeper structures of the anterior neck and trunk.

abdominal aorta as it passes through the aortic hiatus of the diaphragm in the midline at the level of T12 (Moore and Dalley, 1999). The abdominal aorta descends along the anterior surface of the lumbar vertebrae and divides into the common iliac arteries just anterior to the L4 disc, slightly left of the midline.

The aortic arch has three branches. The first is the brachiocephalic trunk. This trunk gives rise to the right common carotid and right subclavian arteries. The left common carotid artery is the second branch of the aortic arch, and the left subclavian artery is the third branch of the aortic arch. The subclavian arteries supply blood to the upper extremities, and the common carotid arteries supply the head and neck region. The common carotid arteries ascend on either side of the anterolateral neck to the level of the C3 disc, where they each split into an internal and external carotid artery. This is the region of the important carotid sinus, which monitors the blood pressure of the body. Therefore care must be taken when palpating these structures, and they should always be palpated only unilaterally.

The pulmonary trunk arises from the right ventricle of the heart and divides into the right and left pulmonary arteries in a plane with T5. The pulmonary arteries enter (and the pulmonary veins exit) their respective lungs via a hilum. The pulmonary artery of the right lung enters in the plane of T5 and that of the left lung at the level of T6 (Williams et al., 1995). The pulmonary veins exit the lungs approximately one vertebral level lower than the arteries enter. There is some variation of these levels with body type, and both of the pulmonary arteries may enter their respective lungs as low as T7 (Gardner, Gray, and O'Rahilly, 1975).

The internal jugular and subclavian veins of each side of the body unite several centimeters lateral to the midline at the level of T1 to form the brachiocephalic veins. The brachiocephalic veins then unite to form the superior vena cava slightly right of the midline at the T2 level (Williams et al., 1995). The superior vena cava runs inferiorly and ends in the upper portion of the right atrium of the heart at approximately the level of T6.

The common iliac veins unite to form the inferior vena cava at the level of the L5 body, a little to the right of the midline. The inferior vena cava then ascends in front of the vertebral column, on the right side of the abdominal aorta. Passing through the caval hiatus of the diaphragm in the horizontal plane of the body of T8 (Moore and Dalley, 1999), the inferior vena cava enters the lower portion of the right atrium just above that level at T7.

Visceral Structures. The respiratory system begins with the nasal cavity, which is separated from the oral cavity by the hard palate. The hard palate lies in the same horizontal plane as the atlas. The nasal cavity becomes continuous with the nasopharynx in the region of the soft palate also at the level of C1. The nasopharynx joins the oropharynx at the inferior border of the posterior margin of the soft palate just anterior to the C2 body, and for several centimeters the alimentary and respiratory systems share a common passageway. At the superior border of the epiglottis, the oropharynx becomes the laryngopharynx. In this region the alimentary and respiratory tracts again become separate. Anteriorly the respiratory tract continues as the larynx. Its lumen is protected during deglutition by the epiglottis, which may be found at the C3 level. The adjacent hyoid bone

provides attachment sites for several muscles involved in deglutition and vocalization, and its greater cornua can be found at the C3 spinous process level. The most anterior projection of the thyroid cartilage, the laryngeal prominence, is at the level of the C4 disc, and the vocal folds, or cords, are slightly lower in the C5 plane. The cricoid cartilage, the lowest portion of the larynx, joins the first tracheal ring, the highest portion of the trachea, at the level of C6. The lobes of the thyroid gland are located anterior and lateral to the larynx and trachea and extend from the C5 to T1 levels. The trachea descends in the midline anterior to the esophagus to the level of the upper border of the T5 body, where it divides into the primary bronchi (Williams et al., 1995). The primary bronchi enter the lungs via their respective hila at around the same levels as the pulmonary arteries, which are T5 on the right and T6 on the left.

The apex of each lung extends superiorly to the level of the T1 body (see Fig. 1-7). On their posterior aspects, the inferomedial angles of both lungs are approximately at T9, and the inferolateral angles, the lowest portion of the lungs, extend inferiorly to near T11. The anterior-inferior border of each lung is approximately one vertebral level higher than the posterior border. With full inspiration these levels may descend nearly two vertebral segments (Williams et al., 1995).

The left lung is divided into upper and lower lobes by an oblique fissure. This fissure extends from the T5 level posterosuperiorly to T10 anteroinferiorly. The right lung not only has an oblique fissure similar to that of the left lung, but also has a horizontal fissure at the level of T7. Therefore the right lung is divided into three lobes: upper, middle, and lower.

The diaphragm extends several vertebral levels superiorly in its center and is shaped like a dome. Therefore the diaphragm makes an impression on the inferior surface of each of the lungs. The right half of the diaphragm, often termed the right hemidiaphragm, reaches the T8 level and because of the underlying liver is approximately 1 cm higher than the level of the left hemidiaphragm (Moore and Dalley, 1999). With full inspiration, these levels may descend as much as two vertebral levels (Williams et al., 1995). Normally the pleural cavity extends slightly lower than the inferolateral angles of the lungs and forms the costodiaphragmatic recesses at the level of T12. Because of the domelike shape of the diaphragm, these recesses represent the lowest points of the thoracic cavity and are potential sites of fluid accumulation in the chest.

The alimentary canal begins as the oral cavity, which becomes the oropharynx in the region of the soft palate at the C1 level. The oropharynx, after being joined by the nasopharynx at the inferior border of the free edge of the soft palate just in front of the C2 body, turns into the laryngopharynx at the superior border of the epiglottis at the level of C3. The laryngopharynx continues inferiorly on the posterior aspect of the larynx and changes into the esophagus at the level of C6. The esophagus runs inferiorly in the chest on the anterior aspect of the vertebral column slightly anterior and to the right of the descending thoracic aorta. Passing through the diaphragm via the esophageal hiatus at the T10 level, the esophagus enters the abdomen (Williams et al., 1995) and ends at the cardiac orifice of the stomach slightly left of the midline at T11.

The stomach is the most dilated portion of the alimentary canal. Curving inferiorly and to the right, the stomach becomes continuous with the small intestine at the pyloric orifice at the level of L1. The duodenum, the first part of the small intestine, is shaped like a U lying on its side and has four parts. The first (superior horizontal) part continues from the pyloric orifice horizontally to the right at the level of L1. The second (descending) part proceeds inferiorly to the horizontal plane of L3, where it turns to the left to become the third (inferior horizontal) part. The third part continues to the left, crosses the midline, and bends slightly superiorly to give rise to the fourth (ascending) part that runs obliquely superior and ends as the duodenal-jejunal junction at the level of L2.

The rest of the small intestine continues as a series of loops and ends by connecting with the large intestine at the junction of the cecum and the ascending portion of the colon in the right lower quadrant of the abdomen at the L5 level. The proximal two fifths and the distal three fifths of the small intestine distal to the duodenum are called the jejunum and ileum, respectively.

The large intestine, or colon, begins as the cecum, which is a cul-de-sac located in the right iliac fossa (see Fig. 1-7). The ileum connects with the upper portion of the cecum at the L5 level. The vermiform appendix usually arises from the cecum approximately one finger breadth (2 cm) inferior to the ileocecal junction. The large intestine continues in a superior direction above the ileocecal junction as the ascending colon. At the level of L2 the ascending colon makes a sharp turn to the left and continues as the transverse colon. This sharp turn is termed the right colic flexure, or hepatic flexure, because it is just below the liver. The transverse colon continues horizontally and slightly superiorly across the midline to the left side of the abdomen, where it turns sharply inferior. This left colic flexure occurs at the L1 level, which is slightly more superior than the right colic flexure. The left colic flexure, located just below the spleen, sometimes is termed the splenic flexure. The large intestine then continues inferiorly on the left side of the abdominal cavity as the descending colon. At the L4 level, the large intestine becomes somewhat tortuous and is called the sigmoid colon. The sigmoid colon then continues into the true pelvis and becomes the rectum in the midline at the S3 level.

The head of the pancreas can be found within the curve of the duodenum. Usually it is described as being located at the level of L2 (Williams et al., 1995). The neck and body of the pancreas extend superiorly and obliquely to the left. The body of the pancreas ends as the tail of the pancreas, which can be found at the lower pole of the spleen in the left upper quadrant at T12. The superior pole of the spleen is adjacent to the left hemidiaphragm at approximately the level of T9.

The liver, the largest gland of the body, is found mostly in the upper right quadrant of the abdomen, but its left lobe does extend somewhat across the midline. Superiorly the liver is in contact with the diaphragm and fills the domelike hollow of the right hemidiaphragm. The superior border of the liver therefore extends up to the T8 level. The inferior border runs diagonally from the right side of the abdomen at the level of L3 to the left hemidiaphragm at the T9 horizontal plane (Williams et al., 1995). The gallbladder rests in a fossa in the inferior border of the right lobe of the liver. The orifice of the gallbladder is usually found at the T12 level.

The urinary system begins with the kidneys. The superior poles of the kidneys lie at the level of T12 and their inferior poles at L3. The right kidney is slightly lower than the left kidney, probably because of its relationship with the liver (Williams et al., 1995). The suprarenal, or adrenal, glands are located on the anterosuperior borders of the kidneys. As with the kidneys, the left suprarenal gland is located somewhat more superior than the right. These endocrine glands can be found at the T11 and T12 levels, respectively. The hilum of the left kidney is just above the level of the L1 disc (transpyloric plane), and that of the right kidney just below it. A ureter arises from the hilum of each kidney, and both run to the bladder in an inferior and slightly medial direction. The bladder is a midline structure in the true pelvis posterior to the pubic symphysis at the coccygeal level. The bladder may expand upward and forward into the abdominal cavity when distended.

In the female the uterus lies posterior to the bladder and anterior to the rectum. Superiorly the uterus extends above the superior border of the bladder to the lower sacral levels, and because of its anteverted and anteflexed position, the superior portion of the uterus usually lies on the posterior portion of the superior surface of the empty bladder. The ovaries are situated one on either side of the uterus near the lateral wall of the true pelvis. The position of the ovaries is variable, especially in parous women, because they are displaced during a woman's first pregnancy and probably never return to their original position (Williams et al., 1995).

This chapter serves as a useful reference as the reader progresses through the rest of this text. Knowledge of the structures of the body that are visible and palpable through the skin and an awareness of the surface locations of deeper structures are important tools in the proper examination and evaluation of patients. Therefore this chapter is designed not only as a beginning reference point for the rest of the text, but also as a quick reference for the health care provider.

REFERENCES

Byfield DC, Mathiasen J, & Sangren C. (1992). The reliability of osseous landmark palpation in the lumbar spine and pelvis. *Eur J Chiro, 40,* 83-88.

Downey BJ, Taylor NF, & Nierce KR. (1999). Manipulative physiotherapists can reliably palpate nominated lumbar spinal levels. *Manipulative Ther, 4,* 351-356.

Fitzgerald MJT. (1985). *Neuroanatomy basic & applied.* London: Bailliere Tindall.

Gardner E, Gray DJ, & O'Rahilly R. (1975). *Anatomy.* Philadelphia: WB Saunders.

Keogh B & Ebbs S. (1984). *Normal surface anatomy.* London: William Heinemann Medical Books.

Moore KL & Dalley AF. (1999). *Clinically oriented anatomy* (4th ed.). Philadelphia: Lippincott Williams & Wilkins.

Oliver J & Middleditch A. (1991). *Functional anatomy of the spine.* Oxford, UK: Butterworth-Heinemann.

Sadler TW. (2000). *Langman's medical embryology* (8th ed.). Philadelphia: Lippincott Williams & Wilkins.

Williams PL et al. (1995). *Gray's anatomy* (38th ed.). Edinburgh: Churchill Livingstone.

CHAPTER 2

General Characteristics of the Spine

Gregory D. Cramer

The purpose of this chapter is to discuss the basic and clinical anatomy of the spine as a whole, that is, to introduce many of the features that are common to the major regions of the spine (cervical, thoracic, and lumbar). Some of the topics listed are discussed in more detail in later chapters.

FUNCTION AND DEVELOPMENT OF THE SPINE

The anatomy of the human spine can be understood best if its functions are considered first. The spine has three primary functions: support of the body, protection of the spinal cord and spinal nerve roots, and movement of the trunk. The vertebral column has the ideal structure to carry out all of these functions simultaneously (Putz and Müller-Gerbl, 1996). These varied functions are carried out by a series of movable bones, called vertebrae, and the soft tissues that surround these bones. A brief explanation of the development of the vertebrae and the related soft tissues is given to highlight the detailed anatomy of these structures. A more thorough discussion of spinal development is presented in Chapter 12.

Development of the Spine

After the early development of the neural groove into the neural tube and neural crest (see Fig. 12-7), paraxial mesoderm condenses to form somites (see Figs. 12-7 and 12-9, *A*). The somites, in turn, develop into dermomyotomes and sclerotomes. Portions of the lateral aspects of the dermomyotomes develop into the dermis and subcutaneous tissue, whereas the majority of the dermomyotomes develop into the axial musculature. The sclerotomes migrate centrally to surround the neural tube and notochord (see Fig. 12-9, *B*). The sclerotomal cells then form the vertebral column and associated ligaments.

While the paraxial mesoderm is developing into somites, the more inferior portion of the neural tube differentiates into the ependymal, mantle, and marginal layers of the future spinal cord. The ependymal layer surrounds the future central canal region of the spinal cord. The mantle layer develops into the cells of the nervous system (neurons and glia), and the outer marginal layer of the tube consists of the axons of tract cells. The neural crest develops into the sensory neurons of the peripheral nervous system and the postganglionic neurons of the autonomic nervous system.

Chondrification Centers and Primary Ossification Centers. Cells of sclerotomal origin condense to form vertebral chondrification centers (one pair in the anterior aspect and at least one center in each half of the posterior aspect of the mesenchymal vertebrae). This results in the development of a cartilage model of each vertebra (see Fig. 12-11). Each vertebra then develops three primary centers of ossification (see Fig. 12-11). One primary center is located in the anterior part of the future vertebra. This region is known as the centrum and helps to form the future vertebral body. The remaining two primary ossification centers are located on each side of the portion of the vertebra that surrounds the developing neural tube. This region is known as the neural or posterior arch. The two ossification centers at the neural arch normally unite posteriorly to form the spinous process. Failure of these centers to unite results in a condition known as spina bifida. This condition is discussed in more detail in Chapter 12.

Anteriorly the left and right sides of the neural arch normally fuse to the centrum. Known as the neurocentral synchondrosis, this region actually is located within the area that becomes the posterior aspect of the vertebral body. The fusion that occurs unites the primary ossification centers of the neural arch with the centrum, consequently forming a vertebral body from both the centrum and a small part of the neural arch. Because of this the vertebral arch is somewhat smaller than its developmental predecessor, the neural arch, and the vertebral body is somewhat larger than its predecessor, the centrum.

The precise time of fusion between the neural arch and centrum at the neurocentral synchondrosis remains a topic of current investigation. Some authors state that closure occurs by 6 years of age (Maat et al., 1996), and other investigators state that the neurocentral cartilage may remain until as late as 16 years of age (Vital et al., 1989). Part of the function of the neurocentral cartilage is to ensure growth of the posterior arch of the vertebrae. Early fusion of the neurocentral synchondrosis has been implicated in the development of scoliosis

(Vital et al., 1989). Scoliosis is discussed in more detail in Chapter 6.

Usually the vertebral body develops from two centers of chondrification, left and right. If one of these centers fails to develop, only one half of the vertebral body remains. This is known as a hemivertebra, or cuneiform vertebra, and can result in lateral curvature of the spine. Frequently a hemivertebra at one level is compensated for by the same condition at another level on the opposite side.

During development the vertebral bodies may appear to be wedge shaped, narrower anteriorly than posteriorly. This can give the appearance of a compression fracture (Fesmire and Luten, 1989). Wedging that occurs in several consecutive vertebrae is seen as an indication of a normal variant. However, a compression fracture of the wedge-shaped vertebra must be considered if it occurs at only one level and the vertebrae above and below are more rectangular in appearance.

Secondary Ossification Centers. Five secondary centers of ossification appear in the vertebral column between the ages of 10 and 13 (see Fig. 12-11). One secondary center of ossification is located on each of the cartilaginous end plates of a typical vertebral body. These centers are known as the anular apophyses or ring apophyses (Williams et al., 1995). A secondary center of ossification also is found on the tips of each of the transverse processes, and another is located on the tip of the single spinous process. The centers on the transverse processes and spinous process enable the rapid growth of these processes that occurs during adolescence.

The two centers of ossification associated with the peripheral rim of the upper and lower surfaces of the vertebral bodies (anular apophyses) do not help with the longitudinal growth of the vertebral bodies and for this reason are frequently termed ring apophyses (Theil, Clements, and Cassidy, 1992; Bogduk, 1997). These centers incorporate the outer layers of the anulus fibrosus (Fardon, 1988), which explains the bony attachment of the outer layers of the anulus, whereas the more central layers are attached to the cartilage of the vertebral end plates (Bogduk, 1997).

All of the secondary ossification centers listed previously fuse with the remainder of the vertebrae between the ages of 14 and 25 (Williams et al., 1995; Bogduk, 1997), and no further growth can occur after their fusion. These centers can be mistaken as sites of fracture before they have fused.

Fully Developed Vertebral Column. The first accurate description of the number of movable vertebrae in the fully developed spine was that of Galen between 100 and 200 AD (Shapiro, 1990). However, perhaps because of the many anatomic errors made by

Galen in other areas, controversy ensued over the precise number of vertebrae until the publication of Vesalius' *De Humani Corporis Fabrica* in 1543 (Shapiro, 1990). This publication showed that the human vertebral column develops into 24 vertebrae (Fig. 2-1), which are divided into 7 cervical, 12 thoracic, and 5 lumbar vertebrae (expressed as C1-7, T1-12, and L1-5). The L5 vertebra rests on the bony sacrum (made of five fused segments). The coccyx (three to five fused segments) is suspended from the sacrum. All of these bones are joined by means of a series of approximately 136 joints (including the joints between vertebrae and ribs) to form the vertebral column.

CURVES OF THE SPINE

The spine develops four anterior to posterior curves, two kyphoses and two lordoses. (See introduction of text for further clarification of the terms lordosis and kyphosis.) Kyphoses are curves that are concave anteriorly, and lordoses are curves that are concave posteriorly. The two primary curves are the kyphoses. These include the thoracic and pelvic curvatures (see Fig. 2-1). They are called primary curves because they are seen from the earliest stages of fetal development. The thoracic curve extends from T2 to T12 and is created by the larger superior to inferior dimensions of the posterior portion of the

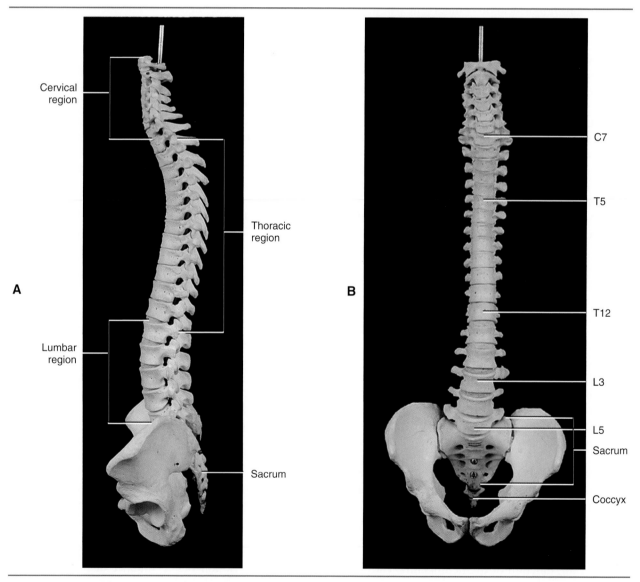

FIG. 2-1 Three views of the vertebral column. **A,** Lateral view showing the cervical, thoracic, lumbar, and sacral regions. Also notice the cervical and lumbar lordoses and the thoracic and sacral kyphoses. **B,** Anterior view.

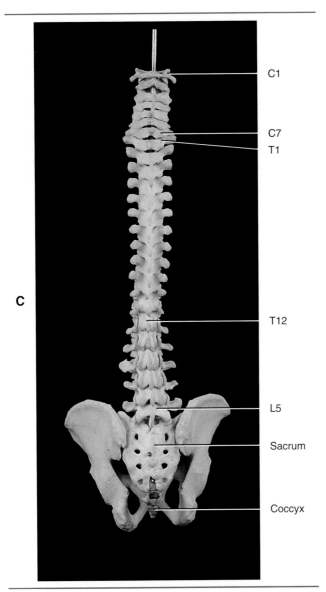

C

C1

C7
T1

T12

L5

Sacrum

Coccyx

FIG. 2-1—cont'd   C, Posterior view of the vertebral column.

into a lordotic curve. The cervical lordosis is further accentuated when the small child begins to sit upright and stabilizes his or her head while looking around in the seated position. This occurs at approximately 9 months of age. In the adult, the cervical curve is maintained by the larger superior to inferior dimensions of the anterior portion of the intervertebral discs. Because this curve is primarily created by the pliable intervertebral discs, traction of the cervical region reduces the cervical lordosis, whereas traction to the thoracic region has little effect on the thoracic kyphosis, because the thoracic curve is primarily created by the shape of the vertebrae. Further details of the cervical curvature are given in Chapter 5.

The action of the erector spinae muscles (see Chapter 4), pulling the lumbar spine erect to achieve the position necessary for walking, creates the posterior concavity known as the lumbar lordosis (see Fig. 2-1). Therefore the lumbar lordosis develops approximately 10 to 18 months after birth as the infant begins to walk upright. The lumbar lordosis extends from T12 to the lumbosacral articulation and is more pronounced in females than males. The region between L3 and the lumbosacral angle is more prominently lordotic than the region from T12 to L2. After infancy, the lumbar lordosis is maintained by a combination of the shape of the intervertebral discs and the shape of the vertebral bodies. Each of these structures is taller anteriorly than posteriorly in the lumbar region of the spine. Therefore the lumbar lordosis is reduced when traction forces are applied to it, but the reduction is less than that found during traction of the cervical region.

A slight lateral curve normally is found in the upper thoracic region. The convexity of the curve is on the left in left-handed people and on the right in right-handed people. Such deviations are probably the result of asymmetric muscle use and tone.

The lumbar lordosis and thoracic kyphosis both increase from the supine to the standing position (Wood et al., 1996). In addition, the cervical lordosis has been found to compensate for the variations in lumbar lordosis that occur during changes in position and during normal motion. For example, lumbar lordosis increases during sitting in the erect position and cervical lordosis decreases during this activity. Lumbar lordosis decreases during lumbar forward flexion and cervical lordosis increases during lumbar flexion, and the opposite occurs during lumbar extension (Black, McClure, and Polansky, 1996).

The kyphoses and lordoses of the spine, along with the intervertebral discs, help to absorb the loads applied to the spine. These loads include the weight of the trunk, along with loads applied through the lower extremities during walking, running, and jumping. In addition, loads are applied by carrying objects with the upper extrem-

thoracic vertebrae (see Chapter 6). The pelvic curve extends from the lumbosacral articulation throughout the sacrum to the tip of the coccyx. The concavity of the pelvic curve faces anteriorly and inferiorly, and is also caused by the greater superior to inferior dimensions of the posterior portion of the sacral segments.

The two secondary curves are the cervical lordosis and lumbar lordosis (see Fig. 2-1). These curves are known as secondary or compensatory curves because, even though they can be detected during fetal development, they do not become apparent until the postnatal period. The cervical lordosis begins late in intrauterine life but becomes apparent when an infant begins to lift his or her head from the prone position (≈3 to 4 months after birth). This forces the cervical spine

ities, the pull of spinal muscles, and the wide variety of movements that normally occur in the spine. The spinal curves, acting with the intervertebral discs and vertebral bodies, dissipate the increased loads that would occur if the spine were shaped like a straight column. Yet even with these safeguards, the vertebrae can be fractured as a result of falling and landing on the feet or buttocks, objects falling onto the head, or diving and landing on the head. Such injuries usually compress the vertebral bodies. Cervical compression usually occurs between C4 to C6 (Foreman and Croft, 1988). When the force comes from below, T9 through L2 are the most commonly affected through compression. Flexion injuries also can result in a compression fracture of vertebral bodies. Again, C4 through C6 are the most commonly affected in the cervical region, whereas T5 and T6 and the upper lumbar vertebrae usually are affected in the thoracic and lumbar regions (White and Panjabi, 1990).

ANATOMY OF A TYPICAL VERTEBRA

A typical vertebra can be divided into two basic regions, a vertebral body and vertebral arch (also called the posterior arch or dorsal arch). The bone in both regions is composed of an outer layer of compact bone and a core of trabecular bone, also known as cancellous, or spongy, bone (Fig. 2-2). The cancellous bone is composed of myriad spicules of bone, known as trabeculae (singular, trabecula). The trabeculae are oriented parallel to the lines of greatest stress (Skedros, Mason, and Bloebaum, 1994; Skedros et al., 1994). Smit, Odgaard, and Schneider (1997) found that the trabecular architecture of the lumbar vertebral bodies was ideal for the loads placed on the spine during axial compression (loads placed on the vertebral bodies from above; for example, to resist gravity) and walking. That is, not only were the trabeculae arranged to withstand axial compression, but they also were quite strong where the pedicles of the posterior arch met the vertebral bodies. This latter finding is consistent with the transfer of loads from the articular processes of the posterior arch to the vertebral bodies during rotational movements in the horizontal plane, and anterior to posterior ("shearing") movements (most closely associated with walking).

The shell of compact bone is thin on the discal surfaces of the vertebral body and is thicker in the vertebral arch and its processes. The outer compact bone is covered by a thin layer of periosteum that is innervated by nerve endings, which transmit both nociception and proprioception (Edgar and Ghadially, 1976). The outer compact bone also contains many small foramina to allow passage for numerous veins and nutrient arteries. The trabecular interior of a vertebra contains red marrow and one or two large canals for the basivertebral vein(s).

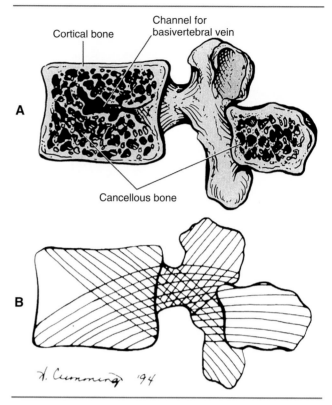

FIG. 2-2   Midsagittal view of a vertebra. **A,** The central cancellous, or trabecular, bone of the vertebral body and spinous process. Also notice the more peripheral cortical bone. **B,** The pattern of trabeculation, which develops along the lines of greatest stress.

The density of bone in the vertebrae varies from individual to individual but seems to increase significantly in most people during puberty and reaches a peak during the mid-twenties, when closure of the growth plates of the secondary centers of ossification occurs (Gilsanz et al., 1988). A decrease in bone mineral density to below normal limits is known as osteoporosis. Osteoporosis also is accompanied by a rearrangement of the trabeculae within the spongy bone (Feltrin et al., 2001). This condition is of particular clinical relevance in the spine because of the weight-bearing function of this region. A decrease in bone mineral density and rearrangement of trabeculae leads to a loss of elasticity in the bone and an increase in bone fragility. These changes, in turn, increase the likelihood of vertebral fracture (Mosekilde and Mosekilde, 1990; Feltrin et al., 2001). Osteoporosis has been associated with aging (Mosekilde and Mosekilde, 1990) and particularly with menopause (Ribot et al., 1988). Ribot et al. (1988) found that spinal bone density in French women remained stable in the young adult years and in women over 70 years of age. An average rate of apparent bone loss of approximately 1% per year was found between the ages of 45 and 65. This represented approximately 75% of the total bone loss occurring within the individuals of their sample population (510 women). Ribot et al. (1988) also found that the bone mineral density in their population of French women appeared to be between 5% and 10% lower than reported values in the United States. Mosekilde and Mosekilde (1990), studying the L2 and L3 vertebrae, found relatively few sex-related differences in vertebral body density. However, Mosekilde (1989) did find a sex-related difference in vertebral trabecular architecture with age. Consistent with the findings of Ribot et al. (1988), Mosekilde (1989) discovered that in both sexes bone density diminished by 35% to 40% from 20 to 80 years of age. She also found that the trabecular center (cancellous bone) of the vertebral body lost more bone mass than the outer cortical rim.

The regions of the vertebral body and vertebral arch are discussed separately in the following sections of this chapter. Elaboration on each component of the vertebra, with special emphasis placed on the characteristics unique to each region of the vertebral column, is included in the chapters on the cervical, thoracic, and lumbar regions of the spine (Chapters 5 through 7). In addition, Table 2-1 compares and contrasts the different parts of cervical, thoracic, and lumbar vertebrae.

Vertebral Body

The vertebral body (Fig. 2-3) is the large anterior portion of a vertebra that acts to support the weight of the human frame. Each vertebral body is designed to provide the greatest amount of strength with the least amount of bone mass (Feltrin et al., 2001). The vertebral bodies are connected to one another by fibrocartilaginous intervertebral discs, and when the bodies are combined with their intervening discs, they create a flexible column or pillar that supports the weight of the trunk and head. The vertebral bodies also must be able to withstand additional forces from contraction of the axial and proximal limb muscles. The bodies are cylindric in shape and have unique characteristics in each named region of the spine. The transverse diameter of the vertebral bodies increases from C2 to L3. This probably results from the fact that each successive vertebral body carries a slightly greater load. There is variation in the width of the last two lumbar vertebrae, but the width steadily diminishes from the first sacral segment to the apex (inferior tip) of the coccyx.

Vertical trabeculae predominate in the vertebral bodies. The vertical trabeculae are supported by horizontal trabeculae that function much like the struts or

Table 2-1   Regional General Characteristics of Typical Vertebrae

Structure	Cervical	Thoracic	Lumbar
Body	Rectangular Uncinate processes	Heart-shaped Taller posterior than anterior Costal demifacets	Kidney-shaped Taller anterior than posterior
Pedicles	Small Superior and inferior vertebral notches	Large, stout No superior vertebral notch	Large, stout Superior (small) and inferior vertebral notches
Transverse processes	Anterior and posterior tubercles Foramen of transverse process	Large Transverse costal facet	Large
Articular processes (orientation [facing] of superior articular facet)	Posteriorly, superiorly, and medially 45 degrees to vertical plane	Posteriorly, superiorly, and laterally 30 degrees to vertical plane	Posteriorly and medially Biplanar Within vertical plane
Laminae	Short from superior-inferior	Tall from superior-inferior	Intermediate from superior-inferior
Spinous process	Bifid	Upper four: posteriorly directed Middle four: long and inferiorly directed Lower four: lumbarlike	Spatulated in shape
Intervertebral foramina	Oval-shaped: one fifth filled with spinal nerve	Inverted pear-shaped: one twelfth filled with spinal nerve	Inverted pear-shaped: one third filled with spinal nerve
Vertebral canal	Trefoil-shaped: largest of vertebral column	Round in shape: smallest of vertebral column	Trefoil-shaped: intermediate in size between cervical and thoracic
Typical vertebrae	C3-6	T2-9	All

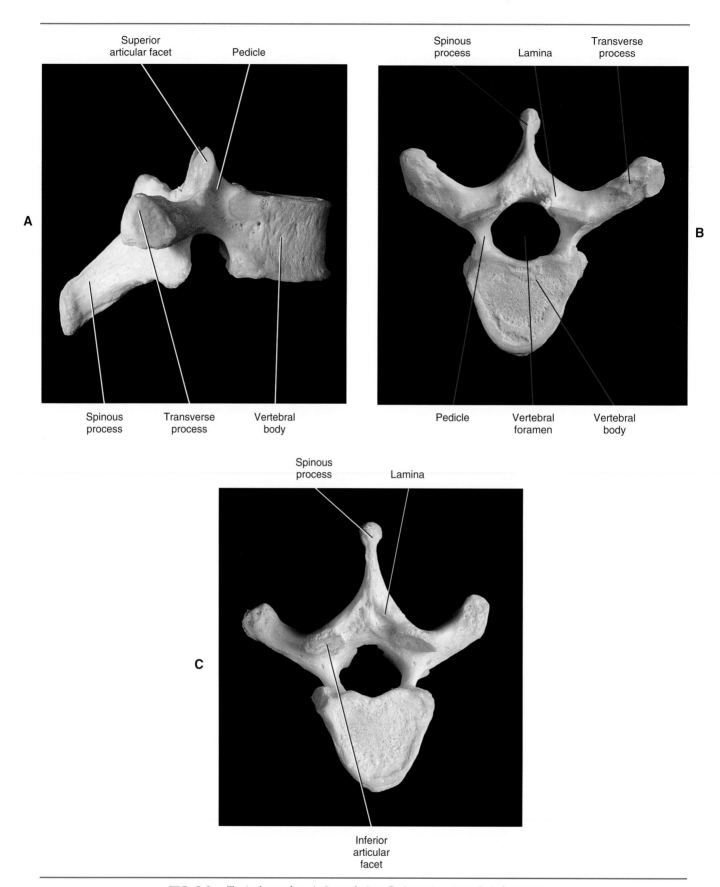

FIG. 2-3   Typical vertebra. **A,** Lateral view. **B,** Superior view. **C,** Inferior view.

support beams in the frame of a building. Animal studies have shown that both the vertical and horizontal trabeculae of a vertebral body increase in number after prolonged (weeks) and increased loading by superior-inferior compression (Issever et al., 2003).

Osteoporosis is associated with a decrease in mass primarily of the *horizontal trabeculae,* leaving less support for the vertical trabeculae when loads are placed on an osteoporotic vertebral body. This lack of horizontal support results in a weakening of the vertebral body beyond that anticipated by the percent reduction in bone mineral content. In fact, a 25% reduction in bone mass is accompanied by a 50% reduction in the ability of a vertebral body to resist loads applied to the spine.

Bone mineral density can vary significantly from one vertebra to another (Curylo et al., 1996). Although determining the presence or absence of osteoporosis by means of x-ray bone densitometry to measure bone mineral density is reliable, fractal analysis of the trabecular pattern within vertebral bodies as imaged by computed tomography (CT) also shows promise (Feltrin et al., 2001).

The vertebral bodies have been found to change (remodel) after degeneration of the intervertebral discs, by adding bone to the region adjacent to the intervertebral disc. This addition of bone is known as subchondral sclerosis, and allows the vertebral bodies to more effectively absorb the additional compressive loads received by the vertebral bodies after intervertebral disc degeneration (Moore et al., 1996).

Mosekilde and Mosekilde (1990) found that the cross-sectional area of vertebral bodies is larger in men than in women. They also found that the cross-sectional area of the vertebral bodies increases with age in men, but no similar finding was discovered in women.

The superior and inferior surfaces of vertebral bodies range from flat, but not parallel (Williams et al., 1995), to interlocking (see Chapter 5). A raised, smooth region around the edge of the vertebral body is formed by the anular apophysis. The vertebral body is rougher inside the anular apophysis.

Most vertebral bodies are concave posteriorly (in the transverse plane), where they help to form the vertebral foramina. Small foramina for arteries and veins appear on the front and sides of the vertebral bodies. Posteriorly there are small arterial foramina and one or two large, centrally placed foramina for the exiting basivertebral vein(s) (Williams et al., 1995).

A series of relatively large arteries pierce the center of the vertebral bodies along their entire circumference (Fig. 2-4). On entering a vertebral body, these large nutrient arteries form a dense plexus of arteries within the central horizontal plane of the vertebral body. From this central plexus, many small branches ascend and descend to reach the superior and inferior margins of the vertebral bodies; these margins are adjacent to the cartilaginous end plates of the intervertebral discs.

Large numbers of small veins drain the superior and inferior margins of the vertebral bodies. These very small veins enter into large tributaries that are oriented in the horizontal plane very close to each superior and inferior vertebral margin. These large tributaries have been called the horizontal subarticular collecting vein system (Crock and Yoshizawa, 1976). Branches of the horizontal subarticular collecting vein system, in turn, drain into large vertically oriented channels that course toward the central horizontal plane of the vertebral body, where a dense venous network is formed. The dense network is drained by the basivertebral vein (occasionally there are two basivertebral veins in the same vertebral body). The subarticular collecting vein system also sends small tributaries laterally. These small tributaries leave the vertebral body and drain into veins of the external vertebral venous plexus (see later information).

Of clinical interest are the findings of Esses and Monro (1992) who found that long-term intraosseous hypertension within the vessels of the vertebral bodies is associated with an increase of pain and severity of osteoarthritis.

Occasionally a vertebral body compression fracture occurs some time (days to years) after an individual suffers trauma to the spine. This condition is known as "delayed posttraumatic vertebral collapse," or Kümmell disease, and is probably the result of damage to the nutrient arteries of the vertebral body during the original injury. Damage to the nutrient arteries then leads to necrosis (ischemic necrosis) of the vertebral body and subsequent vertebral collapse (Van Eenenaam and El-Khoury, 1993).

Osteophytes of the vertebral bodies are protrusions of the superior or inferior aspects of the vertebral bodies that are composed of compact bone and extend toward the adjacent intervertebral disc and vertebral body. Anterior osteophytes of the vertebral bodies generally are more common than posterior ones and usually are larger. A large proportion of vertebral columns have osteophytes by the second decade of life, and by the fourth decade osteophytes are present in almost 100% of vertebral columns. The size of the osteophytes increases with age. There is no significant difference between osteophyte formation on the anterior aspect of the vertebral bodies and race; however, males have more anterior osteophytes than females. Osteophytes on the posterior aspect of the vertebral bodies are most common in the lower cervical and lower lumbar regions and are more common in white than in black males and females. No significant difference exists in the prevalence of posterior osteophytes between males and females of the same racial background (Nathan, 1962).

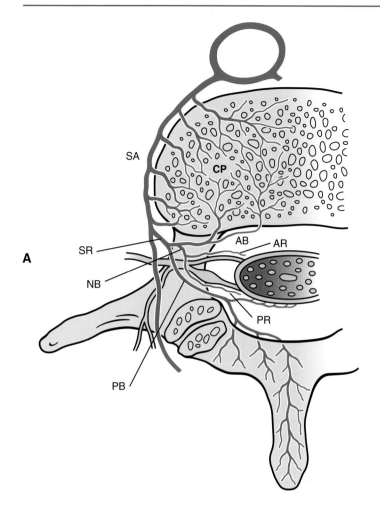

FIG. 2-4 Arterial supply to a typical vertebra and related tissues. **A,** Superior view of a horizontal section through the level of the vertebral body showing, *SA,* a lumbar segmental artery coming off of the abdominal aorta and sending many branches to feed, *CP,* the dense central plexus of arteries formed within this plane of the vertebral body. From this central plexus many small branches ascend and descend to reach the superior and inferior margins of the vertebral bodies (see **B**). Also, notice that, *SR,* the spinal ramus of the segmental artery gives off, *AB,* an anterior branch to the vertebral body and anterior tissues of the vertebral canal; *PB,* a posterior branch to the posterior arch structures and posterior tissues of the vertebral canal; and, *NB,* a neural branch that divides into, *AR,* anterior and, *PR,* posterior radicular arteries to feed the ventral and dorsal roots (and rootlets), respectively. **B,** Midsagittal section showing the superior and inferior branches of the central arterial plexus of the vertebral body. These branches feed the arterial plexuses located subjacent to the cartilaginous end plates. Also notice that the anterior branch (not labeled here) of the spinal ramus is giving off an artery to the center of the vertebral body that helps supply the central arterial plexus as well. The anterior branch also gives off, *AsB,* an ascending and, *DsB,* descending branch, each of which anastomoses with a corresponding artery of adjacent vertebral levels. The posterior branch of the spinal ramus is shown giving off, *L,* a large laminar artery that enters the lamina and then provides, *ALB,* ascending and, *DLB,* descending laminar branches to supply the superior and inferior articular processes, respectively, including the subchondral bone of the articular facets. See Arterial Supply to the Spine for further details.

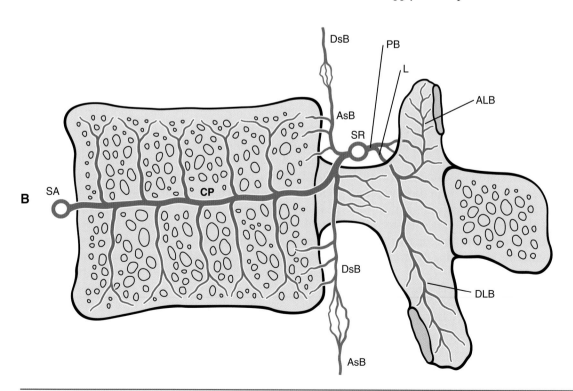

Osteophytes develop slightly earlier in life in the thoracic and lumbar regions than in the cervical and sacral regions. However, in the fifth decade cervical osteophytes develop more rapidly than in the other regions of the spine, and by the seventh decade the incidence is roughly equal among cervical, thoracic, and lumbar osteophytes; osteophytes of the sacral region (only found on the first sacral segment) are the least common (Nathan, 1962).

Anterior osteophytes can result in complete interbody fusion. Such fusion is most common in the mid- to lower-thoracic region and in the lower-cervical region; however, fusion is extremely rare between C7 and T1 and between L5 and the first sacral segment (Nathan, 1962).

Osteophytes are much less common in the region of a vertebral body in contact with the aorta, and they usually develop in the region of the vertebral body that receives the greatest compressive loads during normal stance or common movements. For example, osteophytes tend to develop on the concave side of the normal curves of the spine. Anterior osteophytes, which generally are the most numerous, are most common in the thoracic region, and posterior osteophytes are most common in the cervical and lumbar regions of the spine (Nathan, 1962).

Bony End Plates. The ring apophyses, also known as the ring apophyses, are secondary centers of ossification that develop along the periphery of the superior and inferior aspects of the vertebral bodies before puberty (see Chapter 12). These regions fuse with the remainder of the vertebral bodies usually by the age of 25 years. Some authors refer to the superior- and inferior-most regions of the vertebral body, including the area associated with the superior and inferior ring apophyses (both before and after their fusion with the remainder of the vertebral body), as the vertebral end plates. However, this terminology is confusing because the vertebral end plates (also known as the cartilaginous end plates) refer to the parts of each intervertebral disc that are found superior and inferior to the nucleus pulposus and anulus fibrosus. Therefore the term "bony end plate" is used in this text to describe the superior- and inferior-most regions of the vertebral bodies. During the time of puberty these regions are also associated with the ring apophyses, and the term bony end plate applies to the region of the ring apophyses as well, both before and after their fusion with the remainder of the vertebral bodies. The term vertebral end plate, or cartilaginous end plate, is used in this text to refer to the superior and inferior aspects of each intervertebral disc.

The central region of each bony end plate has a mottled appearance from birth to 6 months of age. This appearance results from vascular markings (holes) formed by small blood vessels that at this early age extend to the cartilaginous end plate from deep within the vertebral body.

Between 6 months and 2.5 years of age the mottled appearance of the central bony end plate disappears (as do the blood vessels), and the end plate retains this smoother appearance for the remainder of the life of the vertebra. However, between 6 months and 25 years of age the peripheral margins of the end plates become prominently scalloped, showing prominent ridges and sulci. This scalloping results in a denticulate, or toothlike, appearance along the vertebral margins, having an appearance similar to that of the outer margins of the epiphyseal plates of other bones of the body. The scalloping of the bony end plate is variable from one vertebra to the next and is most prominent in the lower thoracic and upper lumbar regions, and less pronounced in the cervical and thoracic regions. The scalloping is thought to increase stability during the application of shear forces to the spine (forces that tend to slide one vertebra over the vertebra immediately below). Resistance to shear forces also explains why the scalloping is less prominent in the thoracic and cervical regions, where the ribs and uncinate processes (see Chapter 5), respectively, resist shear forces in these areas. The ridges and sulci of the bony end plates become more prominent until approximately 12 to 25 years of age when the bone of the anular apophysis is laid down over them, creating an enlarging smooth ridge of bone that follows the peripheral margins of the superior and inferior surfaces of the vertebral bodies (Edelson and Nathan, 1988).

Beginning in the latter aspect of the third decade, osteophytes develop on the vertebral bodies, usually just *adjacent* to the bony end plate. That is, an osteophyte usually spares the bony end plate (there is usually a distinct sulcus between each osteophyte and the related bony end plate). The osteophytes then arch across the bony end plate, extending toward the adjacent vertebra (Edelson and Nathan, 1988).

Osteoporotic changes also can occur in the bony end plate. These changes usually begin toward the end of the fifth decade and progress until death. Osteoporotic changes in the bony end plates take on the appearance of lytic, or "punched out" areas of the bone (Edelson and Nathan, 1988).

Vertebral Arch

The vertebral (posterior) arch has several unique structures (see Fig. 2-3). These include the pedicles, laminae, superior articular, inferior articular, transverse, and spinous processes. Each of these subdivisions of the vertebral arch is discussed separately in the following sections.

Pedicles. The pedicles (see Fig. 2-3) create the narrow anterior portions of the vertebral arch. They are short, thick, and rounded and attach to the posterior and lateral aspects of the vertebral body. They also are placed superior to the midpoint of a vertebral body. Because the pedicles are smaller than the vertebral bodies, a groove, or vertebral notch, is formed above and below the pedicles. These are known as the superior and inferior vertebral notches, respectively. The superior vertebral notch is more shallow and smaller than the inferior vertebral notch.

The percentage of compact bone surrounding the inner cancellous bone of the pedicles varies from one region of the spine to another and seems to depend on the amount of motion that occurs at the given region (Pal et al., 1988). More compact, stronger bone is found in regions with more motion. Therefore the pedicles of the middle cervical and upper lumbar regions contain more compact bone than the relatively immobile thoracic region. The thoracic pedicles are made primarily of cancellous bone (Pal et al., 1988).

There are significant differences in the relative size of various parts of vertebrae among various ethnic populations, with those from Western populations generally having larger structures than those from Asia. This is true for the pedicles (Chadha et al., 2003).

Laminae.   The laminae (singular, *lamina*) are continuous with the pedicles. They are flattened from anterior to posterior and form the broad posterior portion of the vertebral arch (see Fig. 2-3). They curve posteromedially to unite with the spinous process, completing the vertebral foramen. Xu et al. (1999) performed a detailed morphometric study of the laminae of the entire vertebral column. They concluded that, generally speaking, the laminae of males are slightly larger than those of females. The laminae generally increase in height from C4, which are the shortest (10.4 + 1.1 mm), to T11, which are the tallest (25.1 + 2.5 mm). The height of the laminae then begin to decrease slowly from T12 to L4, and then more markedly at L5. However, the laminae are widest at L5 (15.7 + 2.0 mm) and narrowest at T4 (5.8 + 0.8 mm). The cervical laminae are wide (rivaling those of L5), the thoracic laminae (with the exception of T11 and T12) are narrow, and the width steadily increases from T11 to L5. The laminae are thickest at T2 (5.0 + 0.2 mm) and least thick at C5 (1.9 + 0.6 mm), with the thickness of the laminae decreasing from the upper to the lower thoracic regions. The lower cervical laminae are the least thick of the vertebral column, and the lumbar laminae are of intermediate thickness (Xu et al., 1999).

Spinous Process.   The spinous process (spine) of each vertebra (see Fig. 2-3) projects posteriorly and often inferiorly from the laminae. The size, shape, and direction of this process vary greatly from one region of the vertebral column to the next (see individual regions). A spinous process also may normally deviate to the left or right of the midline, and this can be a source of confusion in clinical practice. Therefore a deviated spinous process seen on x-ray film or palpated during a physical examination frequently is not associated with a fracture of the spinous process or a malposition of the entire vertebra.

The spinous processes throughout the spine function as a series of levers both for muscles of posture and muscles of active movement (Williams et al., 1995). Most of the muscles that attach to the spinous processes act to extend the vertebral column. Some muscles attaching to the spinous processes also rotate the vertebrae to which they attach.

Lateral to the spinous processes are the vertebral grooves. These grooves are formed by laminae in the cervical and lumbar regions. They are much broader in the thoracic region and are formed by both the laminae and transverse processes. The left and right vertebral grooves serve as gutters. These gutters are filled with the deep back muscles that course the entire length of the spine.

The spinous process of a specific vertebra frequently can be identified by its relationship to other palpable landmarks of the back. Chapter 1 provides a detailed account of the relationship between the spinous processes and other anatomic structures.

Vertebral Foramen and the Vertebral Canal. The vertebral foramen is the opening within each vertebra that is bounded by the structures discussed thus far. Therefore the vertebral body, the left and right pedicles, the left and right laminae, and the spinous process form the borders of the vertebral foramen in a typical vertebra (see Fig. 2-3). The size and shape of the vertebral foramina vary from one region of the spine to the next and even from one vertebra to the next. The vertebral canal is the composite of all of the vertebral foramina. This region houses the spinal cord, nerve roots, meninges, and many vessels. The vertebral canal is discussed in more detail later in this chapter.

Transverse Processes.   The transverse processes project laterally from the junction of the pedicle and lamina (pediculolaminar junction) (see Fig. 2-3). Like the spinous processes, their exact direction varies considerably from one region of the spine to the next. The transverse processes of typical cervical vertebrae project obliquely anteriorly between the sagittal and coronal planes and are located anterior to the articular processes and lateral to the pedicles. The left and right cervical transverse processes are separated from those of the vertebrae above and below by successive intervertebral foramina. The thoracic transverse processes are different and project obliquely posteriorly and are located behind the articular processes, pedicles, and intervertebral foramina (see Fig. 6-1). They also articulate with the ribs. The lumbar transverse processes (see Fig. 7-1) lie in front of the lumbar articular processes and posterior to the pedicles and intervertebral foramina.

The transverse processes serve as muscle attachment sites and are used as lever arms by spinal muscles. The muscles that attach to the transverse processes maintain posture and induce rotation and lateral flexion of single vertebrae and the spine as a whole.

Each transverse process is composed of the "true" transverse process (diapophysis) and a costal element. Each costal element (pleurapophysis) develops as part of the neural arch (see Fig. 12-13). The costal elements of the thoracic region develop into ribs. Elsewhere the costal elements are incorporated with the diapophysis and help to form the transverse process of the fully developed vertebra. The cervical costal elements are composed primarily of the anterior tubercle but also include the intertubercular lamella and a part of the posterior tubercle. The lumbar costal elements are the anterior aspects of the transverse processes, and the left and right sacral alae represent the costal processes of the sacrum. The cervical and lumbar costal processes occasionally may develop into ribs. This occurs most frequently in the lower cervical and upper lumbar regions. These extra ribs may be a cause of discomfort in some individuals. This is particularly true of cervical ribs (see Chapter 5).

Superior Articular Processes. Like the transverse processes, the superior articular processes (zygapophyses) and facets also arise from the pediculolaminar junction (see Fig. 2-3). The left and right superior articular processes project superiorly, and the articular surface (facet) of each articular process faces posteriorly, although the precise direction varies from posteromedial in the cervical and lumbar regions to posterolateral in the thoracic region. (The superior and inferior articular facets are discussed in more detail later in this chapter under Zygapophysial Joints.)

Inferior Articular Processes. The left and right inferior articular processes (zygapophyses) and facets project inferiorly from the pediculolaminar junction, and the articular surface (facet) faces anteriorly (see Fig. 2-3). Again, the precise direction in which they face varies from anterolateral (cervical region) to anteromedial (thoracic and lumbar regions).

Adjoining zygapophyses form zygapophysial joints (Z joints), which are small and allow for limited movement. Mobility at the Z joints varies considerably between vertebral levels. The Z joints also help to form the poste-

rior border of the intervertebral foramina. The anatomy of the Z joint is discussed after the next section.

Functional Components of a Typical Vertebra

Each region of a typical vertebra is related to one or more of the functions of the vertebral column mentioned at the beginning of this chapter (support, protection of the spinal cord and spinal nerve roots, and movement) (Fig. 2-5). In general, the vertebral bodies help with support, whereas the pedicles and laminae protect the spinal cord. The superior and inferior articular processes help determine spinal movement by the facing of their facets. The transverse and spinous processes aid movement by acting as lever arms on which the muscles of the spine act.

The posterior arches also function to support and transfer weight (Pal et al., 1988), and the articular processes of the cervical region form two distinct pillars (left and right) that bear weight. In addition, the laminae of C2, C7, and the upper thoracic region (T1 and T2) help to support weight. Therefore a laminectomy at these levels results in marked cervical instability (Pal et al., 1988), whereas a laminectomy from C3 to C6 is relatively safe.

The pedicles also act to transfer weight from the posterior arch to the vertebral body, and vice versa, in the cervical region (Pal et al., 1988), but only from the posterior arch to the vertebral bodies in the thoracic region. The role of the pedicles in the transfer of loads is yet to be completely determined in the upper lumbar region, but the trabecular pattern of the L4 and L5 pedicles seems to indicate that the majority of load may be transferred from the vertebral bodies to the region of the posterior arch. This is discussed in further detail in Chapter 7, which is devoted to the lumbar spine.

ZYGAPOPHYSIAL JOINTS

The articulating surface of each superior and inferior articular process (zygapophysis) is covered with a 1- to 2-mm-thick layer of hyaline cartilage. This hyaline-lined portion of a superior and inferior articular process is known as the articular facet. The junction found between the superior and inferior articular facets on one side of two adjacent vertebrae is known as a zygapophysial joint. Therefore a left and right Z joint are between each pair of vertebrae. Figure 2-6, *A* shows the Z joints of the cervical, thoracic, and lumbar regions. These joints also are called facet joints or interlaminar joints (Giles, 1992). The Z joints (Fig. 2-6, *B* to *D*) are classified as synovial (diarthrodial), planar joints. They are rather small joints, and although they allow motion to occur, they are perhaps more important in their ability to determine the

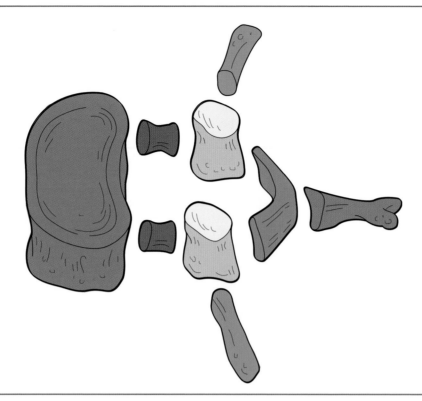

FIG. 2-5   Functional components of a typical vertebra. The vertebral body *(brown)* serves the function of support. The pedicles *(purple)* and laminae *(blue)* serve the function of protection of the spinal cord (cervical and thoracic regions) or cauda equina (below the level of L1). The spinous process *(red)*, transverse processes *(dark green)*, articular processes *(peach)*, and particularly the articular facets *(white)* serve the function of movement.

direction and limitations of movement that can occur between vertebrae. In addition, the Z joints (more specifically, the articular processes) help to carry the loads placed on the spine, particularly during extension and rotation (Schultz et al., 1973). The Z joints are of added interest to those who treat spinal conditions because, as is the case with any joint, loss of motion or aberrant motion may be a primary source of pain (Paris, 1983). In fact, Dreyer and Dreyfuss (1996) estimate that 15% to 40% of chronic low back pain is related to the Z joints.

Each Z joint is surrounded posterolaterally by a capsule. The outer capsule and inner layers of the capsule differ significantly in make-up; this is possibly unique to Z joints (Yamashita et al., 1996). The capsule consists of an outer layer of dense fibroelastic connective tissue, a vascular central layer made up of areolar tissue and loose connective tissue, and an inner layer consisting of a synovial membrane (Giles and Taylor, 1987). Figure 2-6, *B*, shows the previously listed regions of the capsule. The anterior and medial aspects of the Z joint are covered by the ligamentum flavum. The synovial membrane lines the articular capsule, the ligamentum flavum (Xu et al., 1991), and the synovial joint folds (see the following),

but not the hyaline articular cartilage that covers the joint surfaces of the articular processes (Giles, 1992).

The Z joint capsules throughout the vertebral column are thought to do little to limit motion (Onan, Heggeness, and Hipp, 1998), although the capsules probably help to stabilize the Z joints during motions (Boszczyk et al., 2001). Generally, the Z joint capsules are relatively thin and loose and are attached to the margins of the opposed superior and inferior articular facets of the adjacent vertebrae (Williams et al., 1995). Superior and inferior external protrusions of the joint capsules, known as recesses, bulge out from the joint and are filled with adipose tissue. The inferior recess is larger than the superior one (Jeffries, 1988). The capsules are longer and looser in the cervical region than in the lumbar and thoracic regions.

Innervation of the Zygapophysial Joints

The Z joint capsule receives a significant sensory innervation (Cavanaugh, Kallakuri, and Özaktay, 1995; Vandenabeele, Creemers, and Lambrichts, 1996). Ahmed et al. (1993) found both sensory and autonomic fibers in the synovial layer of the Z joint capsules of rats. They also found evidence of nociceptive innervation in the ligamentum flavum proper (that portion of the ligamentum flavum adjacent to the Z joint). The authors concluded that both the sensory and autonomic innervations could play a collaborative role in the pathophysiology of Z joint pain, inflammation, and inflammatory joint disease.

The sensory nerve supply to each Z joint (Fig. 2-7) is derived from the medial branch of the posterior primary division (dorsal ramus) at the level of the joint, and each joint also receives a branch from the medial branch of the posterior primary division of the level above and the level below (Jeffries, 1988). This multilevel innervation is probably one reason why pain from a Z joint frequently has a very broad referral pattern (Jeffries, 1988). Chapter 11 deals with the phenomenon of referred pain in more detail.

The medial branches of the posterior primary divisions innervating a Z joint terminate as one of three types of sensory receptors: free nerve endings (nociceptive), complex unencapsulated nerve endings, and encapsulated nerve endings (Yamashita et al., 1990; Beaman et al., 1993; Cavanaugh, Kallakuri, and Özaktay, 1995). The latter two types are thought to be associated with proprioceptive sense and the modulation of protective muscular reflexes. The free nerve endings are associated with nociception (i.e., signaling potential or real tissue damage). The ultrastructure of these receptors has been described (Vandenabeele et al., 1997; McLain and Pickar, 1998).

In addition, Wyke (1985) categorized the types of sensory receptors in Z joints by their function. These categories are as follows:

◆ *Type I.* Very sensitive static and dynamic mechanoreceptors that fire continually, even to some extent when the joint is not moving
◆ *Type II.* Less sensitive mechanoreceptors that fire only during movement
◆ *Type III.* Mechanoreceptors found in joints of the extremities (Wyke [1985] did not find these in the Z joints.)
◆ *Type IV.* Slow conducting nociceptors

Wyke (1985) asserts that type I and II receptors have a pain suppressive effect (a Melzack and Wall gate control type of mechanism). He also states that there is a reflexogenic effect created by type I and II fibers that causes a normalization of muscle activity on both sides of the spinal column when stimulated. This reflexogenic effect is thought to occur at the level of the site of stimulation, as well as at the levels above and below. Of possible interest is the fact that Isherwood and Antoun (1980) found similar nerve endings within the interspinous and supraspinous ligaments and the ligamentum flavum. These ligaments are discussed in Chapters 5 and 6 on the cervical and thoracic regions.

Innervation by mechanoreceptors is denser in the cervical Z joint capsules than in those of the thoracic and lumbar regions (McLain, 1994; McLain and Pickar, 1998). This may be because the increased mobility of the cervical region may require more proprioceptive input to ensure smooth and accurate head movement and positioning, and also to help prevent injury from inappropriate motions or muscle responses to sudden movements. Innervation by free nerve endings associated with nociception is abundant in all regions of the spine (McLain and Pickar, 1998).

Beaman et al. (1993) found nerves that stained with substance P (associated with pain) in the bone underlying the articular facets of the articular processes (subchondral bone) from specimens of Z joints taken during surgical procedures of patients with low back pain and accompanying degeneration of the Z joints, but not in control specimens. This indicates that the subchondral bone may be an additional source of pain in individuals with arthritis of the spine (including degenerative joint disease, also known as osteoarthritis, or common degenerative arthritis) or with injury to the spine. Because degeneration of the spine can result in an increase in the loads placed on the Z joints by 3% to 47%, depending on the severity of the degeneration, the presence of nociceptive (pain) nerve endings in the subchondral bone of the Z joint articular facets indicates that the subchondral bone in this region may play an active role in back pain. The combined innervation of the Z joint capsules and subchondral bone provides further strong evidence implicating the Z joints as an important source of back pain in many individuals.

Zygapophysial Joint Synovial Folds

Z joint synovial folds are synovium-lined extensions of the capsule that protrude into the joint space to cover part of the hyaline cartilage. The synovial folds vary in size and shape in the different regions of the spine. Figure 2-8 shows a photomicrograph by Singer, Giles, and Day (1990) demonstrating a large Z joint synovial fold.

Kos in 1969 described the typical intraarticular fold (meniscus) (Fig. 2-9) as being attached to the capsule by loose connective tissue. Synovial tissue and blood vessels were distal to the attachment, followed by dense connective tissue (Bogduk and Engel, 1984).

Engel and Bogduk in 1982 reported on a study of 82 lumbar Z joints. They found at least one intraarticular fold within each joint. The intraarticular structures were categorized into three types. The first was described as a connective tissue rim found running along the most peripheral edge of the entire joint. This connective tissue rim was lined by a synovial membrane. The second type of meniscus was described as an adipose tissue pad, and the third type was identified as a distinct, well-defined, fibroadipose meniscoid. This latter type of meniscus usually was found entering the joint from either the superior or inferior pole or both poles of the joint.

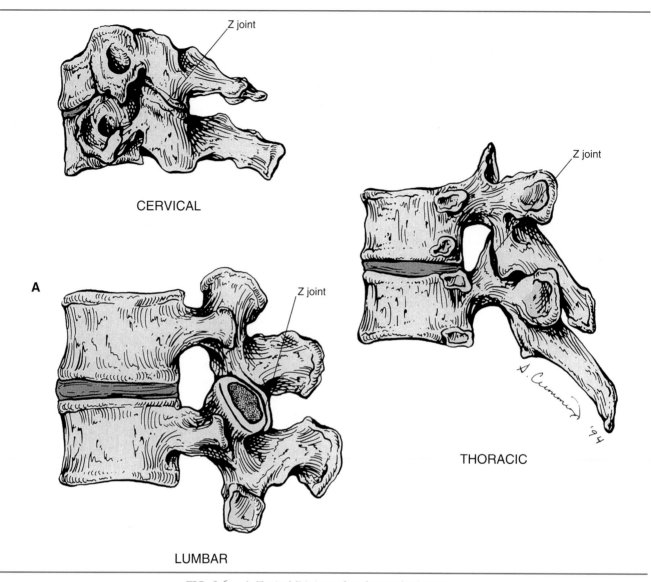

FIG. 2-6   **A,** Typical Z joints of each vertebral region.

Giles and Taylor (1987) studied 30 Z joints, all of which were found to have menisci. The menisci were renamed zygapophysial joint synovial folds because of their histologic make-up. Free nerve endings were found within the folds, and the nerve endings met the criteria necessary for classification as pain receptors (nociceptors). That is, they were distant from blood vessels and were of proper diameter (0.6 to 12 μ). Therefore the synovial folds (menisci) themselves were found to be pain sensitive. This meant that if the Z joint synovial fold became compressed by, or trapped between, the articular facets making up the Z joint, back pain could result (see Fig. 2-9). Other investigators have confirmed the presence of sensory fibers in the Z joint synovial folds (Ahmed et al., 1993; Vandenabeele, Creemers, and Lambrichts, 1996).

Zygapophysial Joints as a Source of Back Pain

Various Clinical Approaches to Pain Management. Damage to the osseous and ligamentous tissues (including the capsule) of a Z joint can result in inflammation, which can cause the release of chemicals that stimulate the nociceptive nerve endings supplying the joint (Cavanaugh, Kallakuri, and Özaktay, 1995; Cavanaugh et al., 1996, 1997). Therefore not surprisingly, the Z joints have been shown to be a source of back pain (Mooney and Robertson, 1976; Lippitt, 1984; Jeffries, 1988; Beaman et al., 1993), and several therapeutic approaches have been designed to treat pain originating from the Z joints. Physical therapy in the form of ice, moist heat, or exercise is used frequently. Acupuncture also has been used. Injection of the Z joints with local anesthetic or

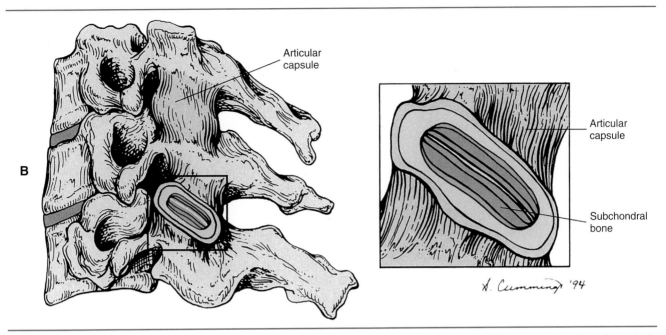

FIG. 2-6—cont'd   **B,** Typical Z joint. The layers of the Z joint as seen in parasagittal section *(inset)* are color coded as follows: *light blue,* joint space; *violet,* articular cartilage; *brown,* subchondral bone; *orange,* synovial lining of articular capsule; *peach,* vascularized, middle layer of the articular capsule; *turquoise,* fibrous, outer layer of the articular capsule.   *Continued*

corticosteroids is carried out with some frequency, and denervation of the Z joints has been performed by a number of clinicians and researchers (Shealy, 1975). Surgical transection of the posterior primary divisions innervating these joints was the first method used to denervate the joint. This technique has been replaced by radiofrequency neurotomy (Shealy, 1975). Others are not yet convinced that this is the method of choice for treating pain arising from these structures (Lippitt, 1984), especially in light of the fact that damage to the medial branch of the posterior primary division during surgical laminectomy has been linked to prolonged postoperative pain, denervation atrophy of paraspinal back muscles, and functional instability that can extend beyond the segments involved in the surgical procedure (Sihvonen et al., 1993; Boelderl et al., 2002). Spinal adjusting (manipulation) to introduce movement into a Z joint suspected of being hypomobile also has been used frequently to treat pain of Z joint origin. Mooney and Robertson (1976) stated that spinal manipulation may produce therapeutic benefit by relieving the Z joint articular capsule or its synovial lining from chronic reaction to trauma. Such chronic reaction to trauma resulting in Z joint pain includes the catching of a synovial fold between the joint capsule and an articular process and also the entrapment of zygapophysial joint menisci (synovial folds) deep within the Z joint (see Fig. 2-9). Entrapped Z joint menisci may be a direct source of

pain because they are supplied by pain-sensitive nerve endings (Giles and Taylor, 1987; Ahmed et al., 1993; Vandenabeele, Creemers, and Lambrichts, 1996). Spinal adjusting (manipulation) separates (gaps) the opposed articular surfaces of the Z joint (Cramer et al., 2000, 2002), and this separation may relieve direct pressure on the meniscus, and also provide traction to the Z joint articular capsule that, by its attachment to the Z joint meniscus, could pull the meniscus peripherally, away from the region of previous entrapment (Kos and Wolf, 1972). Bogduk and Engel (1984) felt that entrapment of a Z joint meniscus would tear it away from its capsular attachment. If this were the case, the nerve endings leading to the synovial fold probably would be torn as well. This could result in transient pain. Bogduk and Engel (1984) also stated that a meniscus that had torn away from its capsular attachment could conceivably result in a loose body being found in the Z joint, similar to those that are sometimes found in the knee. This, they felt, may be amenable to spinal manipulation. However, the frequency with which this scenario actually occurs in clinical practice was questioned (Bogduk and Engel, 1984). Further research is needed to clarify the frequency with which Z joint menisci (synovial folds) actually tear away from their capsular attachments to become loose bodies. Additional study also is needed to determine whether menisci can become entrapped while remaining attached to the capsule and their nerve supply.

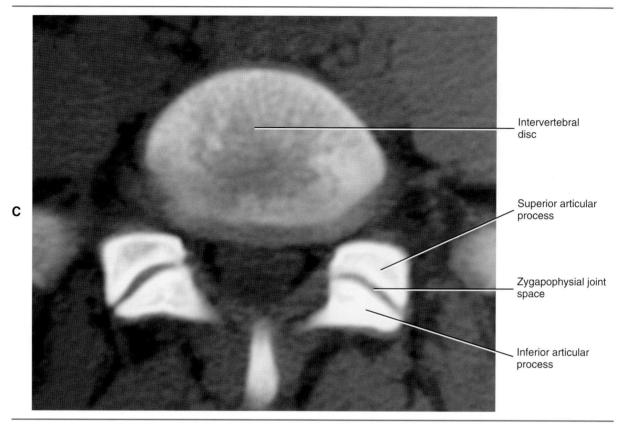

C

Intervertebral disc

Superior articular process

Zygapophysial joint space

Inferior articular process

FIG. 2-6—cont'd   C, Horizontal computed tomography (CT) showing Z joints.

Mooney and Robertson (1976) used facet joint injections of local anesthetic and corticosteroids to treat pain arising from the Z joint. They felt that such injections helped to relieve intraarticular adhesions that had been seen to develop during the degenerative phase of progressive back pain. Because hypomobility results in degenerative changes of the Z joints (Cramer et al., 2004), perhaps the removal of this type of adhesion could be another positive effect of Z joint manipulation.

MOVEMENT OF THE SPINE

Movement between two typical adjacent vertebrae is slight, but when the movement between many segments is combined, the result is a great deal of movement. The movements that can occur in the spine include flexion, extension, lateral flexion (side bending), rotation, and circumduction (Fig. 2-10). Circumduction is a combination of flexion, lateral bending, rotation, and extension. The intervertebral discs help to limit the amount of movement that can occur between individual vertebrae. Therefore the thicker intervertebral discs of the cervical and lumbar regions allow for more movement to occur in these regions. In addition, the shape and orientation of the articular facets determine the movements that can occur between two adjacent segments and also limit the amount of movement that can occur between segments. Interestingly, the beginning and middle stages of degeneration (stages I through IV) of the intervertebral discs increase segmental motion, as the thinning discs allow more "joint play" between the segments. However, once end-stage degeneration is reached (stage V), segmental motion decreases. In addition, the early stages of degeneration of the Z joints (stages I through III; accompanied by erosion of the articular hyaline cartilage) increases rotation (axial rotation) of the spine. However, during the later stages of Z joint degeneration, additional bone is added to the subchondral bone subjacent to the Z joint hyaline cartilage articular facets. This process is known as subchondral sclerosis. Once subchondral sclerosis of the Z joints occurs, axial rotation of the involved segments of the spine decreases to below normal levels (Fujiwara et al., 2000).

The specific ranges of motion of the spine are discussed with each vertebral region (see Chapters 5 through 7). However, this section discusses the factors limiting spinal motion and the phenomenon of coupled motion.

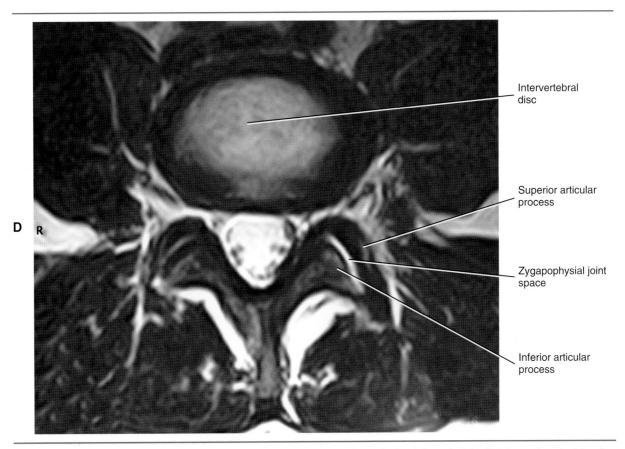

Intervertebral disc

Superior articular process

Zygapophysial joint space

Inferior articular process

D R

FIG. 2-6—cont'd   **D,** Magnetic resonance imaging (MRI) scan through the left and right Z joints of typical lumbar vertebrae. (Images courtesy Dr. Dennis Skogsbergh.)

The Role of Spinal Ligaments

The ligaments of the spine are discussed from superior to inferior with the region in which they first occur (e.g., ligamentum nuchae and anterior longitudinal ligament with the cervical spine; supraspinous ligament with the thoracic spine). Thereafter, the ligaments are mentioned only when they have unique characteristics in a specific region. The intervertebral disc is covered later in this chapter. However, this section discusses some of the characteristics common to the majority of spinal ligaments. In addition, Tables 2-2 and 2-3 summarize the attachment sites and functions (motions restricted) of the most important ligaments of the spine.

The role of the spinal ligaments is to allow smooth motion, with the least amount of resistance and maximum conservation of energy, within the spine's full normal range of motion. The ligaments also help to provide protection to the spinal cord, by limiting too much motion and absorbing a significant amount of the loads placed on the spine during trauma. The functional properties of a ligament are a combination of the physical properties of the ligament (as described by its load

displacement curve; see the following) and also the orientation and location of the ligament with respect to the moving vertebrae.

The ligaments of the vertebral column are most effective in carrying loads along the direction in which their fibers run. They readily resist tensile forces but buckle when subjected to compression.

Although each ligament has a unique combination of stiffness, maximum deformation, and failure load, the similarities of the spinal ligaments with regard to these parameters are striking (i.e., biomechanically speaking, the load-deformation curves for all of the spinal ligaments are similar). For all ligaments of the spine, there is a sharp increase in stiffness once full physiologic motion has been attained (little stiffness up to the end of physiologic motion). Spinal degeneration generally leads to increased motion (in the initial stages). This increased motion can result in increased strain on the ligaments, which in turn can result in ligamentous sprain. Consequently, degenerated spines may carry higher risks for increased ligament sprains during flexion, extension, axial rotation, and lateral flexion.

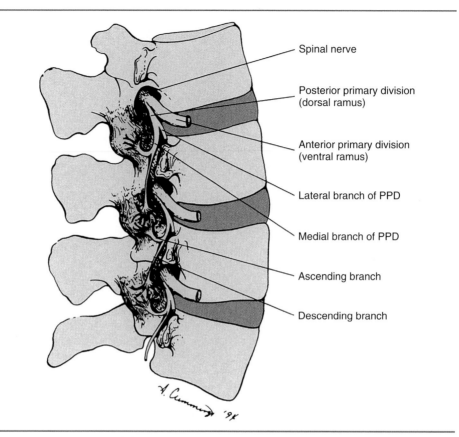

Spinal nerve

Posterior primary division
(dorsal ramus)

Anterior primary division
(ventral ramus)

Lateral branch of PPD

Medial branch of PPD

Ascending branch

Descending branch

FIG. 2-7   Innervation of the Z joints. Each spinal nerve divides into a medial and lateral branch. The medial branch has an ascending division, which supplies the Z joint at the same level, and a descending division, which supplies the Z joint immediately below. Jeffries (1988) states that each medial branch also sends a branch to the Z joint of the level above (not shown in illustration).

Using nerve tracing techniques in an animal model, Jiang (1997) found that stretching of a spinal ligament resulted in "a barrage of sensory feedback from several spinal cord levels on both sides of the spinal cord." The sensory information was found to ascend to many higher centers by way of the dorsal columns and spinocerebellar tracts (see Chapter 9). These higher centers included the thalamus and vestibular nuclei. Jiang's (1997) findings provide provocative evidence that the spinal ligaments, along with the Z joint capsules and the small muscles of the spine (interspinales, intertransversarii, and transversospinalis muscles) play an important role in mechanisms related to spinal proprioception (joint position sense). In addition, Solomonow et al. (1998) found that compression of the supraspinous ligament of cats or electrical stimulation of the same ligament in humans resulted in contraction of the multifidus muscle (see Chapter 4) at the same level as the stimulation and also at the segmental levels above and below the stimulation. These authors concluded that the ligaments of

the vertebral column recruit the help of spinal muscles to achieve general spinal stability.

Structures That Limit Spinal Movement

Spinal motion is limited by a series of bony stops and ligamentous brakes (Louis, 1985). Table 2-4 shows some of the structures limiting spinal motion.

Other factors associated with each type of spinal motion include the following:

- *Flexion.* The anterior longitudinal ligament is relaxed and the anterior aspects of the discs are compressed. The intervals between laminae are widened; the inferior articular processes glide upward on the superior articular processes of the subjacent vertebrae. The lumbar and cervical regions allow for more flexion than the thoracic region (Williams et al., 1995).

- *Extension.* Motion is more restricted in the thoracic region because of thinner discs and the effects of the thoracic skeleton and musculature.

Table 2-2   Ligaments of the Upper Cervical Region*

Ligament	Attachment 1	Attachment 2	Motion Limited
Posterior atlanto-occipital membrane	Posterior arch of atlas	Posterior rim of foramen magnum	Flexion of occiput on atlas
Tectorial membrane	Posterior body C2	Anterior rim of foramen magnum (clivus)	Flexion and extension of atlas and occiput
Cruciform ligament (see below)			
Transverse ligament	Medial tubercle (colliculus atlantis) of lateral mass	Medial tubercle (colliculus atlantis) of contralateral lateral mass	Forms diarthrodial joint with odontoid process, allowing rotation
Superior longitudinal band	Transverse ligament	Anterior rim foramen magnum (clivus)	Holds transverse ligament in place; may limit flexion and extension of occiput
Inferior longitudinal band	Transverse ligament	Body of C2	Holds transverse ligament in place; may limit flexion of occiput and atlas on axis
Alar ligaments	Posterior and lateral aspect of odontoid process	Medial surface of ipsilateral occipital condyle	Contralateral axial rotation
Apical ligament of odontoid process	Posterior and superior aspect of odontoid process	Anterior rim of foramen magnum (clivus)	Prevents some vertical translation and anterior shear of occiput
Anterior atlanto-occipital membrane	Superior aspect anterior arch of atlas	Anterior margin of foramen magnum	Extension of occiput on C1

Cramer G, Gudavalli R, Skogsbergh D. (2000). Functional anatomy of the cervical region. In W Herzog (Ed.). *Clinical biomechanics of the spine.* Philadelphia: Churchill Livingstone.
*See Chapters 5 through 7 for further details.

Table 2-3   Ligaments of the Lower Cervical, Thoracic, and Lumbar Regions*

Ligament	Attachment 1	Attachment 2	Motion Limited
Anterior longitudinal ligament	Body and anterior tubercle of atlas	Sacrum	Extension of vertebral column
Posterior longitudinal ligament	Posterior body C2	Sacrum	Flexion of vertebral column; may help limit posterior intervertebral disc protrusion
Ligamenta flava (paired)	Anterior and inferior aspect of lamina of vertebra above	Posterior and superior aspect of lamina of vertebra below	May aid in extension of spine; slows last few degrees of spinal flexion
Interspinous ligaments	Inferior aspect spinous process of vertebra above	Superior aspect spinous process of vertebra below	Flexion
Ligamentum nuchae	External occipital protuberance; spinous process of C7; dermis of posterior midline of neck	Cervical spinous processes (posterior tip and extending between spinous processes to attach to superior and inferior aspect)	
Intertransverse ligaments	Transverse process of vertebra above	Transverse process of vertebra below	Contralateral lateral flexion

Cramer G, Gudavalli R, Skogsbergh D. (2000). Functional anatomy of the cervical region. In W Herzog (Ed.). *Clinical biomechanics of the spine.* Philadelphia: Churchill Livingstone.
*See Chapters 5 through 7 for further details.

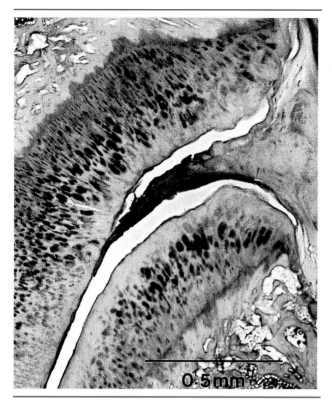

FIG. 2-8 A fibrous synovial fold is shown protruding between the articular surfaces of a Z joint. (From Singer K, Giles D, & Day R. [1990]. Intra-articular synovial folds of thoracolumbar junction zygapophyseal joints. *Anat Rec, 226,* 147-152.)

♦ *Lateral flexion.* Sides of the intervertebral discs are compressed. Lateral flexion is greatest in the cervical region, followed by the lumbar region, and finally the thoracic region (White and Panjabi, 1990).

Rotation with Lateral Flexion ("Coupled Motion")

The main motions of flexion-extension, left and right axial rotation, and left and right lateral bending are accompanied by subtle motions of the vertebrae in the other directions. These subtle motions that attend the main motions of the spine are called "coupled motions." Haher et al. (1992) defined coupled motion more precisely as "consistent association of one motion about an axis with another motion about a second axis." Coupled motions are complex and vary from one vertebral segment to the next. There is little consensus among investigators for many of the coupled motions. These motions are most predictable, and consensus among investigators is highest in the cervical and lumbar regions when the main motion is lateral flexion (Harrison, Harrison, and Troyanovich, 1998).

As a result of the facing of the superior and inferior articular facets, lateral flexion of the cervical and lumbar regions is accompanied by axial rotation (Fig. 2-11). These are coupled motions. However, the direction of the rotation is opposite in these two regions, and more rotation occurs with lateral flexion in the cervical than the lumbar region (Moroney et al., 1988). Lateral flexion of the cervical spine is accompanied by rotation of the vertebral bodies into the concavity of the arch formed by the lateral flexion (vertebral body rotation to the same side as lateral flexion). For example, right lateral flexion of the cervical region is accompanied by right rotation of the vertebral bodies (see Fig. 2-11, *A*). Because the spinous processes move in the direction opposite that of the vertebral bodies during rotation, right lateral flexion of the cervical region is accompanied by left rotation of the spinous processes.

Lateral flexion of the lumbar spine, on the other hand, is accompanied by rotation of the vertebral bodies toward the convexity of the arch formed by lateral flexion (vertebral body rotation away from the side of lateral flexion). For example, left lateral flexion of the lumbar region is accompanied by right rotation of the vertebral bodies and left rotation of the spinous processes (see Fig. 2-11, *B*).

The upper four thoracic vertebrae move in a fashion similar to that of the cervical vertebrae during lateral flexion (i.e., vertebral body rotation into the side of concavity), whereas the lower four thoracic vertebrae mimic the motion of lumbar vertebrae (i.e., vertebral body rotation toward the side of convexity). The middle four thoracic vertebrae have little coupled motion (White and Panjabi, 1990). Other investigators feel that currently there is no strong consensus as to the amount or even the direction of coupled motion of axial rotation when the main motion is lateral bending in the thoracic region (Harrison, Harrison, and Troyanovich, 1998).

INTERBODY JOINT AND INTERVERTEBRAL DISC

The intervertebral discs (IVDs) are structures of extreme clinical importance. IVD disease can be not only a primary source of back pain, but also can result in compression of exiting dorsal and ventral roots and spinal nerves, which can result in radicular symptoms ("radicular pain") and muscle weakness. In addition, pathologic changes within the disc have a strong impact on spinal biomechanics (Humzah and Soames, 1988). Consequently, a thorough knowledge of the IVD is essential for those who treat disorders of the spine. This section discusses those aspects of the IVD common to all regions of the spine. Other chapters discuss those characteristics of the IVD unique to the cervical, thoracic, and lumbar

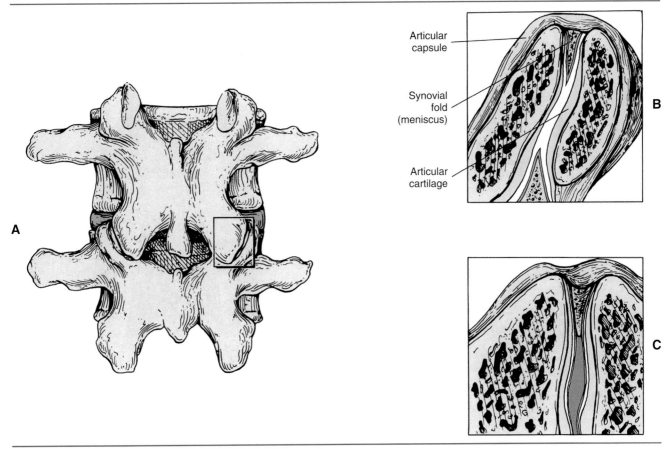

Articular
capsule

Synovial
fold
(meniscus)

Articular
cartilage

B

C

FIG. 2-9   Z joint synovial folds. **A,** Posterior view of the lumbar Z joint. **B,** A coronal section deep to that demonstrated in **A.** This coronal section shows the Z joint synovial folds. Notice the synovial lining of these folds, the articular cartilage, and the joint space. The synovial fold is attached to the articular capsule. **C,** An entrapped synovial fold. The distal portion of the fold is fibrous, and the proximal portion contains vessels and adipose tissue. Giles and Taylor (1987) also have found sensory nerve endings within the Z joint synovial folds.

regions. In addition, a large section of Chapter 11, "Pain of Spinal Origin," is devoted to IVD pathology, and Chapter 14 covers the microscopic anatomy of the IVD in detail.

The IVDs develop from the notochord and from somatic mesenchyme (sclerotome). The somatic mesenchyme surrounds the notochordal cells and differentiates into the 12 to 20 relatively thin layers (in the lumbar region; one large crescent-shaped "chunk" of fibrocartilage in the cervical region) that make up the anulus fibrosus. The notochordal tissue becomes the centrally located nucleus pulposus. Notochordal cells are replaced in the neighboring vertebral body by osteoblasts and in the cartilage end plate primarily by chondroblasts. However, remnants of notochordal cells in the cartilage end plate (see the following discussion) can cause it to weaken. This can lead to herniation of the nucleus pulposus into the cartilage end plate and

vertebral body later in life. This type of herniation is known as a Schmorl's node and can result in more rapid degeneration of the IVD.

During the fetal stage and shortly after birth, the IVDs have a rich vascular supply. However, the blood vessels narrow and diminish in number until the second decade of life, when the IVD is almost completely avascular (Taylor, 1990).

Each IVD is located between adjacent vertebral bodies from C2 to the interbody joint between L5 and the first sacral segment (see Fig. 2-1). The joint formed by two adjacent vertebral bodies and the interposed IVD is classified as a symphysis (Williams et al., 1995). No disc is located between the occiput and the atlas and the atlas and the axis, but a small disc exists between the sacrum and the coccyx. Therefore 24 IVDs are located in the spine: 6 cervical, 12 thoracic, 5 lumbar (including the L5-S1 disc), and 1 between the sacrum and coccyx.

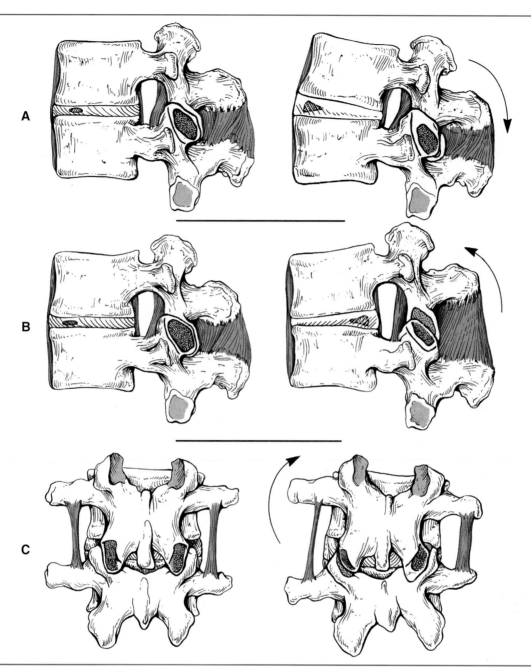

FIG. 2-10   Motion between adjacent vertebrae. **A** through **C** *(left),* Vertebrae in their neutral position. **A** *(right),* Vertebrae in extension. The anterior longitudinal ligament is becoming taut. **B** *(right),* Vertebrae in flexion. Notice that the interspinous and supraspinous ligaments, as well as the ligamentum flavum, are being stretched. **C** *(right),* Vertebrae in lateral flexion. The left intertransverse ligament is becoming taut, and the right inferior articular process is making contact with the right lamina.

Occasionally a small disc remains between the first and second coccygeal segments, and additional discs sometimes are found between the fused sacral segments. Frequently these can be seen well on magnetic resonance imaging (MRI) scans. The IVDs make up 20% to 33% of the height of the vertebral column (Coventry, 1969). Because of the strong and intimate connections

with the vertebral bodies of two adjacent vertebrae, the IVD and the adjacent vertebrae constitute the most fundamental components of the vertebral unit or motor segment.

The function of the disc is to maintain the changeable space between two adjacent vertebral bodies. The disc aids with flexibility of the spine while ensuring that not

Table 2-4	Factors Limiting Spinal Motion
Motion	**Structures Limiting Motion**
Flexion	Posterior longitudinal ligament
	Ligamenta flava
	Interspinous ligament
	Supraspinous ligament
	Posterior fibers of the intervertebral disc
	Articular capsules
	Tension of back extensor muscles
	Anterior surface of inferior articular facet against posterior surface of superior articular facet
Extension	Anterior longitudinal ligament
	Anterior aspect of intervertebral disc
	Approximation of spinous processes, articular processes, and laminae
Lateral flexion	Contralateral side of intervertebral disc and intertransverse ligament
	Approximation of articular processes
	Approximation of uncinate processes (cervical region)
	Approximation of costovertebral joints (thoracic region)
	Antagonist muscles
Rotation	Tightening of lamellar fibers of anulus fibrosus
	Orientation and architecture of articular processes

Williams PL et al. (1995). *Gray's anatomy* (38th ed.). Edinburgh: Churchill Livingstone.

too much motion occurs between spinal segments. In addition, the IVDs simultaneously help properly assimilate compressive loads placed on the spine. The vertebral bodies and articular processes also help the latter role. The mechanical efficiency of the healthy disc appears to improve with use (Humzah and Soames, 1988).

The discs usually are named by using the two vertebrae that surround the disc, for example, the C4-5 disc or the T7-8 disc. A disc also may be named by referring to the vertebra directly above it. For example, the C6 disc is the IVD directly below C6. This can be remembered more easily if the vertebra is pictured as "sitting" on its disc (W. Hogan, personal communication, November 15, 1991).

The shape of an IVD is determined by the shape of the two vertebral bodies to which it is attached. The thickness of the IVDs varies from one part of the spine to the next. The discs are thickest in the lumbar region and thinnest in the upper thoracic region (Williams et al., 1995). The cervical discs are approximately two fifths the height of the vertebral bodies, the thoracic discs approximately one fifth the height of their vertebral bodies, and the lumbar discs approximately one third the height of lumbar vertebral bodies. The discs of the cervical and lumbar regions are thicker anteriorly than posteriorly, helping to create the lordoses found in these regions (Williams et al., 1995). The thoracic discs have a consistent thickness from anterior to posterior.

The discs are connected to the anterior and posterior longitudinal ligaments. The attachment to the posterior longitudinal ligament is firm throughout the spine. The anterior longitudinal ligament generally has a strong attachment to the periosteum of the vertebral bodies, particularly at the most superior and inferior aspects of the anterior vertebral bodies, but this ligament generally has a loose attachment to the anterior aspect of the IVD (Humzah and Soames, 1988). However, regional variations between the cervical, thoracic, and lumbar regions exist. For this reason, Chapters 5 through 7 discuss the specific attachments of the anterior and posterior longitudinal ligaments in further detail. The thoracic discs also are connected to the intraarticular ligaments, which connect the thoracic IVDs to the crests of the heads of the second through the ninth ribs.

Composition of the Intervertebral Disc

Like cartilage elsewhere in the body, the disc is made up of water, cells (primarily chondrocyte-like cells and fibroblasts), proteoglycan aggregates, and type I and II collagen fibers (see Chapter 14). The proteoglycan aggregates are composed of many proteoglycan monomers attached to a hyaluronic acid core. However, the proteoglycans of the IVD are of a smaller size and different composition than the proteoglycans of cartilage found in other regions of the body (e.g., articular cartilage, nasal cartilage, and cartilage of growth plates) (Buckwalter et al., 1989). The cartilaginous IVD is a dynamic structure that has been shown to be able to repair itself and is capable of regeneration (Humzah and Soames, 1988; Nitobe et al., 1988; Mendel et al., 1992), although its ability to regenerate seems to diminish after injury or degeneration (Moore et al., 1996).

The IVD is an osmotic system that is sensitive to load, pressure, and the concentration of proteoglycans within its component parts. When the disc is contained (i.e., no extrusions), loading of the vertebral column leads to an outflow of fluid from the IVD and a loss of IVD height; unloading of the vertebral column results in an uptake of both fluid and nutrient substances, and a corresponding increase in IVD volume. Therefore fluid uptake takes place in lying positions and fluid loss occurs in upright and standard sitting positions. The IVDs thrive on reasonable motion within normal physiologic limits. That is, frequent changes of postures improve and maintain the internal environment of the IVD, whereas high-pressure postures, such as prolonged standing and

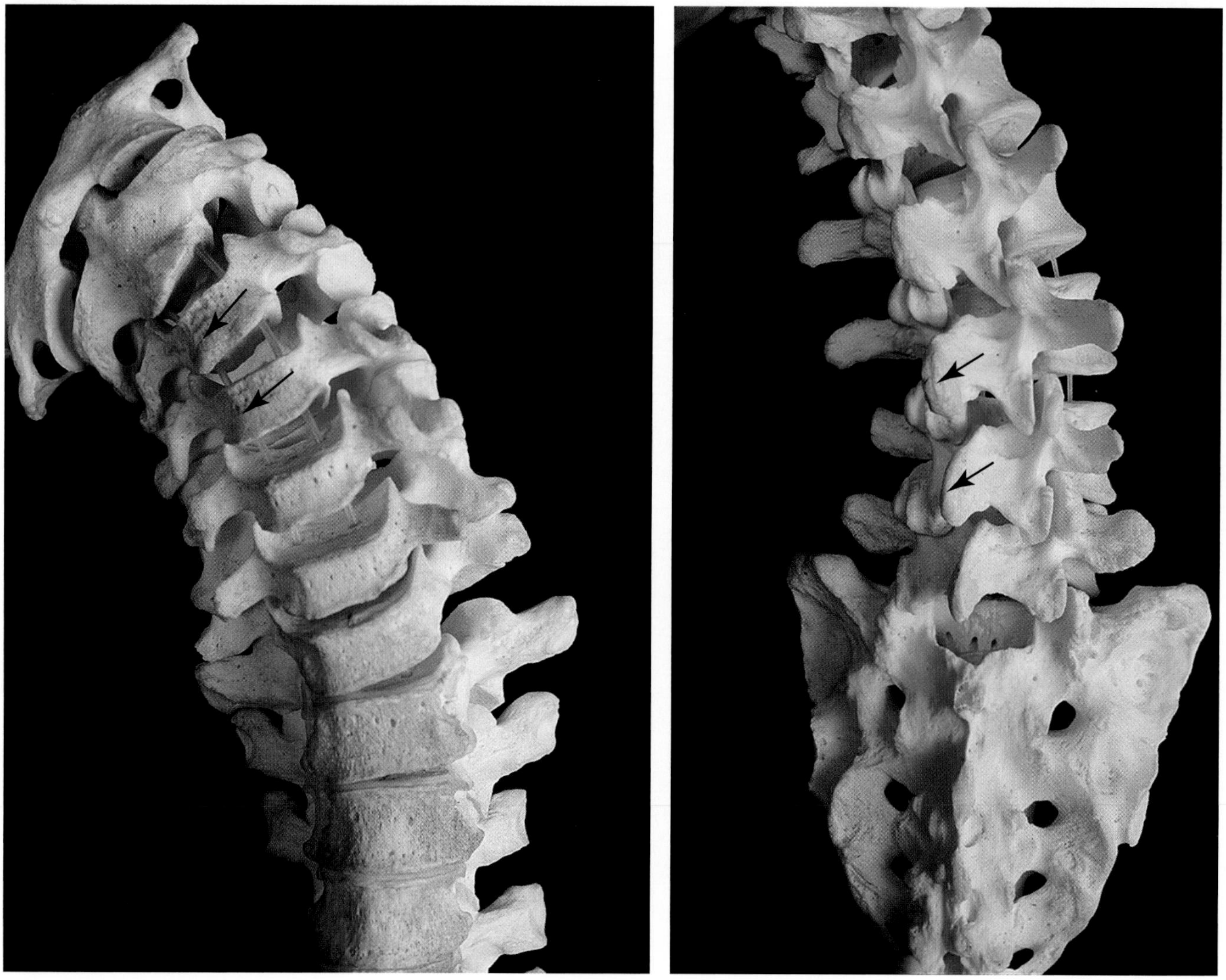

FIG. 2-11   Coupled motion. **A,** Lateral flexion of the cervical region results in concomitant axial rotation of the vertebrae. The cervical vertebral bodies rotate toward the side of lateral flexion *(arrows)*. **B,** Lateral flexion of the lumbar region results in axial rotation to the opposite side. The lumbar vertebral bodies in this case rotate away from the side of lateral flexion, and the spinous processes rotate into the side of lateral flexion *(arrows)*.

sitting, inhibit disc nutrition. A sedentary lifestyle is bad for the IVD and the entire spine (Kraemer, 1995).

Calcification of the IVD during the aging process is much more common than was once thought. Cheng et al. (1996) found such calcification in 58.3% of subjects at autopsy. They concluded that calcification of the IVD is "significantly underestimated" by conventional radiography.

The IVD is composed of three regions (Fig. 2-12) known as the anulus fibrosus, nucleus pulposus, and vertebral (cartilaginous) end plate (Humzah and Soames, 1988). Together the regions make up the anterior interbody joint or intervertebral symphysis. Each region consists of different proportions of the primary materials

that make up the disc (e.g., water, cells, proteoglycan, and collagen). Table 2-5 compares some of the characteristics of the anulus fibrosus with those of the nucleus pulposus.

Although each region of the disc has a distinct composition, the transition between the anulus fibrosus and the nucleus pulposus is rather indistinct. The main difference between the two regions is their fibrous structure (Humzah and Soames, 1988). Type I collagen (typical in tendons) predominates in the anulus fibrosus, and type II collagen (typical for articular cartilage) predominates in the nucleus pulposus. The histologic and biochemical make-up of the IVD is currently an active field of research and has a great deal of potential clinical

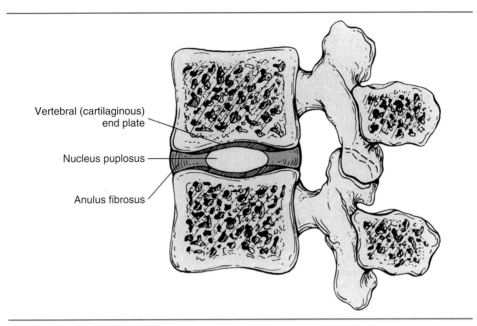

FIG. 2-12 Midsagittal section of two adjacent lumbar vertebrae and the intervertebral disc separating the two vertebral bodies. Notice the components of the intervertebral disc: anulus fibrosus, nucleus pulposus, and vertebral (cartilaginous) end plate.

relevance. As mentioned previously, Chapter 14 discusses the histologic characteristics of the IVD in more detail, and Chapter 11 discusses the clinical relevance of pathology of the IVD in low back pain. The gross morphologic characteristics of the three regions of the disc are discussed in the following sections.

Anulus Fibrosus

The anuli fibrosi (singular, anulus fibrosus) in the lumbar region, and most likely the thoracic region, are each made up of several fibrocartilaginous lamellae, or rings, that are convex externally (Fig. 2-13; see also Fig. 2-12). The lamellae are formed by closely arranged collagen fibers and a smaller percentage (10% of the dry weight) of elastic fibers (Bogduk, 1997). The majority of fibers of each lamella run parallel with one another at approximately a 65-degree angle from the vertical plane. The fibers of adjacent lamellae overlie each other, forming a 130-degree angle between the fibers of adjacent lamellae. The direction of the lamellae can vary considerably from individual to individual and from one vertebra to the next (Humzah and Soames, 1988). The most superficial lamellae of the anulus fibrosus (AF) attach via Sharpey's fibers (see Chapter 14 and Fig. 14-9) directly to the vertebral bodies in the region of the ring apophysis. They anchor themselves to the zone of compact bone that forms the outside of the vertebral rim, as well as the adjacent vertebral body and periosteum that covers it (Humzah and Soames, 1988). The

Table 2-5 Composition of Anulus Fibrosus and Nucleus Pulposus

| Region* | Collagen | | Disc Weight (%) | |
	Percent Water	Type	Collagen†	Proteoglycan‡
Anulus fibrosus	60-70	I, II	50-60	20/50-60
Nucleus pulposus	70-90	II, III	15-20	65/25

*Values are for the lumbar spine (Bogduk, 1997).
†Percentage of dry weight of disc made up of collagen.
‡Percentage of dry weight of disc made up of proteoglycan/percentage of proteoglycan found in aggregated form.

inner lamellae of the AF attach to the cartilaginous vertebral end plate.

The cervical intervertebral discs have been found to differ significantly from the lumbar discs (Mercer and Bogduk, 1999). Rather than being made up of many lamellae, the AF in the cervical region is composed of a single, crescent-shaped piece of fibrocartilage that is thick anteriorly and becomes narrow laterally. Posteriorly the AF is composed of only a single thin lamella. Like the lumbar region, the nucleus pulposus fills the central region of the cervical intervertebral discs and the cartilaginous end plates (CEPs) are found above and below the nucleus pulposus and AF. However, the cervical IVDs of children are similar to those of the lumbar region of children and adults. The changes that distinguish the cervical IVDs from those of the lumbar region begin as clefts in the AF (uncovertebral clefts), and develop adjacent to the uncinate processes during adolescence. During the third and fourth decades of life the shearing forces of cervical movements cause these clefts to extend medially, eroding the posterior AF until it is severely narrowed. This creates the crescent-shaped AF of the adult cervical spine (Taylor, 1999).

Further investigation is needed to precisely determine the makeup of the thoracic IVDs. However, the IVDs of the thoracic region are currently thought to be similar in make-up to those of the lumbar region.

Under normal conditions, the entire IVD is seldom subjected to pure tensile loads (traction forces). Even with clinical traction to the spine, the disc is under some compressive load because of muscle action. The AF is subject to tension stresses in all directions under various movements of the spine and under various conditions. The following list states the movement or condition followed by the region of the anulus that experiences tensile forces during that movement or condition:

♦ Flexion = posterior anulus
♦ Extension = anterior anulus
♦ Side bending = convex side of bend
♦ Axial rotation = tensile stress develops approximately 45 degrees to the plane of the disc
♦ Compressive loading = entire anulus receives tensile loads during compression because of the outward pressure of the nucleus pulposus against the AF during compression

The AF has a significant load-bearing function, which it can perform even when the nucleus has been experimentally removed (Humzah and Soames, 1988). The various movements of the spine also create compressive forces on the IVD. As a result, during flexion the anterior aspect of the AF bulges outward. The opposite occurs during extension (posterior AF bulges outward), and the AF bulges toward the concavity of the curve during left and right lateral flexion. The anterior aspect of the disc is stronger than the rest, whereas the posterolateral aspect of each disc is the weakest region. Therefore the posterolateral aspect of the IVD is the region most prone to protrusion and extrusion.

The most superficial lamellae of the anulus of the lumbar region and the peripheral aspect of the cervical AF are innervated by general somatic afferent nerves and general visceral afferent nerves (which run with sympathetic efferent fibers). Specifically the recurrent meningeal nerve innervates the posterior aspect of the anulus and separate nerves arising from the ventral ramus, and the sympathetic chain innervate the lateral and anterior aspects of the anulus.

CLINICAL IMPLICATIONS

The arrangement of collagen fibers is designed to protect the IVD during bending and torsion, the same motions that place the most stress on the AF (Hickey and Hukins, 1980). Disc saturation (intradiscal pressure) and compression also are related to failure of the AF. Therefore compressive (axial) loading, bending and twisting, and normal disc saturation together can cause failure of the AF, and lack of any one of these factors makes failure of the AF more difficult (Lu, Huttun, and Gharpuray, 1996). The posterior and lateral AF is the most vulnerable to failure (Edwards et al., 2001).

Weinstein, Claverie, and Gibson (1988) investigated the pain associated with discography. Discography is the injection of radiopaque dye into a disc and the subsequent visualization of the disc on x-ray film. They found neuropeptides, which are frequently identified as neurotransmitters associated with inflammation (substance P, calcitonin gene–related peptide, and vasoactive intestinal peptide), in the remaining lamellae of the AF and the dorsal root ganglia of dogs that had undergone surgical removal of an IVD (discectomy). They stated that the dorsal root ganglion may be a mediator of the sensory

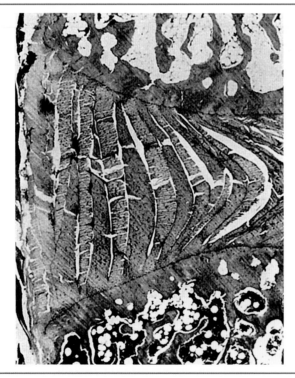

FIG. 2-13   Low-power photomicrograph demonstrating the lamellar arrangement of the anulus fibrosus. (Courtesy Vernon-Roberts. Jayson M. [1992]. *The lumbar spine and back pain* [4th ed.] New York: Churchill Livingstone.)

environment of the motor unit and that discs with anular disruption may be sensitized to further irritation. Therefore fibers whose cell bodies reside in the dorsal root ganglion may release the neurotransmitters listed previously into the region of the AF, making the anulus more sensitive to injury. This may mean that a torn or otherwise diseased disc could be more sensitive to further irritation and therefore more capable of nociceptive (pain) stimulation than the discs of adjacent vertebrae. This may help to explain the heightened sensitivity of patients with disc disorders. Weinstein, Claverie, and Gibson (1988) used their findings to help explain why the chemical irritants found in the radiopaque dye (Renografin) injected into a disc during discography (Fig. 2-14) reproduce the patient's symptoms. However, the procedure generally is not associated with pain when the dye is injected into a neighboring healthy disc of the same individual. A further discussion of neuropeptides and chemokines associated with diseased IVDs is found in Chapter 11.

The lamellae of the AF are subject to tearing. These tears occur in two directions, circumferentially and radially. Many investigators believe that circumferential tears are the most common. This type of tear represents a separation of adjacent lamellae of the anulus, creating vertical clefts in the AF. The separation may cause the lamellae involved to tear away from their vertebral attachments as well. Using an aged rat model, Kuga and Kawabuchi (2001) found this type of disorganization (i.e., circumferential tears) among the protruded anular lamellae in disc protrusions (rather than extrusions). The changes also included widening of lamellae and flaccidity of lamellae. Such changes may help to explain the findings of Lipson (1988) that tissue removed from IVD "herniations" (extrusions) during surgery was frequently found to be mostly AF when examined histologically. Such tissue removed during surgery may be protruded AF that has undergone the type of disorganization just mentioned, and could even be AF undergoing metaplastic change, rather than extruded nucleus pulposus, as is usually assumed to be the tissue removed from an IVD extrusion.

The second type of tear in the AF is radial in direction. These tears run from the deep lamellae of the anulus to the superficial layers, creating horizontal clefts in the AF. Most authors believe that these types of tears follow circumferential tears in chronology and that the circumferential tears make it easier for radial tears to occur (Ito et al., 1991). This is because the radial tears are able to connect the circumferential ones. When the connection occurs, the nucleus pulposus may be allowed to protrude, or even extrude, into the vertebral canal. Radial tears have been associated with IVD degeneration, as well as IVD protrusion and extrusion, and Krismer et al. (2000) found that IVD radial fissures were associated

with a decreased IVD height as seen on x-rays. Herzog (1996) found radial tears in 21% to 35% of cadaveric lumbar IVDs over 40 years of age, but only rarely found such tears in cadavers less than 40 years of age. Chapter 11 discusses pathology of the IVD, including a full discussion of the terminology associated with IVD bulging, protrusion, and extrusion.

Nucleus Pulposus

The nucleus pulposus (NP) is a rounded region located within the center of the IVD (see Fig. 2-12). The NP is thickest from superior to inferior in the lumbar region, followed in thickness by the cervical region; it is the thinnest in the thoracic region. It is most centrally placed within the horizontal plane in the cervical region and is more posteriorly placed in the lumbar region (Humzah and Soames, 1988).

The NP develops from the embryologic notochord. It is gelatinous and relatively large just after birth, and several multinucleated notochordal cells can be found within its substance (Williams et al., 1995). The remnants of the notochord can be recognized in MRI scans as an irregular dark band, usually confined to the NP (Breger et al., 1988). The notochordal tissue has been found to be more apparent in fetal spines than in the spines of infants (Ho et al., 1988). The notochordal cells decrease in number over time and are almost completely replaced by fibrocartilage by approximately the eleventh year of life (Williams et al., 1995), and no notochordal cells normally remain after the mid-teens (Oda, Tamaka, and Tsukuki, 1988). As the notochordal cells are replaced, the outer aspect of the NP blends with the inner layer of the AF, making it more difficult to determine the border between the two regions. Notochordal cells may remain anywhere throughout the spine. These remnants are known as notochordal "rests" and may develop into neoplasms known as chordomas. Chordomas most commonly occur at the base of the skull and in the lumbosacral region (Humzah and Soames, 1988).

The adult disc is an avascular structure, except for the most peripheral region of the AF, and the NP is responsible for absorbing the majority of the fluid received by the disc. The process by which a disc absorbs fluid from the vertebral bodies above and below has been termed imbibition. The size of the NP and its capacity to swell is greatest in the lumbar region, next in the cervical region. The NP is 70% to 90% water and it reaches its peak hydration between the ages of 20 to 30 years, and the process of degeneration begins shortly thereafter (Coventry, 1969). The disc loses water when a load is applied but retains sodium and potassium. This increase in electrolyte concentration creates an osmotic gradient that results in rapid rehydration when the loading of the

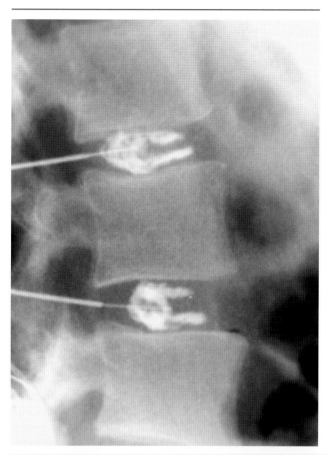

disc is stopped (Kraemer et al., 1985). This osmotic system of the IVD is sensitive to the forces applied to the disc, the pressure within the NP, and the make-up and concentration of the proteoglycan molecules within the IVD (Kraemer, 1995). Frequent changes of posture are beneficial to this osmotic system, and the disc apparently benefits from both activity during the day (Holm and Nachemson, 1983; Kraemer, 1995) and the rest it receives during the hours of sleep. Because of the loss of fluid in the IVD during compression, the total body height is approximately 10 mm less at the end of an average day. This height is completely regained during 8 hours of sleep (Boos et al., 1996; McGill and Axler, 1996). Prolonged bed rest (up to 32 hours) does not significantly increase total body height, but the weightless environment of space can increase total body height by 40 to 60 mm (McGill and Axler, 1996). The diurnal variation in IVD height has been verified with both MRI (Botsford, Esses, and Olgilvie-Harris, 1994) and ultrasound (Boos et al., 1996; Ledsome et al., 1996). However, too much rest may not be beneficial. A decrease in the amount of fluid (hydration) of the IVDs has been noted on MRIs after 5 weeks of bed rest (LeBlanc et al., 1988).

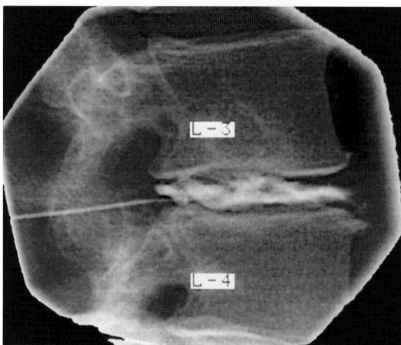

FIG. 2-14 Normal discogram *(top)* and discogram demonstrating protrusion of nuclear material through the lamellae of the anulus fibrosus *(bottom)*. (Images courtesy Dr. Dennis Skogsbergh.)

The NP is a viscoelastic structure that can act as a fluid or solid depending on the rate and magnitude of loading. In addition, the NP can change its shape and position during different motions of the spine and when different loads are placed on the spine (Iatridis et al., 1996). For example, the NP of the lumbar region moves posteriorly during flexion and anteriorly during extension (Fennell, Jones, and Hukins, 1996).

In addition, the pressure within the NP changes as body position changes. When one is lying on the back the pressure within a lower lumbar NP is 20% of the pressure during standing. Leaning forward while sitting or standing substantially increases intradiscal pressure (IDP), and lifting a 20-kg load results in a 4.5-fold increase in IDP. This IDP is reduced by 25% if the knees are bent during lifting. In addition, if the load is held close to the body the IDP is reduced twofold. The IDP is lower in relaxed sitting than in relaxed standing, and slightly slouching while sitting actually decreases IDP, whereas straight sitting and standing both increase IDP. As might be expected, muscle activity increases IDP. During 7 hours of sleep the IDP increases approximately 240% compared with when one initially goes to bed (Wilde et al., 1999). This may support the hypothesis that herniation of the NP is more likely during the beginning of the day than at the end of the day.

Hysteresis is a viscoelastic phenomenon that refers to deformation of a tissue because of short duration loading. Hysteresis helps to protect the spine and nervous system during rapid loadings. For example, the successive vertebrae, intervertebral discs, and other tissues from the feet to the brain absorb the shock of jumping by means of hysteresis. Hysteresis increases as loads increase, is greatest in young tissues, and decreases with age. This phenomenon is lower in the lower thoracic and upper lumbar regions, compared with lower lumbar region of the spine. Hysteresis also decreases when the same disc is loaded a second time, and continues to decrease with repetitive loading. Decreased hysteresis may be a factor in the increased incidence of extruded NP in those with driving occupations (i.e., repetitive loading from subtle and not-so-gentle bouncing).

As the NP ages, it becomes less gelatinous in consistency, its ability to absorb fluid diminishes, and the intradiscal pressure diminishes. The changes in composition and structure that are common to all sources of cartilage with aging occur earlier and to a greater extent in the IVD (Bayliss et al., 1988). In fact, the normal aging process of the IVD is difficult to differentiate from IVD degeneration (Boos et al., 2002). Breakdown of the proteoglycan aggregates and monomers (see Fig. 13-6) is thought to contribute to this process of aging and degeneration. The breakdown of proteoglycans results in a decreased ability of the disc to absorb fluid, which leads to a decrease in the ability of the disc to resist loads placed on it. The degeneration associated with the decrease in ability to absorb fluid (water) has been identified through use of CT (Bahk and Lee, 1988) and MRI and has been correlated with histologic structure and fluid content. As the disc degenerates, it narrows in the superior to inferior dimensions and the adjacent vertebral bodies may become sclerotic (thickened and opaque on x-ray) (Moore et al., 1996). Much of the disc thinning with age seen on x-ray may also be the result of the disc sinking into the adjacent vertebral bodies over the course of many years (Humzah and Soames, 1988).

Pathologic conditions of the IVD are frequently seen in clinical practice. As mentioned, the NP may cause bulging of the outer anular fibers or may protrude (herniate) through some or all of the lamellae of the AF. This was first described by Mixter and Barr (1934). Bulging or protrusion of the disc may be a primary source of pain, or pain may result because of pressure on the exiting nerve roots within the medial aspect of the intervertebral foramen. Such bulging is usually associated with heavy lifting or trauma, although such a history may be absent in as many as 28% of patients with confirmed disc protrusion (Martin, 1978). Some investigators believe that proteoglycan and other molecules leaking out of a tear in the anulus also may cause pain by creating a chemical irritation of the exiting nerve roots. The pain that results from pressure on or irritation of a nerve root radiates in a distribution along the nerves supplied by the compressed nerve root (see Chapter 11). Such pain is termed radicular pain because of its origin from the dorsal root (radix) or dorsal root ganglion. Treatment for protrusion of the NP ranges from excision of the disc (discectomy), to chemical degradation of the disc (chymopapain chemonucleolysis) (Alcalay et al., 1988; Dabezies et al., 1988), to conservative methods (Sanders and Stein, 1988; Brønfort, 1997).

Vertebral (Cartilaginous) End Plates

The vertebral end plates, or cartilaginous end plates (CEPs), limit all but the most peripheral rim of the disc superiorly and inferiorly. They are attached both to the disc and to the adjacent vertebral body (see Fig. 2-12). Although a few authors consider the vertebral end plate to be a part of the vertebral body, most authorities consider it to be an integral portion of the disc (Coventry, 1969; Bogduk, 1991). The CEPs are approximately 1 mm thick peripherally and 3 mm thick centrally. They are composed of both hyaline cartilage and fibrocartilage. The hyaline cartilage is located against the vertebral body, and the fibrocartilage is found adjacent to the remainder of the IVD. The end plates help to prevent the vertebral bodies from undergoing pressure atrophy and, at the same time, contain the AF and NP within their normal anatomic borders.

The CEPs are very important for proper nutrition of the disc (Humzah and Soames, 1988). They are very porous and allow fluid to enter and leave the AF and NP by osmotic action (Humzah and Soames, 1988). Very early in postnatal life, small vascular channels enter the vertebral side of the vertebral end plate and a few channels enter the outermost lamella of the AF. These channels disappear with age and are almost completely gone by the age of 12, leaving the IVD to obtain all of its nutrition by means of imbibition through the CEP (Boos et al., 2002). The end plate is more permeable in the region adjacent to the NP and is relatively impermeable in the region associated with the AF. This may result from morphologic differences in the capillary beds of the bony end plates. These beds are more complex in the region surrounding the NP (Oki et al., 1996).

The first structures to fail with compressive loading of the vertebral column are the CEPs and the adjacent subchondral bone of the vertebral bodies (bony end plates) (Hickey and Hukins, 1980). Such fractures allow the NP to rupture through the CEP, causing a lesion known as a Schmorl's node. These nodes cause the vertebrae surrounding the lesion to move closer together. This movement is thought to increase pressure on the posterior and anterior joints between the vertebrae, increasing the degenerative process of the anterior interbody joint (the remainder of the IVD). In addition, the disc thinning or narrowing that results from these end plate herniations causes more force to be borne by the Z joints and may result in more rapid degeneration of these structures as well.

The CEPs begin to calcify and thin with advancing years. This leaves them more brittle. The central region of the end plate in some vertebrae of certain individuals may be completely lost in the later years of life.

Innervation of the Intervertebral Discs

The entire outer third of the AF has been found to receive both sensory and vasomotor innervation (Bogduk, Tynan, and Wilson, 1981). The sensory fibers probably are both nociceptive (pain sensitive) and proprioceptive in nature, and an extensive distribution of small nerve fibers (both A-delta and C) has been found throughout the peripheral aspect of the AF (Cavanaugh et al., 1995). The vasomotor fibers of the AF are associated with the small vessels located along its most superficial aspect. The posterior aspect of the disc receives its innervation from the recurrent meningeal nerve (sinuvertebral nerve). The posterolateral aspect of the anulus receives both direct branches from the anterior primary division and also branches from the gray communicating rami of the sympathetic chain. The lateral and anterior aspects of the disc receive their innervation primarily from branches of the gray communicating rami and also branches from the sympathetic chain.

Degenerated discs receive increased innervation by sensory fibers conducting nociception. This indicates that injured or degenerated discs are more sensitive to pain (Coppes et al., 1997). Schwann cells of the nerves innervating the outer layers of the AF appear to play a role in this ingrowth of sensory nerves (Johnson et al., 2001).

The fact that the disc has direct nociceptive innervation is clinically relevant. The IVD itself is most likely able to generate pain. Therefore disorders affecting the IVDs alone (e.g., internal disc disruption, tears of the outer third of the AF, and possibly even marked disc degeneration) can be the sole cause of back pain. The disc can also generate pain by compressing (entrapping) an exiting dorsal root. As mentioned, leakage of nerve irritating (histamine-like) molecules from disrupted IVDs also has been found to be a cause of irritation to the exiting dorsal root. These latter conditions cause a sharp, stabbing pain that radiates along the distribution of the nerves receiving fibers from the dorsal root. This type of pain is known as radicular pain because it results from irritation of a nerve root (radix). Chapter 11 covers the differentiation of radicular pain from somatic referred pain. The unique characteristics of the innervation to the IVDs of the specific spinal regions are covered in Chapters 5 through 7.

RELATIONSHIP OF THE SPINAL NERVES TO THE INTERVERTEBRAL DISC

The first seven spinal nerves exit through the intervertebral foramen (IVF) located above the vertebra of the same number (for example, the C5 nerve exits the C4-5 IVF). This relationship changes at the eighth cervical nerve. Because there are eight cervical spinal nerves and only seven cervical vertebrae, the eighth cervical nerve exits the IVF between C7 and T1 (i.e., inferior to C7). All spinal nerves located below the C8 cervical nerve exit inferior to the vertebra of the same number (i.e., the T5 nerve exits below T5, through the T5-6 IVF). Figures 3-7 and 3-8 show this relationship.

The previous information is of clinical importance. Because of the relationships just discussed, a disc protrusion occurring at the level of the C3-4 disc usually affects the exiting C4 nerve. However, a disc protrusion of the T3-4 IVD normally affects the T3 spinal nerve. The anatomic relationships of a disc protrusion in the lumbar spine are unique. As expected, the exiting spinal nerve passes through the IVF located below the vertebra of the same number (L3 nerve through the L3-4 IVF). However, the spinal cord ends between L1 and L2 (see Chapter 3), and below this the lumbar and sacral roots descend inferiorly, forming the cauda equina. To exit an IVF, the sharply descending nerve roots must make a rather dramatic turn laterally, and as each nerve root exits, it "hugs" the pedicle of the most superior vertebra of the IVF (Fig. 2-15). Because they leave at such an angle, the nerve roots are kept out of the way of the IVD at the same level. Even though they are positioned away from the disc at their level of exit, they do pass across the IVD above their level of exit. This is roughly where they enter the dural root sleeve, and this is also where the nerve roots may be compressed by disc protrusions. The other nerve roots of the cauda equina are not as vulnerable at this location because only the nerve beginning to exit the vertebral canal has entered its dural root sleeve. Once in the sleeve, the exiting nerve roots are contained and more or less held in place as they descend to exit the IVF. This more firmly positions the exiting roots against the disc above the level of exit (see Fig. 2-15). The other nerve roots of the cauda equina, within the subarachnoid space of the lumbar cistern, "float" away from a protruding disc. The result is that a lumbar disc protrusion normally affects the nerve roots exiting the subjacent IVF (e.g., an L3 disc protrusion affects the L4 nerve roots).

SYNDESMOSES OF THE SPINE

In addition to the Z joints and the interbody symphysis, the spine also contains a number of joints classified as syndesmoses. Recall that a syndesmosis is a joint consisting of two bones connected by a ligament. The spine is unique in that it has several examples of such joints. The spinal syndesmoses include the following:

◆ Axial-occipital syndesmosis (between odontoid and clivus, ligaments include cruciform, apical-odontoid, and alar)
◆ Ligamentum nuchae (syndesmosis between occiput and C1-7)
◆ Laminar syndesmosis (ligamentum flavum)
◆ Intertransverse syndesmosis (intertransverse ligament)
◆ Supraspinous syndesmosis (supraspinous ligament)
◆ Interspinous syndesmosis (interspinous ligament)

These joints are innervated by the posterior primary division (dorsal ramus) exiting between the two vertebrae connected by the ligaments. The exception to this is the axial-occipital syndesmosis, which is innervated by the anterior primary division (ventral ramus) of the first cervical nerve. Afferent nerves coursing with sym-

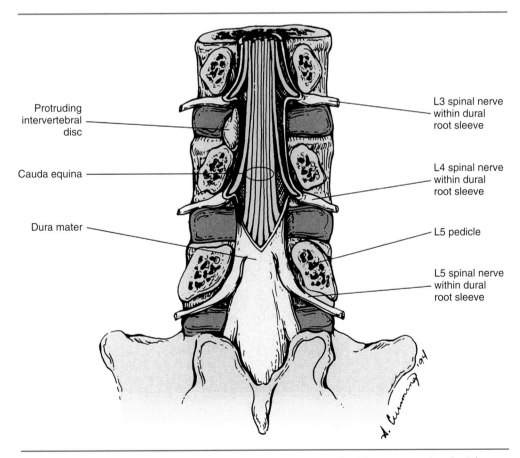

FIG. 2-15 Relationship of exiting nerve roots to the intervertebral discs. Notice that the L4 nerve roots are vulnerable to a protrusion or extrusion of the L3 disc.

pathetic nerves also innervate these joints. The ligaments forming these joints are discussed in Chapters 5 through 7.

VERTEBRAL CANAL

The chapter has thus far been devoted to a discussion of the relatively solid elements of the spine (e.g., bones, ligaments, and joints). The remainder of the chapter is devoted to the "holes" (Latin, *foramen,* singular; *foramina,* plural) of the spine, what runs through them, and the clinical significance of these openings.

A vertebral foramen (see Fig. 2-3, *B*) is the opening within a vertebra through which the spinal cord or cauda equina passes. The vertebral foramen can be best defined by listing its boundaries. The boundaries of a typical vertebral foramen include the following:

♦ Vertebral body
♦ Left and right pedicles
♦ Left and right laminae
♦ Spinous process

The boundaries of a vertebral foramen are shown in Figure 2-3, *B*. Two congenital anomalies can affect the vertebral foramen. The first is failure of the posterior elements of a vertebra to fuse during development. This is known as spina bifida (see Chapter 12). Another congenital anomaly of the vertebral foramen is the development of a fibrous or bony bridge between the vertebral body and the spinous process. Such a bridge may divide the spinal cord midsagittally at that level. This condition, known as diastematomyelia, may go unnoticed throughout life or may become symptomatic later in life or after trauma.

The collection of all of the vertebral foramina is known as the vertebral (spinal) canal. Therefore the IVDs and the posteriorly located ligamenta flava (*ligamentum flavum,* singular) also participate in the formation of the vertebral canal. The ligamenta flava are discussed in detail in Chapter 5.

The vertebral canal is fairly large in the upper cervical region but narrows from C3 to C6. In fact, the spinal cord fills 75% of the vertebral canal at the C6 level. Therefore the lower cervical cord is particularly vulnerable to a wide variety of pathologic entities that can compromise the cord within the vertebral canal. These include IVD protrusion, hypertrophy of the ligamentum flavum, space-occupying lesions, and arteriovenous malformations.

The vertebral canal follows the normal contour of the curves of the spine. It is relatively large and triangular in the cervical (see Fig. 5-1) and lumbar regions (see Fig. 7-2), where there is a great deal of spinal movement. The vertebral canal in the thoracic region is smaller and almost circular in configuration (see Fig. 6-1). This may result from the fact that the thoracic spine undergoes less movement than the other regions of the spine.

Also, the vertebral canal in the thoracic region is not necessarily as large as in the cervical region because the thoracic spinal cord is narrower than the cervical cord, which contains the cervical enlargement.

The size of the vertebral canal (see Chapters 5 and 7 for specific values) has been assessed by several investigators, most of whom were interested in the condition of spinal (vertebral) canal stenosis. This condition is defined as a narrowing of either the anteroposterior or the transverse diameter of the vertebral canal. Some investigators have shown a change in vertebral dimensions and canal size with normal aging (Leiviska, 1985). However, spinal canal stenosis seems to have a strong developmental component and may result, in part, from prenatal and perinatal growth disruption (Clarke et al., 1985). Vertebral canal growth is approximately 90% complete by late infancy. Because canal diameters do not undergo "catch-up growth" (Clarke et al., 1985), factors affecting canal size must occur before infancy. A significant relationship has been found between a decrease in anteroposterior vertebral foramen size and spinal cord constriction. As little as 2 mm in anteroposterior diameter separates persons with or without low back pain, and Clarke et al. (1985) suggest that as many as 53% of low back pain patients may have anteroposterior spinal stenosis. Clarke et al. (1985) believe that spinal stenosis and sciatica may have a developmental basis and that perhaps there is a higher association between canal size and low back pain than was realized previously. They believe that attention to prenatal and neonatal nutrition may play an important role in preventing back pain from this origin. In addition, they state that maternal smoking and other environmental factors have been shown to significantly reduce head circumference. They hypothesize that the same phenomenon may occur with the vertebral canal (Clarke et al., 1985). If this is shown to be the case, reduction in maternal smoking may prevent future back pain in the offspring. Although a link between back pain and smoking has been made, the association is complex and more work is needed to validate the relationship (Leboeuf-Yde, Yashin, and Lauritzen, 1996). However, there is evidence from animal studies that systemic nicotine decreases the bony union of spine surgery fusion sites (intertransverse fusion), suggesting that nicotine may decrease the "biomechanical properties" of new bone formation (Silcox et al., 1995), and many prominent surgeons strongly suggest that a person stop smoking before undergoing a surgical procedure on the spine (Herkowitz et al., 1992).

Spinal canal stenosis also can be caused by the development of bone spurs (osteophytes) along the posterior aspect of the vertebral body, hypertrophy of the uncinate processes of the cervical vertebrae, hypertrophy of the articular processes making up the zygapophysial joints, intervertebral disc protrusion, ossification of the posterior longitudinal ligament, and ligamentum flavum hypertrophy or buckling (Bailey and Casamajor, 1911; Giles, 2000). Further elaboration of the causes and consequences of spinal (vertebral canal) stenosis and foraminal (IVF) stenosis are discussed in more detail in the chapters on the cervical and lumbar regions (Chapters 5 and 7, respectively).

External Vertebral Venous Plexus

Before investigating the contents of the vertebral canal, it is necessary to discuss a plexus of veins that surrounds the outside of the vertebrae and the vertebral canal. This network of veins surrounding the external aspect of the vertebral column is known as the external vertebral venous plexus. The external vertebral venous plexus is associated with both the posterior and anterior elements of the vertebral column and can be divided into an anterior external vertebral venous plexus surrounding the vertebral bodies and a posterior external vertebral venous plexus associated with the posterior arches of adjacent vertebrae. These plexuses communicate with segmental veins throughout the spine (e.g. deep cervical veins, intercostal veins, lumbar veins, and ascending lumbar veins) and also with the internal vertebral venous plexus, which lies within the vertebral canal. The external and internal vertebral plexuses communicate through the IVFs and also directly through the vertebral bodies. The veins that run through the IVFs to connect the two plexuses surround the exiting spinal nerve and form a vascular cuff around the nerve (Humzah and Soames, 1988).

Epidural Space

The region immediately beneath the bony and ligamentous elements forming the vertebral canal is known as the epidural space (see dura mater in Fig. 2-15). Generally throughout the length of the vertebral canal, the epidural space is approximately 4 to 6 mm deep to the osseous and ligamentous anterior and posterior canal borders (Chen et al., 1989; Hackney, 1992). The epidural space is sometimes entered at the L3-4 interspinous space for the purpose of administering anesthetics. The depth to the epidural space at this level is 4.77 ± 0.55 cm in males and 4.25 ± 0.55 cm in females. The range of depth is 3.0 to 7.0 cm (1.2 to 2.8 inches), and there is a positive correlation between both body weight and body height with the depth to the epidural space (Chen et al., 1989).

The epidural space contains a venous plexus embedded in a thin layer of adipose tissue. The adipose tissue is known as the epidural adipose tissue, or epidural fat, and the venous plexus is known as the internal vertebral venous plexus.

Internal Vertebral Venous Plexus

The internal vertebral venous plexus is located beneath the bony elements of the vertebral foramina (e.g., laminae, spinous processes, pedicles, and vertebral body). As mentioned, it is embedded in a layer of loose areolar tissue known as the epidural (extradural) adipose tissue. The internal vertebral venous plexus is a clinically important plexus, and perhaps for this reason it has been given many names. It is known as the internal vertebral venous plexus, the epidural venous plexus, the extradural venous plexus, and also as Batson's channels.

The internal vertebral venous plexus consists of many interconnected longitudinal channels. Several course along the posterior aspect of the vertebral canal, and several course along the anterior aspect of the canal. The posterior channels are rudimentary in the cervical region, but well developed in the thoracic and lumbar regions (Chaynes et al., 1998). The anterior channels drain the vertebral bodies via large basivertebral veins. The basivertebral veins pierce the center of each vertebral body and communicate posteriorly with the internal plexus and anteriorly with the external vertebral venous plexus. The posterior communication of the basivertebral veins with the anterior internal vertebral venous plexus occurs by means of small veins that run from the basivertebral veins and around the posterior longitudinal ligament to reach the anterior internal vertebral venous plexus.

The veins of the internal vertebral venous plexus contain no valves; therefore the direction of drainage is posture and respiration dependent. Inferiorly this plexus is continuous with the prostatic venous plexus of the male, and superiorly (in both sexes) it is continuous with the occipital dura mater venous sinus of the posterior cranial fossa. Therefore prostatic carcinoma may metastasize via this route to all regions of the spine and to the meninges and brain (because of venous communications in the thoracic region, lung and breast cancer can metastasize to these veins as well). However, the veins of the internal vertebral venous plexus eventually (by means of intervertebral, intercostals, and ascending lumbar veins in the cervical, thoracic, and lumbar regions, respectively) drain into large veins. These large veins include the vertebral, for the cervical region; and the azygos, hemiazygos, and right highest intercostal veins, for blood draining the thoracic and lumbar regions. These large veins each have one or two valves at their entrance to the brachiocephalic veins (for the vertebral veins) or at their entrance to the azygos vein (for the right highest intercostal and hemiazygous veins). The azygos vein then drains directly into the superior vena cava, and there is also a valve at this entrance. These valves act as a protective mechanism, preventing reflux of blood (and the accompanying increase in pressure) into the internal vertebral venous plexus and the important neural tissues they serve (Scapinelli, 2000).

The walls of the veins of the internal vertebral venous plexus are thin, and isolated regions of the veins can become dilated (varices of epidural veins). Such varices may rarely compress the exiting spinal nerves and cause radiculopathy (i.e., pain coursing along the distribution of the dorsal root that contributes to the formation of the spinal nerve). Radiculopathy from this cause can mimic that more commonly caused by an IVD protrusion (Wong et al., 2003). In addition, the thin walls of these veins may cause them to collapse from the pressure of an IVD protrusion. This fact has been used in a procedure known as epidural venography (Fig. 2-16) to aid in the diagnosis of IVD disease. In epidural venography, radiopaque dye is injected into the epidural veins and x-ray films are taken. This allows the veins filled with dye to be visualized (Jayson, 1980). Pressure from a disc protrusion prevents the veins from filling and is seen as an area devoid of dye on the x-ray film.

Spinal epidural hematoma is a condition in which bleeding occurs into the space surrounding the dura mater. It is usually the result of a ruptured epidural vein and is rather rare, with only 250 cases reported in the literature. Of these approximately 50% are spontaneous and of unknown cause. The causes of the remainder of the cases include trauma, anticoagulant therapy, and arteriovenous malformation. Spinal epidural hematoma may simulate IVD protrusion but can usually be identified through MRI (Mirkovic and Melany, 1992). Treatment is usually removal of pressure (decompression) by the removal of a lamina (laminectomy), although several cases with spontaneous recovery have been reported (Sei et al., 1991).

Meningeal and Neural Elements within the Vertebral Canal

The meningeal and neural elements of the vertebral canal are thoroughly discussed in Chapter 3. This section focuses on the neural elements that enter and leave the vertebral canal.

Beneath the epidural venous plexus and epidural adipose tissue lie the meninges, which surround the spinal cord (Fig. 2-17). These layers of tissue are known as the dura mater, arachnoid mater, and pia mater. The space between the meninges and the borders of the vertebral canal is known as the epidural space. Recall that this space is approximately 4 to 6 mm anteriorly and posteriorly throughout the length of the vertebral canal (Chen et al., 1989; Hackney, 1992).

The spinal cord lies deep to the dura, arachnoid, and pia mater (see Fig. 2-17). Beneath the transparent pia mater, dorsal and ventral rootlets can be seen attaching to the spinal cord. These rootlets divide the spinal cord into spinal cord segments (see Chapter 3). A spinal cord segment is the region of the spinal cord delineated by those exiting dorsal and ventral rootlets that eventually unite to form a single spinal nerve. Spinal cord segments can be identified easily on a gross specimen of the spinal cord (see Fig. 3-8, *C*). The rootlets combine to form dorsal roots (from dorsal rootlets) and ventral roots (from ventral rootlets). The dorsal and ventral roots then unite to form a spinal nerve. The rootlets are "exceedingly delicate and vulnerable and when implicated in fibrous adhesions from whatever cause, undergo irreversible changes" (Domisse and Louw, 1990).

Formation of the Spinal Nerve and Anterior and Posterior Primary Divisions. The dorsal and ventral roots unite within the IVF to form the spinal nerve (Fig. 2-18; see also Chapter 3). As the spinal nerve exits the IVF, it divides into two parts: a posterior primary division (dorsal ramus) and an anterior primary division (ventral ramus) (see Figs. 2-17 and 2-18). The posterior primary division further divides into a medial branch, which supplies the Z joints and transversospinalis group of deep back muscles; and a lateral branch, which supplies the sacrospinalis group of deep back muscles

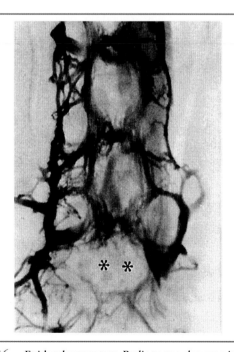

FIG. 2-16 Epidural venogram. Radiopaque dye was injected into the epidural venous plexus, x-ray films were taken, and extraneous tissue was removed using digital subtraction techniques. *Asterisks,* An intervertebral disc protrusion; notice that the dye has not filled the veins in this region. (Courtesy Parke W. From Jayson M. [1980]. *The lumbar spine and back pain.* [2nd ed.] Baltimore: Urban & Schwarzenberg and Pitman Medical Publishing.)

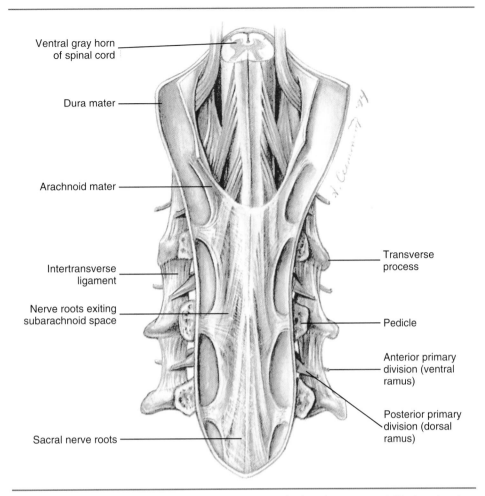

Ventral gray horn of spinal cord

Dura mater

Arachnoid mater

Intertransverse ligament

Nerve roots exiting subarachnoid space

Sacral nerve roots

Transverse process

Pedicle

Anterior primary division (ventral ramus)

Posterior primary division (dorsal ramus)

FIG. 2-17 Vertebral canal with the posterior vertebral arches removed. Notice the dura mater, arachnoid, and neural elements within the canal.

(see Chapter 4). The anterior primary division may unite with other anterior primary divisions to form one of the plexuses of the body. Anterior primary divisions also innervate the body wall; the intercostal nerves serve as a prime example of this function. The plexuses of the anterior primary divisions and the specific innervation of spinal structures by the posterior primary divisions are discussed in the chapters covering the specific regions of the spine (see Chapters 5 through 8). The plexuses are discussed in the chapter dealing with the spinal region from which they arise.

Arterial Supply to the Spine

The external aspect of the vertebral column receives its arterial supply from branches of deep arteries "in the neighborhood" (see Fig. 2-4). The cervical region is supplied by the left and right deep cervical arteries (from the costocervical trunks) and also the right and left ascending cervical arteries (from the right and left

inferior thyroid arteries). The thoracic region of the spine is supplied by posterior intercostal arteries, and the lumbar region is supplied by lumbar segmental arteries.

The internal aspect of the vertebral canal receives its arterial supply from segmental arteries that send spinal branches into the IVFs (see Fig. 2-4). The segmental arteries are branches of the vertebral artery in the cervical region, the intercostal arteries in the thoracic region, and the lumbar segmental arteries in the lumbar region.

On entering the IVF, each spinal branch (ramus) of a segmental artery further divides into three branches. One branch courses posteriorly to supply the laminae and ligamenta flava, and a large branch usually courses to the spinous process, where it enters the base of this process and continues posteriorly to reach its posterior tip. Other arterial twigs from the posterior branch supply the extradural adipose tissue and other small branches course to the posterior spinal dura mater. A large branch enters the lamina close to its junction with the pedicle. On entering the lamina, an ascending and descending

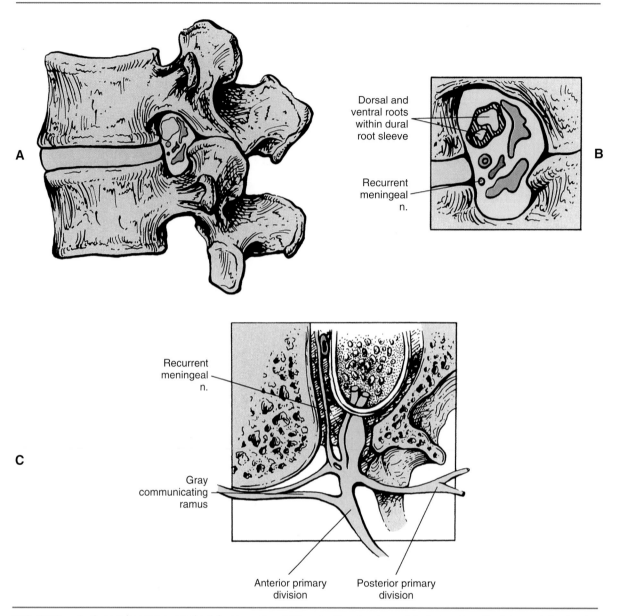

Dorsal and ventral roots within dural root sleeve

Recurrent meningeal n.

Recurrent meningeal n.

Gray communicating ramus

Anterior primary division

Posterior primary division

FIG. 2-18 **A–C,** Lumbar intervertebral foramen. In addition to the structures labeled, notice the intervertebral veins (*blue*), the spinal branch (ramus) of a lumbar segmental artery (*red*), and a lymphatic channel (*green*). **C,** Horizontal section through the intervertebral foramen. Notice that the recurrent meningeal nerve originates from the most proximal portion of the anterior primary division and receives a branch from the gray communicating ramus. It then passes medially to enter the intervertebral foramen.

(the longer of the two) branch course through the superior and inferior articular processes, respectively, to reach the subchondral bone of the articular facets (Crock and Yoshizawa, 1976).

Another branch of the spinal ramus of a segmental artery courses anteriorly. This anterior branch gives off large offshoots to the center of the posterolateral aspect of the vertebral body and then divides into an ascending and a descending branch. The ascending branch crosses

the IVD above and joins the descending branch of the level above. The descending branch courses near the pedicle, sending branches to it. The ascending and descending branches both supply the posterior aspect of the vertebral bodies and also send twigs to the posterior longitudinal ligament (Crock and Yoshizawa, 1976).

The third branch of each spinal ramus of a segmental artery, known as the neural branch, courses to the spinal nerve. The neural branch then divides into an anterior and a posterior radicular artery to supply the ventral and dorsal nerve roots and rootlets, respectively. The spinal cord, the vasculature of the cord (including radiculomedullary arteries), and its meningeal coverings are discussed in detail in Chapter 3, and the unique characteristics of the blood supply to each region of the spine are discussed in further detail in the chapters on specific regions of the spine (Chapters 5 through 8).

INTERVERTEBRAL FORAMEN

The second major opening, or foramen, of the spine is the intervertebral foramen. The IVF is an area of great biomechanical, functional, and clinical significance (Williams et al., 1995). Much of its importance stems from the fact that the IVF provides an osteoligamentous boundary between the central nervous system and peripheral nervous system. This foramen is unlike any other in the body in that the spinal nerve and vessels running through it are passing through an opening formed by two movable bones (vertebrae) and two joints (anterior interbody joint and the Z joint) (Amonoo-Kuofi et al., 1988a). Because of this the IVFs change size during movement. They become larger in spinal flexion and smaller in extension (Amonoo-Kuofi et al., 1988a; Awalt et al., 1989; Mayoux-Benhamou et al., 1989). Compression of the exiting spinal nerves or other foraminal contents has been reported to be an important cause of back pain and pain radiating into the extremities (Amonoo-Kuofi et al., 1988a). Hasue et al. (1983) found evidence that osseous tissue can constrict neurovascular tissue in the nerve root tunnel (IVF). Such osseous tissue can include the uncinate processes in the cervical region; the ribs and their vertebral attachments forming the costocorporeal (costovertebral) joints in the thoracic region; and the intervertebral discs (Hadley, 1948), vertebral bodies, and articular processes of the Z joints (Bailey and Casamajor, 1911) in the lumbar region. Therefore knowledge of the specific anatomy of this clinically important area is important in the differential diagnosis of back and extremity pain and can help with the proper management of individuals with compromise of this region.

A pair (left and right) of IVFs are located between all of the adjacent vertebrae from C2 to the sacrum. The sacrum also has a series of paired dorsal and ventral foramina (see Chapter 8). There are no IVFs between C1 and C2. Where present, the IVFs lie posterior to the vertebral bodies and between the inferior and superior vertebral notches of adjacent vertebrae. Therefore the pedicles of adjacent vertebrae form the roof and floor of this region. The width of the pedicles in the horizontal plane gives depth to these openings, actually making them neural canals (Czervionke et al., 1988) rather than foramina, but the name intervertebral foramina remains.

Six structures form the boundaries of the IVF (see Fig. 2-18, *A* and *B*). Beginning from the most superior border (roof) and continuing anteriorly in a circular fashion, the boundaries include the following:

1. The pedicle of the vertebra above (more specifically, its periosteum)
2. The vertebral body of the vertebra above (again, its periosteum)
3. The IVD (posterolateral aspect of the AF)
4. The vertebral body of the vertebra below, and in the cervical region, the uncinate process (periosteum)
5. The pedicle of the vertebra below forms the floor of the IVF (periosteum). A small part of the sacral base (between the superior articular process and the body of the S1 segment) forms the floor of the L5-S1 IVF.
6. The Z joint forms the "posterior wall." Recall that the Z joint is made up of: (a) the inferior articular process (and facet) of the vertebra above, (b) the superior articular process (and facet) of the vertebra below, and (c) the anterior articular capsule, which is composed of the ligamentum flavum (Xu et al., 1991; Giles, 1992).

The IVFs are smallest in the cervical region, and generally there is a gradual increase in IVF dimensions to the L4 vertebra. The left and right IVFs between L5 and S1 are unique in size and shape (see the following discussion). The different characteristics of the cervical, thoracic, and lumbar IVFs are covered in the chapters on regional anatomy of the spine (Chapters 5 through 7).

As mentioned, the IVFs are actually canals. These canals vary in width from approximately 5 mm (Hewitt, 1970) in the cervical region to 18 mm (Pfaundler, 1989) at the L5-S1 level.

Many structures traverse the IVF (see Fig. 2-18). They include the following:

◆ The spinal nerve (union of dorsal and ventral roots)
◆ The dural root sleeve
◆ Lymphatic channel(s)
◆ The spinal branch (ramus) of a segmental artery. Recall that this artery divides into three branches: one to the posterior aspect of the vertebral body, one to the posterior arch, and one to the spinal nerve (neural branch).
◆ Communicating (intervertebral) veins between the internal and external vertebral venous plexuses
◆ Two to four recurrent meningeal (sinuvertebral) nerves

Adipose tissue surrounds all of the listed structures.

The dorsal and ventral roots unite to form the spinal nerve in the region of the IVF, and the spinal nerve is surrounded by the dural root sleeve. The dural root sleeve is attached to the borders of the IVF by a series of fibrous bands. The dural root sleeve becomes continuous with the epineurium of the spinal nerve at the lateral border of the IVF (see Fig. 2-15). The arachnoid blends with the perineurium proximal to the dorsal root ganglion and at an equivalent region of the ventral root (Hewitt, 1970). Occasionally the arachnoid extends more distally, and in such cases the subarachnoid space extends to the lateral third of the IVF.

Each recurrent meningeal nerve (sinuvertebral nerve of von Luschka) originates from the most proximal portion of the ventral ramus. It receives a branch from the nearest gray communicating ramus of the sympathetic chain before traversing the IVF. This nerve provides sensory innervation (including nociception) to the posterior aspect of the AF, posterior longitudinal ligament, anterior epidural veins, periosteum of the posterior aspect of the vertebral bodies, and anterior aspect of the spinal dura mater. Usually several recurrent meningeal nerves enter the same IVF. These nerves are discussed in more detail in Chapters 5 and 11.

Since the beginning of the twentieth century, the IVF has been a region that has received much attention for a variety of reasons from those engaged in the treatment of the spine. The effects of spinal adjusting on the nerve roots and spinal nerves is an area of acute interest and much debate. In addition, lumbar IVFs have received much scrutiny because of their extreme clinical importance in lumbar IVD protrusion and lumbar intervertebral foraminal (canal) stenosis. In the words of Lancourt, Glenn, and Wiltse (1979), "The importance of the nerve root entrapment in the nerve root canals cannot be overemphasized." The arteries, veins, lymphatics, and particularly the neural elements may be adversely affected by pathologic conditions of one or more of the following structures (Williams et al., 1995):

Fibrocartilage of the AF
NP (especially in earlier decades)
Red bone marrow of the vertebral bodies
Compact bone of the pedicles
Z joints
Capsules
Synovial membranes
Articular cartilage
Fibroadipose meniscoids
Fat pads
Connective tissue rim (fibrous labra)
Costocorporeal joints (in the thoracic region)

CT and MRI allow for accurate evaluation of the IVF in the living. Previous studies have shown both methods to be reliable in measuring the IVF in the sagittal plane (Cramer et al., 1992).

Figure 2-19 shows three parameters measured from MRI scans of the lumbar IVFs of normal human subjects. Table 2-6 shows the average values obtained from the left lumbar IVFs of 95 subjects (46 females and 49 males), and Table 2-7 gives the same values for the right side. Figure 2-20 shows the values displayed graphically. (*Note:*

Because the values for the left and right IVFs shown in Tables 2-6 and 2-7 are statistically the same, one graph can display the values for both sides.) The greatest superior to inferior dimension of the IVF is at L2. This IVF dimension then diminishes until L5, where it is the smallest. The anteroposterior dimensions are smaller than the vertical dimension and remain quite constant throughout the lumbar region, with the more superior of the two anteroposterior measurements shown in Figures 2-19 and 2-20 being larger. Therefore the IVFs from L1 to L4 are similar in shape. They are shaped similar to an inverted pear. The L5 IVF is distinct in shape. It is more oval than the others, with the superior to inferior dimension being greater than the anteroposterior dimension (Cramer et al., 2003).

The width of the IVF is normally the same in males and females. However, the height is approximately 0.5 mm less in females versus males. As one ages, the height of the IVF significantly decreases, whereas the upper anterior to posterior dimension increases. All of the IVF dimensions increase with an increase in overall height of an individual. However, as the weight of an individual increases, the width of the IVF decreases. Figure 2-21 demonstrates these relationships (Cramer et al., 2003).

The databases shown in the previous tables and figures may be used as a source of comparison when studying the IVF in healthy and diseased states such as suspected intervertebral foraminal stenosis (narrowing). Such stenosis can occur as the result of disc degeneration (Crock, 1976), ligamentum flavum hypertrophy, or Z joint arthrosis (i.e., increased bone formation because of increased weight-bearing or torsional stress). Of further interest to clinicians is the fact that the dimensions of the IVF have been found to be significantly related to anteroposterior vertebral canal diameters. However, transverse diameters of the vertebral canals and vertebral body heights do not correlate with IVF dimensions (Clarke et al., 1985). Clarke et al. (1985) speculate that prenatal and neonatal growth disruption may be a primary cause of abnormally small vertebral canal and IVF size. This remains an important area for future investigation.

Accessory Ligaments of the Intervertebral Foramen

Accessory ligaments of the IVF were first studied in the early nineteenth century (Bourgery, 1832). However, these structures received very little attention until the mid- to late-twentieth century, when Golub and Silverman (1969) first used the term *transforaminal ligaments* (TFLs) in the description of ligamentous bands crossing the IVFs. Since then, several investigators have studied these structures in the cervical (Bakkum

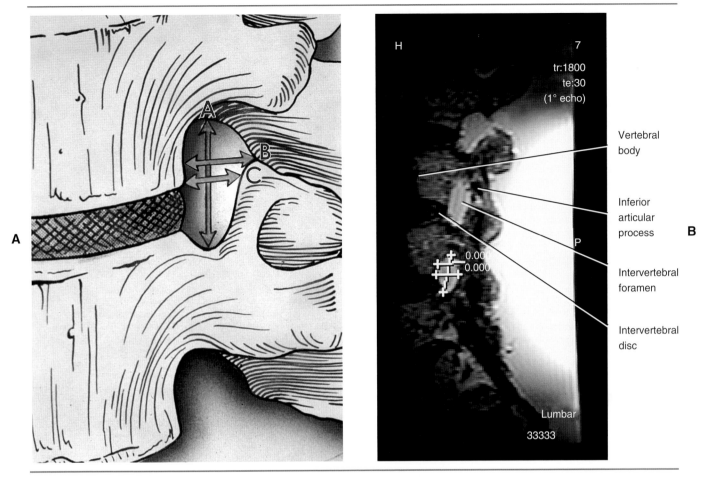

FIG. 2-19 **A,** Illustration and, **B,** magnetic resonance imaging (MRI) scan demonstrating the three measurements made on the parasagittal MRI scans of 95 individuals. **A,** *A* = superior-inferior (SI) measurement, *B* = upper (superior) anterior-posterior (SAP) measurement, *C* = lower (inferior) anterior-posterior (IAP) measurement. Summaries of the data from these measurements are shown in Tables 2-6 and 2-7 and Figure 2-20. **B,** The measurements read "0.00" because the scale was set to zero before this photograph was taken. This was done to avoid a distracting overlap of numbers on the screen. (**A,** From Cramer G et al. [2003]. Dimensions of the lumbar intervertebral foramina as determined from the sagittal plane magnetic resonance imaging scans of 95 normal subjects. *J Manipulative Physiol Ther 26,* 160-170.)

and Berthiaume, 1994), thoracic (Bakkum and Mestan, 1994), and lumbar (Amonoo-Kuofi et al., 1988a,b; Cramer et al., 2002; Nowicki and Haughton, 1992a,b; Bakkum and Mestan, 1994) regions of the spine. These ligaments are much more common in the lower thoracic and lumbar regions (Bakkum and Mestan, 1994) than in the cervical region (Bakkum and Berthiaume, 1994), and are now considered to be normal structures within the lumbar IVFs. However, the reported incidence of TFLs in the lumbar region varies considerably (Table 2-8). One reason for the difference in reported findings is that there is considerable variation in size, shape, and location of TFLs from one IVF to another. Also some investigators evaluated different regions of the IVFs (i.e., medial, lateral, or both), and some authors only identified very

thick and substantial structures as TFLs, whereas others were less restrictive in their definition of TFLs.

Amonoo-Kuofi et al. (1988a) also studied TFLs of the IVFs, and mapped out the relationship of the spinal nerve, segmental veins and arteries, and the recurrent meningeal nerve through the openings between the TFLs. They concluded that these accessory ligaments tend to hold the previously mentioned structures in their proper position within the IVF.

Transforaminal ligaments have been identified on both CT (Nowicki and Haughton, 1992b) and MRI scans (Nowicki and Haughton, 1992b; Cramer et al., 2002). Cramer et al. (2002) conducted a reliability study to evaluate the ability of trained radiologists to identify TFLs on MRI. The study was performed on cadaveric spines

Table 2-6	Dimensions of Left Lumbar Intervertebral Foramina*		
IVF	Superior to Inferior Dimension (Measurement "A")	SAP (Measurement "B")	IAP (Measurement "C")
LL1	19.7 (1.9)	9.5 (1.5)	8.3 (1.7)
LL2	21.0 (2.1)	10.2 (1.7)	7.9 (1.6)
LL3	20.5 (2.1)	10.5 (2.0)	7.8 (1.7)
LL4	19.3 (2.1)	10.5 (1.9)	7.4 (1.8)
LL5	17.0 (2.6)	10.9 (2.1)	8.7 (2.1)

From Cramer G et al. (2003). Dimensions of the lumbar intervertebral foramina as determined from the sagittal plane magnetic resonance imaging scans of 95 normal subjects. *J Manipulative Physiol Ther 26,* 160-170.

IAP, Inferior anterior-posterior measurement taken at the level of the inferior vertebral end plate (measurement "C" Fig. 2-19); *IVF,* intervertebral foramina; *SAP,* Superior anterior-posterior measurement taken at the level of the Z joint (measurement "B" Fig. 2-19).

*The average size of the left L1-5 IVFs for three measured parameters (Figs. 2-19 and 2-20). Values given in millimeters with standard deviations in parentheses. Values calculated from 95 human subjects: 46 females and 49 males.

Table 2-7	Dimensions of Right Lumbar Intervertebral Foramina*		
IVF	Superior to Inferior Dimension (Measurement "A")	SAP (Measurement "B")	IAP (Measurement "C")
RL1	20.2 (1.9)	9.4 (1.6)	8.2 (1.6)
RL2	21.2 (2.0)	10.1 (1.7)	7.9 (1.7)
RL3	20.8 (2.1)	10.6 (2.1)	7.9 (1.8)
RL4	18.8 (2.3)	10.9 (1.9)	7.5 (1.8)
RL5	17.1 (2.5)	10.6 (1.8)	8.4 (1.9)

From Cramer G et al. (2003). Dimensions of the lumbar intervertebral foramina as determined from the sagittal plane magnetic resonance imaging scans of 95 normal subjects. *J Manipulative Physiol Ther 26,* 160-170.

IAP, Inferior anterior-posterior measurement taken at the level of the inferior vertebral end plate (measurement "C" Fig. 2-19); *IVF,* intervertebral foramina; *SAP,* Superior anterior-posterior measurement taken at the level of the Z joint (measurement "B" Fig. 2-19).

*The average size of the left L1-5 IVFs for three measured parameters (Figs. 2-19 and 2-20). Values given in millimeters with standard deviations in parentheses. Values calculated from 95 human subjects: 46 females and 49 males.

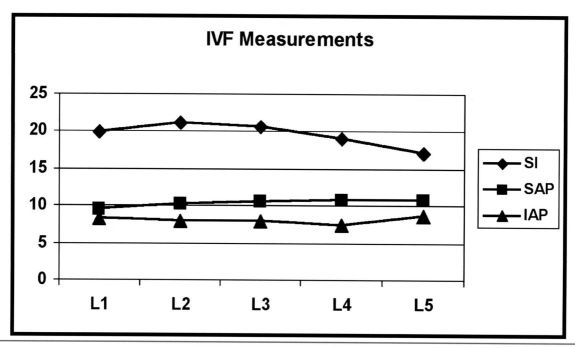

FIG. 2-20   Dimensions of the lumbar intervertebral foramina of 95 normal human subjects. Notice that the two anteroposterior measurements (superior and inferior anterior-posterior) remain almost the same throughout the lumbar region. The superior-inferior (S-I) dimension is the greatest at L2 and then becomes progressively smaller. (From Cramer G et al. [2003]. Dimensions of the lumbar intervertebral foramina as determined from the sagittal plane magnetic resonance imaging scans of 95 normal subjects. *J Manipulative Physiol Ther, 26,* 160-170.)

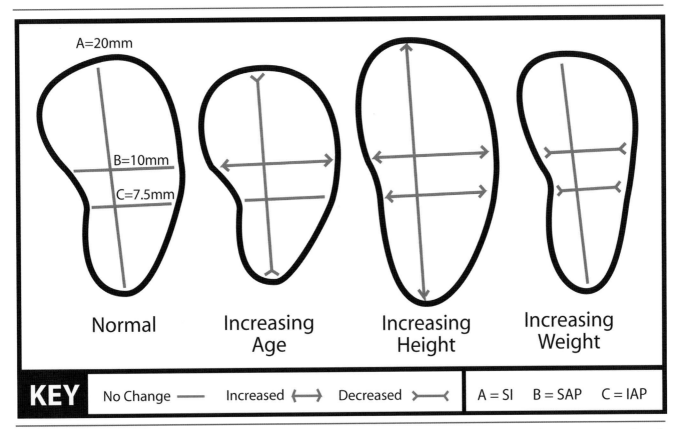

FIG. 2-21   Illustration demonstrating changes in IVF dimensions with increasing age, height, and weight. (From Cramer G et al. [2003]. Dimensions of the lumbar intervertebral foramina as determined from the sagittal plane magnetic resonance imaging scans of 95 normal subjects. *J Manipulative Physiol Ther 26,* 160-170.)

that were carefully dissected to identify all TFLs. The spines were then embedded in gelatin and MRI scanned. Three radiologists were trained to identify TFLs on MRI scans and then evaluated the MRI scans of the cadaveric spines to identify the presence or absence of TFLs. The radiologists were blinded to the results of one another and to the anatomic specimens. The results showed that if a radiologist, trained to identify TFLs on MRI, determined that a TFL was present at a given IVF, there was approximately an 87% chance that one was actually pre-

sent (i.e., a positive predictive value of 86.7%). However, if a trained radiologist said a TFL was not present in an IVF, there remained approximately a 50% chance that one was present (i.e., a negative predictive value of 50.8%).

TFLs have been implicated as both a cause of low back pain and nerve root entrapment (Bachop and Janse, 1983; Giles, 1988; Macnab and McCulloh, 1990; Olsewski et al., 1991; Transfeldt, Robertson, and Bradford, 1993). Bakkum and Mestan (1994) found that when TFLs were

Table 2-8   Comparison of Results of Several Studies Evaluating Percentage of Intervertebral Foramina with Transforaminal Ligaments

IVFs with TFLs	Bachop and Hilgendorf (1981)*	Amonoo-Kuofi et al. (1988a, b)	Giles (1992)	Transfeldt et al. (1993)	Bakkum and Mestan (1994)	Cramer et al. (2002)
Overall L1-2 to L5-S1	17.3%	100%	N/A	N/A	67.5%	60.0%
L1-2 to L4-5	10.8%	100%	61% L4-5	N/A	68.8%	58.3%
L5-S1	43.3%	100%	43%	76.5%	62.5%	66.7%

From Cramer G et al. (2002). Evaluation of transforaminal ligaments by magnetic resonance imaging. *J Manipulative Physiol Ther 25,* 199-208.
IVFs, Intervertebral foramina; *TFLs,* transforaminal ligaments.
*Very rigorous criteria.

present, the superior to inferior dimension of the compartment transmitting the anterior primary division of the spinal nerve was significantly decreased as compared with the osseous IVF (the mean decrease in size was 31.5%). They concluded that there is often less space at the exit zone of the IVF for the emerging anterior primary division than was traditionally thought to be the case. Furthermore, they felt that the decreased space may contribute to the incidence of neurologic symptoms in the region at times, especially after trauma or secondary to degenerative arthritic changes in the region of the IVF. Bachop and Janse (1983) reported that the higher a TFL is located within the IVF, the less space remains for the intervertebral vessels, which conceivably could lead to ischemia or venous congestion. They also postulated that lower placement of the ligament would increase the possibility of sensory and motor deficits. Figure 2-22, *A* and *B*, shows examples of TFLs, and Figure 2-22, *C*, shows a composite drawing demonstrating the TFLs that have been reported in the literature.

The term *corporotransverse ligament* is used when referring to a TFL that courses between the vertebral body and the transverse process at the L5-S1 junction (Bachop and Janse, 1983). The lumbar spinal ramus of the segmental artery, intervertebral veins, and gray sympathetic ramus course above this structure, and the anterior primary division courses underneath it (Golub and Silverman, 1969; Bachop and Ro, 1984).

Corporotransverse ligaments can be either broad and flat or rodlike (McNab, 1971; Bachop and Hilgendorf, 1981). The rodlike ligaments are usually tougher (firmer) than the flat type. Wang et al. (1999) found that corporotransverse ligaments have the histologic make-up of other ligaments of the spine. In addition, calcification often is found in corporotransverse ligaments. Therefore the corporotransverse ligaments are sturdy ligamentous bands that can calcify (Wang et al., 1999).

Like TFLs, the corporotransverse ligaments can be seen on CT (Church and Buehler, 1991) and MRI (Nowicki and Haughton, 1992b; Cramer et al., 2002), but not on standard x-rays (Winterstein and Bachop, 1990). Figure 2-23 shows a corporotransverse ligament at the L5-S1 level of a cadaveric spine. Figure 2-24 shows two MRIs of the same cadaveric spine. The TFL is shown on the MRI of Figure 2-24, *B*.

As with TFLs, the corporotransverse ligaments are also thought to be clinically significant. They may have a constricting effect on the anterior primary division (ventral ramus) as that nerve courses under the ligamentous band (McNab, 1971; Bachop and Janse, 1983). That is, in patients with sciatica, as the leg is raised, the anterior primary division could be stretched across the ligament, possibly mimicking the thigh and leg pain of a disc protrusion. In addition, Breig and Troup (1979) and Rydevik et al. (1984) have reported on increased sensi-

tivity of inflamed nerve roots. Factors such as facet arthrosis, disc protrusion, and ligamentum flavum hypertrophy could conceivably increase intraforaminal pressure. The presence of a corporotransverse ligament could further increase this pressure and possibly cause a subclinical problem to become clinical.

Other accessory ligaments of the spine that might impinge on nerves and blood vessels have been described by Bogduk (1981) and Nathan, Weizenbluth, and Halperin (1982).

ADVANCED DIAGNOSTIC IMAGING

One of the most important clinical applications of the anatomy of the spine and spinal cord is in the field of advanced diagnostic imaging. The imaging modalities of CT and MRI frequently allow for extremely clear visualization of the normal and pathologic anatomy of spinal structures. Examples of these images are included in other chapters to demonstrate various anatomic structures and show how some of the structures discussed in the text appear on these images. A general understanding of the advantages and disadvantages of the most commonly used advanced imaging techniques helps the reader gain more information from these images. Therefore the first purpose of this section, which is written for those who do not specialize in diagnostic imaging, is to review the general application and uses of procedures. The second purpose is to discuss which anatomic structures and spinal disorders can best be imaged with a specific type of modality. Areas of relevant research also are discussed when the results affect currently used imaging procedures. The final purpose is to provide a brief review of the literature for the student, clinician, and researcher whose major field is not related to diagnostic imaging. Because most of the principles discussed in this section are applicable to all spinal regions, diagnostic imaging included in this chapter is related to general characteristics of the spine rather than to specific spinal regions, which are discussed later in the text.

Because the advanced imaging modalities most commonly used are MRI and CT, the majority of this review deals with these two imaging modalities. Other methods, including ultrafine flexible fiberoptic scopes, myelography, discography, angiography, ultrasonography, three-dimensional computed tomography, radionuclide imaging, and digital imaging, also are discussed.

Magnetic Resonance Imaging

MRI has become an important component of spinal imaging. MRI shows soft tissue especially well and represents a quantum leap in the evaluation of patients with disc disease (Woodruff, 1988). It has been found to be more sensitive than contrast-enhanced CT in demon-

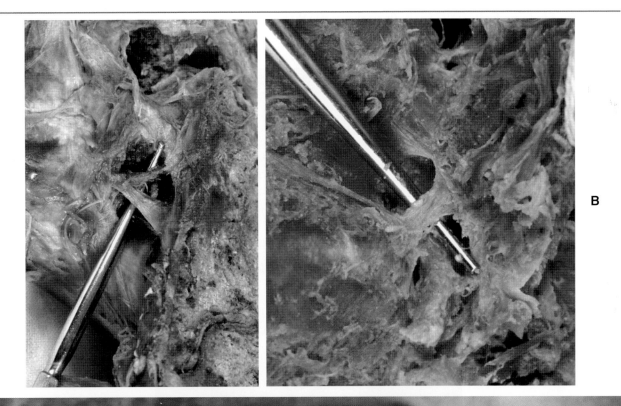

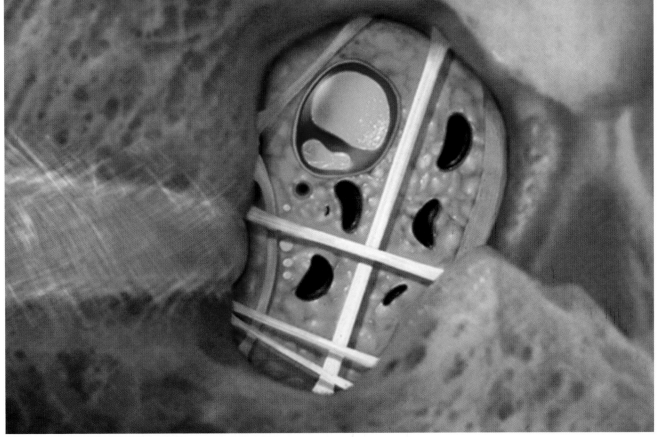

FIG. 2-22   Transforaminal ligaments (TFLs) in two different cadaveric specimens. **A,** Two TFLs coursing over a probe placed within the left L5-S1 intervertebral foramina (IVFs). Anteriorly, the two TFLs almost attach together onto the posterior aspect of the body of L5. Posteriorly, the two TFLs diverge, both attaching to the posterior border of the IVF. **B,** A different specimen. The probe is placed behind a broad flat TFL that is coursing from the body of L3 to the posterosuperior aspect of the IVF. The posterior–superior attachment is on the ligamentum flavum that is covering the junction of the superior and inferior articular processes of L3. **C,** A composite illustration demonstrating TFLs (white bands traversing intervertebral foramen in illustration) that have been reported in the literature. (From Cramer G et al. [2002]. Evaluation of transforaminal ligaments by magnetic resonance imaging. *J Manipulative Physiol Ther, 25,* 199-208.)

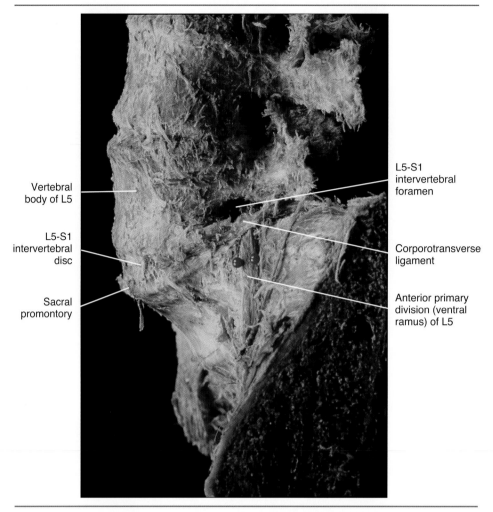

Vertebral
body of L5

L5-S1
intervertebral
disc

Sacral
promontory

L5-S1
intervertebral
foramen

Corporotransverse
ligament

Anterior primary
division (ventral
ramus) of L5

FIG. 2-23   Lateral view of a cadaveric lumbar spine. The red pins pass beneath a corporotransverse ligament that spans the left L5-S1 intervertebral foramen. Notice the anterior primary division (ventral ramus) passing beneath this ligament (between the red pins).

strating disc degeneration (Schnebel et al., 1989), and is currently the imaging modality of choice in the evaluation of lumbar disc protrusion and extrusion (Forristall, Marsh, and Pay, 1988; Jackson et al., 1989). MRI can also detect some tears of the AF (Herzog, 1996). However, MRI alone is not enough to determine the cause of back pain (Borenstein et al., 2001), and correlations with patient history, physical examination findings, and if necessary findings of laboratory and other diagnostic procedures (e.g., electromyography) are essential to establish the most likely cause of back pain.

MRI also can detect disruption of the posterior longitudinal ligament secondary to extrusion of the NP. Not only does MRI allow for visualization of the discs, cerebrospinal fluid, spinal cord, and the perimeter of the spinal canal, but it also allows visualization of these structures in several planes without the use of intravenous contrast media. For these reasons MRI is currently the method of choice for detecting disorders of the spinal canal and spinal cord (Woodruff, 1988). Edema of bone marrow, spinal cord tumors, syringomyelia, extramedullary tumors (e.g., meningiomas), early detection of metastatic disease and primary malignancies of the vertebrae, and spina bifida (dysraphism) are all evaluated exceptionally well with this technology (Alexander, 1988; Woodruff, 1988; An et al., 1995; Buckwalter and Brandser, 1997). MRI also has been found to be effective in the evaluation of failed back surgery syndrome by differentiating fibrotic scar formation secondary to spinal surgery from disc herniation (Frocrain et al., 1989; Kricun, Kricun, and Danlinka, 1990) and is becoming the most important modality for all imaging of the postoperative spine (Djukic et al., 1990). Discitis also can be evaluated with MRI (Woodruff, 1988). MRI and conventional films are considered adequate for the pre-neurosurgical evaluation of cervical radiculopathy and

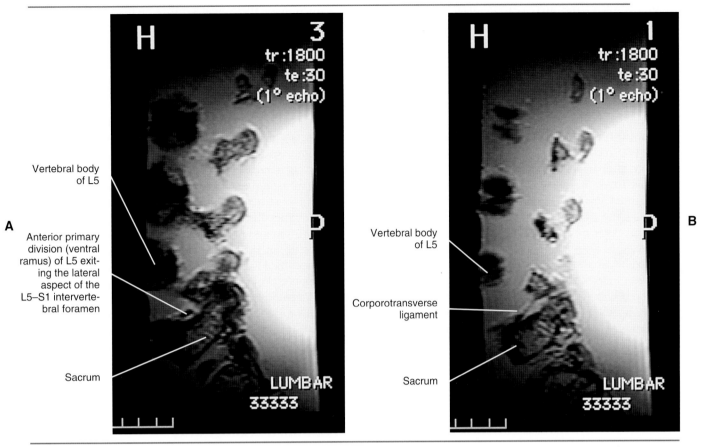

FIG. 2-24 Parasagittal magnetic resonance imaging scans of the same cadaveric spine shown in Figure 2-20. **A,** The anterior primary division (ventral ramus). **B,** Corporotransverse ligament in a scan lateral to that of **A.**

myelopathy, with CT myelography being the follow-up procedure of choice (Brown et al., 1988).

A discrete area of high signal, known as a "high-intensity zone", has been identified as a marker for painful tears of the outer AF of the IVD, especially tears related to internal disc disruption (Aprill and Bogduk, 1992; Schellhas et al., 1996). (See Chapter 11 for a discussion of internal disc disruption.) Perhaps a related finding is that the high-intensity zone also has been related to decreased stiffness of the IVD, especially in axial rotation (Schmidt et al., 1998). Saifuddin, McSweeney, and Lehovsky (2003) found that the high-intensity zone became more apparent when MRI scans were taken during axial loading of the spine (loads causing compression of the IVDs; e.g., standing). However, other research questions the clinical relevance of the high-intensity zone (Narvani, Tsiridis, and Wilson, 2003).

MRI continues to be a rapidly developing field, and the many technical advances should continue to improve its clinical utility. One such advance is the ability to decrease cerebrospinal fluid (CSF) flow artifact. This development results in better visualization of the spinal cord and the cord–CSF interface. Other advances are

related to an increased variety of new imaging protocols used by radiologists. The imaging protocols of gradient-echo imaging (e.g., GRASS, FLASH, FISP, MPGR) allow for greater contrast between anatomic structures while decreasing scan time. Such gradient-echo techniques are the procedures of choice in patients with suspected cervical radiculopathy (Kricun, Kricun, and Danlinka, 1990), giving information of greater or equal value to that obtained from myelography or CT myelography (Hedberg, Dayer, and Flom, 1988).

Two of the primary properties of MR images are related to the various responses of different tissues to the radiofrequency applied during the MRI evaluation. These two characteristics are known as T1 and T2. Various MRI protocols can highlight either of these characteristics and thereby selectively enhance different tissues. T1-weighted images are better for depicting anatomic detail. Adipose tissue has a high signal (is bright) on T1-weighted images, and these images are particularly useful in the evaluation of the spinal cord, bone marrow of vertebrae, IVDs, osteophytes, and ligaments (Woodruff, 1988; Kricun, Kricun, and Danlinka, 1990).

As a result of the increased acquisition time of the second echo, the resolution of T2-weighted images is not as good as that of T1-weighted images. However, T2-weighted images allow for better visualization of fluid and edema, and often reveal subtle, significant spinal cord pathology. T2-weighted images are also the most sensitive at showing a decreased signal intensity resulting from degeneration and desiccation of the disc (Woodruff, 1988; Herzog, 1996), and a decreased signal of the IVD on T2-weighted images may either precede or come after histologic evidence of IVD degeneration (Herzog, 1996). Because CSF has a very high signal on T2-weighted images, these images also are valuable in evaluating the amount of narrowing of the subarachnoid space in cases of spinal stenosis. T2-weighted images also create a "myelographic effect" related to the bright appearance of CSF on these films. This myelographic effect can help with the detection and characterization of subtle disc bulges and protrusions. T2-weighted images also are useful in the detection of multiple myeloma of the vertebral column (Avrahami, Tadmor, and Kaplinsky, 1993). Even with all of these advantages, in general, T1-weighted images are more valuable than T2-weighted images in the evaluation of the majority of spinal disorders (Moffit et al., 1988).

The contrast medium of gadolinium (Gd-DTPA) can be used in conjunction with MRI and has been found to be safe and effective in increasing the contrast of certain pathologic conditions. Differentiation of scar formation (epidural fibrosis) from disc herniation in failed back surgery syndrome (recurrent postoperative sciatica) is improved with the use of Gd-DTPA (Hueftle et al., 1988). Gd-DTPA also may be useful in depicting disc protrusions and extrusions surrounded by scar tissue and free disc fragments. It also can be useful in identifying acute healing compression fractures and differentiating whether a compression fracture of the vertebral body is the result of a benign or malignant process. Gd-DTPA also is useful in evaluating patients with intradural tumors, but it is less useful in evaluating tumors external to the dura mater.

Advances in MRI technology include developments in the hardware of the MRI unit, such as coil configurations (Woodruff, 1988). These changes allow large areas of the spine to be viewed at once, which is particularly useful in the evaluation of metastatic disease and syringomyelia. Other advances include three-dimensional reconstruction of spinal images with a video display that allows images to be rotated 360 degrees for viewing. Axial loaded (standing) MRI of the lumbar spine, which images the spine in a more physiologic state, may help to more accurately assess the dimensions of the spinal canal, when compared with routinely performed supine examinations with the hips and knees flexed (Saifuddin, Blease, and McSweeney, 2003). In addition, functional MRI (fMRI)

evaluation of the spinal cord, which maps MRI signal changes after a specific stimulus designed to change neural activity, may become fundamental in the future work-up of spinal cord injury (Stroman et al., 2002).

Research is also being done involving morphometry of the spine by means of MRI (Cramer et al., 2003). Morphometry means the measurement of an organism or its parts. The digital images available from MRI (and CT) scans may be used to accurately quantify certain anatomic structures of the spine. This is the first time many such measurements can be made in the living. Such measurements allow for an increased ability to study the structures influenced by a variety of therapeutic procedures (Cramer et al., 2002, 2003).

Diffusion and perfusion MRI allows information to be gained about the structure and function of tissue at a microscopic level. These procedures have an increasingly prominent clinical role, especially in neurovascular imaging (Valentini et al., 2003). Finally, extraordinary opportunities for advances in the clinical applications of MRI exist as imaging at the molecular level becomes possible (Rollo, 2003). Advances in spinal research will undoubtedly make use of such important applications as the imaging of the chemical mediators of back pain. (See Chapter 11 for a discussion of these chemical mediators.)

Computed Tomography

Conventional CT remains effective in the evaluation of many conditions. It is especially valuable when accurate depiction of osseous tissues is important. Pathologic conditions including spinal stenosis, tumors of bone, congenital anomalies, degenerative changes, trauma, spondylolysis, and spondylolisthesis can all be accurately evaluated by CT (Wang, Wesolowski, and Farah, 1988). Images reformatted to the sagittal or coronal plane may help with the evaluation of complicated bone anatomy. Arachnoiditis ossificans, a rare ossification of the arachnoid mater as a consequence of trauma, hemorrhage, previous myelogram, or spinal anesthesia, can be better visualized on CT than MRI (Wang, Wesolowski, and Farah, 1988). Criteria for the diagnosis of intraspinal hemangiomas by means of CT also have been established (Salamon and Freilich, 1988). Although lumbar disc disease can be evaluated adequately by means of CT, "beam hardening" artifacts lead to inadequate evaluation of disc disease in the thoracic and, to a lesser extent, the lower cervical canal (Woodruff, 1988).

CT is especially valuable in the evaluation of lumbar spinal stenosis, although artifacts sometimes make the evaluation of cervical and thoracic spinal stenosis difficult (Wang, Wesolowski, and Farah, 1988). The evaluation of facet joint disease and calcification of the ligamentum flavum is currently more efficient with CT than with MRI (Wang, Wesolowski, and Farah, 1988).

CT is also quite effective in the evaluation of bone destruction and new bone formation secondary to neoplasia. It demonstrates the vertebral bony cortex and vertebral bodies well (Buckwalter and Brandser, 1997). In addition, CT is excellent in allowing the identification of osseous changes subsequent to spinal trauma. For example, CT is particularly good at identifying the presence of bony fragments in the spinal canal after posterior arch fracture (Wang, Wesolowski, and Farah, 1988).

Intrathecal contrast-enhanced CT (CT myelography) results in a more complete depiction of the spinal canal, the IVD relative to the spinal canal, and the perimeter of the spinal cord (Woodruff, 1988). Contrast-enhanced CT and MRI are comparable in their abilities to demonstrate spinal stenosis (Schnebel et al., 1989). CT and MRI have a complementary role in the evaluation of such disorders as spinal canal stenosis, congenital disorders, facet disorders, and acute spinal injury (Wang, Wesolowski, and Farah, 1988; Tracy, Wright, and Hanigan, 1989). Extraforaminal (far lateral and anterior) disc herniations can also be readily identified on both CT and MRI if scans include L2 through S1, and if the IVF and paravertebral spaces are closely examined (Osborn et al., 1988).

Other Imaging Modalities

Ultrafine Flexible Fiberoptic Scopes. Ultrafine flexible fiberoptic scopes ("fiberscopes") have been used to provide direct visualization of the epidural space and the subarachnoid space with exceptional clarity of visual detail. In fact, using fiberscopes, Tobita et al. (2003) made new diagnoses in 12 of 55 chronic low back pain subjects who had previously been imaged with other advanced diagnostic procedures. The most common new diagnosis was chronic arachnoiditis.

Myelography. Myelography is the injection of radiopaque dye into the subarachnoid space of the lumbar cistern followed by spinal x-ray examinations. Myelography for the evaluation of lumbar disc herniation is rapidly being replaced by CT and MRI. However, it may be useful when the level of the lesion is clinically unclear or when the entire lumbar region and thoracolumbar junction are to be examined (Fagerlund and Thelander, 1989).

Discography. Discography is the injection of radiopaque dye into the IVD. This technique is useful as an adjunct in the evaluation of symptomatic disorders of the disc. Discography in conjunction with CT (CT/discography) allows delineation and classification of anular disc disruption not possible with plain discography (i.e., discography used in conjunction with conventional radiographs) and, in some cases, identifies such disruption when not seen on T2-weighted MR images. Discography may be particularly useful in evaluating chronic low back pain patients with suspected disc disorders (McFadden, 1988; Herzog, 1996) when the patient's pain is at a significant level of intensity (stress discography). Although discography remains a controversial diagnostic procedure, current literature supports the use of discography in select situations (Guyer and Ohnmeiss, 2003).

Angiography. Spinal angiography is the imaging of the vasculature after the injection of a radiopaque contrast medium. This technique is used to evaluate the arterial supply of spinal tumors (e.g., aneurysmal bone cyst) to assist the surgeon in operative planning (Wang, Wesolowski, and Farah, 1988). Magnetic resonance angiography is gaining widespread use in the evaluation of spinal and intracranial vascular pathology.

Ultrasonography. Ultrasonography (sonography) is currently being used in the evaluation of posterior arch defects in spina bifida (dysraphism), in the intraoperative and postoperative evaluation of the spinal cord, and in the evaluation of the fetal and neonate spine (Wang, Wesolowski, and Farah, 1988). Three-dimensional ultrasound is becoming an important adjunct imaging procedure in this regard as well. This technique has the ability to show the alignment of the posterior spinal elements and the integrity of the vertebral bodies (Hughes et al., 2003). Ultrasound is also useful in the evaluation of tumors of the cauda equina (Friedman, Wetjen, and Atkinson, 2003).

Three-Dimensional Computed Tomography. Three-dimensional CT uses the digital data obtained from conventional CT and reprocesses the information to create a three-dimensional display that can be rotated 360 degrees on a video console. This technique is useful as an adjunct to conventional CT in the evaluation of complex spinal fractures, spondylolisthesis, postoperative fusion, and in some cases of spinal stenosis (Pate, Resnick, and Andre, 1986). Three-dimensional CT is excellent for the assessment of degenerative stenosis of the vertebral canal, lateral recess stenosis, and foraminal stenosis (Krupski, 2002).

Radionuclide Imaging. Single photon emission CT (SPECT) uses tomographic slices obtained with a gamma camera to evaluate radionuclide uptake. This modality has been shown to be a useful adjunct to planar bone scintigraphy (i.e., bone scans, which are very effective in identifying primary and metastatic neoplasia of bone) in the identification and localization of spinal lesions, especially those responsible for low back pain (Kricun, Kricun, and Danlinka, 1990). SPECT is also effective in the evaluation of spondylolysis. Positron emission tomography (PET) is useful in the differentiation of degenerative and infectious end plate abnormalities in the lumbar spine (Stumpe et al., 2002), and is becoming an important physiologic imaging modality in the staging of malignant tumors and for the monitoring of the results of cancer therapy (Jerusalem et al., 2003).

Digital Imaging. Digital imaging uses a conventional x-ray source and a very efficient x-ray detector to digitize and immediately obtain images. This technique is being used currently in the follow-up evaluation of scoliosis because of its relatively small radiation dose. However, because of the lack of adequate spatial resolution, conventional radiographs should be used at the initial evaluation of scoliosis with osseous etiologic components, such as congenital anomalies (Kushner and Cleveland, 1988; Kricun, Kricun, and Danlinka, 1990). Imaging applications of all types are rapidly becoming digitally based. Digitally based imaging aids in the rapid transport of images for interpretation and also reduces the space and cost of archiving images.

REFERENCES

Ahmed M et al. (1993). Sensory and autonomic innervation of the facet joint in the rat lumbar spine. *Spine, 18,* 2121-2126.

Alcalay M et al. (1988). Traitement par nucleolyse a la chymopapaine des hernies discales a forme purement lombalgique. *Revue du Rhumatisme, 55,* 741-745.

Alexander A. (1988). Magnetic resonance imaging of the spine and spinal cord tumors. In Bisese JH (Ed.). *Spine, state of the art reviews, spinal imaging: Diagnostic and therapeutic applications.* Philadelphia: Hanley & Belfus.

Amonoo-Kuofi HS et al. (1988a). Ligaments associated with lumbar intervertebral foramina. I. L1 to L4. *J Anat, 156,* 177-183.

Amonoo-Kuofi HS et al. (1988b). Ligaments associated with lumbar intervertebral foramina, 2. The fifth lumbar level. *J Anat, 159,* 1-10.

An HS et al. (1995). Can we distinguish between versus malignant compression fractures of the spine by magnetic resonance imaging? *Spine, 20,* 1776-1782.

Andersson GBJ & Weinstein JN. (1996). Disc herniation. *Spine, 21,* 1S.

Aprill C & Bogduk N. (1992). High-intensity zone: A diagnostic sign of painful lumbar disc on magnetic resonance imaging. *Br J Radiol, 65,* 361-369.

Avrahami E, Tadmor R, & Kaplinsky N. (1993). The role of T2 weighted gradient echo in MRI demonstration of spinal multiple myeloma. *Spine, 18,* 1812-1815.

Awalt P et al. (1989). Radiographic measurements of intervertebral foramina of cervical vertebra in forward and normal head posture. *J Craniomand Pract, 7,* 275-285.

Bachop W & Hilgendorf C. (1981). Transforaminal ligaments of the human lumbar spine. *Anat Rec, 199* (abstract).

Bachop W & Janse J. (1983). The corporotransverse ligament at the L5 intervertebral foramen. *Anat Rec, 205* (abstract).

Bachop WE & Ro CS. (1984). A ligament separating the nerve from the blood vessels at the L5 intervertebral foramen. *J Bone Joint Surg, 8,* 437.

Bahk YW & Lee JM. (1988). Measure-set computed tomographic analysis of internal architectures of lumbar disc: Clinical and histologic studies. *Invest Radiol, 23,* 17-23.

Bailey P & Casamajor L. (1911). Osteo-arthritis of the spine as a cause of compression of the spinal cord and its roots. *J Nerve Ment Dis, 38,* 588-609.

Bakkum BW & Berthiamue B. (1994). Transforaminal ligaments of the human cervical spine. *Proceedings of the Eleventh Annual Meeting of the American Association of Clinical Anatomists, 22.*

Bakkum BW & Mestan M. (1994). The effects of transforaminal ligaments on the sizes of T11 to L5 human intervertebral foramina. *J Manipulative Physiol Ther, 17,* 517-522.

Bayliss M et al. (1988) Proteoglycan synthesis in the human intervertebral disc: Variation with age, region, and pathology. *Spine, 13,* 972-981.

Beaman DN et al. (1993). Substance P innervation of lumbar spine facet joints. *Spine, 18,* 1044-1049.

Black KM, McClure P, & Polansky M. (1996). The influence of different sitting positions on cervical and lumbar posture. *Spine, 21,* 65-70.

Bogduk N. (1981). The lumbar mamillo-accessory ligament: Its anatomical and neurosurgical significance. *Spine, 6,* 162-167.

Bogduk N. (1997). *Clinical anatomy of the lumbar spine* (3rd ed.). London: Churchill Livingstone.

Bogduk N & Engel R. (1984). The menisci of the lumbar zygapophyseal joints. *Spine, 9,* 454-460.

Bodguk N, Tynan W, & Wilson A. (1981). The nerve supply to the human lumbar intervertebral discs. *J Anat, 132,* 39-56.

Boelderl A et al. (2002). Danger of damaging the medial branches of the posterior rami of spinal nerves during a dorsomedian approach to the spine. *Clin Anat, 15,* 77-81.

Boos N et al. (1996). A new magnetic resonance imaging analysis method for the measurement of disc height variations. *Spine, 21,* 563-570.

Boos N et al. (2002). Classification of age-related changes in lumbar intervertebral discs: 2002 Volvo award in basic science. *Spine, 27,* 2631-2644.

Borenstein DG et al. (2001). The value of magnetic resonance imaging of the lumbar spine to predict low-back pain in asymptomatic subjects. *J Bone Joint Surg, 83a,* 1306-1311.

Boszczyk BM et al. (2001). Related an immunohistochemical study of the dorsal capsule of the lumbar and thoracic facet joints. *Spine, 26(15),* E338-E343.

Botsford DJ, Esses SI, & Olgilvie-Harris DJ. (1994). In vivo diurnal variation in intervertebral disc volume and morphology. *Spine, 19,* 935-945.

Bourgery J. (1832). *Traite commplet de l'Anatomie del'Homme, comprenant la medicine operatiore.* Tome 1.C. Paris: Delauney, 449-450.

Breger R et al. (1988). Truncation artifact in MR images of the intervertebral disc. *AJRN, 9,* 825-828.

Breig A & Troup J. (1979). Biomechanical considerations in the straight leg raising test. *Spine, 4,* 242-250.

Brønfort G. (1997). *Efficacy of manual therapies of the spine.* Amsterdam: Thesis Publishers Amsterdam.

Brown BM et al. (1988). Preoperative evaluation of cervical radiculopathy and myelopathy by surface-coil MRI imaging. *AJR, Am J Roentgenol, 151,* 1205-1212.

Buckwalter J et al. (1989). Articular cartilage and intervertebral disc proteoglycans differ in structure: An electron microscopic study. *J Orthop Res, 7,* 146-151.

Buckwalter JA & Brandser EA. (1997). Metastatic disease of the skeleton. *Am Fam Physician, 55,* 1761-1768.

Cavanaugh JM et al. (1996). Lumbar facet pain: Biomechanics, neuroanatomy and neurophysiology. *J Biomech, 29(9),* 1117-1129.

Cavanaugh JM et al. (1997). Mechanisms of low back pain: A neurophysiologic and neuroanatomic study. *Clin Orthop, 335,* 166-180.

Cavanaugh JM, Kallakuri S, & Özaktay AC. (1995). Innervation of the rabbit lumbar intervertebral disc and posterior longitudinal ligament. *Spine, 20,* 2080-2085.

Chadha M et al. (2003). Pedicle morphology of the lower thoracic, lumbar, and S1 vertebrae: An Indian perspective. *Spine, 28,* 744-749.

Chaynes P et al. (1998). Microsurgical anatomy of the internal vertebral venous plexuses. *Surg Radiol Anat, 20,* 47-51.

Chen KP et al. (1989). The depth of the epidural space. *Anaesth Sinica, 27,* 353-356.

Cheng XG et al. (1996). Radiological prevalence of lumbar intervertebral disc calcification in the elderly: An autopsy study. *Skeletal Radiol, 25,* 231-235.

Church CP & Buehler MT. (1991). Radiographic evaluation of the corporotransverse ligament at the L5 intervertebral foramen: A cadaveric study. *J Manipulative Physiol Ther, 14(4),* 240-248.

Clarke GA et al. (1985). Can infant malnutrition cause adult vertebral stenosis? *Spine, 10,* 165-170.

Coppes MH et al. (1997). Innervation of "painful" lumbar discs. *Spine, 22,* 2342-2349.

Coventry MB. (1969). Anatomy of the intervertebral disc. *Clin Orthop, 67,* 9-15.

Cramer G et al. (1992). Comparative evaluation of the lumbar intervertebral foramen by computed tomography and magnetic resonance imaging. *Clin Anat, 5*, 238.

Cramer G et al. (2003). Dimensions of the lumbar intervertebral foramina as determined from the sagittal plane magnetic resonance imaging scans of 95 normal subjects. *J Manipulative Physiol Ther, 26*, 160-170.

Cramer GD et al. (2004). Degenerative changes following spinal fixation in a small animal model. *J Manipulative Physiol Therap, 27*, 141-154.

Cramer GD et al. (2000). Effects of side-posture positioning and side-posture adjusting on the lumbar zygapophysial joints as evaluated by magnetic resonance imaging: A before and after study with randomization. *J Manipulative Physiol Ther, 23*, 380-394.

Cramer GD et al. (2002). Evaluation of transforaminal ligaments by magnetic resonance imaging. *J Manipulative Physiol Ther, 25*, 199-208.

Crock HV. (1976). Isolated lumbar disk resorption as a cause of nerve root canal stenosis. *Clin Orthop, 115*, 109-115.

Crock HV & Yoshizawa H. (1976). The blood supply of the lumbar vertebral column. *Clin Orthop, 115*, 6-21.

Curylo IJ et al. (1996). Segmental variations of bone mineral density in the cervical spine. *Spine, 21*, 319-322.

Czervionke L et al. (1988). Cervical neural foramina: Correlative anatomic and MR imaging study. *Radiology, 169*, 753-759.

Dabezies E et al. (1988). Safety and efficacy of chymopapain (Discase) in the treatment of sciatica due to a herniated nucleus pulposus: Results of a double-blind study. *Spine, 13*, 561-565.

Djukic S et al. (1990). Magnetic resonance imaging of the postoperative lumbar spine. *Radiol Clin North Am, 28*, 341-360.

Domisse GF & Louw JA. (1990). Anatomy of the lumbar spine. In Y Floman (Ed.). *Disorders of the lumbar spine.* Rockville, Md: Aspen Publishers.

Dreyer SJ & Dreyfuss PH. (1996). Low back pain and the zygapophysial (facet) joints. *Arch Phys Med Rehabil, 77*, 290-300.

Edelson JG & Nathan H. (1988). Stages in the natural history of the vertebral end plates. *Spine, 13*, 21-26.

Edgar M & Ghadially J. (1976). Innervation of the lumbar spine. *Clin Orthop, 115*, 35-41.

Edwards WT et al. (2001). Peak stresses observed in the posterior lateral annulus. *Spine, 26*, 1753-1759.

Engel R & Bogduk N. (1982). The menisci of the lumbar zygapophysial joints. *J Anat, 135*, 795-809.

Esses SI & Moro JK. (1992). Intraosseous vertebral body pressures. *Spine, 17*, s155-s159.

Fagerlund MKJ & Thelander UE. (1989). Comparison of myelography and computed tomography in establishing lumbar disc herniation. *Acta Radiol, 30*, 241-246.

Fardon DF. (1988). The name of the ring. *Spine, 13*, 713-715.

Feltrin GP et al. (2001). Fractal analysis of lumbar vertebral cancellous bone architecture. *Clin Anat, 14*, 414-417.

Fennell AJ, Jones AP, & Hukins DWL. (1996). Migration of the nucleus pulposus within the intervertebral disc during flexion and extension of the spine. *Spine, 21*, 2753-2757.

Fesmire F & Luten R. (1989). The pediatric cervical spine: Development anatomy and clinical aspects. *J Emerg Med, 7*, 133-142.

Foreman SM & Croft AC (1988). *Whiplash injuries: The cervical acceleration/deceleration syndrome.* Baltimore: Williams & Wilkins.

Forristall R, Marsh H, & Pay N. (1988). Magnetic resonance imaging and contrast CT of the lumbar spine: Comparison of diagnostic methods of correlation with surgical findings. *Spine, 13*, 1049-1054.

Friedman JA, Wetjen NM, & Atkinson JL. (2003). Utility of intraoperative ultrasound for tumors of the cauda equine. *Spine, 28*, 288-291.

Frocrain L et al. (1989). Recurrent postoperative sciatica: Evaluation with MR imaging and enhanced CT. *Radiology, 170*, 531-533.

Fujiwara A et al. (2000). The effect of disc degeneration and facet joint osteoarthritis on the segmental flexibility of the lumbar spine. *Spine, 25*, 3036-3044.

Giles LG. (1988). Human zygapophyseal joint inferior recess synovial folds: A light microscopic examination. *Anat Rec, 220*, 117-124.

Giles LG. (1992). The surface lamina of the articular cartilage of human zygapophyseal joints. *Anat Rec, 233*, 350-356.

Giles LG & Taylor JR. (1987). Human zygapophyseal joint capsule and synovial fold innervation. *Br J Rheumatol, 26*, 93-98.

Giles LGF. (2000). Mechanisms of neurovascular compression within the spinal and intervertebral canals. *J Manipulative Physiol Ther, 23*, 107-111.

Gilsanz V. (1988). Vertebral bone density in children: Effects of puberty. *Radiology, 166*, 847-850.

Gilsanz V et al. (1988). Peak trabecular vertebral density: A comparison of adolescent and adult females. *Calcif Tissue Int, 43*, 260-262.

Golub B & Siverman B. (1969). Transforaminal ligaments of the lumbar spine. *J Bone Joint Surg, 51*, 947-956.

Guyer RD & Ohnmeiss DD. (2003). Lumbar discography. *Spine J, 3(3 suppl)*, 11S-27S.

Hackney DB. (1992). Normal anatomy. *Top Magn Reson Imaging, 4*, 1-6.

Hadley L. (1949). Intervertebral foramen constriction. *JAMA, 140*, 473-476.

Hadley LA. (1948). Apophysial subluxation. *J Bone Joint Surg*, 428-433.

Haher TR et al. (1992). Instantaneous axis of rotation as a function of the three columns of the spine. *Spine, 17*, S149-S154.

Harrison DE, Harrison DD, & Troyanovich SJ. (1998). Three-dimensional spinal coupling mechanics: Part 1. A review of the literature. *J Manipulative Physiol Ther, 21*, 101-113.

Hasue M et al. (1983). Anatomic study of the interrelation between lumbo-sacral nerve roots and their surrounding tissues. *Spine, 8*, 50-58.

Hedberg MC, Dayer BP, & Flom RA. (1988). Gradient echo (GRASS) MR imaging in cervical radiculopathy. *AJNR, 9*, 145-151.

Herkowitz HN et al. (1992). Discussion on cigarette smoking and the prevalence of spinal procedures. *J Spin Disord, 5*, 135-136.

Herzog RJ. (1994). Imaging corner: The goal of spinal imaging. *Spine, 19*, 2486-2488.

Herzog RJ. (1996). The radiologic assessment for a lumbar disc herniation. *Spine, 21*, 19S-38S.

Hewitt W. (1970). The intervertebral foramen. *Physiotherapy, 56*, 332-336.

Hickey DS & Hukins DWL. (1980). Relation between the structure of the annulus fibrosus and the function and failure of the intervertebral disc. *Spine, 5*, 106-116.

Ho PSP et al. (1988). Progressive and regressive changes in the nucleus pulposus. Part I. The neonate. *Radiology, 169*, 87-91.

Holm S & Nachemson A. (1983). Variations in the nutrition of the canine intervertebral disc induced by motion. *Spine, 8*, 866-874.

Hueftle M et al. (1988). Lumbar spine: Postoperative MR imaging with Gd-DTPA. *Radiology, 167*, 817-824.

Hughes JA et al. (2003). Three-dimensional sonographic evaluation of the infant spine: Preliminary findings. *J Clin Ultrasound, 31*, 9-20.

Humzah MD & Soames RW. (1988). Human intervertebral disc: Structure and function. *Anat Rec, 220*, 337-356.

Iatridis JC et al. (1996). Is the nucleus pulposus a solid or a fluid? Mechanical behaviors of the nucleus pulposus of the human intervertebral disc. *Spine, 21*, 1174-1184.

Issever AS et al. (2003). Micro-computed tomography evaluation of trabecular bone structure on loaded mice tail vertebrae. *Spine, 28*, 123-128.

Isherwood I & Antoun NM. (1980). CT scanning in the assessment of lumbar spine problems. In M Jayson (Ed.). *The lumbar spine and back pain* (2nd ed.). London: Pitman Publishing.

Ito S et al. (1991). An observation of ruptured annulus fibrosus in lumbar discs. *J Spine Disord, 4*, 462-466.

Jackson R et al. (1989). The neuroradiographic diagnosis of lumbar herniated nucleus pulposes. II. A comparison of computed tomography (CT), myelography, CT-myelography, and magnetic resonance imaging. *Spine, 14*, 1362-1367.

Jayson M. (1980). *The lumbar spine and back pain* (2nd ed.). Baltimore: Urban & Schwarzenberg and Pitman Medical Publishing.

Jeffries B. (1988). Facet joint injections. *Spine: State of the art Reviews, 2*, 409-417.

Jerusalem G et al. (2003). PET scan imaging in oncology. *Eur J Cancer, 39*, 1525-1534.

Jiang H. (1997). Identification of the location, extent, and pathway of sensory neurologic feedback after mechanical stimulation of a lateral spinal ligament in chickens. *Spine, 22(1)*, 17-25.

Johnson WEB et al. (2001). Immunohistochemical detection of Schwann cells in innervated and vascularized human intervertebral discs. *Spine, 26*, 2550-2557.

Kos J. (1969). Contribution a l'etude de l'anatomie et de la vascularisation des ariticulations intervertebrales. *Bulletin de l'Association des Anatomistes, 142*, 1088-1105.

Kos J & Wolf J. (1972). Les menisques intervertebraux et le role possible dans les blocages vertebraux (translation), *J Orthop Sports Phys Ther, 1*, 8-9.

Kraemer J. (1995). Presidential address: Natural course and prognosis of intervertebral disc diseases. *Spine, 20*, 635-639.

Kraemer J et al. (1985). Water and electrolyte content of human intervertebral discs under variable load. *Spine, 10*, 69-71.

Kricun R, Kricun M, & Danlinka M. (1990). Advances in spinal imaging. *Radiol Clin North Am, 28*, 321-339.

Krismer M et al. (2000). Motion in lumbar functional spine units during side bending and axial rotation moments depending on the degree of degeneration. *Spine, 25*, 2020-2027.

Krupski W et al. (2002). Degenerative changes of the vertebral column in spatial imaging of 3D computed tomography. *Ann Univ Mariae Curie Sklodowska, 57*, 459-465.

Kuga N & Kawabuchi M. (2001). Histology of intervertebral disc protrusion: An experimental study using an aged rat model. *Spine, 26(17)*, E379-E384.

Kushner DC & Cleveland RH. (1988). Digital imaging in scoliosis. In ME Kricun (Ed.). *Imaging modalities in spinal disorders.* Philadelphia: WB Saunders.

Lancourt JE, Glenn WV, & Wiltse LL. (1979). Multiplanar computerized tomography in the normal spine and in the diagnosis of spinal stenosis: A gross anatomic-computerized tomographic correlation. *Spine, 4*, 379-390.

LeBlanc AD et al. (1988). The spine: Changes in T2 relaxation times from disuse. *Radiology, 169*, 105-107.

Leboeuf-Yde C & Yashin A. (1995). Smoking and low back pain: Is the association real? *J Manipulative Physiol Ther, 18*, 457-463.

Ledsome JR et al. (1996). Diurnal changes in lumbar intervertebral distance, measured using ultrasound. *Spine, 21*, 1671-1675.

Leiviska T et al. (1985). Radiographic versus direct measurements of the spinal canal at the lumbar vertebrae L3-L5 and their relations to age and body stature. *Acta Radiol, 26*, 403-411.

Lippitt AB. (1984). The facet joint and its role in spine pain: Management with facet joint injections. *Spine, 9*, 746-750.

Lipson SJ. (1988). Metaplastic proliferative fibrocartilage as an alternative concept to herniated intervertebral disc. *Spine, 13*, 1055-1060.

Louis R. (1985). Spinal stability as defined by the three-column spine concept. *Anatomia Clinica, 7*, 33-42.

Lu J & Ebraheim N. (1998). Anatomic considerations of C2 nerve root ganglion. *Spine, 23*, 649-652.

Lu YM, Hutton WC, & Gharpuray VM. (1996). Do bending, twisting, and diurnal fluid changes in the disc affect the propensity to prolapse? A viscoelastic finite model. *Spine, 21*, 2570-2579.

Maat GJR, Matricali M, & van Perijn van Meerten EL. (1996). Postnatal development and structure of the neurocentral junction. *Spine, 21*, 661-666.

Martin G. (1978). The role of trauma in disc protrusion. *NZ Med J, March*, 208-211.

Mayoux-Benhamou MA et al. (1989). A morphometric study of the lumbar foramen: Influence of flexion-extension movements and of isolated disc collapse. *Surg Radiol Anat, 11*, 97-102.

McFadden JW. (1988). The stress lumbar discogram. *Spine, 13*, 931-933.

McGill SM & Axler CT. (1996). Changes in spine height throughout 32 hours of bedrest. *Arch Phys Med Rehabil, 77*, 1071-1073.

McLain RF. (1994). Mechanoreceptor endings in human cervical joints. *Spine, 19*, 495-501.

McLain RF & Pickar JG. (1998). Mechanoreceptor endings in human thoracic and lumbar facet joints. *Spine, 23*, 168-173.

McNab I. (1971). Negative disc exploration: An analysis of the cause of nerve-root involvement in sixty-eight patients. *J Bone Joint Surg, 53A*, 891-903.

Mendel T et al. (1992). Neural elements in human cervical intervertebral discs. *Spine, 17*, 132-135.

Mercer S & Bogduk N. (1999). The ligaments and anulus fibrosis of the human adult cervical intervertebral discs. *Spine, 24*, 619-628.

Mirkovic S & Melany M. (1992). A thoracolumbar epidural hematoma simulating a disc syndrome. *J Spin Disord, 5*, 112-115.

Mixter WJ & Barr JS. (1934). Rupture of the intervertebral disc with involvement of the spinal canal. *N Engl J Med, 211*, 210-215.

Moffit B et al. (1988). Comparison of T1 and T2 weighted images of the lumbar spine. *Comp Med Imaging Graph, 12*, 271-276.

Mooney V & Robertson J. (1976). The facet syndrome. *Clin Orthop Res, 115*, 149-156.

Moore RJ et al. (1996a). Remodeling of vertebral bone after outer anular injury in sheep. *Spine, 21*, 936-940.

Moore RJ et al. (1996b). The origin and fate of herniated lumbar intervertebral disc tissue. *Spine, 21*, 2149-2155.

Moroney S et al. (1988). Load displacement properties of lower cervical spine motion segments. *J Biomech, 21*, 769-779.

Mosekilde L. (1989). Sex differences in age-related loss of vertebral trabec-

ular bone mass and structure biomechanical consequences. *Bone, 10*, 425-432.

Mosekilde L & Mosekilde L. (1990). Sex differences in age-related changes in vertebral body size, density and biomechanical competence in normal individuals. *Bone, 11*, 67-73.

Narvani AA, Tsiridis E, & Wilson LF. (2003). High-intensity zone, intradiscal electrothermal therapy, and magnetic resonance imaging. *J Spinal Disord Tech, 16*, 130-136.

Nathan H. (1962). Osteophytes of the vertebral column: An anatomical study of their development according to age, race, and sex with considerations as to their etiology and significance. *J Bone Joint Surg, 44-A*, 243-268.

Nathan H, Weizenbluth M, & Halperin N. (1982). The lumbosacral ligament (LSL), with special emphasis on the "lumbosacral tunnel" and the entrapment of the 5th lumbar nerve. *Int Orthop, 6*, 197-202.

Nitobe T et al. (1988). Degradation and biosynthesis of proteoglycans in the nucleus pulposus of canine intervertebral disc after chymopapain treatment. *Spine, 11*, 1332-1339.

Nowicki BH & Haughton VM. (1992a). Ligaments of the lumbar neural foramina: A sectional anatomic study. *Clin Anat, 5*, 126-135.

Nowicki BH & Haughton VM. (1992b). Neural foraminal ligaments of the lumbar spine: Appearance at CT and MR imaging. *Radiology, 183(1)*, 257-264.

Oda J, Tamaka H, & Tsukuki N. (1988). Intervertebral disk changes with aging of human cervical vertebra: From the neonate to the eighties. *Spine, 13*, 1205-1211.

Oki S et al. (1996). Morphologic differences of the vascular buds in the vertebral end plate: Scanning electron microscopic study. *Spine, 21*, 174-177.

Olsewski JM et al. (1991). Evidence from cadavers suggestive of entrapment of fifth lumbar spinal nerves by lumbosacral ligaments. *Spine, 16*, 336-347.

Onan OA, Heggeness MH, & Hipp JA. (1998). A motion analysis of the cervical facet joint. *Spine, 23*, 430-439.

Osborn A et al. (1988). CT/MR spectrum of far lateral and anterior lumbosacral disk herniations. *AJNR, 9*, 775-778.

Pal GP et al. (1988). Trajectory architecture of the trabecular bone between the body and the neural arch in human vertebrae. *Anat Rec, 222*, 418-425.

Paris S. (1983). Anatomy as related to function and pain. Symposium on Evaluation and Care of Lumbar Spine Problems. *Orthop Clin North Am, 14*, 476-489.

Pate D, Resnick D, & Andre M. (1986). Perspective: Three-dimensional imaging of the musculoskeletal system. *AJNR, 147*, 545-551.

Pfaundler S. (1989). Pedicle origin and intervertebral compartment in the lumbar and upper sacral spine. *Acta Neurochir, 97*, 158-165.

Putz RL & Müller-Gerbl M. (1996). The vertebral column: A phylogenetic failure? A theory explaining the function and vulnerability of the human spine. *Clin Anat, 9*, 205-212.

Ribot C et al. (1988). Influence of the menopause and aging on spinal density in French women. *Bone Miner, 5*, 89-97.

Rollo FD. (2003). Molecular imaging: An overview and clinical applications. *Radiol Manage, 25*, 28-32.

Rydevik B et al. (1984). Pathoanatomy and physiology of nerve root compression. *Spine, 9*, 7-15.

Saifuddin A, Blease S, & McSweeney E. (2003). Axial loaded MRI of the lumbar spine. *Clin Radiol, 58*, 661-671.

Saifuddin A, McSweeney E, & Lehovsky J. (2003). Development of lumbar high intensity zone on axial loaded magnetic resonance imaging. *Spine, 28*, 449-452.

Salamon O & Freilich M. (1988). Calcified hemangioma of the spinal canal: Unusual CT and MR presentation. *AJNR, 9*, 799-802.

Sanders M & Stein K. (1988). Conservative management of herniated nucleus pulposes: Treatment approaches. *J Manipulative Physiol Ther, 11*, 309-313.

Scapinelli R. (2000). Antireflux mechanisms in veins draining the upper territory of the vertebral column and spinal cord in man. *Clin Anat, 13*, 410-415.

Schellhas KP et al. (1996a). Lumbar disc high-intensity zone: Correlation of magnetic resonance imaging and discography. *Spine, 21*, 79-86.

Schellhas KP et al. (1996b). Cervical discogenic pain: Prospective correlation of magnetic resonance imaging and discography in asymptomatic subjects and pain sufferers. *Spine, 21*, 300-311.

Schmidt TA et al. (1998). The stiffness of lumbar spinal motion segments with a high-intensity zone in the annulus fibrosus. *Spine, 23*, 2167-2173.

Schnebel B et al. (1989). Comparison of MRI to contrast CT in the diagnosis of spinal stenosis. *Spine, 14*, 332-337.

Schultz AB et al. (1973) Analog studies of forces in the human spine: Mechanical properties and motion segment behavior. *Biomechanics, 6,* 373-383.

Sei A et al. (1991). Cervical spinal epidural hematoma with spontaneous remission. *J Spin Disord, 4,* 234-237.

Shapiro R. (1990). Talmudic and other concepts of the number of vertebrae in the human spine. *Spine, 15,* 246-247.

Shealy CN. (1975). Facet denervation in the management of back and sciatic pain. *Clin Orthop, 115,* 157-164.

Sihvonen T et al. (1993). Local denervation atrophy of paraspinal muscles in postoperative failed back syndrome. *Spine, 18,* 575-591.

Silcox DH et al. (1995). The effect of nicotine on spinal fusion. *Spine, 20,* 1549-1553.

Singer K, Giles L, & Day R. (1990). Intra-articular synovial folds of thoraco-lumbar junction zygapophyseal joints. *Anat Rec, 226,* 147-152.

Skedros JG et al. (1994). Analysis of a tension/compression skeletal system: Possible strain-specific differences in the hierarchical organization of bone. *Anat Rec, 239,* 396-404.

Skedros JG, Mason MW, & Bloebaum RD. (1994). Differences in osteonal micromorphology between tensile and compressive cortices of a bending skeletal system: Indications of potential strain-specific differences in bone microstructure. *Anat Rec, 239,* 405-413.

Smit TH, Odgaard A, & Schneider E. (1997). Structure and function of vertebral trabecular bone. *Spine, 24,* 2823-2833.

Solomonow M et al. (1998). The ligamento-muscular stabilizing system of the spine. *Spine, 23,* 2552-2562.

Stroman PW et al. (2002). Mapping of neuronal function in the healthy and injured human spinal cord with spinal fMRI. *Neuroimage, 17,* 1854-1860.

Stumpe KD et al. (2002). FDG position emission tomography for differentiation of degenerative and infectious end plate abnormalities in the lumbar spine detected on MR imaging. *AJR Am J Roentgenol, 179,* 1151-1157.

Taylor J. (1990). The development and adult structure of lumbar intervertebral discs. *J Man Med, 5,* 43-47.

Taylor JR. (1999). Ligaments and annulus fibrosus of cervical discs. *Spine, 24,* 627-628.

Theil HW, Clements DS, & Cassidy JD. (1992). Lumbar apophyseal ring fractures in adolescents. *J Manipulative Physiol Ther, 15,* 250-254.

Tobita T et al. (2003). Diagnosis of spinal disease with ultrafine flexible fiberscopes in patients with chronic pain. *Spine, 28,* 2006-2012.

Tracy PT, Wright RM, & Hanigan WC. (1989). Magnetic resonance imaging of spinal injury. *Spine, 14,* 292-301.

Transfeldt EE, Robertson D, & Bradford DS. (1993). Ligaments of the lumbosacral spine and their role in possible extraforaminal spinal nerve entrapment and tethering. *J Spin Disord, 6(6),* 507-512.

Valentini V et al. (2003). Diffusion and perfusion MR imaging. *Rays, 28,* 29-43.

Vandenabeele F et al. (1997). Encapsulated Ruffini-like endings in human lumbar facet joints. *J Anat, 191(Pt 4),* 571-583.

Vandenabeele F, Creemers J, & Lambrichts I. (1996). Ultrastructure of the human spinal arachnoid mater and dura mater. *J Anat, 189(Pt 2),* 417-430.

Van Eenenaam DP & El-Khoury GY. (1993). Delayed post-traumatic vertebral collapse (Kümmell's disease): Case report with serial radiographs, computed tomographic scans, and bone scans. *Spine, 18,* 1236-1241.

Vital J et al. (1989). The neurocentral vertebral cartilage: Anatomy, physiology, and physiopathology. *Surg Radiol Anat, 11,* 323-328.

Wang A, Wesolowski D, & Farah J. (1988). Evaluation of posterior spinal structures by computed tomography. In JH Bisese (Ed.). *Spine, state of the art reviews, spinal imaging: Diagnostic and therapeutic applications.* Philadelphia: Hanley & Belfus.

Wang J et al. (1999). Composition of the corporotransverse ligaments of the lumbar L5-S1 IVFs. *1999 Proceedings of the Fifth World Federation of Chiropractic Congress, May 18-22, Auckland, New Zealand, 150-151.*

Weinstein J, Claverie W, & Gibson S. (1988). The pain of discography. *Spine, 13,* 1344-1348.

White AA & Panjabi MM. (1990). *Clinical biomechanics of the spine* (2nd ed.). Philadelphia: JB Lippincott.

Williams PL et al. (1995). *Gray's anatomy* (38th ed.). Edinburgh: Churchill Livingstone.

Winterstein JF & Bachop WE. (1990). The corporotransverse ligament at the L5/S1 intervertebral foramen: A gross anatomical-radiographic comparison. *Anat Rec, 226,* 111A.

Wong C et al. (2003). Symptomatic spinal epidural varices presenting with nerve impingement: Report of two cases and review of the literature. *Spine, 28,* 347-350.

Wood KB et al. (1996). Effect of patient position on the sagittal-plane profile of the thoracolumbar spine. *J Spin Disord, 9,* 165-169.

Woodruff W Jr. (1988). Evaluation of disc disease by magnetic resonance imaging. In JH Bisese (Ed.). *Spine, state of the art reviews, spinal imaging: Diagnostic and therapeutic applications.* Philadelphia: Hanley & Belfus.

Wyke B. (1985). Articular neurology and manipulative therapy. In EF Glasgow et al. (Eds.). *Aspects of manipulative therapy* (2nd ed.). London: Churchill Livingstone.

Xu G et al. (1991). Normal variations of the lumbar facet joint capsules. *Clin Anat, 4,* 117-122.

Xu R et al. (1999). The quantitative anatomy of the laminas of the spine. *Spine, 24,* 107-113.

Yamashita T et al. (1990). Mechanosensitive afferent units in the lumbar facet joint. *J Bone Joint Surg, 72-A,* 865-870.

Yamashita T et al. (1996). A morphological study of the fibrous capsule of the human lumbar facet joint. *Spine, 21,* 538-543.

CHAPTER 3

General Anatomy of the Spinal Cord

Susan A. Darby

The purpose of this chapter is to describe in detail the gross anatomy of the external spinal cord, its coverings, and its vasculature. To help the reader acquire a general appreciation of the spinal cord as a complete entity, this chapter also provides a cursory description of the organization and physiology of the internal aspect of the spinal cord. Subsequent chapters expand on the generalities presented here. The intimate relationship of the spinal cord to the vertebral column makes the anatomy of the spinal cord extremely important to those who treat disorders of the spine.

OVERVIEW OF SPINAL CORD ORGANIZATION

The spinal cord, which is located in the vertebral (spinal) canal, is a cylindric-shaped structure with a tapered inferior end. The cord is well protected by the vertebrae and the ligaments associated with the vertebrae. In addition to these bones and ligaments, cerebrospinal fluid (CSF) and a group of membranes, collectively called the meninges, also provide protection. The spinal cord does not lie immediately adjacent to the bone and ligaments but is separated from them by fluid, meninges, fat, and a venous plexus (Fig. 3-1, A and B).

The spinal cord and brain develop from the same embryologic structure, the neural tube, and together they form the central nervous system (CNS). One end of the neural tube becomes encased in the skull, whereas the remainder of the neural tube becomes encased in the vertebral column. Size alone suggests that the higher centers making up the brain process information more thoroughly and complexly than the processing that occurs in the spinal cord. For the CNS to respond to the environment, it requires input from structures peripheral to the CNS and, in turn, a means to send output to structures called effectors. The sensory input begins in peripheral receptors found throughout the entire body in skin, muscles, tendons, joints, and viscera. These receptors send electrical currents (action potentials) toward the spinal cord of the CNS via the nerves that make up the peripheral nervous system (PNS). The sensory receptors respond to general sensory information such as pain, temperature, touch (including the submodalities of vibration and pressure), or proprioception (awareness of body position and movement). The PNS also is used when the CNS sends output to the body's effectors, which are the smooth muscle, cardiac muscle, skeletal muscle, and glands of the body. Thus the PNS consists of the body's peripheral nerves and is the means by which the CNS communicates with its surrounding environment.

Within a peripheral nerve, the individual fibers are classified as either a part of the somatic division of the nervous system or the visceral division of the nervous system. Somatic fibers (both sensory/afferent and motor/efferent) innervate skin, joints, tendons, and skeletal

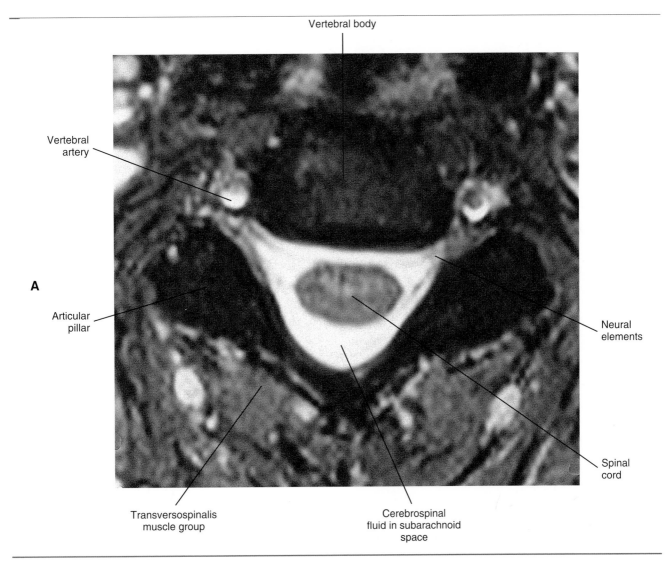

Vertebral body

Vertebral artery

Articular pillar

A

Transversospinalis muscle group

Cerebrospinal fluid in subarachnoid space

Neural elements

Spinal cord

FIG. 3-1   **A,** Magnetic resonance image (MRI) showing a horizontal section of the cervical spinal cord within the vertebral canal.
Continued

muscle located in the extremities and body wall. Visceral (or autonomic) fibers carry sensory/afferent information from the viscera to the CNS and provide motor/efferent control of smooth muscle, cardiac muscle, and glands. Twelve pairs of these nerves are associated with the brain (10 of which are attached to the brain stem) and innervate structures primarily in the head. These nerves, called cranial nerves, also convey special sense information such as hearing, vision, and taste. In the context of this chapter, another group of peripheral nerves is more pertinent. These 31 pairs of nerves attach to the spinal cord; communicate with structures primarily located in the neck, trunk, and extremities; and are called the spinal nerves. In general, once input reaches the

spinal cord via the spinal nerves, spinal cord neurons integrate and modulate the information and then send information back to the periphery as a motor response (i.e., reflexive, postural, or voluntary). In addition, such input to the spinal cord may result in the transmission of sensory input to higher brain centers for further processing. The higher centers then may send information down to the spinal cord neurons, which in turn relay it to the periphery, again via spinal nerves (Fig. 3-2).

A spinal nerve is formed by the merger of two roots within the intervertebral foramen (IVF). One root, called the dorsal root, contains fibers that convey sensory information. The cell bodies of these sensory fibers are located in the dorsal root ganglion. The cell bodies are

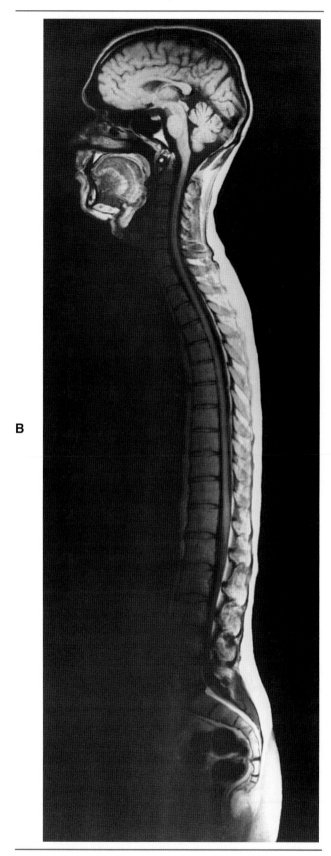

B

FIG. 3-1—Cont'd   **B,** Midsagittal MRI demonstrating the entire spinal cord within the vertebral canal. (**B,** From Nolte J. [2002. *The human brain: An introduction to its functional anatomy* [5th ed.]. St Louis: Mosby.)

not found in the spinal cord because they developed from neural crest (see Chapter 12). Each sensory neuron of the PNS is pseudounipolar because two processes diverge from one common stem (see Fig. 3-2). One of the processes is called the peripheral process and is continuous with a peripheral receptor. The other process is the central process, which courses in the dorsal root and enters the spinal cord (CNS). The dorsal root contains fibers of various diameters and conduction velocities that convey all types of sensory information. For example, some fibers in the dorsal root convey cutaneous sensory information from a specific area of skin called a dermatome. As the dorsal root approaches the spinal cord within the individual vertebral foramen, it divides into approximately six to eight dorsal rootlets, or filaments. These rootlets attach in a vertical row to the cord's dorsolateral sulcus. The other root, which helps form a spinal nerve, is called the ventral root and contains fibers that convey motor information to the body's effectors, that is, all muscle tissue and glands. The cell bodies of these axons are located in the spinal cord. The axons emerge from the cord's ventrolateral sulcus as ventral rootlets and unite to form one ventral root. Within the IVF the dorsal and ventral roots form the spinal nerve, which subsequently divides into its two major components: the *dorsal* and *ventral rami* (also known as the posterior primary division and anterior primary division, respectively) (Fig. 3-3).

From this description, it can be seen that the spinal nerve and nerves formed distal to it (including the dorsal ramus and the ventral ramus) are mixed because they contain fibers conveying sensory input and fibers conveying motor output. However, proximal to the IVF, sensory and motor information are segregated in the fibers forming separate dorsal and ventral roots. This segregation of dorsal and ventral root fibers, and therefore of root function, was discussed and demonstrated by Bell and Magendie in the early 1800s and later was called the law of separation of function of spinal roots (law of Bell and Magendie) (Coggeshall, 1980).

At the level of the skull's foramen magnum, the spinal cord becomes continuous with the medulla oblongata of the brain stem (Fig. 3-4). Although in cross section it is impossible to delineate the exact beginning of the cord and the end of the brain stem, grossly the beginning of the cord is easily distinguished by the definitive presence of the skull and vertebrae. As discussed in Chapter 12, a period during development occurs when the spinal cord extends the length of the vertebral column. However, while the vertebral column continues to develop in length, the spinal cord lags behind so that it comes to occupy the upper two thirds of the vertebral (spinal) canal (Fig. 3-1, *B*). It has been reported that at birth the cord ends at roughly the level of the L3 vertebra. Malas et al. (2000) used ultrasonography on full-term neonates (40 ± 2 weeks) and found the termination level of the

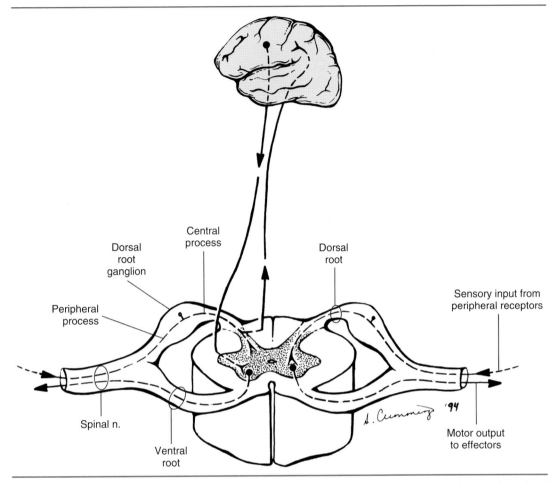

FIG. 3-2   General functions of the spinal cord. *Right,* Two-way communication between the spinal cord and the periphery. *Left,* Information within the cord traveling to and from higher centers in the brain.

cord to range anywhere from the L1-2 disc space to the L2-3 disc space. The spinal cord terminated at the L2-3 disc space in 50% (7 out of 14) of the neonates. In adults, because of continued greater growth of the vertebral column, the spinal cord ends at the level of the L1 vertebra. In some individuals, however, the spinal cord may end as high as the disc between the T11 and T12 vertebrae or as low as the L3 vertebra (see Meninges and Table 3-1 for further description). At roughly the level of the caudal part of the T12 vertebral body, the cord tapers down to a cone, which is known as the conus medullaris (Fig. 3-5, *B*). The overall length of the spinal cord to the inferior tip of the conus medullaris is approximately 42 cm in an average-sized woman and 45 cm in an average-sized man. The spinal cord's weight is approximately 30 to 35 g. Remember that in most individuals the spinal cord does not extend inferior to the L2 vertebra. Therefore a lesion such as a herniated disc or trauma occurring below the L2 vertebra does not directly affect the spinal cord in most individuals.

EXTERNAL MORPHOLOGY

The external surface of the spinal cord is not a smooth surface but instead shows grooves of various depths called sulci and fissures. (When discussing cord anatomy, understand that the terms *dorsal* and *ventral* can be used interchangeably with *posterior* and *anterior,* respectively.) The spinal cord's dorsal surface includes a midline dorsal median sulcus, right and left dorsal intermediate sulci (located from the midthoracic cord region superiorly), and right and left dorsolateral sulci. The cord's ventral surface includes a midline ventral median fissure (approximately 3 mm deep) and right and left ventrolateral sulci. When inspecting the cord's external surface, the dorsal and ventral rootlets are readily apparent, and the outward attachment to the cord of the paired (left and right) dorsal rootlets and paired ventral rootlets that serve one pair of spinal nerves defines one spinal cord segment (Fig. 3-6; see also Fig. 3-11, *C*).

Therefore one pair of spinal nerves is associated with one cord segment; because 31 pairs of spinal nerves

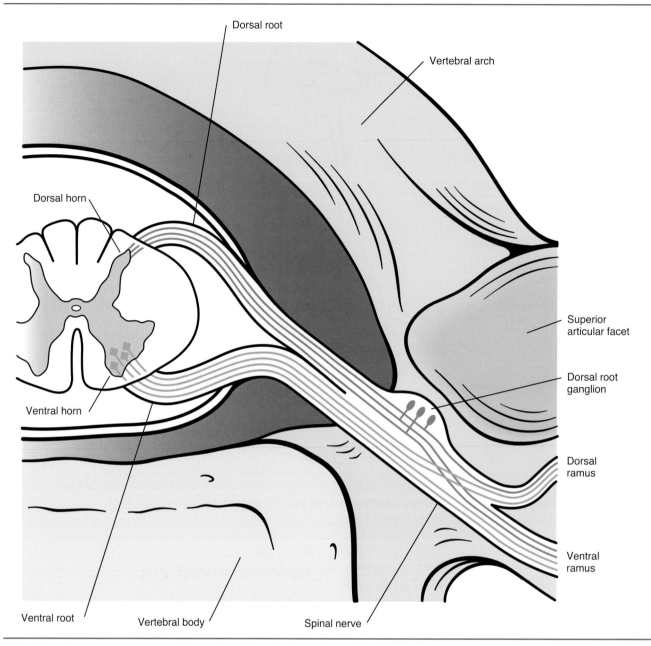

Dorsal root

Vertebral arch

Dorsal horn

Ventral horn

Superior articular facet

Dorsal root ganglion

Dorsal ramus

Ventral ramus

Ventral root

Vertebral body

Spinal nerve

FIG. 3-3 Components and somatic branches of a typical spinal nerve. The dorsal and ventral roots unite within the intervertebral foramen to form a spinal nerve. The spinal nerve branches into a dorsal ramus and ventral ramus. Each ramus contains motor and sensory fibers. Note: Sympathetic fibers are not shown.

exist, there are also 31 spinal cord segments. These cord segments are numbered similar to the numbering of the spinal nerves: eight cervical, twelve thoracic, five lumbar, five sacral, and one coccygeal cord segment. (Note that the first seven cervical nerves exit the IVF above their corresponding vertebra, and the remaining nerves exit below their corresponding vertebra. This allows one more cervical spinal nerve than cervical vertebrae.) Therefore the coccygeal segment is found at the very tip of the conus medullaris, which, as mentioned, is usually

at the level of the L1 vertebra (Fig. 3-7). This means that cord segments are not necessarily located at the same level as their corresponding vertebrae (Fig. 3-8). The relationship between cord segments and vertebral levels is always an approximation because cord length may vary among individuals.

Although cervical cord segments and cervical vertebrae correspond closely to one another (i.e., the cervical cord segments are at the level of the spinous processes of C1-6); this is not true for the remaining cord segments.

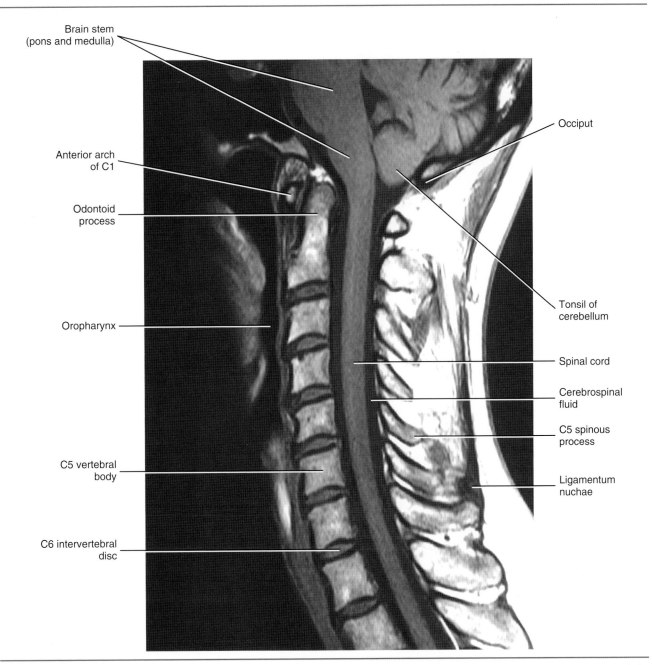

Brain stem (pons and medulla)

Anterior arch of C1

Odontoid process

Oropharynx

C5 vertebral body

C6 intervertebral disc

Occiput

Tonsil of cerebellum

Spinal cord

Cerebrospinal fluid

C5 spinous process

Ligamentum nuchae

FIG. 3-4   Sagittal magnetic resonance image of the brain stem, cerebellum, and cervical spinal cord. Note the continuation of the spinal cord with the brain stem at the level of the foramen magnum.

The segments' lengths change such that the L1 through coccygeal cord segments are housed at approximately vertebrae T9 through L1, and the segments responsible for the innervation of the lower extremities are found at the vertebral level of spinous processes T9 to T12. This anatomic relationship of cord segment to vertebra is important to remember for clinical reasons. For example, a patient with a fractured L1 vertebra does not experience the same lower extremity signs and symp-

toms as a patient with a fractured T10 vertebra, because a T10 fracture typically injures upper lumbar segments and an L1 fracture injures the lower sacral and coccygeal segments. Although the spinal cord ends at the L1 vertebra, each root that corresponds to a cord segment forms a spinal nerve and exits at its corresponding IVF. This includes the IVFs below the L2 vertebra. Therefore the rootlets and roots of the more inferior cord segments are longer and descend to their respective IVFs at a more

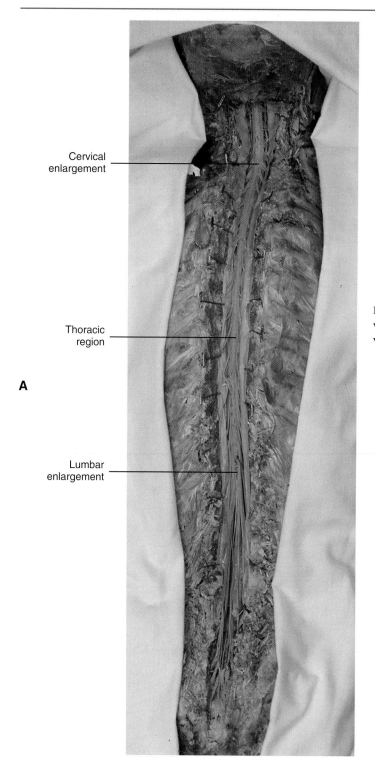

Cervical enlargement

Thoracic region

A

Lumbar enlargement

FIG. 3-5 Dorsal view of the spinal cord within the vertebral canal. The dura mater has been reflected laterally with pins. **A,** Spinal cord in its entirety.

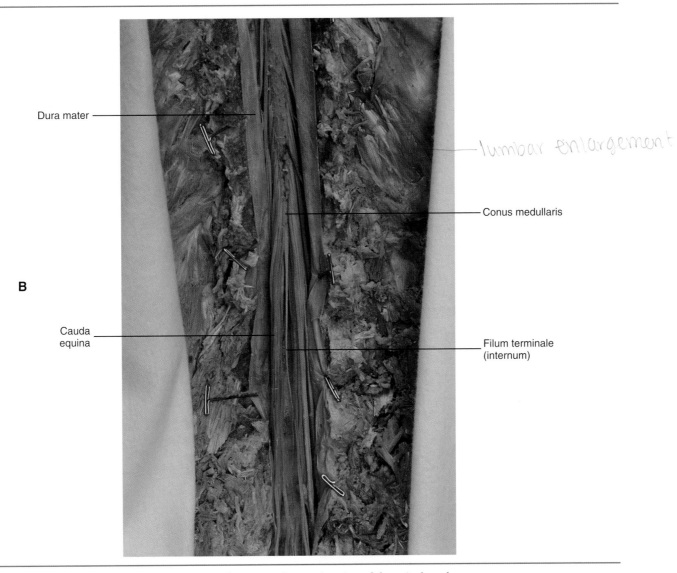

Dura mater

lumbar enlargement

Conus medullaris

B

Cauda equina

Filum terminale (internum)

FIG. 3-5—Cont'd   **B,** Lumbosacral region of the spinal cord.

oblique angle than the rootlets and roots of cervical segments, which are shorter and almost at right angles to the spinal cord. The lumbosacral roots therefore become the longest and most oblique. The collection of these elongated lumbosacral roots making their way inferiorly to their corresponding IVFs is called the cauda equina (see Figs. 3-7, 3-8, and 3-11, *B*) because of its resemblance to a horse's tail (the literal English translation of the term in Latin).

In addition to the sulci and fissures, another anatomic characteristic seen on gross inspection of the spinal cord is the presence of two enlarged areas. One area is the cervical enlargement seen in cord segments C4 to T1. These cord segments are responsible for the input from and output to the upper extremities. The other cord enlargement is the lumbar enlargement, which is visible

from segments L2 to S3. These segments are responsible for the input from and output to the lower extremities. Because many more structures must be innervated in the extremities than the trunk, it is necessary to have more neuron cell bodies in the cord, and thus these two regions are enlarged (Fig. 3-9; see also Figs. 3-5, *A,* and 3-6).

MENINGES

Surrounding and providing protection and support to the spinal cord is a group of three membranes that are collectively called the meninges. The meninges surrounding the spinal cord are a continuation of the meninges surrounding the brain and consist of the dura mater (pachymeninx) and the leptomeninges; the latter being composed of the arachnoid mater and pia mater

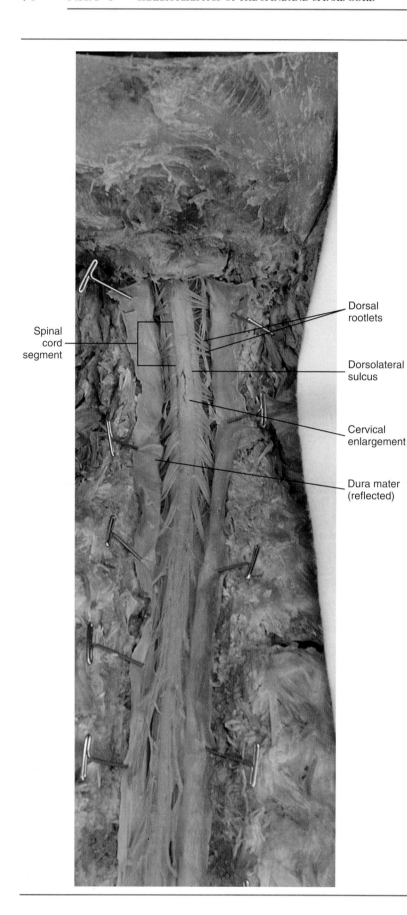

Spinal cord segment

Dorsal rootlets

Dorsolateral sulcus

Cervical enlargement

Dura mater (reflected)

FIG. 3-6 Dorsal view of the spinal cord. The cord segments are delineated by the attachment of rootlets to the spinal cord.

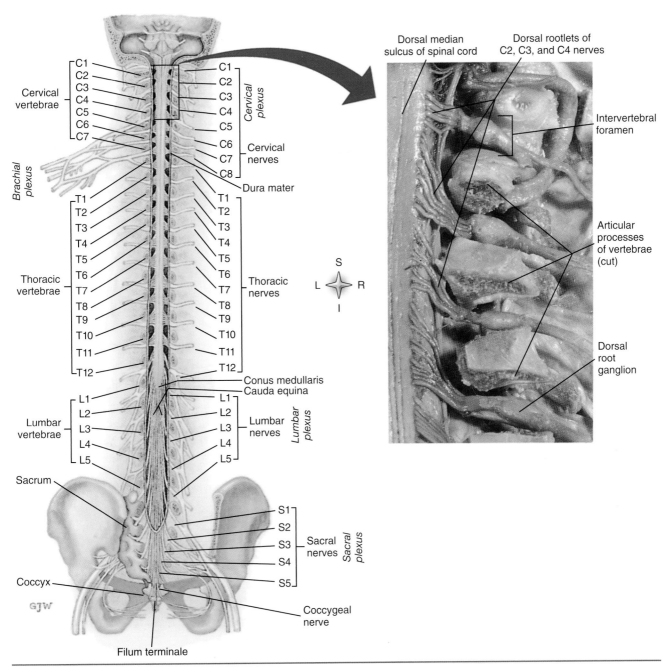

FIG. 3-7   Dorsal view of the external morphology of the spinal cord within the vertebral canal and the spinal nerves exiting within the intervertebral foramina. The tip of the cord (conus medullaris) is located approximately at the level of the L1 vertebra. The roots of the lumbar and sacral cord segments form the cauda equina, which is found in the lumbar cistern. The *inset* shows the cervical region, dorsal rootlets, and the location of the dorsal root ganglia in the exposed intervertebral foramina. (From Thibodeau GA & Patton KT. [2003]. *Anatomy & physiology* [5th ed.]. St Louis: Mosby.)

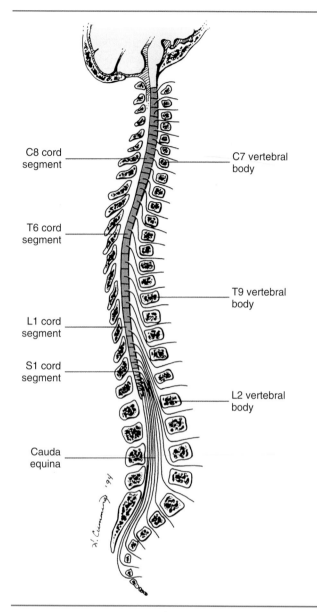

FIG. 3-8 Relationship of spinal cord segments and spinal nerves to vertebrae.

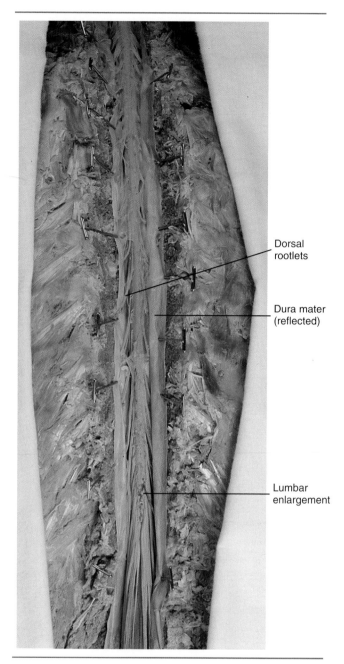

FIG. 3-9 Dorsal view of the spinal cord showing the lumbar enlargement. Cervical enlargement is shown in Figure 3-6.

(Figs. 3-10, 3-11, and 3-12). During development, mesenchyme surrounding the neural tube thickens to form the primordial meninx. The outermost layer thickens and becomes the dura mater. The thin, innermost layer becomes infiltrated with neural crest cells and forms the leptomeninges. CSF fills spaces that coalesce (the future subarachnoid space) within, and subsequently separate the leptomeninges into two layers, the arachnoid mater and pia mater (Moore and Persaud, 1998) (see the following). As they separate, tiny strands called trabeculae remain and can still be identified in the adult subarachnoid space (Figs. 3-10 and 3-12). The trabeculae are composed of a collagenous core and are surrounded by leptomeningeal cells (Williams et al., 1995). The trabeculae become concentrated and form septa in the vertebral subarachnoid space.

The fully developed dura mater (pachymeninx) of the cord is the tough, outermost membrane and is a continuation of the inner layer or meningeal layer of dura mater surrounding the brain. It is separated from the vertebrae by the epidural space, which contains epidural fat, loose connective tissue, and an extensive internal vertebral venous plexus (see Chapter 2). The spinal dura mater attaches to the edge of the foramen magnum, the posterior aspect of the C2-3 vertebral bodies, and the

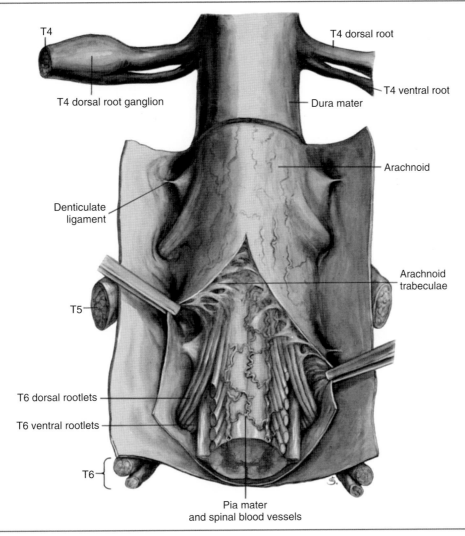

T4

T4 dorsal root ganglion

T4 dorsal root

T4 ventral root

Dura mater

Arachnoid

Denticulate ligament

Arachnoid trabeculae

T5

T6 dorsal rootlets

T6 ventral rootlets

T6

Pia mater and spinal blood vessels

FIG. 3-10   The meninges surrounding the spinal cord. Notice the arachnoid trabeculae and the denticulate ligament attaching to the dura mater and anchoring the spinal cord. (From Mettler FA. [1948]. *Neuroanatomy* [2nd ed.]. St Louis: Mosby.)

posterior longitudinal ligaments (Williams et al., 1995) by fibrous bands of tissue. This elongated dural sac is held in place to the borders of the vertebral canal by the filum terminale externum and many other thickenings of connective tissue that vary in type in different regions of the vertebral canal (Barbaix et al., 1996; Fricke, Andres, and Von During, 2001; Dean and Mitchell, 2002; Humphreys et al., 2003). These connective tissue attachments to the dura mater are discussed in detail in Chapters 5 and 7.

The recurrent meningeal nerve (or sinuvertebral nerve of von Luschka), which is formed outside the IVF and reenters the vertebral canal, provides a significant innervation to the anterior aspect of the spinal dura mater. Although a few nerves sparsely innervate the posterolateral dura mater, the posteromedial region appears to have no innervation, which may explain why a patient

feels no pain when the dura mater is pierced during a lumbar puncture (Groen, Baljet, and Drukker, 1988).

The dura mater has been analyzed microscopically and has been found to be composed of outer and inner parts. The outer portion contains layers of fibroblasts, collagen fiber bundles (providing tensile strength and protection), and some elastic fibers. The latter afford flexibility for mechanical changes during movements and postural adjustments. The fibers are not arranged in a longitudinal or parallel fashion but are oriented in a variety of directions (Haines, Harkey, and Al-Mefty, 1993; Vandenabeele, Creemers, and Lambrichts, 1996; Reina et al., 1997, 1998; Fricke, Andres, and Von During, 2001).

The inner portion of the dura mater lies adjacent to the arachnoid mater and consists of layers of cells called dural border, subdural, or neurothelial cells. These flattened cells are described as being sinuous with

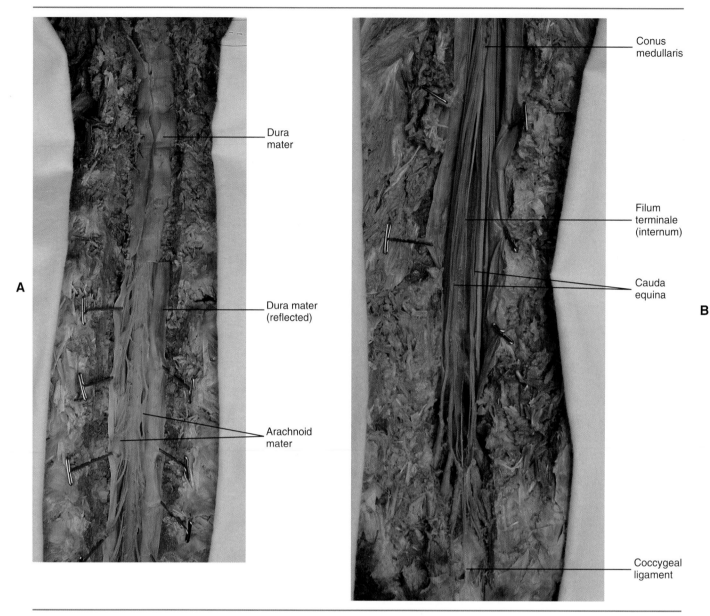

FIG. 3-11 Dorsal view of the spinal cord showing the meninges. **A,** Cervical and thoracic regions. **B,** Lumbar cistern and its contents.

interdigitating processes that create extracellular spaces and few intercellular junctions (Haines, Harkey, and Al-Mefty, 1993; Vandenabeele, Creemers, and Lambrichts, 1996; Reina et al., 1998; Fricke, Andres, and Von During, 2001; Reina et al., 2002).

Deep to the dura mater is the arachnoid mater, which is a vascular, delicate, and loosely arranged membrane (see Figs. 3-10 and 3-11, *A*). The outer portion consists of layers of flattened cells (arachnoid barrier cells) that form an anatomic and functional barrier between the dural blood supply and CSF in the subarachnoid space. Underneath the barrier cells is the arachnoid reticular layer, which is composed of cells and collagen fibers. The

innermost portion is the trabecular arachnoid, which is located in the subarachnoid space and consists of strands of densely packed, thick collagen fiber bundles covered by fibroblast-like arachnoid cells (Haines, Harkey, and Al-Mefty, 1993; Vandenabeele, Creemers and Lambrichts, 1996; Reina et al., 1998; Fricke, Andres, and Von During, 2001; Nolte, 2002; Reina et al., 2002).

Numerous studies (Haines, Harkey, and Al-Mefty, 1993; Vandenabeele, Creemers, and Lambrichts, 1996; Reina et al., 1998; Nolte, 2002; Reina et al., 2002) suggest that there is continuity between the inner surface of the dura mater and the arachnoid barrier cell layer such that there is no naturally occurring subdural space. Because the

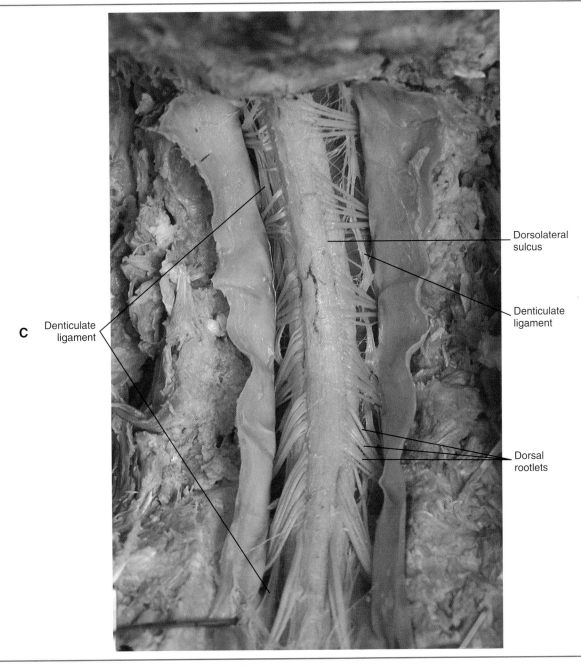

C

Denticulate ligament

Dorsolateral sulcus

Denticulate ligament

Dorsal rootlets

FIG. 3-11—Cont'd   **C**, Cervical cord segments.

cellular characteristics of the dural border (neurothelial) cell layer create a structurally weak plane and an area of low resistance, disruption of this layer during surgery or by trauma, for example, can create an artificial subdural space.

Both the dura and arachnoid (collectively forming the dural sac, or thecal sac) have typically been described as extending to the lower border of the S2 vertebra, well below the end of the spinal cord (conus medullaris). However, Macdonald et al. (1999) studied magnetic resonance imaging (MRI) scans of the lumbosacral region of 136 adults and found that the level of termination ranged from the upper border of S1 to the upper border of S4, with the median level being the middle one third of S2. They also noticed a gender difference in the termination level, with the median level for males being the upper one third of S2, and the middle one third of S2 the median level for females. This is supported by the work of Hansasuta, Tubbs, and Oakes (1999).

In addition to typically extending inferiorly to the S2 level, the dura and arachnoid also extend laterally and invest the nerve roots in a manner similar to a coat

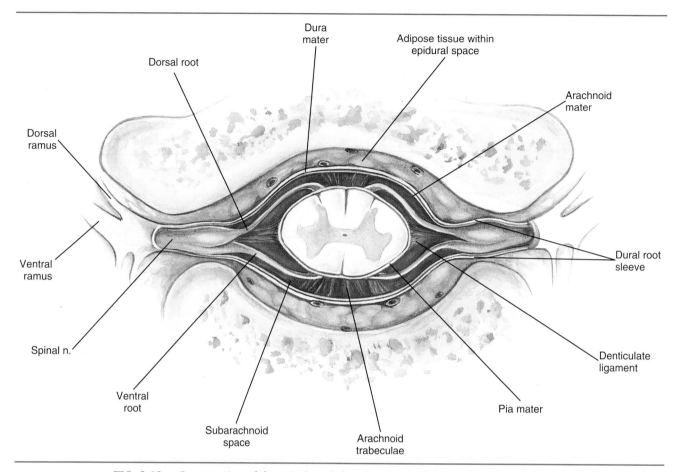

FIG. 3-12   Cross section of the spinal cord showing the meninges and dural root sleeves.

sleeve, as the roots travel distally toward the IVF to form their spinal nerve (see Fig. 3-12). At that point the dura blends in with the epineurial connective tissue surrounding the newly formed spinal nerve, whereas the arachnoid merges with the perineurium (Hewitt, 1970; Williams et al., 1995; Snell, 2001; FitzGerald and Folan-Curran, 2002).

The subarachnoid space is under the arachnoid (see Fig. 3-12). This space is filled with CSF. At various locations throughout the CNS, the subarachnoid space becomes enlarged, forming regions known as cisterns. The subarachnoid space inferior to the conus medullaris is such an enlargement and is called the lumbar cistern (see Figs. 3-7 and 3-11, *B*). At this level the lumbar cistern contains not only CSF, but also the cauda equina and filum terminale (see the following discussion). CSF is actively secreted, via various transport mechanisms, by the choroid plexus. The choroid plexus is specialized tissue located in the ventricles within the brain. Although CSF is often compared with plasma, its ionic composition is different; therefore CSF is not considered to be an ultrafiltrate of blood. CSF has numerous functions: it provides buoyancy and protection for the CNS against

mechanical trauma; it provides a route for the removal of products of neuronal metabolism (sometimes referred to as "acting as a large metabolic sink") (Benarroch et al., 1999; Nolte, 2002); it provides and regulates a stable chemical microenvironment to ensure normal functioning of neurons and glial cells; and it is a route by which neuroactive hormones may travel through the nervous system. Such neuroactive hormones include hypothalamic hormones that bind to distant target cells in the brain (Laterra and Goldstein, 2000) and pineal secretions traveling to the pituitary gland (Snell, 2001; Nolte, 2002).

The CSF flows inferiorly in one direction within the ventricles located in the brain. At a level just rostral to the foramen magnum, most CSF leaves the most caudal (fourth) ventricle, enters the subarachnoid space, and flows superiorly over the brain and inferiorly around the spinal cord. In addition, a very small amount of CSF remains within the central canal of the cord. The CSF in the subarachnoid space gradually and slowly flows inferiorly into the lumbar cistern and then makes its way back superiorly. Pulsation of large spinal arteries within the subarachnoid space, respiratory movements, movements of the vertebral column, changing of body positions, and intrathoracic and intraabdominal pressure changes contribute to the flow of the CSF. Some CSF surrounding the cord flows superiorly and into the subarachnoid space surrounding the brain. Because of a pressure gradient, this CSF eventually flows from the subarachnoid space through arachnoid granulations (i.e., multiple villi that serve as one-way valves) and into the venous sinuses of the cranial dura mater. The CSF around the spinal cord also is absorbed through arachnoid villi that penetrate the dural root sleeves and project into small spinal veins leaving the IVF (Afifi and Bergman, 1998; Laterra and Goldstein, 2000; FitzGerald and Folan-Curran, 2002; Johnston and Papaiconomou, 2002; Nolte, 2002). Emptying into the venous system completes the one-way circulation of the CSF. Human and animal studies also suggest that CSF drains into lymphatic vessels and subsequently into regional lymph nodes (Boulton et al., 1996; Miura, Kato, and von Ludinghausen, 1998; Fricke, Andres, and Von During, 2001; Snell, 2001; Johnston and Papaiconomou, 2002).

The innermost membrane of the meninges is called the pia mater. This layer consists of one to two layers of flattened cells that are joined by desmosomes and gap junctions. They are continuous with the leptomeningeal cells of the trabeculae. Separating this layer from the neural tissue of the external surface of the spinal cord (the astrocytic glia limitans) is the subpial space. This space contains collagen fiber bundles, fibroblast-like cells, and blood vessels, such as the anterior spinal artery. The pia mater invests the spinal cord and forms a fold within the ventral median fissure. It also surrounds the rootlets and roots as they course into the IVF. In addition to serving as a separation between the subarachnoid and subpial spaces, it has been suggested that the pia mater surrounding the brain may serve as a regulatory interface between the two spaces by means of the pinocytotic action of the pial cells (Williams et al., 1995).

Two specializations of pia mater that function to stabilize the spinal cord within the vertebral canal are the left and right denticulate ligaments and filum terminale. Each denticulate ligament is a collagenous, triangular-shaped serrated ribbon coursing the length of the cord. It consists of a medial border that is continuous with the subpial connective tissue of the spinal cord, and a lateral apical border that attaches to the dura mater in an even distribution at approximately 21 points on each side along the cord's length. Because of its location, the denticulate ligament forms a shelf within the vertebral canal between the dorsal and ventral roots (see Figs. 3-10, 3-11, C, and 3-12) and divides the canal into anterior and posterior compartments. Superiorly the ligament attaches to the dura mater above the lateral rim of the foramen magnum and behind the hypoglossal nerve. The ligament lies between the anteriorly placed vertebral artery (which separates the ligament from the first

cervical ventral root) and the ascending spinal root of the spinal accessory nerve. The most inferior portion ends at the level of the conus medullaris where the last lateral attachment to the dura mater lies between the roots of the T12 and L1 cord segments. The denticulate ligament continues inferiorly as a narrow oblique band that descends laterally and fuses with the filum terminale (Williams et al., 1995). In the cervical region, the lateral apical attachments of the left and right denticulate ligaments attach to the dura further away from the exiting nerve roots than those of the lower thoracic region (Kershner and Binhammer, 2002). Tubbs et al. (2001) dissected 12 cadavers and described the morphology of the ligament in detail. They described the lateral apices of most ligaments as consisting of a superior and inferior prong that were approximately 1 mm in length. These two pronged ligaments were most prominent in the cervical and upper thoracic region; the lower thoracic ligaments were not pronged. The lateral apical attachments in the cervical region were found to be thicker than those found in the thoracic and lumbar regions. Based on gross inspection and electron microscopy of 56 cadavers, Kershner and Binhammer (2002) suggested that developmental remnants of the lateral apex of denticulate ligaments formed "intrathecal ligaments" that were associated with the cauda equina. An average of 18 such ligaments per cadaver were found within the lumbar cistern. These dense collagenous intrathecal ligaments were covered with a thin layer of leptomeningeal cells and varied in thickness (0.13 to 0.35 μm) and length (3 mm to 3.5 cm). Some of the ligaments randomly connected dorsal nerve roots of the cauda equina to the dura mater, and occasionally the ligaments joined dorsal and ventral roots. These intrathecal ligaments are thought to be derived from the denticulate ligaments because the spinal cord ascends relative to the rest of the vertebral column during development. The clinical significance of these structures is unknown.

The other special component of pia mater is a bluish-white structure called the filum terminale. This slender filament consists of glial cells and ependyma (ependyma cells line the central canal of the spinal cord), and is covered by pia mater. The first 5 to 6 mm of the filum terminale includes a central canal. The filum extends approximately 20 cm from the tip of the conus medullaris within the lumbar cistern to the dorsum of the coccyx, where it blends into the connective tissue covering this bone (see Fig. 3-11, B). The portion of the filum terminale between the conus medullaris and the inferior tip of the dural sac is known as the filum terminale *internum* (≈15 cm long). Because the filum terminale pierces the dura and arachnoid at the S2 level on its way to the dorsum of the coccyx (thereby exiting the lumbar cistern), the filum terminale picks up two additional layers (dura and arachnoid); thus from S2 to the coccyx, it is usually called the coccygeal ligament (filum terminale *externum*). A few strands of nerve fibers adhere to the upper part of the filum. It has been suggested that these are likely to be rudimentary roots of the second and third coccygeal spinal nerves (Williams et al., 1995).

The filum terminale may seem to be an unassuming remnant that only functions to stabilize the cord longitudinally. However, it does have clinical significance in its contribution to a condition known as tethered cord syndrome (TCS). This syndrome is characterized by an abnormally low conus medullaris that is "tethered or anchored" by one or more forms of intradural abnormalities. Such intradural abnormalities include a short, thickened filum terminale, fibrous bands, adhesions, and intradural lipomas that represent a form of occult spinal dysraphism. TCS can be seen in children because of a congenital dural defect. In this situation the cord becomes anchored because of its contact with subcutaneous tissue and is prevented from ascending within the vertebral canal (Afifi and Bergman, 1998; Pinto et al., 2002). However, TCS can also occur in adults. In this case a subclinical degree of spinal cord traction is present. The traction can become clinically apparent when abrupt cord traction occurs because of sudden flexion of the vertebral canal (e.g., the abdominal flexion movements and trauma resulting from motor vehicle accidents) (Pinto et al., 2002). The sudden traction leads to neurologic deficits caused by anatomic and metabolic changes in the spinal cord. The most common neurologic deficit is pain in the lower back and pain radiating into the lower limbs. This pain is exacerbated by physical activity involving flexion and extension of the trunk. Other findings include sensory deficits in the lower extremities, lower extremity deformities, musculoskeletal deformities such as scoliosis, and urinary incontinence. Adults who present with these types of deficits, but are asymptomatic as children, often are misdiagnosed with "failed back syndrome" or other unrelated problems of the spine (Yamada and Lonser, 2000). The radiologic criteria that have been established to aid in diagnosing this condition are a filum terminale that has a diameter greater than 2 mm or a spinal cord that terminates lower than the L2 or L3 vertebral body levels, and a conus medullaris displaced posteriorly with the filum in contact with the dural sac at or near the L5 lamina (Yamada and Lonser, 2000; Pinto et al., 2002). However, because of considerable anatomic variation of the conus medullaris and filum terminale, the patient's history, examination, and radiologic findings are important in diagnosing TCS. The surgical treatment for TCS is to perform a laminectomy at a level that will expose the filum and conus and subsequently untether the cord (Hansasuta, Tubbs, and Oakes, 1999; Pinto et al., 2002).

The vast majority (89%) of fila fuse on the dorsal midline of the dura, with 11% fusing to the left or right of the midline. The level of fusion varies anywhere from the lower L5 vertebral body to the upper S3 body. The majority (approximately 85%) of fila fuse at or below S1, and approximately 15% fuse above the S1 level. Forty-four percent of the time the fusion is at the same level as the termination of the dural sac (Hansasuta, Tubbs, and Oakes, 1999). The work of Pinto et al. (2002) supports these findings.

The diameter of the filum terminale decreases in a superior to inferior direction; the mean thickness at the midpoint of the filum is 0.76 ± 0.39 mm and the mean thickness at the initial point of origin is 1.38 ± 0.56 mm. In addition to the variation in the anatomy of the filum and its relationship with the dural sac, anatomic variations of the conus medullaris are still being documented. The accepted view was that the mean level of termination of the conus medullaris was at the level of the L1-2 intervertebral disc (Reimann and Anson, 1944). However, the majority of recent MRI studies of human spines report the mean level of termination to be at a slightly higher level (i.e., the mid- to lower L1 vertebral body), although there is variation among the results of the studies and among individuals (Table 3-1). Interestingly there appears to be no difference in termination levels with increasing age (Saifuddin, Burnett, and White, 1998; Arai et al., 2001; Demiryürek et al., 2002), although Arai et al. (2001) reported a more caudal distribution of the termination of the conus medullaris in children less than 11 years of age. In addition, the majority of authors have found no difference in termination levels between males and females (Safuddin, Burnett, and White, 1998; Macdonald et al., 1999; Arai et al., 2001). However, Demiryürek et al. (2002) reported that the termination level in females was lower than in males (L1-2 IVD vs. T12-L1 IVD, respectively). Although the conus medullaris generally is centrally located within the lumbar subarachnoid cistern, it slants ventrally 10% of the time and dorsally 30% of the time (Arai et al., 2001).

The discrepancies in the data among various investigators may result from racial differences, statistical analysis, the presence of transitional lumbosacral vertebra, and the limitations of cadaveric and MRI studies (Choi, Carroll, and Abrahams, 1996; Saifuddin, Burnett, and White, 1998; Macdonald et al., 1999; Demiryürek et al., 2002).

Knowing the vertebral level in which the majority of spinal cords terminate and being aware that the sites of termination vary among individuals is important. For example, neurologic deficits seen in patients who have experienced vertebral fractures, especially burst fractures, and osteoporotic vertebral collapse at the thoracolumbar level differ depending on the location of the conus. Also, noting variations is important when an invasive procedure such as a lumbar puncture (spinal tap) is performed. In this procedure, a long needle is inserted in the midline between adjacent lower lumbar vertebrae

Table 3-1 Termination Level of the Conus Medullaris as Determined by Magnetic Resonance Imaging Scans

Author	Range	Mean	Number and Age of Subjects/ Magnetic Resonance Imaging Method
Arai et al., 2001	T11-12 disc to center of L3 body	Middle ⅓ and distal ⅓ of L1	$n = 602$ Age = 8 mo–84 yr T1* 5 mm†
Demiryurek et al., 2002	T11-12 disc to upper ⅓ of L3	T12-L1 disc	$n = 639$ Age = 20–69 yr T1 4 mm
Macdonald et al., 1999	Mid ⅓ T11 to mid ⅓ of L3	Median level: mid ⅓ of L1	$n = 136$ Age = 30–70 yr T2 4 mm
Malas et al., 2000	T12-L2	Most frequently seen: L1-2 disc	$n = 25$ Age = 22–72 yr T1 and T2 5 mm
Saifuddin et al., 1998	Mid ⅓ of T12 to upper ⅓ of L3	Lower ⅓ of L1	$n = 504$ Age = 16–85 yr T1 5 mm

Macdonald et al. (1999) did not use the disc spaces as a possible point of termination. The intervertebral disc (IVD) was considered to be a part of the vertebral level above or below based on whether the conus ended at the upper or lower half of the disc (e.g., conus ending at upper part of the L1-2 IVD considered to end at L1 level).
*T1 and T2, T1- and T2-weighted images.
†Slice thickness in millimeters.

(L3-4 or L4-5) and into the lumbar cistern. Because the cauda equina is floating in the CSF, the roots usually are avoided by the needle. Once the needle is inserted, agents can be injected into the region for diagnostic imaging and anesthetic purposes. For example, in myelography, a radiopaque iodinated contrast medium is injected to outline the spinal cord and roots. Anesthetics occasionally may be injected into the subarachnoid space (spinal anesthesia) for abdominal, pelvic, or lower extremity surgery. Hamandi et al. (2002) and Reynolds (2001) reported on a total of 12 cases in which spinal anesthesia alone or in combination with epidural anesthesia was used on eight patients undergoing obstetric operations and four undergoing surgical operations. Direct damage from needle insertion to the cord was seen on MRI scans in these patients, resulting in long-term neurologic deficits in the lower extremity such as pain, muscle atrophy weakness, foot drop, decreased sensation, and absent ankle muscle stretch reflexes. Because of the seriousness of these deficits, the authors of both studies indicate the importance of inserting the needle in the interspace of lower lumbar vertebrae.

The volume, pressure, and contents of CSF also are clinically relevant; for example, although not done routinely, the removal and analysis of typically 5 to 15 ml of CSF by means of lumbar puncture, when indicated, can be used as an important neurodiagnostic test. The total volume of CSF ranges from 80 to 150 ml, and CSF is produced sufficiently to replace itself four to five times daily. Notice that there is a dramatic variation in CSF volume in different individuals (Hogan et al., 1996). In addition, the volume of CSF has been found to decrease in relatively obese individuals as a result of increased abdominal pressure (a condition seen in obese and pregnant individuals). This decrease was greater at the levels of the IVFs, which suggested that CSF was displaced by the inward movement of soft tissue from the IVF into the vertebral canal.

CSF pressure ranges from 80 to 180 mm (of water) and is measured on a patient lying in a curled, lateral recumbent position. CSF is normally clear, colorless, and slightly alkaline. It contains approximately six white blood cells (WBCs), usually lymphocytes, per milliliter and no red blood cells (RBCs). As with plasma, it includes sodium, potassium, magnesium, and chloride ions. It also contains glucose and protein, but the concentrations are substantially less than in plasma.

CSF volume may become altered as a result of a pathologic state. The Monro-Kellie hypothesis states that the sum of brain tissue, intracranial blood, and CSF volumes is constant, and that if one of these volumes increases, the other volumes must compensate because the bony confines do not. If no compensatory readjustment occurs, intracranial pressure (ICP) increases. Interference in CSF circulation in the cranium by a space-occupying lesion such as a tumor or hematoma can increase CSF pressure. If an increase in ICP is suspected, a lumbar puncture (spinal tap) is contraindicated. Removal of CSF in such cases could produce a vacuum and cause herniation of the cerebellum into the foramen magnum, with serious consequences, including death. Increased CSF pressure also can cause swelling of the optic disc (papilledema) of the retina. Because the retina can be observed easily by an ophthalmoscope, papilledema could contraindicate the performance of a lumbar puncture. Although the condition of increased intracranial pressure presents very serious clinical sequelae, the Monro-Kellie hypothesis also is applicable to a decrease in intracranial pressure and reduced CSF volume. The necessary compensation that occurs is to affect the intracranial blood volume, resulting in intracranial (usually venous) hyperemia and changes in the cranium that can be seen on MRI scans. A decrease in CSF volume also results in changes in the spinal canal, such as an engorgement of the epidural venous plexus that compensates for a moderate degree of collapse of the dura mater, which is also observed on MRI scans (Mokri, 2001).

In addition to pressure changes, the appearance, cell content, levels of gamma globulins (antibodies), and protein and glucose concentrations in CSF may be altered in patients with some pathologic conditions. For example, in bacterial meningitis (inflammation of the leptomeninges) the CSF is cloudy, pressure is increased, WBC count is elevated, protein concentration is increased, and glucose concentration is decreased (Daube et al., 1986). The CSF in a patient with a subarachnoid hemorrhage appears cloudy, and RBCs are present. Therefore the alterations of certain characteristics of the CSF become useful in diagnosing certain pathologic conditions.

INTERNAL ORGANIZATION OF THE SPINAL CORD

Having discussed the external morphology of the spinal cord and its coverings, the internal morphology is now described to provide an understanding of spinal cord anatomy in its entirety. In Chapter 9, a more detailed description of the internal aspect of the spinal cord and its functions is given.

The overall internal organization of the spinal cord can be observed in a transverse or horizontal cross section. This view shows the spinal cord as being clearly divided into a butterfly- or H-shaped central area of gray matter and a peripheral area of white myelinated axons.

Gray Matter

Each half of the H-shaped gray matter consists of a dorsal horn, ventral horn, and intermediate area between the horns (Fig. 3-13). In thoracic segments the intermediate zone includes a lateral horn. The crossbar of the gray matter unites the two laterally placed halves and is called the gray commissure. The gray commissure can be divided into dorsal and ventral components, based on their relationship to the central canal. The gray commissure is thinnest in the thoracic segments and thickest in the conus medullaris and contains two longitudinal veins. Coursing through the dorsal aspect of the commissure are transverse myelinated axons that are sometimes called the dorsal white commissure (Williams et al., 1995). The gray commissure also contains the central canal. This canal is the remnant of the lumen of the embryologic neural tube and is a continuation of the fourth ventricle of the brain stem. Lined by a single layer of ependymal cells, it extends the length of the spinal cord and continues into the filum terminale for approximately 5 to 6 mm. Within the conus medullaris it expands into a triangular-shaped, 8- to 10-mm-long structure called the terminal ventricle. The location of the canal relative to the midpoint of the spinal cord varies among the regions of the cord. It is slightly ventral in the cervical and thoracic segments, central in the segments of the lumbar enlargement, and dorsal in the conus medullaris. Immediately adjacent to the canal lies the substantia gelatinosa centralis, which is a region containing neurons, neuroglia, and a reticulum of fibers. Coursing through this area are processes radiating from the basal aspects of the ependymal cells lining the canal. Peripheral to the substantia gelatinosa centralis is the gray commissure (Williams et al., 1995).

The central canal is frequently involved with cavitary lesions of the spinal cord, such as syringomyelia. The pathogenesis of this condition, which is a dilation of the central canal causing a syrinx, appears to be related to a hydrodynamic mechanism relating to the CSF. Studies on kaolin-induced hydrocephalic animals indicated that the distending forces of a downward movement of CSF from ventricles in the brain into the central canal caused spinal cord cavitation including central canal distention and disruption into the cord parenchyma (Yasui et al., 1999).

After birth the central canal becomes progressively occluded (typically with ependymal cells) as one ages. Histologic studies of the canal indicate that ependymal cell breakdown during the aging process contributes to the canal occlusion. The ependymal cell changes result in glial bundle formation, proliferation of ependymal cells and astrocytes, formation of ependymal rosettes or microcanals, proliferation of subependymal gliovascular buds, and intracanalicular gliosis (Milhorat, Kotzen, and

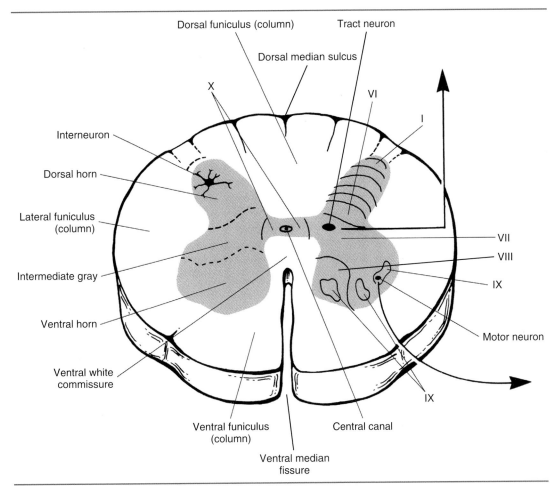

FIG. 3-13   Cross section of the spinal cord. *Left,* Organization of gray matter into regions. *Right,* Lamination of the gray matter. Motor and tract neurons and interneurons also are shown.

Anzil, 1994; Yasui et al., 1999). Interestingly, Milhorat, Kotzen, and Anzil (1994) suggest that central canal stenosis is an acquired pathologic lesion rather than a degenerative process related to aging. They postulate that the cause is recurring episodes of ependymitis caused by the common virus infections one is exposed to throughout life.

Using a computerized three-dimensional histologic study on a small sample of spinal cords, Storer et al. (1998) demonstrated a variety of anatomic features of the central canal. They observed forking within the lower conus medullaris near the terminal ventricle with outpouchings of each fork of the canal into the filum terminale. They also noticed an extension of ependymal cells from the lumen of the canal to the surface of the pia mater that suggested a possible functional communication between the canal and the subarachnoid space. The ependymal lining of the canal was also in close proximity to the pial surface throughout most of the length of the extrusion of the central canal into the filum terminale. This region was found to have openings into

the subarachnoid space at two levels within the caudal filum. The researchers postulated that this connection may provide a physiologically important fluid communication that may play a role in the "sink" function of the canal. Other data also suggest that the canal functions like a "sink" based on its capability of clearing substances such as vital dyes, horseradish peroxidase, and cellular elements from cord parenchyma (Milhorat, Kotzen, and Anzil, 1994). However, Yasui et al. (1999) believe that this proposed function of the human central canal is insignificant after birth. They found that the patency rate of the central canal was 100% in infants under 1 year of age. A marked decrease was seen in the percentage of individuals with patent central canals in the second decade and by the fourth decade all levels were occluded except in the cervical cord, where the patency rate remained high. The canals were occluded in the vast majority of all the segments after the seventh decade. The T6 and L5-S2 levels occluded earliest, and the upper cervical segments were the last to occlude. The progressive nature and segment location of the canal stenosis most likely affects the clinical presentation of syringomyelia, and, in fact, Yasui et al. (1999) suggest that because the canal is obliterated, it is not involved in the development of the adult form of syringomyelia.

The large dense gray area of the cord (gray matter) consists of neurons, primarily cell bodies; neuroglia; and capillaries. Microscopically this region appears to be a tangle of neuron processes and their synapses and neuroglial processes, all of which form the neuropil. This network forms the cord's amazingly complex circuitry. The neurons of the gray matter consist of four general types: motor, tract, interneuron, and propriospinal. The larger motor and tract neurons, which have long axons (1 m or more in length), are sometimes called Golgi type I cells. Interneurons and propriospinal neurons, which have shorter axons, may be called Golgi type II cells. These are the more numerous of the two (Carpenter, 1991; Williams et al., 1995). The neurons are not distributed equally throughout the gray matter but instead are found in clusters.

Axons of motor neuron cell bodies leave the spinal cord, enter the ventral root, and ultimately innervate the body's effector tissues, that is, skeletal muscle, smooth muscle, cardiac muscle, and glands. Skeletal muscle is innervated by alpha and gamma motor neurons. Smooth muscle, cardiac muscle, and glands are innervated by autonomic motor fibers. Motor neuron cell bodies are located in either the ventral horn or the intermediate gray area and are densely covered with presynaptic terminals of axons from higher centers, incoming sensory afferent fibers, propriospinal neurons, and interneurons. It is believed that each of the large alpha motor neurons that innervates a skeletal muscle may have at least 20,000 synapses on its surface (Davidoff and Hackman, 1991; Kiernan, 1998).

Axons of tract neurons in the gray matter emerge from the gray matter and ascend in the white matter to higher centers. These axons help to form the ascending tracts of the cord's white matter. The cell bodies of these neurons are located in the dorsal horn and intermediate gray area.

The third type of neuron is the interneuron. Interneurons make up the vast majority of the neuronal population, and their cell bodies are found in all parts of the gray matter. They conduct the important "business" of the CNS by forming complex connections. Although various types of interneurons exist, their processes are all relatively short. They usually are located within the limits of one cord segment, although the axons may include collateral branches that terminate both contralaterally and ipsilaterally. The interneurons receive input from each other, incoming sensory afferents, propriospinal neurons, and descending fibers from higher centers. Through their elaborate synaptic circuitry, the interneurons transform this input and disseminate it

to other neurons, including the motor neurons. For example, some interneurons play a crucial role in motor control by their actions in motor reflexes involving peripheral proprioceptive input from neuromuscular spindles and Golgi tendon organs (see Chapter 9).

Other "motor" interneurons called Renshaw cells provide a negative feedback mechanism to adjacent motor neurons. This intricate circuitry may be necessary for synchronizing events such as the force, rate, timing, and coordination of contraction of muscle antagonists, synergists, and agonists that must occur in the complex motor activities performed by humans. In addition, other interneurons located in the dorsal horn are involved in the circuitry that modifies and edits pain input conveyed into the dorsal horn by afferent fibers (see Chapter 9).

The fourth type of neuron located in the gray matter is the propriospinal neuron. This neuron's axon leaves the gray matter at one level, ascends or descends, and terminates in the gray matter at a different cord level. The majority of the axons are located in the white matter immediately adjacent to the gray matter (fasciculus proprius), although some axons are spread diffusely within the white matter funiculi. The classification of propriospinal neurons is based on the length of their axons. Short propriospinal neurons travel ipsilaterally over a distance of approximately six to eight segments; intermediate neurons course ipsilaterally more than eight segments but less than the entire length of the cord; and long propriospinal neurons project the length of the cord, descending bilaterally and ascending contralaterally.

These neurons allow communication to occur among cord segments for the coordination of skeletal muscle contraction and regulation of autonomic functions such as sudomotor (to sweat glands) and vasomotor activities, and bladder and bowel control (Williams et al., 1995).

As mentioned, in cross section the gray matter resembles a butterfly- or H-shaped area. Each half is subdivided into a dorsal horn, an intermediate area that in certain segments includes a lateral horn, and a ventral horn (see Fig. 3-13). The dorsal horn functions as a receiving area for both descending information from higher centers and sensory afferents from the dorsal roots. The cell bodies of the sensory afferents are located in the dorsal root ganglia. The sensory afferents bring information from receptors in the skin (exteroceptors); muscles, tendons, and joints (proprioceptors, i.e., mechanoreceptors for proprioception); and the viscera (interoceptors). These afferent fibers synapse on interneurons, propriospinal neurons, and tract neurons, depending on the type of information carried and the resulting action needed.

The intermediate region, which is actually the central core of each half of the gray matter, receives proprioceptive input from sensory afferents, input from the dorsal horn, and descending input from higher centers, thus becoming an area in which interaction of sensory and descending input can occur. In general, the intermediate area comprises interneurons, tract neurons, propriospinal neurons, and the cell bodies of neurons innervating smooth muscle, cardiac muscle, and glands. These cell bodies are located in cord segments T1 to L2-3 and make up the lateral horn.

The ventral horn of the gray matter includes interneurons, propriospinal neurons, and the cell bodies of motor neurons. The axons of these motor neurons, also called alpha and gamma motor neurons or anterior horn cells, leave via the ventral roots to innervate skeletal muscle. Descending tracts from the brain, axons from propriospinal neurons in other cord segments, intrasegmental interneurons, and primary afferents from mechanoreceptors (proprioceptors) involved with monosynaptic muscle stretch reflexes terminate in this region of ventral gray matter.

As is the case throughout the nervous system, neurons communicate with each other and form circuits within the gray matter of the spinal cord by means of synapses and chemical substances. A synapse is the junction between two neurons. The average neuron is thought to have as many as 10,000 synapses on its surface and to give rise to approximately 1000 synaptic connections (Kandel and Siegelbaum, 2000). The chemical substances called neuromediators are released at the synapse from the terminal of a presynaptic neuron. These mediators cross the synaptic cleft and bind to receptors on the postsynaptic neuron, causing either a depolarization or hyperpolarization of the cell membrane (via neurotransmitters), or a structural or functional change in the neuron (via neuromodulators). Through use of techniques such as autoradiography and immunohistochemistry, much new information concerning the neural circuitry of the spinal cord is emerging. Through use of antibody labeling techniques, neuromediators have been localized in neuronal cell bodies of the gray matter and in axon terminals of neurons, including descending fibers and primary afferent fibers. Examples of neuromediators that have been found in the dorsal horn are enkephalins, somatostatin, substance P, cholecystokinin, dynorphin, gamma-aminobutyric acid (GABA), glycine, glutamate, and calcitonin gene-related peptide (CGRP). The intermediate gray matter and ventral horn include neuromediators such as cholecystokinin, enkephalins, serotonin, vasoactive intestinal polypeptide (VIP), glycine, GABA, and CGRP. These chemicals bind to specific receptors, some of which also have been located through labeling techniques. Examples of receptors located in various regions of the gray matter include opiate receptors, muscarinic cholinergic receptors, and receptors for GABA, CGRP, and thyrotropin-releasing hormone (Schoenen, 1991; Willis and Coggeshall, 1991).

In addition to the types of neurons comprising the spinal cord gray matter, each half is also described microscopically by its longitudinal laminar cytoarchitectural pattern. These longitudinal laminae contain combinations of motor, tract, propriospinal, and interneurons. In some instances, neuron cell bodies of one of the four types may form a cluster, called a nucleus (i.e., an aggregation of neuron cell bodies found within the CNS). The neurons of each nucleus are similar morphologically, and the axons have a common termination and function. Numerous nuclei have been identified in the gray matter. Some are located in all cord segments, whereas others are limited to specific cord segments.

The laminar cytoarchitectural organization of the spinal cord gray matter was proposed by Rexed in 1952. Studying the size, density, staining characteristics, and connections of the neurons in feline spinal cords, he identified 10 layers within the gray matter. This has since been accepted as standard in human spinal cords as well. Rexed's gray matter laminae proceed sequentially from dorsal to ventral (see Fig. 3-13). Lamina I is the tip of the dorsal horn, and lamina IX is in the ventral horn. Lamina X corresponds to the gray commissures (dorsal and ventral) surrounding the central canal. Each lamina contains specific types of neurons and, in some cases, nuclei, which indicate a function for that layer of cells. The neuronal populations of each lamina and the functional significance of the laminae, relative to the connections between the cord and brain and between the CNS and the periphery, are described in more detail in Chapter 9.

White Matter

A cross section of the spinal cord demonstrates that peripheral to the gray matter of the cord is a well-defined area of white matter (see Fig. 3-13). White matter includes a longitudinal arrangement of predominantly myelinated axons (which gives the area the white appearance), neuroglia, and blood vessels. The white matter is divided into three major areas called columns or funiculi. The dorsal funiculus or column is located between the dorsal horns, the lateral funiculus or column between each dorsal and ventral horn, and the ventral funiculus or column between the ventral horns (see Fig. 3-13). The white area connecting the two halves of the cord and surrounding the gray commissure forms the dorsal and ventral white commissures. The dorsal white commissure is small. The ventral commissural area includes clinically important decussating axons of pain and temperature tract neurons. The neuronal cell bodies of the axons that course in the funiculi are found in various locations. The cell bodies of axons that interconnect cord segments or ascend to the brain are located in the cord's gray matter or dorsal root ganglia. The cell bodies of axons that descend in the spinal cord to synapse in the gray matter are located in the brain.

The long ascending and descending axons are not randomly mixed together but are organized into bundles called tracts or fasciculi (see Chapter 9, Fig. 9-8). The axons of each tract or fasciculus share a common origin and convey similar information to a common destinaion. For example, axons that are conveying impulses for pain and temperature are found in an anterolateral position in the cord. Although the tracts are well organized, they still overlap somewhat, and boundaries are often arbitrary. The axons that make up the funiculi vary in diameter (Williams et al., 1995). Makino et al. (1996) studied the morphometry of the C7 cord segment in seven adult cadavers. They found that myelinated axons in the dorsal funiculus (DF) (location of the dorsal columns), marginal zone of the lateral funiculus (M-LF) (location of the spinocerebellar tracts), and the dorsal half of the lateral funiculus (LF) (location of the lateral corticospinal tract) consist of small-diameter fibers (<5 μm in the DF and <7 μm in the M-LF and LF) and large-diameter fibers (>5 μm in the DF and >7 μm in the M-LF and LF). The fiber density was greatest in the LF, followed by the DF, which was denser than the M-LF. There was considerable variation among the specimens concerning the density of small fibers, but not of large-diameter fibers. The density of small fibers appears to determine the total myelinated fiber density. A large variation also was noted among specimens relative to the total area of all funiculi (ventral, lateral, and dorsal) and the hemilateral area of the cord. In thick cords (large cross-sectional area) the absolute number of large diameter fibers was greater than in the thin cords (small cross-sectional areas). Research on peripheral nerve fibers suggests that ischemia or compression selectively injure large-diameter fibers. Therefore it is possible that a thin cord with a small cross-sectional area in which the absolute number of large-diameter fibers is less could be more susceptible to neural injury caused by chronic compressive myelopathy (Makino et al., 1996).

Regional Characteristics

Although the characteristics of gray and white matter are generally the same in all cord segments, some identifying features are seen in cross section that distinguish the cervical, thoracic, lumbar, and sacral regions of the spinal cord (Fig. 3-14 and Table 3-2). For example, differences

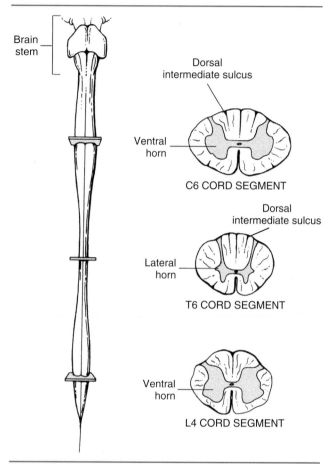

FIG. 3-14 Cross sections of the spinal cord at cervical, thoracic, and lumbar levels showing regional characteristics of gray and white matter.

Table 3-2	Distinguishing Features of Spinal Cord Regions			
Feature	**Cervical**	**Thoracic**	**Lumbar**	**Sacral**
Shape	Oval	Round	Round	Round to almost square
Gray matter	Enlarged ventral horn (C4-8)	Lateral horn present; narrow dorsal and ventral horns	Large dorsal and ventral horns	Ipsilateral dorsal and ventral horns form almost continuous oval mass
White matter	Large amount of white relative to gray Dorsal intermediate sulcus present	Large amount of white relative to gray Dorsal intermediate sulcus present T1-6	Almost equal amount of white relative to gray	Small amount of white relative to gray

exist in the appearance and amount of white matter because of the presence and absence of certain tracts at different levels such that the volume of white matter increases as cord segments progress cranially. Also, the gray matter changes its appearance because of regional differences in the number of autonomic motor neuron cell bodies (the axons of which innervate smooth muscle, cardiac muscle, and glands) and somatic sensory and motor neuron cell bodies associated with the innervation of the extremities and trunk. Because the density of sensory receptors is greater in the extremities than in the trunk, more neurons are needed to process this information, which results in a larger dorsal horn. Also, the extremities have more muscles than the trunk, so there are more somatic motor neurons and associated interneuronal pools to regulate limb movement, which results in a larger ventral horn.

Numerous investigators have measured the human spinal cord using cadaveric specimens and also using computed tomography (CT) myelography and MRI techniques on patients (Elliott, 1945; Nordqvist, 1964; Fujiwara et al., 1988; Carpenter, 1991; Choi, Carroll, and Abrahams, 1996; Kameyama, Hashizume, and Sobue, 1996; Fountas et al., 1998; Schoenen, 1991). The specific data for measurements of individual cord segments in these studies differ significantly. This may result from the variability in cord size among individuals or the techniques and methodologies used, which are inherently different. Because of this, the regional characteristics of the cord are described in more general terms (see the preceding references for detailed descriptions). However, for reference purposes, all of the sagittal and transverse diameters of the cord are in the range of 5 to 15 mm.

Kameyama, Hashizume, and Sobue (1996) measured the transverse (side-to-side) and sagittal (dorsal-to-ventral) diameters and the cross-sectional area of the entire normal cadaveric cord. Their data indicate that the transverse diameter increases from C2 (10.5 ± 0.8 mm), peaks at approximately C6 (12.6 ± 0.7 mm), and then dramatically decreases to the T2 level (9.2 ± 0.6 mm). In the thoracic segments there was a gradual decrease, with the smallest diameter being at the T8 and T9 segments (7.4 ± 0.5 mm). At this point, the diameter increases until it peaks again, but to a lesser degree, at L4 (8.7 ± 0.4 mm). It then decreases until the S3 level (5.2 ± 0.7 mm). The sagittal diameter gradually decreases from C2 (6.4 ± 0.4 mm) to the thoracic levels T3-9, where it levels off (5.0 ± 0.5 mm). From here the sagittal diameter increases, forming a small peak at L4 (6.4 ± 0.6 mm), and then decreases until the S3 level (4.0 ± 0.4 mm). The cross-sectional area measurements mirror the measurements of the transverse diameters in that the cross-sectional area is largest at C6 (58.5 ± 7.2 mm^2), decreases and levels off, and then peaks again at L4 (43.4 ± 5.1 mm^2).

Cervical cord segments are nearly circular in shape in the upper region but become oval shaped in the mid- and lower segments (as well as the T1 segment). At almost all levels, the transverse diameter is greater than the sagittal diameter and the increased transverse diameter forms the cervical enlargement (Kameyama, Hashizume, and Sobue, 1996). Because all ascending and descending axons to and from the brain must traverse the cervical region, the amount of white matter is greater here than in other regions. The increase in white matter content, rather than gray matter, is the basis for the cervical enlargement (Kameyama, Hashizume, and Sobue, 1996). However, the gray matter does contribute to this enlargement. The gray matter cross-sectional area is greatest in the C7 segment and the ventral horn of gray matter found in the segments forming the cervical enlargement bulges laterally because of the increased number of interneurons and motor neuron cell bodies. The axons of these motor neurons innervate upper extremity skeletal muscles (see Fig. 3-14).

Thoracic segments are most easily distinguished by their small amount of gray matter relative to white matter. Because the thoracic segments are not involved with innervating the muscles of the extremities, the lateral enlargement of the ventral horn is absent. Compared with cervical segments, both the transverse and the sagittal diameters of the thoracic spinal cord are smaller. One distinguishing feature of the thoracic segments is the presence of a lateral horn. This horn is located on the lateral aspect of the intermediate gray matter and is the residence of sympathetic neuronal cell bodies, the axons of which innervate smooth muscle, cardiac muscle, and glands. In addition, from midthoracic levels superiorly, the dorsal funiculus includes a dorsal intermediate sulcus (see Fig. 3-14).

Lumbar segments are distinguished by their nearly round appearance. Although they contain relatively less white matter than cervical regions, the dorsal and ventral horns are very large. The ventral horns of the lumbar segments are involved with the innervation of lower extremity skeletal muscles, and the additional neuron cell bodies for the motor axons are located laterally in those ventral horns. Therefore this lumbar enlargement (also including the S1-3 segments) is the result of an increase in gray matter (not white matter), and is formed by an increase in both the sagittal and transverse diameters (Kameyama, Hashizume, and Sobue, 1996). The cross-sectional area of gray matter is greatest in the L5 segment. Although the T12 and L1 cord segments are indistinguishable, the large dorsal and ventral horns make lumbar segments easy to identify compared with cervical and thoracic segments (see Fig. 3-14).

Sacral segments are recognized by their predominance of gray matter and relatively small amount of white matter. The short and wide shape of the dorsal horns is also characteristic of these segments. Interestingly although cervical and lumbar segments have large transverse and sagittal diameters, the thoracic segments are the greatest in length (superior to inferior) and the sacral the shortest. The average superior-to-inferior dimensions of various cord segments are cervical, 13 mm; midthoracic, 26 mm; lumbar, 15 mm; and sacral, 5 mm (Schoenen, 1991).

Advances in imaging techniques allow greater precision in identifying neuroradiographic anatomical structures. Having an understanding of the morphologic characteristics of the normal human spinal cord provides accuracy in interpreting imaging findings, diagnosing various cord pathologies such as degenerative syndromes and compressive cervical myelopathies, and providing treatment (Fujiwara et al., 1988; Hackney, 1992; Kameyama, Hashizume, and Sobue, 1996). Table 3-2 summarizes the regional characteristics of the spinal cord.

ARTERIAL BLOOD SUPPLY OF THE SPINAL CORD

Spinal Arteries

The spinal cord is vascularized by branches of the vertebral artery and branches of segmental vessels. The vertebral artery, a branch of the subclavian artery, courses superiorly through the foramina of the transverse processes of the upper six cervical vertebrae to enter the posterior cranial fossa via the foramen magnum (see Chapter 5 for further details). Within the posterior fossa of the cranial cavity, one small ramus from each of the vertebral arteries anastomose in a Y-shaped configuration to form the anterior spinal artery (Fig. 3-15, *A*). Usually this configuration occurs within 2 cm from their origin but may occur as far inferiorly as the C5 cord segment (Turnbull, Brieg, and Hassler, 1966). Gövsa et al. (1996) looked at the anatomic variations of the origin of the anterior spinal artery in 80 cadaveric brains and found that the majority (75%) did indeed originate from two rami. Of these, the caliber of the right ramus was greater in 17.5%, whereas the caliber of the left ramus was greater in 15%. Only one ramus was present in 11.3% of the brains, and in 13.8% the anterior spinal artery originated from a transverse intervertebral anastomosis. They also noted that in 82% of the 65 brains with bilateral rami, the fusion of the two rami occurred at the intersection of the medulla oblongata and spinal cord, although in 15% of the specimens the rami fused as far inferior as the C2 and C3 cord segments. The contributing branches to the anterior spinal artery by the left and right vertebral arteries help to supply the anterior and inferior aspect of the medulla oblongata before uniting at the ventral median tissue of the spinal cord. The anterior spinal artery continues inferiorly within the

pia mater covering the ventral median fissure. This artery is usually straight, tapering as it courses inferiorly in the midline until it becomes extremely small, and often barely evident, just superior to the level of the artery of Adamkiewicz usually between the T8-L3 cord segments (see Anterior Radiculomedullary Arteries) (Gillilan, 1958; Schoenen, 1991). It may alter to one side as the anterior radiculomedullary arteries anastomose with it. The diameter of the anterior spinal artery varies from approximately 0.2 to 0.5 mm in the cervical and thoracic cord segments to 0.5 to 0.8 mm in the lumbar cord. Its diameter has been reported in a preliminary study to be approximately 0.47 mm above and 1.12 mm below its anastomosis with the artery of Adamkiewicz (Biglioli et al., 2000).

Also branching from each vertebral artery, and less frequently from the posterior inferior cerebellar artery, is the posterior spinal artery (Fig. 3-15, *B*). Each posterior spinal artery supplies the dorsolateral region of the caudal medulla oblongata. As it continues on the spinal cord, each artery forms two longitudinally irregular, anastomotic channels that course inferiorly on both sides of the dorsal rootlet attachment to the spinal cord. The medial channel is larger than the lateral (Schoenen, 1991). The two anastomotic channels are interconnected across the midline by numerous small vessels forming a plexiform network of small arteries that contribute to the pial plexus on the cord's posterior surface.

At the level of the conus medullaris, a loop or basket is formed as the anterior spinal artery anastomoses with the two posterior spinal arteries (Lazorthes et al., 1971). At this location the artery of the filum terminale branches off and courses on the filum's ventral surface (Djindjian et al., 1988).

Although the spinal arteries originate in the cranial cavity, segmental vessels, which help to supply blood to the cord, originate outside the vertebral column. The segmental arteries in the cervical region include branches of the cervical part of the vertebral artery, which vascularize most of the cervical cord, and branches of ascending and deep cervical arteries. The latter arteries originate from the subclavian artery's thyrocervical and costocervical trunks, respectively. Segmental branches that help to supply the rest of the cord arise from intercostal and lumbar arteries, which are branches of the aorta, and lateral sacral arteries, which are branches of the internal iliac artery. These vessels provide spinal branches (spinal rami) that enter the vertebral canal through the IVF; vascularize the meninges, ligaments, osseous structures, roots, and rootlets; and reinforce the spinal arteries.

As each of the 31 pairs (Lazorthes et al., 1971) of spinal branches of the segmental spinal arteries enters its respective IVF, it divides into three branches. Anterior and posterior branches vascularize the dura mater, liga-

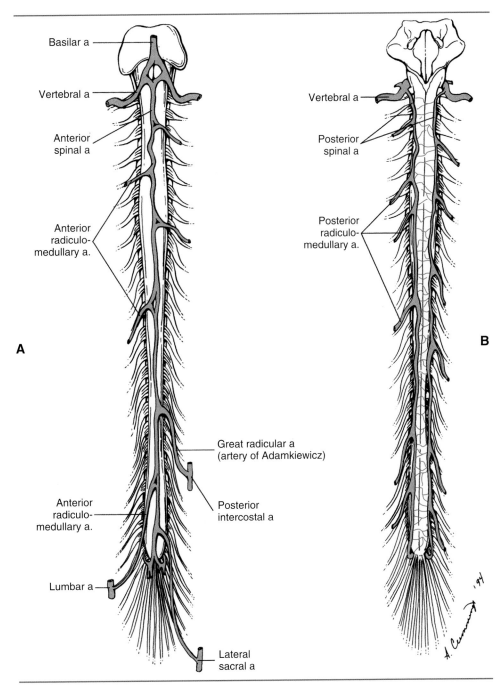

FIG. 3-15 Arterial blood supply of the spinal cord showing spinal and radiculomedullary arteries. **A,** Anterior view. **B,** Posterior view.

ments, and osseous tissue of the vertebral canal (see Chapter 2). The third branch, called the neurospinal artery (of Kadyi) (Schoenen, 1991), courses with the spinal nerve and divides into anterior and posterior branches that give off branches that either supply the roots or anastomose with the spinal arteries associated with the cord. Those small (<0.2 mm diameter) branches that vascularize the roots and their meningeal coverings are called radicular arteries. Each anterior and posterior

radicular artery also supplies small branches to its neighboring root. The posterior radicular arteries also supply branches to the dorsal root ganglion. These small branches enter the ganglion at both the proximal and distal poles and form a dense capillary bed supplying the ganglion cells. On the surface, other branches form a delicate network of vessels (the periganglionic plexus) that communicates with the deeper capillaries (Parke and Whalen, 2002).

The other (larger) branches of the neurospinal artery vary in number and anastomose with and reinforce the anterior or posterior spinal arteries, thus enhancing the circulation of the cord. Unfortunately, there is no consensus as to the name of these vessels. Some authors (Zhang et al., 1995; Bowen and Pattany, 1999; Krauss, 1999; Milen et al., 1999; Greathouse, Halle, and Dalley, 2001) consider these vessels to be separate branches and call them medullary arteries (the term medulla, L., middle, refers to the spinal cord). These authors believe that the medullary arteries contribute minimally or not at all to the vascularization of the roots. Others (Brockstein, Johns, and Gewertz, 1994; Lu et al., 1996; Tator and Koyanagi, 1997; Lo et al., 2002; White and Le-Khoury, 2002) refer to the vessels that supply nerve roots and rootlets and then continue medially to reinforce the anterior or posterior spinal arteries as radiculomedullary arteries, because they are considered to be radicular branches that continue to anastomose with spinal arteries (Brockstein, Johns, and Gewertz, 1994) (see Figs. 3-15 and 3-16). This latter nomenclature is used in this text. Usually the anterior and posterior radiculomedullary arteries do not reach their respective spinal arteries at the same segmental level (Gillilan, 1958; Turnbull, Brieg, and Hassler, 1966).

Anterior Radiculomedullary Arteries

Anterior radiculomedullary (feeder) arteries (defined here as those that reach the anterior spinal artery) vary in number from 5 to 10. Because the anterior spinal artery sufficiently supplies the first two or three cervical segments, the anterior radiculomedullary arteries of the vertebral, ascending and deep cervical, and highest intercostal arteries in general vascularize the lower cervical and upper thoracic segments, that is, the cervical enlargement (Lazorthes et al., 1971). Turnbull, Brieg, and Hassler (1966) did microdissection and microangiographic studies on the C3 to T1 cord segments of 43 cadavers. They discovered a range of one to six anterior radiculomedullary arteries, which were found as often on the left as on the right sides. Of the 43 spinal cords studied, 13 had a total of only two anterior radiculomedullary arteries, and another 13 had a total of four arteries reinforcing the cord. However, 39 of 43 had at least one anterior radiculomedullary artery at the C7 or C8 segment.

Anterior radiculomedullary arteries from the intercostal and lumbar arteries are found primarily on the left side (Turnbull, 1973; Carpenter, 1991), possibly because the aorta is on the left. Although the thoracic cord segments are the longest, usually just one to four anterior radiculomedullary arteries are present. As an anterior radiculomedullary artery approaches the ventral median fissure, it often sends a branch into the pial plexus on the

cord's lateral side. It then bifurcates, usually branching gently up and sharply down before uniting with the anterior spinal artery. If both right and left anterior radiculomedullary arteries join the anterior spinal artery at the same level, the anastomosis becomes diamond shaped (Turnbull, Brieg, and Hassler, 1966).

The largest anterior radiculomedullary artery was first described in 1882 by Albert Adamkiewicz and subsequently named the artery of Adamkiewicz. It is also called the arteria radicularis magna of Adamkiewicz, great anterior medullary artery, segmental medullary artery, great radicular artery, arteria radiculo-medullaris, or the artery of the lumbar enlargement because of its area of distribution (Turnbull, 1973; Zhang et al., 1995; Bowen and Pattany, 1999; Krauss, 1999; Milen et al., 1999; Pawlina and Maciejewska, 2002). Within the IVF, the artery of Adamkiewicz is located at the rostral or middle region, ventral and slightly rostral to the union of the dorsal root ganglion and ventral root (Alleyne et al., 1998). Although most anterior radiculomedullary arteries range from 0.2 to 0.8 mm in diameter, the diameter of the artery of Adamkiewicz is typically larger. Various reports describe it to range from 0.5 to 1.49 mm (Turnbull, 1973; Alleyne et al., 1998; Koshino et al., 1999; Biglioli et al., 2000). In general the artery enters the vertebral canal most frequently (68% to 80% of the time) on the left side (Turnbull, 1973; Alleyne et al., 1998; Koshino et al., 1999; Biglioli et al., 2000) as a branch of a posterior intercostal or lumbar artery within the range of lower thoracic and upper lumbar levels (i.e., from T8 to L3) (Turnbull, 1973; Alleyne et al., 1998; Koshino et al., 1999; Biglioli et al., 2000). It also has been located with a midthoracic T5 to T8 root (15%), in which case a lower lumbar anterior radiculomedullary artery is present and is called the artery of the conus medullaris. Lo et al. (2002) reported an anatomic variation of the artery of Adamkiewicz (three cases out of 4000 angiographies) in which the fourth lumbar artery supplied the anterior spinal artery of the conus medullaris. Before reaching the anterior spinal artery, the artery of Adamkiewicz supplements the posterior spinal artery by providing an anastomotic branch. When it reaches the anterior spinal artery, the artery of Adamkiewicz makes an abrupt caudal ("hairpin" in appearance) turn dividing into a large descending and small ascending branch (Lazorthes et al., 1971; Turnbull, 1973; Bowen and Pattany, 1999; Biglioli et al., 2000). This artery is the predominant source of blood to the lower two thirds or one half of the cord (deGroot and Chusid, 1988; Williams et al., 1995; Zhang et al., 1995). Zhang et al. (1995) calculated that the arterial resistance would be 14.8 times greater in the anterior spinal artery above the anastomosis with the artery of Adamkiewicz than below. This puts the lower thoracic cord, which relies on its blood supply from the artery of Adamkiewicz flowing in a cephalad direction, at a higher risk of ischemic damage than lumbar segments, if the artery of Adamkiewicz is compromised.

Posterior Radiculomedullary Arteries

Posterior radiculomedullary arteries (defined here as those that reach the posterior spinal arteries) vary in number from 10 to 23 and outnumber the anterior radiculomedullary arteries. They range in diameter from 0.2 to 0.5 mm (Turnbull, 1973), which generally is smaller than an average anterior radiculomedullary artery, and they are largest in the cervical and lumbar cord segments (Bowen and Pattany, 1999). Turnbull, Brieg, and Hassler (1966) showed that in the C3 to T1 segments of 43 cadavers, the number of posterior radiculomedullary arteries ranged from zero to eight. Only two or three posterior radiculomedullary arteries were found in 75% of the cadavers, and of those, most were found coursing with lower cervical roots. No relationship seemed to exist between anterior and posterior

radiculomedullary arteries concerning their number and position. Although posterior radiculomedullary arteries often enter on the left side, they are less prone to do so than the anterior radiculomedullary arteries (Carpenter, 1991). Also, as it nears the posterior spinal artery, which it reinforces, the posterior radiculomedullary artery often gives a small branch to the pial plexus on the cord's lateral side.

Arterial Supply of the Internal Cord

Having discussed the location of the spinal arteries on the external surface of the spinal cord, it is pertinent to elaborate on the vascularization of the underlying nervous tissue. The spinal cord tissue is vascularized by branches of the anterior spinal artery, posterior spinal anastomotic channels, and their interconnecting vessels. The unpaired anterior spinal artery that lies in the ventral median fissure periodically gives off a single branch, which is called the *central*, or *sulcal, branch* (Fig. 3-16).

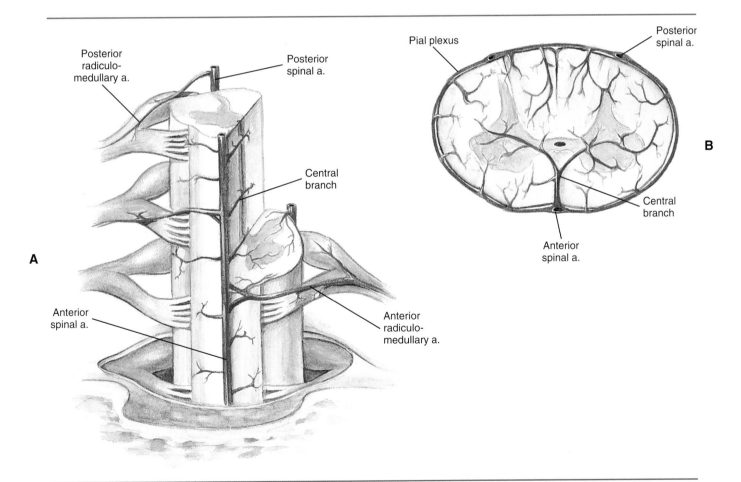

FIG. 3-16   Cross section of the spinal cord showing the arterial blood supply. **A,** Radiculomedullary arteries reinforce the spinal arteries. The anterior spinal artery gives off central branches. **B,** Note the spinal cord areas vascularized by the anterior spinal artery and by the posterior spinal arteries.

Compared with the distance between central branches in the cervical cord, the distance is greater between these branches in thoracic segments and is less between branches in lumbar and sacral segments (Hassler, 1966). The central branch comes off at right angles in the lumbar and sacral segments, but comes off at an acute superior or inferior angle in the cervical and thoracic cord (Hassler, 1966; Turnbull, 1973). Its length is approximately 4.5 mm, and the central branch courses deep into the fissure, alternately turning to the left or right.

In addition, the central branches are more numerous and larger in the cervical and lumbar regions and less frequent in the thoracic region (Gillilan, 1958; Turnbull, 1973; Carpenter, 1991; Kiernan, 1998). In the human cord these arteries number between 250 and 300 (Gillilan, 1958). The anterior spinal artery produces five to eight central branches per centimeter in the cervical region, two to six branches per centimeter in the thoracic region, and five to twelve branches per centimeter in the lumbar and sacral regions (Turnbull, 1973). The widest average diameter of the central branch is in the lumbar region (0.23 mm), followed by cervical (0.21 mm), upper sacral (0.20 mm), and thoracic (0.14 mm). As the branches of the central arteries vascularize the cord, they extend superiorly and inferiorly and overlap each other, particularly in the lumbar and sacral segments. Tator and Koyangi (1997) studied a small sample of cervical cords and determined that the overlap was such that each segment of gray matter was vascularized by capillaries from two to three central arteries.

In addition to the vascularization of the deep tissue, an interconnecting plexus of arteriolar size vessels called the pial peripheral plexus, or vasocorona, is located in the pia mater encircling the spinal cord. The dorsal and ventral aspects of the pial plexus are formed from small branches of the posterior and anterior spinal arteries, respectively. The lateral aspects of the pial plexus are formed by branches from both spinal arteries and occasionally from small branches of the radicular (radiculomedullary) arteries (Gillilan, 1958; Turnbull, 1973; Carpenter, 1991; Kiernan, 1998). The pial plexus vascularizes a band of white matter on the periphery of the spinal cord. Much overlap occurs between the distributions of the central arteries and the peripheral plexus. When one considers all branches, the anterior spinal artery vascularizes roughly the ventral two thirds of the cross-sectional area of the spinal cord. This area includes the ventral horn, lateral horn, central gray matter, base of the dorsal horn, and the majority of the ventral and lateral funiculi. The posterior spinal artery, in conjunction with the pial plexus, vascularizes the remainder of the cord. This includes the bulk of the dorsal horn and dorsal funiculus and outer rim of the lateral and ventral funiculi (Tator and Koyanagi, 1997; Afifi and Bergman, 1998; Bowen and Pattany, 1999; Krauss, 1999; Nolte,

2002) (Fig. 3-16, B). In the C3 to T1 segments, the top of the dorsal horn is particularly well vascularized (Turnbull, Brieg, and Hassler, 1966).

When one studies the details of the arterial supply, it is apparent that at any given level of the spinal cord, a direct relationship exists between the size of the anterior spinal artery and radiculomedullary artery and the amount of gray matter, as seen in cross section (Gillilan, 1958). Because gray matter has a higher metabolic rate than white matter (Gillilan, 1958) and includes the regions of highest neuronal density, the capillaries are denser in gray matter, especially around the top of the dorsal horn and the ventral horn cells, than in the white matter. In addition, studies suggest that because there are more neurons in cervical and lumbosacral regions and that those neurons have a high metabolic rate because they innervate the extremities, these levels contain a richer capillary bed than the midthoracic region (Duggal and Lach, 2002). Concerning the white matter of the cord, the dorsal and lateral white funiculi have a more extensive capillary supply than the ventral white funiculus (Turnbull, 1973).

The distribution of the anterior and posterior spinal arteries to the cross-sectional area of the spinal cord is clinically important and much research has been devoted to this topic. Any interruption of the vascular supply to the spinal cord (aorta, segmental arteries, radiculomedullary branches, spinal arteries, and intrinsic vessels) can cause ischemia and cell necrosis, resulting in serious functional deficits.

Because the spinal arteries alone are unable to supply the spinal cord sufficiently, the radiculomedullary supply is critical. In the mid- to upper thoracic spinal cord segments, especially around T4-6, reinforcing radiculomedullary arteries originating from intercostal segmental arteries are scarce; therefore this area has been described as a watershed zone of ischemic vulnerability. For example, ischemia can develop if one radiculomedullary artery is occluded and another is insufficient. Duggal and Lach (2002) studied 66 human spinal cords demonstrating global ischemic changes resulting from cardiac arrest or a severe hypotensive episode. In all cases, histologic changes were seen in the gray matter (in the large neurons in the ventral horn and in Clarke's nucleus of the low thoracic and lumbar segments), but only in the most severe cases was a narrow rim of white matter affected. In addition, their data showed that the area that most commonly revealed ischemic change was the lumbosacral region (69.7%). The thoracic cord was affected only 7.6% of the time and always in association with another cord region. It is possible that the large number of metabolically active neurons in the ventral horn of the lumbosacral region explains these results, even though the thoracic cord is called the watershed zone based on the anatomic studies of its regional blood supply.

Because the artery of Adamkiewicz is typically the only artery to supply a significant amount of blood to the lumbosacral cord, it is of supreme clinical, surgical, and radiologic importance. Unfortunately, the blood flow in this artery, and in any radiculomedullary artery, can be directly or indirectly disrupted for various reasons, including the following: during surgical treatment of descending thoracic and thoracoabdominal aortic aneurysms (Alleyne et al., 1998; Koshino et al., 1999; Biglioli et al., 2000; FitzGerald and Folan-Curran, 2002); thoracic aortic dissection causing an expanding blood clot in the aortic wall (Snell, 2001); leaking aneurysm putting direct pressure on the lumbar arteries (Snell, 2001); acute aortic dissection (which commonly presents as an abrupt onset of pain localized to the chest, neck, or back with additional signs of systemic distress) (Patel, Curtis, and Weiner, 2002); elective coronary artery bypass grafting resulting in microembolization of atherosclerotic plaques or cholesterol emboli that then enter a segmental artery (Geyer, Maik, and Pillai, 2002); hereditary protein S deficiency (a congenital deficiency in coagulation inhibitors) (Ramelli et al., 2001); and postural compression of the second right lumbar artery by the diaphragmatic crus (Rogopoulos et al., 2000). Also, any obstruction to venous return resulting in spinal cord edema (FitzGerald and Folan-Curran, 2002), and any operation in which severe hypotension occurs (Snell, 2001), can compromise blood flow to the spinal cord, resulting in loss of cord function.

Although less common, direct occlusion of the anterior spinal artery may occur from such circumstances as thrombosis, embolus, herniated disc compression, and tumors. Such occlusion results in spinal cord ischemia (Gillilan, 1958; Turnbull, 1973; Morris and Phil, 1989). Lesions affecting the anterior spinal arterial region of distribution are more common than those affecting the posterior spinal arterial region (Gillilan, 1958; Daube et al., 1986).

The consequences of an infarct are devastating in terms of the loss of function. Damage is to the areas that house cell bodies of motor neurons (ventral horn), descending motor pathways (lateral white matter), and the ascending pain and temperature pathways (ventrolateral white matter) (see Chapter 9). In these cases the posterior spinal arterial distribution to the dorsal one third of the spinal cord, which includes the pathway for vibration, position sense, and discriminatory touch (dorsal white funiculus), is left intact. Several cases in the late 1800s and early 1900s established that a lesion causing insufficient vascularization to the area of distribution of the anterior spinal artery could frequently and clearly be diagnosed clinically (Gillilan, 1958). This lesion has subsequently been called the *anterior spinal artery syndrome* and presents with sudden bilateral loss of pain and temperature sense below the level of the lesion with a preservation of vibratory and position sense (dissociated sensory loss), motor deficits (usually paraplegia) below the level of the lesion, and loss of bladder and bowel control. Painful dysesthesia develops in some patients approximately 6 to 8 months after the onset of symptoms. This phenomenon is explained by either the misinterpretation of sensory input by the brain resulting from the imbalance created between the lesioned ventrolateral white matter and normal dorsal white matter, or by a sparing of the spinoreticulothalamic tract, which allows nociceptive impulses to pass to the reticular formation and thalamus (Afifi and Bergman, 1998).

VENOUS DRAINAGE OF THE SPINAL CORD

The venous system found within the vertebral canal consists of an epidural, or internal, vertebral venous plexus, located in the epidural space (see Chapter 2), and also an irregular venous plexus lying on the cord. This entire venous system is devoid of valves and anastomoses freely with itself.

The venous system of the cord is a tortuous plexus that consists of six variable longitudinal veins: three anterior and three posterior (Fig. 3-17, *A*). The anteromedian vein is located deep in the ventral median fissure and has an average diameter ranging between 0.5 to 1.5 mm. It is a single vessel in the lumbar region but is accompanied by two anterolateral veins in the thoracic and cervical segments (Bowen and Pattany, 1999). These anterior venous channels receive blood from the neural tissue via sulcal veins and subsequently drain into anterior radiculomedullary veins. (Note: The nomenclature used for these vessels is inconsistent [Brockstein, Johns, and Gewertz, 1994; Bowen and Pattany, 1999; Krauss, 1999]. This text uses radiculomedullary to identify the veins draining the cord [which are variable in number] and roots [which are present at every level].) The anterior radiculomedullar vessels range in number from 10 to 20 (Bowen and Pattany, 1999), and empty into the epidural venous plexus. In the lumbar region, there may be one large anterior radiculomedullary vein, the vena radicularis magna (Carpenter, 1991; Brockstein, Johns, and Gewertz, 1994; Bowen and Pattany, 1999; Krauss, 1999), which usually courses with one of the left nerve roots located between the T11 and L3 spinal cord segments. The posterior aspect of the cord has a similar venous pattern. A midline posteromedian vein is the dominant vessel in the lumbar area with two posterolateral veins accompanying it in other regions. These drain the dorsal funiculus, dorsal gray horns, and their adjacent lateral white matter. These posteromedian and posterolateral veins in turn become tributaries of posterior radiculomedullary veins, which number the same as, or more than, the anterior radiculomedullary veins (Bowen and Pattany, 1999). The posterior radiculomedullary veins

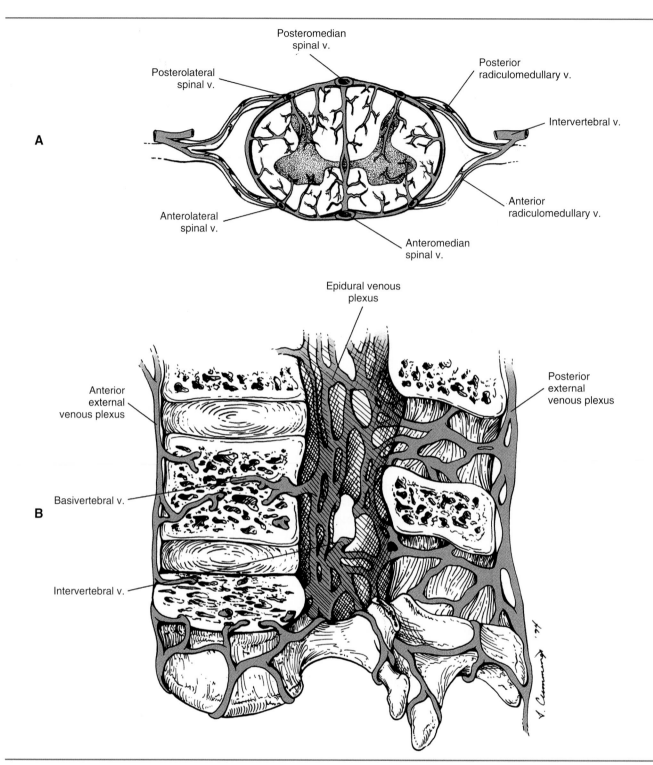

FIG. 3-17 Venous drainage of the spinal cord. **A,** Cross section of the spinal cord. **B,** Median view of the vertebral canal. The spinal cord has been removed to show the epidural venous plexus

empty into the epidural venous plexus. At the level of the dorsal root ganglion, the posterior radiculomedullary vein receives blood from the parenchyma of the dorsal root ganglion via a periganglionic venous plexus located on the surface of the ganglion (Parke and Whalen, 2002). A large posterior radiculomedullary vein also is found in the lumbar region, and usually is seen accompanying a L1 or L2 root. Using MR angiography images, the intersection of either an anterior or posterior radiculomedullary vein with a spinal vein (e.g., anteromedian vein) can be identified by its "coat hook" appearance, which distinguishes it from the "hairpin" look of the artery of Adamkiewicz (Bowen and Pattany, 1999). As also seen in the arterial system, an encompassing venous vasocorona interconnects the six longitudinal veins.

The epidural (internal vertebral) venous plexus, which drains blood not only from the cord but also from bone and red bone marrow, consists of several anterior and posterior longitudinal and interconnecting vessels. At the level of the foramen magnum, it forms a dense network that communicates with vertebral veins. In addition, it is continuous with the dural venous sinuses (occipital and sigmoid) and venous channels (basilar plexus, venous plexus of the hypoglossal canal, and the emissary veins of the condyles [Williams et al., 1995]) within the skull (see Chapter 2). This plexus also drains into intervertebral veins in the IVFs and also into another longitudinally arranged plexus, the external vertebral venous plexus (Fig. 3-17, B). From intervertebral veins, venous blood drains into segmental veins such as the vertebral, intercostal, lumbar, and lateral sacral veins (Williams et al., 1995). These segmental veins lie outside the vertebral column. Chapter 2 provides a full description of the external and internal vertebral venous plexuses.

A metastatic tumor in the epidural space may damage the cord by impeding venous return and cause vasogenic edema (Grant et al., 1991). Also, because the internal and external vertebral venous plexuses lack valves, allowing blood flow through the intervertebral veins (which communicate with segmental veins) to be reversed, the opportunity exists for cancer to metastasize from such areas as the prostate, lung, breast, and thyroid gland to the brain and vertebral bodies (Williams et al., 1995; FitzGerald and Folan-Curran, 2002) (see Chapter 2).

REFERENCES

Afifi AK & Bergman RA. (1998). *Functional neuroanatomy: Text and atlas*. St Louis: McGraw-Hill.

Alleyne CH Jr et al. (1998). Microsurgical anatomy of the artery of Adamkiewicz and its segmental artery. *J Neurosurg, 89*, 791-795.

Arai Y et al. (2001). Magnetic resonance imaging observation of the conus medullaris. *Bull Hosp Jt Dis, 60*, 10-12.

Barbaix E et al. (1996). Anterior sacrodural attachments: Trolard's ligaments revisited. *Man Ther, 2*, 88-91.

Benarroch EE et al. (1999). *Medical neurosciences: An approach to anatomy, pathology, and physiology by systems and levels* (4th ed.). Baltimore: Lippincott Williams & Wilkins.

Biglioli P et al. (2000). The anterior spinal artery: The main arterial supply of the human spinal cord: A preliminary anatomic study. *J Thorac Cardiovasc Surg, 119*, 376-379.

Boulton M et al. (1996). Drainage of CSF through lymphatic pathways and arachnoid villi in sheep: Measurement of 125I-albumin clearance. *Neuropathol Appl Neurobiol, 22*, 325-333.

Bowen BC & Pattany PM. (1999). Vascular anatomy and disorders of the lumbar spine and spinal cord. *Magn Reson Imaging Clin North Am, 7*, 555-571.

Brockstein B, Johns L, & Gewertz BL. (1994). Blood supply to the spinal cord: Anatomic and physiologic correlations. *Ann Vasc Surg, 8*, 394-399.

Carpenter MB. (1991). *Core text of neuroanatomy* (4th ed.). Baltimore: Williams & Wilkins.

Choi D, Carroll N, & Abrahams P. (1996). Spinal cord diameters in cadaveric specimens and magnetic resonance scans, to assess embalming artefacts. *Surg Radiol Anat, 18*, 133-135.

Coggeshall RE. (1980). Law of separation of function of the spinal roots. *Physiol Rev, 60*, 716-755.

Daube JR et al. (1986). *Medical neurosciences* (2nd ed.). Boston: Little, Brown.

Davidoff RA & Hackman JC. (1991). Aspects of spinal cord structure and reflex function. *Neurol Clin, 9*, 533-550.

Dean NA & Mitchell BS. (2002). Anatomic relation between the nuchal ligment (ligamentum nuchae) and the spinal dura mater in the craniocervical region. *Clin Anat, 15*, 182-185.

deGroot J & Chusid JG. (1988). *Correlative neuroanatomy* (20th ed.). East Norwalk, Conn: Appleton & Lange.

Demiryürek D et al. (2002). MR imaging determination of the normal level of conus medullaris. *Clin Imag, 26*, 375-377.

Djindjian M et al. (1988). The normal vascularization of the intradural filum terminale in man. *Surg Radiol Anat, 10*, 201-209.

Duggal N & Lach B. (2002). Selective vulnerability of the lumbosacral spinal cord after cardiac arrest and hypotension. *Stroke, 33*, 116-126.

Elliott HC. (1945). Cross-sectional diameters and areas of the human spinal cord. *Anat Rec, 93*, 287-293.

FitzGerald MJT & Folan-Curran J. (2002). *Clinical neuroanatomy and related neuroscience* (4th ed.). Edinburgh: WB Saunders.

Fountas KN et al. (1998). Cervical spinal cord: Smaller than considered? *Spine, 23*, 1513-1516.

Fricke B, Andres KH, & Von During M. (2001). Nerve fibers innervating the cranial and spinal meninges: Morphology of nerve fiber terminals and their structural integration. *Microsc Res Tech, 53*, 96-105.

Fujiwara K et al. (1988). Morphometry of the cervical spinal cord and its relation to pathology in cases with compression myelopathy. *Spine, 13*, 1212-1216.

Geyer TE, Maik MJ, & Pillai R. (2002). Anterior spinal artery syndrome after elective coronary artery bypass grafting. *Ann Thorac Surg, 73*, 1971-1973.

Gillilan LA. (1958). The arterial blood supply of the human spinal cord. *J Comp Neurol, 110*, 75-103.

Gövsa F et al. (1996). Origin of the anterior spinal artery. *Surg Radiol Anat, 18*, 189-193.

Grant R et al. (1991). Changes in intracranial CSF volume after lumbar puncture and their relationship to post-LP headache. *J Neurol Neurosurg Psychiatry, 54*, 440-442.

Greathouse DG, Halle JS, & Dalley II AF. (2001). Blood supply to the spinal cord. *Phys Ther, 81*, 1264-1265.

Groen GJ, Baljet B, & Drukker J. (1988). The innervation of the spinal dura mater: Anatomy and clinical implications. *Acta Neurochir (Wien), 92*, 39-46.

Hackney DB. (1992). Normal anatomy. *Top Magn Reson Imaging, 4*, 1-6.

Haines DE, Harkey HL, & Al-Mefty O. (1993). The "subdural" space: A new look at an outdated concept. *Neurosurgery, 32*, 111-120.

Hamandi K et al. (2002). Irreversible damage to the spinal cord following spinal anesthesia. *Neurology, 59*, 624-626.

Hansasuta A, Tubbs RS, & Oakes WJ. (1999). Filum terminale fusion and dural sac termination: Study in 27 cadavers. *Pediatr Neurosurg, 30*, 176-179.

Hassler O. (1966). Blood supply to the human spinal cord. *Arch Neurol, 15*, 302-307.

Hewitt W. (1970). The intervertebral foramen. *Physiotherapy, 56*, 332-336.

Hogan QH et al. (1996). Magnetic resonance imaging of cerebrospinal fluid volume and the influence of body habitus and abdominal pressure. *Anesthesiology, 84,* 1341-1349.

Humphreys BK et al. (2003). Investigation of connective tissue attachments to the cervical spinal dura mater. *Clin Anat, 16,* 152-159.

Johnston M & Papaiconomou C. (2002). Cerebrospinal fluid transport: A lymphatic perspective. *News Physiol Sci, 17,* 227-230.

Kameyama T, Hashizume Y, & Sobue G. (1996). Morphologic features of the normal human cadaveric spinal cord. *Spine, 21,* 1285-1290.

Kandel ER & Siegelbaum SA. (2000). Overview of synaptic transmission. In ER Kandel, JH Schwartz, & TM Jessell. (Eds.). *Principles of neural science* (4th ed.). St Louis: McGraw-Hill.

Kiernan JA. (1998). *Barr's the human nervous system* (7th ed.). Philadelphia: JB Lippincott.

Kershner D & Binhammer R. (2002). Lumbar intrathecal ligaments. *Clin Anat, 15,* 82-87.

Koshino T et al. (1999). Does the Adamkiewicz artery originate from the larger segmental arteries? *J Thorac Cardiovasc Surg, 117,* 898-905.

Krauss WE. (1999). Vascular anatomy of the spinal cord. *Neurosurg Clin N Am, 10,* 9-15.

Laterra J & Goldstein GW. (2000). Ventricular organization of cerebrospinal fluid: Blood-brain barrier, brain edema, and hydrocephalus. In ER Kandel, JH Schwartz, & TM Jessell (Eds.). *Principles of neural science* (4th ed.). St Louis: McGraw-Hill.

Lazorthes G et al. (1971). Arterial vascularization of the spinal cord. *J Neurosurg, 35,* 253-262.

Lo D et al. (2002). Unusual origin of the artery of Adamkiewicz from the fourth lumbar artery. *Neuroradiology, 44,* 153-157.

Lu J et al. (1996). Vulnerability of great medullary artery. *Spine, 21,* 1852-1855.

Macdonald A et al. (1999). Level of termination of the spinal cord and the dural sac: A magnetic resonance study. *Clin Anat, 12,* 149-152.

Makino M et al. (1996). Morphometric study of myelinated fibers in human cervical spinal cord white matter. *Spine, 21(9),* 1010-1016.

Malas MA et al. (2000). The relationship between the lumbosacral enlargement and the conus medullaris during the period of fetal development and adulthood. *Surg Radiol Anat, 22,* 163-168.

Milen MT et al. (1999). Albert Adamkiewicz, 1850–1921: His artery and its significance for the retroperitoneal surgeon. *World J Urol, 17,* 168-170.

Milhorat TH, Kotzen RM, & Anzil AP. (1994). Stenosis of central canal of spinal cord in man: Incidence and pathological findings in 232 autopsy cases. *J Neurosurg, 80,* 716-722.

Miura M, Kato S, & von Ludinghausen M. (1998). Lymphatic drainage of the cerebrospinal fluid from monkey spinal meninges with special reference to the distribution of the epidural lymphatics. *Arch Histol Cytol, 61,* 277-286.

Mokri B. (2001). The Monro-Kellie hypothesis. *Neurology, 56,* 1746-1748.

Moore KL & Persaud TVN. (1998). *The developing human: Clinically oriented embryology,* (6th ed.). Philadelphia: WB Saunders.

Morris JH & Phil D. (1989). The nervous system. In RS Cotran, V Kumar, & SL Robbins (Eds.). *Robbins pathologic basis of disease,* (4th ed.). Philadelphia: WB Saunders.

Nolte J. (2002). *The human brain: An introduction to its functional anatomy* (5th ed.). St Louis: Mosby.

Nordqvist L. (1964). The sagittal diameter of the spinal cord and subarachnoid space in different age groups. A roentgenographic post-mortem study. *Acta Radiol, 227,* 1-96.

Parke WW & Whalen JL. (2002). The vascular pattern of the human dorsal root ganglion and its probable bearing on a compartment syndrome. *Spine, 27,* 347-352.

Patel NM, Curtis R, & Weiner BK. (2002). Aortic dissection presenting as an acute cauda equina syndrome: A case report. *J Bone Joint Surg Am, 84-A,* 1430-1432.

Pawlina W & Maciejewska I. (2002). Albert Wojciech Adamkiewicz, 1850–1921. *Clin Anat, 15,* 318-320.

Pinto FCG et al. (2002). Anatomic study of the filum terminale and its correlations with the tethered cord syndrome. *Neurosurgery, 51,* 725-730.

Ramelli GP et al. (2001). Anterior spinal artery syndrome in an adolescent with protein S deficiency. *J Child Neurol, 16,* 134-135.

Reimann AF & Anson BJ. (1944). Vertebral level of termination of the spinal cord with report of a case of sacral cord. *Anat Rec, 88,* 127-138.

Reina MA et al. (1997). New perspectives in the microscopic structure of human dura mater in the dorsolumbar region. *Reg Anesth, 22,* 161-166.

Reina MA et al. (1998). Does the subdural space exist? *Rev Esp Anestesiol Reanim, 45,* 367-376.

Reina MA et al. (2002). The origin of the spinal subdural space: Ultrastructure findings. *Anesth Analg, 94,* 991-995.

Rexed B. (1952). The cytoarchitectonic organization of the spinal cord in the cat. *J Comp Neurol, 96,* 415-495.

Reynolds F. (2001). Damage to the conus medullaris following spinal anaesthesia. *Anaesthesia, 56,* 238-247.

Rogopoulos A et al. (2000). Lumbar artery compression by the diaphragmatic crus: A new etiology for spinal cord ischemia. *Ann Neurol, 48,* 261-264.

Saifuddin A, Burnett SJD, & White J. (1998). A magnetic resonance imaging study. *Spine, 23,* 1452-1456.

Schoenen J. (1991). Clinical anatomy of the spinal cord. *Neurol Clin, 9,* 503-532.

Snell RS. (2001). *Clinical neuroanatomy for medical students* (5th ed.). Baltimore: Lippincott Williams & Wilkins.

Storer KP et al. (1998). The central canal of the human spinal cord: A computerised 3-D study. *J Anat, 192,* 565-572.

Tator CH & Koyanagi I. (1997). Vascular mechanisms in the pathophysiology of human spinal cord injury. *J Neurosurg, 86,* 483-492.

Tubbs RS et al. (2001). The denticulate ligament: Anatomy and functional significance. *J Neurosurg Spine, 94,* 271-275.

Turnbull IM. (1973). Blood supply of the spinal cord: Normal and pathological considerations. *Clin Neurosurg, 20,* 56-84.

Turnbull IM, Brieg A, & Hassler O. (1966). Blood supply of cervical spinal cord in man. *J Neurosurg, 24,* 951-966.

Vandenabeele F, Creemers J, & Lambrichts I. (1996). Ultrastructure of the human spinal arachnoid mater and dura mater. *J Anat, 189,* 417-430.

White ML & El-Khoury GY. (2002). Neurovascular injuries of the spinal cord. *Eur J Rad, 42,* 117-126.

Williams PL et al. (1995). *Gray's anatomy* (38th ed.). Edinburgh: Churchill Livingstone.

Willis WD Jr & Coggeshall RE. (1991). *Sensory mechanisms of the spinal cord* (2nd ed.). New York: Plenum Press.

Yamada S & Lonser RR. (2000). Adult tethered cord syndrome. *J Spin Disord, 13,* 319-323.

Yasui K et al. (1999). Age-related morphologic changes of the central canal of the human spinal cord. *Acta Neuropathol, 97,* 253-259.

Zhang T et al. (1995). The size of the anterior spinal artery in relation to the arteria medullaris magna anterior in humans. *Clin Anat, 8,* 347-351.

CHAPTER 4

Muscles That Influence the Spine

Barclay W. Bakkum
Gregory D. Cramer

Second only to the vertebral column and spinal cord, the muscles of the spine are the most important structures of the back. A thorough understanding of the back muscles is fundamental to a comprehensive understanding of the spine and its function. The purpose of this chapter is to discuss the muscles of the back and other muscles that have an indirect influence on the spine. The intercostal muscles provide an example of the latter category. These muscles do not actually attach to the spine, but their action can influence the spine by virtue of their attachment to the ribs. The abdominal wall muscles, diaphragm, hamstrings, and others can be placed into this same category. These muscles have a less direct yet important influence on the spine. Chapter 5 discusses the sternocleidomastoid, scalene, suprahyoid, and infrahyoid muscles.

The musculature of the spine and trunk plays an important role in the normal functioning of the vertebral column. Beside their obvious ability to create the variety of spinal movements, many of these muscles also help to maintain posture. In addition, the back and trunk muscles function as shock absorbers, acting to disperse loads applied to the spine. The shear bulk of these muscles also protects the spine and viscera from outside forces.

Although it is beyond the scope of this text to detail the kinesiology of the muscles influencing the spine, a few generalities are in order. There is a complicated interplay of many muscles when a motion of the body, especially of the spine, is produced. Sometimes this is termed muscle coordination. Some of the specifics of this complex interplay are only beginning to be understood, especially in asymmetric motions of the trunk (van Dieen, 1996; Danneels et al., 2001; Andersson et al., 2002). Muscles known as prime movers are the most important. Other muscles, known as synergists, assist the prime movers. For example, the psoas major and rectus abdominis muscles are prime movers of the spine during flexion of the lumbar spine from a supine position, as in the performance of a sit-up. However, the erector spinae muscles also undergo an eccentric contraction toward the end of the sit-up. This contraction of the erector spinae helps to control the motion of the trunk and allows a graceful, safe accomplishment of the movement. The erector spinae muscles are acting as synergists in this instance.

Besides producing motion, muscle contraction also stabilizes the spine by making it stiffer. This is important not only for posture (Cholewicki et al., 1997; Quint et al., 1998), but also for providing a stable base for other motions of the body, such as appendicular motions (Lorimer Moseley et al., 2002).

Muscle coordination seems to be under the control of the central nervous system. The central nervous system is constantly receiving afferent information from the muscles and other surrounding tissues, such as ligaments and tendons. On the basis of this information, the central nervous system appears to use reflex pathways to finely control muscle activity. Some of the details of this process are beginning to be understood (Kang et al., 2002). Interestingly, the specifics of the interplay of the muscles in producing a motion of the body are not always constant. In other words, the same motion may not always be produced by the same muscles working together in the same way. The central nervous system can alter muscle activity depending on the circumstances, such as muscle fatigue, to accomplish the same goal (Clark et al., 2003). This appears to be especially true when there is an abnormality in the system, such as pain or abnormal joint function (McPartland et al., 1997; Hirayama et al., 2001; Lehman et al., 2001; van Dieen et al., 2003).

The muscles of the spine and other muscles associated with the back can, and frequently do, sustain injury. Other painful conditions of muscles (or fascia) are commonly seen by clinicians besides frank injury or pathology of muscles. One of these is myofascial trigger points, sometimes known as myofascial pain syndrome (Travell and Simons, 1983, 1992). Another condition is fibromyalgia or fibromyalgia syndrome (Krsnich-Shriwise, 1997). Both of these conditions are not well understood but are being increasingly accepted as true syndromes. They are similar in presentation but are distinct entities (Schneider, 1995). A complete understanding of the anatomy of the muscles associated with the spine aids in the differential diagnosis of pain arising from muscles versus pain arising from neighboring ligaments or other structures.

The back muscles are discussed from superficial to deep. This is accomplished by dividing the muscles into six layers, with layer one the most superficial and layer six the deepest. Other important muscles of the spine are described after a discussion of the six layers of back muscles. These include the suboccipital muscles, anterior and lateral muscles of the cervical spine, and iliac muscles. The muscles that have an indirect yet important influence on the spine are discussed last.

SIX LAYERS OF BACK MUSCLES

First Layer

The first layer of back muscles consists of the trapezius and latissimus dorsi muscles (Fig. 4-1). These two muscles course from the spine (and occiput) to either the shoulder girdle (scapula and clavicle) or the humerus, respectively.

Trapezius Muscle. The trapezius muscle is the most superficial and superior back muscle (see Fig. 4-1). It is a large, strong muscle that is innervated by the accessory nerve (cranial nerve XI). In addition to its innervation from the accessory nerve, the trapezius muscle receives some proprioceptive fibers from the third and fourth cervical ventral rami. Because the trapezius muscle is so large, it originates from and inserts on many structures. This muscle originates from the superior nuchal line, external occipital protuberance, ligamentum nuchae of the posterior neck, spinous processes of C7 to T12, and supraspinous ligament between C7 and T12. It inserts onto the spine of the scapula, acromion, and distal third of the clavicle. Detailed morphometric measurements have been performed on this muscle (Kamibayashi and Richmond, 1998).

Because of its size and the many locations of its attachments, the trapezius muscle also has many actions. Most of these actions result in movement of the neck and scapula (i.e., the "shoulder girdle" as a whole). The function of the trapezius depends on which region of the muscle is contracting (upper, middle, or lower). The middle portion retracts the scapula, whereas the lower portion depresses the scapula and at the same time rotates the scapula so that its lateral angle moves superiorly (i.e., rotates the point of the shoulder up). The actions of the upper part of the trapezius also depend on whether the head or neck or the scapula is stabilized. When moving the head and neck, the actions of the upper trapezius also are determined by whether the muscle is contracting unilaterally or bilaterally. There is some conflicting evidence as to whether or not the upper fibers of the trapezius muscle help in elevation of the scapula. Based upon information gathered from cadaveric dissections of the attachment points and directions of the upper fibers of the trapezius muscle, Johnson et al. (1994) concluded that these fibers do not aid in elevation of the scapula. On the other hand there is good electromyographic evidence that the upper fibers of the trapezius muscle are active during elevation of the shoulder (Campos et al., 1994; Guazzelli et al., 1994). Table 4-1 summarizes the actions of the trapezius muscle.

Latissimus Dorsi Muscle. The latissimus dorsi muscle is the most inferior and lateral of the two muscles that make up the first layer of back muscles (see Fig. 4-1). This large muscle has an extensive origin. The origin of the latissimus dorsi includes the following:

◆ Spinous processes and supraspinous ligament of T6-L5 (supraspinous ligament ends between L2 and L4)

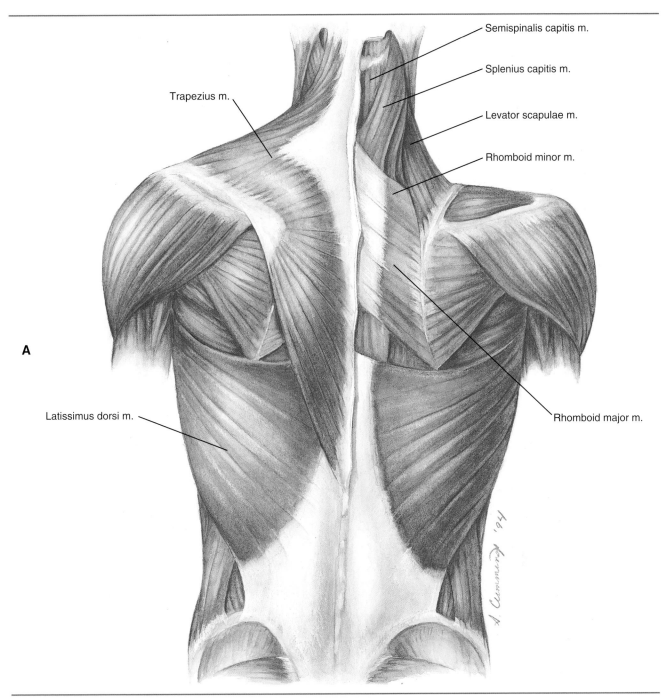

FIG. 4-1   **A,** First *(left)* and second *(right)* layers of back muscles.

Continued

- Thoracolumbar fascia
- Posterior sacrum (median sacral crest) (see Chapter 8)
- Iliac crests
- Lower four ribs

The latissimus dorsi muscle derives much of its origin from the thoracolumbar fascia. This is a tough and extensive aponeurosis (see the following discussion). The latissimus dorsi muscle passes superiorly and laterally to insert into the floor of the intertubercular groove of the humerus, between the laterally located attachment of the pectoralis major muscle and the medially located attachment of the teres major muscle. Contraction of the latissimus dorsi results in adduction, medial rotation, and extension of the humerus.

The latissimus dorsi is innervated by the thoracodorsal nerve, which is a branch of the posterior cord of

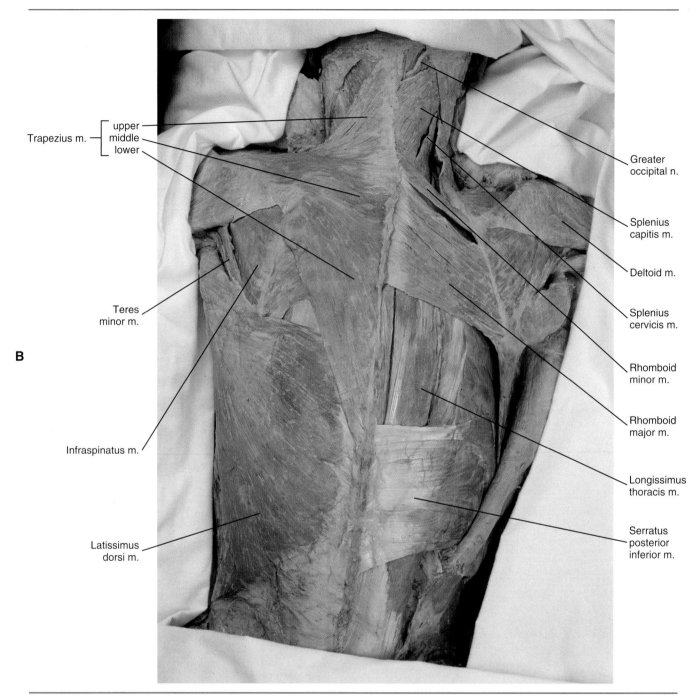

B

Trapezius m. — upper, middle, lower

Teres minor m.

Infraspinatus m.

Latissimus dorsi m.

Greater occipital n.

Splenius capitis m.

Deltoid m.

Splenius cervicis m.

Rhomboid minor m.

Rhomboid major m.

Longissimus thoracis m.

Serratus posterior inferior m.

FIG. 4-1—cont'd   **B,** Dissection of these same two layers.

the brachial plexus. The thoracodorsal nerve is derived from the anterior primary divisions of the sixth through eighth cervical nerves.

Thoracolumbar (or Lumbodorsal) Fascia. Because of its clinical significance, the anatomy of the thoracolumbar fascia deserves further discussion. This fascia extends from the thoracic region to the sacrum. It forms a thin covering over the erector spinae muscles in

the thoracic region, whereas in the lumbar region the thoracolumbar fascia is strong and is composed of three layers. The posterior layer attaches to the lumbar spinous processes, interspinous ligaments between these processes, and median sacral crest. This layer has its own superficial and deep laminae (Macintosh and Bogduk, 1987a). The middle layer attaches to the tips of the lumbar transverse processes and intertransverse ligaments and extends superiorly from the iliac crest to the twelfth

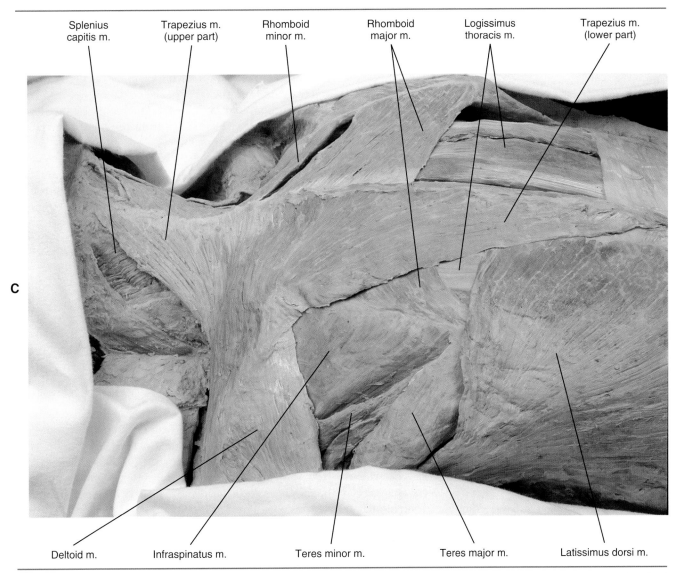

Splenius capitis m. Trapezius m. (upper part) Rhomboid minor m. Rhomboid major m. Logissimus thoracis m. Trapezius m. (lower part)

C

Deltoid m. Infraspinatus m. Teres minor m. Teres major m. Latissimus dorsi m.

FIG. 4-1—cont'd **C,** Close-up, taken from a left posterior oblique perspective. The serratus posterior inferior muscle of the third layer can also be seen in **B** and in Figure 4-2, *A* and *B.*

rib. The anterior layer covers the anterior aspect of the quadratus lumborum muscle and attaches to the anterior surfaces of the lumbar transverse processes. Superiorly the anterior layer forms the lateral arcuate ligament (see Diaphragm). The anterior layer continues inferiorly to the ilium and iliolumbar ligament. The posterior and middle layers surround the erector spinae muscles posteriorly and anteriorly, respectively (see Fifth Layer), and meet at the lateral edge of the erector spinae, where these two layers are joined by the anterior layer (Williams et al., 1995). Barker and Briggs (1999) have demonstrated in a cadaveric study that the thoracolumbar fascia may continue more superiorly than classically described. They found that the superficial lamina of the posterior layer ran superiorly to be continuous with the rhomboid muscles, whereas the deep lamina of the posterior layer

was continuous superiorly with the splenius muscles. These superior extensions of the fascia were of variable thickness, but seemed thick enough to transmit tension. This means that the thoracolumbar fascia may have a more global influence on biomechanics than thought previously.

The lateral union of the three principal layers of the thoracolumbar fascia serves as a posterior aponeurosis for origin of the transversus abdominis muscle. The direction of the fibers within each lamina of the posterior layer makes the thoracolumbar fascia stronger along its lines of greatest stress. When the thoracolumbar fascia is tractioned laterally by the action of the abdominal muscles, the distinct direction of fibers of the posterior layer's two laminae aids in extension of the spine and the maintenance of an erect posture.

Table 4-1   Functions of Trapezius Muscle

| Region of Muscle | Head and Neck Stabilized during Muscle Contraction | With Scapula Stabilized | |
		Contraction of One Side (Unilateral)	Contraction of Both Sides (Bilateral)
Upper	Elevates scapula	Extends head and neck; rotates face to opposite direction	Extends head and neck
Middle	Retracts scapula	—	—
Lower	Retracts, depresses scapula; rotates lateral angle of scapula superiorly	—	—

Some investigators believe that because the posterior and middle layers surround the erector spinae muscles, injury to these muscles at times may lead to a "compartment" type of syndrome within these two layers of the thoracolumbar fascia (Peck et al., 1986). This syndrome results from edema within the erector spinae muscles. The edema stems from injury and increases the pressure in the relatively closed compartment composed of the erector spinae muscles wrapped within the posterior and middle layers of the thoracolumbar fascia. This may result in increased pain and straightening of the lumbar lordosis (Peck et al., 1986). However, further research is necessary to determine the best approach available to diagnose this condition and the frequency with which it occurs.

Second Layer

The second layer of back muscles includes three muscles that, along with the first layer, connect the upper limb to the vertebral column. All three muscles lie deep to the trapezius muscle and insert onto the scapula's medial border. They include the rhomboid major, rhomboid minor, and levator scapulae muscles (see Fig. 4-1). Detailed morphometric measurements have been performed on them (Kamibayashi and Richmond, 1998).

Rhomboid Major and Minor Muscles. The rhomboid major muscle originates by tendinous fibers from the spinous processes of T2 through T5 and the supraspinous ligament at those levels. The muscle fibers run in an inferolateral direction and insert via a tendinous band on the medial border of the scapula between the root of the spine and the inferior angle.

The rhomboid minor muscle is located immediately superior to the rhomboid major; its fibers also run in an inferolateral direction. Beginning from the lower portion of the ligamentum nuchae and the spinous processes of C7 and T1, the rhomboid minor ends on the scapula's medial border at the level of the spinal root.

Both rhomboid muscles are innervated by the dorsal scapular nerve, which arises from the anterior primary division of the C5 spinal nerve.

Because the fibers of these two muscles are parallel, their actions are similar. In addition to the other muscles that insert on the scapula, they help stabilize its position and movement during active use of the upper extremity. Specifically, the rhomboids retract and rotate the scapula such that the lateral angle moves inferiorly (i.e., rotates the point of the shoulder down).

Levator Scapulae Muscle. The levator scapulae muscle arises by tendinous slips from the transverse processes of the atlas and axis and the posterior tubercles of the transverse processes of C3 and C4. Its fibers descend and insert onto the scapula's medial border between the spinal root and the superior angle. It is innervated by branches from the ventral rami of the C3 and C4 spinal nerves and the dorsal scapular nerve (C5). If the cervical spine is fixed, the levator scapulae helps in elevating and rotating the scapula such that the lateral angle moves inferiorly (i.e., rotates the point of the shoulder down). When the scapula is stabilized, contraction of this muscle laterally flexes and rotates the neck to the same side. Bilateral contraction helps in extension of the cervical spine.

Third Layer

The third layer of back muscles is sometimes called the intermediate layer of back muscles. This is because the two small muscles of this group lie between layers one and two (the superficial back muscles) and layers four through six (the deep back muscles).

The third layer of back muscles consists of two thin, almost quadrangular muscles: the serratus posterior superior and serratus posterior inferior (Fig. 4-2, A and B).

Serratus Posterior Superior and Serratus Posterior Inferior. The serratus posterior superior muscle originates from the spinous processes of C7 through T3 and the supraspinous ligament that runs between them. It inserts onto the posterior and superior aspect of the second through the fifth ribs. This muscle is innervated by the anterior primary divisions (ventral rami) of the second through the fifth thoracic nerves (intercostal nerves).

The serratus posterior inferior originates from the spinous processes and intervening supraspinous ligament

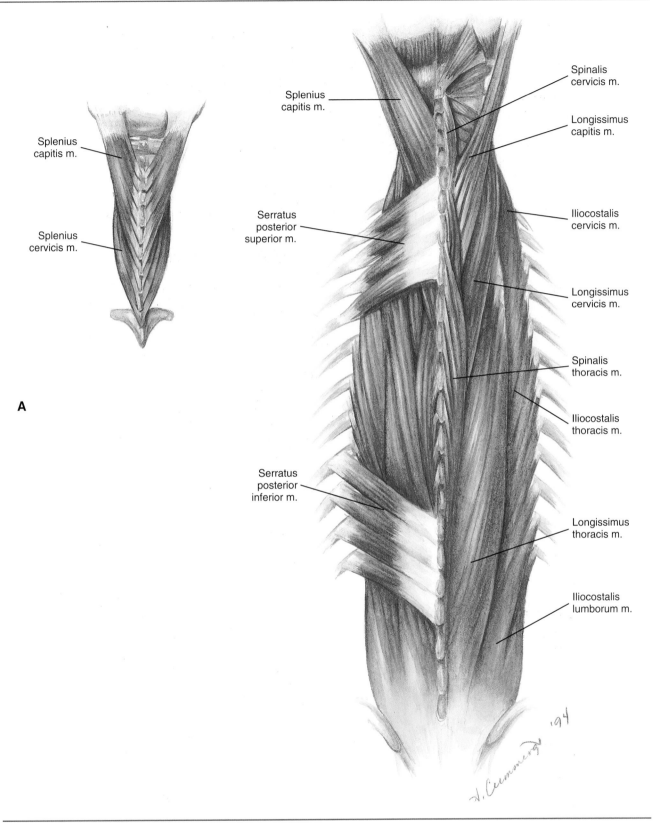

A

Splenius capitis m.

Splenius cervicis m.

Splenius capitis m.

Spinalis cervicis m.

Longissimus capitis m.

Serratus posterior superior m.

Iliocostalis cervicis m.

Longissimus cervicis m.

Spinalis thoracis m.

Iliocostalis thoracis m.

Serratus posterior inferior m.

Longissimus thoracis m.

Iliocostalis lumborum m.

FIG. 4-2   A, Third, fourth (also see inset), and fifth layers of back muscles.

Continued

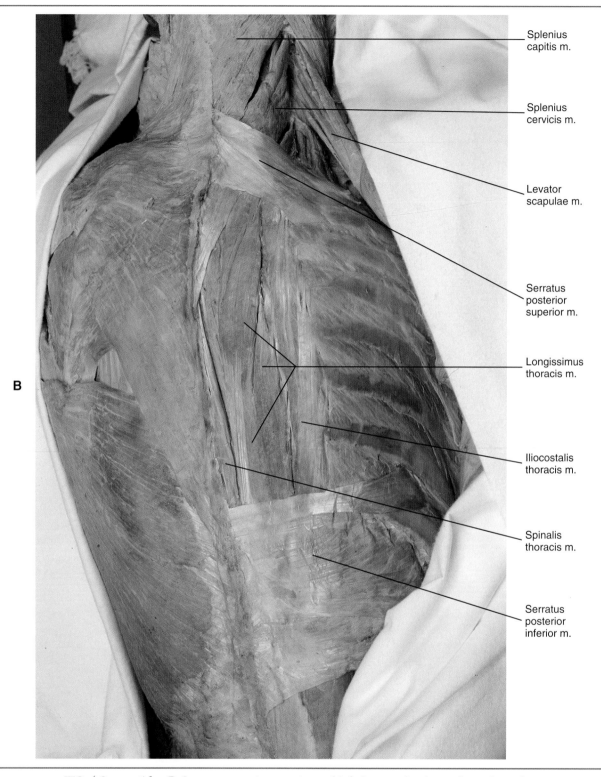

B

Splenius
capitis m.

Splenius
cervicis m.

Levator
scapulae m.

Serratus
posterior
superior m.

Longissimus
thoracis m.

Iliocostalis
thoracis m.

Spinalis
thoracis m.

Serratus
posterior
inferior m.

FIG. 4-2—cont'd **B,** Serratus posterior superior and inferior muscles that make up layer three.

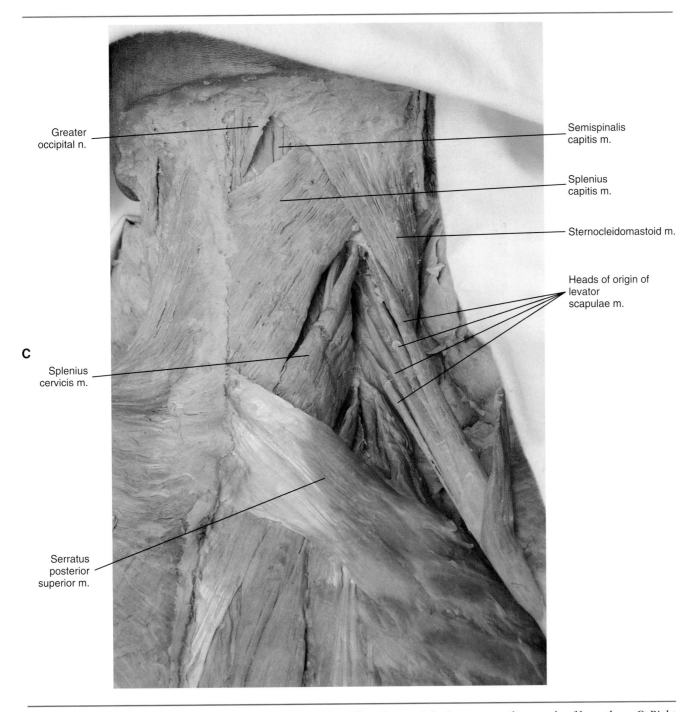

Greater
occipital n.

Semispinalis
capitis m.

Splenius
capitis m.

Sternocleidomastoid m.

Heads of origin of
levator
scapulae m.

C

Splenius
cervicis m.

Serratus
posterior
superior m.

FIG. 4-2—cont'd   **C-E,** Splenius capitis and cervicis muscles of layer four and the levator scapulae muscle of layer three. **C,** Right
posterior view.

Continued

of T11 to L2. It inserts onto the posterior and inferior surfaces of the lower four ribs and is innervated by the lower three intercostal nerves (T9 to T11) and the subcostal nerve. These nerves are all anterior primary divisions of their respective spinal nerves. The serratus posterior superior and inferior muscles may help with respiration. More specifically, the serratus posterior superior raises the second through fourth ribs, which may aid with inspiration. The serratus posterior inferior lowers the ninth through twelfth ribs, which may help with forced expiration. However, electromyographic evidence refutes a respiratory function for these muscles (Vilensky et al., 2001); they may function primarily in proprioception.

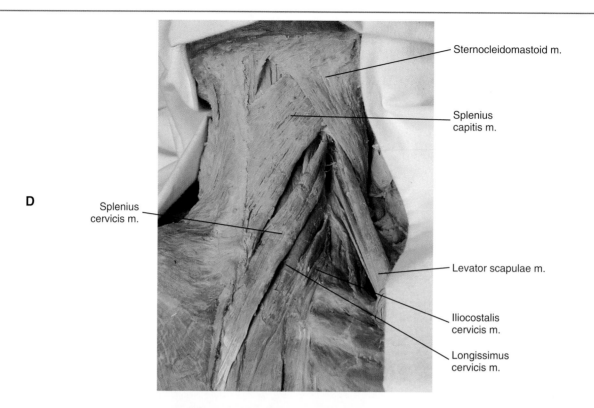

D

Sternocleidomastoid m.

Splenius
capitis m.

Splenius
cervicis m.

Levator scapulae m.

Iliocostalis
cervicis m.

Longissimus
cervicis m.

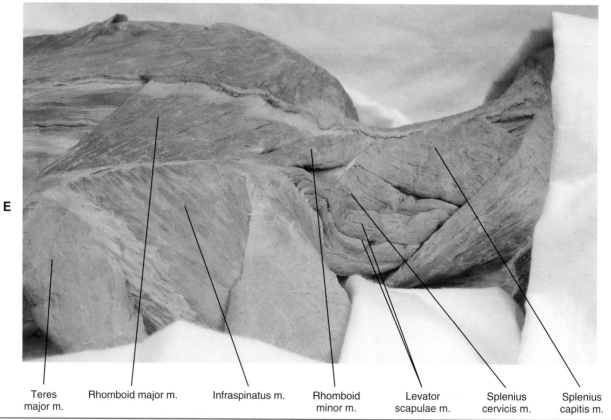

E

Teres
major m.

Rhomboid major m.

Infraspinatus m.

Rhomboid
minor m.

Levator
scapulae m.

Splenius
cervicis m.

Splenius
capitis m.

FIG. 4-2—cont'd   D, Right posterior view with the serratus posterior superior muscle removed. E, Right lateral view.

Fourth Layer

The most superficial layer of deep back muscles is the fourth layer, which consists of two muscles whose fibers ascend in a superolateral direction. This layer is composed of the splenius capitis and splenius cervicis muscles (Fig. 4-2, *C* to *E*). Detailed morphometric measurements have been performed on these muscles (Kamibayashi and Richmond, 1998).

Splenius Capitis and Splenius Cervicis Muscles.

The splenius capitis muscle begins from the lower half of the ligamentum nuchae and the spinous processes of C7 through T3 or T4. It attaches superiorly to the mastoid process of the temporal bone and to the occiput just inferior to the lateral third of the superior nuchal line.

The splenius cervicis muscle originates from the spinous processes of T3 through T6 and inserts onto the transverse processes of the atlas and axis and the posterior tubercles of the transverse processes of C3 and sometimes C4. These insertions are deep to the origins of the levator scapulae. The splenius capitis and cervicis are innervated by lateral branches of the posterior primary divisions (dorsal rami) of the midcervical and lower cervical spinal nerves, respectively. When the splenius muscles of both sides act together, they extend the head and neck. When the muscles of one side contract, they laterally flex the head and neck and slightly rotate the face toward the side of contraction.

Fifth Layer

The largest group of back muscles is the fifth layer. This layer is composed of the erector spinae group of muscles (Fig. 4-3, *A*; see also Fig. 4-2, *A* and *B*). This erector spinae group is also collectively known as the sacrospinalis muscle. The muscles that make up this group are a series of longitudinal muscles that course the length of the spine, filling a groove lateral to the spinous processes. Because of this location, these muscles generally have a similar function, which is to extend and laterally flex the spine. The erector spinae are all innervated by lateral branches of the posterior primary divisions (dorsal rami) of the nearby spinal nerves and are covered posteriorly in the thoracic and lumbar regions by the thoracolumbar fascia. These longitudinal muscles can be divided into three groups. These three groups are, from lateral to medial, the iliocostalis, the longissimus, and the spinalis groups of muscles. Each of these groups, in turn, is made up of three subdivisions. The subdivisions are named according to the area of the spine to which they insert (e.g., lumborum, thoracis, cervicis, capitis). The erector spinae muscles are discussed from the most lateral group to the most medial, and each group is discussed from inferior to superior.

Iliocostalis Muscles.

The iliocostalis (iliocostocervicalis) group of muscles is subdivided into lumborum, thoracis, and cervicis muscles (see Fig. 4-3, *A* and *B*). Inferiorly the iliocostalis muscles derive from the common origin of the erector spinae muscles.

Iliocostalis lumborum.

The iliocostalis lumborum muscle is the most inferior and lateral of the erector spinae muscles. It originates from the common origin of the erector spinae muscles, which includes the following:
- Spinous processes and supraspinous ligament of T11 through L5 (supraspinous ligament ends between L2 and L4)
- Median sacral crest
- Sacrotuberous ligament
- Long posterior sacroiliac ligament
- Lateral sacral crest
- Posteromedial iliac crest

The iliocostalis lumborum muscle runs superiorly to insert onto the posterior and inferior surfaces of the angles of the lower six to nine ribs. This muscle extends and laterally flexes the thoracolumbar spine and is innervated by lateral branches of the posterior primary divisions of lumbar and lower thoracic spinal nerves.

Macintosh and Bogduk (1987b) further described the anatomy of the iliocostalis lumborum muscle based on a series of elegant dissections. They found that part of this muscle originates from the posterior superior iliac spine and the posterior aspect of the iliac crest and inserts into the lower eight or nine ribs. They called this part the iliocostalis lumborum pars thoracis. Another part of the classically described iliocostalis lumborum originates from the tips of the lumbar spinous processes and associated middle layer of the thoracolumbar fascia of L1 to L4 (see Thoracolumbar Fascia) and inserts onto the anterior edge of the iliac crest. They called this part the iliocostalis lumborum pars lumborum and found that it formed a considerable mass of muscle. More recent evidence from the Visible Human Project corroborates this classification (Daggfeldt et al., 2000).

Iliocostalis thoracis.

The iliocostalis thoracis muscle originates from the superior aspect of the angles of the lower six ribs and inserts onto the angles of roughly the upper six ribs and transverse process of the C7 vertebra. This muscle extends and laterally flexes the thoracic spine and is innervated by the lateral branches of the posterior primary divisions (dorsal rami) of the thoracic spinal nerves.

Iliocostalis cervicis.

The iliocostalis cervicis originates from the superior aspect of the angle of the third through sixth ribs and inserts onto the posterior tubercles of the transverse processes of the C4 to C6 verte-

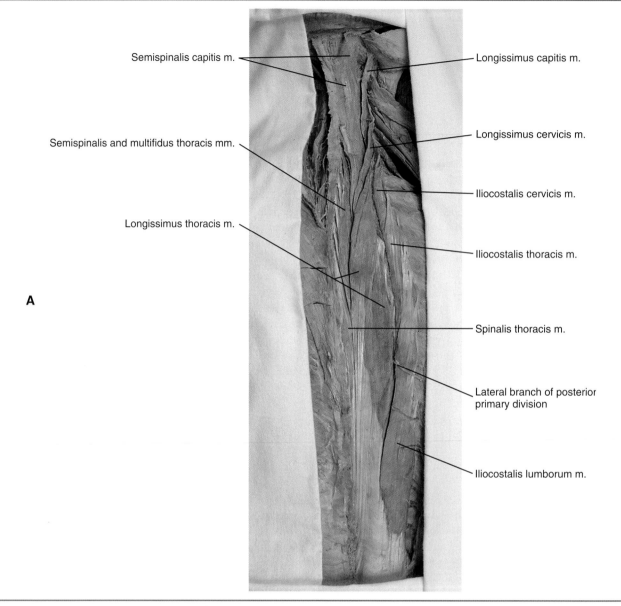

Semispinalis capitis m.

Semispinalis and multifidus thoracis mm.

Longissimus thoracis m.

A

Longissimus capitis m.

Longissimus cervicis m.

Iliocostalis cervicis m.

Iliocostalis thoracis m.

Spinalis thoracis m.

Lateral branch of posterior primary division

Iliocostalis lumborum m.

FIG. 4-3   **A,** Fifth layer of back muscles of the right side.

brae. It laterally flexes and extends the lower cervical region and is innervated by the dorsal rami of the upper thoracic and lower cervical spinal nerves.

Longissimus Muscles. The longissimus muscles are located medial to the iliocostalis group. The longissimus group is made up of thoracis, cervicis, and capitis divisions. The lateral branches of the posterior primary divisions (dorsal rami) of the spinal nerves exit the thorax and then course laterally and posteriorly between the iliocostalis muscles and longissimus thoracis muscle (see Fig. 4-3, *A*). This fact is used in the gross anatomy laboratory not only to quickly find the lateral branches of the posterior primary divisions, but also to demon-

strate the separation between these two large muscle masses. After providing motor and sensory innervation to the sacrospinalis muscle, the lateral branches continue to the skin of the back, providing cutaneous sensory innervation.

Longissimus thoracis. The longissimus thoracis is the largest of the erector spinae muscles. It arises from the common origin of the erector spinae muscles (see Iliocostalis lumborum). In addition, many fibers originate from the transverse and accessory processes of the lumbar vertebrae. This muscle is the longest muscle of the back, thus the name longissimus. It inserts onto the third through twelfth ribs, between their angles and tubercles.

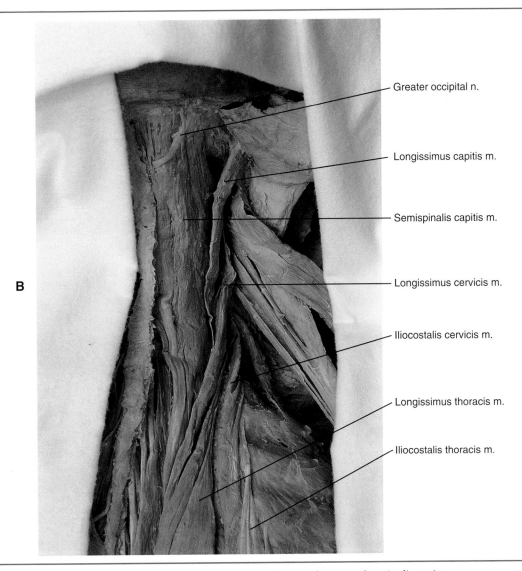

B

Greater occipital n.

Longissimus capitis m.

Semispinalis capitis m.

Longissimus cervicis m.

Iliocostalis cervicis m.

Longissimus thoracis m.

Iliocostalis thoracis m.

FIG. 4-3—cont'd   **B,** Right semispinalis capitis muscle of the sixth layer from a cadaveric dissection.   *Continued*

The longissimus thoracis also inserts onto the transverse processes of all 12 thoracic vertebrae. This muscle functions to hold the thoracic and lumbar regions erect, and laterally flexes the spine when it acts unilaterally. It is innervated by lateral branches of the thoracic and lumbar posterior primary divisions.

Macintosh and Bogduk (1987b) found fibers of the longissimus thoracis that are confined to the lumbar and sacral regions. These fibers originated from lumbar accessory and transverse processes and inserted onto the medial surface of the posterior superior iliac spine. The authors called these fibers the longissimus thoracis pars lumborum.

Longissimus cervicis. The longissimus cervicis muscle originates from the transverse processes of the upper thoracic vertebrae (T1 to T5) and inserts onto the posterior tubercle of the transverse processes and the articular processes of C3 through C6 and onto the posterior aspect of the transverse process and the articular process of C2. Unilateral contraction produces a combination of extension and lateral flexion of the neck to the same side. The longissimus cervicis is innervated by lateral branches of the upper thoracic and lower cervical posterior primary divisions.

Longissimus capitis. The longissimus capitis muscle derives from upper thoracic transverse processes (T1 to T5) and articular processes of C4 through C7. It inserts onto the mastoid process of the temporal bone, and its action is to extend the head. If it acts unilaterally, the longissimus capitis can laterally flex the head and rotate

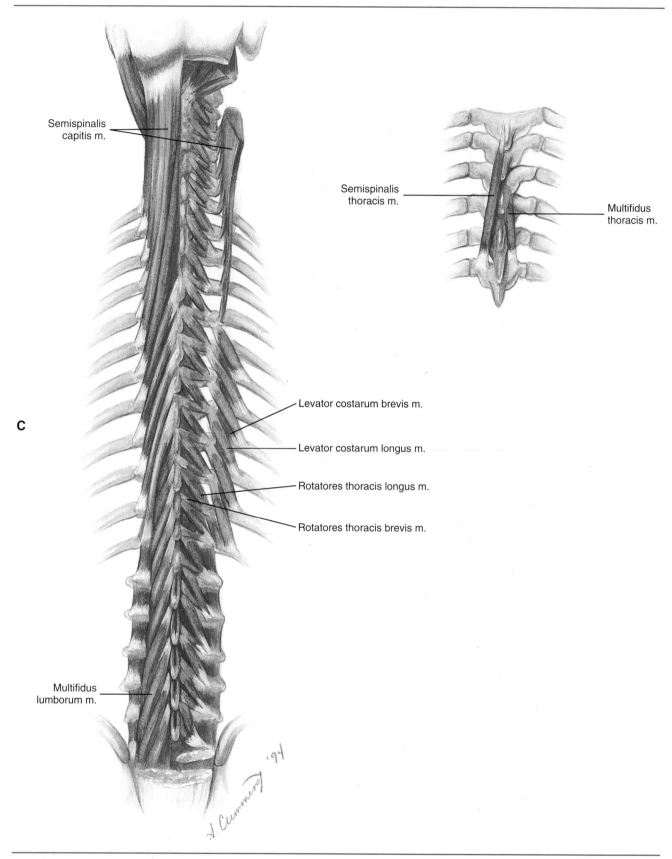

C

FIG. 4-3   C, Sixth layer of back muscles. *Left,* Semispinalis capitis and thoracis and multifidus lumborum muscles. *Right,* Semispinalis capitis has been cut from its superior attachment and folded laterally to display, rotatores, intertransversarii, interspinales, and levator costarum longus and brevis muscles. *Inset,* Multifidus and rotatores muscles.

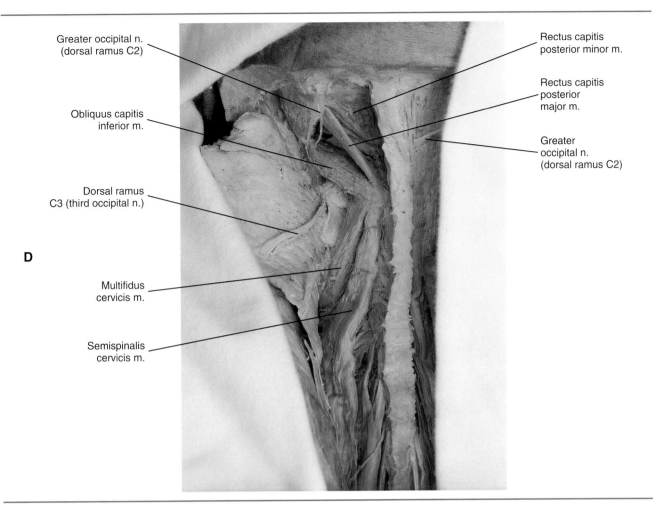

Greater occipital n. (dorsal ramus C2)

Obliquus capitis inferior m.

Dorsal ramus C3 (third occipital n.)

D

Multifidus cervicis m.

Semispinalis cervicis m.

Rectus capitis posterior minor m.

Rectus capitis posterior major m.

Greater occipital n. (dorsal ramus C2)

FIG. 4-3—cont'd   **D,** Semispinalis cervicis and multifidus cervicis muscles in a left posterior view of the upper cervical region.

Continued

it to the same side. It is innervated by the posterior primary divisions of upper thoracic and cervical spinal nerves.

Spinalis Muscles. The spinalis muscle group originates from spinous processes and inserts onto spinous processes, except for the spinalis capitis muscle. This muscle group is made up of thoracis, cervicis, and capitis divisions.

Spinalis thoracis. The spinalis thoracis muscle fibers are the most highly developed of this muscle group. It originates from the lower thoracic and upper lumbar spinous processes (T11 to L2) and inserts onto the upper thoracic spinous processes (T1 to T4 and perhaps down to T8). Laterally the fibers of this muscle blend with the fibers of the longissimus thoracis. The spinalis thoracis muscle functions to extend the thoracic spine. It is innervated by posterior primary divisions of thoracic nerves.

Spinalis cervicis. The spinalis cervicis muscle originates from upper thoracic spinous processes (T1 to T6) and inserts onto the spinous processes of C2 (occasionally C3 and C4). Maintaining the tradition of the erector spinae muscles, the spinalis cervicis extends the cervical region. This muscle usually is quite small and frequently absent.

Spinalis capitis. The spinalis capitis muscle differs from the other spinalis muscles in that it does not typically originate from or insert onto spinous processes. This muscle is difficult to differentiate from the more lateral semispinalis capitis muscle (see the following discussion). Its origin is blended with that of the semispinalis capitis from the transverse processes of the C7 to the T6 or T7 vertebra, the articular processes of C4 to C6, and sometimes from the spinous processes of C7 and T1. The fibers of this muscle blend with those of the semispinalis capitis and insert with the latter muscle onto the occiput between the superior and inferior nuchal

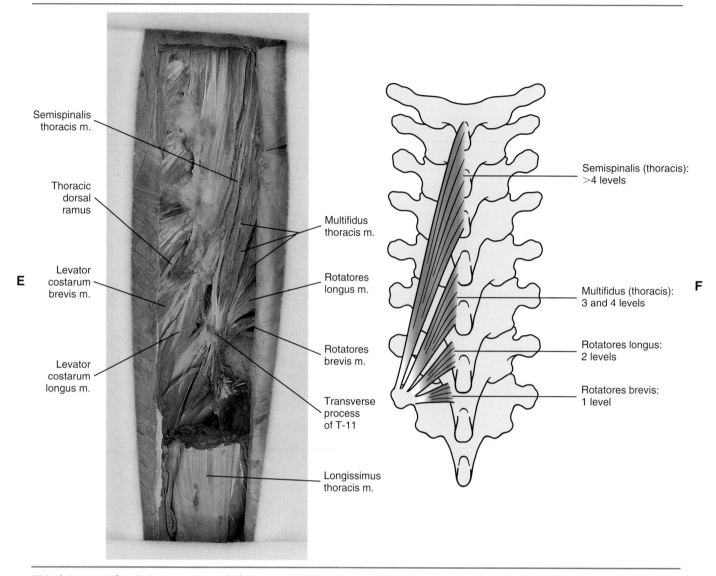

E

F

FIG. 4-3—cont'd   **E,** Semispinalis, multifidus, and rotatores longus and brevis muscles as they arise from a single left lower thoracic transverse process (transverse process of T11). **F,** Illustration demonstrating origin from a single transverse process of semispinalis, multifidus, and rotatores longus and brevis muscles. The number of vertebral segments ascended before inserting is listed for each muscle.

lines. The spinalis capitis muscle is sometimes called the biventer cervicis muscle because an incomplete tendinous intersection passes across it. When the left and right spinalis capitis muscles contract together, the result is extension of the head. Unilateral contraction results in lateral flexion of the head and neck and also rotation of the head away from the side of contraction. This muscle is innervated by upper thoracic and lower cervical posterior primary divisions.

Sixth Layer

The sixth layer of back muscles includes the deep back muscles with fibers that course superiorly and medially.

They are sometimes called the transversospinalis group because they generally originate from transverse processes and insert onto spinous processes (see Fig. 4-3, *B* to *F*). The muscles in this layer are arranged such that the length of the muscles becomes progressively shorter from superficial to deep. Although the actions of these muscles are described separately, remember that these muscles (especially the shorter ones) function primarily in a postural role as stabilizers rather than as prime movers. This group is made up of the semispinalis, multifidus, and rotatores muscles.

Semispinalis Muscles. The semispinalis muscles are located only in the thoracic and cervical regions and are divided into three parts: semispinalis thoracis, semispinalis cervicis, and semispinalis capitis muscles (see Fig. 4-3, *B* to *F*).

Semispinalis thoracis. The semispinalis thoracis consists of thin muscular fasciculi located between long tendons that attach inferiorly to the transverse processes of the lower six thoracic vertebrae and superiorly to the spinous processes of C6 to T4 (see Fig. 4-3, *C*). The semispinalis thoracis is innervated by the medial branches of the posterior primary divisions of the upper six thoracic spinal nerves.

Semispinalis cervicis. The semispinalis cervicis is a thicker mass of muscle that begins from the transverse processes of the upper five or six thoracic vertebrae (see Fig. 4-3, *D*). It may arise from the articular processes of the lower four cervical vertebrae also. This muscle mainly inserts onto the spinous process of the axis, but also attaches to the spinous processes of C3 to C5. It derives its innervation from the posterior primary divisions (dorsal rami) of the C6 to C8 spinal nerves.

Semispinalis capitis. The semispinalis capitis is a thick, powerful muscle and represents the best-developed portion of the semispinalis muscle group (see Fig. 4-3, *B* to *D*). Detailed morphometric measurements have been performed on this muscle (Kamibayashi and Richmond, 1998). It arises from the transverse processes of C7 to T6 and the articular processes of C4 to C6. The semispinalis capitis muscle inserts onto the medial part of the area between the occiput's superior and inferior nuchal lines. Usually it is blended with the spinalis capitis muscle, which is supplied by the dorsal rami of the first through sixth cervical spinal nerves.

When the muscles of both sides act together, the semispinalis thoracis and cervicis function to extend the thoracic and cervical portions of the spine, respectively, whereas unilateral contraction of these muscles not only slightly extends the spine but also rotates the vertebral bodies to the opposite side. The semispinalis capitis muscles together function to extend the head and, working separately, slightly rotate the head to the opposite side.

Multifidus Muscles

Multifidus lumborum, thoracis, and cervicis. The multifidus muscles lie deep to the semispinalis muscles, where they fill the groove between the transverse and spinous processes of the vertebrae. This group consists of multiple muscular and tendinous fasciculi that originate from the mamillary processes of the lumbar vertebrae, transverse processes of the thoracic vertebrae, and articular processes of the lower four cervical vertebrae. These fasciculi ascend two to four (or sometimes five) vertebral segments before inserting onto a spinous

process. Multifidi insert onto all the vertebrae except the atlas. The multifidus muscles produce extension of the vertebral column. They also produce some rotation of the vertebral bodies away from the side of contraction, and they are also active in lateral flexion of the spine.

This muscle group has been found to contract during axial rotation of the trunk in either direction (Oliver and Middleditch, 1991). When the oblique abdominal muscles contract to produce trunk rotation, some flexion of the trunk is produced as well. The multifidus muscles oppose this flexion component and maintain a pure axial rotation, thereby acting as stabilizers during trunk rotation. The multifidus muscles are innervated segmentally by the medial branches of the posterior primary divisions of the spinal nerves.

In the lumbar spine, where the multifidus group is best developed, it is arranged into five bands, each attaching superiorly to one lumbar spinous process (Macintosh et al., 1986). In each band the deepest fascicles actually run from the mamillary process below to the lamina of the vertebra two segments above. The more superficial fascicles are longer and run from mamillary processes to spinous processes three to five segments above. In the lower lumbar spine the inferior attachments of the fascicles include the posterior aspect of the sacrum lying adjacent to the spinous tubercles, posterior sacroiliac ligaments, posterosuperior iliac spine, and deep surface of the erector spinae aponeurosis.

Each band of multifidus lumborum is actually a myotome arranged such that the fibers that move a particular lumbar vertebra (e.g., those that attach superiorly to a single spinous process) are innervated by the medial branch of the dorsal ramus of that segment's spinal nerve. For example, the multifidus inserting onto the spinous process of L2 is innervated by the medial branch of the dorsal ramus (posterior primary division) of L2. Specifically in the lumbar region, the multifidus produces primarily extension (Macintosh and Bogduk, 1986). Rotation of the lumbar spine is seen only secondarily, in conjunction with extension.

Rotatores Muscles

Rotatores lumborum, thoracis, and cervicis. The rotatores muscles are located deep to the multifidus group. They constitute the deepest muscle fasciculi located in the groove between the spinous and transverse processes. This groove runs the entire length of the vertebral column from sacrum to axis. The two groups of rotatores are determined by their length. The fascicles of the rotatores brevis begin on transverse processes and attach to the root of the vertebral spinous process immediately superior. The fascicles of the rotatores longus have similar origins but insert on the root of the spinous process of the second vertebra above. The rotatores muscles are best developed in the thoracic region and are only poorly developed in the cervical and lumbar regions, where they are difficult to distinguish from multifidus muscles. Acting bilaterally, these muscles help in extension of the spine, although unilateral contraction helps produce rotation of the spine such that the vertebral bodies move away from the side contracted. The rotatores muscles' main function probably is to stabilize the vertebral column. These muscles are segmentally innervated by the medial branches of the posterior primary divisions of the spinal nerves.

The muscles of the fifth and sixth layers may be torn (strained) during hyperflexion of the spine or while lifting heavy loads. The muscles of these layers are made up of many individual strands that may tear near their musculotendinous junction. This tearing results in pain and tenderness, which may refer to neighboring regions (see Chapter 11). Localizing the torn muscle during physical examination may be difficult because many attachment sites of these muscles are deep. However, the costal attachments of the iliocostalis lumborum and the iliac attachment of the longissimus thoracis are close to the surface, and pain from these muscles may be localized to these attachment sites during examination (Bogduk, 1997).

OTHER MUSCLES DIRECTLY ASSOCIATED WITH THE SPINE

Suboccipital Muscles

The suboccipital muscles are a group of four small muscles located inferior to the occiput in the most superior portion of the posterior neck. They are the deepest muscles in this region, located under the trapezius, splenius capitis, and semispinalis capitis muscles. The suboccipital muscles consist of two rectus muscles (major and minor) and two obliquus muscles (superior and inferior). These muscles are concerned with extension of the head at the atlanto-occipital joint and rotation of the head at the atlanto-axial articulations. All are innervated by the posterior primary division of the C1 spinal nerve, which is also called the suboccipital nerve. The small number of muscle fibers per neuron for this group of muscles ranges from three to five (Oliver and Middleditch, 1991). This high degree of innervation allows these muscles to rapidly change tension, thus fine tuning the movements of the head and controlling head posture with a considerable degree of precision. Detailed morphometric measurements have been performed on these muscles (Kamibayashi and Richmond, 1998).

Rectus Capitis Posterior Major Muscle. The rectus capitis posterior major muscle (Fig. 4-4) begins at the spinous process of C2, widens as it ascends, and attaches superiorly to the lateral portion of the occiput's

inferior nuchal line. When acting bilaterally, the rectus capitis posterior muscles (both major and minor) produce extension of the head. Unilateral contraction turns the head so that the face rotates toward the side of the shortening muscle.

Rectus Capitis Posterior Minor Muscle. The rectus capitis posterior minor muscle is located just medial to and partly under the rectus capitis posterior major (see Fig. 4-4). It attaches inferiorly to the posterior tubercle of the atlas and becomes broader as it ascends. It inserts on the medial portion of the occiput's inferior nuchal line and the area between that line and the foramen magnum.

A connective tissue bridge between the rectus capitis posterior minor muscle and dorsal spinal dura at the atlanto-occipital junction has been consistently observed in cadavers (Hack et al., 1995). These bridges are also observable on magnetic resonance imaging (MRI) (Humphreys et al., 2003). They may serve to anchor the dura posteriorly. Contraction of the rectus capitis posterior minor muscle produces extension of the head.

Obliquus Capitis Inferior Muscle. The obliquus capitis inferior muscle is the larger of the two obliquus muscles (see Fig. 4-4). It originates on the spinous process of the axis and passes laterally and slightly superiorly to insert onto the transverse process of C1. This muscle rotates the atlas such that the face is turned to the same side of contraction. The length of the transverse processes of the atlas gives this muscle a considerable mechanical advantage (Williams et al., 1995).

Obliquus Capitis Superior Muscle. The obliquus capitis superior arises from the transverse process of the atlas (see Fig. 4-4). It becomes wider as it runs superiorly and posteriorly. This muscle inserts onto the occiput between the superior and inferior nuchal lines, lateral to the attachment of the semispinalis capitis, overlapping the insertion of the rectus capitis posterior major. Head extension and lateral flexion to the same side are produced by contraction of this muscle. The left and right obliquus capitis superior muscles, in conjunction with the two rectus muscles of each side, probably act more frequently as postural muscles than as prime movers (Williams et al., 1995).

Three of the four suboccipital muscles on each side of the upper cervical region form the sides of a suboccipital triangle. The boundaries of each suboccipital triangle are: (a) the obliquus capitis inferior, below and laterally; (b) the obliquus capitis superior, above and laterally; and (c) the rectus capitis posterior major, medially and somewhat above. The roof of this triangle is composed of the splenius capitis laterally and semispinalis capitis medially. Deep to these muscles is a layer of dense fibrofatty

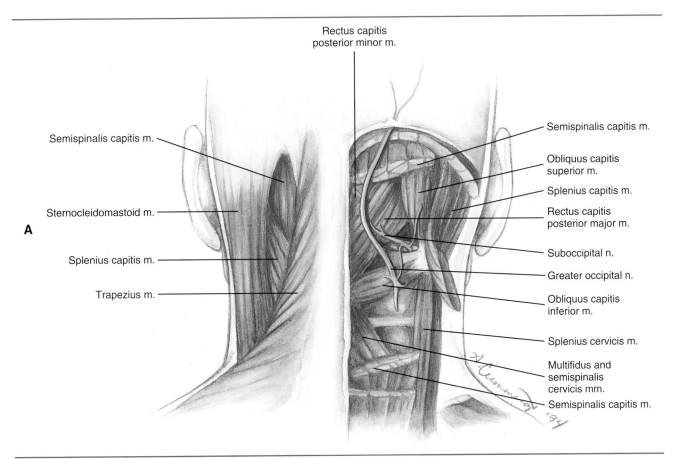

Rectus capitis
posterior minor m.

Semispinalis capitis m.

Sternocleidomastoid m.

Splenius capitis m.

Trapezius m.

A

Semispinalis capitis m.

Obliquus capitis
superior m.

Splenius capitis m.

Rectus capitis
posterior major m.

Suboccipital n.

Greater occipital n.

Obliquus capitis
inferior m.

Splenius cervicis m.

Multifidus and
semispinalis
cervicis mm.

Semispinalis capitis m.

FIG. 4-4 **A,** Illustration and, **B,** photograph of the suboccipital region. Three of the suboccipital muscles—the rectus capitis posterior major, obliquus capitis inferior, and obliquus capitis superior—form the suboccipital triangle. The remaining suboccipital muscle, the rectus capitis posterior minor, lies medial to the triangle. Notice the vertebral artery and the posterior arch of the atlas deep within the suboccipital triangle. **A** and **B,** Suboccipital muscles of the right and left sides, respectively.   *Continued*

tissue that also helps to form the roof. The floor of the triangle is made up of the posterior arch of the atlas and posterior atlanto-occipital membrane. The suboccipital triangle contains the horizontal portion (third part) of the vertebral artery, dorsal ramus of the C1 spinal nerve (suboccipital nerve), and suboccipital plexus of veins.

Intertransversarii Muscles

The intertransversarii muscles (Fig. 4-5) extend between adjacent transverse processes. These muscles are most highly developed in the cervical region. The cervical intertransversarii usually begin at C1 (although the muscle between C1 and C2 often is absent) and continue to T1. They consist of anterior and posterior subdivisions that run between adjacent anterior and posterior tubercles, respectively. The ventral ramus of the spinal nerve exits between each pair of anterior and posterior intertransversarii muscles and innervates each anterior intertransversarius muscle. Each posterior intertransversarius muscle in the cervical region is further subdivided into a medial and lateral part. The posterior

primary division (dorsal ramus) of the spinal nerve frequently pierces the medial part of a posterior intertransversarius muscle and innervates that part of the muscle. The anterior primary division (ventral ramus) innervates the lateral part of the posterior intertransversarius muscle and anterior intertransversarius muscle, as mentioned. The intertransversarii muscles function to flex the spine laterally by approximating adjacent transverse processes. They also help to stabilize adjacent vertebrae during large spinal movements.

The thoracic intertransversarii muscles are small and are usually only present in the lower thoracic region. They are not divided into subdivisions and are innervated by the dorsal rami (posterior primary divisions).

The lumbar intertransversarii muscles are found between all lumbar vertebrae. As with the posterior portion of the cervical intertransversarii, the lumbar group of muscles divides into medial and lateral divisions. Each medial division passes from the accessory process, mamillo-accessory ligament, and mamillary process of the vertebra above to the mamillary process of the vertebra below (see Fig. 4-5). Each lateral

Obliquus capitis
superior m.

Vertebral artery and
posterior arch of C1

Obliquus capitis
inferior m. and
greater occipital n.
(dorsal ramus C2)

B

Rectus capitis
posterior major m.

Rectus capitis
posterior minor m.

Greater
occipital n.

Ligamentum nuchae
(funicular portion)

Multifidus cervicis

Semispinalis
cervicis m.

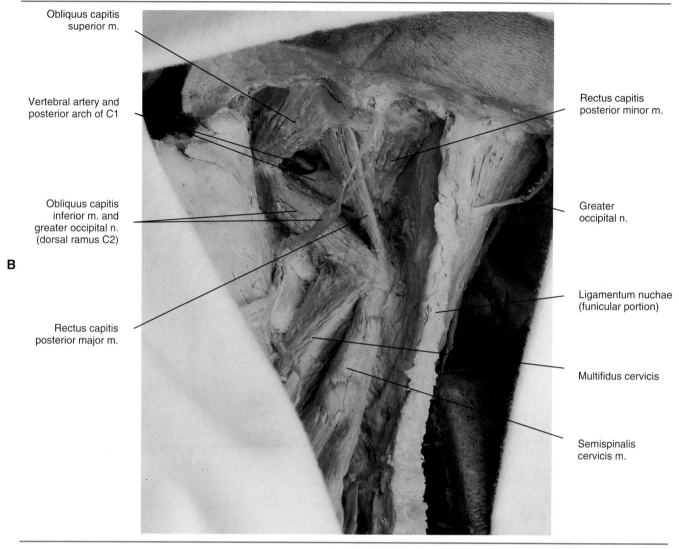

FIG. 4-4—cont'd

intertransversarius muscle in the lumbar region can be further subdivided into an anterior and posterior division. The anterior division runs between adjacent transverse processes, and the posterior division runs from the accessory process of the vertebra above to the transverse process of the vertebra below. Both the anterior and posterior divisions of the lateral intertransversarii muscles are innervated by lumbar anterior primary divisions (ventral rami). The medial intertransversarii muscles are innervated by lumbar posterior primary divisions.

The intertransversarii muscles generally are thought to laterally flex the lumbar region and stabilize adjacent vertebrae during spinal movement. However, the intertransversarii muscles are short and lie close to the axes of motion for lateral flexion and rotation of the spine, which places them at a considerable biomechanical disadvantage. Thus their usefulness as lateral flexors or sta-

bilizers has been questioned (Bogduk, 1997). In addition, the intertransversarii and interspinales muscles have been found to possess up to six times more muscle spindles than the other deep back muscles. The large number of muscle spindles in these muscles has led Bogduk (1997) to speculate that the intertransversarii muscles function as proprioceptive transducers, providing afferent information for spinal and supraspinal circuits. These circuits help to maintain posture and produce smooth and accurate movements of the spine by adjusting and regulating neural activity to the back muscles.

Interspinales Muscles

The interspinales muscles (see Fig. 4-5) are small muscles that extend between adjacent spinous processes. They are located on each side of the interspinous ligament. Interspinales muscles are present as small, distinct bundles of fibers throughout the cervical region, beginning at the spinous processes of C2 and continuing to the spinous process of T1. The thoracic interspinales muscles are variable and are located only in the upper and lower few segments. The lumbar region, as with the cervical region, has interspinales muscles running between all the spinous processes of that spinal region. The interspinales muscles are innervated by the medial branches of the posterior primary divisions of spinal nerves. The interspinales muscles function to extend the spine and may act as proprioceptive organs.

Levator Costarum Muscles

The levator costarum (see Fig. 4-3, *C*) are muscular fasciculi that arise from the tips of the transverse processes of C7 to T11 and run inferiorly and laterally, parallel with the posterior borders of the external intercostal muscles. The levator costarum brevis attaches to the superior surface, between the tubercle and angle, of the rib immediately inferior to its level of origin. Sometimes, especially in the lower thoracic levels, fasciculi attach to the second rib below. These fasciculi are known as levator costarum longus muscles and are located medial to the brevis muscle originating from the same transverse process. The levator costarum muscles elevate the ribs and may help laterally flex and rotate the trunk to the same side. They are segmentally innervated by lateral branches of the posterior primary divisions (dorsal rami) of the spinal nerves.

Muscles Associated with the Anterior Aspect of the Cervical Vertebrae

The muscles associated with the anterior aspect of the cervical vertebrae include the longus colli, longus capitis, rectus capitis anterior, and rectus capitis lateralis (Fig. 4-6). These muscles are responsible for flexing the neck and occiput and may be injured during extension injuries of the cervical region. Detailed morphometric measurements have been performed on these muscles (Kamibayashi and Richmond, 1998).

Longus Colli Muscle. The left and right longus colli muscles (see Fig. 4-6) are located along the anterior aspect of the cervical vertebral bodies. Each of these muscles is made up of three parts: vertical, inferior oblique, and superior oblique. Together the three parts of this muscle flex the neck. The superior and inferior oblique parts also may aid with lateral flexion. The inferior oblique part also rotates the neck to the opposite side. The longus colli muscle is innervated by branches of the anterior primary divisions of C2 to C6. This muscle is probably one of the muscles responsible for reversal of the cervical lordosis after extension injuries of the neck.

The longus colli muscle has been found to contain a high density of muscle spindles. This implies an important proprioceptive function for this muscle (Boyd-Clark et al., 2002). The origins, insertions, and unique characteristics of the three parts of the longus colli muscle are listed next.

Vertical portion. The vertical portion of the longus colli originates from and inserts onto vertebral bodies. More specifically, this muscle originates from the anterior aspect of the vertebral bodies of C5 to T3 and inserts onto the vertebral bodies of C2 to C4.

Inferior oblique portion. The inferior oblique portion of the longus colli muscle originates from the vertebral bodies of T1 to T3 and passes superiorly and laterally to insert onto the anterior tubercles of the transverse processes of C5 and C6.

Superior oblique portion. The superior oblique portion of the longus colli muscle originates from the anterior tubercles of the transverse processes of C3 to C5. Its fibers course superiorly and medially and converge to insert onto the anterior tubercle of the atlas by means of a narrow tendon. This tendinous insertion can be torn during an extension injury of the neck. Such an injury can be followed by the deposition of calcium in the region, a condition known as retropharyngeal calcific tendonitis. The calcium may be seen on x-ray film approximately 3 weeks after injury and usually appears as an irregular and sometimes subtle region of increased radiopacity located just anterior to the atlas. Usually the calcium is resorbed as the injury heals and then is no longer visible on x-ray film.

Longus Capitis Muscle. The longus capitis muscle is located anterior and slightly lateral to the longus colli muscle (see Fig. 4-6). It originates as a series of thin tendons from the anterior tubercles of the transverse processes of C3 to C6. The tendinous origins unite to form a distinct muscular band that courses superiorly toward the occiput. This muscular band inserts onto the region of the occiput anterior to the foramen magnum and posterior to the pharyngeal tubercle. The longus capitis muscle functions to flex the head and is innervated by branches of the anterior primary divisions of C1 to C3.

Rectus Capitis Anterior Muscle. The rectus capitis anterior is a small muscle located deep to the inserting fibers of the longus capitis muscle (see Fig. 4-6). It originates from the anterior aspect of the lateral mass and the most medial part of the transverse process of the atlas. The rectus capitis anterior muscle inserts onto the occiput just in front of the occipital condyle. This muscle

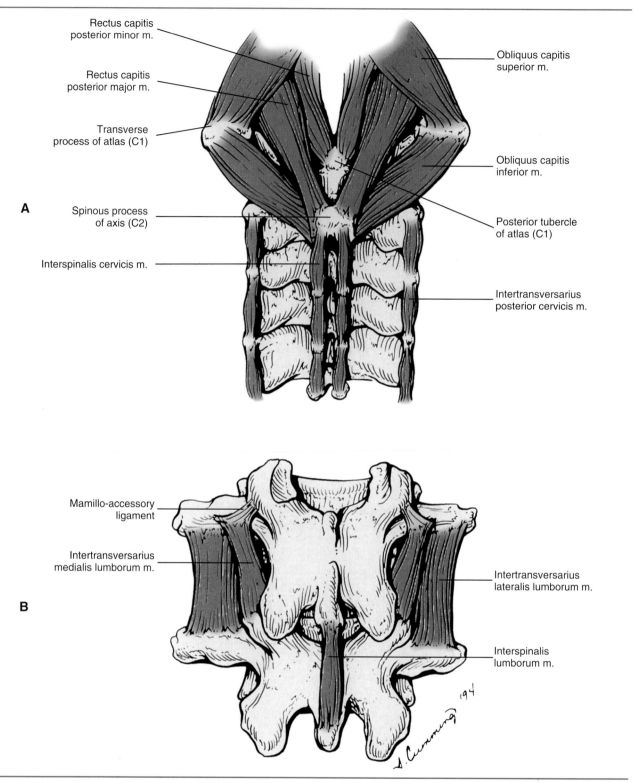

FIG. 4-5   A, Suboccipital, cervical interspinales, and cervical intertransversarii muscles. **B,** Lumbar interspinalis and left and right lumbar intertransversarii muscles. Also illustrated is the mamillo-accessory ligament. Notice the intertransversarii mediales lumborum muscles on each side, taking part of their origin from the left and right mamillo-accessory ligaments.

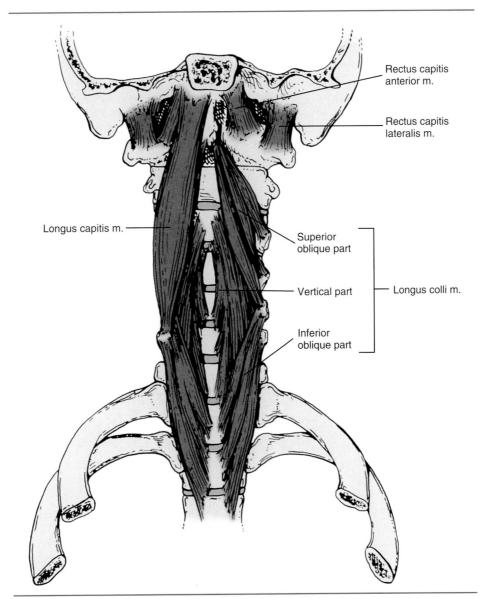

FIG. 4-6   Muscles associated with the anterior aspect of the cervical vertebrae and the occiput. *Right,* Three parts of the longus colli muscle (vertical, inferior oblique, superior oblique). *Left,* Longus capitis muscle. The rectus capitis anterior and lateralis also can be seen as they pass from the atlas to the occiput.

functions to flex the head at the atlantooccipital joints and is innervated by the anterior primary divisions of the first and second cervical nerves.

Rectus Capitis Lateralis Muscle.   The rectus capitis lateralis muscle is another small muscle. It originates from the anterior aspect of the transverse process of the atlas and courses superiorly to insert onto the jugular process of the occiput (see Fig. 4-6). It laterally flexes the occiput on the atlas and is innervated by the anterior primary division of the first and second cervical nerves.

Iliac Muscles

The muscles of the iliac region—the psoas major, psoas minor, and quadratus lumborum (Fig. 4-7)—sometimes are called the posterior abdominal wall muscles. However, they may be classified properly as spinal muscles because they all have direct action on the vertebral column and are attached to the lumbar region. All three of these muscles attach inferiorly onto either the pelvis or the femur; therefore they also help connect the lower limb to the spine.

Psoas Major and Iliacus Muscles. The psoas major muscle (see Fig. 4-7) arises from the anterolateral portion of the bodies of T12 to L5, the intervertebral discs between these bones, and the transverse processes of all the lumbar vertebrae. It descends along the pelvic brim, passes deep to the inguinal ligament and in front of the hip capsule, and inserts via a tendon onto the femur's lesser trochanter. The lateral side of the tendon of the psoas major muscle receives the bulk of the fibers of the iliacus muscle. Together they form what is sometimes loosely called the iliopsoas muscle. The iliacus originates from the inner lip of the iliac crest, upper two thirds of the iliac fossa, and superolateral portion of the sacrum. It inserts with the psoas major onto the femur's lesser trochanter.

The psoas major muscle, along with the iliacus muscle, functions primarily to flex the thigh at the hip. If the lower limb is stabilized, these muscles are concerned primarily with flexing the trunk and pelvis. They are important in raising the body from the supine to the sitting position. Electromyographic evidence further suggests that the psoas major is involved in balancing the trunk when in the sitting position (Williams et al., 1995). When the neck of the femur is fractured, this muscle acts as a lateral rotator of the thigh, which results in the characteristic laterally rotated position of the lower limb after such a fracture. Both the psoas major and the iliacus muscles usually are innervated by fibers arising from the L2 and L3 spinal cord levels. The iliacus muscle receives branches of the femoral nerve, and the psoas major

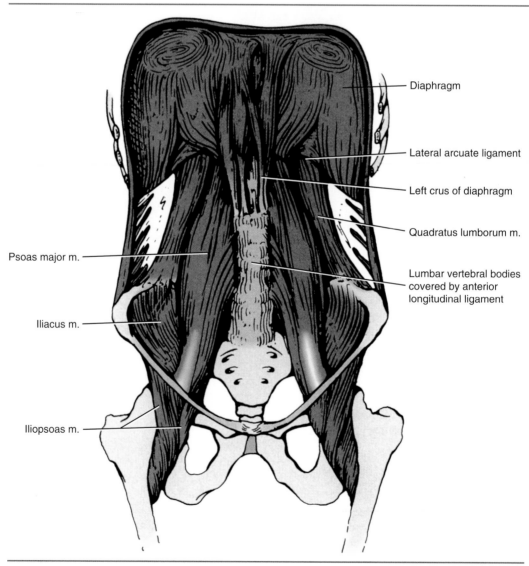

Diaphragm

Lateral arcuate ligament

Left crus of diaphragm

Quadratus lumborum m.

Lumbar vertebral bodies covered by anterior longitudinal ligament

Psoas major m.

Iliacus m.

Iliopsoas m.

FIG. 4-7   Iliac muscles and the diaphragm. The left and right crura of the diaphragm are prominently displayed. Also notice the left and right quadratus lumborum, psoas major, and iliacus muscles.

muscle is supplied by direct fibers from the ventral rami of the L2-3 spinal nerves. Sometimes the L1 and L4 spinal nerves also send branches into the psoas major muscle.

Psoas Minor Muscle. The psoas minor is a variable muscle, absent in approximately 40% of the population (Williams et al., 1995). When present, it is located on the anterior surface of the psoas major muscle. The psoas minor muscle attaches superiorly to the lateral aspect of the bodies of T12 and L1 and the interposing intervertebral disc. It descends to attach inferiorly by a long tendon to the pecten pubis and iliopubic eminence. The psoas minor acts as a weak trunk flexor and is innervated by fibers arising from the anterior primary division of the L1 spinal nerve.

Quadratus Lumborum Muscle. The quadratus lumborum (see Fig. 4-7) lies along the tips of the transverse processes of the lumbar vertebrae and is irregularly quadrangular in shape. It attaches inferiorly to the transverse process of L5, iliolumbar ligament, and posterior aspect of the iliac crest adjacent to that ligament. Superiorly the quadratus lumborum is attached to the lower border of the twelfth rib and the tips of the transverse processes of L1 to L4. If the pelvis is fixed, this muscle laterally flexes the lumbar spine. When both muscles contract, they help with extension of the spine. Each quadratus lumborum muscle also depresses the twelfth rib and aids in inspiration by stabilizing the origin of the diaphragm to the twelfth rib. It is innervated by fibers from the ventral rami of the T12 to L3 (sometimes L4) spinal nerves.

MUSCLES THAT INDIRECTLY INFLUENCE THE SPINE

Muscles of Respiration

All the muscles of respiration have attachments to ribs. In addition to aiding respiration, all these muscles are involved to some extent with stabilizing the thoracic cage during trunk movements. The muscles of respiration are composed of the following: those that connect adjacent ribs (intercostals), those that span across more than one rib (subcostals), those that attach ribs to the sternum (transverse thoracis), those connecting ribs to vertebrae (levator costarum and serratus posterosuperior and posteroinferior), and the diaphragm. Because the levator costarum and posterior serratus muscles have vertebral attachments, they are considered true back muscles and are discussed in previous sections.

Diaphragm. The diaphragm is the principal muscle of respiration (see Fig. 4-7). It is a domelike musculotendinous sheet that is convex superiorly. It completely separates the thoracic and abdominal cavities, except where it has apertures that allow for the passage of the esophagus, aorta, inferior vena cava, sympathetic trunks, and splanchnic nerves. This sheet consists of muscle fibers that attach to the entire border of the thoracic outlet. These fibers converge superiorly and medially and end as a central tendon. From anterior to posterior, muscle fibers arise from the posterior surface of the xiphoid process, the deep surface of the lower six ribs and their costal cartilages, interdigitations with the origin of the transversus abdominis muscle, lateral and medial lumbocostal arches, and first three lumbar vertebrae. The origins from the lumbar vertebrae form the left and right crura.

The lateral lumbocostal arch, also known as the lateral arcuate ligament, is a thickening of the fascia of the quadratus lumborum muscle. It attaches medially to the transverse process of L1, arches over the upper portion of the quadratus lumborum, and ends laterally on the lower border of the twelfth rib.

The medial lumbocostal arch, or medial arcuate ligament, is a similar structure, except that it is associated with the psoas major muscle. This arch also is attached to the transverse process of L1, but arches medially over the psoas major and is connected to the lateral aspect of the body of L1 or L2.

The crura of the diaphragm originate from the anterolateral surfaces of the upper two (on the left) or three (on the right) lumbar vertebrae, their discs, and the anterior longitudinal ligament. The two crura meet in the midline and arch over the aorta's anterior aspect to form what is sometimes called the median arcuate ligament.

The lower ribs are fixed when the diaphragm first contracts; then the central tendon is drawn inferiorly and anteriorly. The abdominal contents provide resistance to further descent of the diaphragm, which leads to protrusion of the anterior abdominal wall ("abdominal" breathing) and elevation of the rib cage ("thoracic" breathing). The diaphragm is innervated by the left and right phrenic nerves, which arise from the ventral rami of C3 to C5. Also, some afferent fibers from the peripheral aspect of this muscle are carried in the lower six or seven intercostal nerves. These nerves, and the sensory fibers of the phrenic nerves, are responsible for the referred pain patterns seen with some diaphragmatic pathology.

External, Internal, and Innermost Intercostal Muscles. The intercostal muscles (Fig. 4-8, *A*) comprise three sets of superimposed muscles located between adjacent ribs. These sets of muscles consist of the external intercostal, internal intercostal, and innermost intercostal muscles.

The external intercostal muscles, 11 on each side, have attachments that extend along the shafts of the ribs from the tubercles to just lateral to the costal cartilages.

More anteriorly, each is replaced by an aponeurosis, called the external intercostal membrane, which continues to the sternum. Each external intercostal originates from the lower border of one rib and inserts onto the upper border of the adjacent rib below. The fibers of each are directed obliquely; in the posterior chest, they run inferolaterally, although at the front, they course inferomedially and somewhat anteriorly.

The 11 pairs of internal intercostal muscles are located immediately deep to the external intercostals. Their attachments begin anteriorly at the sternum, or at the costal cartilages for ribs 8 through 10, and continue posteriorly to the costal angles. At that point, they are replaced by an aponeurotic layer, termed the internal intercostal membrane, which continues posteriorly to the anterior fibers of the superior costotransverse ligament. Each internal intercostal muscle attaches superiorly to the floor of the costal groove and corresponding portion of the costal cartilage and runs obliquely inferior to its attachment on the superior surface of the adjacent rib below. The fibers of the internal intercostal muscles are arranged orthogonally to those of the external intercostals.

The fibers of the innermost intercostal muscles lie just deep to and run parallel with those of the internal intercostals. They are poorly developed in the upper thoracic levels but become progressively more pronounced in the lower levels. They are attached to the deep surfaces of adjacent ribs and are best developed in the middle two fourths of the intercostal space. The intercostal veins, arteries, and nerves (from superior to inferior) can be found in the superior aspect of the intercostal space passing between the fibers of the internal and innermost intercostal muscles.

Although the intercostal muscles play a role in respiration, their exact function is still controversial (Williams et al., 1995). Conflicting evidence exists as to the actions of the various layers of the intercostals during inspiration and expiration. Results from studies using electromyography show differences in the activity of upper versus lower intercostals during the different phases of respiration. In addition, activity has been recorded in the intercostal muscles during many trunk movements, and they appear to act as stabilizers of the thoracic cage (Oliver and Middleditch, 1991). The intercostal muscles are innervated by branches of the adjacent intercostal nerves.

Subcostal Muscles. The subcostal muscles (Fig. 4-8, *D*) are musculotendinous fasciculi that usually are best developed only in the lower thorax. Each arises from the inferior border of one rib, near the angle, and runs obliquely inferior to the second or third rib below. The fibers of the subcostal muscles are parallel to those of the internal intercostals. They probably help depress

the ribs and are innervated by branches from adjacent intercostal nerves.

Transversus Thoracis Muscle. The transversus thoracis, or sternocostalis, muscle is located on the deep surface of the anterior thoracic wall (Fig. 4-8, *B*). It originates from the posterior surface of the inferior one third of the sternal body, posterior surface of the xiphoid process, and the posterior surfaces of the costal cartilages of the lower three or four true ribs. It inserts onto the inferior and deep surfaces of the costal cartilages of the second through sixth ribs. The fibers of the muscle form a fanlike arrangement, with the upper fibers being almost vertically oriented and the intermediate fibers more obliquely oriented. The lowermost fibers not only are horizontal, but also are continuous with the most superior fibers of the transversus abdominis muscle. The transversus thoracis muscle pulls the costal cartilages, to which it inserts in an inferior direction, and is innervated by the adjacent intercostal nerves.

Anterolateral Abdominal Muscles

Although the four muscles composing the anterolateral abdominal wall do not have direct attachments to the spine, they are involved in producing several movements of the trunk, including flexion, lateral flexion, and rotation. They are also important as postural muscles and in increasing intraabdominal pressure. These muscles include the external abdominal oblique, internal abdominal oblique, transversus abdominis, and rectus abdominis muscles.

External Abdominal Oblique Muscle. The external abdominal oblique (obliquus externus abdominis) (see Fig. 4-8, *A*) is the largest and most superficial of these muscles. It originates as eight muscular slips from the inferior borders of the lower eight ribs. The upper slips attach near the cartilages of the ribs, whereas the lower ones attach at a progressively greater distance from the costal cartilages. The serratus anterior, latissimus dorsi, and sometimes pectoralis major muscles interdigitate with these slips. The lower fibers descend almost vertically, attaching to roughly the anterior half of the outer lip of the iliac crest. The upper and middle fibers pass inferomedially and become aponeurotic by the time they pass a line connecting the umbilicus and anterior superior iliac spine. The external oblique aponeurosis is a strong sheet of connective tissue whose fibers continue inferomedially to the midline, where they blend with the linea alba. The linea alba is a tendinous raphe running in the midline from the xiphoid process to the pubic symphysis. The inferior portion of the aponeurosis of the external oblique forms the inguinal ligament, the reflected portion of that ligament, and the lacunar ligament. It also has an opening, the superficial inguinal ring, which allows passage of the spermatic cord in the male and the round ligament of the uterus in the female. The external abdominal oblique muscle is innervated by the ventral rami of the T7 to T12 spinal nerves.

Internal Abdominal Oblique Muscle. The internal abdominal oblique (obliquus internus abdominis) (see Fig. 4-8, *A*), located immediately deep to the external oblique, originates from the lateral two thirds of the inguinal ligament, anterior two thirds of the iliac crest, and the thoracolumbar fascia. The uppermost fibers insert onto the lower borders of the lower three or four ribs and are continuous with the internal intercostal muscles. The lowest fibers become tendinous and attach to the pubic crest and the medial portion of the pecten pubis. Here they are joined by the transversus abdominis aponeurosis, and together their united insertion forms the conjoint tendon, or inguinal falx. The intermediate fibers diverge from their origin and become aponeurotic. The internal oblique aponeurosis continues toward the midline, where it blends with the linea alba. In the upper two thirds of the abdomen, this aponeurosis splits into two laminae at the lateral border of the rectus abdominis. These laminae pass on either side of that muscle before reuniting at the linea alba. In the lower one third of the abdomen, the entire aponeurosis, along with the inserting aponeurosis of the transversus abdominis, passes anterior to the rectus abdominis. The internal abdominal oblique muscle is innervated by branches of the ventral rami of T7 to L1 spinal nerves.

Transversus Abdominis Muscle. The transversus abdominis muscle is located deep to the internal abdominal oblique muscle. It arises from the lateral one third of the inguinal ligament or adjacent iliac fascia, anterior two thirds of the outer lip of the iliac crest, the thoracolumbar fascia between the iliac crest and twelfth rib, and the internal aspects of the lower six costal cartilages, where it blends with the diaphragm. The fibers of the transversus abdominis run basically in a horizontal direction and become aponeurotic. The lowest fibers of the transversus abdominis aponeurosis curve inferomedially and, along with the fibers from the internal oblique aponeurosis, form the conjoint tendon (see the preceding discussion). The rest of the fibers of this aponeurosis pass horizontally to the midline, where they blend with the linea alba. The upper three fourths of the fibers run posterior to the rectus abdominis, whereas the lower one fourth course anterior to this muscle. The transversus abdominis is innervated by the anterior primary divisions of the T7 to L1 spinal nerves.

Rectus Abdominis Muscle. The rectus abdominis muscle (see Fig. 4-8, *A*) is a long, straplike muscle

extending the entire length of the anterior abdominal wall. The linea alba forms the medial border of this muscle and separates the two (right and left). The lateral border of the rectus usually can be seen on the surface of the anterior abdominal wall and is termed the linea semilunaris. This muscle attaches inferiorly to the pubic crest (sometimes as far laterally as the pecten pubis) and also to ligamentous fibers anterior to the symphysis pubis. The left and right rectus abdominis muscles may interlace in this region. Superiorly this muscle attaches to the fifth through seventh costal cartilages and the xiphoid process. Sometimes the most lateral fibers may reach the fourth or even third costal cartilages. The rectus abdominis muscle is crossed by three horizontal fibrous bands called the tendinous intersections. Usually they are found at the level of the umbilicus, the inferior tip of the xiphoid process, and halfway between these two points.

The rectus abdominis muscle is enclosed by the aponeurosis of the abdominal obliques and transversus abdominis muscles. Sometimes this aponeurosis is called the rectus sheath. In the upper portion of the anterior abdominal wall, the external oblique and anterior lamina of the internal oblique aponeuroses pass anterior to the rectus, whereas the posterior lamina of the internal oblique and transverse aponeuroses lie posterior to the rectus. This arrangement changes roughly halfway between the umbilicus and pubic symphysis, forming a curved line known as the arcuate line. Inferior to this line all three aponeurotic layers are found anterior to the rectus, and only the transversalis fascia (the layer of fascia deep to the anterolateral abdominal muscles) separates this muscle from the parietal peritoneum, although this traditional description of the rectus sheath may be too simplistic (Williams et al., 1995). The rectus abdominis muscle is supplied by the anterior primary divisions of the lower six or seven thoracic spinal nerves.

The abdominal muscles act to retain the abdominal viscera in place and oppose the effects of gravity on them in the erect and sitting positions. When the thorax and pelvis are fixed, these muscles, especially the obliques, increase the intraabdominal pressure. This is important for childbirth, expiration, emptying the bladder and rectum, and vomiting. It is also the basis of the Valsalva maneuver (increasing abdominal pressure for diagnostic purposes). The external abdominal oblique can further aid expiration by depressing the lower ribs. If the pelvis is fixed, these muscles, primarily the recti, bend the trunk forward and flex the lumbar spine. If the thorax is fixed, the lumbar spine still flexes, but the pelvis is brought upward. With unilateral contraction the trunk is laterally flexed to that side. In addition, the external oblique can help produce rotation of the trunk away from the side of contraction, whereas the internal oblique turns it to the same side. The transversus abdominis muscle probably

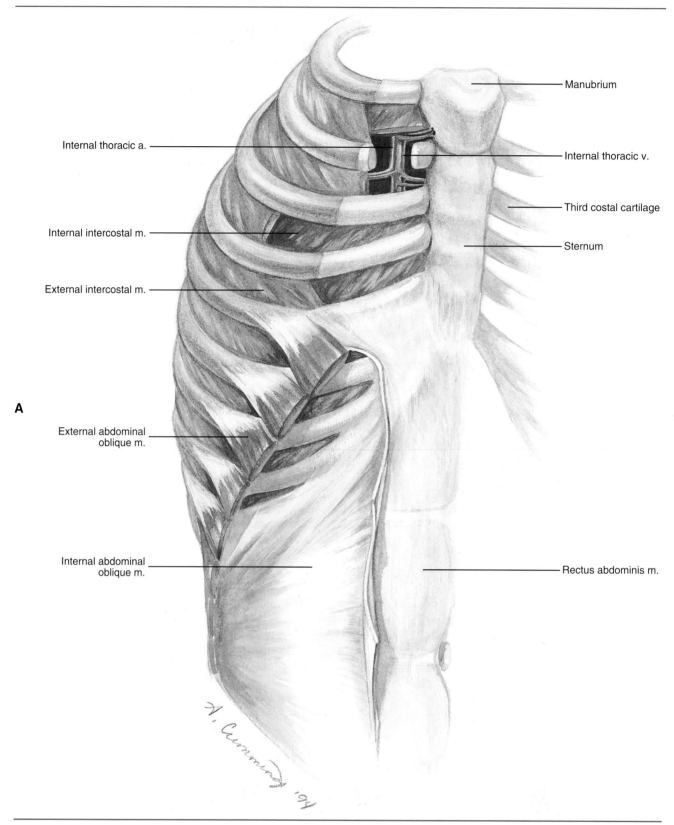

Manubrium

Internal thoracic a.

Internal thoracic v.

Third costal cartilage

Internal intercostal m.

Sternum

External intercostal m.

A

External abdominal
oblique m.

Internal abdominal
oblique m.

Rectus abdominis m.

FIG. 4-8   A, Anterolateral view of the thoracic and abdominal walls. *Upper aspect,* Cutaway view of the medial intercostal spaces demonstrating the internal thoracic artery and vein. The external intercostal muscle has been reflected between two ribs to show the internal intercostal muscle to best advantage. The external abdominal oblique muscle also has been reflected and cut away to reveal the internal abdominal oblique muscle.

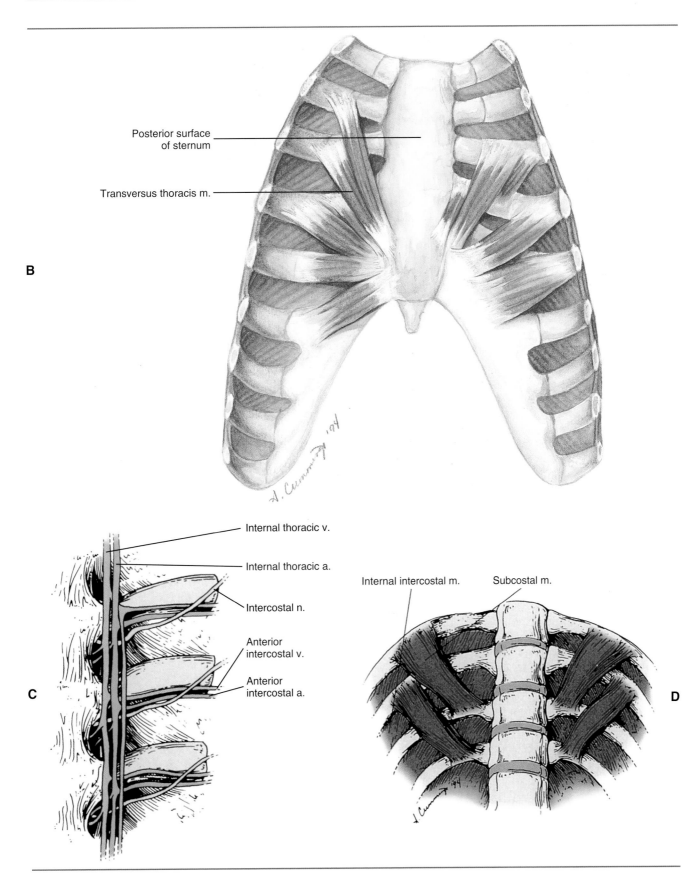

Posterior surface of sternum

Transversus thoracis m.

B

Internal thoracic v.

Internal thoracic a.

Intercostal n.

Anterior intercostal v.

Anterior intercostal a.

Internal intercostal m.   Subcostal m.

C

D

FIG. 4-8—cont'd   B, Internal view of the *anterior* thoracic wall showing the transversus thoracis muscle. **C,** Detail of **B** showing several intercostal spaces just lateral to the sternum. **D,** Internal view of the *posterior* thoracic wall showing several subcostal muscles.

has an effect only on the abdominal viscera and does not produce any appreciable movement of the vertebral column, although rotational movements are a distinct possibility (Williams et al., 1995). Contraction of the transversus abdominis muscle has been shown to significantly decrease laxity (or rather increase stiffness) of the sacroiliac joint, implying a stabilizing role of the transversus abdominis muscle for the sacroiliac joints (Richardson et al., 2002).

OTHER MUSCLES THAT HAVE CLINICAL RELEVANCE TO THE BACK

The tilting of the pelvis on the heads of the femurs in an anteroposterior direction is an important component of posture and locomotion. Movement of the anterior portion of the pelvis in a proximal direction (e.g., bringing the pubic symphysis toward the umbilicus) is termed *backward tilting* and involves flexion of the lumbar spine. Tilting of the pelvis in the opposite direction tends to extend the lumbar spine. This forward tilting of the pelvis is accomplished by contraction of the erector spinae and psoas major muscles. Backward tilting of the pelvis is accomplished not only by the rectus abdominis and the two oblique abdominal muscles, but also by the hamstring and gluteus maximus muscles (Fig. 4-9). Imbalance of the muscles responsible for pelvic tilt is often seen in people with low back pain. These individuals may have shortened and tight psoas major and erector spinae muscles combined with weakened gluteal and abdominal muscles (Oliver and Middleditch, 1991).

Hamstring Muscles

The posterior group of thigh muscles, commonly known as the hamstrings, acts to extend the hip and flex the knee joints. The three muscles in this group are the semitendinosus, semimembranosus, and biceps femoris. The latter muscle has two heads of origin, long and short (see Fig. 4-9).

With the exception of the short head of the biceps femoris, all three of these muscles attach proximally to the ischial tuberosity. The short head of the biceps femoris arises from the lateral lip of the linea aspera and lateral supracondylar line of the femur. The semitendinosus and semimembranosus muscles are located posteromedial in the thigh, whereas the biceps femoris is posterolateral.

Semitendinosus Muscle. The semitendinosus, as its name implies, becomes tendinous approximately halfway along its course (see Fig. 4-9). This long tendon curves around the medial tibial condyle, passes superficial to the tibial collateral ligament, and ends by attaching to the superior portion of the medial surface of the

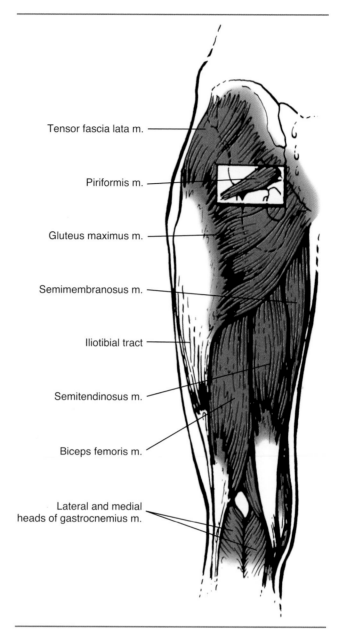

FIG. 4-9   Muscles of the posterior thigh. *Inset,* Piriformis muscle.

tibia immediately below and posterior to the attachment sites of the sartorius and gracilis muscles. This grouping of muscular insertions sometimes is known as the pes anserine. The semitendinosus muscle is innervated by the tibial portion (L5, S1, and S2) of the sciatic nerve.

Semimembranosus Muscle. The semimembranosus muscle (see Fig. 4-9) arises as a tendon and expands into an aponeurosis that is deep to the semitendinosus. The muscular fibers arise from this aponeurosis. The semimembranosus ends primarily on the posterior aspect of the medial tibial condyle via a short tendon. It also sends slips laterally and superiorly, some of which help form the oblique popliteal ligament. The semimembranosus muscle is innervated by the tibial portion (L5, S1, and S2) of the sciatic nerve.

Biceps Femoris Muscle. The short head of the biceps femoris joins the belly of the long head of the biceps femoris on its deep surface as it descends in the thigh. After the two heads unite, the biceps femoris muscle gradually narrows to a tendon that attaches to the head of the fibula, the fibular collateral ligament, and the lateral tibial condyle (see Fig. 4-9). The long head of the biceps femoris muscle is innervated by the tibial portion (L5, S1, and S2) and the short head by the common fibular (peroneal) portion (L5, S1, S2) of the sciatic nerve.

These muscles produce flexion at the knee and extension at the hip when they contract. When the thigh is flexed, the hamstring muscles (especially the biceps femoris) help tilt the pelvis backward. Tight hamstrings sometimes are associated with low back pain.

Gluteus Maximus Muscle

The gluteus maximus is the most superficial muscle in the gluteal region (see Fig. 4-9). It is considered the body's largest muscle. Its large size is a characteristic feature of the human musculature and is thought to be a result of its role in attaining an upright posture (Williams et al., 1995). It originates from the area of the ilium posterior to the posterior gluteal line. It also takes origin from the erector spinae aponeurosis, posterior and inferior sacrum, lateral coccyx, sacrotuberous ligament, and the fascial covering of the gluteus medius. The fibers of the gluteus maximus run inferolaterally and attach distally to the iliotibial tract and gluteal tuberosity of the femur between the attachment sites of the vastus lateralis and adductor magnus.

The gluteus maximus can extend the thigh from a flexed position when the pelvis is fixed. It also helps in strong lateral rotation of the thigh. Its upper fibers are active in strong abduction at the hip. If the thigh is stabilized, this muscle, along with the hamstrings, helps rotate the pelvis posteriorly on the femur heads, as in rising from a stooped position. By virtue of its attachment to the iliotibial tract, the gluteus maximus aids in stabilizing the femur on the tibia. It is also important for its intermittent action in various phases of normal gait. This muscle is innervated by the inferior gluteal nerve (L5 to S2).

Piriformis Muscle

The piriformis is a pear-shaped muscle lying deep to the gluteus medius (see Fig. 4-9). It arises from the antero-lateral sacrum by three musculotendinous slips. It also originates from the gluteal surface of the ilium (in proximity to the posterior inferior iliac spine), the ventral sacroiliac ligament, and sometimes from the anterior surface of the sacrotuberous ligament. The piriformis exits the pelvis via the greater sciatic foramen. The piriformis is the largest structure within that foramen. It attaches distally by a tendon to the upper border of the femur's greater trochanter. Normally this muscle lies immediately superior to the sciatic nerve as it exits the greater sciatic foramen, but sometimes (≈10%) the common fibular (peroneal) portion of the sciatic nerve pierces the piriformis and splits it (Moore and Dalley, 1999). Entrapment or irritation of the sciatic nerve (or a portion of it) in the region of the piriformis muscle sometimes is termed *piriformis syndrome* (Rodrigue and Hardy, 2001). With contraction, this muscle produces lateral rotation of the extended thigh. If the thigh is flexed, abduction at the hip occurs. It is innervated by branches from the ventral rami of the L5 to S2 spinal nerves.

Rectus Femoris Muscle

The quadriceps femoris is the great extensor muscle of the leg. This muscle consists of four parts: vastus lateralis, vastus intermedius, vastus medialis, and rectus femoris muscles. The three vasti muscles originate on the femur, but the rectus femoris arises from the pelvis. The rectus femoris muscle begins as two (or three) heads. The straight head attaches to the anterior inferior iliac spine, and the reflected head attaches to the superior rim of the acetabulum and capsule of the hip. Sometimes a recurrent head that arises from the anterosuperior angle of the femur's greater trochanter is described (Segal and Jacob, 1983). All the heads join, and the belly of the muscle then runs down the anterior thigh to attach by a broad aponeurosis to the base of the patella. By virtue of its proximal attachment sites, the rectus femoris muscle not only extends the knee, but also flexes the hip. If the thigh is fixed, contraction of this muscle helps to tilt the pelvis forward. The rectus femoris, along with the rest of the quadriceps femoris, is innervated by the femoral nerve (L2 to L4).

SUMMARY OF MUSCLES AFFECTING THE SPINE

Table 4-2 provides a summary of the muscles that influence the spine. This table does not give a complete account of all the points of origin and insertion of some of the more complex muscles. A more detailed description of each muscle appears in the text of this chapter. Box 4-1 organizes the muscles that influence the spine according to the motion produced by their contraction.

Table 4-2   Summary of Muscles Affecting the Spine

Muscle	Origin	Insertion	Action	Innervation
Layer One				
Trapezius	Superior nuchal line, external occipital protuberance, ligamentum nuchae, spinous processes and supraspinous ligament of C7-T12	Spine of the scapula, acromion, distal third of clavicle	See Table 4-1	Motor: spinal portion of accessory (spinal accessory [cranial nerve XI]) Sensory (proprioception): ventral rami of C3-4
Latissimus dorsi	Spinous processes and supraspinous ligament of T6-15, thoracolumbar fascia, median sacral crest, iliac crests, lower four ribs	Intertubercular groove of the humerus (between insertion of pectoralis major and teres major)	Adduction, internal rotation, and extension of the humerus	Thoracodorsal (C6-8)
Layer Two				
Rhomboid major	Spinous processes and supraspinous ligament (T2-5)	Medial border of scapula inferior to root of scapular spine	Retract scapula, rotate point of shoulder down	Dorsal scapular (C5)
Rhomboid minor	Lower portion of ligamentum nuchae, spinous processes (C7 and T1)	Medial border of scapula at level of root of scapular spine	Retract scapula, rotate point of shoulder down	Dorsal scapular (C5)
Levator scapulae	Transverse processes (C1-4)	Medial border of scapula above root of scapular spine	If neck stabilized: elevate scapula, rotate point of shoulder down If scapula stabilized bilaterally—extend neck; unilaterally—lateral flex and rotate neck to same side	Ventral rami of C3-4, dorsal scapular (C5)
Layer Three				
Serratus posterior superior	Spinous processes and supraspinous ligament (C7-T3)	Posterior and superior aspect of second through fifth ribs	Aids respiration, raises second through fifth ribs	Ventral rami of T2-5 (intercostal nerves)
Serratus posterior inferior	Spinous processes and supraspinous ligament of T11-L2(3)	Posterior and inferior surfaces of lower four ribs (T9-12)	Aids respiration, lowers ninth through twelfth ribs	Ventral rami of T9-12 (lower three intercostal nerves and subcostal nerve)
Layer Four				
Splenius capitis	Lower part of ligamentum nuchae and spinous processes of C7-T3(4)	Mastoid process, temporal bone, and occiput below lateral part of superior nuchal line	Bilaterally: extend head Unilaterally: lateral flex and rotate face to same side	Lateral branches of dorsal rami of midcervical spinal nerve (C3-5)
Splenius cervicis	Spinous processes (T3-6)	Transverse processes of C1-3(4)	Bilaterally: extend neck Unilaterally: lateral flex and rotate face toward same side	Lateral branches of dorsal rami of lower cervical spinal nerves (C5-7)

Table 4-2   Summary of Muscles Affecting the Spine—cont'd

Muscle	Origin	Insertion	Action	Innervation
Layer Five				
Iliocostalis lumborum	Common origin of erector spinae muscles: spinous processes and supraspinous ligament of T11-L5, median sacral crest, sacro-tuberous ligament, posterior sacroiliac ligament, lateral sacral crest, posteromedial iliac crest	Angles of lower six to nine ribs	Extend and laterally flex spine	Lateral branches of dorsal rami of nearby spinal nerves
Iliocostalis thoracis	Angles of lower six ribs	Angles of upper six ribs and transverse process of C7	Extend and laterally flex spine	Lateral branches of dorsal rami of nearby spinal nerves
Iliocostalis cervicis	Angles of third through sixth ribs	Posterior tubercles of transverse processes of C4-6	Extend and laterally flex spine	Dorsal rami of nearby spinal nerves
Longissimus thoracis	Common origin of erector spinae muscles (see iliocostalis lumborum), also transverse and accessory processes of all lumbar vertebrae	Third through twelfth ribs, transverse processes of all 12 thoracic vertebrae	Extend and laterally flex spine	Lateral branches of dorsal rami of nearby spinal nerves
Longissimus cervicis	Transverse processes of upper thoracic vertebrae (T1-5)	Transverse processes and articular processes of C2-6	Extend and laterally flex spine	Lateral branches of dorsal rami of nearby spinal nerves
Longissimus capitis	Upper thoracic transverse processes (T1-5) and articular processes of C4-7	Mastoid process temporal bone	Extend and laterally flex head	Lateral branches of dorsal rami of nearby spinal nerves
Spinalis thoracis	Lower thoracic and upper lumbar spinous processes (T11-L2)	Upper thoracic spinous processes (T1-4, sometimes down to T8)	Extend spine	Dorsal rami of nearby spinal nerves
Spinalis cervicis	Upper thoracic spinous processes (T1-6)	Spinous processes of C2 (occasionally C3 and C4)	Extend spine	Dorsal rami of nearby spinal nerves
Spinalis capitis	Transverse process of C7-T6(7), articular processes of C4-6, sometimes spinous processes of C7 and T1	Occiput between superior and inferior nuchal lines	Extend head	Dorsal rami of upper thoracic and lower cervical spinal nerves
Layer Six				
Semispinalis thoracis	Transverse processes (T7-12)	Spinous processes of four to six vertebrae above (C6-T4)	Bilaterally: extend thoracic spine Unilaterally: extend, laterally flex, and rotate vertebral bodies of thoracic spine to opposite side	Medial branches of dorsal rami of T1-6

Continued

Table 4-2   Summary of Muscles Affecting the Spine—cont'd

Muscle	Origin	Insertion	Action	Innervation
Layer Six—cont'd				
Semispinalis cervicis	Transverse processes (T1-5), articular processes (C4-7)	Spinous processes of four to six vertebrae above (C2-3)	Bilaterally: extend neck Unilaterally: extend, laterally flex, and rotate neck to opposite side	Dorsal rami of C6-8
Semispinalis capitis	Transverse processes (C7-T6), articular processes (C4-6)	Occiput between medial portions of superior and inferior nuchal lines	Bilaterally: extend head Unilaterally: slight rotation of face to opposite side	Dorsal rami of C1-6
Multifidus (lumborum, thoracis, cervicis)	Posterior sacrum, L1-5 mamillary processes, T1-12 transverse processes, C4-7 articular processes*	Spinous processes two to four segments above (C2-15)*	Bilaterally: extend spine Unilaterally: extend, laterally flex, and rotate vertebral bodies to opposite side	Medial branches of dorsal rami of spinal nerves
Rotatores (lumborum, thoracis, cervicis)	Transverse processes	Spinous processes; longus ascends two vertebral segments, brevis ascends one vertebral segment	Bilaterally: extend spine Unilaterally: rotate vertebral bodies to opposite side	Medial branches of dorsal rami of spinal nerves
Suboccipital Muscles				
Rectus capitis posterior major	Spinous process (C2)	Lateral portion of inferior nuchal line	Bilaterally: extend head Unilaterally: rotate face toward same side	Suboccipital (dorsal ramus of C1)
Rectus capitis posterior minor	Posterior tubercle (C1)	Medial portion of inferior nuchal line	Extend head	Suboccipital (dorsal ramus of C1)
Obliquus capitis inferior	Spinous process (C2)	Transverse process (C1)	Rotate face toward same side	Suboccipital (dorsal ramus of C1)
Obliquus capitis superior	Transverse process (C1)	Occiput between lateral portions of superior and inferior nuchal lines	Bilaterally: extend head Unilaterally: lateral flex head to same side	Suboccipital (dorsal ramus of C1)
Small Muscles of the Spine				
Intertransversarius*	Transverse process	Transverse process of adjacent vertebra	Lateral flexion of vertebra (approximates transverse processes)	Medial part of posterior intertransversarius: dorsal ramus of spinal nerve Anterior intertransversarius and lateral part of posterior intertransversarius: ventral ramus
Interspinalis	Spinous process	Spinous process of adjacent vertebra	Extend spine (approximate spinous processes)	Medial branch of dorsal rami
Levator costarum (longus and brevis)	Lateral aspect of transverse processes (C7-T11)	Brevis: rib immediately below Longus: second rib below	Elevate ribs, may help laterally flex and rotate trunk to same side	Sementally innervated by lateral branches of dorsal rami of spinal nerve

Table 4-2   Summary of Muscles Affecting the Spine—cont'd

Muscle	Origin	Insertion	Action	Innervation
Muscles of the Anterior Aspect of the Cervical Vertebrae				
Longus colli (vertical part)	Anterior aspect vertebral bodies (C5-T3)	Anterior aspect vertebral bodies (C2-4)	Flex neck	Ventral rami of C2-6 spinal nerves
Logus colli (inferior oblique part)	Vertebral bodies (T1-3)	Anterior tubercles of transverse processes (C5 and C6)	Flex neck, aid with lateral flexion of neck to same side, rotate neck to opposite side	Ventral rami of lower cervical spinal nerves
Longus colli (superior oblique part)	Anterior tubercles of transverse processes (C3-5)	Anterior tubercle (C1)	Flex neck, aid with lateral flexion of neck to same side	Ventral rami of upper cervical spinal nerves
Longus capitis	Anterior tubercles of transverse processes (C3-6)	Anterior occiput	Flex head	Ventral rami of C1-3
Rectus capitis anterior	Anterior aspect of lateral mass of atlas	Occiput (anterior to occipital condyle)	Flex head at atlanto-occipital joints	Ventral rami of C1 and C2
Rectus capitis lateralis	Anterior aspect of transverse process (C-I)	Occiput (jugular process)	Laterally flex occiput on atlas	Ventral rami of C1 and C2
Iliac Muscles				
Psoas major	Anterolateral bodies (T12-L5), discs (T12-L4), transverse processes (L1-5)	Lesser trochanter (with iliacus)	If spine stabilized: flex thigh. If thigh stabilized: flex trunk, tilt pelvis forward	Ventral rami of L2-3
Iliacus	Medial lip of iliac crest, iliac fossa, superolateral sacrum	Lesser trochanter (with psoas major)	See psoas major	Femoral (L2-3)
Psoas minor	Bodies (T12-L1), disc (T12)	Pecten pubis, iliopubic eminence	Flex trunk	Ventral ramus of L1
Quadratus lumborum	Transverse process (L5), iliolumbar ligament, posterior portion of iliac crest	Lower border of twelfth rib, transverse processes (L1-4)	Bilaterally: extend spine, depress twelfth rib, stabilize origin of diaphragm to twelfth rib. Unilaterally: lateral flex spine	Ventral rami of T12-L3
Muscles of Respiration				
Diaphragm	Xiphoid process, deep surface of lower six ribs and their costal cartilages, lateral and medial lumbocostal arches and bodies (L1-3)	Central tendon	Inspiration, stabilize thorax	Phrenic (C3-5), lower six intercostals (afferent only)
External intercostals	Lower border ribs (1-11) from tubercles to costal cartilages	Upper border of adjacent rib below from tubercles to costal cartilages	Respiration, stabilize thorax	Adjacent intercostals
Internal intercostals	Lower border ribs (1-11) from sternum/costal cartilage to angle	Upper border of adjacent rib below from sternum/costal cartilage to angle	Respiration, stabilize thorax	Adjacent intercostals

Continued

Table 4-2 Summary of Muscles Affecting the Spine—cont'd

Muscle	Origin	Insertion	Action	Innervation
Muscles of Respiration—cont'd				
Innermost intercostals	Lower border ribs (1-11) in middle two fourths of intercostal space	Upper border of adjacent rib below in middle two fourths of intercostal space	Respiration, stabilize thorax	Adjacent intercostals
Subcostal	Inferior border ribs (1-10) near angle	Superior border of second rib below	Depress ribs	Adjacent intercostals
Transversus thoracis	Deep surface of inferior sternal body, xiphoid process, costal cartilages (4-7)	Deep surface of costal cartilages (2-6)	Depress costal cartilages	Adjacent intercostals
Anterolateral Abdominal Muscles				
External abdominal oblique	Inferior borders of lower eight ribs*	Linea alba, iliac crest*	Bilaterally: flex spine, tilt pelvis backward Unilaterally: lateral flex spine to same side, rotate spine to opposite side	Ventral rami of T7-12
Internal abdominal oblique	Lateral two thirds of inguinal ligament, anterior iliac crest, thoracolumbar fascia	Pecten pubis, pubic crest, linea alba*	Bilaterally: flex spine, tilt pelvis backward Unilaterally: lateral flex and rotate spine to same side	Ventral rami of T7-L1
Transversus abdominis	Lateral two thirds of inguinal ligament, anterior illiac crest, thoracolumbar fascia, lower six costal cartilages	Linea alba*	Unilaterally: rotate spine to same side	Ventral rami of T7-L1
Rectus abdominis	Pubic crest, symphysis pubis	Costal cartilages (5-7), xiphoid process	Bilaterally: flex spine, tilt pelvis backward Unilaterally: lateral flex spine	Ventral rami of T7-12
Hamstring Muscles				
Semitendinosus	Ischial tuberosity	Medial tibia (pes anserine)	If leg stabilized: extend thigh, tilt pelvis backward If thigh stabilized: flex leg	Tibial division of sciatic nerve (L5, S1, S2)
Semimembranosus	Ischial tuberosity	Posterior aspect of medial tibial condyle*	If leg stabilized: extend thigh, tilt pelvis backward If thigh stabilized: flex leg	Tibial division of sciatic nerve (L5, S1, S2)
Biceps femoris	Long head: ischial tuberosity Short head: linea aspera, lateral supracondylar line of femur	Fibular head, fibular collateral ligament, lateral tibial condyle	Long head: if leg stabilized—extend thigh, tilt pelvis backward Both heads: if thigh stabilized—flex leg	Long head: tibial division of sciatic nerve (L5, S1, S2), Short head: common fibular (peroneal) division of sciatic nerve (L5, S1, S2)

Table 4-2   Summary of Muscles Affecting the Spine—cont'd

Muscle	Origin	Insection	Action	Innervation
Muscles Attaching to the Sacrum and Ilium				
Gluteus maximus	Ilium, posterior-to-posterior gluteal line, aponeurosis of erector spinae, posterior sacrum, lateral coccyx, sacrotuberous ligament	Gluteal tuberosity, iliotibial tract	If pelvis stabilized: extend, abduct, and laterally rotate thigh If thigh stabilized: tilt pelvis backward, stabilize knee	Inferior gluteal (L5-S2)
Rectus femoris	Straight head: anteroinferior iliac spine Reflected head: acetabulum, capsule of hip*	Base of patella	If thigh stabilized: extend leg, tilt pelvis forward If pelvis stabilized: flex hip	Femoral (L2-4)
Piriformis	Anterolateral sacrum, gluteal surface of ilium, capsule of sacroiliac joint	Greater trochanter	If thigh extended: laterally rotate hip If thigh flexed: abduct hip	Ventral rami of L5-S2

*See text for further details.

BOX 4-1
SUMMARY OF ACTIONS OF SPINAL MUSCLES

MUSCLES ACTING ON THE HEAD AT THE ATLANTO-AXIAL AND ATLANTO-OCCIPITAL JOINTS

Extension
Trapezius
Semispinalis capitis
(Spinalis capitis)
Rectus capitis posterior major
Rectus capitis posterior minor
Obliquus capitis superior
Splenius capitis
Longissimus capitis

Flexion
Longus capitis
Rectus capitis anterior
Sternocleidomastoid

Lateral flexion
Trapezius
Sternocleidomastoid
Splenius capitis
Longissimus capitis
Semispinalis capitis
Rectus capitis lateralis
Obliquus capitis superior

Rotation
Splenius capitis, same side
Longissimus capitis, same side
Obliquus capitis inferior, same side
Longus capitis, same side
Rectus capitis posterior major, same side
Trapezius, opposite side
Sternocleidomastoid, opposite side

MUSCLES ACTING ON THE CERVICAL REGION

Extension
Levator scapulae
Splenius capitis
Splenius cervicis
Longissimus capitis
Longissimus cervicis
(Spinalis capitis)
(Spinalis cervicis)
Iliocosalis cervicis
Semispinalis capitis
Semispinalis cervicis
Multifidus
Interspinales

Flexion
Sternocleidomastoid
Longus capitis
Longus colli
Scalenus anterior

Continued

BOX 4-1
SUMMARY OF ACTIONS OF SPINAL MUSCLES—cont'd

MUSCLES ACTING ON THE CERVICAL REGION—cont'd

Lateral flexion
Sternocleidomastoid
Scalenus anterior
Scalenus medius
Scalenus posterior
Splenius capitis
Splenius cervicis
Levator scapulae
Longissimus capitis
Longissimus cervicis
Iliocostalis cervicis
Semispinalis cervicis
Trapezius
Intertransversarii

Rotation
Splenius capitis, same side
Splenius cervicis, same side
Longissimus cervicis, same side
Iliocostalis cervicis, same side
Sternaocleidomastoid, opposite side
Semispinalis cervicis, opposite side
Multifidus, opposite side
Rotatores, opposite side
Scalenus anterior, opposite side
Trapezius, opposite side

MUSCLES ACTING ON THE TRUNK

Flexion
Psoas major
Psoas minor
Rectus abdominis
External abdominal oblique
Internal abdominal oblique

Extension
Quadratus lumborum
Multifidus
Rotatores
Semispinalis thoracis
Spinalis thoracis
Longissimus thoracis
Iliocostalis thoracis
Iliocostalis lumborum
Interspinales

Lateral flexion
External abdominal oblique
Internal abdominal oblique
Rectus abdominis
Iliocostalis lumborum
Iliocostalis thoracis
Longissimus thoracis
Semispinalis thoracis
Multifidus
Quadratus lumborum
Intertransversarii
Psoas major

Rotation
Internal abdominal oblique, same side
Iliocostalis thoracis, same side
Iliocostalis lumborum, same side
External abdominal oblique, opposite side
Multifidus, opposite side
Rotatores, opposite side

MUSCLES PRODUCING ANTEROPOSTERIOR TILTING OF THE PELVIS

Forward tilting
Erector spinae
Psoas major
Rectus femoris

Backward tilting
Rectus abdominis
External abdominal oblique
Internal abdominal oblique
Gluteus maximus
Biceps femoris (long head)
Semitendinosus
Semimembranosus

REFERENCES

Andersson EA et al. (2002). Diverging intramuscular activity patterns in back and abdominal muscles during trunk rotation. *Spine, 27(6),* E152-E160.

Barker PJ & Briggs CA. (1999). Attachments of the posterior layer of lumbar fascia. *Spine, 24,* 1757-1766.

Bogduk N. (1997). *Clinical anatomy of the lumbar spine* (3rd ed.). London: Churchill Livingstone.

Boyd-Clark LC et al. (2002). Muscle spindle distribution, morphology, and density in longus colli and multifidus muscles of the cervical spine. *Spine, 27(7),* 694-701.

Campos GE et al. (1994) Electromyographic study of the trapezius and deltoideus in elevation, lowering, retraction and protraction of the shoulders. *Electromyogr Clin Neurophysiol, 34(4),* 243-7.

Cholewicki J et al. (1997). Stabilizing function of trunk flexor-extensor muscles around a neutral spine posture. *Spine, 22(19),* 2207-2212.

Clark BC et al. (2003). Derecruitment of the lumbar musculature with fatiguing trunk extension exercise. *Spine, 28(3),* 282-287.

Daggfeldt K et al. (2000). The visible human anatomy of the lumbar erector spinae. *Spine, 25(21),* 2719-2725.

Danneels LA et al. (2001). A functional subdivision of hip, abdominal, and back muscles during asymmetric lifting. *Spine, 26(6),* E114-E121.

Guazzelli FH et al. (1994). Electromyographic study of the trapezius muscle in free movements of the shoulder. *Electromyogr Clin Neurophysiol, 45(5),* 279-83.

Hack GD. (1995). Anatomic relation between the rectus capitis posterior minor muscle and the dura mater. *Spine, 20(23),* 2484-2486.

Hirayama J et al. (2001). Effects of electrical stimulation of the sciatic nerve on background electromyography and static stretch reflex activity of the trunk muscles in rats. *Spine, 26(6),* 602-609.

Humphreys BK. (2003). Investigation of connective tissue attachments to the cervical spinal dura mater. *Clin Anat, 16(2),* 152-159.

Kamibayashi LK & Richmond FJR. (1998). Morphometry of human neck muscles. *Spine, 23(12),* 1314-1323.

Kang Y-M et al. (2002). Electrophysiologic evidence for an intersegmental reflex pathway between lumbar paraspinal tissues. *Spine, 27(3),* E56-E63.

Krsnich-Shriwise S. (1997). Fibromyalgia syndrome: An overview. *Phys Ther, 77,* 68-75.

Lehman GJ et al. (2001). Effects of a mechanical pain stimulus on erector spinae activity before and after a spinal manipulation in patients with back pain: A preliminary investigation. *J Manipulative Physiol Ther, 24(6),* 402-406.

Lorimer Moseley G et al. (2002). Deep and superficial fibers of the lumbar multifidus muscle are differentially active during voluntary arm movements. *Spine, 27(2),* E29-E36.

Macintosh JE & Bogduk N. (1986). The biomechanics of the lumbar multifidus. *Clin Biomech, 1,* 205-213.

Macintosh JE & Bogduk N. (1987a). The biomechanics of the thoracolumbar fascia. *Clin Biomech, 2,* 78-83.

Macintosh JE & Bogduk N. (1987b). The morphology of the lumbar erector spinae. *Spine, 12,* 658-668.

Macintosh JE et al. (1986). The morphology of the human lumbar multifidus. *Clin Biomech, 1,* 196-204.

McPartland JM et al. (1997). Chronic neck pain, standing balance, and suboccipital muscle atrophy: A pilot study. *J Manipulative Physiol Ther, 20(1),* 24-29.

Moore KL & Dalley AF. (1999). *Clinically oriented anatomy* (4th ed.). Philadelphia: Lippincott Williams & Wilkins.

Oliver J & Middleditch A. (1991). *Functional anatomy of the spine.* Oxford, UK: Butterworth-Heinemann.

Peck D et al. (1986). Are there compartment syndromes in some patients with idiopathic back pain? *Spine, 11,* 468-475.

Quint U et al. (1998). Importance of the intersegmental trunk muscles for the stability of the lumbar spine. *Spine, 23(18),* 1937-1945.

Richardson CA et al. (2002). The relation between the transverses abdominis muscles, sacroiliac joint mechanics, and low back pain. *Spine, 27(4),* 399-405.

Rodrigue T & Hardy RW. (2001). Diagnosis and treatment of piriformis syndrome. *Neurosurg Clin N Am, 12(2),* 311-319.

Schneider MJ. (1995). Tender points/fibromyalgia vs. trigger points/myofascial pain syndrome: A need for clarity in terminology and differential diagnosis. *J Manipulative Physiol Ther, 18(6),* 398-406.

Segal P & Jacob M. (1983). *The knee.* Chicago: Year Book.

Travell JG & Simons DG. (1983). *Myofascial pain and dysfunction: The trigger point manual* (vol. 1.). Baltimore: Williams & Wilkins.

Travell JG & Simons DG. (1992). *Myofascial pain and dysfunction: The trigger point manual* (vol. 2.). Baltimore: Williams & Wilkins.

van Dieen JH. (1996). Asymmetry of erector spinae muscle activity in twisted postures and consistency of muscle activation patterns across subjects. *Spine, 21(22),* 2651-2661.

van Dieen JH et al. (2003). Trunk muscle activation in low-back pain patients: An analysis of the literature. *J Electromyogr Kinesiol, 13(4),* 333-351.

Vilensky JA et al. (2001). Serratus posterior muscles: Anatomy, clinical relevance, and function. *Clin Anat, 14(4),* 237-241.

Williams PL et al. (Eds.). (1995). *Gray's anatomy* (38th ed.). Edinburgh: Churchill Livingstone.

CHAPTER 5

The Cervical Region

Gregory D. Cramer

The cervical region is possibly the most distinct region of the spine. The fact that so many structures, spinal and otherwise, are packed into such a small cylinder, connecting the head to the thorax, makes the entire neck an outstanding feat of efficient design. The cervical spine is the most complicated articular system in the body, comprising 37 separate joints (Bland, 1989). It allows more movement than any other spinal region and is surrounded by a myriad of nerves, vessels, and many other vital structures. However, such complexity can come at a high cost; more than 50% of individuals suffer from significant neck pain at some time in their lives (SBU Project Group, 2000). All clinicians who have spent significant time working with patients suffering from pain of cervical origin have been challenged and sometimes frustrated with this region of immense clinical importance. Understanding the detailed anatomy of this area helps clinicians make more accurate assessments of their patients, which in turn results in the establishment of more effective treatment protocols.

This chapter begins by covering the general characteristics of the cervical spine as a whole. This is followed by a discussion of the region's typical and atypical vertebrae. The external aspect of the occiput is included because of its intimate relationship with the upper two cervical segments. Then the ligaments of the cervical region are covered, followed by a discussion of the cervical spine's ranges of motion. The most important structures of the anterior neck and cervical viscera also are included.

CHARACTERISTICS OF THE CERVICAL SPINE AS A WHOLE

Cervical Curve (Lordosis)

The cervical curve is the least distinct of the spinal curves. It is convex anteriorly (lordosis) and is a secondary (compensatory) curvature (see Chapter 2). The cervical curve begins to develop before birth at as early as 9 weeks of prenatal life. Onset of fetal movements plays an important role in the early development of the cervical lordosis (Bagnall, Harris, and Jones, 1977; Williams et al., 1995). However, the curve becomes much more marked when the child begins to lift the head at approximately 3 to 4 months after birth, and the curve increases as the child begins to sit upright at approximately 9 months of age (Williams et al., 1995).

The amount of cervical lordosis can be measured reliably from standard x-rays if rigorous, standardized methods of evaluation are used (Côté et al., 1997). The cervical lordosis increases significantly with age in both sexes. In males, the change is rather gradual until the age of 70, when a dramatic increase in lordosis occurs. In females, in whom the cervical lordosis is greater throughout life, the curve increases gradually until a time of several years of marked increase begins near the age of 50; the rate of change then becomes more gradual but continues throughout the remainder of life (Doual, Ferri, and Laude, 1997).

Some authors state that the cervical curve actually is composed of two curves, upper and lower (Kapandji, 1974; Oliver and Middleditch, 1991). The upper cervical curve is described as a distinct primary curve that extends from the occiput to the axis and is concave anteriorly (kyphotic). The lower cervical curve is the classically described lordosis, but in this case begins at C2 rather than C1. This description helps to explain the dramatic differences seen between the upper and lower cervical vertebrae, such as the independent movements that can occur in the two regions (e.g., flexion of the lower cervicals and simultaneous extension of occiput on atlas and atlas on axis).

The lack of a normal cervical lordosis is a frequent finding in children and adolescents under age 17, but a lack of cervical lordosis in the adult may be a sign of ligamentous injury (Fesmire and Luten, 1989) or anterior cervical muscular hypertonicity. However, some controversy exists on this topic. Some authors (G. Schultz, personal communication) consider a hypolordotic or even kyphotic cervical curve to be clinically insignificant, especially if a tendency toward the establishment of a lordosis can be demonstrated during extension of the cervical region. Methods used to evaluate such a tendency include palpation at the spinous processes during extension, lateral projection x-ray films taken with the patient holding the neck in extension, and cineradiography studies in which a series of x-ray films are taken while the patient moves the neck. Another cause of decreased cervical lordosis is the presence of hyperplastic articular pillars (see Articular Processes). Hyperplastic articular pillars are considered to be a common normal variation of the typical cervical vertebrae (C3-6) and are associated with a reduction of the cervical lordosis (Peterson et al., 1999).

Total cerebrospinal (CS) height decreases significantly from early adulthood to senescence in both sexes, but the rate of change is different in males and females. In males, the change is more gradual, whereas in females, in whom the overall decrease in height is greater than in males, there is a marked change near the age of 50, presumably associated with menopause. As described, the cervical lordosis also markedly increases during this time. The rate of decrease in height of the cervical region then slows again after the fifth decade (Doual, Ferri, and Laude, 1997).

Degenerative joint disease (DJD; bone spur, or osteophyte formation, and intervertebral disc narrowing) occurs earlier in males (31 to 40 years of age) than females. However, the incidence of female DJD of the cervical region catches up as a sharp rise in DJD occurs at 51 to 60 years of age. After 60 years of age the incidence between males and females is roughly equal (Wiegand et al., 2003).

Typical Cervical Vertebrae

The typical cervical vertebrae are C3 through C6. These are some of the smallest but most distinct vertebrae of any vertebral region. C1 and C2 are considered to be atypical vertebrae, and C7 is unique. These three vertebrae are discussed later in this chapter.

The individual components of the typical cervical vertebrae are discussed in the following section. Special emphasis is placed on those characteristics that distinguish typical cervical vertebrae from the other spinal vertebrae.

Vertebral Bodies. Each cervical vertebra is made up of a vertebral body and a posterior arch (Fig. 5-1). The vertebral bodies of the cervical spine are small and are more or less rectangular in shape when viewed from above, with the transverse (left-to-right) diameter greater than the anteroposterior diameter. The exception to this is C7, which is almost square. The transverse and anterior to posterior diameters both increase from C2 to C7. This allows the lower vertebrae to support the greater weights they are required to carry. In addition, the vertebral bodies of males have been found to be larger than those of females (Liguoro, Vandermeersch, and Guerin, 1994; Lu et al., 1999).

The thickness of the outer cortex of the superior and inferior aspects of the vertebral bodies increases from C3 to C7. In addition, the superior aspect of each C3-7 vertebral body (superior bony end plate) is thickest posteriorly and thinnest anteriorly; the opposite is true for the inferior end plate (i.e., thickest anteriorly). The center of the inferior bony end plate also is thicker than the center of the superior bony end plate in the C3-7 vertebrae. Finally, the heights (superior to inferior

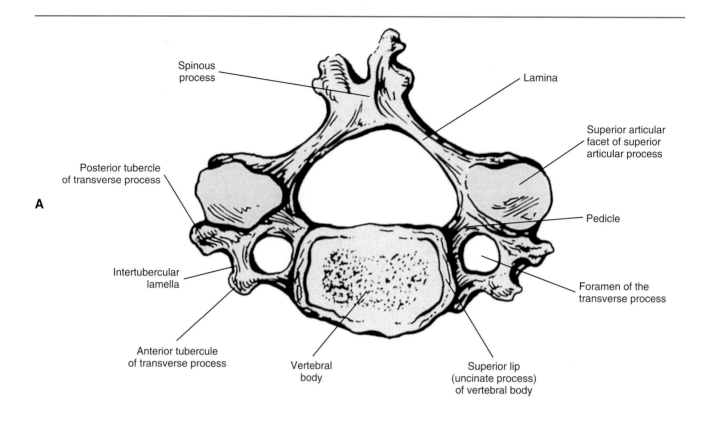

A

Spinous process

Lamina

Superior articular facet of superior articular process

Posterior tubercle of transverse process

Pedicle

Intertubercular lamella

Foramen of the transverse process

Anterior tubercule of transverse process

Vertebral body

Superior lip (uncinate process) of vertebral body

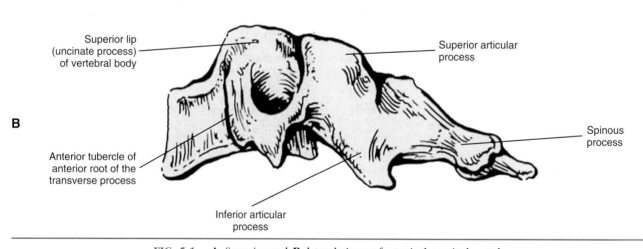

B

Superior lip (uncinate process) of vertebral body

Superior articular process

Anterior tubercle of anterior root of the transverse process

Spinous process

Inferior articular process

FIG. 5-1   **A,** Superior and, **B,** lateral views of a typical cervical vertebra.

dimensions) of both the anterior and posterior aspects of the cervical vertebral bodies generally increase from C3 to C7 (Panjabi et al., 2001a).

The anterior surface of the cervical vertebral body is convex from side to side. However, these same surfaces are concave from superior to inferior (Panjabi et al., 2001a) because of prominent ridges at the superior and inferior borders (discal margins) formed by the attachment sites of the anterior longitudinal ligaments. Indentations seen on the left and right of the anterior midline of the vertebral bodies are for attachment of the vertical fibers of the longus colli muscle.

The anterior aspects of the vertebral bodies can develop bony spurs (osteophytes). Asymptomatic osteophytes may occur in 20% to 30% of the population. Pressure on the more anteriorly located esophagus or trachea from osteophytes may lead to difficulty with swallowing (dysphagia) and speech (dysphonia), although such consequences are rare (Kissel and Youmans, 1992).

The posterior surface of a typical cervical vertebral body is slightly indented (Panjabi et al., 2001a) and possesses two or more foramina for exit of the basivertebral veins (Williams et al., 1995). The posterior longitudinal ligament attaches to the superior and inferior margins of the posterior aspect of the cervical vertebral bodies.

The superior and inferior surfaces of the vertebral bodies typically are described as being sellar or saddle shaped. More specifically, the superior surface is concave from left to right as a result of the raised lateral lips (uncinate processes). The superior surface is also convex from front to back because of the beveling of its anterior aspect. The inferior surface is convex from left to right and concave from anterior to posterior. Much of the concavity is created by the anterior lip of the inferior surface. This concavity is greatest at C3 and C4 and then becomes shallower as one moves inferiorly from C5 to C7 (Panjabi et al., 2001a). The inferior aspects of the vertebral bodies of C5 and C6 have the greatest anteroposterior dimension (Lu et al., 1999). Osteophyte (bone spur) formation is also most common at the C5-6 levels (Wiegand et al., 2003).

The anteroinferior aspect of each vertebral body usually protrudes inferiorly to overlap the anterior portion of the intervertebral disc (IVD) and occasionally the vertebra below. When the latter occurs, the anterosuperior aspect of the vertebra below is more beveled than would otherwise be the case. This increased beveling allows the vertebra to receive the projecting portion of the body above during flexion of the cervical spine.

Raised Lips at the Superior Aspect of the Vertebral Bodies and the Uncovertebral Joints. When viewed from the lateral or anterior aspect, several unique characteristics of the vertebral bodies become apparent (see Fig. 5-1, *B*). Lateral lips (uncinate processes) project from the superior surface of each typical cervical vertebra. These structures arise as elevations of the lateral and posterior rims on the top surface of the vertebral bodies (Dupuis et al., 1985). The posterior components of the uncinate processes tend to become more prominent in the lower cervical vertebrae. Normally the uncinate processes allow for flexion and extension of the cervical spine and help to limit lateral flexion. In addition, the uncinate processes serve as barriers to posterior and lateral IVD protrusion. The relationship of the left and right uncinate processes to the IVD has led at least one investigator to state that IVD herniation in the cervical region may occur less frequently than previously thought (Bland, 1989).

The uncinate processes of one vertebra may articulate with the small indentations found on the inferior surface of the vertebra above by means of small synovial joints. These joints are sometimes called the uncovertebral joints (of von Luschka). They consist of oblique clefts that develop at approximately 9 to 10 years of age. The clefts are limited medially by the IVD and laterally by capsular ligaments (Williams et al., 1995); the latter are derived from the anulus fibrosus of the IVD. Some investigators do not believe that the uncovertebral joints can be classified as synovial joints (Tondury, 1943; Orofino, Sherman, and Schecter, 1960; Bland, 1989), whereas others believe they do possess a synovial lining (Cave, Griffiths, and Whiteley, 1955). Regardless of their true classification, the distance between the apposing bony structures in the uncovertebral region is only approximately one third of that of the remainder of the interbody space (Hadley, 1957). In addition, the uncovertebral joints frequently undergo degeneration with resulting bony outgrowth (osteophyte formation) of the uncinate processes. These osteophytes may encroach on neighboring structures such as the vertebral artery and exiting cervical spinal nerves within the intervertebral foramen (Hadley, 1957; Bland, 1989). The uncinate processes are significantly higher at C4 to C6 (5.8 ± 1.1 mm to 6.1 ± 1.3 mm) than at C3 or C7 levels, and the length of the exiting dorsal and ventral roots and spinal nerve from the dura mater to the lateral border of the intervertebral foramina increases from C3 to C7. The higher uncinate processes at C4-6 and the longer nerves in this region may help to explain the higher incidence of neural compression syndromes associated with the C4-6 vertebral levels (Ebraheim et al., 1997c). Furthermore, dense fibrous tissue attaches to the uncinate process and this tissue then encases the spinal nerve and vertebral artery in the intertransverse space at the same level. The vertebral artery may become vulnerable to irritation, or in extreme cases perforation, from osteophytes projecting from the uncinate processes, because in essence the vertebral artery is held in a relatively close relationship to the uncinate process by this uncinate–spinal nerve–vertebral artery fibrous complex (Ebraheim et al., 1998; Yilmazlar et al., 2003a,b). Because the vertebral artery courses closer to the uncinate processes in the midcervical region than in the lower cervical region, the vertebral artery in the midcervical region is potentially more vulnerable than the vertebral artery in the lower cervical region to damage from osteophytes arising from the uncinate processes (Ebraheim et al., 1997c).

Injury to the Vertebral Bodies. Injury to the vertebral bodies frequently, but not always, results in swelling of the prevertebral soft tissues (Miles and Finlay, 1988). Therefore swelling of the prevertebral tissues seen on standard x-ray films after trauma is an indication for further diagnostic studies such as computed tomography (CT).

Pedicles. The left and right pedicles of a typical cervical vertebra (see Fig. 5-1) are small and project posterolaterally from the vertebral bodies at approximately a 60-degree angle to the frontal (coronal) plane. They form the medial boundary of the left and right foramina of the transverse processes, respectively. The length of the pedicles is similar in the C3 to C7 vertebrae, and the pedicles of C2 are shorter than those of the rest of the cervical region (Karaikovic et al., 1997). The pedicles of typical cervical vertebrae are placed more or less midway between the superior and inferior margins of the vertebral body. Therefore the superior and inferior vertebral notches are of roughly equal size (Williams et al., 1995). The spinal nerve, surrounded by a sleeve of dura, courses just above (superior to) the pedicle of each typical cervical vertebra.

The cervical pedicles have a relatively thick layer of cortical bone (also known as compact bone) that surrounds a central core of cancellous bone (also known as trabecular, or spongy, bone). Generally, the cortex of the lateral aspect of the pedicle (the region closest to the vertebral artery) is thinner than that of the medial side. However, approximately 4% of pedicles are composed entirely of cortical bone with no medullary cavity. In the remainder of pedicles, the central trabecular bone is continuous with that of the articular processes. This allows transfer of loads from the vertebral body to the articular pillar (discussed later in this chapter) during flexion and from the articular pillar to the vertebral body during extension (Pal et al., 1988).

Transverse Processes. The left and right transverse processes (TPs) of a typical cervical vertebra are each composed of two roots, or bars, one anterior and one posterior (see Fig. 5-1). The two roots end laterally as tubercles (anterior and posterior). Occasionally an anterior tubercle of one vertebra is significantly longer than those of its neighbors. This usually occurs at C5 or C6 and has been associated with a lack of segmentation (congenital fusion) of the vertebral body of the segment with the long anterior tubercle to the vertebral body directly above or below (Ehara, 1996). The two tubercles are joined to one another by an intertubercular lamella, which is less correctly known as a costotransverse lamella (bar) (Williams et al., 1995). The distance between the lateral tips of the left and right TPs is greatest at C1. This same distance, although smaller, remains relatively constant from C2 through C6 and then increases greatly at C7.

In the typical cervical vertebrae a gutter, or groove, for the spinal nerve is formed between the anterior and posterior roots of each TP (Fig. 5-2). This groove serves as a passage for exit of the spinal nerve and its largest branch, the anterior primary division (ventral ramus). The neural grooves form approximately a 50-degree anterior angle with the midsagittal plane, except for C7 where the angle is larger, usually 56 to 57 degrees. Generally, there is no significant difference between the length of the neural grooves in males and females. The depth of the neural grooves gradually increases from C3 (≈3 mm ± 1.0 mm deep) to C7 (≈5 mm ± 0.7 mm deep) (Ebraheim, Biyani, and Salpietro, 1996). The intertubercular lamellae of C3 and C4 have an oblique course, descending from the anterior root and passing laterally as they reach the posterior root of the TP. Therefore the anterior tubercles (roots) of these vertebrae are shorter than the posterior ones, and the grooves for the spinal nerves are deeper posteriorly than anteriorly. The left and right intertubercular lamellae of C6 are wide (from left to right) and shallow (from superior to inferior) (Williams et al., 1995).

A dural root sleeve, which surrounds each spinal nerve, as well as its continuation as the epineurium of the ventral ramus (anterior primary division) are held to the gutter of the TP by fibrous tissue. This strong attachment to the TP is unique to the cervical region. The C4, C5, and C6 spinal nerves and anterior primary divisions (ventral rami) are held in place to the groove for the spinal nerve by means of tough connective tissue attachments. The nerves at the other levels are not as tightly bound to the bone of the groove for the spinal nerve. Lateral traction of the dura (more specifically the "dural funnel") pulls it laterally into an intervertebral foramen (IVF) until it plugs the foramen. This prevents further traction on the nerve roots and rootlets and their attachment to the spinal cord. In addition, traction of nerves also tractions the denticulate ligament, which in turn causes the spinal cord to move laterally toward the traction force, thus removing tension on the spinal cord from the nerve roots undergoing traction (Sunderland, 1974).

The dural root sleeves in the cervical region receive more sensory innervation than any other region of cervical dura, and the fibers innervating the dural root sleeves originate directly from the dorsal root ganglia, not the recurrent meningeal nerves (Yamada et al., 1998). This means significant traction or compression of the cervical dural root sleeves could result in the production of pain.

A dorsal ramus leaves each spinal nerve shortly after the spinal nerve is formed by the union of the dorsal and ventral roots. The dorsal ramus (posterior primary division) courses posteriorly and laterally along the zygapophysial joint (see next section), supplying the joint with sensory innervation. The ramus then passes posteriorly to supply the cervical parts of the deep back

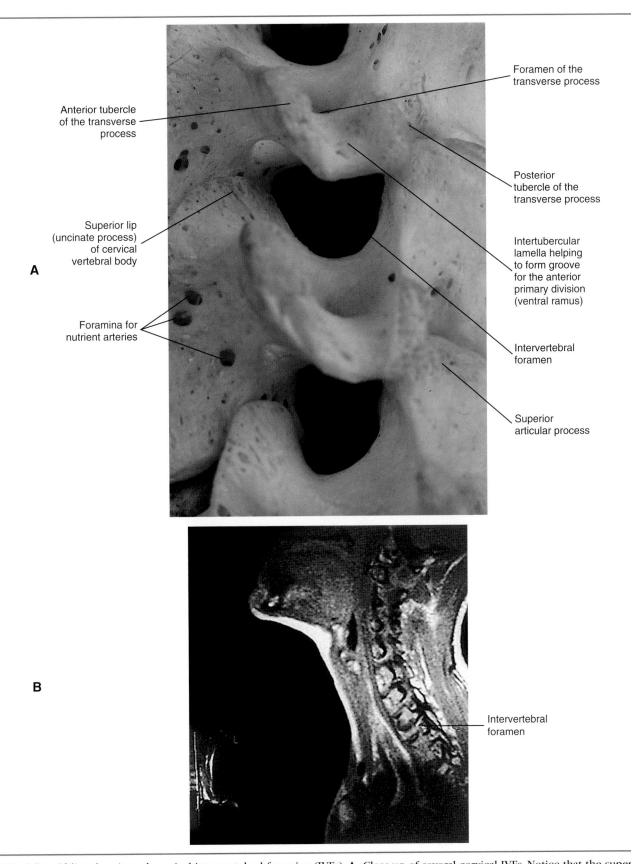

Foramen of the
transverse process

Anterior tubercle
of the transverse
process

Posterior
tubercle of the
transverse process

Superior lip
(uncinate process)
of cervical
vertebral body

A

Intertubercular
lamella helping
to form groove
for the anterior
primary division
(ventral ramus)

Foramina for
nutrient arteries

Intervertebral
foramen

Superior
articular process

B

Intervertebral
foramen

FIG. 5-2 Obliquely oriented cervical intervertebral foramina (IVFs). **A,** Close-up of several cervical IVFs. Notice that the superior lip (uncinate process) of a typical cervical vertebral body helps to form the anterior border of the IVF. **B,** Standard parasagittal magnetic resonance imaging (MRI) scans of the cervical region frequently show only the lower cervical IVFs. (**B,** Courtesy Dr. Dennis Skogsbergh.)

Continued

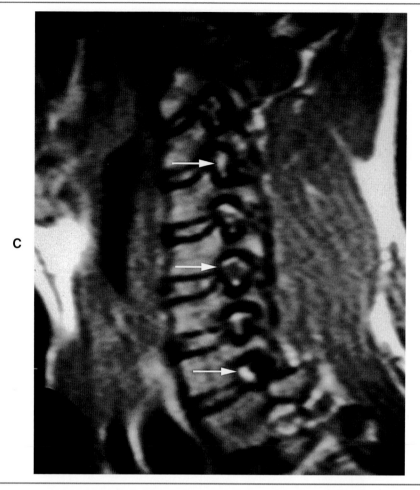

FIG. 5-2—cont'd   **C,** Because the cervical IVFs face anteriorly as well as laterally, MRI scans taken at a 40- to 45-degree angle to a sagittal plane show the cervical IVFs to better advantage. Notice that in this direct oblique sagittal MRI the C2-3 through T1-2 IVFs all can be seen (arrows are pointing to the C3-4, C5-6, and C7-T1 IVFs). (From Cramer G et al. [2002]. Oblique MRI of the cervical intervertebral foramina: A comparison of three techniques. *J Neuromusculoskel Syst 10,* 41-51.)

muscles with motor, nociceptive, and proprioceptive innervation; and then continues posteriorly to reach the dermal and epidermal layers of the back to supply them with sensory innervation. The nerves of the cervical region are discussed in more detail later in this chapter.

The anterior aspect of the TPs of C4 to C6 end in roughened tubercles that serve as attachments for the tendons of the scalenus anterior, longus colli (superior and inferior oblique fibers), and longus capitis muscles. The posterior tubercles extend further laterally and slightly more inferiorly than their anterior counterparts (except for C6, where they are level). The splenius cervicis, longissimus cervicis, iliocostalis cervicis, levator scapulae, and scalenus medius and posterior muscles attach to the posterior tubercles.

As the name implies, the foramen of the TP is an opening within the TP. This foramen is present in the left and right TPs of all cervical vertebrae. It was previously called the foramen transversarium, but the currently preferred term is simply *foramen of the transverse process.* The boundaries of this foramen are formed by four structures: the pedicle, anterior root of the TP, posterior root of the TP, and intertubercular lamella. The sizes of left and right foramina of the TPs of a single vertebra frequently are asymmetric, and occasionally the foramen of a single TP is double (Taitz, Nathan, and Arensburg, 1978). The vertebral artery normally enters the foramen of the TP of C6 and continues superiorly through the corresponding foramina of C5 through C1. The vertebral artery of each side loops posteriorly and then medially around the superior articular process of the atlas on the corresponding side. The artery then continues superiorly to pass through the foramen magnum. The ventral rami of the C3 to C7 spinal nerves pass posterior to the vertebral artery as they exit the gutter (groove) for the spinal nerve of the TP (see Fig. 5-2).

Several vertebral veins on each side also pass through the foramina of the TPs. These veins begin in the atlanto-occipital region and continue inferiorly through the foramina of the TPs of C1 through C7 and then enter the subclavian vein. The vertebral veins receive branches from both the epidural venous plexus and the external vertebral venous plexus. In addition to the veins, a plexus of sympathetic nerves also accompanies the vertebral artery as it passes through the foramina of the TPs of C1 through C6 (see Fig. 5-22). The vertebral artery and sympathetic plexus associated with it are discussed in more detail later in this chapter.

As mentioned in Chapter 2, the vertebrae of each region of the spine possess specific sites that are capable of developing ribs. Such regions are known as costal elements, costal processes, or pleurapophyses. The cervical region is no exception. The costal process of a typical cervical vertebra makes up the majority of its TP. In fact, all but the most medial aspect of the posterior root of the TP participates in the formation of the costal process. The costal processes may develop into cervical ribs in some individuals (Williams et al., 1995). This occurs most frequently at the level of C7. A cervical rib at C7 may be present and may compress underlying portions of the brachial plexus and the subclavian artery. The symptom complex that results from compression of these structures is commonly known as the thoracic outlet syndrome, and a cervical rib is one cause of this syndrome (Bland, 1987). (Thoracic outlet syndrome is discussed in detail in Chapter 6.) A cervical rib may develop as a small projection of the TP or may be a complete rib that attaches to the manubrium of the sternum or the first thoracic rib. However, the cervical rib usually is incomplete, and a bridge of fibrous tissue usually connects the tip of the cervical rib to either the manubrium or first thoracic rib. The osseous extension of the cervical TP frequently can be detected on standard x-ray films, but the fibrous band is much more difficult to evaluate radiographically.

Articular Processes and Zygapophysial Joints.
The general characteristics of the articular processes and the zygapophysial joints (Z joints) are discussed in Chapter 2. The unique characteristics of the cervical Z joints are discussed here. The superior articular processes and their hyaline cartilage-lined facets face posteriorly, superiorly, and slightly medially (see Fig. 5-1), and the cervical Z joints lie approximately 45 degrees to the horizontal plane (White and Panjabi, 1990; Panjabi et al., 1991). More specifically, the facet joints of the upper

cervical spine lie at approximately a 35-degree angle to the horizontal plane, and the lower cervical Z joints form a 65-degree angle to the horizontal plane (Oliver and Middleditch, 1991). The articular processes and their hyaline cartilage–lined facets of the typical cervical vertebrae are more horizontally oriented at birth (averaging approximately 34 degrees to the horizontal plane) than in the adult. The articular processes then gradually become more vertically oriented until approximately 10 years of age, reaching an angle averaging approximately 45 to 53 degrees. They maintain this angle throughout the remainder of life. The seventh cervical vertebra follows the same pattern, but throughout life is more vertically oriented than the typical vertebrae. The more horizontally oriented articular processes of children (when compared with adults) lead to an increased anterior-to-posterior translation among the typical cervical vertebrae (Kasai et al., 1996).

Right-to-left asymmetry of the plane of articulation of the cervical articular processes is common. This is particularly true at the junction of the cervical and thoracic regions. An asymmetry of greater than 10 degrees in the coronal (frontal) plane occurs 24% of the time at C6, 10% of the time at C7, and 16% of the time at T1. There is no significant difference in asymmetry of the spatial orientation of the articular processes between men and women (Boyle, Singer, and Milne, 1996).

The heights of the superior articular facets of C3-7 range from 10.0 to 8.7 mm, decreasing in height from C3 to C7. The widths are approximately 11.0 mm from C3 to C6 and increase to 12.3 mm at C7. The height and width of the superior articular processes of males are again greater than that of females (Ebraheim et al., 1997b).

The heights (superior-to-inferior dimension) of the inferior articular facets range from 9.0 to 9.6 mm from C3 to C7; C3 has the greatest height and C5 the smallest. There is a steady decrease in height from C3 to C5, then a slight increase at C6, and again at C7. Therefore unlike the superior articular processes, there is no steady trend in height of the inferior articular processes. The width of the inferior articular processes ranges from 11.2 to 12.1 mm, and there is a small, steady increase from C3 to C7. The height and width of the inferior articular processes of males are greater than that of females (Ebraheim et al., 1997b).

The appearance of the cervical Z joints changes significantly with age. Before age 20 the articular cartilage is smooth, approximately 1.0 to 1.3 mm thick, and the subarticular bone is regular in thickness. The articular cartilage thins with age, and most adult cervical Z joints possess an extremely thin layer of cartilage with irregularly thickened subarticular cortical bone. These changes of articular cartilage and the subchondral bone usually go undetected on CT and magnetic resonance imaging (MRI) scans. Osteophytes (bony spurs) projecting from the articular processes and sclerosis (thickening) of the bone within the articular processes occur often in adult cervical Z joints (Fletcher et al., 1990). Osteophytes of the superior articular processes can extend into the intervertebral foramen and compress the neural elements coursing through this region (Hackney, 1992).

The Z joint capsules probably do little to limit motion in the cervical region (Onan, Heggeness, and Hipp, 1998). They are thicker along the lateral aspect of the joint compared with the posterior aspect, and become even thicker from posterior to anterior along the lateral aspect of the capsule, making the anterolateral aspect the thickest region of the Z joint capsule (Tonetti et al., 1999). However, overall the Z joint articular capsules of the cervical region are thin (Panjabi et al., 1991) and are longer and looser than those of the thoracic and lumbar regions. The collagen fibers, which make up the capsules, course from the region immediately surrounding the articular facet of the inferior articular process of the vertebra above to the corresponding region of the superior articular process of the vertebra below (Fig. 5-3; see also Figs. 5-11 and 5-16). The bands of collagen fibers are approximately 9 mm long and course perpendicular to the plane created by the Z joint (Panjabi et al., 1991).

Z joint synovial folds (menisci) project into the Z joints at all levels of the cervical spine. There are four distinct types of cervical Z joint menisci, which are also known as synovial folds (Yu, Sether, and Haughton, 1987) (Fig. 5-4). Type I menisci are thin and protrude far into the Z joints, covering approximately 50% of the joint surface. They are found only in children. Type II menisci are relatively large wedges that protrude a significant distance into the joint space and are found almost exclusively at the lateral C1-2 Z joints. Type III folds are small nubs found throughout the C2-3 to C6-7 cervical Z joints of most healthy adults. Type IV menisci are large and thick and usually are only found in degenerative Z joints. Types II and IV have been seen on MRI scans (Yu, Sether, and Haughton, 1987).

When the individual vertebrae are united, the articular processes of each side of the cervical spine form an articular pillar that bulges laterally at the pediculolaminar junction (Williams et al., 1995). This pillar is conspicuous on lateral x-ray films. The cervical articular pillars (left and right) help to support the weight of the head and neck (Pal et al., 1988). Therefore weight bearing in the cervical region is carried out by a series of three longitudinal columns: one anterior column, which runs through the vertebral bodies, and two posterior columns, which run through the right and left articular pillars (Louis, 1985; Pal et al., 1988).

Articular pillar fracture is fairly common in the cervical spine and frequently goes undetected (Renaudin and Snyder, 1978). This type of fracture is usually a chip frac-

ture of a superior articular facet and process. The patient often experiences transient radicular pain (see Chapter 11), which usually is followed by mild to intense neck pain. Persistent radiculopathy in such patients indicates displacement of the fractured facet and articular process onto the dorsal root within the intervertebral foramen (Czervionke et al., 1988) (see Fig. 5-2).

The posterior primary division (dorsal ramus) of the spinal nerve provides sensory innervation by means of both mechanoreceptors and free nerve endings to the Z joint capsule. This indicates that the Z joint capsules are important for providing information on both joint position and tissue damage to the central nervous system (McLain, 1994). The Z joints are a source of pain in a substantial number of patients with neck pain (Aprill and Bogduk, 1992). Pain arising from pathologic conditions or dysfunction of the cervical Z joints can refer to regions distant from the affected joint (Bogduk, 1989b; Aprill, Dwyer, and Bogduk, 1990; Dwyer, Aprill, and Bogduk, 1990). The two most common types of pain referral are neck pain and head pain (headache) arising from the C2-3 Z joints, and neck pain and shoulder pain arising from the C5-6 Z joints (Bogduk and Marsland, 1988).

Laminae. The laminae of the cervical region are fairly narrow from superior to inferior. Therefore a gap can be seen between the laminae of adjacent vertebrae in a dried specimen (see Fig. 5-3, *C*). However, this gap is filled by the ligamentum flavum in the living (see Fig. 7-20). The upper border of each cervical lamina is thin, and the anterior surface of the inferior border is roughened by the attachment of the ligamentum flavum. The ligamentum flavum is discussed in detail later in this chapter.

Vertebral Canal. A vertebral foramen of a typical cervical vertebra is triangular (trefoil) in shape (see Fig. 5-1). It is also large, allowing it to accommodate the cervical enlargement of the spinal cord.

Recall that the collection of all the vertebral foramina is known as the vertebral (spinal) canal. Therefore the IVDs and ligamenta flava also participate in the formation of the vertebral canal. The internal vertebral venous plexus lies within the epidural adipose tissue of the vertebral canal. The left and right longitudinal channels of the cervical anterior internal vertebral venous plexus are kept in the most anterior and lateral regions of the epidural space by a thin fibrous membrane on each side of the vertebral canal. These venous channels anastomose with one another behind each vertebral body via retrocorporeal veins that course between the posterior longitudinal ligament and vertebral bodies (Chaynes et al., 1998).

The vertebral canal is fairly large in the upper cervical region but narrows from C3 to C6. More specifically, the

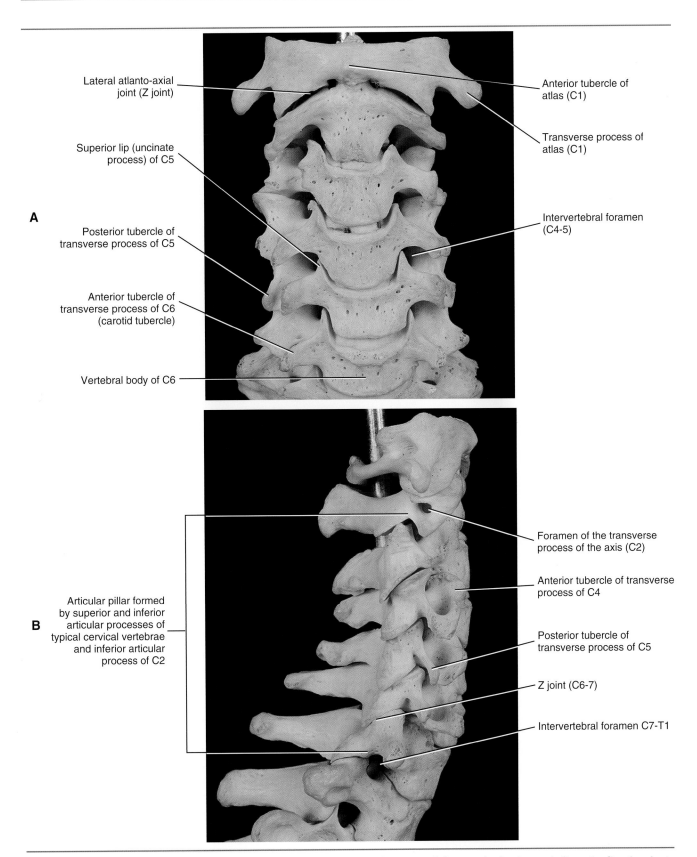

Lateral atlanto-axial joint (Z joint)

Superior lip (uncinate process) of C5

A

Posterior tubercle of transverse process of C5

Anterior tubercle of transverse process of C6 (carotid tubercle)

Vertebral body of C6

Anterior tubercle of atlas (C1)

Transverse process of atlas (C1)

Intervertebral foramen (C4-5)

Articular pillar formed by superior and inferior articular processes of typical cervical vertebrae and inferior articular process of C2

B

Foramen of the transverse process of the axis (C2)

Anterior tubercle of transverse process of C4

Posterior tubercle of transverse process of C5

Z joint (C6-7)

Intervertebral foramen C7-T1

FIG. 5-3   **A,** Anterior, **B,** lateral, and, **C,** posterior views of the cervical portion of the vertebral column. **A,** Superior lips (uncinate processes) of the C3 to C6 vertebral bodies are shown to advantage. **B,** Note the articular pillar, formed by the C3 through C6 superior and inferior articular processes.

Continued

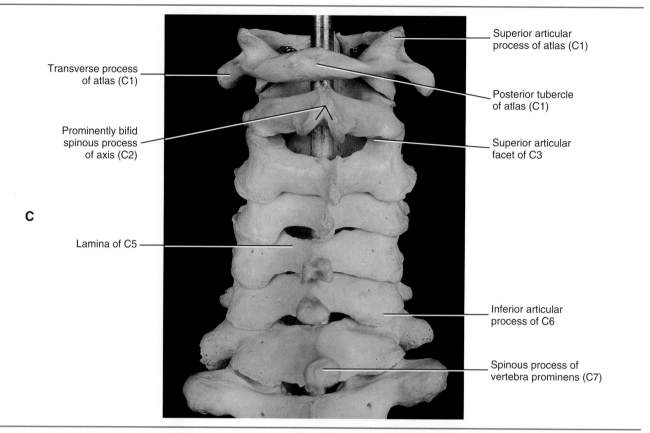

C

Transverse process of atlas (C1)

Prominently bifid spinous process of axis (C2)

Lamina of C5

Superior articular process of atlas (C1)

Posterior tubercle of atlas (C1)

Superior articular facet of C3

Inferior articular process of C6

Spinous process of vertebra prominens (C7)

FIG. 5-3—cont'd   **C,** Posterior view of the cervical portion of the vertebral column.

transverse (left-to-right) dimension remains relatively constant at approximately 24.6 mm. However, the sagittal dimension becomes smaller; therefore the shape of the trefoil becomes relatively wider as one descends the vertebral canal in the cervical region (Hackney, 1992). In fact, the spinal cord takes up 75% of the space available within the vertebral canal at the C6 level. The volume of cerebrospinal fluid in the subarachnoid space in the cervical vertebral canal is least in extension and greatest in flexion, and the total change in volume of the cervical subarachnoid space (C2 to C7 levels) during full extension to full flexion is approximately 1.9 ml (Holmes et al., 1996). Table 5-1 summarizes the general characteristics of the cervical vertebral canal.

Connective tissue attachments to the posterior spinal dura mater. Connective tissue attachments to the posterior aspect of the spinal dura arising from the foramen magnum, posterior arch of C1, spinous process of C2 (Von Lanz, 1929), rectus capitis posterior minor muscle (Hack et al., 1995a,b; Zumpano, Jagos, and Hartwell-Ford, 2002), ligamentum nuchae (Mitchell, Humphreys, and O'Sullivan, 1998; Humphreys et al., 2003), and ligamenta flava between C1-2 and C6-7 (Shinomiya et al., 1995, 1996) have been described.

These attachments may hold the dura mater posteriorly during cervical extension (to prevent buckling of the dura mater into the spinal cord) and flexion (to prevent the dura from moving forward and compressing the cord). Some authors have speculated that increased tension of the cervical paraspinal muscles may traction the connection between the rectus capitis posterior minor muscle and the dura, leading to headaches secondary to dural tension (Alix and Bates, 1999). Others have proposed that tearing of these connective tissue attachments during the flexion component of flexion-extension (whiplash) type of injuries or other trauma to the cervical region could lead to buckling of the dura mater into the cervical segments of the spinal cord. Such dural buckling could potentially result in chronic neck pain, headaches, disorders of balance, and signs and symptoms of cervical myelopathy experienced by some patients who have had trauma to the cervical region (Mitchell, Humphreys, and O'Sullivan, 1998). However, these theories remain conjecture until further basic science and clinical studies are performed to investigate the relationships between connective tissue attachments of the spinal dura mater and clinical conditions. In this regard, Shinomiya et al. (1995, 1996) have identified connective tissue attachments between the ligamenta flava

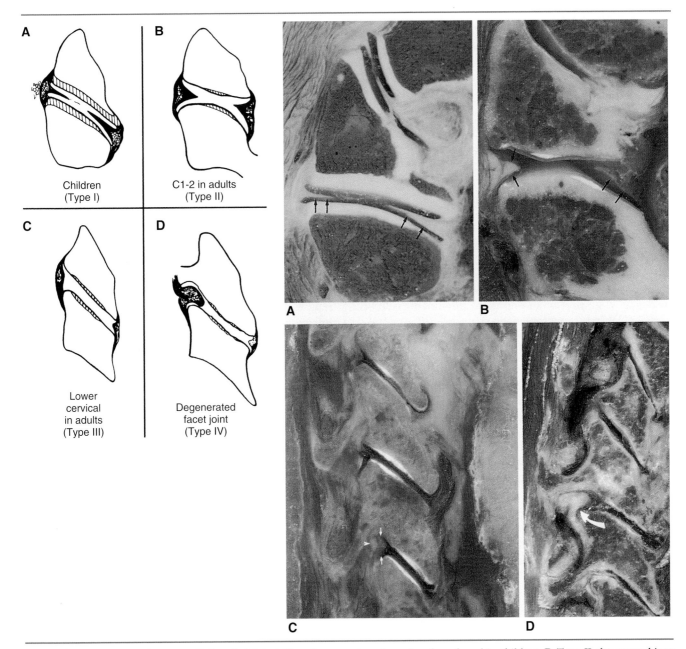

FIG. 5-4   Four types of menisci (*left* and *right*). **A,** Type I are washer shaped and are found in children. **B,** Type II also extend into the joint spaces and can be found in the lateral atlanto-axial joints of adults. **C,** Type III do not extend into the joint spaces and are found in the typical C2-3 to C6-7 Z joints of adults. **D,** Type IV are composed of collagen, fat, and cartilage and may extend into degenerated Z joints. *Right,* Menisci from sagittal sections of cadaveric cervical spines *(arrow).* (From Yu S et al. [1987]. Facet joint menisci of the cervical spine: Correlative MR imaging and cryomicrotomy study. *Radiology,* 164, 79-82.)

at C1-2 and C6-7, which they call epidural ligaments. Using MRI scans of humans and spinal cord blood flow measurements and electrophysiologic recordings of the nerves innervating upper extremity muscles and from the spinal cord in an animal model (cat), they have identified a relationship between tearing or absence of the epidural ligaments at C6-7 and Hirayama-type amyotrophy. This condition is characterized by isolated muscle

paralysis and atrophy of hand muscles resulting from segmental degenerative changes of the spinal cord gray matter. The authors found that absence or tearing of the epidural ligaments caused the spinal dura to press against the posterior aspect of the spinal cord during flexion of the spine. This compressed the spinal cord and its arterial supply, and led to a reduced blood flow to the anterior aspect of the spinal cord. The decreased blood flow to

Table 5-1	General Characteristics of the Cervical Vertebral Canal
Region	**Dimensions**
Upper cervical vertebral canal	Upper canal is infundibular in shape, wider superiorly than inferiorly; less than half the available space is occupied by the spinal cord at C1
C4	Narrowing of the vertebral canal begins
C6	Cord occupies 75% of the vertebral canal
C1-7	Critical anteroposterior dimension is 12–13 mm

the spinal cord subsequently decreased motor activity of peripheral nerves to the upper extremity, and also decreased neuronal activity in the spinal cord at the C7 and C8 spinal cord segments. Their work provides strong evidence in support of an important physiologic role of connective tissue attachments to the posterior aspect of the spinal dura mater.

Cervical myelopathy. Pathology of the spinal cord is termed cervical myelopathy. The development of bone spurs (osteophytes) from the posterior aspect of the vertebral bodies, and articular processes close to the Z joints and uncinate processes have long been accepted as potential causes of compression of the spinal cord and spinal nerve roots, respectively (Bailey and Casamajor, 1911; Boulos and Lovely, 1996). Other potential causes of spinal cord and nerve root compression include IVD protrusion, spinal cord tumor, Z joint hypertrophy, ossification of the posterior longitudinal ligament, buckling of a ligamentum flavum in a congenitally narrow vertebral canal, and a displaced fracture of a lamina, pedicle, or vertebral body. The critical anteroposterior dimension of the cervical vertebral canal is approximately 12 to 13 mm before symptoms occur. A vertebral canal this narrow usually is the result of one of the mentioned pathologic conditions combined with a congenitally narrow canal. However, the minimum dimension before symptoms occur may be slightly lower in blacks than whites. The transverse and midsagittal diameter of the cervical vertebral canal is significantly smaller in black than white South Africans, although determining if the difference in dimensions results from heredity, environment, or prenatal and childhood nutrition is difficult. However, white South Africans have more bone spurs (spondylosis or osteophyte formation) affecting the size of the vertebral canal than black South Africans (Taitz, 1996).

When increased bone formation (spondylosis) of the vertebral bodies, articular processes, or the uncinate processes contributes to cervical myelopathy, the term *cervical spondylotic myelopathy* (CSM) is appropriate.

CSM develops slowly, is progressive, and also may be related to a congenitally narrow vertebral canal (Crawford, Cassidy, and Burns, 1995; Hukuda et al., 1996). Less common causes of the condition are ossification of the posterior longitudinal ligament, ossification of the ligamentum flavum, and calcium pyrophosphate dehydrate deposition disease (Omura et al., 1996). In addition, Hukuda et al. (1996) found that large vertebral bodies (an increase of both the transverse and sagittal diameters) were significantly related to CSM. They assumed this was because the large vertebral bodies resulted in larger osteophytes and larger disc bulges; therefore increasing the chances of clinically significant narrowing of the vertebral canal that would result in compression of the spinal cord. Cervical myelopathy in elderly persons frequently results from anterior or posterior translation of adjacent vertebrae (anterolisthesis or retrolisthesis), secondary to narrowing of the IVDs or injury to the cervical region (Kawaguchi et al., 2003). Inflammation, initiated by arachnoid cells, may occur in the arachnoid mater in certain cases of CSM (Frank, 1995).

The progression of spinal cord changes in CSM begins with neuronal loss in the anterior gray horn. This progresses to the intermediate gray matter. Degeneration then occurs in the lateral and posterior funiculi of white matter. The changes in the white matter are consistent with demyelination and remyelination similar to what occurs in compression neuropathies of peripheral nerves, such as carpal tunnel syndrome. Finally, atrophy is seen throughout the entire gray matter and more severe degeneration is found in the lateral funiculus (Ito et al., 1996). These changes lead to decreased processing of afferent (sensory) input and efferent (motor) output of the affected spinal cord levels (Chistyakov et al., 1995).

CSM usually is associated with diffuse neck pain accompanied by varying degrees of neurologic deficit and can mimic multiple sclerosis, amyotrophic lateral sclerosis, intervertebral disc protrusion, and less commonly spinal cord tumor and subacute combined degeneration of the spinal cord (Cusick, 1988; Crawford, Cassidy, and Burns, 1995).

Vertebral canal measurements taken from the level of the superior border of the pedicle on standard lateral x-rays can be done reliably, and can be used before more advanced imaging procedures are employed to evaluate the size of the vertebral canal (Senol et al., 2001). Metrizamide myelography (injection of radiopaque dye followed by x-ray examination) and computer-assisted myelography (injection of dye followed by CT scanning) have been shown to be useful in the evaluation of cervical spondylotic myelopathy (Yu, Sether, and Haughton, 1987). Measurement (morphometry) of the cervical cord by means of MRI has been shown to correlate well with the severity of cord compression (Fujiwara et al., 1988).

Neurapraxia of cervical nerves. The neurapraxia (i.e., injury to a nerve resulting in paralysis that recovers completely in a short period of time) known as "stingers" or "burners" that occurs in contact sports, is thought to result from injury to the cervical nerve roots (usually thought to be C5 or C6) or the brachial plexus. Narrowing of the vertebral canal (spinal stenosis) of the cervical region (defined as a Torg ratio <0.8) results in a threefold increase in the risk of stingers from an extension-compression mechanism in football players (Meyer et al., 1994). The Torg ratio is the anterior to posterior distance between the vertebral body and the spinous process-laminar junction at the narrowest region of the cervical vertebral canal, divided by the anterior to posterior dimension of the vertebral body at the same level (Torg et al., 1986). The measurements are made from lateral extension x-rays. The presence of stenosis also increases the incidence of a complicated recovery from these injuries (Meyer et al., 1994).

Spinous Process. The spinous process of a typical cervical vertebra is short and bifid posteriorly. It is bifid because it develops from two separate secondary centers of ossification. This morphology is unique to cervical spinous processes. The "terminal tubercles" of the bifid spinous process are frequently of unequal size and allow for attachment of the ligamentum nuchae (Williams et al., 1995) and many of the deep extensor muscles of the spine (semispinalis thoracis and cervicis, multifidi cervicis, spinalis cervicis, and interspinalis cervicis muscles).

Cervical spinous processes, as with spinous processes throughout the spine, may deviate from the midline, making the determination of structural defects, fractures, and dislocations more challenging (Williams et al., 1995). The length of the spinous processes decreases from C2 to C4 and then increases from C4 to C7 (Panjabi et al., 1991).

Intervertebral Foramina. The left and right intervertebral foramina (IVFs) in the cervical region lie between the inferior and superior vertebral notches of adjacent cervical vertebrae (see Fig. 5-2). They face obliquely anteriorly at approximately a 45-degree angle from the midsagittal plane for the upper and middle cervical IVFs and approximately a 55-degree angle to the midsagittal plane for the lower cervical IVFs (Marcelis et al., 1993). The IVFs also are directed inferiorly at approximately a 10-degree angle to a horizontal plane passing through the superior vertebral end plate. The specific borders and contents of the IVF are discussed in Chapter 2. However, the uncinate processes, which help to form the anterior border of the IVFs, are unique to the cervical region. The cervical IVFs, as with those of the thoracic and lumbar regions, can best be considered as neural

canals because they are 4 to 6 mm in length. They are almost oval in shape. The average height of the cervical IVFs is 8.1 mm and the average width is 5.6 mm. Foraminal height increases from C3-4 (7.4 ± 1.1 mm) to C7-T1 (8.6 ± 1.0 mm), as does width (C3-4 = 4.5 ± 0.8, C7-T1 = 7.0 ± 1.1). The dimensions of C2-3 left and right IVFs are more similar to those of the mid- to lower cervical IVFs (height = 8.1 ± 1.2, width = 5.2 ± 0.9) (Ebraheim, Biyani, and Salpietro, 1996).

The IVFs change dimensions with movement. Flexion of 20 degrees, 30 degrees, and full flexion from the neutral position increases the superior to inferior IVF diameter by 8%, 10%, and 31%, respectively; and extension of 20 degrees, 30 degrees, and full extension from the neutral position decreases IVF diameter by 10%, 13%, and 20%, respectively (Yoo et al., 1992; Muhle et al., 2001). The pressure within the IVF also increases during extension, and elevation (abduction) of the upper extremity decreases pressure within the IVF (Farmer and Wisneski, 1994). Relief of pain radiating down the upper extremity after abduction of the arm is known as a positive Bakody's sign, and the decreased IVF pressures associated with abduction of the upper extremity may explain the mechanism of this sign. Ipsilateral axial rotation of 20 and 40 degrees results in foraminal narrowing of up to 15% and 23%, respectively; and contralateral axial rotation of 20 and 40 degrees results in foraminal widening of up to 9% and 20%, respectively (Muhle et al., 2001).

The dorsal and ventral roots (medially) or the spinal nerve (laterally) and the dural root sleeve account for 35% to 50% of the cross-sectional area of a typical cervical IVF (Sunderland, 1974). When the cervical spine is in the neutral position, the dorsal and ventral roots are located in the inferior portion of the IVF at or below the disc level (Pech et al., 1985). Epidural fat and blood vessels are found in the superior aspect of the IVF. The dorsal root and dorsal root ganglion are located posterior to and slightly above the ventral root. The dorsal root is also in contact with the superior articular process. The dorsal root ganglion is associated with a small notch on the anterior surface of the superior articular process in the cervical region. The ventral root contacts the uncinate process, and the dorsal and ventral roots are separated from each other by adipose tissue (Pech et al., 1985). This adipose-filled region between the dorsal and ventral roots has been called the interradicular foramen or cleft and can be seen on MRI (Yenerich and Haughton, 1986).

Stenosis of the intervertebral foramina. Narrowing (stenosis) of the IVFs can occur for a variety of reasons. Such stenosis can result in compression of the dorsal and ventral rootlets or roots, or dorsal root ganglion. This can lead to decreased muscle strength in the muscles innervated by the affected ventral roots, or pain radiating along the distribution of the nerves composed of the peripheral processes of the neurons found in the dorsal roots. Pain that results from compression of the dorsal rootlets, roots, or the dorsal root ganglion is known as radicular pain (see Chapter 11). Recall that the rootlets and roots are surrounded by the meninges, and more specifically, the dorsal and ventral roots and dorsal root ganglion are surrounded by a dural root sleeve. As mentioned, the cervical dural root sleeves are infundibular (funnel-shaped), being widest proximally, and compression of the neural elements usually occurs within the proximal IVF. The structures that most frequently cause stenosis and compression of the neural elements from the anterior are the IVDs, and bone spurs (osteophytes) from the uncinate processes or vertebral bodies. Structures that most frequently cause foraminal stenosis and compress the neural elements from the posterior are fibrous tissue in the IVF, thickening or buckling of the ligamentum flavum, and osteophytes from the superior or inferior articular process (Bailey and Casamajor, 1911; Hadley, 1957; Bland, 1989; Humphreys et al., 1998; Tanaka et al., 2000). Other possible causes of cervical IVF stenosis and radicular pain include fibrous adhesions within the IVF and inflammation of the nerve roots caused by the adhesions, edema, and congestion of the blood vessels within the cervical IVFs (Hadley, 1957). Radicular pain of the cervical dorsal roots is most common in the C6, C7, and C8 roots, with C6 accounting for 26%, C7 accounting for 61%, and C8 accounting for 8% of radicular pain of cervical origin (Murphy, Simmons, and Brunson, 1973). One reason for the lower incidence of radiculopathy from the C8 nerve roots is that they lie above the C7-T1 IVDs, whereas the C6 and C7 nerve roots are located directly posterior to the C5-6 and C6-7 IVDs, respectively (Tanaka et al., 2000).

Stenosis of the IVFs can be evaluated with standard x-rays, CT scanning, or MRI. Direct oblique MRI provides more accurate assessment of all of the borders of the cervical IVFs than standard sagittal images (Cramer et al., 2002) (Fig. 5-2, *C*). Kinalski and Kostro (1971) found the area of the cervical IVFs (as recorded from plain oblique radiographs) to correlate with age and patient symptoms. Individuals 20 to 40 years of age had larger IVFs than those older than 40. Also, a smaller IVF size was found among patients with chronic neck pain. These findings were confirmed by Humphreys et al. (1998), who found that the left-to-right width of the IVFs decreased with age and that this dimension also was smaller in individuals with chronic neck pain with radiculopathy.

Enlargement of the intervertebral foramina. An IVF may enlarge as a result of various pathologic conditions. The most common cause of significant pathologic enlargement of the IVF is the presence of a neurofibroma. Less frequently enlargement may be caused by meningioma, fibroma, lipoma, herniated meningocele, a tortuous vertebral artery (Danziger and Bloch, 1975), congenital absence of the pedicle with malformation of the TP (Schimmel, Newton, and Mani, 1976), and chordoma (Wang et al., 1984).

EXTERNAL ASPECT OF THE OCCIPITAL BONE

The external surface of the occipital bone is so intimately related to the spine (direct articulation and ligamentous attachments with the atlas and ligamentous attachments with the axis) that it is included in this section on the cervical region.

The external aspect of the occipital bone consists of three different regions: squamous, left and right lateral, and basilar. These three regions are discussed separately.

Squamous Part

The squamous part of the occipital bone (occipital squama) is located posterior to the foramen magnum (Fig. 5-5). The most prominent aspect of the occipital squama is the external occipital protuberance (EOP). This mound, whose summit is known as the inion, serves as the attachment site for the medial insertion of the trapezius muscle. The external occipital crest extends inferiorly from the EOP.

The squamous part of the occipital bone also has several markings formed by muscular and ligamentous attachments. Extending laterally from the EOP are two pairs of nuchal lines. The first is present only occasionally and is known as the highest (supreme) nuchal line. The second is almost always present and is known as the superior nuchal line. The highest nuchal line, when present, extends superiorly and laterally from the EOP. It is formed by attachment of the occipital belly of the occipitofrontalis (epicranius) muscle. The superior nuchal line extends almost directly laterally from the EOP and is formed by the attachment of the trapezius and sternocleidomastoid (SCM) muscles. A third nuchal line called the inferior nuchal line extends laterally from the external occipital crest approximately midway between the EOP and foramen magnum. Several muscles attach above and below the inferior nuchal line (Table 5-2). The posterior atlanto-occipital membrane attaches to the most inferior aspect of the occipital squama, which is the posterior border of the foramen magnum.

Lateral Parts

The left and right lateral portions of the occipital bone are located to the sides of the foramen magnum. They include the left and right occipital condyles, jugular processes, and jugular notches.

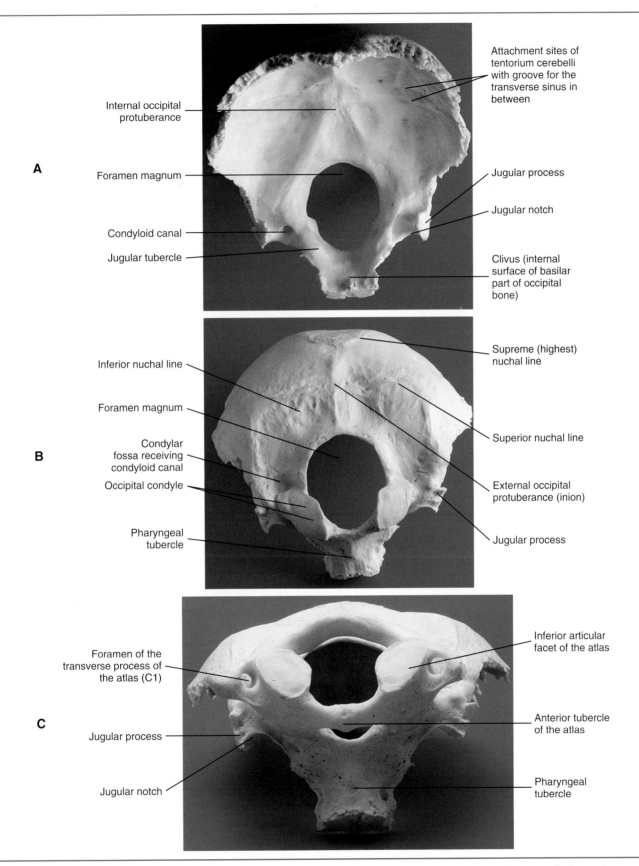

A, Internal occipital protuberance

Foramen magnum

Condyloid canal

Jugular tubercle

Attachment sites of tentorium cerebelli with groove for the transverse sinus in between

Jugular process

Jugular notch

Clivus (internal surface of basilar part of occipital bone)

B, Inferior nuchal line

Foramen magnum

Condylar fossa receiving condyloid canal

Occipital condyle

Pharyngeal tubercle

Supreme (highest) nuchal line

Superior nuchal line

External occipital protuberance (inion)

Jugular process

C, Foramen of the transverse process of the atlas (C1)

Jugular process

Jugular notch

Inferior articular facet of the atlas

Anterior tubercle of the atlas

Pharyngeal tubercle

FIG. 5-5 **A,** Superior, or internal, and, **B,** inferior, or external, views of the occiput. **C,** Atlas articulating with the occiput.

Table 5-2	Attachments to the Occiput
Region	**Muscles and Ligaments Attached**
Squamous	Trapezius
	Sternocleidomastoid
	Occipital belly of occipitofrontalis
	Splenius capitis
	Semispinalis capitis
	Obliquus capitis superior
	Rectus capitis posterior major and minor
	Posterior atlanto-occipital membrane
Lateral	Rectus capitis lateralis
	Alar ligament
Basilar	Rectus capitis anterior
	Longus capitis
	Superior constrictor
	Anterior atlanto-occipital membrane
	Apical ligament of the odontoid process
	Superior (upper) band of the cruciform ligament
	Tectorial membrane

The two occipital condyles are convex structures located on each side of the foramen magnum. Each condyle follows the contour of the large foramen and protrudes inferiorly, anteriorly, and medially (see Fig. 5-5). Each possesses a hyaline cartilage–lined articular facet. The left and right occipital condyles fit snugly into the superior articular facets of the atlas, and the left and right atlanto-occipital articulations allow for flexion, extension, and lateral flexion of the occiput on the atlas. The facetal surface of occipital condyles may be constricted in the center and occasionally may be completely divided (bipartite). When this occurs, the superior articular facet of the atlas matches the articular facet of the corresponding occipital condyle and also is constricted or bipartite (Gottleib, 1994).

The jugular notch is a groove along the lateral margin of each side of the occiput. This groove helps to form the large jugular foramen of the same side by lying in register with the jugular fossa of the temporal bone.

The jugular notch is bounded laterally by the jugular process. The jugular process is an anterior projection on the lateral aspect of each side of the occiput. Each one helps to form the posterolateral margin of the jugular foramen of the same side. The rectus capitis lateralis muscle, which helps to laterally flex the occiput on the atlas, attaches to this process.

Basilar Part

The basilar region of the occipital bone extends anteriorly from the foramen magnum. It meets the basilar portion of the sphenoid bone, and together the internal surface of the two basilar processes is known as the clivus.

The superior constrictor muscle of the pharynx attaches to the distinct pharyngeal tubercle, which is located in the center of the external surface of the basiocciput. The rectus capitis anterior muscle attaches just in front of the occipital condyle, and the longus capitis muscle attaches anterior and lateral to the pharyngeal tubercle. The anterior atlanto-occipital membrane attaches just in front of the foramen magnum. The apical ligament of the odontoid process attaches to the rim of the foramen magnum, and the superior (upper) band of the cruciform ligament attaches to the surface of the clivus, covered posteriorly by the clival attachment of the tectorial membrane. The transition of the spinal dura to the meningeal layer of the cranial dura occurs just posterior to the tectorial membrane.

Congenital Anomalies of the Occiput and Clinical Considerations. The craniovertebral region is associated with many variants and anomalies. These variations in normal anatomy and related anomalies are thought to primarily result from genetic transmission, although environmental factors may influence their development (Taitz, 2000).

Normally the occipital sclerotomes and the first cervical sclerotome are incorporated into the occiput (see Chapter 12). If these sclerotomes are incompletely incorporated, then remnants of an occipital vertebra may develop. These remnants can result in a variety of structures in the fully developed skull, including a paracondylar process, epitransverse process, hypocondylar arch, or third occipital condyle.

A paracondylar process is a bony process that protrudes inferiorly from the occiput just lateral to an occipital condyle. This type of process can cause decreased or aberrant motion of the upper cervical region and has been listed as a cause of cervical torticollis of skeletal origin. An epitransverse process is a bony projection from the transverse process of the atlas that extends superiorly toward the occiput. In some cases an epitransverse process can form a crude joint (pseudarthrosis) with a paracondylar process descending from the occiput. A hypocondylar arch is a prominent ridge coursing along the anterior margin of the foramen magnum. If the ridge is incomplete, the term "third occipital condyle" is used to describe the elevation along the anterior margin of the foramen magnum. The third occipital condyle can form a pseudarthrosis with the odontoid process or anterior arch of the atlas (Taitz, 2000).

Other common anomalies of the craniovertebral region are associated with a lack of segmentation of the occipital and upper cervical somites, and include various degrees of assimilation, or fusion, of the atlas with the occiput. Such assimilations can be almost complete fusions, but usually take the form of asymmetric fusion of one lateral mass to the adjacent occipital condyle. However, both lateral masses and the anterior arch of C1 may fuse with the occiput, but the posterior arch usually is spared from such fusion, allowing room for the vertebral artery to enter the foramen magnum.

The various forms of fusion of the atlas with the occiput frequently are accompanied by ascension of the odontoid process either into the foramen magnum or to just the inferior border of the foramen magnum. These locations of the odontoid process can result in partial compression of the inferior aspect of the medulla or the first cervical spinal cord segment (Taitz, 2000).

The various forms of atlantal fusions also can be accompanied by superior deviation of the inferior aspect of the occiput, known as basilar invagination, or basilar impression. Basilar invagination can result in neurologic signs and symptoms of cerebellar and lower cranial nerve dysfunction. In fact, anomalies of the occipitocervical region in general are not infrequently associated with neurologic disorders related to the region of the medulla and upper cervical spinal cord segments. These disorders usually manifest themselves later in life (after 30 years of age), unless they are triggered by trauma to the upper cervical region in earlier years (Taitz, 2000).

Because the somites (see Chapter 12), branchial arches, and mesonephros are developing at roughly the same time, anomalies of the craniovertebral region frequently are accompanied by additional anomalies of the face, ear, and other cervical vertebrae. Less frequently anomalies of the craniovertebral region are accompanied by anomalies of the thoracic and lumbar vertebrae (e.g., supernumerary thoracic vertebra and transitional lower lumbar segments) and with congenital disorders of the urinary system (Taitz, 2000).

ATYPICAL AND UNIQUE CERVICAL VERTEBRAE

The atypical cervical vertebrae are C1 and C2. C7 is unique. C6 is considered to have unique characteristics but remains typical. The distinctive features of these vertebrae are discussed in the following sections.

Atlas (First Cervical Vertebra)

The most superior atypical vertebra of the spine is the first cervical vertebra (Fig. 5-6). Given the name atlas, after the Greek god, this vertebra actually does function to support a round sphere (the head). The fully developed atlas comprises two arches (anterior and posterior) separated by two laterally placed pieces of bone known as the lateral masses. The lateral masses, in turn, have a TP projecting from their sides. The atlas develops from three primary centers of ossification, one in each lateral mass

and one in the anterior arch (see Fig. 13-9). The centers located in the lateral masses are the first to appear, and are formed by approximately the seventh week after conception. These centers develop posteriorly into the future posterior arch of the atlas, where they usually unite with one another by approximately the fourth year of life. Occasionally these ossification centers fail to unite posteriorly, leaving a cartilaginous bridge. This cartilaginous bridge is radiolucent on standard x-ray films. Such radiolucency must be differentiated from a fracture in trauma patients.

Anterior Arch. The anterior arch of the atlas develops from a bridge of tissue that connects the two lateral masses of the atlas in the embryo. This bridge is known as the hypochordal arch, and although the hypochordal arch is found throughout the spine embryologically, the anterior arch of the atlas is the only place where it persists into adulthood. The primary ossification center of the anterior arch usually appears by the end of the first year of postnatal life and fuses with the left and right lateral masses between the ages of 7 and 9 years (Fesmire and Luten, 1989).

The anterior arch is the smaller of the two atlantal arches (see Fig. 5-6). It possesses an elevation on its anterior surface known as the anterior tubercle. This tubercle serves as the attachment site for the anterior longitudinal ligament centrally and the superior oblique fibers of the longus colli muscle slightly laterally.

The posterior surface of the anterior arch (see Fig. 5-6) contains a smooth articulating surface known as the facet for the dens (odontoid). This facet is covered with hyaline cartilage and articulates with the anterior surface of the odontoid process as a diarthrodial joint. Because the atlas has no vertebral body, the odontoid process of the axis occupies the region homologous to the body of the atlas. Consequently the atlas is oval in shape and can pivot easily around the odontoid process at the diarthrodial joint between this process and the anterior arch of C1.

Posterior Arch. The posterior arch is larger than the anterior arch and forms approximately two thirds of the ring of the atlas. The larger posterior arch contains an elevation on its posterior surface known as the posterior tubercle. This tubercle may be palpated in some individuals. It serves centrally as an attachment site for the ligamentum nuchae (Williams et al., 1995) and also as the origin for the rectus capitis posterior minor muscle.

The first left and right ligamenta flava attach to the lower border of the posterior arch of the atlas. The ligamenta flava are discussed in more detail later in this chapter. The lateral aspects of the superior surface of the posterior arch are extremely thin and "dug out." These dug-out regions are known as the left and right grooves

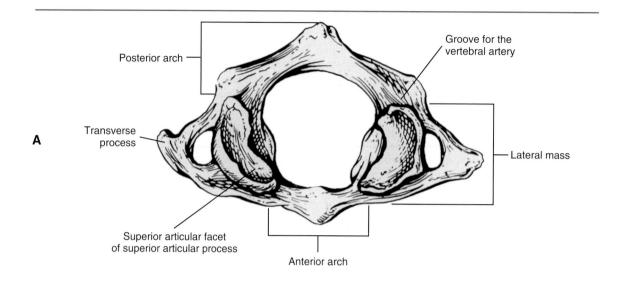

A

Posterior arch

Groove for the vertebral artery

Transverse process

Lateral mass

Superior articular facet of superior articular process

Anterior arch

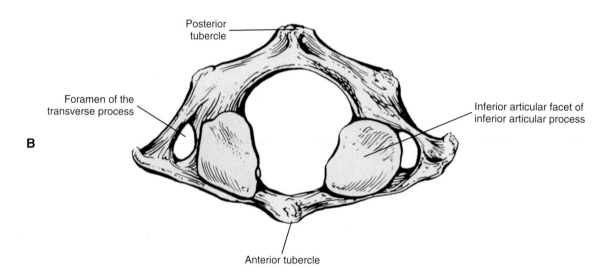

B

Posterior tubercle

Foramen of the transverse process

Inferior articular facet of inferior articular process

Anterior tubercle

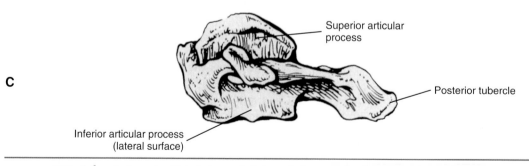

C

Superior articular process

Posterior tubercle

Inferior articular process (lateral surface)

FIG. 5-6   **A,** Superior, **B,** inferior, and, **C,** lateral views of the first cervical vertebra, the atlas.

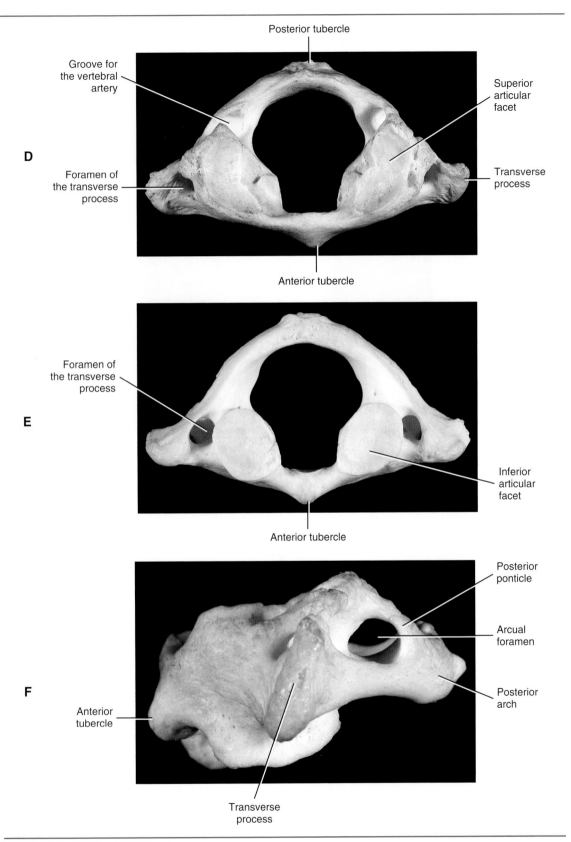

Posterior tubercle

Groove for
the vertebral
artery

Superior
articular
facet

D

Foramen of
the transverse
process

Transverse
process

Anterior tubercle

Foramen of
the transverse
process

E

Inferior
articular
facet

Anterior tubercle

Posterior
ponticle

Arcual
foramen

F

Posterior
arch

Anterior
tubercle

Transverse
process

FIG. 5-6—cont'd   **D,** Superior; **E,** inferior; and, **F,** lateral views of the first cervical vertebra, the atlas.

Continued

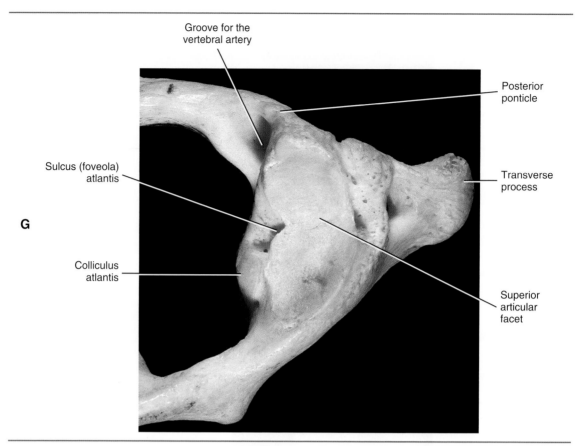

FIG. 5-6—cont'd   **G,** Close-up (superior view) of the lateral mass of the atlas. Notice the colliculus atlantis and sulcus (foveola) on the medial surface of the lateral mass.

for the vertebral arteries. Each groove allows passage of the vertebral artery, vertebral veins, and suboccipital nerve of the same side. The suboccipital nerve is the dorsal ramus of C1 and is located between the vertebral artery and posterior arch. The groove for the vertebral artery has been found to be covered by an arch of bone in approximately 32% to 37% of subjects studied (Taitz and Nathan, 1986). This results in the formation of a foramen, sometimes called the arcuate or arcual foramen (Fig. 5-6, *F*). Each vertebral artery reaches its respective groove as it courses around the superior articular process and comes to lie on top of the posterior arch. The posterior atlanto-occipital membrane attaches to each side of the groove, and it is the lateral and inferior edge of this membrane that may ossify to create an arcuate foramen (see Fig. 5-10). When ossification occurs, the bone bridge that is created is known as a posterior ponticle (Fig. 5-6, *F*). A study of 672 atlas vertebrae found that 25.9% had a partial posterior ponticle and 7.9% had a complete posterior ponticle (Taitz and Nathan, 1986). Interestingly these authors reported that a much higher number of atlases (57%) from a Middle Eastern population showed partial or complete ponticle formation, possibly because this population customarily carried heavy loads on their heads. However, these authors stated that further study is necessary to determine with certainty the cause of the high incidence of posterior ponticles in this population.

A significant relationship has been found between the presence of a posterior ponticle and migraine headache without aura. However, the reason for this relationship is unclear. Speculation includes ischemic compression of the vertebral artery or tension on the dura mater in the region of the occiput and atlas (Wight, Osborne, and Breen, 1999).

Occasionally a bone bridge for the vertebral artery develops laterally between the superior articular process of the atlas and the TP. Such a process is known as a lateral ponticle (ponticulus lateralis) (Buna et al., 1984). Taitz and Nathan (1986) found such a ponticle in 3.8% of the atlases they studied. Regardless of whether the ponticle is posteriorly or laterally placed, they are usually more than 12 mm in length and thicker than 1 mm. Some controversy surrounds whether posterior and lateral ponticles are congenital or are a part of the aging process. Taitz and Nathan (1986) found that partial ponticles were predominant in the specimens of 10- to 30-year-old individuals, and complete posterior ponticles usually were found in specimens from 30- to 80-year-old individuals. This indicates that at least posterior ponticles are created by ossification of the lateral-most portion of the posterior atlanto-occipital membrane as some people age. Even though these ponticles also have been implicated in some cases of vertebrobasilar arterial insufficiency (Buna et al., 1984), their clinical significance remains a matter of debate.

Lateral Masses. Located between the anterior and posterior arches are the left and right lateral masses. Each mass consists of a superior articular process, an inferior articular process, and a transverse process. The average superior to inferior height of a lateral mass is 14.09 mm (±1.92 mm) (Dong et al., 2003). Each superior articular process (SAP) is oriented so that the anterior aspect is more medially positioned than the posterior aspect. Recall that the anterior aspect of each lateral mass serves as the origin for the rectus capitis anterior muscle. The medial surface of each lateral mass has a small tubercle for attachment of the transverse atlantal ligament. This tubercle has been called the colliculus atlantis (see Fig. 5-6, *G*), and usually develops by the age of 13 years. A prominent depression that has been called the sulcus atlantis (foveola atlantis) is found immediately posterior to the colliculus. A nutrient artery to the lateral mass that branches from the third part of the vertebral artery usually enters the lateral mass through a nutrient foramen in the sulcus atlantis. The sulcus atlantis can be seen on CT scans taken in the horizontal (axial) plane and the colliculus atlantis can be seen on both axial CT scans and standard anteroposterior open mouth radiographs of the atlas (Weiglein and Schmidberger, 1998).

The SAP of each lateral mass has an average maximum left-to-right width of 15.47 mm (±1.19 mm) and an average anterior to posterior dimension of 17.21 mm (±0.93 mm) (Dong et al., 2003). The SAPs are irregular in shape. In fact, the hyaline-lined superior articular facet of each SAP usually has the appearance of a peanut. That is, it is narrow centrally and wider anteriorly and posteriorly. The SAP is quite concave superiorly and faces slightly medially to accommodate the convex occipital condyle of the corresponding side. The joint between the occiput and atlas is categorized as a condyloid, diarthrodial joint, although some authors describe it as being ellipsoidal in type because of its shape (Williams et al., 1995). The primary motion at this joint is anteroposterior rocking (flexion and extension). In addition, a small amount of lateral flexion occurs at this articulation.

Asymmetry of the left and right SAPs of the atlas is the rule rather than the exception. Approximately 63% of SAPs of atlases are "grossly asymmetric", and approximately 11% are slightly asymmetric. Approximately 37% of grossly asymmetric SAPs have three or four distinct articular facets (two on one side and one on the other or two on each side). In addition, the depth of the concavity of the SAPs is quite variable, ranging from being almost flat (<3-mm maximum depression) to being very concave (≥5-mm maximum depression) (Gottleib, 1994). Further investigation is necessary to determine the effects of asymmetry on motion between the occiput and atlas.

The inferior articular process of each lateral mass of the atlas presents as a regularly shaped oval. In fact, it is almost circular in many cases. This process is flat or slightly concave (Williams et al., 1995) and faces slightly medially. Hyaline cartilage lines the slightly smaller inferior articular facet of the articular process. The average maximum left-to-right width of the inferior articular facet is 17.90 mm (±1.18 mm) (Dong et al., 2003). The inferior articular facet articulates with the superior articular facet of C2. A loose articular capsule attaches to the rim of the corresponding articular facets, surrounding the lateral C1-2 joint. This loose capsule allows approximately 45 degrees of unilateral rotation to occur at each atlanto-occipital joint. This joint is categorized as a planar diarthrodial articulation (typical joint type for Z joints).

The large vertebral foramen of C1 usually has a greater anteroposterior than transverse diameter (Le Minor, Kahn, and Di Paola, 1989). The anteroposterior dimensions of the C1 vertebral foramen can be divided into thirds, with one third filled with the odontoid process of C2, one third filled with the spinal cord, and one third being free space. The free space actually is filled with epidural adipose tissue, vessels, ligaments, meninges, and the subarachnoid space. This division of the vertebral foramen of the atlas into three parts is sometimes known as Steele's rule of thirds (Foreman and Croft, 1992).

Transverse Processes. The left and right TPs of the atlas are large and may be palpated between the mastoid process and the angle of the mandible (see Chapter 1). Each projects laterally from the lateral mass and acts as a lever by which the muscles that attach to it may rotate the head. Because of the large size of the TPs, the atlas is wider than all the cervical vertebrae except C7. The width ranges from approximately 65 to 76 mm in females and 74 to 90 mm in males (Williams et al., 1995). Although they are composed of only a single lateral process (rather than having anterior and posterior tubercles, as is the case with typical cervical vertebrae), the atlantal TPs are almost completely homologous to the posterior roots, or bars, of the other cervical vertebrae. In fact, the TP of the atlas can be considered to be composed of a posterior root and a small portion of the intertubercular lamella (Williams et al., 1995). A foramen for the vertebral artery, which also provides passage for the vertebral veins and the vertebral artery sympathetic nerve plexus, also is found within each transverse process. This foramen of the TP of C1 is the largest of the cervical spine (Taitz, Nathan, and Arensburg, 1978).

In addition to its relationship with the vertebral vessels, each TP of the atlas is also the site of muscle attachments. These muscles include the rectus capitis lateralis, obliquus capitis superior, obliquus capitis inferior, levator scapulae, splenius cervicis, and scalenus medius muscles. Each TP also is related to the C1 spinal nerve. Although the dorsal ramus of this spinal nerve (the suboccipital nerve) provides motor innervation to the suboccipital muscles, the ventral ramus passes laterally around the lateral mass, remaining medial to the vertebral artery and the rectus capitis lateralis muscle. It courses between the rectus capitis lateralis and anterior muscles and then descends anterior to the atlas and is joined by the ascending branch of the ventral ramus of C2. The nerves of the cervical region are discussed in more detail later in this chapter.

Axis (Second Cervical Vertebra)

The second cervical vertebra, the axis or epistropheus, also is atypical. This vertebra develops from five primary and five secondary centers of ossification. The primary centers are distributed as follows: one in the vertebral body, two in the neural arch (one on each side), and two in the dens (odontoid process, see the following section). One secondary center of ossification is associated with the odontoid process, another is associated with the inferior aspect of the vertebral body, two are associated with the transverse processes (one for each, left and right), and one is located at the posterior tip of the spinous process.

The major distinguishing features of the axis are the prominent odontoid process, superior articular processes, and transverse processes (Fig. 5-7). In addition, the vertebral foramen of C2 is large. These distinguishing features are discussed in the following sections.

Dens (Odontoid Process). Also known as the odontoid process, the dens develops from two laterally placed primary centers of ossification and an apical secondary center of ossification (see Fig. 13-10). The two primary centers appear in utero and usually fuse in the midline by the eighth fetal month (Fesmire and Luten, 1989). The united primary ossification centers then normally fuse along their inferior outer rim to the vertebral body of C2 by approximately age 3 to 6 years. The fusion line between the odontoid and the body of C2 usually is visible on x-ray film until approximately age 11, and one third of individuals retain the line of fusion throughout life. This line is frequently confused with a fracture (Fesmire and Luten, 1989). Inside the rim of attachment between the dens and the body of C2 a small disc is present, which persists until late in life. This disc frequently can be seen on sagittal MRI scans. This area of

fusion between the odontoid and the body of C2 is known as the subdental synchondrosis.

The apical secondary center of ossification first appears at 3 to 6 years of age. It is V or cuneiform in shape, forming a deep cleft between the primary centers of ossification (see Fig. 13-10, *D*). This secondary center unites with the remainder of the odontoid process usually by age 12. When seen on x-ray film before fusion occurs or if fusion does not occur, the small bone fragment is known as a persistent ossiculum terminale (or simply ossiculum terminale, if before age 12) and also can be difficult to distinguish from a fracture.

The fully developed odontoid process (dens) is peg shaped with a curved superior surface. The height of the odontoid process is 15.5 mm (±1.8 mm) in males and 14.6 mm (±1.5 mm) in females. Its anterior-to-posterior diameter is 10.3 mm (±0.7 mm) in males and 9.6 mm (±0.9 mm) in females (Xu et al., 1995). The dens has a hyaline-lined articular facet on its anterior surface. This facet articulates with the corresponding facet on the posterior surface of the anterior arch of the atlas. The posterior surface of the dens has a groove at its base formed by the transverse atlantal ligament (transverse portion of the cruciform ligament). The transverse ligament forms a synovial joint with the groove on the posterior surface of the dens. Together the complex of anterior and posterior joints between the atlas, odontoid, and transverse ligament is classified as a trochoid (pivot) diarthrodial joint. This joint allows the atlas to rotate on the axis through approximately 45 degrees of motion in each direction (left and right). The sides of the odontoid process above the groove formed by the transverse ligament are flat and serve as attachment sites for the left and right alar ligaments. The apical odontoid ligament attaches to the top of the odontoid process. The ligaments and joints of the cervical spine are discussed later in this chapter.

Os odontoideum. Rarely the odontoid is not properly fused with the body of C2 or is united by only a rim of cartilage. Therefore its appearance on x-ray film is that of a free and unattached odontoid. This unfused odontoid is known as an os odontoideum (OO). The precise incidence of OO is unknown, although it is considered to be a rather rare phenomenon. Previously OO was thought to result from a lack of fusion of the odontoid process with the body of the axis during early childhood development; however, this condition is now thought usually to result from a fracture of the base of the odontoid (type II odontoid fracture) during the early postnatal period (Lefebvre et al., 1993; Lohiya, 1993; Verska and Anderson, 1997). The natural history of OO is unknown, and OO can exist without symptoms. However, relatively minor trauma can cause a previously pain-free OO to become symptomatic (Lohiya, 1993; Sosner, Fast, and Kahan, 1996). In some cases, OO can lead to severe neurologic deficits. However, limited neck motion and neck pain in the upper cervical region are the most common signs and symptoms of an unstable OO, and less often torticollis (neck laterally flexed and rotated to the same side) and headache may be present as well. X-ray examination is an important part of the accurate diagnosis of an unstable OO. Although OO appears as a translucent line at the base of the dens on standard x-rays, such a translucent line seen in the x-rays of children corresponds to the normal appearance of the cartilaginous attachment (growth plate) of the dens to the body of C2. This growth plate closes in 50% of children by the age of 4 years and should be closed in all children by 6 years of age. Therefore further investigation with lateral projection and flexion-extension x-rays is warranted in both adults and children suspected of having an OO, to reveal whether or not the odontoid is unstable. The space between the anterior aspect of the dens and anterior arch of the atlas (atlanto-odontal interspace) is normal in an unstable OO. However, the distance between lines drawn along the posterior aspect of the anterior arch of the atlas and anterior aspect of the body (not the odontoid) of C2 increases in flexion as compared with the neutral position in an unstable OO, and an unstable OO causes the odontoid-to-spinous process distance to decrease during extension (Lefebvre et al., 1993).

Fracture of the odontoid process. The odontoid process can fracture, and any fracture of the odontoid is serious because of the close relationship between the odontoid process and spinal cord. Fracture of the odontoid superior to its attachment to the body of C2 is known as a type I fracture. Fracture along the attachment of the odontoid process to the body of C2 is known as a type II fracture, and fracture of the odontoid inferior to its attachment to the body of C2 that includes part of the body of C2 is known as a type III odontoid fracture. Type II fractures usually have the most difficulty reestablishing bony union at the fracture site, and surgical fusion generally is necessary in type II (Bednar, Parikh, and Hummel, 1995) and unstable type III fractures (Chiba et al., 1996). Type I fractures usually are treated with specialized plaster casts and cervical braces and stable type III fractures can be treated with halo braces (cervical stabilization braces that are attached by bone screws into the calvarium) (Chiba et al., 1996).

Body of the Axis. The body of C2 contains less cancellous bone than the dens (Williams et al., 1995). The body has a prominent inferior indentation and a subtle posterior one (Panjabi et al., 2001a). The anterior surface of the body is hollowed out because of the attachment of the longus colli muscle. As occurs throughout the cervical spine, the anterior longitudinal ligament attaches to the inferior border of the vertebral body of C2 in close association with the attachment of the anterior fibers of the anulus fibrosus. Another similarity of the inferior or discal border of C2 with the same border of the other cervical vertebrae is that its anterior aspect projects inferiorly. The posterior aspect of the vertebral body serves as an important attachment for the posterior longitudinal ligament and its superior continuation as the tectorial membrane. Specifically these structures attach to the posterior and inferior borders of the vertebral body. Also associated with the vertebral body is the first IVD of the spine, which is found between the inferior surface of the vertebral body of C2 and the superior surface of the vertebral body of C3.

Pedicles. The pedicles of the axis are thick from medial to lateral and from superior to inferior (see Fig. 5-7, *B* and *E*). Significant asymmetry between the left and right pedicles of C2 exists in the transverse (left to right) width and the angle formed between the C2 pedicles and vertebral body of C2 (Kazan et al., 2000). The left and right inferior vertebral notches of C2 are large, whereas the superior vertebral notches are almost nonexistent.

Superior Articular Processes. The superior articular processes of the axis can be thought of as smoothed out regions of the left and right pedicles of C2. That is, the superior articular processes do not project superiorly from the pediculolaminar junction, as occurs with the typical cervical vertebrae. Instead, they lie almost flush with the pedicle (see Fig. 5-7). This configuration, along with the very loose articular capsule at this level, allows much axial rotation (approximately 45 degrees unilaterally) to occur between C1 and C2. The articular cartilage of the superior articular process of C2 is convex superiorly, with a transverse ridge running from medial to lateral along the central region of the process. This ridge allows the anterior and posterior aspects of the facet to slope inferiorly, aiding in more effective rotation between C1 and C2 (Koebke and Brade, 1982) (see Atlanto-Axial Articulations). The articulation between the superior articular facet of C2 with the inferior articular facet of C1 is located anterior to the rest of the Z joints of the cervical spine. Therefore the superior articular processes of C2 and inferior articular processes of C1 are not a part of the articular pillars, as is the case with the lower cervical spine's articular processes.

Laminae. The laminae of C2 are taller and thicker than those found in the rest of the cervical vertebrae. Because of the distinct architecture of the axis, the forces applied to it from above (by carrying the head) are

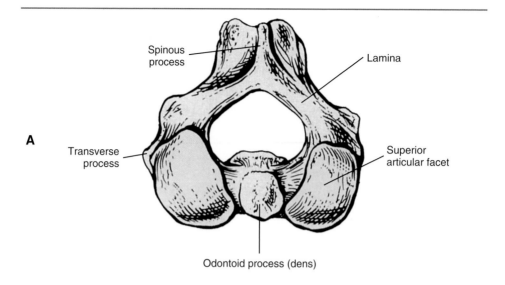

A

Spinous process

Lamina

Transverse process

Superior articular facet

Odontoid process (dens)

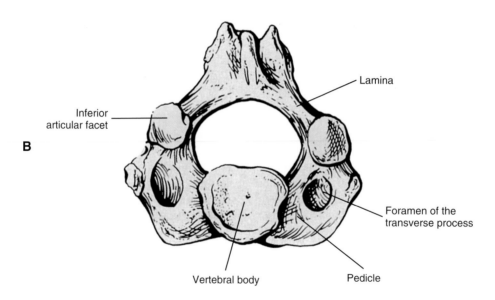

B

Lamina

Inferior articular facet

Foramen of the transverse process

Vertebral body

Pedicle

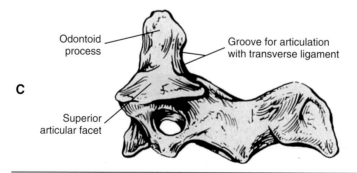

C

Odontoid process

Groove for articulation with transverse ligament

Superior articular facet

FIG. 5-7   **A,** Superior, **B,** inferior, and, **C,** lateral views of the second cervical vertebra, the axis.

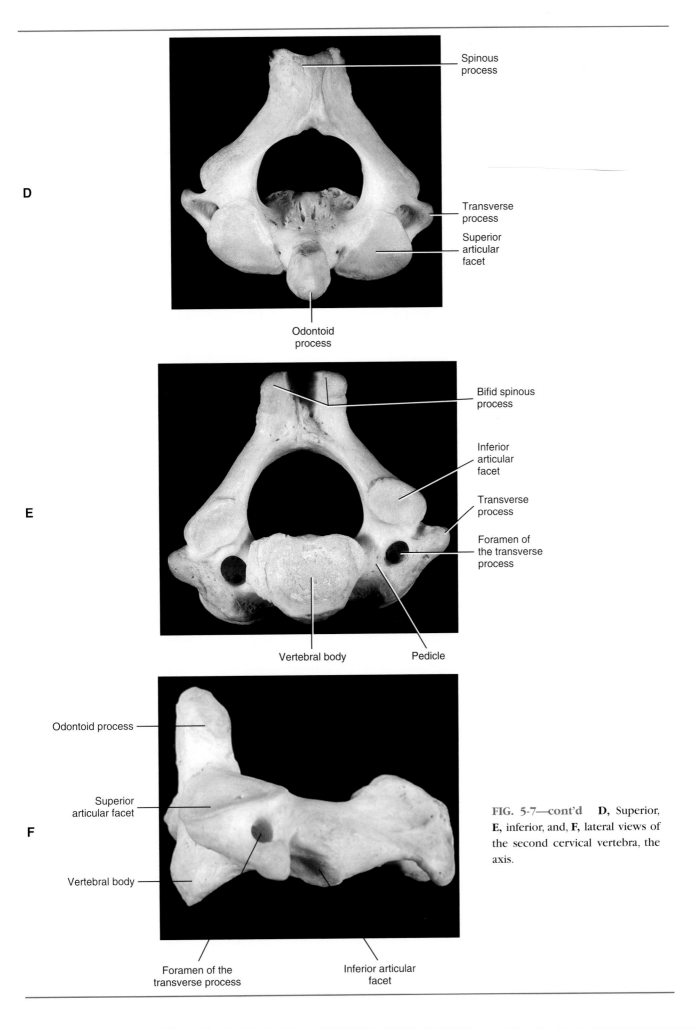

D

Spinous process

Transverse process

Superior articular facet

Odontoid process

E

Bifid spinous process

Inferior articular facet

Transverse process

Foramen of the transverse process

Vertebral body

Pedicle

F

Odontoid process

Superior articular facet

Vertebral body

Foramen of the transverse process

Inferior articular facet

FIG. 5-7—cont'd **D,** Superior, **E,** inferior, and, **F,** lateral views of the second cervical vertebra, the axis.

transmitted from the superior articular processes to both the inferior articular processes and the vertebral body via the pedicle. Because the superior and inferior facets of the axis are arranged in different planes, the forces transmitted to the inferior articular processes are, by necessity, transferred through the laminae. This is accomplished by a rather complex arrangement of bony trabeculae (Pal et al., 1988). The laminae of the axis therefore are quite strong compared with the laminae of the rest of the cervical vertebrae.

Transverse Processes. The TPs of C2 are quite small and, like the TPs of C1 but unlike those of the rest of the cervical spine, *do not* possess distinct anterior and posterior tubercles. Developmentally they are considered to be homologues of the posterior roots or bars of the TPs, although minute homologues of the anterior tubercles are associated with the junction of the anterior aspect of the TPs with the vertebral body of C2.

The small left and right TP of C2 face obliquely superiorly and laterally. Each has a foramen of the TP that, at C2, is an angular canal with two openings, one inferior and one lateral (Taitz, Nathan, and Arensburg, 1978). Therefore the vertebral artery courses laterally from the foramen of the TP of C2 to proceed to the more lateral foramen of the TP of C1.

Even though they are very small, the TPs of the axis serve as attachment sites for many muscles. Table 5-3 lists the muscles that attach to C2.

Spinous Process and Inferior Articular Processes. The spinous process of C2 is more prominently bifid than the other spinous processes of the cervical vertebrae because of the many muscles attaching to it (see Table 5-3). The inferior articular processes of C2 are typical for the cervical region. They arise from the

junction of the pedicle and lamina and face anteriorly, inferiorly, and laterally.

Carotid Tubercles and Articular Processes of the Sixth Cervical Vertebra

Although the C6 vertebra is considered typical, its left and right anterior tubercles of the TPs are unique. These tubercles are prominent and are known as the carotid tubercles because each is so closely related to the overlying common carotid artery of the corresponding side. The common carotid artery may be compressed in the groove between the carotid tubercle and vertebral body of C6 (Williams et al., 1995).

In addition, the left and right articular pillars of C6 are unique to other cervical vertebrae in three ways. The first two features can be seen in the vertebrae of both children and adults, and the third feature is unique to adults only. First, each superior articular process and facet is distinctly more anterior in position than the inferior articular process and facet (rather than being almost "stacked" one above the other as found in C3-5). Second, the sulcus for the posterior primary division of C6 usually is a deep incisure that is distinct and can be seen from both the lateral and posterior views of the vertebra. Finally, a prominent "muscular process" protrudes from the posterior aspect of adult C6 articular pillars. This process is found just inferior to the incisure for the posterior primary division (Herrera and Puchades-Ortis, 1998).

Vertebra Prominens (Seventh Cervical Vertebra)

Spinous Process. The seventh cervical vertebra is known as the vertebra prominens because of its prominent spinous process (Fig. 5-8). The spinous process of C7 is the most prominent of the cervical region, although occasionally C6 is more prominent (C6 is the last cervical vertebra with palpable movement in flexion and extension). Also, the spinous process of T1 may be more prominent than that of C7 in some individuals. The spinous process of C7 usually projects directly posteriorly. Unlike typical cervical vertebrae, the spinous process of C7 is not bifid. The funicular portion of the ligamentum nuchae attaches to the single posterior tip of the spinous process of C7. This ligament is discussed in more detail later in this chapter.

Because of its large spinous process and its location at the base of the neck, C7 serves as an attachment site for many muscles. Table 5-4 lists the muscular attachments of C7.

Transverse Processes. The TPs of C7 are also unique. The anterior tubercle of each TP of C7 is small and short. The posterior tubercle is large, making the

Table 5-3	Muscular Attachments to the Axis
Region	**Muscles Attached**
Vertebral body	Longus colli
Transverse processes	Levator scapula
	Scalenus medius
	Splenius cervicis
	Intertransversarii (to upper and lower surfaces)
Spinous process	Obliquus capitis inferior
	Rectus capitis posterior major
Notch of spinous	Semispinalis cervicis
	Spinalis cervicis
	Interspinalis cervicis
	Multifidus
	(also ligamentum nuchae, when present)

entire TP large. The anterior tubercle is the costal element of C7, and is unique because it develops from an independent primary center of ossification. This center usually unites with the TP by the fifth or sixth year of life. However, it may remain distinct and develop into a cervical rib. The formation of a cervical rib may also occur at C4 to C6 by the same mechanism, although this is less common. The intertubercular lamella usually is grooved by the ventral ramus of C7 anterior and lateral to the foramen of the TP (Williams et al., 1995). The suprapleural membrane, or cupola, which is the protective layer of connective tissue that reinforces the apical pleura of each lung, is attached to the posterior tubercle of the C7 TP.

Similar to the rest of the cervical region, the left and right C7 TPs contain a foramen. This foramen is usually the smallest of the cervical spine. Occasionally a double foramen is found in one of the TPs of C7 (Taitz, Nathan, and Arensburg, 1978) (Figs. 5-8, *C* and *D*). Frequently branches of the stellate ganglion run through the foramen of the TP of C7, although normally the only structures that course through this opening are accessory arteries and veins (Jovanovic, 1990). The accessory vessels comprise branches of the deep or ascending cervical arteries and their accompanying veins. The remainder of the C7 TP foramen is filled with areolar connective tissue. Recall that the vertebral artery and its associated sympathetic plexus run with the vertebral veins through the C6 foramen of the TP and the more superior vertebrae. Approximately 5% of the time, the vertebral artery and vein(s) traverse the foramen of the TP of C7 (Jovanovic, 1990).

ARTICULATIONS OF THE UPPER CERVICAL REGION

The Z joints of the cervical region are covered earlier in this chapter. The atlanto-occipital and atlanto-axial joints are discussed here.

The articulations (joints) of the upper cervical spine are extremely important. These joints allow much of the flexion and extension that occurs in the cervical region and at least one half of the axial (left and right) rotation of the cervical spine. In addition, the proprioceptive input from the atlanto-occipital and atlanto-axial joints, as well as proprioception from the suboccipital muscles, are responsible for the control of head posture (Panjabi et al., 1991).

Left and Right Atlanto-Occipital Articulations

The joints between the left and right superior articular surfaces of the atlas and the corresponding occipital condyles have been described as ellipsoidal (Williams et al., 1995) and condylar (Gates, 1980) in shape and type. The superior articular processes of the atlas are concave superiorly and face medially (see Fig. 5-6). Recall that the facets are narrow in their center, resulting in their peanut shape. The occiput and the atlas are connected by articular capsules and the anterior and posterior atlanto-occipital membranes (see Figs. 5-10 and 5-15). The fibrous capsules surround the occipital condyles and the superior articular facets of the atlas. These capsules are thickest posterolaterally. Each capsule is further reinforced in the posterolateral region by a ligamentous band that passes between the jugular processes of the occiput and the lateral mass of the atlas. This band has been called the lateral atlanto-occipital ligament (Oliver and Middleditch, 1991). The atlanto-occipital joint capsules are thin and sometimes completely nonexistent medially. When present, this medial deficiency frequently allows the synovial cavity of the atlanto-occipital joint to connect with the bursa or joint cavity between the dens and the transverse atlantal ligament (Cave, 1934; Williams et al., 1995).

More than 1 mm of anterior-to-posterior translation of the occiput on the atlas (as measured from the anterior rim of the foramen magnum, or basion, to the posterior aspect of the anterior arch) on flexion and extension lateral radiographs is considered to be related to instability of this region. However, the value for the lower limit of normal can be considered slightly higher in children and translation of less than 3 mm should not be considered as serious in children with Down syndrome (Matsuda et al., 1995).

Atlanto-Axial Articulations

The atlas and axis articulate with one another at three synovial joints: two lateral joints and a single median joint complex (Fig. 5-9, *B*).

Lateral atlanto-axial joints. The lateral atlanto-axial joints are planar joints that are oval in shape. The atlantal surfaces are concave, and the axial surfaces are convex. Asymmetry between the shapes of the left and right articular facets making up these joints and asymmetry of the plane of articulation of the left and right lateral atlanto-axial joints is common (Ross, Bereznick, and McGill, 1999). The fibrous capsule of each lateral joint is thin and loose and attaches to the outermost rim of the articular margins of the atlas and axis (inferior articular facet of the atlas and superior articular facet of the axis). Each capsule is lined by a synovial membrane. A posteromedial accessory ligament attaches inferiorly to the body of the axis near the base of the dens and courses superiorly to the lateral mass of the atlas near the attachment site of the transverse ligament. This ligament is known as the accessory atlanto-axial ligament (see Ligaments of the Cervical Region).

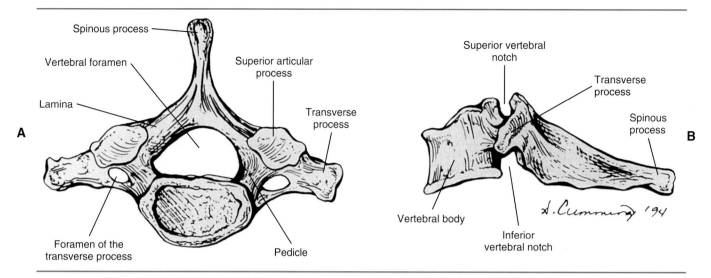

FIG. 5-8   **A,** Superior, and, **B,** lateral views of the seventh cervical vertebra, the vertebra prominens.

Median Atlanto-Axial Joint. The median atlanto-axial joint is a pivot (or trochoid) joint between the dens and a ring of structures that encircles the dens. These structures are the anterior arch of the atlas anteriorly and the transverse ligament posteriorly (see Cruciform Ligament and Fig. 5-13 later in this chapter). The hyaline articular cartilages on the atlas and the odontoid process, making up the median atlanto-axial joint, are oval, but the facet on the odontoid process has its longest axis oriented longitudinally and that of C1 oriented horizontally. The *posterior* facet of the dens (that articulates with the transverse ligament of the atlas) is also oval and is oriented longitudinally. The area of the articular cartilage of the atlas is 58.2 mm^2, and that of the anterior surface of the dens is 55.1 mm^2. The thickness of the articular cartilage on C1 and both the anterior and posterior articular surfaces of the odontoid process is approximately 0.80 mm (Ebraheim et al., 1997a).

The anterior and posterior components of the median atlanto-axial articulation both have synovial-lined fibrous capsules forming distinct joint cavities. The synovial-lined capsules attach to the outer edge of the articular cartilages of the opposing surfaces, and the capsules have slack in them to allow for significant movement (Ebraheim et al., 1997a). The posterior joint cavity is the larger of the two, and sometimes it has a bursa associated with it. In either case it is located between the anterior surface of the transverse ligament and the posterior grooved surface of the odontoid process. This posterior joint is often continuous with one of the atlanto-occipital joints (Williams et al., 1995).

CLINICAL APPLICATIONS

Eighty-six percent of patients with rheumatoid arthritis have involvement of the cervical region. In addition, the median atlanto-axial joint is affected in approximately 20% to 25% of these patients. Pathologic horizontal displacement of the atlas on the axis occurs in a significant number of these patients. These displacements are caused by erosive synovitis of the capsules, extending into the joints and affecting the articular cartilages, including the fibrocartilage of the transverse ligament of the atlas. The erosions of the articular cartilages can be seen on CT and MRI. Signs and symptoms of myelopathy secondary to these horizontal subluxations are relatively frequent. In addition, approximately 7% of patients with rheumatoid arthritis have a small vertical subluxation (i.e., ascension of the odontoid process toward the foramen magnum), although symptoms related to these relatively subtle vertical displacements in patients with rheumatoid arthritis are rare (Ebraheim et al., 1997a).

Also, degenerative changes of the median atlanto-axial joint in individuals *without* rheumatoid arthritis can begin at 50 years of age and can progress to completely obliterate the anterior and posterior joint spaces (Ebraheim et al., 1997a; Milz et al., 2001).

Children frequently have increased ligamentous laxity, which leads to increased spinal motion. This occurs most often in the cervical region. Increased motion seen during physical or x-ray examination should be differentiated from pathologic subluxation (Fesmire and Luten, 1989). For example, the space between the anterior arch of the atlas and odontoid process, known as the preden-

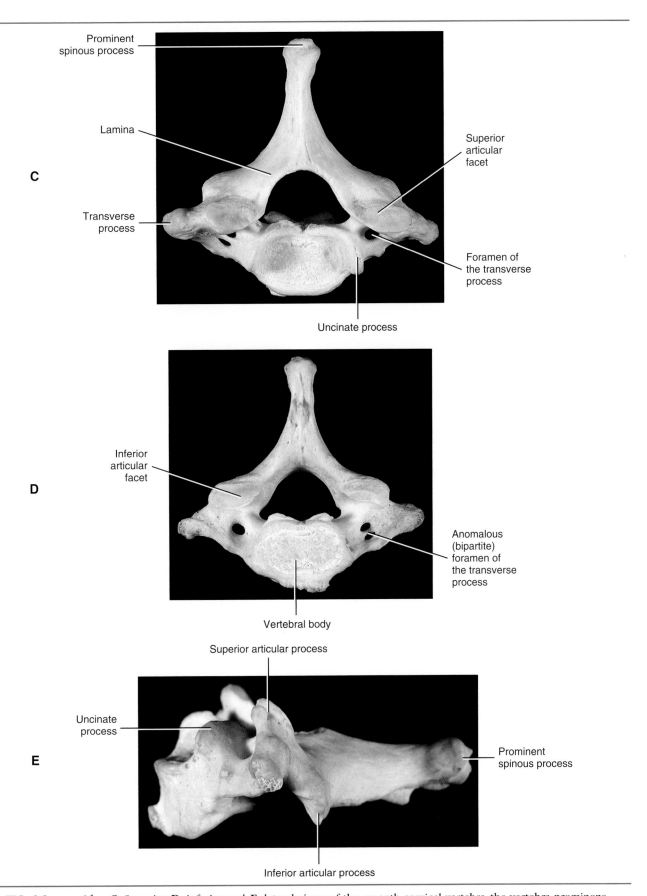

FIG. 5-8—cont'd **C,** Superior, **D,** inferior, and, **E,** lateral views of the seventh cervical vertebra, the vertebra prominens.

Table 5-4   Muscular Attachments of C7

Region	Muscles Attached
Spinous process	Trapezius
	Rhomboid minor
	Serratus posterior superior
	Splenius capitis
	Spinalis cervicis
	Semispinalis thoracis
	Multifidus thoracis
	Interspinales
Transverse process	Middle scalene
	Spinalis capitis
	Intertransversarii
	Levator costarum (first pair)
	(also the suprapleural membrane [cupola])
Articular process	Longissimus capitis
Vertebral body	Longus colli

tal space or atlanto-odontal interspace, usually does not exceed 3 mm. A predental space greater than 3 mm generally is considered to indicate a tear of the transverse ligament (see later discussion) or pathologic subluxation of C1 on C2. However, a 3-mm or greater predental space has been found in 20% of normal patients less than 8 years of age (Fesmire and Luten, 1989). Although a space of greater than 3.5 mm usually is considered abnormal in children, spaces of up to 5 mm have been seen in normal children (Fesmire and Luten, 1989). Therefore x-ray evaluation of atlanto-axial stability in children should be tempered with sound clinical judgment.

Pathologic subluxation of the atlas on the axis resulting in compromise of the spinal cord (compressive myelopathy) has been associated not only with rheumatoid arthritis (Kaufman and Glenn, 1983) but also less frequently with ankylosing spondylitis. Displacement of the atlas on the axis also has been found in 9% of 5- to 21-year-old patients with Down syndrome. In addition, significant degeneration of the entire cervical spine with osteophyte formation, narrowing of foramina, and narrowing of the disc space has been found with increasing incidence in the adult Down syndrome population. The premature aging process that occurs in individuals with this syndrome may be one possible explanation for this latter finding (Van Dyke and Gahagan, 1988).

LIGAMENTS OF THE CERVICAL REGION

The ligaments of the cervical region can be divided into upper and lower cervical ligaments. The upper ligaments are those associated with the occiput, atlas, and the anterior and lateral aspect of the axis. The lower cervical ligaments encompass all other ligaments of the cervical region. The ligaments of both categories are discussed in the following sections. The points of insertion and the function of each are discussed, beginning with those located most posteriorly and progressing to those located most anteriorly.

Upper Cervical Ligaments

Posterior Atlanto-Occipital Membrane. The posterior atlanto-occipital membrane is a rather thin structure that attaches to the posterior arch of the atlas and the posterior rim of the foramen magnum (Fig. 5-10). It is usually closely adherent to the posterior aspect of the spinal dura mater, and together these structures have been called the posterior atlanto-occipital membrane–spinal dura complex (Hack et al., 1995a). The posterior atlanto-occipital membrane functions to limit flexion of the occiput on the atlas. The ligament is so broad from left to right that the term *membrane* applies. It spans the distance between the left and right lateral masses. Laterally this ligament arches over the left and right grooves for the vertebral artery on the posterior arch of the atlas (see Fig. 5-10). This allows passage of the vertebral artery, vertebral veins, and the suboccipital nerve. These structures are covered in more detail later in this chapter. This lateral arch of the posterior atlanto-occipital membrane occasionally ossifies, creating a foramen for the previously mentioned structures. (See previous section on the atlas for elaboration on the arcuate, or arcual, foramen created by the ossified posterior atlanto-occipital membrane.)

Tectorial Membrane. The tectorial membrane is the superior extension of the posterior longitudinal ligament (Fig. 5-11). It begins by attaching to the posterior aspect of the vertebral body of C2. It then crosses over the odontoid process and inserts onto the anterior rim of the foramen magnum (specifically the upper region of the basilar part of the occipital bone, or clivus). The tectorial membrane has superficial and deep fibers. The deep fibers have a median band that extends all the way to the basilar portion of the occipital bone. Two lateral bands of deep fibers pass medial to the atlanto-occipital joints before attaching to the occiput. The superficial fibers extend even more superiorly than the deep fibers and blend with the cranial dura mater at the upper region of the basilar part of the occipital bone (clivus). This ligament limits both flexion and extension of the atlas and occiput (Williams et al., 1995).

Accessory Atlanto-Axial Ligaments. Each of the accessory atlanto-axial ligaments (left and right) course from the base of the odontoid process to the infero-medial surface of the lateral mass of the atlas on the same side (Figs. 5-11 and 5-12). They help to strengthen the

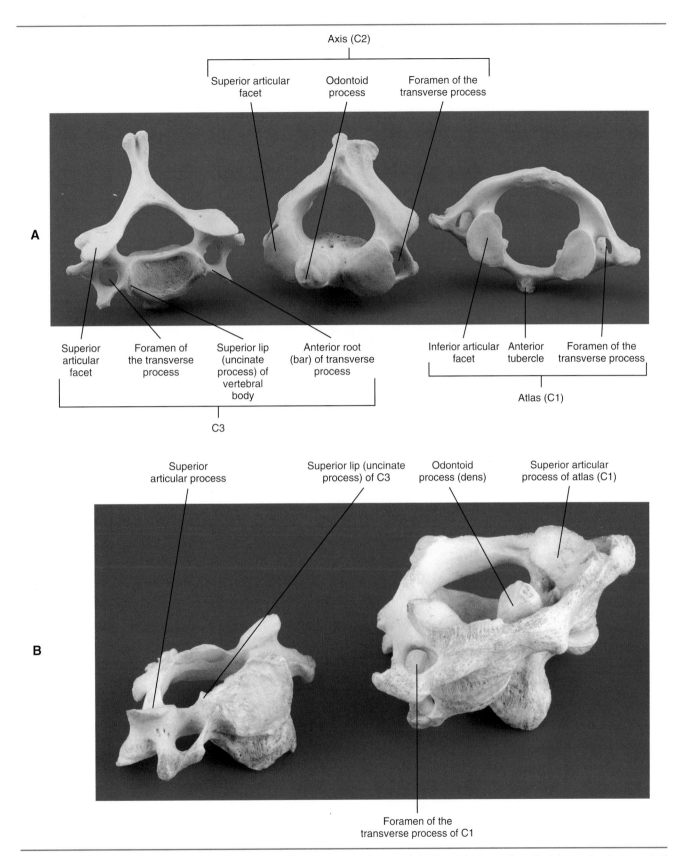

FIG. 5-9   A, Inferior view of the atlas and a superior view of the axis and third cervical vertebra. **B,** Atlas and axis in typical anatomic relationship, with C3 to the side.

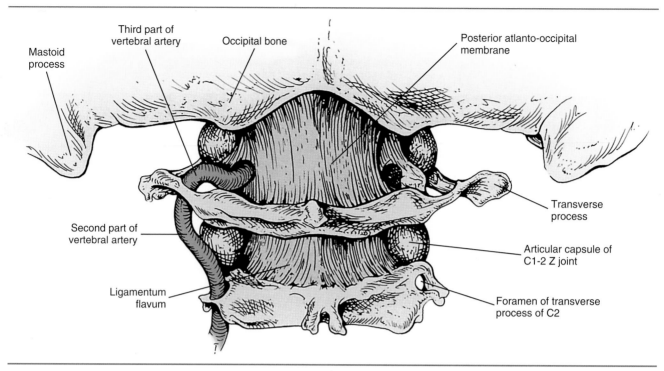

FIG. 5-10   Posterior ligaments of the upper cervical region.

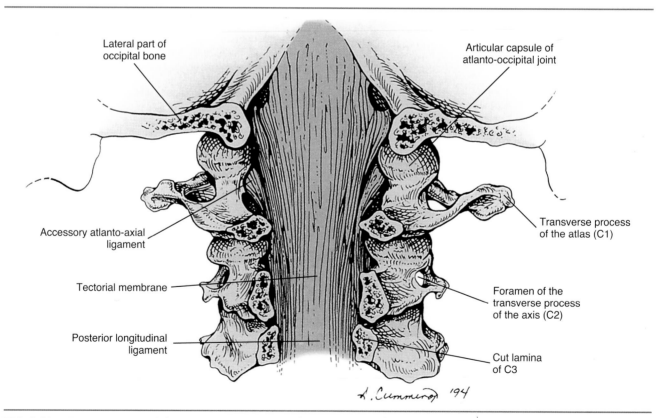

FIG. 5-11   Posterior aspect of the occiput, posterior arch of the atlas, laminae and spinous processes of C2 and C3, neural elements, and meninges have all been removed to show the ligaments of the anterior aspect of the upper cervical vertebral canal and foramen magnum.

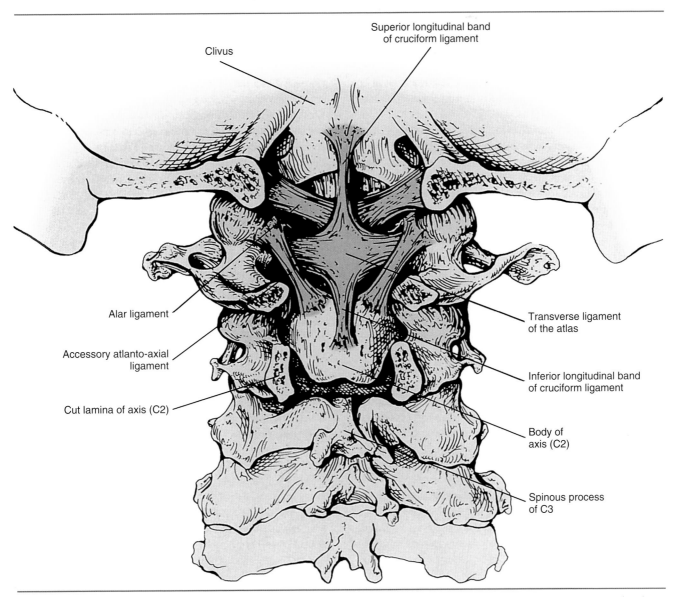

Superior longitudinal band
of cruciform ligament

Clivus

Alar ligament

Accessory atlanto-axial
ligament

Cut lamina of axis (C2)

Transverse ligament
of the atlas

Inferior longitudinal band
of cruciform ligament

Body of
axis (C2)

Spinous process
of C3

FIG. 5-12   Anterior aspect of the vertebral canal and foramen magnum as seen from behind. The tectorial membrane has been removed, and many of the upper cervical ligaments can be seen. Notice the centrally located cruciform ligament with its narrow superior and inferior longitudinal bands and its stout transverse ligament. The alar and accessory atlanto-axial ligaments also can be seen.

posteromedial aspect of the capsule of the lateral atlanto-axial joints. They are considered to be deep fibers of the tectorial membrane.

Cruciform Ligament. The cruciform ligament is named such because of its cross shape. Actually it may be divided into several parts: a large transverse ligament, superior longitudinal band, and inferior longitudinal band (Fig. 5-12). Each portion is discussed next.

Transverse ligament. The transverse ligament of the atlas (TLA), or transverse portion of the cruciform

ligament, has been called the most important ligament of the occiput–C1-2 complex of joints (White and Panjabi, 1990). It is a strong ligament that runs from a small medial tubercle of one lateral mass of the atlas (colliculus atlantis, Fig. 5-6, *G*) to the same tubercle on the opposite side. The TLA lies in the horizontal plane. However, approximately a 21-degree angle with the frontal (coronal) plane is created from the origin of the transverse ligament to the region where it passes behind the odontoid process (Panjabi, Oxland, and Parks, 1991a). It courses approximately 5 mm inferior to the odontal attachments of the apical odontoid ligament and the left and right alar ligaments (Ebraheim et al., 1997a). The superoinferior width of this ligament is greatest at its center, where it passes posterior to the odontoid process. Anteriorly the TLA is lined by a thin layer of fibrocartilage (Ebraheim et al., 1997a). This enables it to form a diarthrodial joint with the odontoid as it passes posterior to this structure.

The TLA allows the atlas to pivot on the axis (Fig. 5-13). It also holds the atlas in its proper position, thereby preventing compression of the spinal cord during flexion of the head and neck. Because the transverse ligament fits into the groove on the posterior surface of the odontoid, it holds the atlas in proper position even when all other ligaments are severed (Williams et al., 1995). Panjabi, Oxland, and Parks (1991a) found that this ligament appears to exist in two distinct layers, superficial and deep.

Fibrocartilage frequently develops in regions of ligaments that are constantly compressed against bone. Examples of this include portions of the Achilles tendon, tendons of the rotator cuff, and extensor tendons of the fingers and toes. Similarly, the region of the TLA that passes posterior to the odontoid process also develops fibrocartilage. However, this region is unique in that a fibrous capsule surrounds the fibrocartilage facet on the transverse ligament, forming a diarthrodial (synovial) joint with the posterior articular facet of the odontoid process. The fibrocartilage of the TLA possesses substances also found in typical articular cartilage (e.g., link protein, aggrecan, and type II collagen). Some cases of rheumatoid arthritis are related to an autoimmune response to these substances. Such autoimmune responses could erode the TLA, resulting in the upper cervical instability seen in a significant number of patients with rheumatoid arthritis. Furthermore, fibrocartilage has less ability to repair than typical ligaments, complicating the healing of erosions affecting the TLA. This slower rate of healing may help to explain why calcium deposition or ossification frequently is seen in TLAs of arthritic median atlanto-axial joints (Milz et al., 2001).

Superior longitudinal band. The superior longitudinal band of the cruciform ligament runs from the transverse ligament to the anterior lip of the foramen magnum (see Fig. 5-12). More specifically it attaches to the superior aspect of the basilar part of the occipital bone (clivus). It is interposed between the apical ligament of the odontoid process, which is anterior to it, and the tectorial membrane, which is posterior to it. Although it may limit both flexion and extension of the occiput, its primary function may be to hold the transverse ligament in its proper position, thus aiding the transverse ligament in holding the atlas against the odontoid process.

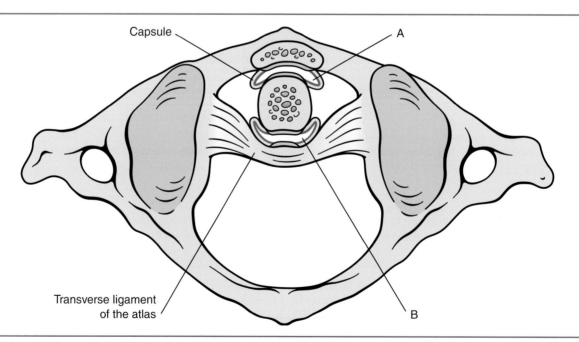

Capsule

A

Transverse ligament of the atlas

B

FIG. 5-13 Median atlanto-axial joint. Notice the role played by the transverse ligament of the atlas in allowing the atlas to pivot around the odontoid process. The two parts of the joint are distinct, each with its own joint capsule (Ebraheim et al., 1997a). The synovial lining of the capsules is shown in red. *A,* Anterior part of the joint, between the anterior arch of the atlas and the odontoid. *B,* Posterior part of the joint, between the odontoid process and the transverse ligament of the atlas.

Inferior longitudinal band. The inferior longitudinal band of the cruciform ligament attaches the TLA to the body of C2, preventing the transverse ligament from riding too far superiorly (see Fig. 5-12). It also helps to limit flexion of the occiput and atlas on the axis (with the aid of the superior band and transverse ligament).

Alar Ligaments. The left and right alar ligaments originate from the posterior and lateral aspect of the odontoid process with some of the fibers covering the entire posterior surface of the dens (Panjabi et al., 1991a). Each alar ligament passes anteriorly and superiorly to insert onto a roughened region of the medial surface of the occipital condyle of the same side (Fig. 5-14; see also Fig. 5-12). The alar ligaments are approximately the width of a pencil and are strong.

The functions of the alar ligaments are complex and are not understood completely. However, each alar ligament limits contralateral axial rotation (Dvorak and Panjabi, 1987). For example, the left alar ligament primarily limits right rotation. More specifically, the fibers of the left alar ligament, which attach to the odontoid process posterior to the axis of movement, act in concert with those fibers of the right alar ligament, which attach to the odontoid in front of the axis of movement. Both of these segments of the alar ligaments act together to limit right axial rotation. The opposite is also true: Right posterior odontal fibers and left anterior odontal fibers limit left rotation (Williams et al., 1995). Because the alar ligaments limit or check rotation, they are also known as the check ligaments.

The alar ligaments also limit flexion of the upper cervical spine after the tectorial membrane and cruciform ligaments have torn. The alar ligaments themselves are most vulnerable to tearing during the combined movements of axial rotation and flexion. This combination of movements may occur during a motor vehicle accident (e.g., hit from the front while looking in the rearview mirror) (Foreman and Croft, 1992). Injury as a result of this same pair of movements also can irreparably stretch the alar ligaments while sparing the cruciform ligament. When an alar ligament is torn or stretched, increased rotation occurs at the atlanto-occipital and atlanto-axial joint complexes, and increased lateral displacement occurs between the atlas and the axis during lateral flexion (Dvorak and Panjabi, 1987).

Dvorak and Panjabi (1987) found that in addition to attaching to the occipital condyle of the same side, a portion of each alar ligament usually attaches to the lateral mass of the atlas on the same side as well (see Fig. 5-13, *A*). They also occasionally found fibers coursing from the odontoid process to the anterior arch of the atlas. They named these latter fibers the anterior atlanto-dental ligament and believed that this ligament, when present, gives functional support to the transverse ligament. They stated that the alar ligaments also help to limit lateral flexion at the atlanto-occipital joint. The atlantal fibers of the alar ligament on the side of lateral flexion tighten first during this motion, followed by tightening of the occipital fibers of the alar ligament on the opposite side.

Apical Ligament of the Odontoid Process. The apical ligament of the odontoid process is thin, approximately 1 inch in length, and runs from the posterior and superior aspects of the odontoid process to the anterior wall of the foramen magnum (inferior aspect of the clivus) (see Fig. 5-13, *A*). Its fibers of insertion blend with the deep fibers of the superior longitudinal band of the cruciform ligament. Its course from the odontoid to the clivus results in approximately a 20-degree anterior tilt of the apical odontoid ligament. Its insertion is wider than its origin, giving it a V shape (Panjabi et al., 1991a). Embryologically this ligament develops from the core of the centrum of the proatlas (see Chapter 12) and contains traces of the notochord (Williams et al., 1995). The apical odontoid ligament probably functions to prevent some vertical translation and anterior shear of the occiput (Panjabi et al., 1991a).

Anterior Atlanto-Occipital Membrane. The anterior atlanto-occipital membrane is located in front of the apical odontoid ligament and courses from the superior aspect of the anterior arch of the atlas to the anterior margin of the foramen magnum (Fig. 5-15). It is composed of densely woven fibers (Williams et al., 1995) and is so broad that it can best be described as a membrane. The anterior atlanto-occipital membrane blends laterally with the capsular ligaments of the atlanto-occipital articulation (see Fig. 5-15). It functions to limit extension of the occiput on C1. Fibers continuous with the anterior longitudinal ligament strengthen the anterior atlanto-occipital ligament medially and form a tough central band between the anterior tubercle of the atlas and the occiput (Williams et al., 1995) (see Fig. 5-15). The anterior longitudinal ligament is discussed in more detail in the following section.

Lower Cervical Ligaments

Anterior Longitudinal Ligament. The anterior longitudinal ligament (ALL) is wide and covers the anterior aspect of the vertebral bodies and IVDs from the occiput to the sacrum. Superiorly the ALL thickens medially to form a cord that attaches to the body of the axis and the anterior tubercle of the atlas (see Fig. 5-15). Some of the atlantal fibers diverge laterally as the ALL fibers attach to the inferior aspect of the anterior arch of the atlas. Further superiorly the ALL becomes continuous with the medial portion of the anterior atlanto-occipital

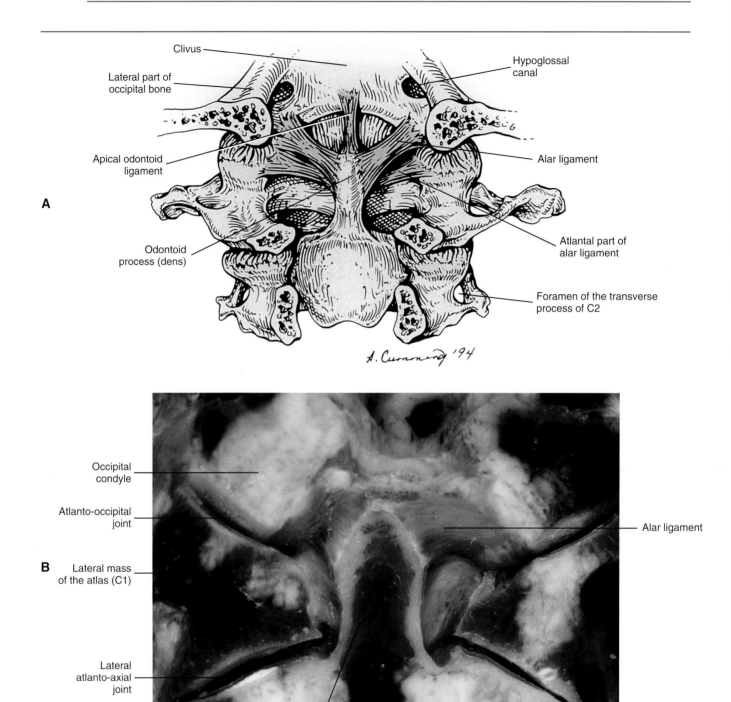

Clivus

Hypoglossal canal

Lateral part of occipital bone

Apical odontoid ligament

Alar ligament

A

Odontoid process (dens)

Atlantal part of alar ligament

Foramen of the transverse process of C2

A. Cumming '94

Occipital condyle

Atlanto-occipital joint

Alar ligament

B Lateral mass of the atlas (C1)

Lateral atlanto-axial joint

Odontoid process

FIG. 5-14   **A,** Alar and apical odontoid ligaments. This is the same view as that of Figures 5-11 and 5-12. The tectorial membrane and cruciform ligament have been removed. Notice that some fibers of each alar ligament attach to the lateral mass of the atlas. These fibers have been described by Dvorak and Panjabi (1987). **B,** Coronal section of upper cervical region demonstrating the alar ligaments.

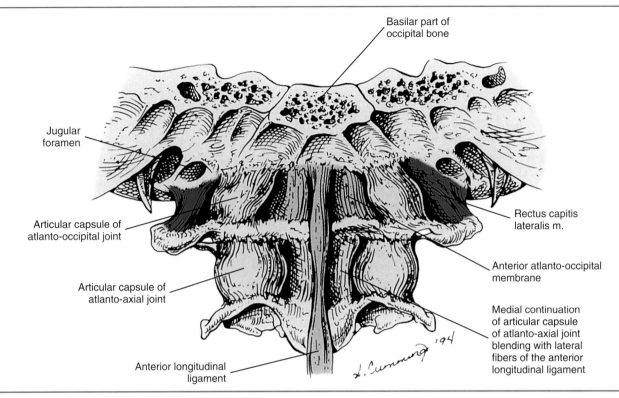

FIG. 5-15 Anterior view of the occiput, atlas, axis, and related ligaments. The anterior longitudinal ligament narrows considerably between the atlas and occipital bone and blends with the anterior atlanto-occipital membrane. The articular capsules of the atlanto-occipital and lateral atlanto-axial joints also are seen clearly in this figure.

membrane (see previous discussion). The ALL is approximately 3.8 mm wide at C1-2, is somewhat wider at C2-3, and increases in width to 7.5 mm from C3 to T1. The ALL is firmly attached to a significant portion of the superior and inferior bony end plates in all regions of the spine. However, regional differences exist for the ALL attachment sites. The ALL is firmly attached to the central region of the vertebral bodies 40% of the time in the cervical region, but is firmly attached to the center of the thoracic or lumbar vertebral bodies only rarely. In contrast, the ALL is almost never firmly attached to the IVD in the lumbar region and is firmly attached to this structure infrequently in the cervical region (20% of the time); however, the ALL is firmly attached to the IVD roughly half the time (50%) in the thoracic region (Cramer et al., 1996, 1998). Laterally the ALL is sometimes difficult to distinguish from the anterolateral fibers of the anulus fibrosus.

Several layers are associated with the ALL. The superficial fibers span several vertebrae, whereas the deep fibers course from one vertebra to the next. This ligament tends to be thicker from anterior to posterior in the regions of the vertebral bodies rather than the areas over the IVDs. Therefore the ALL helps to smooth the contour of the anterior surface of the vertebral bodies by filling the natural concavity of the anterior vertebral bodies. The ALL functions to limit extension and frequently is damaged in extension injuries to the cervical region (Bogduk, 1986a). However, during extension injuries to the spine, fibers of the anterior anulus fibrosus of the IVDs frequently tear before those of the more anteriorly located ALL because the fibers of the anulus fibrosus are shorter than those of the ALL and reach their failure loads before the fibers of the ALL do (Taylor, 1999).

Posterior Longitudinal Ligament. The posterior longitudinal ligament (PLL) is the inferior continuation of the tectorial membrane (see Fig. 5-11). It courses from the posterior aspect of the body of C2, inferiorly to the sacrum, and possibly to the coccyx (Behrsin and Briggs, 1988). The ALL and PLL have similar tensile properties (Przybylski et al., 1996). That is, they can withstand similar loads applied to the spine, although the ALL limits forces applied in extension and the PLL resists forces applied in flexion. The PLL is wide and regularly shaped in the cervical and upper thoracic regions and is also three to four times thicker, from anterior to posterior, in the cervical region than in the thoracic or lumbar regions (Bland, 1989). Its superficial fibers span several vertebrae, and its deep fibers course between adjacent vertebrae. Panjabi, Oxland, and Parks (1991b) found the cervical PLL to be firmly attached to both the vertebral bodies and the IVDs, whereas Bland (1989) found the PLL to have a stronger discal attachment. In either case, the PLL probably functions to help prevent posterior IVD protrusion. Although the PLL is attached to the entire length of the vertebral bodies in the cervical region (Przybylski et al., 1998), it is more loosely attached to the central region of the vertebral bodies to allow the exit of the basivertebral veins from the vertebral bodies (Williams et al., 1995). The PLL in the middle and lower thoracic and lumbar regions differs from the PLL in the cervical region in that it becomes narrow over the vertebral bodies and then widens considerably over the IVDs in the thoracic and lumbar areas.

The PLL receives a significant nociceptive and vasomotor innervation. The nociceptive innervation may make this ligament one of the most pain sensitive of the spine. The vasomotor fibers probably help to increase regional blood flow to promote healing after ligamentous damage (Imai et al., 1999).

The PLL occasionally ossifies. This occurs most frequently in the cervical region and occasionally occurs in the lumbar region. (Do not confuse this with ossification of the ligamenta flava, which occurs most frequently in the thoracic region.) Ossification of the PLL (OPLL) is clinically relevant because it may be a source of compression of the spinal cord in the cervical region, and has been associated with radicular symptoms in the lumbar region (Hasue et al., 1983). OPLL is found primarily in the middle or lower cervical spine of middle-aged and elderly men (almost 3.5:1 more than women) of Japanese origin, living in Japan (Yamada et al., 2003). Japanese people also have a higher incidence of ossification of other spinal ligaments than other ethnic populations. The incidences of OPLL, ossification of the ALL, and ossification of the ligamentum nuchae in Japanese men 48 to 57 years old are 4.1%, 23.1%, and 23.3%, respectively (Shingyouchi, Nagahama, and Niida, 1996). A close association of OPLL and diffuse idiopathic skeletal hypertrophy (DISH) has also been found, and OPLL is now considered to be a variant of DISH (Yamada et al., 2003). DISH has been associated with obesity and glucose intolerance (Shingyouchi, Nagahama, and Niida, 1996). Although the etiology of OPLL is unknown and undoubtedly complex, mechanical stress, genetic factors, dietary factors, and vitamin K_2 (menaquinone) metabolism all have been associated with this condition (Matsunaga et al., 1996; Shingyouchi, Nagahama, and Niida, 1996; Yamada et al., 2003). Estrogen levels also play a role in OPLL. (Estrogen promotes osteoblastic activity.) With respect to diet, OPLL and ossification of the ALL also have been significantly linked to obesity and diabetes or impaired glucose tolerance, whereas ossification of the ligamentum nuchae (OLN) has been linked to obesity only (Shingyouchi, Nagahama, and Niida, 1996). Furthermore, OPLL also may be associated with the high-salt, low-meat diets of Japanese and Taiwanese (Wang et al., 1999). Hypertrophy of the PLL (HPLL) is a distinct condition that is a pathologic thickening of the PLL, and HPLL may or may not be a precursor to OPLL. Both HPLL and OPLL show unique cellular characteristics. Cells of both HPLL and OPLL ligaments seem to possess similar regulatory mechanisms (perhaps secreting a similar growth factor) that may allow for accelerated growth and division of cells in the PLL (Motegi et al., 1998).

Ligamenta Flava. The ligamenta flava (*singular,* ligamentum flavum) are paired ligaments (left and right) that run between the laminae of adjacent vertebrae (see Fig. 5-10). They are found throughout the spine beginning with C1-2 superiorly and ending with L5-S1 inferiorly. The posterior atlanto-occipital membrane is the homologue of the ligamenta flava at the level of occiput-C1. Each ligamentum flavum is approximately 5 mm thick from anterior to posterior (Panjabi, Oxland, and Parks, 1991b). These ligaments are thinnest in the cervical region, become thicker in the thoracic region, and are thickest in the lumbar region.

Each ligament passes from the anterior and inferior aspect of the lamina of the vertebra above to the posterior and superior aspect of the lamina of the vertebra below. The ligamenta flava increase in length from C2-3 to C7-T1. This implies that the distance between the laminae also increases in a similar manner. Laterally each ligamentum flavum helps to support the anterior aspect of the Z joint capsule. Although each ligament is considered to be distinct, a ligamentum flavum frequently blends with the ligamentum flavum of the opposite side (Panjabi et al., 1991b) and also blends with the interspinous ligament. Small gaps exist between the left and right ligamenta flava, allowing for the passage of veins that unite the posterior internal (epidural) vertebral venous plexus with the posterior external vertebral venous plexus. The ligamentum flavum between C1 and C2 is usually thin and membranous and is pierced by the C2 spinal nerve. In fact, Panjabi, Oxland, and Parks (1991b) were unable to find ligamenta flava between C1 and C2 in their study of six cervical spines.

The ligamentum flavum is unique in that it contains yellow-colored elastin, which causes it to constrict naturally. Therefore this ligament actually may do work; that is, it may aid in extension of the spine. It also slows the last few degrees of spinal flexion. However, the most important function of the elastin may be to prevent buckling of the ligamentum flavum into the spinal canal during extension.

The ligamentum flavum may undergo degeneration with age or after trauma. Under such circumstances, it usually increases in thickness and may calcify or become infiltrated with fat (Ho et al., 1988). These changes may cause the ligament to lose its elastic characteristics, which can result in buckling of the thickened ligamentum flavum into the vertebral canal or medial aspect of the IVF. This further results in narrowing of these regions, which can compromise the neural elements running within them (e.g., spinal cord, cauda equina [lumbar region], or exiting nerve roots). Ossification of the ligamentum flavum is reported to occur most often in the thoracic and thoracolumbar regions of the spine, where it may compress either the posterior aspect of the spinal cord or the exiting nerve roots (Hasue et al., 1983) (see Chapter 6).

Interspinous Ligaments. The interspinous ligaments are a series of ligaments that course between the spinous processes of each pair of vertebrae from C2-3 to L4-5. Some authors consider this ligament to be the anterior aspect of the ligamentum nuchae in the cervical region (see following discussion). The interspinous ligaments are poorly developed in the cervical region, typically consisting of a thin, membranous, translucent septum (Panjabi et al., 1991). They are short from superior to inferior and broad from anterior to posterior in the thoracic region and more rectangular in shape in the lumbar region (Williams et al., 1995). Because these ligaments are more fully developed in the thoracic region, they are discussed in more detail in Chapter 6.

Ligamentum Nuchae. The ligamentum nuchae (LN) is a flat, membranous structure that runs from the region between the cervical spinous processes anteriorly to the skin of the back of the neck posteriorly (Fig. 5-16), and spans the region between the occiput superiorly to the spinous process of C7 inferiorly. The posterior portion is its thickest and most distinct part and is sometimes called the funicular portion of the LN (or the dorsal nuchal raphe). This funicular part extends from the external occipital protuberance to the spinous process of C7. It is formed, at least in part, by the intertwining fibers of origin of the left and right trapezius, splenius capitis, and rhomboid minor muscles (Johnson, Zhang, and Jones, 2000; Mercer and Bogduk, 2003). The thinner, larger, and more membranous anterior portion of this ligament sometimes is known as the lamellar portion. This midline fascial lamellar portion of the LN is the portion that extends anteriorly between the cervical spinous processes. The lamellar portion also is continuous with the dense cervical fascia that extends laterally to separate the left and right semispinalis capitis muscles from the underlying semispinalis cervicis, multifidus cervicis, and suboccipital muscles. This dense cervical fascia extends superiorly and laterally to attach to the entire width of the occiput in the region of the inferior nuchal line (Mitchell, Humphreys, and O'Sullivan, 1998). The LN is considered to be the homologue of the supraspinous and interspinous ligaments of the thoracic and lumbar regions.

Between the occiput and C1 and between C1 and C2, the LN extends anteriorly all of the way to the dura mater, to which it attaches (Mitchell, Humphreys, and O'Sullivan, 1998; Dean and Mitchell, 2002; Humphreys et al., 2003). The attachment from the LN to the posterior dura mater between C1 and C2 can be seen on MRI (Humphreys et al., 2003). Figure 5-17 demonstrates the attachment between the LN and the posterior aspect of the spinal dura mater between C1 and C2 and its MRI appearance. These attachments may hold the dura mater posteriorly during cervical extension (to prevent buckling of the dura mater into the spinal cord) and flexion (to prevent the dura from moving forward and compressing the cord). Similar connective tissue attachments also connect the rectus capitis posterior minor muscle with the posterior aspect of the dura mater/posterior atlanto-occipital membrane complex (see Fig. 5-17). These latter attachments course between the occiput and the posterior arch of the atlas (see Chapter 4). Other connective tissue attachments to the posterior spinal dura mater have been identified and were described in the section entitled Vertebral Canal.

In addition, between the occiput and the atlas the LN has a firm attachment along the entire posterior border of the rectus capitis posterior minor muscle (Humphreys et al., 2003).

Intertransverse Ligaments. Each intertransverse ligament passes from one transverse process to the transverse process of the vertebra below. These ligaments are not well defined in the cervical region and frequently are replaced by the posterior intertransverse muscles. The thoracic intertransverse ligaments are rounded cords closely related to the deep back muscles (Williams et al., 1995). Some authors describe the lumbar intertransverse ligaments as being thin membranous bands. Others consider them to be discrete and well defined. Still others consider them to consist of two distinct lamellae (Bogduk, 1997) (see Chapter 7).

General Considerations Related to the Role of Spinal Ligaments in Limiting Specific Motions. Notice from the preceding sections that in flexion, significant strains (tension) exist in all spinal ligaments, except the ALL. In extension, the ALL is under the most strain (the most stretched). In axial rotation the same-sided capsular ligament is maximally stretched (e.g., left axial rotation results in the highest strain being placed on the left capsular ligament). In lateral flexion, the

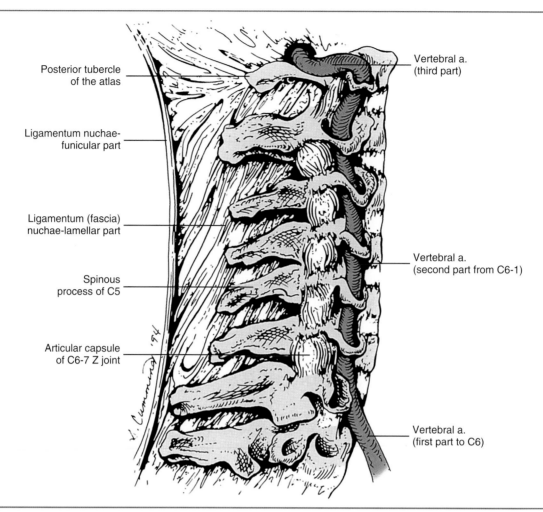

Posterior tubercle
of the atlas

Ligamentum nuchae-
funicular part

Ligamentum (fascia)
nuchae-lamellar part

Spinous
process of C5

Articular capsule
of C6-7 Z joint

Vertebral a.
(third part)

Vertebral a.
(second part from C6-1)

Vertebral a.
(first part to C6)

FIG. 5-16   Lateral view of the cervical portion of the vertebral column. The ligamentum (fascia) nuchae and the articular capsules of the C1-2 through C6-7 Z joints are seen. The vertebral artery can be seen entering the foramen of the transverse process (TP) of C6 and ascending through the remaining foramina of the TPs of C5 through C1. Then it can be seen passing around the superior articular process of C1. The vertebral artery disappears from view as it courses beneath the posterior atlanto-occipital membrane.

contralateral ligament flavum and intertransverse ligament have the highest strains.

Flexion-Extension (Whiplash) Types of Injuries. Flexion-extension (whiplash) automobile injuries occur with some frequency. Even an 8-mile-per-hour rear end collision can cause injury to structures of the cervical region. Head rests are of limited value in preventing flexion-extension injuries, and in certain situations the head rest can actually act as a fulcrum and increase injury (Croft, 1993). In addition, the incidence of neck pain after flexion-extension injuries has been reported to be higher among those wearing seat belts (Lohiya, 1993). Although the brain is more susceptible to injury from side-to-side trauma (broadside accident) than from flexion-extension trauma (rear end collision), flexion-extension injuries can sprain the ligaments of the cervi-

cal region and lead to acute neck pain. In addition, flexion-extension injuries also can lead to chronic pain arising from the Z joints, temporomandibular joints, IVDs, and other structures of the neck (Croft, 1993; Barnsley et al., 1995; Lord et al., 1996). Croft (1993) reports that 45% to 83% of patients involved in flexion-extension injuries have symptoms that persistent for more than 2 years after litigation related to their case has been settled (i.e., these symptoms are not related to pending litigation). Disc pathology seems to contribute to chronic neck pain after flexion-extension (whiplash) injuries (Pettersson et al., 1997), and Loudon, Ruhl, and Field (1997) found evidence of decrease in proprioceptive ability after flexion-extension injuries. They speculate that this results from damage to cervical neck muscles and to the Z joint capsules, resulting in abnormal proprioception from these structures.

CERVICAL INTERVERTEBRAL DISCS

The IVDs of the cervical spine make up more than 25% of the superior-to-inferior length of this region, and they help to allow the large amount of motion that occurs here. Recall that there are no IVDs between the occiput and atlas and between the atlas and axis. The C2-3 interbody joint is the first such joint to possess an IVD. Therefore the C3 spinal nerve is the most superior nerve capable of being affected by IVD protrusion.

Mendel et al. (1992) studied the innervation of the cervical IVDs and found sensory nerve fibers throughout the anulus fibrosus. No nerves were found in the nucleus pulposus. The sensory fibers were most numerous in the middle third (from superior to inferior) of the anulus. The structure of many of the nerve fibers and their end receptors was consistent with those that transmit pain. In addition, pacinian corpuscles and Golgi tendon organs were found in the posterolateral aspect of the disc. These authors' findings help to confirm that the anulus fibrosus is a pain-sensitive structure. Furthermore, their findings indicate that the cervical discs are involved in proprioception, thereby enabling the central nervous system to monitor the mechanical status of the IVDs. These authors hypothesized that the arrangement of the sensory receptors may allow the IVD to sense peripheral compression or deformation and also alignment between adjacent vertebrae.

The posterior aspect of each cervical IVD has less height from superior-to-inferior than the anterior aspect of the IVD (Lu et al., 1999). In addition, the IVDs of the cervical region become thinner with age. This is because the cervical IVDs dehydrate earlier in life than those of the thoracic and lumbar regions, and by the age of 45 the nucleus pulposus is difficult to distinguish from the anulus fibrosus. Evaluation of such IVD thinning with degeneration can be done reliably from standard x-rays if rigorous, standardized methods of evaluation are used (Côté et al., 1997). Furthermore, horizontal and vertical clefts can develop in these aging cervical IVDs. These clefts cause bulging and protrusion of the hardened cervical cartilaginous end plates. These end plate herniations are the predominant type of IVD herniations in the cervical region (Kokubun, Sakurai, and Tanaka, 1996). Like IVD herniations in the lumbar region, cervical disc herniations usually regress with time (Bush et al., 1997). However, the higher the concentration of cartilaginous end plates in the herniation, the slower is the process of IVD resorption.

As the cervical IVDs narrow, the uncinate processes enlarge. As a result, by age 40 the uncinate processes help to create a barrier that in turn helps to prevent lateral and posterolateral herniation of the IVD (Bland, 1989). However, the uncinate processes can develop osteophytes that can cause stenosis of the vertebral canal and IVF, leading to radiculopathy of osteophytic origin (Bland, 1989).

MRI has been shown to be effective in evaluating the status of the IVD (Forristall, Marsh, and Pay, 1988). Viikari-Juntara et al. (1989) also found that ultra–low-field MRI is useful in identifying posterior disc displacement below the level of C4. These MRI units are less expensive, and as resolution improves, they may be more frequently used in place of standard x-ray procedures. However, tears of the anulus fibrosus frequently go undetected on cervical MRI (Schellhas et al., 1996), and the importance of a thorough and accurate clinical history and physical examination are essential for the correct diagnosis of cervical pain of discogenic origin, with or without radiculopathy.

The basic anatomy of the cervical IVDs differs from that of the IVDs throughout the remainder of the spine. The anulus fibrosus is a single crescent-shaped piece of fibrocartilage that is thick anteriorly and extremely thin posteriorly (Fig. 5-18). Those interested in the detailed anatomy of the IVDs should refer to the sections of Chapters 2 and 14 devoted to the gross and microscopic anatomy of these clinically relevant structures.

RANGES OF MOTION OF THE CERVICAL SPINE

Although cervical ranges of motion can be measured reliably (Nilsson, Christensen, and Hartvigsen, 1996), one must keep in mind that measurements made on different days of both active (performed by an individual's own muscular activity) and passive (performed by another person holding the subject's head and moving the spine through the range of motion to be measured) ranges of motion of the same individual can vary considerably. Variations of 12 to 20 degrees can be found in flexion-extension, lateral flexion, and axial rotation (Christensen and Nilsson, 1998).

Atlanto-Occipital Joint

The right and left atlanto-occipital joints together form an ellipsoidal joint that allows movement in flexion, extension, and, to a lesser extent, left and right lateral flexion (Table 5-5). A little rotation also occurs between occiput and atlas (Williams et al., 1995). Extension is limited by the opposition of the posterior aspect of the superior articular processes of the atlas with the bone of the occiput's condylar fossa. Flexion is limited by soft-tissue stops, such as the posterior atlanto-occipital membrane.

Table 5-6 lists the muscles that produce the most flexion, extension, and lateral flexion between the occiput and atlas and between the atlas and axis.

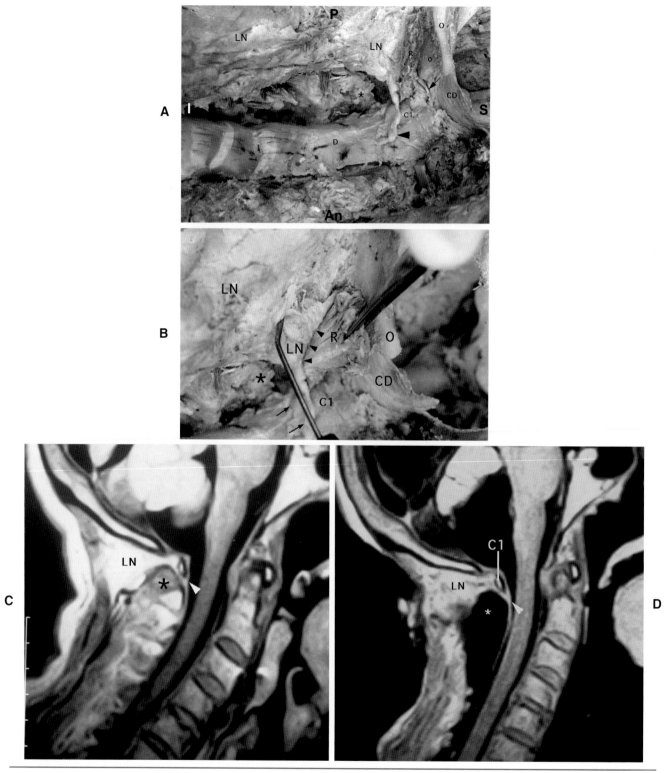

FIG. 5-17

For legend see opposite page.

FIG. 5-17   **A–D,** Right lateral dissection of a cadaveric specimen. The spinous processes of the C2-6 vertebrae have been removed. The asterisk is located in the region normally occupied by the C2 spinous process. The attachment between the ligamentum (fascia) nuchae (LN) and, **D,** the dura mater of the cervical vertebral canal is identified with the large black arrowhead. The smaller black arrow demonstrates the attachment between, **R,** the rectus capitis posterior minor muscle (RCPM) and the superior-most aspect of the dura mater of the vertebral canal. **A,** Vertebral artery; **An,** anterior; **C1,** posterior arch of the atlas; **CD,** dura mater within the posterior cranial fossa; **I,** inferior; **O,** occiput (note that a portion of the occiput has been sectioned in the midsagittal plane and the region labeled with a small "O" lies deep to and to the left of the plane of section); **P,** posterior; **S,** superior. **B,** Arrowheads demonstrate the attachment between the LN, being distracted posteriorly by the probe, and **R,** the posterior aspect of the RCPM being grasped by the forceps. This attachment is composed of a continuous series of firm connective tissue bridges coursing between the LN and RCPM. The small arrows and the region between the arrows at the bottom of this figure represent the attachment site of the LN to the dura mater. Pulling on the RCPM results in movement of the LN beginning in the region of the arrowheads. This movement continues to the region between the two arrows and results in tugging of the dura mater at this location. **C,** Magnetic resonance imaging (MRI) of the specimen in **B** before dissection was performed. Note the connection *(arrowhead)* between the LN and dura mater between the posterior arch of the atlas and spinous process of C2 *(asterisk).* **D,** MRI taken of this specimen after dissection. The spinous processes of the C2-6 vertebrae have been removed. The region normally occupied by the spinous process of C2 is indicated by an asterisk, and the posterior arch of the atlas is labeled **C1.** No contrast enhancement was used to produce this image. Notice that the LN retains the same appearance as in the predissection MRI **(C)** as it passes between the posterior arch of the atlas and the region of the spinous process of C2. The connection of the LN with the dura mater *(arrowhead)* also retains the same appearance in the predissection and postdissection MRIs. By comparing this image with the same dissected specimen in **A,** one can observe that the LN is the only tissue inferior to, **Cl,** the posterior arch of the atlas as it passes inferior to the posterior arch of the atlas to attach to the dura mater. This helps confirm the MRI appearance of the LN in this region and, more specifically, the MRI appearance of the LN–dura mater attachment. (From Humphreys BK et al. [2003]. Investigation of connective tissue attachments to the cervical spinal dura matter. *Clin Anat, 16,* 152-159.)

Atlanto-Axial Joints

Motion occurs at all three (median and left and right lateral) atlanto-axial joints simultaneously. The most motion occurs in axial rotation (Table 5-7), which is limited by the alar ligaments (see earlier discussion). Because the superior articular process of C2 is convex superiorly and the inferior articular facet of C1 is only slightly concave inferiorly, the anterior and posterior gliding that accompanies axial rotation also is accompanied by descent of the atlas. This moves the upper joint surface (i.e., inferior facet of C1) inferiorly, which conserves the amount of capsule necessary to accommodate the large amount of unilateral axial rotation that can occur at this joint. In addition, the descent of the atlas, as its inferior articular processes move along the superior articular processes of the axis, allows added rotation to occur between the two segments (Williams et al., 1995).

Muscles that produce rotation at this joint include the following: obliquus capitis inferior, rectus capitis posterior major, splenius capitis, and the contralateral sternocleidomastoid.

Lower Cervicals

The ranges of motion for the cervical region from C2-3 through C7-T1 are given in Table 5-8.

Usually extension is somewhat greater than flexion. Extension is limited below by the inferior articular processes of C7 entering a groove below the superior articular processes of T1. Flexion is limited by the lip on the anterior and inferior aspects of the cervical vertebral bodies pressing against the beveled surface of the anterior and superior aspects of the vertebral bodies immediately below (Williams et al., 1995).

Rotation with Lateral Flexion

Lateral flexion of the cervical spine is accompanied by rotation of the C2-7 vertebral bodies (the occiput-atlas and atlas-axis articulations perform uniquely) into the concavity formed by the lateral flexion (vertebral body rotation to the same side as lateral flexion) (Panjabi et al., 2001b). For example, right lateral flexion of the cervical region is accompanied by right rotation of the vertebral bodies. This phenomenon is known as *coupled motion*

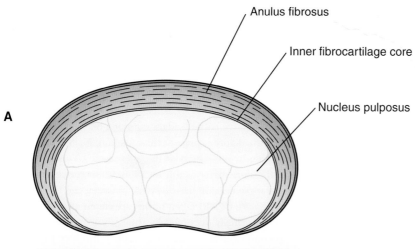

A

Anulus fibrosus

Inner fibrocartilage core

Nucleus pulposus

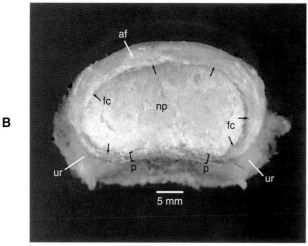

B

FIG. 5-18 **A,** Illustration and, **B,** dissection showing superior view of a cervical intervertebral disc demonstrating the crescent-shaped anulus fibrosus in the cervical region. Notice that the anulus is extremely thin posteriorly. *af,* Anulus fibrosus; *fc,* inner fibrocartilage core; *np,* nucleus pulposus; *p,* posterior aspect of the anulus fibrosus (the posterior longitudinal ligament has been removed); *ur,* uncinate region. (**B,** From Mercer S & Bogduk N. [1999]. The ligaments and anulus fibrosis of the human adult cervical intervertebral discs. *Spine, 24,* 619-628.)

Table 5-5	Approximate Ranges of Motion at the Atlanto-Occipital Joints

Direction	Amount
Combined flexion and extension	25°
Unilateral lateral flexion	5°
Unilateral axial rotation	5°

From White AW & Panjabi MM (1990). *Clinical biomechanics of the spine.* Philadelphia: JB Lippincott; and Panjabi et al. (2001a). The cortical shell architecture of human cervical vertebral bodies. *Spine, 26,* 2478-2484.

and occurs because the superior articular processes of cervical vertebrae face not only superiorly, but also are angled slightly medially. This arrangement forces some rotation with any attempt at lateral flexion. A more thorough discussion of coupled motion is found in Chapter 2.

NERVES, VESSELS, ANTERIOR NECK MUSCLES, AND VISCERA OF THE CERVICAL REGION

Vertebral Artery

The vertebral artery is so closely related to the cervical spine that it is discussed before the nerves of the neck. The remaining arteries of the neck are covered later in this chapter.

The vertebral artery is the first branch of the subclavian artery. It enters the foramen of the TP of C6 and ascends through the remaining foramina of the TPs of the cervical vertebrae (Fig. 5-19; see also Fig. 5-16). Continuing, it passes through the foramen of the TP of C1, winds medially around the superior articular process of the atlas, and passes beneath the posterior atlanto-occipital membrane (see Fig. 5-10). The vertebral artery then pierces the dura and arachnoid and courses

Table 5-6 Muscles Producing Flexion, Extension, and Lateral Flexion at Occiput, C1-2

Movement	Muscles
Flexion	Longus capitis
	Rectus capitis anterior
Extension	Rectus capitis posterior major and minor
	Obliquus capitis superior
	Semispinalis and spinalis capitis
	Longissimus capitis
	Splenius capitis
	Trapezius
	Sternocleidomastoid
Lateral flexion	Rectus capitis lateralis
	Semispinalis capitis
	Longissimus capitis
	Splenius capitis
	Sternocleidomastoid
	Trapezius

Table 5-7 Approximate Ranges of Motion at the Atlanto-Axial Joint

Direction	Amount
Combined flexion and extension	20°
Unilateral lateral flexion	5°
Unilateral axial rotation	28°–40°

From White AW & Panjabi MM (1990). *Clinical biomechanics of the spine.* Philadelphia: JB Lippincott; and Panjabi et al. (2001a). The cortical shell architecture of human cervical vertebral bodies. *Spine, 26,* 2478-2484.

Table 5-8 Total Range of Motion of Cervical Vertebrae (C2-T1)*

Direction	Amount
Combined flexion and extension	91°
Unilateral lateral flexion	51°
Unilateral axial rotation	33°

Values calculated from White AW & Panjabi MM (1990). *Clinical biomechanics of the spine.* Philadelphia: JB Lippincott.
*Ranges are for C2-3 through C7-T1 and do not include occiput, C1 and C1-2 (see Tables 5-5 and 5-7 for upper cervical ranges of motion).

superiorly through the foramen magnum to unite with the vertebral artery of the opposite side. The union of the two vertebral arteries forms the basilar artery.

Each vertebral artery is approximately 4.5 mm in diameter. The left and right arteries often are asymmetric, with one artery much larger than the other. When this is the case the larger artery is called the "dominant artery" and the smaller artery is called the "minor artery" (George and Laurian, 1987). George and Laurian (1987) reported that the left vertebral artery is dominant 35.8% of the time, the right vertebral artery is dominant 23.4% of the time, and they are of roughly equal diameter 40.8% of the time. The minor artery can be small and occasionally is absent (in which case a well-developed anastomosis is found).

The First Part of the Vertebral Artery. The vertebral artery can be divided into four parts (Williams et al., 1995). The first part of the vertebral artery begins at the artery's origin from the subclavian artery and continues until it passes through the foramen of the TP of C6. The first part courses between the longus colli and scalenus anterior muscles before reaching the TP of C6. In a study of 36 vertebral arteries, Taitz and Arensburg (1989) found that 18 (50%) were tortuous to some degree in the first segment. Currently there is debate as to whether or not tortuosity of a vertebral artery may cause a decrease in flow to the structures supplied by it. However, to date no clinical significance has been ascribed to mild-to-moderate tortuosity of the vertebral artery. True anomalies of the origin of the vertebral artery are relatively rare. However, the most common anomaly is an origin from the aortic arch (4%), with the anomalous vertebral artery usually arising between the left common carotid and left subclavian arteries.

The first part of the vertebral artery is accompanied by several venous branches that become the vertebral vein in the lower cervical region. It is also accompanied by a large branch and several small branches from the more posteriorly located inferior cervical ganglion or, when present, the cervicothoracic ganglion (stellate ganglion, present 80% of the time). These branches form a plexus of nerves around the vertebral artery. This plexus is discussed in more detail later in this chapter.

The Second Part of the Vertebral Artery. The second part of the vertebral artery is the region that passes superiorly through the foramina of the TPs of C6 to C1 (Fig. 5-20; see also Figs. 5-16 and 5-19). It usually enters the foramen of the TP of C6 (89.8% of the time), but may enter at any level (e.g., C5, 6.3%; C7, 3.0%). The entrance is symmetric from left to right 85% of the time and is asymmetric 15% of the time (Francke et al., 1980). When asymmetry is present, the arteries have only very rarely been found to enter the foramina of the TPs more than two levels apart, and the right artery almost always has been found to enter at the lower level (Francke et al., 1980; Gluncic et al., 1999). When the vertebral artery originates from the arch of the aorta it usually enters the foramen of the TP at C5 or C4.

In its ascent through the foramina of the TPs of the C6 to C1 vertebrae, the second part of the vertebral artery passes approximately 1 mm posterior and lateral to the uncinate processes of C2 to C6 vertebrae. More specifi-

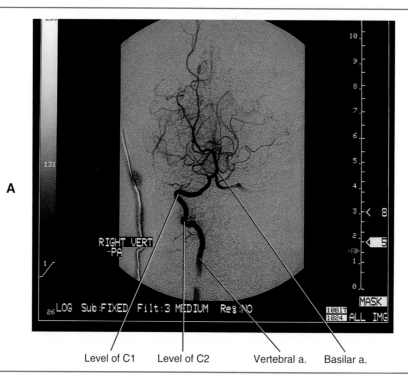

Level of C1   Level of C2   Vertebral a.   Basilar a.

FIG. 5-19   **A,** Posteroanterior and, **B,** lateral angiograms of the right vertebral artery. A radiopaque dye has been injected into the vertebral artery, and x-ray films have been taken. The vertebral artery can be seen as it courses superiorly through the foramina of the TPs of C6 through C1. Notice the normal tortuosity seen as the vertebral artery passes laterally at C2 to reach the foramen of the TP of C1. The vertebral artery also is tortuous as it passes around the superior articular process of C1 and then passes superiorly to enter the foramen magnum. It then unites with the vertebral artery of the opposite side to form the basilar artery. Several branches of the basilar artery can be seen, and its termination as the posterior cerebral arteries also can be seen.

cally, the distance of the vertebral artery from the uncinate processes gradually decreases during the ascent of the vertebral artery from C6 to C3. This may predispose the vertebral artery to compression from bone spurs (osteophytes) of the uncinate processes in the midcervical region (Ebraheim et al., 1997c). In addition, the second part of the vertebral artery passes anterior to the C2 to C6 cervical spinal nerves and ventral rami, which course from medial to lateral in the grooves (gutters) for the spinal nerves of their respective cervical TPs (see Fig. 5-23).

Occasionally the second part of the vertebral artery may become tortuous between any two TPs. Such tortuousness increases with age. Whether this tortuosity is congenital, acquired (secondary to atherosclerosis), or a combination of both has yet to be determined. However, Oga et al. (1996) found that severe disc degeneration, as sometimes seen in cervical spondylotic myelopathy, causes the distance between adjacent vertebrae to decrease. This decreased intervertebral dis-

tance occasionally can result in an increase in tortuosity of the second part of the vertebral artery. On rare occasions a tortuous vertebral artery causes a widening of the foramen of the TP (Taitz and Arensburg, 1989; Schima et al., 1993). Severe trauma to the cervical region leading to partial or complete anterior dislocation of one vertebra on another can lead to complete occlusion of flow through the second part of the vertebral artery (Giacobetti et al., 1997).

The second part of the vertebral artery normally makes a rather dramatic lateral curve (usually 45 degrees but up to 90 degrees) after passing through the foramen of the TP of the axis (see Figs. 5-10 and 5-20). This allows the artery to reach the more laterally placed TP of the atlas. Taitz and Arensburg (1989) found that 4 of 36 vertebral arteries (11%) showed marked kinking or tortuosity at the foramen of the TP of the axis.

A sympathetic nerve plexus surrounds the second through fourth parts of the vertebral artery. External to the sympathetic plexus, a dense connective tissue sheath

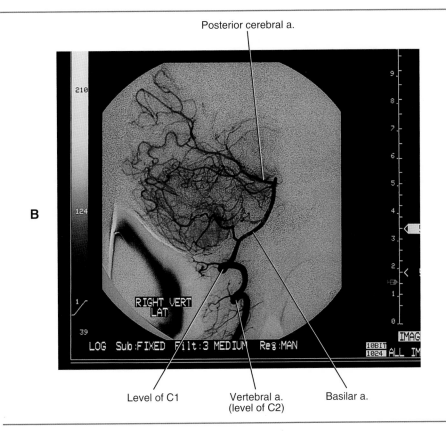

Posterior cerebral a.

B

RIGHT VERT
LAT

LOG Sub:FIXED Filt:3 MEDIUM Reg:MAN

Level of C1   Vertebral a.   Basilar a.
                     (level of C2)

FIG. 5-19—cont'd

covers the second part of the vertebral artery. Irritation of the vertebral artery sympathetic plexus (as can occur from hypertrophy of the closely related uncinate processes) has been associated with posterior occipital headaches, dizziness, and various pupillary changes, but not with a change of blood flow through the vertebral artery or any of the intracranial vessels (George and Laurian, 1987). The second part of the vertebral artery is accompanied by an interconnected venous plexus, which is most highly developed at the superior and inferior-most ends of this part of the artery (Schmidt and Pierson, 1934; Meyer, Yoshida, and Sakamoto, 1967; Nagashima and Iwama, 1972).

The dynamics of blood flow through the left and right vertebral arteries between the atlas and the axis remain rather poorly understood. Until recently, the general consensus was that extension combined with rotation of the head to one side normally impaired blood flow through the second part of the vertebral artery of the opposite side; the constriction occurring between the axis and atlas (Taitz, Nathan, and Arensburg, 1978). However, Haynes et al. (2002) found that usually there is no compression or stenosis of the vertebral artery with atlanto-axial rotation. Yi-Kai et al. (1999) found that extreme extension, and extension with rotation resulted in decreased flow in both vertebral arteries. Licht et al.

(1998) found a decrease in flow in the vertebral artery contralateral to rotation and for the first time documented an increase in flow on the ipsilateral side of rotation. Mitchell (2003) found a decrease in flow through both the left and right vertebral arteries (more in the contralateral vessel) with maximal rotation, especially in those arteries with underlying pathology (e.g., atherosclerosis). Therefore maximal rotation and extension seem to decrease flow through the vertebral arteries, but submaximal rotation seems to have less of an effect.

The Third Part of the Vertebral Artery. The third part of the vertebral artery normally has a tortuous course. It begins as the artery passes through the foramen of the TP of the atlas (see Fig. 5-20). Here it is located posterior and medial to the rectus capitis lateralis muscle. Immediately the vertebral artery curves farther posteriorly and medially around the superior articular process of C1. It reaches the posterior arch of the atlas, where it lies in the groove for the vertebral artery of the posterior arch. The dorsal ramus of the first cervical nerve (suboccipital nerve) passes between the vertebral artery and the posterior arch of the atlas in this region. The artery then passes inferior to the posterior atlanto-occipital membrane (see Fig. 5-10). This

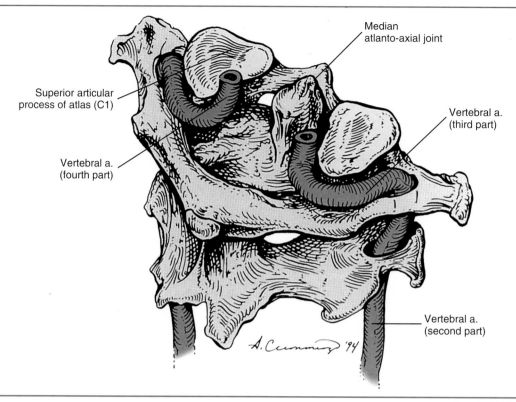

Superior articular
process of atlas (C1)

Median
atlanto-axial joint

Vertebral a.
(fourth part)

Vertebral a.
(third part)

Vertebral a.
(second part)

FIG. 5-20   The second, third, and fourth parts of the left and right vertebral arteries. Notice that each vertebral artery courses laterally between C2 and C1. It then courses posteriorly and medially at the level of C1, and finally passes superiorly and medially to reach the foramen magnum.

membrane may form an ossified bridge for the artery, which, when present, passes from the posterior arch of the atlas to the lateral mass. This bony bridge is known as a posterior ponticle and is discussed earlier in this chapter (see Fig. 5-6, *F*).

The Fourth Part of the Vertebral Artery. The fourth part of the vertebral artery begins as the artery passes beneath the bridge of the posterior atlanto-occipital membrane. It continues anteriorly, superiorly, and medially from the posterior atlanto-occipital membrane, and ascends along the anterolateral aspect of the spinal dura mater. At the level of the foramen magnum, each vertebral artery pierces the dura and arachnoid mater and continues ascending within the subarachnoid space. The left and right vertebral arteries continue to gradually course medially along the anterior aspect of the medulla and inferior pons, where they unite to form the single basilar artery. The basilar artery ascends along the anterior aspect of the pons and midbrain, until it helps to form the cerebral arterial circle (of Willis) by ending as the left and right posterior cerebral arteries.

Along its course, each vertebral artery gives off muscular branches, osteoarticular branches, meningeal branches, and spinal rami; the latter enter the IVFs to

help supply the vertebral body, posterior arch, and soft-tissue structures within the vertebral canal (including the nerve roots and rootlets). The fourth part of the vertebral artery has several branches. Each vertebral artery gives off a branch that unites with its pair from the opposite side to form a single anterior spinal artery. The anterior spinal artery supplies the anterior aspect of the spinal cord throughout its length. Each vertebral artery then gives off a posterior spinal artery. The left and right posterior spinal arteries remain separate as they course along the posterior aspect of the spinal cord (see Chapter 3 for both anterior and posterior spinal arteries). Each vertebral artery then gives off a posterior inferior cerebellar artery that supplies the inferior aspect of the cerebellum and a portion of the medulla.

As mentioned, the right and left vertebral arteries unite at the level of the inferior pons to form the basilar artery. The basilar artery gives off the left and right posterior superior cerebellar arteries. These arteries course posteriorly around the medulla to supply the medulla, inferior pons, and inferior one half to two thirds of the cerebellum. The basilar artery also sends the left and right internal acoustic (auditory) arteries to the internal acoustic meatus of each side. After passing through the meatus, each of these arteries supplies the middle and inner ear structures of each side. As the basilar artery ascends along the anterior aspect of the pons, it sends many small pontine branches to the pons. The basilar artery then gives off the left and right superior cerebellar arteries that course posteriorly, supplying the superior pons and inferior aspect of the cerebral peduncles before continuing posteriorly to supply the superior aspect of the cerebellum. The basilar artery ends at the level of the superior pons by dividing into the left and right posterior cerebral arteries. The posterior cerebral arteries participate in the cerebral arterial circle (of Willis) and then continue posteriorly to supply the occipital lobes of the cerebral cortex and the inferior portion of the temporal lobes.

Microscopic Anatomy. Each vertebral artery is thin walled, but its structure is quite similar to all other arteries (Wilkinson, 1972). As with all typical arteries, the vertebral artery is composed of three layers. From internal to external these layers are as follows: tunica intima, tunica media, and tunica adventitia. An internal elastic lamina separates the intima from the media, and an external elastic lamina separates the media from the adventitia. The tunica intima is the most delicate layer; the tunica media is more rugged and has elastic fibers within it. The tunica media and external elastic lamina are well developed in the vertebral artery below the foramen magnum. After piercing the dura and arachnoid mater at roughly the level of the foramen magnum, the adventitia decreases in thickness, the external elastic lamina disappears, and the tunica media loses most of its elastic fibrils.

As with all large arteries, much potential pathology can affect the walls of the vertebral artery; primary among these is atherosclerosis. The usual lesion of atherosclerosis is a smooth plaque that can be found anywhere within the first and second parts of the artery. These plaques may calcify. Hemorrhage in plaques has been observed in the vertebral artery, but ulceration of plaques only occurs in approximately 4% of the lesions, and is less common than such ulceration found in the carotid arteries. Possible complications to atherosclerosis include local thrombosis, ischemia to structures supplied downstream of the lesion, embolism, and stenosis leading to decreased flow.

As mentioned, the intima is the most delicate layer of any artery and severe trauma or plaque formation may cause this layer to tear and separate from the media. Such tearing of the intima causes rapidly flowing blood to be forced between the intima and media, causing dissection of the intima from the media. The vertebral artery is not exempted from such pathology. Causes of dissection include trauma, dissection associated with preexisting arterial disease (e.g., atherosclerosis, which is the most common cause of vertebral artery dissection), and spon-taneous dissection. With respect to trauma, there are four regions of the vertebral artery where such lesions have been identified. These are as follows: at the entrance of the vertebral artery to the foramen of the TP of C6, as the artery passes through the foramina of the TPs of C6 to C2, at the C1 foramen of the TP, and as the vertebral artery perforates the dura mater (George and Laurian, 1987). An intimal tear also may lead to the formation of a thrombus at the site of the tear. The thrombus can extend proximally or distally from the tear, and embolism formation from the thrombus is possible. Alternatively, a local hematoma also may form at the tear site. Such hematoma formation can result in subsequent stenosis or occlusion of the artery. If dissection causes only narrowing, as opposed to complete occlusion, the condition usually either improves or completely resolves. If complete occlusion occurs, the condition will usually not resolve (George and Laurian, 1987). Like most intracranial arteries, the thinner walls of the portion of the vertebral artery distal to its entrance to the dura mater predispose this portion of the vertebral artery to aneurysm formation after dissection.

Difference between the Vertebral Artery and Other Arteries. Intracranial arteries have thinner walls than extracranial arteries of comparable size. More specifically, the media and adventitial layers of intracranial arteries are narrower and have fewer elastic fibers in them. Wilkinson (1972) found that the structure of the vertebral artery changed dramatically just proximal to its point of penetration through the dura mater. Up to this point the structure of the vertebral artery was found to be similar to most extracranial vessels, and distal to this point its structure resembled that of intracranial vessels. More precisely, the adventitia and media of the intracranial portion of the vertebral artery were found to be thinner and had fewer elastic fibrils, and the external elastic lamina "was either absent completely or represented by sparse single elastic fibrils only" (Wilkinson, 1972). The changes were not found to be complete until approximately 5 mm "past the point of dural perforation" (Wilkinson, 1972). The intima and internal elastic lamina were found to be similar in the extracranial and intracranial regions of the vertebral artery. These findings are similar to those reported for the intracranial and extracranial portions of the internal carotid artery (Ratinov, 1964).

Nerves of the Cervical Region

A thorough understanding of patients presenting with neck pain can be achieved only if clinicians know those structures capable of nociception (pain perception). Also, clinicians first must understand how pathologic conditions, aberrant movement, or pressure affecting these structures can result in nociception, and then how the patient perceives that nociception. Knowledge of the innervation of the cervical region gives clinicians an understanding of the structures that are pain sensitive and the way in which this nociceptive information is transmitted to the central nervous system. This topic is significant to clinicians dealing with pain of cervical origin.

Rootlets, Roots, Dorsal Root Ganglia, Spinal Nerves, and Rami. The dorsal and ventral rootlets of the cervical region leave the spinal cord and unite into dorsal and ventral roots (see Chapter 3). The lengths of cervical nerve roots increase from C4 to C8 (Yabuki and Kikuchi, 1996), and the positions of the dorsal root ganglia vary from being proximally to distally located within the IVF. No relationship has been found among the varying positions of the dorsal root ganglia within the cervical IVFs and patients' symptoms (Yabuki and Kikuchi, 1996). The dorsal and ventral roots unite within the region of the IVF to form the spinal nerve (Fig. 5-21). The spinal nerve is short and almost immediately divides into a dorsal ramus (posterior primary division) and a ventral ramus (anterior primary division).

Unique rootlets, roots, and dorsal root ganglia. The posterior rootlets of C1 are unique. They are so thin that frequently they are mistaken for arachnoidal strands during dissection (Edmeads, 1978). Stimulation of the C1 rootlets has been found to cause orbital pain (superior rootlets of C1), frontal pain (middle rootlets), and vertex pain (lower rootlets). Conditions such as tumors of the posterior cranial fossa, herniations of the cerebellar tonsils through the foramen magnum, bony anomalies of the craniovertebral junction, and possibly prolonged muscle tightness can cause irritation of the sensory rootlets or root of C1. Irritation of these rootlets or root may, in turn, refer pain to the regions just mentioned (Edmeads, 1978; Darby and Cramer, 1994).

Great variation exists in the distribution of rootlets in the cervical region. More specifically, anastomoses frequently exist between rootlets of adjacent spinal cord segments. These anastomoses occur 61% of the time in the cervical spinal cord, compared with 7% in the thoracic region and 22% in the lumbar cord (Moriishi et al., 1989; Tanaka et al., 2000). This is clinically significant because sensory impulses conducting nociceptive (pain) sensations through the dorsal root ganglion at one vertebral level may enter the spinal cord at the next spinal cord segment above or below. The pain sensations in such cases may be perceived one segment "off," adding to the body's already difficult task of pain localization (Darby and Cramer, 1994). These anastomoses also complicate the presentation of radicular pain by disrupting the normal dermatomal pattern of innervation by dorsal roots and dorsal root ganglia (see Chapter 11).

Recall that the cell bodies of all afferent nerve fibers are located in the dorsal root ganglia (DRG), which are also known as the spinal ganglia. These ganglia, with the exception of those of the C1 and C2 cord segments, are located within the IVFs. The C1 DRG may be absent; however, when present, it usually is found lying on the posterior arch of the atlas (Williams et al., 1995).

The C2 DRG is located between the posterior arch of the atlas and the lamina of C2; more exactly, it is located posterior and medial to the lateral atlanto-axial joint. It contains the cell bodies of sensory fibers innervating the median atlanto-axial joint, the lateral atlanto-axial joint, and a large part of the neck and scalp, extending from the posterior occipital region to the vertex and occasionally even to the coronal suture of the skull (Bogduk, 1982). Another unique characteristic of the C2 DRG is that it is the only such ganglion normally located outside the dura. The ganglion normally fills 76% of the superior-to-inferior space between the posterior arch of the atlas and the lamina of C2. It is vulnerable to compression in this location. In addition to compression during prolonged extension of the upper cervical region, spondylosis of the lateral atlanto-axial joint may contact the C2 DRG and further increase its vulnerability to compression. The morphologic changes that occur in this ganglion after compression have been shown to be similar to those associated with compressive neuropathy of peripheral nerves (Lu and Ebraheim, 1998). The prominent and predictable location of the C2 DRG also has enabled investigators to study the effects of localized anesthesia on the C2 DRG (Bogduk, 1989a), allowing for a better understanding of the importance of the second cervical nerve in suboccipital headaches.

Dorsal rami. The dorsal rami (posterior primary divisions) generally are smaller than the ventral rami (anterior primary divisions). Recall that each dorsal ramus exits the spinal nerve just lateral to the IVF (see Fig. 5-21). After exiting the IVF, the dorsal ramus curves posteriorly, close to the anterolateral aspect of the articular pillar. In fact, the dorsal rami of C4 and C5 produce a groove on the lateral aspect of the articular pillars of the C4 and C5 vertebrae. On reaching the posterior and lateral aspect of the superior articular process, each dorsal ramus quickly divides into a medial and lateral branch (see Fig. 5-21).

Some of the most important structures innervated by the dorsal rami are the deep back muscles. The deeper and more segmentally oriented transversospinalis muscles receive innervation from the medial branch of the dorsal rami. The longer and more superficial erector spinae muscles are innervated by the lateral branch of the dorsal rami. Other structures innervated by the medial branch include the Z joints and the interspinous ligaments. The lateral branch of the dorsal rami of the upper

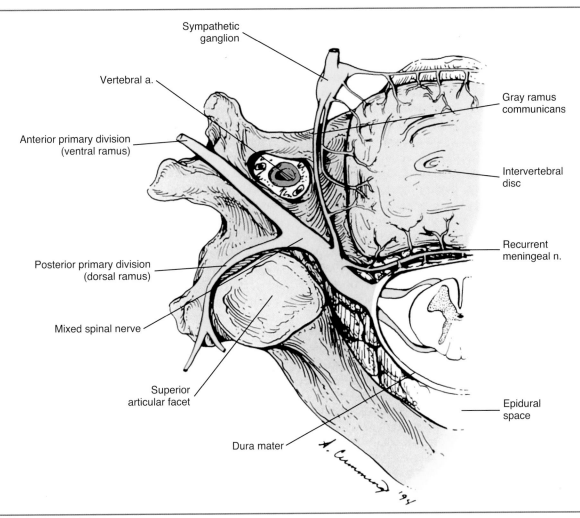

FIG. 5-21   Superior view of a typical cervical segment showing the neural elements. Notice the dorsal and ventral roots, spinal nerve, and posterior and anterior primary divisions (dorsal and ventral rami). The posterior primary division can be seen dividing into a medial and lateral branch. The recurrent meningeal nerve is shown entering the intervertebral foramen. Fibers arising from the middle cervical ganglion and the gray communicating ramus also are shown. Notice that these fibers supply the anterior and lateral aspects of the intervertebral disc, vertebral body, and anterior longitudinal ligament. The sympathetic plexus that surrounds the vertebral artery is shown in Figure 5-22.

cervical nerves (except C1) continue posteriorly, after innervating the erector spinae and splenius capitis and cervicis muscles, to supply sensory innervation to the skin of the neck. The dorsal rami of C6, C7, and C8 usually do not have cutaneous branches (Kasai et al., 1989).

The dorsal ramus of the C1 spinal nerve is unique. The C1 nerve exits the vertebral canal by passing above the posterior arch of the atlas. It quickly divides into a ventral and dorsal ramus. The dorsal ramus (suboccipital nerve) runs between the posterior arch of the atlas and the vertebral artery. It does not divide into a medial and lateral branch, but rather curves superiorly for a short distance (≈1 cm) and terminates by providing motor innervation to the suboccipital muscles. It also sends a communicating branch to the dorsal ramus of C2. Some

authors have described an inconsistent cutaneous branch that runs to the posterolateral scalp (Williams et al., 1995), although other detailed studies have not reproduced this finding (Bogduk, 1982).

The C2 spinal nerve branches into a dorsal and ventral ramus posterior to the lateral atlanto-axial joint. The dorsal ramus loops superiorly around the inferior border of the obliquus capitis inferior muscle and then divides into medial, lateral, superior communicating, inferior communicating, and a branch to the obliquus capitis inferior. The lateral branch of the dorsal ramus of C2 helps to supply motor innervation to the longissimus capitis, splenius capitis, and semispinalis capitis muscles (Bogduk, 1982). The medial branch of the dorsal ramus of C2 is large and is called the greater occipital nerve.

This nerve receives a communicating branch from the third occipital nerve before piercing the large semi-spinalis capitis muscle. The greater occipital nerve always pierces the semispinalis capitis muscle and pierces the trapezius muscle 20% of the time. However, the distance from the midline that this nerve pierces the neck muscles to reach the subcutaneous tissue of the scalp is variable (5 to 28 mm from the midline) (Becser, Bovim, and Sjaastad, 1998). As it pierces the semispinalis muscle, the greater occipital nerve usually is accompanied by the occipital artery. As the nerve reaches the scalp it is sometimes (when the nerve does not pierce the trapezius muscle) thought to be protected from compression during contraction of the trapezius muscle by passing through a protective aponeurotic sling. This sling is associated with the insertions of the trapezius and SCM muscles onto the superior nuchal line (Bogduk, 1982). After passage through the sling, the greater occipital nerve courses superiorly and divides into several terminal branches. These branches provide a broad area of sensory innervation extending from the occipital region medially to the region superior to the mastoid process and posterior to the ear laterally. Superiorly they supply sensory innervation to the scalp from the region of the posterior occiput to as far as the skull's coronal suture (Bogduk, 1982). Terminal branches of the greater occipital nerve also provide sensory branches to the occipital and transverse facial arteries.

Disorders of the upper cervical spine, including irritation of the greater occipital nerve or the C2 ganglion, definitely can cause headaches (Edmeads, 1978; Bogduk et al., 1985, 1986b, 1989a). Causes of irritation to the nerve or ganglion include direct trauma to the posterior occiput and entrapment between traumatized or hypertonic cervical muscles, particularly the semispinalis capitis (Edmeads, 1978). Hyperextension injuries to the neck, especially during rotation, also can compress the C2 ganglion between the posterior arch of the atlas and the lamina of the axis.

The C3 spinal nerve is the most superior nerve to pass through an IVF. Within the lateral aspect of the IVF the C3 nerve branches into a dorsal and ventral ramus. The dorsal ramus of C3 passes posteriorly between the C2 and C3 TPs, where it divides into deep and superficial medial branches, a lateral branch, and a communicating branch with the C2 dorsal ramus (Bogduk, 1982). The superficial medial branch of the dorsal ramus is known as the third occipital nerve. This nerve courses around the lower part of the C2-3 Z joint from anterior to posterior. The deep surface of the third occipital nerve provides articular branches to the C2-3 Z joint (Bogduk and Marsland, 1986). Because of its close relationships with the bony elements of the C2-3 IVF, the third occipital nerve has been implicated by one investigator as the cause of the headaches that frequently accompany

generalized osteoarthritis of the cervical spine (Trevor-Jones, 1964). After supplying the C2-3 Z joint, the third occipital nerve courses superiorly; pierces the semispinalis capitis, splenius capitis, and trapezius muscles; then assists the greater occipital nerve (C2) in its sensory innervation of the suboccipital region (Bogduk, 1982).

The deep medial branch of the C3 dorsal ramus helps to supply the uppermost multifidus muscles. The lateral branch of the C3 dorsal ramus helps to supply the more superior of the fourth through sixth layers of neck muscles (e.g., longissimus capitis, splenius capitis, semispinalis capitis). In addition, the C3 dorsal ramus also helps to supply the C2-3 (via the dorsal ramus itself, the third occipital nerve, or a communicating branch) and the C3-4 (via the deep medial branch) Z joints. The atlanto-occipital joints and the median and lateral atlanto-axial joints are innervated by the C1 and C2 ventral rami, respectively (Bogduk, 1982). Bogduk and Marsland (1986) reported on the relief of occipital and suboccipital headaches by local anesthetic block of the third occipital nerve in 10 consecutive patients with headaches of suspected cervical origin. They suggested that the cause of the headaches was traumatic arthropathy or degenerative joint disease of the C2-3 Z joints and stated that their findings "may reflect an actual high incidence in the community of a condition that has remained unrecognized by specialists dealing with headache, and perhaps misdiagnosed as tension headache." They also mentioned that C1-2 joints may be another cause of cervical headache but thought that further investigation was necessary before differentiation between C1-2 and C2-3 headaches could be performed accurately.

Injury to structures of the upper cervical spine can result in pain referral to the occipital regions innervated by the dorsal rami of the upper three cervical nerves. Upper cervical injury can also refer to regions of the head innervated by the trigeminal nerve, because the central processes of the upper three cervical sensory nerves enter the upper cervical spinal cord and converge on neurons of the spinal tract and spinal nucleus of the trigeminal nerve. This region has been called the trigemino-cervical nucleus (Bogduk et al., 1985). The specific location of pain referral depends on the central neurons stimulated by the incoming cervical fibers. Therefore after injury to the upper cervical region, pain can be interpreted as arising from as far away as the anterior aspect of the head (trigeminal nerve, C2 ventral ramus) or the suboccipital region to the scalp above the vertex of the skull (region innervated by [C1] C2 and C3 dorsal rami).

The spinal nerves of C4 through C8 exit through their respective IVFs (e.g., C4 through the C3-4 IVF, C8 through the C7-T1 IVF). The dorsal rami are quickly given off and pass posteriorly, medial to the posterior intertransversarii muscles, which they supply. They then divide into medial and lateral branches. The medial branches of C4 and C5 (occasionally C6) divide into a superficial and deep branch. The dorsal rami of (C6) C7 and C8 do not divide and only have deep medial branches. The superficial branches help to supply the semispinalis cervicis and capitis muscles and then send cutaneous fibers to provide sensory innervation to the skin of the posterior neck. The deep medial branches of the dorsal rami course to the multifidi muscles, where they provide a specific innervation. Each nerve supplies those muscle fibers that attach to the spinous process of a segmental level numbered one less than the nerve. Therefore the C5 deep medial branch supplies those multifidus fibers that insert onto the C4 spinous process (Bogduk, 1982). The deep medial branches of C4 to C8 also supply the Z joints. Each deep medial branch sends a rostral branch to the Z joint above and a caudal branch to the Z joint below. These branches run along the dorsal aspect of the joints within the pericapsular fibrous tissue (Bogduk, 1982). The lateral branches of the C4 to C8 dorsal rami help to supply the semispinalis capitis, longissimus cervicis, splenius cervicis, and iliocostalis cervicis muscles (C8).

Because many structures of the cervical region that can produce pain receive their sensory supply from dorsal rami, certain diagnostic procedures and therapies for neck and head pain have been directed specifically at these nerves (Bogduk, 1989a,b).

Ventral rami. Each ventral ramus of the cervical region leaves its spinal nerve of origin and then exits the spine by passing posterior to the vertebral artery and then between the anterior and posterior intertransversarii muscles. The cervical ventral rami innervate the anterior muscles of the cervical spine, including the longus capitis, longus colli, and rectus capitis anterior and lateralis muscles. The atlanto-occipital joints and the median and lateral atlanto-axial joints are innervated by the C1 and C2 ventral rami, respectively (Bogduk, 1982).

Bogduk (1981) stated that abnormal position (subluxation) of a lateral atlanto-axial joint, compressing the C2 ventral ramus, is the most likely cause of neck-tongue syndrome. This syndrome includes suboccipital pain with simultaneous numbness of the tongue on the same side. The author explained the tongue numbness by the fact that some proprioceptive fibers to the tongue accompany the hypoglossal nerve and then pass through the ventral ramus of C2. Such "numbness" is analogous to that reported in Bell palsy, in which the proprioceptive fibers of the seventh cranial nerve give the sensation of numbness over a region of the face that receives its sensory innervation from the trigeminal nerve.

The cervical ventral rami also help to supply the vertebral bodies, ALL, and anterior aspect of the IVD with sensory innervation. These latter structures also receive sensory innervation from fibers arising from the sympathetic chain (see Fig. 5-21) and from the autonomic fibers associated with the vertebral artery (Bogduk, Windsor, and Inglis, 1988; Groen, Baljet, and Drukker, 1990). A thorough understanding of the specific sensory innervation to the anterior structures of the spine is important because these structures can be damaged during an extension injury or during the acceleration portion of an acceleration-deceleration injury (Foreman and Croft, 1992). Therefore the autonomic fibers associated with the recurrent meningeal nerve, the sympathetic chain itself, and the vertebral artery are listed in the following discussion.

The ventral rami of cervical spinal nerves also form the cervical and brachial plexuses, which innervate the anterior neck and upper extremities. These neural elements are discussed at the end of this section.

Recurrent Meningeal Nerve. The recurrent meningeal nerves also are known as the sinuvertebral nerves. In the cervical region, each nerve originates from the ventral ramus and then receives a contribution from the gray communicating ramus and other sympathetic nerves that run with the vertebral artery (Groen, Baljet, and Drukker, 1990) (Fig. 5-22; see also Fig. 5-21). The recurrent meningeal nerve then courses medially, through the medial aspect of the IVF and anterior to the spinal dura. This nerve supplies the posterior aspect of the IVD, PLL, anterior spinal dura mater (Williams et al., 1995), posterior vertebral bodies, and uncovertebral joints (Xiuqing, Bo, and Shizhen, 1988). Usually the recurrent meningeal nerve supplies these structures at the level at which it enters the vertebral canal and then continues superiorly to innervate the same structures at the vertebral level above, although the distribution varies (Groen, Baljet, and Drukker, 1990).

More than one recurrent meningeal nerve usually is present at each vertebral level (Groen, Baljet, and Drukker, 1990). The recurrent meningeal nerves of the cervical region probably carry both vasomotor fibers, derived from the sympathetic contribution, and general somatic afferent fibers (including nociceptive fibers), arising from the ventral rami (Bogduk, Windsor, and Inglis, 1988).

The recurrent meningeal nerves of C1, C2, and C3 have relatively large meningeal branches that ascend to the posterior cranial fossa. As they course superiorly to reach the posterior cranial fossa, they supply the atlanto-axial joint complex (also supplied by the ventral ramus of C2), tectorial membrane, components of the cruciform ligament, and alar ligaments (Bogduk, Windsor, and Inglis, 1988). Once in the posterior cranial fossa, they help to supply the cranial dura mater, including that in the region of the clivus, which is supplied by the recurrent meningeal nerve of C3 (Bogduk, Windsor, and Inglis, 1988). These meningeal branches probably are related

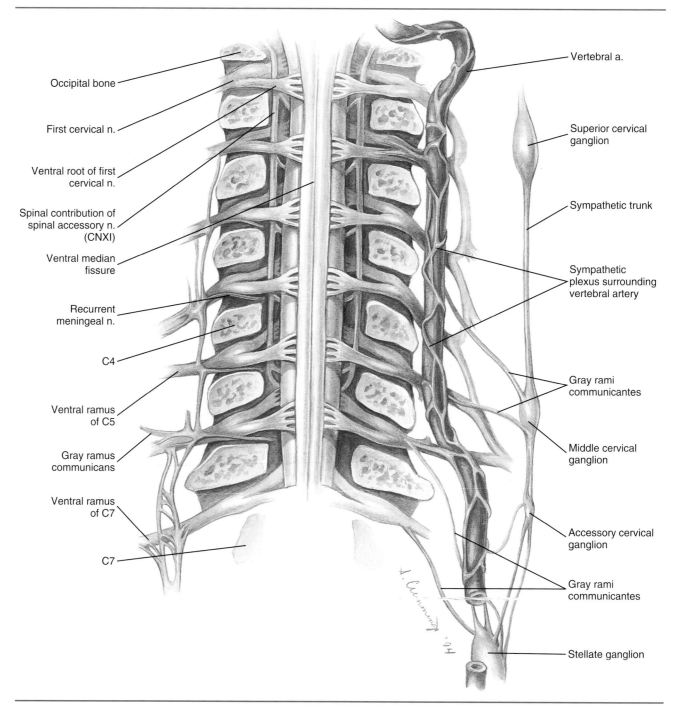

Occipital bone

First cervical n.

Ventral root of first
cervical n.

Spinal contribution of
spinal accessory n.
(CNXI)

Ventral median
fissure

Recurrent
meningeal n.

C4

Ventral ramus
of C5

Gray ramus
communicans

Ventral ramus
of C7

C7

Vertebral a.

Superior cervical
ganglion

Sympathetic trunk

Sympathetic
plexus surrounding
vertebral artery

Gray rami
communicantes

Middle cervical
ganglion

Accessory cervical
ganglion

Gray rami
communicantes

Stellate ganglion

FIG. 5-22   Sympathetic plexus surrounding the vertebral artery. The pedicles have been cut coronally, and the vertebral bodies and transverse processes have been removed to reveal an anterior view of the neural elements. *Right,* One vertebral artery was spared. Notice several branches from the stellate ganglion coursing to this vertebral artery. The largest of these branches is sometime known as the vertebral nerve. Also, notice several gray communicating rami (GR) contributing to the vertebral artery sympathetic plexus. *Left,* Components of this plexus after the vertebral artery has been removed. Notice that the GR branches considerably and sends twigs to join branches of adjacent GR. In addition, the GR sends twigs to ventral rami of the same level, the level above, and the level below. Other twigs of the plexus unite with branches of the ventral rami to form recurrent meningeal nerves. The recurrent meningeal nerves, in turn, course medially to enter the vertebral canal. Branches of the plexus also innervate the vertebral artery itself by passing into the arterial walls (see text for further details). The ventral rami of the spinal nerves can be seen uniting to form the cervical and brachial plexuses on the right side of the illustration. Notice that the vertebral artery is sending a small arterial branch to the C2 spinal nerve. This branch can be seen dividing into anterior and posterior radicular arteries. These branches, which are normally found at each vertebral level, have been removed from the remaining levels to display the neural elements more clearly.

to the pain referral patterns associated with disorders of the upper cervical spine and occipital headache (Williams et al., 1995).

Cervical Sympathetics. This section focuses on those aspects of the sympathetic nervous system most closely related to the general anatomy of the cervical spine. The specific anatomy of the cervical sympathetics is discussed in Chapter 10. The cervical sympathetic chain lies anterior to the longus capitis muscle. The sympathetic trunk takes a slight medial to lateral course (10.4 degrees ± 3.8 degrees) as it ascends the cervical region (Ebraheim et al., 2000). It is composed of three ganglia: superior, middle, and inferior. The superior ganglion is by far the largest, and it is positioned inferior to the occiput and anterior to the TPs of C2 and C3. The middle cervical ganglion is not always present. When it is present, it lies anterior to the TP of C6. Usually the inferior ganglion unites with the first thoracic ganglion to form the cervicothoracic (stellate) ganglion, located just inferior to the TP of C7.

The relationships at the sympathetic plexus surrounding the vertebral artery are complex (see Fig. 5-22). Because of the intimate relationship of this plexus with the vertebral artery and the spinal structures innervated by this plexus, it is discussed here. Chapter 10 also discusses this plexus in the context of the entire autonomic nervous system.

The plexus surrounding the vertebral artery has been called the vertebral nerve (Edmeads, 1978). Other authors (Gayral and Neuwirth, 1954; Xiuqing et al., 1988) state that of the nerves surrounding the vertebral artery, the vertebral nerve is the largest of the several branches that arise from the cervicothoracic (stellate) ganglion to follow the vertebral artery through the foramen of the TP of C6. This discussion uses the term *vertebral nerve* only when discussing the previously mentioned large branch of the stellate ganglion. The term *vertebral plexus* of nerves is used to refer to the neural network surrounding the vertebral artery.

In addition to the branches of the cervicothoracic ganglion that reach the vertebral artery, a branch (or branches) from the middle cervical ganglion and sometimes branches from intermediate ganglia join the vertebral plexus of nerves above the level of C6 (Xiuqing, Bo, and Shizhen, 1988). The branch from the middle cervical ganglion runs laterally to either the C5-6 or C4-5 uncovertebral joint before reaching the vertebral artery. The superior part of the plexus surrounding the vertebral artery is joined by branches directly from the ventral rami of C1 and C2 (Bogduk, Lambert, and Duckworth, 1981) and C3 (Xiuqing, Bo, and Shizhen, 1988). Most of the large nerves accompanying the vertebral artery are gray rami communicantes that follow the artery superiorly to join the ventral rami of C3 to C6 (see Fig. 5-22).

Other branches of the vertebral artery nerve plexus supply sensory innervation to the lateral aspects of the cervical IVDs (Bogduk, Windsor, and Inglis, 1988). A deeper and denser plexus of nerves also surrounds the vertebral artery. This deeper plexus is derived from smaller branches of the vertebral nerve, the stellate ganglion, middle and intermediate cervical ganglia, and cervical ventral rami. These fibers form vascular branches that create a dense neural plexus around the vertebral artery. The vertebral arteries themselves have been found to be capable of producing pain. The afferents for their nociceptive sensation course with the autonomic fibers. Therefore irritation of these fibers by degenerative spur formation of the upper cervical uncovertebral or Z joints may be a cause of headaches (Edmeads, 1978).

Nerves of the Anterior Neck. This section and the sections that follow discuss the neural, muscular, vascular, and visceral structures of the anterior neck. Even though an extensive description of the anatomy of this region is beyond the scope of this text, the mentioned structures are so intimately related to the cervical spine that covering them in adequate detail is important. Also, flexion and extension injuries to the cervical region, commonly known as whiplash injuries, are prevalent (Foreman and Croft, 1992). Such injuries vary considerably in severity and can result in damage to a variety of anatomic structures. Injury to the ALL, PLL, interspinous ligament (ligamentum nuchae), IVDs, vertebral end plates, odontoid process, spinous processes, Z joints, muscles, esophagus, sympathetic trunk, temporomandibular joint, cranium, and brain all have been reported, either through experimental studies or during clinical examination, after flexion and extension injury to the cervical region (Bogduk, 1986a). In addition, proper examination of the cervical region includes an examination of the anterior neck. Therefore the following sections describe the most clinically relevant relationships of the anterior neck, beginning with the nerves.

The nerves of the anterior neck include the ventral rami of the cervical nerves. These ventral rami make up the cervical and brachial (including T1) plexuses (Fig. 5-23). Also, several cranial nerves (CNs) are found in the anterior neck. These include the glossopharyngeal (CN IX), vagus (CN X), accessory (CN XI), and hypoglossal (CN XII) nerves. The cervical and brachial plexuses are discussed in modest detail, and the most relevant points of CNs IX through XII are covered.

Ventral ramus of C1. This ramus passes laterally around the superior articular process of the atlas. It lies anterior to the vertebral artery in this region and runs medial to the artery as the nerve passes medial to the rectus capitis lateralis muscle (which it supplies) to exit

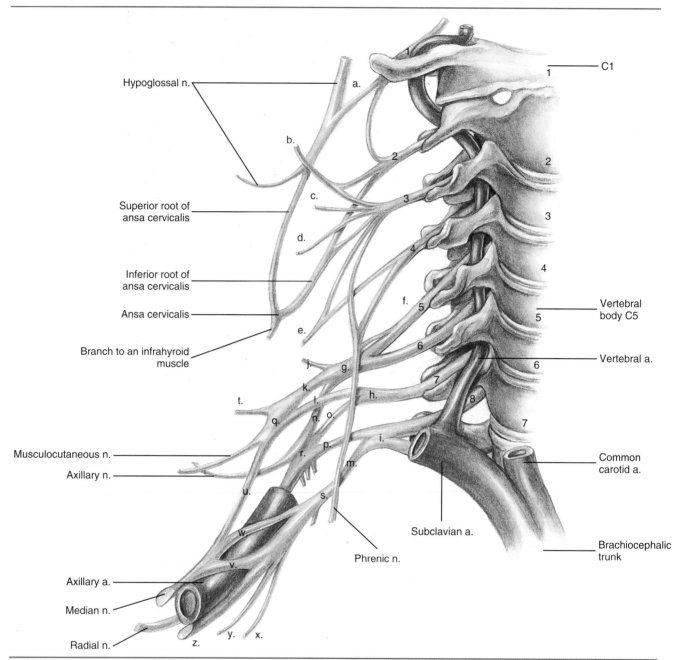

FIG. 5-23   Nerves of the cervical region, including the cervical plexus and the brachial plexus. Notice that the anterior primary divisions (ventral rami) exit posterior to the vertebral artery. The anterior primary divisions of C1 through C4 (with a contribution from C5 to the phrenic nerve) form the cervical plexus, and the anterior primary divisions of C5 through T1 form the roots of the brachial plexus. The following structures are identified: *a,* anterior primary division (ventral ramus) of C1, uniting with the hypoglossal nerve; *b,* lesser occipital nerve; *c,* great auricular nerve (receives contributions from both C2 and C3 ventral rami); *d,* transverse cervical nerve, also known as the transverse cutaneous nerve of the neck (also receives contributions from both C2 and C3 ventral rami); *e,* supraclavicular nerve (common trunk of origin for lateral, intermediate, and medial supraclavicular nerves); *f,* dorsal scapular nerve from C5 ventral ramus would be given off here; *g,* upper trunk of the brachial plexus; *h,* middle trunk; *i,* lower trunk; *j,* suprascapular nerve; *k,* anterior division of upper trunk of the brachial plexus; *l,* anterior division of middle trunk; *m,* anterior division of lower trunk; *n,* posterior division of upper trunk of the brachial plexus; *o,* posterior division of middle trunk; *p,* posterior division of lower trunk; *q,* lateral cord of the brachial plexus; *r,* posterior cord; *s,* medial cord; *t,* lateral pectoral nerve; *u,* contribution of the lateral cord to the median nerve; *v,* contribution of the medial cord to the median nerve; *w,* variant additional contribution of medial cord to the median nerve; *x,* medial brachial cutaneous nerve (medial cutaneous nerve of the arm); *y,* medial antebrachial cutaneous nerve (medial cutaneous nerve of the forearm); *z,* ulnar nerve. The medial pectoral nerve is shown arising from the inferior aspect of, *s,* the medial cord. From proximal to distal, the upper subscapular, thoracodorsal, and lower subscapular nerves are shown arising from, *r,* the posterior cord. The long thoracic nerve, which arises from the ventral rami of C5, C6, and C7, is not shown in this illustration.

above the TP of the atlas. The ventral ramus of C1 receives some fibers from the ventral ramus of C2, and together these fibers join the hypoglossal nerve. Some fibers of the ventral ramus of C1 follow the hypoglossal nerve proximally and help provide sensory innervation to the dura mater of the posterior cranial fossa (Agur, 1991). However, most fibers of the ventral ramus of C1 continue distally along CN XII and then give several branches that leave CN XII. The first such branch participates in the ansa cervicalis and is known as the superior (upper) root of the ansa cervicalis (descendens hypoglossi). The next branch is the nerve to the thyrohyoid, which innervates the thyrohyoid muscle. The nerve to the geniohyoid is the last branch. It innervates the muscle of the same name.

Cervical plexus. The cervical plexus can be divided into a sensory and motor portion. The sensory portion of the cervical plexus is more superficially placed than the motor portion. The named nerves of the sensory portion (see Fig. 5-23) are formed deep to the SCM by the union of individual C2 to C4 ventral rami. The named nerves course around the posterior surface of the SCM and emerge from behind its midpoint in proximity to one another. They then proceed in different directions to reach their respective destinations. The named nerves of the sensory (superficial) part of the cervical plexus and their ventral rami of origin are reviewed in Table 5-9 (see also Fig. 5-23).

The motor portion of the cervical plexus lies deep to the sensory portion and is located within the anterior triangle of the neck. The motor portion makes up the ansa cervicalis (see Fig. 5-23). The two limbs (roots) of the ansa cervicalis are the following:

♦ *C1 ventral ramus (see preceding discussion).* Provides separate motor innervation to the thyrohyoid and geniohyoid muscles and also forms the superior root of the ansa cervicalis (descendens hypoglossi)

♦ *C2 and C3 rami.* Combine to form the inferior root of the ansa cervicalis (descendens cervicalis)

Table 5-9	Sensory Portion of Cervical Plexus	
Nerve	**Cord Segments**	**Destination**
Lesser occipital nerve	C2, C3	Mastoid region and superior aspect of ear
Great auricular nerve	C2, C3	Ear and region overlying angle of mandible
Transverse cervical nerve	C2, C3	Anterior neck
Supraclavicular nerve	C3, C4	Medial, intermediate, and lateral branches to skin over clavicle and deltoid muscle

Together the superior and inferior roots combine to form the ansa cervicalis. Branches of this neural loop provide motor innervation to all of the infrahyoid (strap) muscles (i.e., both bellies of the omohyoid, sternohyoid, and sternothyroid), except the thyrohyoid muscle, which is supplied by the ventral ramus of C1.

The phrenic nerve also is considered to be a part of the cervical plexus. It arises from the ventral rami of C3, C4, and C5, with C4 providing the most significant contribution. The phrenic nerve provides motor and sensory innervation to the diaphragm. Occasionally an accessory phrenic nerve arises from the ventral rami of C5 and C6. When present, the accessory phrenic nerve branches from the nerve to the subclavius and courses to the diaphragm.

Brachial plexus. The brachial plexus (see Fig. 5-23) is formed by the ventral rami of C5 through T1. The ventral rami that participate in forming the brachial plexus are called the "roots" of the brachial plexus. The ventral rami (or roots of the plexus) form trunks, the trunks form anterior and posterior divisions, the divisions form cords, and the cords end as terminal branches. The brachial plexus is discussed in more detail in the following section. Where appropriate, the spinal cord segments that contribute to the formation of the individual named nerves are included in parentheses following the named nerves, for example, radial nerve (C5,6,7,8,T1).

The ventral rami of C5 and C6 form the upper trunk of the brachial plexus. The ventral ramus of C7 remains free of the complex relationships seen in the other rami and forms the middle trunk by itself. The C8 and T1 ventral rami converge to form the lower trunk. A few important branches arise from the ventral rami before they form trunks. The first is the dorsal scapular nerve, which branches from the C5 ramus and provides motor innervation to the rhomboid major and minor muscles and occasionally to the levator scapulae muscle. Branches of the fifth, sixth, and seventh ventral rami form the long thoracic nerve (of Charles Bell), which innervates the serratus anterior muscle.

The suprascapular nerve branches from the upper trunk. (Therefore it is derived from C5 and C6.) It courses through the scapular notch (beneath the superior transverse scapular ligament) to innervate the supraspinatus and infraspinatus muscles. The suprascapular nerve also sends articular twigs to the shoulder joint and the acromioclavicular joint. The nerve to the subclavius muscle (C5,6), which also branches from the upper trunk (C5 and C6), supplies the small muscle of the same name. The nerve to the subclavius usually sends a communicating branch to the phrenic nerve (usually from the C5 contribution).

The trunks divide into anterior and posterior divisions. The anterior divisions of the upper and middle trunks unite to form the lateral cord. The anterior division of the lower trunk remains alone to form the medial cord, and all the posterior divisions unite to form the posterior cord.

The cords of the brachial plexus are named according to their anatomic relationship to the axillary artery (e.g., lateral cord is lateral to the artery). The cords themselves have branches. The lateral cord has a branch called the lateral pectoral nerve (C5,6,7), which innervates both the pectoralis major and minor muscles. The medial cord gives off the medial pectoral nerve (C8,T1), which innervates the pectoralis minor muscle, and a few branches may help to supply the pectoralis major (Williams et al., 1995). The posterior cord gives off the superior or upper (C5,6) and inferior or lower (C5,6) subscapular nerves and the thoracodorsal (middle subscapular) nerve (C6,7,8). The upper subscapular nerve supplies the subscapularis muscle. The thoracodorsal nerve supplies the latissimus dorsi muscle, and the inferior subscapular nerve supplies the teres major muscle and helps to supply the subscapularis muscle.

The cords end as terminal branches of the brachial plexus. The lateral cord divides into the musculocutaneous nerve (C5,6,7) and a large contributing branch to the median nerve (C[5],6,7). The musculocutaneous nerve provides motor innervation to the flexor muscles of the arm and sensory innervation to the lateral forearm. The median nerve is discussed in more detail in the following section.

The medial cord provides the medial brachial (C8,T1) and medial antebrachial (C8,T1) cutaneous nerves (sensory to arm and forearm, respectively) before dividing into the ulnar nerve (C[7],8,T1) and the medial cord contribution to the median (C8,T1) nerve. The ulnar nerve sends articular branches to the elbow and wrist, motor fibers to one and a half muscles of the forearm, and the majority of the intrinsic muscles of the palm. The ulnar nerve is also sensory to the medial distal forearm and medial hand (medial palm, fifth digit, ulnar side of the fourth digit).

Recall that both the lateral and medial cords participate in the formation of the median nerve (C[5],6,7,8,T1). This nerve provides articular branches to the elbow and wrist joints, motor innervation to the majority of the muscles of the anterior forearm, and innervation to five muscles of the palm (three thenar muscles, first two lumbricals). In addition, the median nerve provides sensory innervation to the lateral aspect (radial side) of the palm, the anterior aspect of the first three and a half digits, and the distal aspect of the posterior surface of the first three and a half digits. However, the sensory innervation to the hand is subject to significant variation.

The posterior cord ends by dividing into the axillary (C5,6) and radial nerves (C5,6,7,8,T1). The axillary nerve

courses through the quadrangular space (i.e., space between the teres minor, teres major, long head of the triceps muscles, and surgical neck of the humerus), supplying motor innervation to the teres minor and the deltoid muscles. In addition, the axillary nerve provides sensory innervation to the upper lateral aspect of the arm.

The radial nerve provides motor and sensory innervation to the posterior arm and forearm. It also gives articular branches to the elbow and wrist joints. In addition, the radial nerve provides sensory innervation to the lateral aspect of the dorsum of the hand and the dorsal aspect of the first three and a half digits (except for the distal portions of these digits that are innervated by the median nerve). Chapter 9 provides additional information on the large terminal branches of the brachial plexus.

Vagus nerve. The vagus nerve exits the jugular foramen of the posterior cranial fossa and courses inferiorly throughout the entire length of the neck. Accompanying the vagus nerve in its course through the neck are the internal jugular vein and the internal and common carotid arteries. These structures are wrapped in a fibrous tissue sheath known as the carotid sheath. The vagus nerve is located within the posterior aspect of the carotid sheath between the internal jugular vein, which is lateral to it, and the internal carotid artery, which is medial to it. Inferiorly the vagus nerve lies between the internal jugular vein and the common carotid artery.

The vagus nerve has several branches in the neck:

- *Pharyngeal branch.* This nerve participates in the pharyngeal plexus, which supplies motor and sensory innervation to the pharynx.
- *Superior laryngeal nerve.* This nerve divides into two branches. The first, the internal laryngeal nerve, pierces the thyrohyoid membrane to provide sensory innervation to laryngeal structures above the true vocal folds. The second branch, the external laryngeal nerve, runs inferiorly to innervate the cricothyroid muscle and also helps to supply the inferior constrictor muscle with motor innervation.
- *Nerve to the carotid body.* This nerve supplies sensory innervation to the chemoreceptor of the same name. It also may help to innervate the carotid sinus, the baroreceptor located at the bifurcation of the common carotid artery into the internal and external carotid arteries.
- *Cardiac nerves.* Several cardiac nerves enter the thorax and participate in the cardiac plexus of nerves. The cervical cardiac nerves of the vagus provide parasympathetic innervation to the heart.
- *Recurrent laryngeal nerve.* This nerve loops around the subclavian artery (from anterior to posterior) on the right to run in the groove between the trachea and

the esophagus (tracheo-esophageal groove). It provides motor innervation to all the muscles of vocalization with the exception of the cricothyroid muscle, which is innervated by the external laryngeal nerve. The left recurrent laryngeal nerve wraps around the arch of the aorta (from anterior to posterior) just lateral to the ligamentum arteriosum and continues superiorly in the left tracheo-esophageal groove.

Cranial nerves IX, XI, and XII. As with the vagus nerve, the glossopharyngeal nerve (CN IX) exits the posterior cranial fossa by passing through the jugular foramen. It courses along the posterior pharynx just lateral to the stylopharyngeus muscle, which it supplies. CN IX enters the pharynx together with the stylopharyngeus muscle by passing between the superior and middle constrictor muscles and terminates on the posterior third of the tongue. This branch supplies both general sensation and taste sensation to this region of the tongue. The glossopharyngeal nerve also participates in the pharyngeal plexus of nerves. This plexus supplies both motor and sensory innervation to the pharynx. In addition, CN IX with the vagus nerve supplies sensory fibers to the carotid body and sinus. It also provides the parasympathetic fibers that eventually become the lesser petrosal nerve. This nerve synapses in the otic ganglion, and the postganglionic fibers supply secretomotor fibers to the parotid gland.

The accessory and hypoglossal nerves (CNs XI and XII) are located in the superior neck just behind the posterior belly of the digastric muscle. The accessory (spinal accessory) nerve enters the carotid triangle by coursing behind the posterior belly of the digastric and enters the posterior aspect of the SCM. It innervates this muscle before continuing posteriorly to supply the trapezius muscle.

The hypoglossal nerve (CN XII) enters the neck dorsal to the posterior belly of the digastric, courses anteriorly and slightly inferiorly, and then exits the neck by passing medial to the intermediate tendon of the digastric muscle. It continues deep to the mylohyoid muscle and supplies the intrinsic and extrinsic (except the palatoglossus muscle, supplied by CN X-pharyngeal branch) muscles of the tongue.

Muscles of the Anterior Neck

The muscles of the anterior neck (Fig. 5-24) can conveniently be divided into those below the hyoid bone (*infrahyoid muscles*) and those above the hyoid bone (*suprahyoid muscles*). The salient features of these two groups of muscles are listed in Tables 5-10 and 5-11 for easy reference.

In addition to the infrahyoid and suprahyoid muscles, the SCM and scalene muscles also are associated with

the anterior aspect of the cervical spine and neck (Figs. 5-25 and 5-26). The principal features of the scalene muscles are listed in Table 5-12 and illustrated in Figure 5-26. Because of its importance, the SCM is discussed next.

Sternocleidomastoid Muscle. The SCM, or sternomastoid muscle, is a prominent and important muscle of the cervical region (see Fig. 5-25). Its origin, insertion, innervation, and function are listed in Table 5-10. As shown in the table, when it contracts unilaterally, the SCM laterally flexes the neck to the same side and rotates the face to the opposite side. Occasionally this muscle becomes abnormally tight, holding the neck in the laterally flexed and contralaterally rotated position. This is known as torticollis, or "wry neck." Torticollis is caused by a variety of factors, including prolonged exposure (e.g., a night of sleep) in the presence of a cool breeze, congenital torticollis, neurologic torticollis, and torticollis of unknown causes (idiopathic). The pain arising from neurologic and idiopathic torticollis most likely results from more than nociception arising from the muscles or the Z joints, but probably also has a mechanism involving the central nervous system (Kutvonen, Dastidar, and Nurmikko, 1997).

In addition to its innervation from the accessory nerve (CN XI), the SCM receives some fibers of innervation from the ventral rami of C2-4. These are thought to be primarily proprioceptive, although some authors believe that a small proportion of motor fibers also may be present. The presence of motor fibers from cervical ventral rami explain reports of individuals retaining some SCM function after their CN XI had been severed.

Vascular Structures of the Anterior Neck

Lymphatics of the Head and Neck. Lymphatics of the face and head drain inferiorly into the pericervical lymphatic collar. This collar is made up of a series of connected lymph nodes, which form a chain that encircles the junction of the head and the neck. The collar consists of the following groups of nodes (from posterior to anterior): occipital, postauricular (retroauricular), preauricular, submandibular, and submental. These lymph nodes are drained by lymphatic channels that eventually drain into the deep cervical lymph nodes, located along the internal jugular vein. The deep cervical lymph nodes empty into the thoracic duct on the left side and the right lymphatic duct on the right side.

Major Arteries of the Anterior Neck. The major arteries of the anterior neck (Fig. 5-27) begin in the base (root) of the neck. The root of the neck lies between the neck and thorax. This region is bounded by the first thoracic vertebra, first rib, and manubrium of the

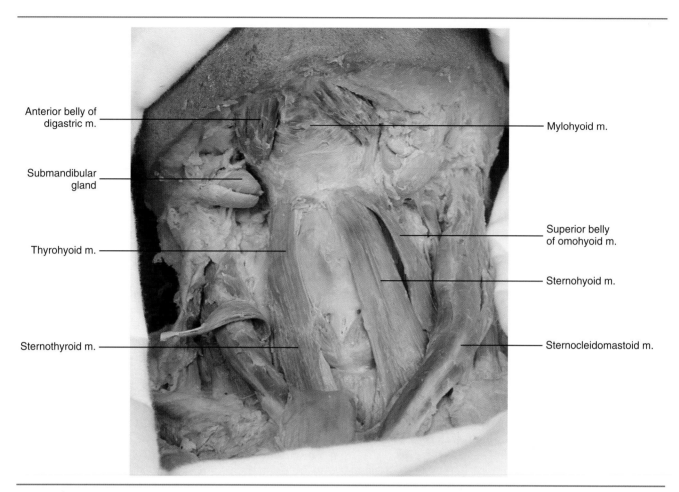

Anterior belly of digastric m.

Submandibular gland

Thyrohyoid m.

Sternothyroid m.

Mylohyoid m.

Superior belly of omohyoid m.

Sternohyoid m.

Sternocleidomastoid m.

FIG. 5-24 Anterior dissection of the neck. The suprahyoid and infrahyoid muscles are shown. The sternohyoid muscle has been removed on the right side of the cadaver to demonstrate the sternothyroid and thyrohyoid muscles more clearly.

Table 5-10 Infrahyoid Muscles and Sternocleidomastoid Muscle

Muscle	Origin	Insertion	Nerve	Function	Notes
Sternocleidomastoid	Manubrium, proximal clavicle	Mastoid process	Accessory (CN XI), ventral rami (C2,3[4])	Bilaterally flex neck, extend head	Unilaterally, laterally flex same side, rotate head to opposite side
Omohyoid	Scapular notch	Hyoid bone	Ansa cervicalis (C1-3)	Depress hyoid bone	Superior and inferior bellies divided by intermediate tendon
Sternohyoid	Posterior manubrium	Hyoid bone	Ansa cervicalis (C1-3)	Depress or stabilize hyoid bone	—
Sternothyroid	Posterior manubrium	Thyroid cartilage	Ansa cervicalis (C1-3)	Depress or stabilize thyroid cartilage	—
Thyrohyoid	Thyroid cartilage	Hyoid bone	C1	Elevate thyroid cartilage, depress hyoid bone	—

Table 5-11   Suprahyoid Muscles

Muscle	Origin	Insertion	Nerve	Function	Notes
Digastric	Mastoid process	Digastric fossa of mandible	Posterior belly, CN VII; anterior belly, CN V3 (nerve to mylohyoid)	Elevate hyoid, move hyoid anteriorly or posteriorly	Anterior and posterior bellies separated by an intermediate tendon
Mylohyoid	Mylohyoid line of mandible	Median raphe, hyoid bone	CN V3 (nerve to mylohyoid)	Elevate hyoid and floor of oral cavity	—
Geniohyoid	Genial spine of mandible	Hyoid bone	Ventral ramus C1	Elevate hyoid bone	—

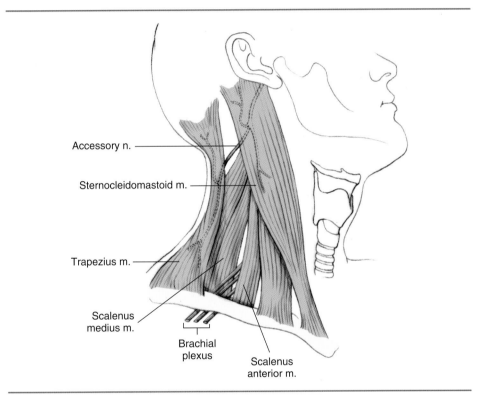

FIG. 5-25   Anterolateral view of the neck demonstrating the sternocleidomastoid muscle. (From Mathers LH. [1996]. *Clinical anatomy principles.* St Louis: Mosby.)

sternum. The principal arteries of this region are the right and left subclavian and the right and left common carotid. The right subclavian and right common carotid arteries are branches of the brachiocephalic trunk from the aortic arch. The left subclavian and left common carotid arteries branch directly from the aortic arch.

Subclavian arteries. The branches of the first part of the subclavian artery (from its origin to the medial border of the anterior scalene muscle) are listed next:

1. *Vertebral artery.* This artery enters the foramen of the TP of C6 and ascends the cervical region through the foramina of the TPs of the remaining five cervical vertebrae. This artery is discussed in detail earlier in this chapter.

2. *Internal thoracic artery.* Also known as the internal mammary artery, this vessel passes inferiorly into the thorax along the posterior aspect of the anterior thoracic wall.

3. *Thyrocervical trunk.* This artery has several branches:

   a. *Inferior thyroid artery.* This branch provides the ascending cervical artery before supplying the inferior aspect of the thyroid gland. The ascending

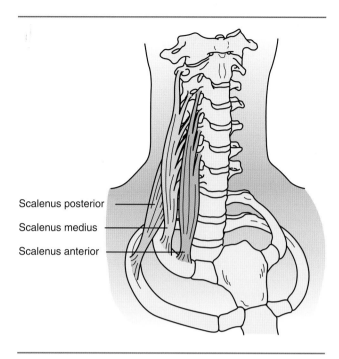

Scalenus posterior

Scalenus medius

Scalenus anterior

FIG. 5-26 Anterior, middle, and posterior scalene muscles. (From Salvo S. [2003]. *Massage therapy principles and practice* [2nd ed.]. Philadelphia: WB Saunders.)

cervical artery helps to supply the neck musculature and the posterior elements of the cervical vertebrae.

   b. *Superficial (transverse) cervical artery.* This artery supplies the superficial and deep back muscles of the cervical and upper thoracic regions.

   c. *Suprascapular artery.* This artery supplies several muscles of the scapula.

The following are branches of the second part of the subclavian artery (between the medial and lateral borders of the anterior scalene muscle).

4. *Costocervical trunk.* This short artery divides into two branches:

   a. *Deep cervical artery.* This branch helps to supply the posterior neck musculature and the posterior arches of the cervical vertebrae.

   b. *Highest intercostal artery.* This branch courses to the first two intercostal spaces.

5. *Dorsal scapular artery.* This is a branch from the third part of the subclavian (between the lateral aspect of the anterior scalene muscle and the first rib) and is only present when there is no deep branch of the superficial (transverse) cervical artery. It supplies the superficial and deep back muscles of the upper thoracic region.

   Carotid arteries. The common carotid artery divides into the internal and external carotid arteries (see Fig. 5-27). Before its bifurcation, the common carotid artery expands to form the carotid sinus, which contains baroreceptors to monitor blood pressure. At the bifurcation of the common carotid artery into its internal and external branches, the carotid body is found. The carotid body is responsible for monitoring oxygen and carbon dioxide concentration in the blood. The carotid sinus and body are innervated by CNs IX and X.

   Each internal carotid artery ascends the neck to enter the cranial cavity via the carotid foramen (canal). The

Table 5-12	Scalene Muscles			
Origin	**Insertion**	**Nerve**	**Function**	**Notes**
Anterior Scalene				
Anterior tubercles of C3-6 TPs	Anterior aspect of first rib (scalene tubercle)	Anterior primary divisions of C4-6	Combination of flexion and lateral flexion of neck, rotate neck to opposite side, elevate first rib	Subclavian vein passes anterior to this muscle
Middle Scalene				
TP of C2 (sometimes C1), posterior tubercles of C3-7 TPs	Anterior aspect of first rib, posterior to insertion of anterior scalene	Anterior primary divisions of C3-8	Combination of flexion and lateral flexion of neck, rotate neck to opposite side, elevate first rib	Largest of scalene muscles; subclavian artery and roots of brachial plexus pass between this muscle and anterior scalene
Posterior Scalene				
Posterior tubercles of C4-6 TPs	Lateral aspect of second rib	Anterior primary divisions of C6-8	Lateral flexion of neck, elevate second rib	Smallest of scalene muscles

TPs, Transverse processes.

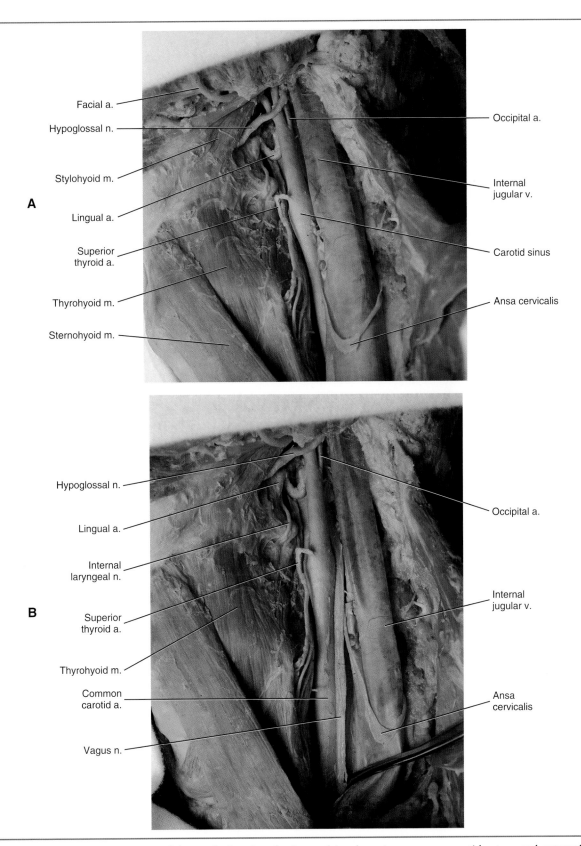

Facial a.

Hypoglossal n.

Stylohyoid m.

A

Lingual a.

Superior
thyroid a.

Thyrohyoid m.

Sternohyoid m.

Occipital a.

Internal
jugular v.

Carotid sinus

Ansa cervicalis

Hypoglossal n.

Lingual a.

Internal
laryngeal n.

B

Superior
thyroid a.

Thyrohyoid m.

Common
carotid a.

Vagus n.

Occipital a.

Internal
jugular v.

Ansa
cervicalis

FIG. 5-27   Anterolateral dissection of the neck showing the internal jugular vein, common carotid artery, and external carotid artery and several of its branches. **B,** The internal jugular vein has been moved laterally to reveal the left vagus nerve, which lies between the internal jugular vein and common carotid artery. Superior to the bifurcation of the common carotid artery, the vagus nerve lies between the internal jugular vein and internal carotid artery. **A** and **B,** The ansa cervicalis can be seen looping across the internal jugular vein.

internal carotid artery then supplies the orbit, pituitary gland, and a large part of the frontal, parietal, and temporal lobes of each cerebral hemisphere.

The external carotid artery is responsible for the blood supply to the neck and face (both the superficial and deep face) (see Fig. 5-27). The branches of the external carotid artery are listed next:

1. *Superior thyroid artery.* This artery courses to the thyroid gland. The superior laryngeal artery branches from the superior thyroid artery. This artery pierces the thyrohyoid membrane with the internal laryngeal nerve and helps supply the larynx.
2. *Ascending pharyngeal artery.* This is a long artery of small diameter that ascends between the internal and external carotid arteries and supplies the pharynx.
3. *Lingual artery.* This is a tortuous artery that runs to the tongue by passing deep to the mylohyoid and hyoglossus muscles.
4. *Facial artery.* This is another tortuous artery that courses to the anterior face; it runs deep to the submandibular gland. (*Note:* Sometimes the lingual and facial arteries arise from a common faciolingual [linguofacial] trunk.)
5. *Occipital artery.* This branch courses to the occiput. It is "held" against the external carotid artery by the hypoglossal nerve (CN XII).
6. *Posterior auricular artery.* This artery runs to and supplies the region posterior to the ear.
   The external carotid artery ends by dividing into the:
7. *Superficial temporal artery.* This large artery courses superiorly to the temporal region and divides into frontal and parietal branches.
8. *Maxillary artery.* This artery supplies the structures within the infratemporal fossa (deep face), nasal cavity, palate, maxilla, and superior aspect of the pharynx.

Major Veins of the Anterior Neck. A large part of the scalp and the superior and lateral face are drained by the external jugular vein. This vein is formed by the union of the posterior auricular vein and the posterior division of the retromandibular vein. The external jugular vein empties into the subclavian vein.

The veins in the central region of the face and the deep structures of the head and neck drain into the internal jugular vein (see Fig. 5-27). This vein is formed at the jugular foramen by the union of the sigmoidal and inferior petrosal dura mater venous sinuses of the cranial cavity.

More specifically, the central region of the face is drained by the facial vein (anterior facial vein). This vein ends by passing in front of the submandibular gland to join the anterior branch of the retromandibular vein (posterior facial vein). The union of these two veins forms the common facial vein. The common facial vein, in turn, empties into the internal jugular vein. The internal jugular vein joins the subclavian vein to form the brachiocephalic vein. The right and left brachiocephalic veins then unite to form the superior vena cava, which empties into the right atrium.

The anterior jugular veins (right and left) drain the anterior neck. They may communicate in the midline low in the neck close to the region between the left and right clavicular heads (the jugular fossa). The anterior jugular vein drains into either the external jugular or the subclavian vein.

Viscera of the Anterior Neck

The pharynx and esophagus lie in the midline and allow for passage of food from the oral cavity through the thorax and eventually to the abdomen. The larynx and trachea lie anterior to the esophagus and function in vocalization and passage of air to and from the lungs.

The thyroid gland lies in contact with the anterolateral aspect of the inferior larynx and superior trachea. This gland has two lobes, a right and a left, which are united in the midline by the isthmus. The isthmus covers the anterior aspect of the second to fourth tracheal rings. The superior and inferior thyroid arteries provide the blood supply to the thyroid gland. Sympathetics (vasomotor) reach the gland via the middle cervical ganglion. Parasympathetics (uncertain function) are supplied by the laryngeal branches of the vagus nerve.

The four small parathyroid glands (two on each side), are located on the posterior aspect of the thyroid gland.

REFERENCES

Agur AM. (1991). *Grant's atlas of anatomy* (9th ed.). Baltimore: Williams & Wilkins.

Alix ME & Bates DK. (1999). A proposed etiology of cervicogenic headache: The neurophysiologic basis and anatomic relationship between dura mater and the rectus posteriorcapitis minor muscle. *JMPT, 22,* 534-539.

Aprill C & Bogduk N. (1992). The prevalence of cervical zygapophyseal joint pain. *Spine, 17,* 744-747.

Aprill C, Dwyer A, & Bogduk N. (1990). Cervical zygapophyseal joint pain patterns II: A clinical evaluation. *Spine, 15,* 458-461.

Bagnall KM, Harris PF, & Jones PRM. (1977). A radiographic study of the human fetal spine. 2. The sequence of development of ossification centres in the vertebral column. *J Anat, 124,* 791-802.

Bailey P & Casamajor L. (1911). Osteo-arthritis of the spine as a cause of compression of the spinal cord and its roots. *J Nerv Ment Dis,* 588-609.

Barnsley L et al. (1995). The prevalence of chronic cervical zygapophysial joint pain after whiplash. *Spine, 20,* 20-26.

Becser N, Bovim G, & Sjaastad O. (1998). Extracranial nerves in the posterior part of the head: Anatomic variations and their possible clinical significance. *Spine, 23,* 1435-1441.

Bednar DA, Parikh J, & Hummel J. (1995). Management of type-2 odontoid process fractures in geriatric patients; a prospective study of sequential cohorts with attention to survivorship. *J Spinal Disord, 8,* 166-169.

Behrsin J & Briggs C. (1988). Ligaments of the lumbar spine: A review. *Surg Radiol Anat, 10,* 211-219.

Bland J. (1987). *Disorders of the cervical spine.* Philadelphia: WB Saunders.

Bland J. (1989). The cervical spine: From anatomy to clinical care. *Med Times, 117,* 15-33.

Bogduk N. (1981). An anatomical basis for the neck-tongue syndrome. *J Neurol Neurosurg Psychiatry, 44,* 202-208.

Bogduk N. (1982). The clinical anatomy of the cervical dorsal rami. *Spine, 7,* 319-330.

Bogduk N. (1986a). The anatomy and pathophysiology of whiplash. *Clin Biomech, 1,* 92-101.

Bogduk N. (1986b). Headaches and the cervical spine (editorial). *Cephalalgia 4,* 7-8.

Bogduk N. (1989a). Local anesthetic blocks of the second cervical ganglion: A technique with application in occipital headache. *Cephalalgia, 1,* 41-50.

Bogduk N. (1989b). The rationale for patterns of neck and back pain. *Patient Management, 13,* 17-28.

Bogduk N. (1997). *Clinical Anatomy of the lumbar spine* (3rd ed.). London: Churchill Livingstone.

Bogduk N et al. (1985). Cervical headache. *Med J Aust, 143,* 202-207.

Bogduk N, Lambert G, & Duckworth J. (1981). The anatomy and physiology of the vertebral nerve in relation to cervical migraine. *Cephalalgia, 1,* 11-24.

Bogduk N & Marsland A. (1986). On the concept of third occipital headache. *J Neurol Neurosurg Psychiatry, 49,* 775-780.

Bogduk N & Marsland A. (1988). The cervical zygapophysial joints as a source of neck pain. *Spine, 13,* 610-617.

Bogduk N, Windsor M, & Inglis A. (1988). The innervation of the cervical intervertebral discs. *Spine, 13,* 2-8.

Boulos AS & Lovely TJ. (1996). Degenerative cervical spondylolisthesis: Diagnosis and management in five cases. *J Spinal Disord, 9,* 241-245.

Boyle JJW, Singer KP, & Milne N. (1996). Morphological survey of the cervicothoracic junctional region. *Spine, 21,* 544-548.

Buna M et al. (1984). Ponticles of the atlas: A review and clinical perspective. *J Manipulative Physiol Ther, 7,* 261-266.

Bush K et al. (1997). The pathomorphologic changes that accompany the resolution of cervical radiculopathy: A prospective study with repeat magnetic resonance imaging. *Spine, 22,* 183-186.

Cave AJE. (1934). On the occipito-atlanto-axial articulations. *J Anat, 68,* 416-423.

Cave AJE, Griffiths JD, & Whiteley MM. (1955). Osteo-arthritis deformans of Luschka joints. *Lancet, 1,* 176-179.

Chaynes P et al. (1998). Microsurgical anatomy of the internal vertebral venous plexuses. *Surg Radiol Anat, 20,* 47-51.

Chiba K et al. (1996). Treatment protocol for fractures of the odontoid process. *J Spinal Disord, 9,* 267-276.

Chistyakov AV et al. (1995). Motor and somatosensory conduction in cervical myelopathy and radiculopathy. *Spine, 20,* 2135-2140.

Christensen HW & Nilsson N. (1998). Natural variation of cervical range of motion: A one-way repeated-measures design. *J Manipulative Physiol Ther, 21,* 383-387.

Côté P et al. (1997). Apophysial joint degeneration, disc degeneration, and sagittal curve of the cervical spine. *Spine, 22,* 859-864.

Cramer G et al. (1996). Identification of the anterior longitudinal ligament on cadaveric spines and comparison with appearance on MRI. *Proceedings of the 1996 International Conference on Spinal Manipulation (ICSM),* 151-152.

Cramer G et al. (1998). Morphometric evaluation of the anterior longitudinal ligament on cadaveric spines by means of magnetic resonance imaging. *J Chiropract Educ, 11,* 141.

Cramer G et al. (2002). The effects of side posture positioning and spinal adjusting on the lumbar Z joints: A randomized controlled trial of 64 subjects. *Spine, 27,* 2459-2466.

Crawford CM, Cassidy JD, & Burns S. (1995). Cervical spondylotic myelopathy: A report of two cases. *Chiropract J Aust, 25,* 101-110.

Croft AC. (1993). Cervical acceleration/deceleration trauma: A reappraisal of physical and biochemical events. *J Neuromusculo Syst, 1,* 45-51.

Cusick J. (1988). Monitoring of cervical spondylotic myelopathy. *Spine, 13,* 877-880.

Czervionke L et al. (1988). Cervical neural foramina: Correlative anatomic and MR imaging study. *Radiology, 169,* 753-759.

Danziger J & Bloch S. (1975). The widened cervical intervertebral foramen. *Radiology, 116,* 671-674.

Darby S & Cramer G. (1994). Chapter 3: Pain generators and pain pathways of the head and neck. In D Curl (Ed.). *Chiropractic approach to head pain.* Baltimore: Williams & Wilkins, 55-73.

Dean NA & Mitchell BS. (2002). Anatomic relation between the nuchal ligament (ligamentum nuchae) and the spinal dura mater in the craniocervical region. *Clin Anat, 15,* 182-185.

Dong Y et al. (2003). Quantitative anatomy of the lateral mass of the atlas.

Spine, 28, 860-863.

Doual JM, Ferri J, & Laude M. (1997). The influence of senescence on cranio-facial and cervical morphology in humans. *Surg Radiol Anat, 19,* 175-183.

Dupuis PR et al. (1985). Radiologic diagnosis of degenerative lumbar spinal instability. *Spine, 10,* 262-276.

Dvorak J & Panjabi M. (1987). Functional anatomy of the alar ligament. *Spine, 12,* 183-189.

Dwyer A, Aprill C, & Bogduk N. (1990). Cervical zygapophyseal joint pain patterns. I. A study in normal volunteers. *Spine, 15,* 453-457.

Ebraheim NA, Biyani A, & Salpietro B. (1996). Zone III fractures of the sacrum: A case report. *Spine, 21,* 2390-2396.

Ebraheim NA et al. (1997a). Cartilage and synovium of the human atlanto-odontoid joint. *Acta Anat, 159,* 48-56.

Ebraheim NA et al. (1997b). Quantitative anatomy of the cervical facet and the posterior projection of its inferior facet. *J Spinal Disord, 10,* 308-316.

Ebraheim NA et al. (1997c). Anatomic considerations for uncovertebral involvement in cervical spondylosis. *Clin Orthop Rel Res, 334,* 200-206.

Ebraheim NA et al. (1998). Anatomic basis if the anterior surgery on the cervical spine: Relationships between uncus-artery-root complex and vertebral artery injury. *Surg Radiol Anat, 20,* 389-392.

Ebraheim N et al. (2000). Vulnerability of the sympathetic trunk during the anterior approach to the lower cervical spine. *Spine, 25,* 1603-1606.

Edmeads J. (1978). Headaches and head pains associated with diseases of the cervical spine. *Med Clin North Am, 62,* 533-544.

Ehara S. (1996). Relationship of elongated anterior tubercle to incomplete segmentation in the cervical spine. *Skeletal Radiol, 25,* 243-245.

Farmer JC & Wisneski RJ. (1994). Cervical spine nerve root compression. *Spine, 19,* 1850-1855.

Fesmire F & Luten R. (1989). The pediatric cervical spine: Development anatomy and clinical aspects. *J Emerg Med, 7,* 133-142.

Fletcher G et al. (1990). Age-related changes in the cervical facet joints: Studies with cryomicrotomy, MR and CT. *AJNR, 11,* 27-30.

Foreman SM & Croft AC. (1992). *Whiplash injuries: The cervical acceleration/deceleration syndrome.* Baltimore: Williams & Wilkins.

Forristall R, Marsh H, & Pay N. (1988). Magnetic resonance imaging and contrast CT of the lumbar spine: Comparison of diagnostic methods of correlation with surgical findings. *Spine, 13,* 1049-1054.

Francke JP et al. (1980). The vertebral arteries: Atlanto-axial and intracranial segments. *Anatom Clin (Surg Radiol Anat), 2,* 229-242.

Frank E. (1995). HLA-DR expression on arachnoid cells. *Spine, 20,* 2093-2096.

Fujiwara K et al. (1988). Morphometry of the cervical spinal cord and its relation to pathology in cases with compression myelopathy. *Spine, 13,* 1212-1216.

Gates D. (1980). *Correlative spinal anatomy.* Lakemont, Ga: CHB Printing and Binding.

Gayral L & Neuwirth E. (1954). Oto-neuro-ophthalmologic manifestations of cervical origin, posterior cervical sympathetic syndrome of Barré-Lieou. *NY State J Med, 54,* 1920-1926.

George B & Laurian C. (1987). *The vertebral artery: Pathology and surgery.* New York: Springer-Verlag, 258.

Giacobetti FB et al. (1997). Vertebral artery occlusion associated with cervical spine trauma. *Spine, 22,* 188-192.

Gluncic V et al. (1999). Anomalous origin of both vertebral arteries. *Clin Anat, 12,* 281-284.

Gottleib MS. (1994). Absence of symmetry in superior articular facets on the first cervical vertebra in humans: Implications for diagnosis and treatment. *J Manipulative Physiol Ther, 17,* 314-320.

Groen G, Baljet B, & Drukker J. (1990). Nerves and nerve plexuses of the human vertebral column. *Am J Anat, 188,* 282-296.

Hack GD et al. (1995a). Anatomic relation between the rectus capitis posterior minor muscle and the dura mater. *Spine, 20,* 2484-2486.

Hack GD et al. (1995b). In response. *Spine, 20,* 925-926.

Hackney DB. (1992). Normal anatomy. *Top Magn Reson Imaging, 4,* 1-6.

Hadley LA. (1957). The covertebral articulations and cervical foramen encroachment. *J Bone Joint Surg, 39-A,* 910-920.

Hasue M et al. (1983). Anatomic study of the interrelation between lumbosacral nerve roots and their surrounding tissues. *Spine, 8,* 50-58.

Haynes MJ et al. (2002). Vertebral arteries and cervical rotation: Modeling and magnetic resonance angiography studies. *J Manipulative Physiol Ther, 25,* 370-382.

Herrera M & Puchades-Ortis A. (1998). Correspondence: Morphology of the articular process of the sixth cervical vertebra in humans. *J Anat, 192,* 309-311.

Ho PS et al. (1988). Ligamentum flavum: Appearance on sagittal and coronal MR images. *Radiology, 168,* 469-472.

Holmes A et al. (1996). Changes in cervical canal spinal volume during in vitro flexion-extension. *Spine, 21,* 1313-1319.

Hukuda S et al. (1996). Large vertebral body, in addition to narrow spinal canal, are risk factors for cervical myelopathy. *J Spinal Disord, 9,* 177-186.

Humphreys BK et al. (2003). Investigation of connective tissue attachments to the cervical spinal dura mater. *Clin Anat, 16,* 152-159.

Humphreys SC et al. (1998). The natural history of the cervical foramen in symptomatic and asymptomatic individuals aged 20–60 years as measured by magnetic resonance imaging. *Spine, 23,* 2180-2184.

Imai S et al. (1997). An ultrastructural study of calcitonin gene-related peptide-immunoreactive nerve fibers innervating the rat posterior longitudinal ligament. *Spine, 22,* 1941-1947.

Ito T et al. (1996). Cervical spondylotic myelopathy. *Spine, 21,* 827-833.

Johnson GM, Zhang M, & Jones G. (2000). The fine connective tissue architecture of the human ligamentum nuchae. *Spine, 25,* 5-9.

Jonsson E. (2000). Back pain, neck pain. *SBU Project Group 2000, Summary & Conclusions, Report 145.*

Jovanovic M. (1990). A comparative study of the foramen transversarium of the sixth and seventh cervical vertebrae. *Surg Radiol Anat, 12,* 167-172.

Kapandji IA. (1974). *The physiology of the joints. Annotated diagrams of the mechanics of the human joints* (2nd ed.). Edinburgh: Churchill Livingstone.

Karaikovic EE et al. (1997). Morphologic characteristics of human cervical pedicles. *Spine, 22,* 493-500.

Kasai T et al. (1989). Cutaneous branches from the dorsal rami of the cervical nerves, with emphasis on their positional relations to the semispinalis cervicis. *Okajimas Folia Anat Jpn, 66,* 153-160.

Kasai T et al. (1996). Growth of the cervical spine with special reference to its lordosis and mobility. *Spine, 21,* 2067-2073.

Kaufman R & Glenn W. (1983). Rheumatoid cervical myelopathy evaluation by computerized tomography with multiplanar reconstruction. *J Rheumatol, 10,* 42-54.

Kawaguchi Y et al. (2003). Pathomechanism of myelopathy and surgical results of laminoplasty in elderly patients with cervical spondylosis. *Spine, 28,* 2209-2214.

Kazan S et al. (2000). Anatomical evaluation of the groove for the vertebral artery in the axis vertebrae for atlanto-axial transarticular screw fixation technique. *Clin Anat, 13,* 237-243.

Kinalski R & Kostro B. (1971). Planimetric measurements of intervertebral foramina in cervical spondylosis. *Polish Med J, 10,* 737-742.

Kissel P & Youmans J. (1992). Post-traumatic anterior cervical osteophyte and dysphagia: Surgical report and literature review. *J Spinal Disord, 5,* 104-107.

Koebke J & Brade H. (1982). Morphological and functional studies on the lateral joints of the first and second cervical vertebrae in man. *Anat Embryol, 161,* 265-275.

Kokubun S, Sakurai M, & Tanaka Y. (1996). Cartilaginous end plate in cervical disc herniation. *Spine, 21,* 190-195.

Kutvonen O, Dastidar P, & Nurmikko T. (1997). Pain in spasmodic torticollis. *Pain, 69,* 279-286.

Lefebvre S et al. (1993). Unstable os odontoideum in young children. *J CCA, 37,* 141-144.

Le Minor J, Kahn E, & Di Paola R. (1989). Osteometry by computer aided image analysis: Application to the human atlas. *Gegenbaurs morphol jahrb (Leipzig), 135,* 865-874.

Licht PB et al. (1999). Vertebral artery flow and cervical manipulation: An experimental study. *J Manipulative Physiol Ther, 22,* 431-435.

Licht P et al. (1998). Triplex ultrasound of vertebral artery flow during cervical rotation. *J Manipulative Physiol Ther, 21,* 27-31.

Liguoro D, Vandermeersch B, & Guerin J. (1994). Dimensions of cervical vertebral bodies according to age and sex. *Surg Radiol Anat, 16,* 149-155.

Lohiya GS. (1993). Os odontoideum: Chronic neck pain after car accident; failure of two posterior atlanto-axial arthrodeses-medicolegal issues in the occupational setting. *J Manipulative Physiol Ther, 16,* 475-480.

Loudon JK, Ruhl M, & Field E. (1997). Ability to reproduce head position after whiplash injury. *Spine, 22,* 865-868.

Louis R. (1985). Spinal stability as defined by the three column spine concept. *Anat Clin, 7,* 33-42.

Lord SM et al. (1996). Chronic cervical zygapophysial joint pain after whiplash. *Spine, 21,* 1737-1745.

Lu J et al. (1999). Anatomic basis for anterior spinal surgery: Surgical anatomy of the cervical vertebral body and disc space. *Surg Radiol Anat, 21,* 235-239.

Lu J & Ebraheim N. (1998). Anatomic considerations of C2 nerve root ganglion. *Spine, 23,* 649-652.

Marcelis S et al. (1993). Cervical spine: Comparison of 45° and 55° antero-posterior oblique radiographic projections. *Radiology, 188,* 253-256.

Matsuda Y et al. (1995). Atlanto-occipital hypermobility in subjects with Down's syndrome. *Spine, 20,* 2283-2286.

Matsunaga S et al. (1996). Effects of strain distribution in the intervertebral discs on the progression of ossification of the posterior longitudinal ligaments. *Spine, 21,* 184-189.

McCormack BM & Weinstein PR. (1996). Cervical spondylosis. *WJM, 165,* 43-51.

McLain RF. (1994). Mechanoreceptor endings in human cervical facet joints. *Spine, 19,* 495-501.

Mendel T et al. (1992). Neural elements in human cervical intervertebral discs. *Spine, 17,* 132-135.

Mercer SR & Bogduk N. (2003). Clinical anatomy of ligamentum nuchae. *Clin Anat, 16,* 484-493.

Meyer SA et al. (1994). Cervical spinal stenosis and stingers in collegiate football players. *Am J Sports Med, 22,* 158-166.

Meyer JS, Yoshida K, & Sakamoto K. (1967). Autonomic control of cerebral blood flow measured by electromagnetic flowmeters. *Neurology, 17,* 638-648.

Milz S et al. (2001). Fibrocartilage in the transverse ligament of the human atlas. *Spine, 26,* 1765-1771.

Miles KA & Finlay D. (1988). Is prevertebral soft tissue swelling a useful sign in injury of the cervical spine? *Injury, 19,* 177-179.

Mitchell BS, Humphreys BK, & O'Sullivan E. (1998). Attachments of the ligamentum nuchae to cervical posterior spinal dura and the lateral part of the occipital bone. *J Manipulative Physiol Ther, 21,* 145-148.

Mitchell JA. (2003). Changes in vertebral artery blood flow following normal rotation of the cervical spine. *J Manipulative Physiol Ther, 26,* 347-351.

Moriishi J et al. (1989). The intersegmental anastomoses between spinal nerve roots. *Anat Rec, 224,* 110-116.

Motegi H et al. (1998). Proliferating cell nuclear antigen in hypertrophied spinal ligaments. *Spine, 23,* 305-310.

Muhle C et al. (2001). In vivo changes in the neuroforaminal size at flexion-extension and axial rotation of the cervical spine in healthy persons examined using kinematic magnetic resonance imaging. *Spine, 26,* e287-e293.

Murphy F, Simmons JC, & Brunson B. (1973). Ruptured cervical discs, 1939–1972. *Clin Neurosurg, 20,* 9-17.

Nagashima C & Iwama K. (1972). Electrical stimulation of the stellate ganglion and the vertebral nerve. *J Neurosurg, 36(6),* 756-762.

Nilsson N, Christensen HW, & Hartvigsen J. (1996). The interexaminer reliability of measuring passive cervical range of motion, revisited. *J Manipulative Physiol Ther, 19,* 302-305.

Oga M et al. (1996). Tortuosity of the vertebral artery in patients with cervical spondylotic myelopathy: Risk factor for the vertebral artery injury during anterior cervical decompression. *Spine, 21,* 1085-1089.

Oliver J & Middleditch A. (1991). *Functional anatomy of the spine.* Oxford, UK: Butterworth Heinemann.

Omura K et al. (1996). Cervical myelopathy caused by calcium pyrophosphate dehydrate crystal deposition in facet joints. *Spine, 21,* 2372-2375.

Onan OA, Heggeness MH, & Hipp JA. (1998). A motion analysis of the cervical facet joint. *Spine, 23,* 430-439.

Orofino C, Sherman MS, & Schecter D. (1960). Luschka's joint: A degenerative phenomenon. *J Bone Joint Surg, 42A,* 853-858.

Pal GP et al. (1988). Trajectory architecture of the trabecular bone between the body and the neural arch in human vertebrae. *Anat Rec, 222,* 418-425.

Panjabi M et al. (1991). Flexion, extension, and lateral bending of the upper cervical spine in response to alar ligament transections. *J Spinal Disord, 4,* 157-167

Panjabi MM et al. (2001a). The cortical shell architecture of human cervical vertebral bodies. *Spine, 26,* 2478-2484.

Panjabi MM et al. (2001b). Mechanical properties of the human cervical spine as shown by three-dimensional load-displacement curves. *Spine, 26,* 2692-2700.

Panjabi M, Oxland T, & Parks E. (1991a). Quantitative anatomy of cervical spine ligaments. Part I. Upper cervical spine. *J Spinal Disord, 4,* 270-276.

Panjabi M, Oxland T, & Parks E. (1991b). Quantitative anatomy of cervical spine ligaments. Part II. Middle and lower cervical spine. *J Spinal Disord, 4,* 277-285.

Pech P et al. (1985). The cervical neural foramina: Correlation on microtomy and CT anatomy. *Radiology, 155,* 143-146.

Peterson C et al. (1999). Prevalence of hyperplastic articular pillars in the cervical spine in relationship with cervical lordosis. *J Manipulative Physiol Ther, 22,* 390-394.

Pettersson K et al. (1997). Disc pathology after whiplash injury. *Spine, 22,* 283-288.

Przybylski GJ et al. (1996). Human anterior and posterior cervical longitudinal ligaments possess similar tensile properties. *J Orthop Res, 14,* 1005-1008.

Przybylski GJ et al. (1998). Quantitative anthropometry of the subatlantal cervical longitudinal ligaments. *Spine, 23,* 893-898.

Ratinov G. (1964). Extradural intracranial portion of the carotid artery. *Arch Neurol, 10,* 66-73.

Renaudin J & Snyder M. (1978). Chip fracture through the superior articular facet with compressive cervical radiculopathy. *J Trauma, 18,* 66-67.

Ross JK, Bereznick DE, & McGill SM. (1999). Atlas-axis facet asymmetry: Implications in manual palpation. *Spine, 24,* 1203.

Schellhas KP et al. (1996). Cervical discogenic pain: Prospective correlation of magnetic resonance imaging and discography in asymptomatic subjects and pain sufferers. *Spine, 21,* 300-311.

Schima W et al. (1993). Case report; cervical intervertebral foramen widening caused by vertebral artery tortuosity. Diagnosis with MR and colour-coded doppler sonography. *Br J Radiol, 66,* 165-167.

Schimmel D, Newton T, & Mani J. (1976). Widening of the cervical intervertebral foramen. *Neuroradiology, 12,* 3-10.

Schmidt HP & Pierson JC. (1934). The intrinsic regulation of the blood vessels of the medulla oblongata. *Am J Physiol, 10,* 241-263.

Senol U et al. (2001). Anteroposterior diameter of the vertebral canal in cervical region: Comparison of anatomical, computed tomographic, and plain film measurements. *Clin Anat, 14,* 15-18.

Shingyouchi Y, Nagahama A, & Niida M. (1996). Ligamentous ossification of the cervical spine in late middle-aged Japanese men. *Spine, 21,* 2474-2478.

Shinomiya K et al. (1995). Isolated muscle atrophy of distal upper extremity in spinal compression disorders. *J Spinal Disord, 7,* 311-316.

Shinomiya K et al. (1996). An analysis of the posterior epidural ligament role on the cervical spinal cord. *Spine, 21,* 2081-2088.

Sunderland S. (1974). Meningeal-neutral relations in the intervertebral foramen. *J Neurosurg, 40,* 756-763.

Sosner J, Fast A, & Kahan BS. (1996). Odontoid fracture and c1-c2 subluxation in psoriatic cervical spondyloarthropathy. *Spine, 21,* 519-521.

Taitz C. (1996). Anatomical observations of the developmental and spondylotic cervical spinal canal in South African blacks and whites. *Clin Anat, 9,* 395-400.

Taitz C. (2000). Bony observations of some morphological variations and anomalies of the craniovertebral region. *Clin Anat, 13,* 354-360.

Taitz C & Arensburg B. (1989). Erosion of the foramen transversarium of the axis. *Acta Anat, 134,* 12-17.

Taitz C & Nathan H. (1986). Some observations on the posterior and lateral bridge of the atlas. *Acta Anat, 127,* 212-217.

Taitz C, Nathan H, & Arensburg B. (1978). Anatomical observations of the foramina transversaria. *J Neurol Neurosurg Psychiatry, 41,* 170-176.

Tanaka N et al. (2000). The anatomic relation among the nerve roots, intervertebral foramina, and intervertebral discs of the cervical spine. *Spine, 25,* 286-291

Taylor JR. (1999). Ligaments and annulus fibrosus of cervical discs. *Spine, 24,* 627-628.

Tondury G. (1943). Zur anatomie der Halswirbelsaule. Gibt es Uncovertebralgelenke? *Z Anat EntwGesch, 112,* 448-459.

Tonetti J et al. (1999). Elastic reinforcement and thickness of the joint capsules of the lower cervical spine. *Surg Radiol Anat, 21,* 35-39.

Torg JS et al. (1986). Neurapraxia of the cervical spinal cord with transient quadriplegia. *J Bone Joint Surg, 68A,* 1354-1370.

Trevor-Jones R. (1964). Osteo-arthritis of the paravertebral joints of the second and third cervical vertebrae as a cause of occipital headaches. *S Afr Med J, May,* 392-394.

Van Dyke D & Gahagan C. (1988). Down's syndrome cervical spine abnormalities and problems. *Clin Pediatr, 27,* 415-418.

Verska JM & Anderson PA. (1997). Os odontoideum. *Spine, 22,* 706-709.

Viikari-Juntara E et al. (1989). Evaluation of cervical disc degeneration with ultralow field MRI and discography: An experimental study on cadavers. *Spine, 14,* 616-619.

Von Lanz T. (1929). Uber die Ruckenmarkshaute. I. Die konstruktive Form der harten Haut des menschlichen Ruckenmarkes und ihrer Bander. *Arch Entwickl Mech Org, 118,* 252-307.

Wang A et al. (1984). Cervical chordoma presenting with intervertebral foramen enlargement mimicking neurofibroma CT findings. *J Comput Assist Tomogr, 8,* 529-532.

Wang P et al. (1999). Ossification of the posterior longitudinal ligament of the spine. *Spine, 24,* 142-144.

Weiglein AH & Schmidberger HR. (1998). The radio-anatomic importance of the colliculus atlantis. *Surg Radiol Anat, 20,* 209-214.

Wiegand R et al. (2003). Cervical spine geometry correlated to cervical degenerative disease in a symptomatic group. *J Man Physiol Ther, 26,* 341-346.

White AW & Panjabi MM. (1990). *Clinical biomechanics of the spine.* Philadelphia: JB Lippincott.

Wight S, Osborne N, & Breen AC. (1999). Incidents of ponticulus posterior of the atlas in migraine and cervicogenic headache. *J Manipulative Physiol Ther, 22,* 15-20.

Wilkinson IMS. (1972). The vertebral artery. *Arch Neurol, 27,* 392-396.

Williams PL et al. (1995). *Gray's anatomy* (38th ed.). Edinburgh: Churchill Livingstone.

Xiuqing C, Bo S, & Shizhen Z. (1988). Nerves accompanying the vertebral artery and their clinical relevance. *Spine, 13,* 1360-1364.

Xu R et al. (1995). Morphology of the second cervical vertebra and the posterior projection of the C2 pedicle axis. *Spine, 20,* 259-263.

Yabuki S & Kikuchi S. (1996). Positions of dorsal root ganglia in the cervical spine. *Spine, 21,* 1513-1517.

Yamada H et al. (1998). Direct innervation of sensory fibers from the dorsal root ganglion of the cervical dura mater of rats. *Spine, 23,* 1524-1530.

Yamada K et al. (2003). High serum levels of menatetrenone in male patients with ossification of the posterior longitudinal ligament. *Spine, 28,* 1789-1793.

Yenerich DO & Haughton VM. (1986). Oblique plane MR imaging of the cervical spine. *J Comput Assist Tomogr, 5,* 823-826.

Yi-Kai L et al. (1999). Changes and implications of blood flow velocity of the vertebral artery during rotation and extension of the head. *J Manipulative Physiol Ther, 22,* 91-95.

Yilmazlar S et al. (2003a). Clinical importance of ligamentous and osseous structures in the cervical uncovertebral foraminal region. *Clin Anat, 16,* 404-410.

Yilmazlar S et al. (2003b). Details of fibroligamentous structures in the cervical unco-vertebral region: An obscure corner. *Surg Radiol Anat, 25,* 50-53.

Yoo JU et al. (1992). Effect of cervical spine motion on the neuroforaminal dimensions of the human cervical spine. *Spine, 17,* 1131-1136.

Yu S, Sether L, & Haughton VM. (1987). Facet joint menisci of the cervical spine: Correlative MR imaging and cryomicrotomy study. *Radiology, 164,* 79-82.

Zumpano MP, Jagos CS, & Hartwell-Ford S. A cadaveric survey exploring the variation, prevalence, sex bias, and tissue type of the soft tissue bridge between rectus capitis posterior minor and the posterior atlanto-occipital membrane. *J Neuromusculoskeletal Syst, 10,* 133-140.

CHAPTER 6

The Thoracic Region

Gregory D. Cramer

The thoracic region contains the most vertebrae (12) of any of the movable regions of the spine. Consequently it is the longest region of the spine. However, because of its relationship with the ribs, which attach anteriorly to the sternum, the thoracic region has relatively little movement. Many of the unique characteristics of the thoracic region result from its anatomic relationships with the ribs. The typical thoracic vertebrae are T2 through T8. T1, T9 (occasionally), T10, T11, and T12 perhaps can best be described as unique rather than "atypical." The size of the thoracic vertebrae generally increases from the superior to the inferior vertebrae, just as the load they are required to carry increases from superior to inferior.

This chapter first discusses the typical thoracic curve, vertebrae, ribs, and sternum. This is followed by a discussion of the thoracic vertebrae that have unique features (T1, T9 to T12). Next, ligaments with distinctive features in the thoracic region are covered. Many ligaments are described with the cervical region in Chapter 5 and are not covered again here. This chapter also includes a brief discussion of lateral curves that may develop in the thoracic region (scoliosis). The last section is devoted to nerves, vessels, and visceral structures associated with the thoracic vertebrae and the thoracic cage.

THORACIC CURVE (KYPHOSIS)

As stated in Chapter 2, the normal thoracic curve is a rather prominent kyphosis, which extends from T2 to T12. It is created by the larger superior-to-inferior dimensions of the posterior portion of the thoracic vertebrae.

Prolonged changes in the forces received by the thoracic region can result in postural changes and pain. For example, carrying book bags on one shoulder has been found to adversely affect posture and gait (Pascoe et al., 1997).

Occasionally the thoracic kyphosis is almost completely absent. This is logically called the straight back syndrome. This syndrome is associated with systolic heart murmurs and a distorted cardiac silhouette on x-ray film; as a result it can simulate organic heart disease. The straightening of the thoracic kyphosis results in a narrowing of the anterior-to-posterior dimension of the thoracic cage, which decreases the space available for the heart. The heart is forced to shift to the left, which leads to kinking of the great vessels. This results in a variety of heart murmurs. The straight back syndrome also has been associated with idiopathic mitral valve prolapse, a potentially life-threatening condition (Spapen et al., 1990).

Scheuermann's Disease

Another clinical condition that can affect the thoracic kyphosis is Scheuermann's disease. This disease is found in 0.4% to 8.3% of adolescents; its cause is unknown. The condition has two forms based almost entirely on the location of the disease, classical Scheuermann's disease (affecting the thoracic region and seen in two thirds of cases), and Scheuermann's disease of the lumbar region (one third of cases). Both types usually occur during adolescence. Scheuermann's disease is characterized by disruption of the cartilaginous end plate and fragmentation of the anular apophyses and the adjacent bone of the vertebral bodies (bony end plate) of many adjacent vertebral segments. The vertebral bodies become wedge-shaped (shorter anteriorly than posteriorly) if the disease is left untreated. This results in an increase in the thoracic kyphosis, or in the case of the lumbar form of the disease, a continuation of the thoracic kyphosis into the upper lumbar region. As a result, the condition is the most common cause of a pathologic increase in the kyphosis of adolescents. Scheuermann's disease affects males and females with equal frequency (Lemire et al., 1996).

Scheuermann's disease usually is thought to begin at 10 to 12 years of age; however, no radiologic changes usually are seen at this stage. The individual typically seeks treatment at 12 to 15 years of age because of aching back pain, an increase in thoracic kyphosis, or both. Irregularity and fragmentation of the bony end plates usually can be seen on x-rays at this time. The apex of the curve is at T8 in two thirds of the cases. The apex is usually in the upper lumbar region in the remainder of cases (lumbar type). Progression of the condition is slow in the beginning, increases as skeletal maturity of the spine occurs, and ends when vertebral growth is complete (up to 25 years of age). Multiple Schmorl's nodes (end plate fractures) are another hallmark of the con-

dition. Schmorl's nodes typically are found in approximately 36% of all spines, but in up to 93% of spines with an increase in kyphosis resulting from Scheuermann's disease. In addition, the intervertebral disc spaces usually narrow, especially in the segments affected by Schmorl's nodes (Lemire et al., 1996).

In the classical form of Scheuermann's disease, the affected individual may develop a stooped and round-shouldered appearance, with the general posture appearing to be poor. Not all patients have pain; in those who do, the pain is frequently aching rather than constant and incapacitating. The pain almost always disappears as skeletal maturity is reached. The increased kyphosis that develops usually is rigid or fixed rather than flexible in nature (Lemire et al., 1996).

The severity of the condition typically is tracked by measuring the kyphosis and the vertebral wedging of affected vertebrae. The kyphosis is measured by drawing lines anteriorly from the bony end plates at the superior and inferior boundaries of the kyphosis and then measuring the angle between these lines. The normal average is approximately 25 degrees (range, 10 to 40 degrees). A kyphosis greater than 45 degrees is indicative of Scheuermann's disease. Vertebral wedging is measured by drawing a line anteriorly from the bony end plates of an individual vertebra. One or more vertebrae with wedging of greater than 5 degrees also is indicative of Scheuermann's disease (Lemire et al., 1996).

Complications can occur in Scheuermann's disease. The spinal cord may become compressed against the posterior surfaces of the vertebral bodies forming the peak of the kyphosis, leading to signs and symptoms of myelopathy (signs of a bilateral upper motor neuron lesion). In addition, in rare instances the condition may progress to form a significant deforming kyphosis (Lemire et al., 1996).

Treatment for Scheuermann's disease includes bracing the spine in extension and palliative treatment for pain and discomfort. Exercise also has been found to be beneficial. Most patients respond well to such treatment (Lemire et al., 1996).

TYPICAL THORACIC VERTEBRAE, RIBS, AND STERNUM

Typical Thoracic Vertebrae

Vertebral Bodies. The vertebral bodies of the typical thoracic vertebrae (T2 to T8) are larger than those of the cervical region (Fig. 6-1). They appear to be heart shaped when viewed from above, and their antero-posterior dimensions are roughly equal to their lateral dimensions. Dupuis et al. (1985) report that the posterior edge of the superior surface of upper thoracic vertebral bodies exhibit small remnants of the cervical uncinate

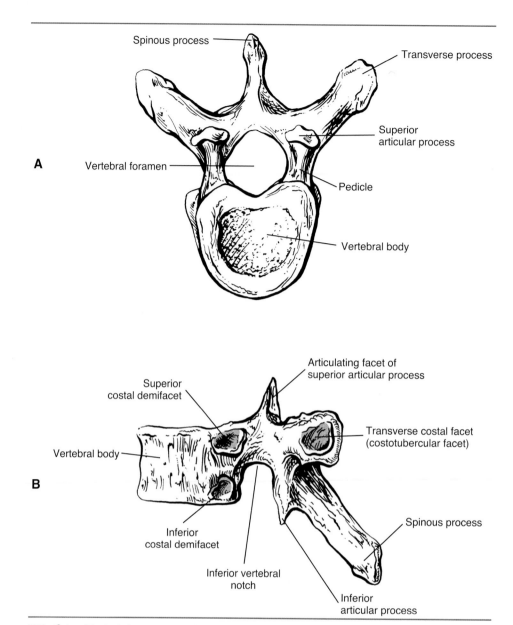

A

Spinous process
Transverse process
Superior articular process
Vertebral foramen
Pedicle
Vertebral body

B

Articulating facet of superior articular process
Superior costal demifacet
Transverse costal facet (costotubercular facet)
Vertebral body
Inferior costal demifacet
Spinous process
Inferior vertebral notch
Inferior articular process

FIG. 6-1 Typical thoracic vertebra. **A,** Superior view. **B,** Lateral view.

processes. The posterior aspect of a typical thoracic vertebra is approximately five times the height of the posterior aspect of the intervertebral disc immediately above the vertebra (Harrison et al., 2003).

The T2 vertebral body is somewhat cervical in appearance, being slightly larger in transverse than anteroposterior diameter. The body of the T3 vertebra is the smallest of the thoracic region; the vertebral bodies gradually increase in size below this level. The vertebral bodies of T5 through T8 become more and more heart shaped. This means that the concavity of the posterior aspect of the vertebral bodies becomes more prominent. The heart-shaped appearance also is accentuated

because the anteroposterior dimension of the vertebral bodies increases, whereas the transverse dimension remains approximately the same. Typical thoracic vertebrae also are more flattened on their left than right surfaces because of pressure from the thoracic aorta. The T9 through T12 vertebral bodies begin to acquire lumbar characteristics (see the following discussion) and enlarge more in their transverse than anteroposterior dimension. The T12 vertebral body is similar in shape to that of a lumbar vertebra. Experimental studies have shown that the vertebral bodies of the thoracic vertebrae become stronger from upper to lower thoracic vertebrae. This results from an increase in bone density that is

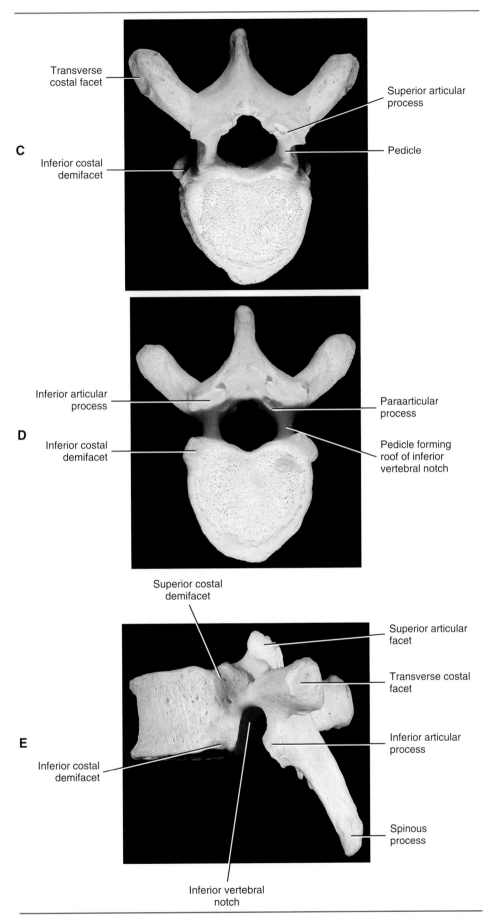

FIG. 6-1—cont'd   Photograph of a typical thoracic vertebrae. **C,** Superior view. **D,** Inferior view. **E,** Lateral view.

probably a response to the increase in compressive forces placed on the successively lower vertebral bodies (Humzah and Soames, 1988).

The neurocentral synchondrosis (see Chapter 12), found between the neural arches and centra of developing vertebrae, fuses first in the lumbar and cervical regions and last in the thoracic region. This fusion may be incomplete in the thoracic region, even in adults (Edelson and Nathan, 1988).

Osteophytes are more prominent at T9-10 than other thoracic levels. Generally, the aorta decreases the formation of osteophytes (bone spurs) on the thoracic vertebral bodies. Recall that the thoracic aorta courses along the left side of the thoracic vertebral bodies. It then begins to move to the anterior surface of the lower thoracic vertebrae, before passing through the aortic hiatus of the diaphragm. Consequently, osteophytes are found more on the right than left sides of the typical thoracic vertebral bodies (Edelson and Nathan, 1988).

Typical thoracic vertebral bodies have four small facets, two on each side, for articulation with the heads of two adjacent ribs. These facets are known as costal demifacets (literally, "half-facets") because the head of each rib articulates with both the superior demifacet of the vertebra with the same number and the inferior demifacet of the vertebra above (see Fig. 6-8). For example, the head of the sixth rib articulates with the superior demifacet of T6 and the inferior demifacet of T5. A ridge on the head of each rib, known as the crest of the head, is located between the two articular surfaces of the rib head. The crest of the head of each rib has a ligamentous attachment (intraarticular ligament) to the intervertebral disc (IVD) between adjacent thoracic vertebrae. A fibrous capsule surrounds each vertebral demifacet and continues to the rib surrounding the articular surface on the corresponding half of the rib head. The capsule is lined by synovium, making the costovertebral joint (costocorporeal joint) a synovial joint (diarthrosis). The radiate ligament extends from the head of each rib to the adjoining vertebral bodies and the surface of the intervening IVD (see Costocorporeal Articulations). Several structures attach to the thoracic vertebral bodies. Table 6-1 summarizes these attachments.

Pedicles. The pedicles of the thoracic spine are long and stout (Fig. 6-1). The size of the thoracic pedicles varies considerably from individual to individual and vertebra to vertebra, but the left and right pedicles of the same vertebra usually are similar (McLain, Ferrara, and Kabins, 2002). Unlike the pedicles of the cervical vertebrae, cancellous bone, rather than cortical bone, predominates in the thoracic pedicles. However, like the cervical pedicles, the cortical bone of the lateral wall of a typical thoracic pedicle is thinner than that of the medial wall (Kothe et al., 1996).

Table 6-1	Attachments to Thoracic Vertebral Bodies	
Region	**Structure(s) Attached**
Anterior surface	Anterior longitudinal ligament, origin of longus colli muscle (T1, T2, T3, lateral to anterior longitudinal ligament)
Posterior surface	Posterior longitudinal ligament
Lateral surface	Origin of psoas major and minor muscles from T12

The thoracic pedicles become larger along their inferior surface from T1 to T12. Also, unlike the cervical pedicles, which attach at a significant lateral angle with the cervical vertebral bodies, the thoracic pedicles form only a slight lateral angle in the transverse plane with the thoracic vertebral bodies (and T12 forms no angle with the vertebral body in this plane). The thoracic pedicles incline slightly superiorly in the sagittal plane (Marchesi et al., 1988). They also attach very high on their respective vertebral bodies; as a result, no superior vertebral notch is associated with typical thoracic vertebrae. T1, which is atypical, does have a superior vertebrae notch (see First Thoracic Vertebra later in this chapter). On the other hand, the inferior vertebral notches of the typical thoracic vertebrae are very prominent.

Transverse Processes. The transverse processes (TPs) of typical thoracic vertebrae project obliquely posteriorly (see Chapter 2) (Fig. 6-1). They also lie in a more posterior plane than those of the cervical or lumbar regions, being located behind the pedicles, intervertebral foramina, and articular processes of the thoracic vertebrae (Williams et al., 1995). The TPs also become progressively shorter from T1 to T12; therefore the distance between the tips of the left and right TPs is the greatest at T1 and then decreases incrementally until T12, where the TPs are very small. This distance increases in the lumbar region (see Chapter 7).

Each thoracic TP possesses a facet for articulation with the articular tubercle of the corresponding rib (e.g., the TP of T6 articulates with the sixth rib). This facet is appropriately named the transverse costal facet, or costal facet of the transverse process, and is located on the anterior surface of the TP.

The first six transverse costal facets are concave and not only face *anteriorly* but also slightly *laterally*. The transverse costal facets inferior to T6 are more planar (flatter) in shape and face *anteriorly, laterally,* and *superiorly*. The forces applied to the ribs during movements, load carrying, or muscular contraction are transmitted through the TPs to the laminae of the thoracic vertebrae (Pal et al., 1988).

The TPs serve as attachment sites for many muscles and ligaments. Table 6-2 lists the most important attachments to the TPs of thoracic vertebrae.

Articular Processes. The superior articular processes of the thoracic spine are small superior projections of bone oriented in a plane that lies approximately 60 degrees to the horizontal plane (White and Panjabi, 1990). This makes them much more vertically oriented than the cervical superior articular processes. The thoracic superior articular processes face posteriorly, slightly superiorly, and laterally (see Fig. 6-1). The inferior articular processes and their facets face anteriorly, slightly inferiorly, and medially.

The capsules of the thoracic zygapophysial (Z) joints are similar to those of the cervical and lumbar regions. Z joint synovial folds have been found to protrude into all thoracic Z joints (Ley, 1974). However, there are fewer mechanoreceptors in the Z joint capsules of the thoracic region than in the cervical or lumbar regions (McLain and Pickar, 1998). However, further investigation is needed to quantify the number of mechanoreceptors in the costocorporeal and costotransverse articulations related to the thoracic vertebrae.

The orientation of the thoracic articular processes and their articulating facets allows a significant amount of rotation to occur in this region (see Ranges of Motion in the Thoracic Spine). Flexion and extension are limited primarily by the orientation of the thoracic facets (Oda et al., 1996), and lateral flexion is limited partly by the orientation of the facets. However, the firm attachments of the thoracic vertebrae to the relatively immobile thoracic cage, by means of the costocorporeal and costo-

Table 6-2	Attachments to Thoracic Transverse Processes
Region	**Structure(s) Attached**
Anterior surface	Costotransverse ligament (medial to transverse costal facet)
Apex	Lateral costotransverse ligament
Posterior apex	Levator costarum muscle
Inferior surface	Superior costotransverse ligament
Superior border	Intertransversarius muscle (or remnant) Intertransverse ligament
Inferior border	Intertransversarius muscle (or remnant) Intertransverse ligament
Posterior surface	Deep back muscles (longissimus thoracis, semispinalis thoracis and cervicis, multifidus thoracis, rotatores thoracis longus and brevis)

From Williams PL et al. (1995). *Gray's anatomy* (38th ed.). Edinburgh: Churchill Livingstone.

transverse articulations, are the primary constraints to axial rotation and lateral flexion of the thoracic spine.

Laminae. The laminae in the thoracic region are short from medial to lateral, broad from superior to inferior, and thick from anterior to posterior. They completely protect the vertebral canal from behind. Therefore no space exists between the laminae of adjacent vertebrae in a dried preparation. This is unique to thoracic vertebrae. The rotators longus and brevis muscles partially insert on the laminae of the thoracic vertebrae.

Paraarticular processes. Paraarticular processes are spurlike calcifications on the anterior and inferior aspect of the laminae of thoracic vertebrae (Figs. 6-1, *D*, and 6-6, *B*). They also have been called "laminar spurs" or "spicules," and represent spur formations of the lateral-most attachment sites of the ligamentum flavum (LF) (Nathan, 1959). They are rarely found in the lumbar region, and they are almost never found in the cervical region. However, paraarticular processes are thought to be normal findings on thoracic vertebrae and are distinct from the condition known as ossification of the LF. Paraarticular processes have a relatively wide base and then taper to a dull point or blunt end inferiorly. They usually are paired and the left and right processes generally are of similar size, although they can be found unilaterally and also can be asymmetric in size. They are found throughout the thoracic region of the vertebral column, and their frequency increases as one descends the thoracic region from T1 to T10; the latter is the vertebra where they are most commonly found. The processes are also found at T11 and T12, but less frequently than at T10. Paraarticular processes occur with increasing frequency from 16 to 30 years of age, when they reach the maximum incidence; the incidence remains roughly the same throughout all succeeding age groups. The presence of paraarticular processes in younger age groups distinguishes them from osteophytes. The processes are thought to reinforce the attachment of the LF, adding strength to the attachment site. Nathan (1959) felt that their presence reflected increased strains placed on the LF as a result of the kyphotic architecture of the thoracic region.

More specifically, paraarticular processes attach to the lamina at the junction between the pedicle and inferior articular process and extend obliquely inferiorly and slightly anteriorly, forming a notch that opens inferiorly. The superior tip of the superior articular process of the vertebra below fits into this notch. Occasionally a bone spur extending from the *superior articular process* ascends and almost comes in contact with the paraarticular process. This latter process is a calcification of the *inferior* attachment of the LF. Other similar but smaller superior projections are found occasionally where the LF attaches along the superior margin of the laminae (Nathan, 1959).

The paraarticular processes vary in size from 1 to 15 mm in length, and the width of their attachment to the laminae ranges from 1 to 10 mm. They are found in 74.7% of spines, and are more common in whites than blacks or native Africans (whites, 82.1%; blacks, 63.8%; native Africans: Bantus, 62%; East Africans, 65%) (Nathan, 1959).

Occasionally paraarticular processes become quite large. These large processes could compress the exiting spinal nerve. However, a more likely scenario is that large paraarticular processes would predispose the exiting nerve to compression from either posterior osteophytes projecting from the vertebral body, or possibly from IVD protrusion (Nathan, 1959).

Vertebral Canal. The vertebral canal in the thoracic region is more rounded in shape than any other region (Fig. 6-1, *A, C,* and *D*). It is also smaller in the thoracic region than either the cervical or lumbar regions. The thoracic spinal cord also is smaller than the other regions of the spinal cord.

Spinous Processes. The spinous processes of thoracic vertebrae generally are large (Fig. 6-1, *B* and *E*). The upper four thoracic spinous processes project almost directly posteriorly. The next four (T5 through T8) project dramatically inferiorly. The spinous process of T8 is the longest of this group. The last four thoracic spinous processes begin to acquire the characteristics of lumbar spinous processes by projecting more directly posteriorly and being larger in their superior-to-inferior dimension (see Unique Thoracic Vertebrae). The spinous processes of thoracic vertebrae serve as attachment sites for many muscles and ligaments. Because of the length of the thoracic region, attachments vary somewhat from the upper to lower thoracic vertebrae. Table 6-3 lists the attachments to the spinous processes of the upper and lower thoracic spinous processes.

Intervertebral Foramina. The intervertebral foramina (IVFs) are covered in detail in Chapter 2. The IVFs in the thoracic region differ from those of the cervical region by facing directly laterally rather than obliquely anterolaterally. The lateral orientation of the thoracic IVFs is similar to that found in the lumbar region.

Unique to the thoracic region is that the T1 through T10 IVFs are associated with the ribs. The eleventh and twelfth ribs are not directly associated with IVFs. More precisely, the following structures are associated with the T1 through T10 IVFs: the head of the closest rib (e.g., T5-6 IVF associated with head of sixth rib), the articulation between the rib head and the demifacets of the vertebral bodies, including the associated ligamentous

Table 6-3	Attachments to Thoracic Spinous Processes
Region	**Structure(s) Attached**
Upper thoracic region	Ligaments: supraspinous, interspinous Muscles: trapezius, rhomboid major and minor, serratus posterior superior, deep back muscles (erector spinae and transversospinalis)
Lower thoracic region	Ligaments: supraspinous, interspinous Muscles: trapezius, latissimus dorsi, serratus posterior inferior, deep back muscles (erector spinae and transversospinalis)

From Williams PL et al. (1995). *Gray's anatomy* (38th ed.). Edinburgh: Churchill Livingstone.

and capsular attachments with the vertebral bodies and the interposed IVD (see Costocorporeal Articulations). All these structures help to form the anterior and inferior boundaries of the first 10 thoracic IVFs. Pathologic conditions of these articulations may compromise the contents of the thoracic IVFs (Williams et al., 1995). For example, osteoarthritis (development of osteophytes) of the costocorporeal articulations may cause stenosis of the thoracic intervertebral foramina (Bailey and Casamajor, 1911).

Approximately one twelfth of the IVF contains spinal nerve in the thoracic region, whereas approximately one fifth of the IVF contains spinal nerve in the cervical region, and approximately one third of the IVF is filled with spinal nerve in the lumbar region. This may be one reason why radiculopathy as a result of IVD protrusion is much less common in the thoracic region than the lumbar or cervical areas. Thoracic disc protrusion is also less common than cervical or lumbar disc protrusion. One reason may be that the thoracic spine is rendered less movable than the cervical and lumbar regions. This is because the thoracic region is strongly supported by the ribs and sternum. The reduced motion may result in a reduction of stress on the thoracic IVDs.

Thoracic Cage

Discussing the bony elements of the thoracic cage here is appropriate because they are so intimately involved with the thoracic vertebrae. However, because the primary focus of this book is the spine, the ribs and sternum are not discussed in as much detail as the vertebrae. The intercostal muscles of the thoracic wall are covered in Chapter 4.

Components of the Thoracic Cage. The components of the thoracic cage (Fig. 6-2) include the following:

◆ Anteriorly: sternum, costal cartilages
◆ Laterally: ribs
◆ Posteriorly: T1 through T12

Superior Thoracic Aperture (Thoracic Inlet). The thoracic cage is bounded superiorly by the superior thoracic aperture and inferiorly by the inferior thoracic aperture. The superior thoracic aperture is bounded by the following: T1, first ribs (left and right), and superior aspect of the sternum. The superior thoracic aperture allows anatomic structures of the thorax and the neck to connect.

The term *thoracic inlet* has a slightly different meaning. It refers to the superior thoracic aperture, the region just above the first rib, and the opening between the clavicle and the first rib. Ironically the term *thoracic outlet syndrome* is frequently used to describe symptoms and signs arising from compromise of the neural or vascular structures as they pass through the region of the thoracic *inlet*. The symptoms associated with this syndrome typically are felt in the distal aspect of the upper extremity rather than the area of neurovascular

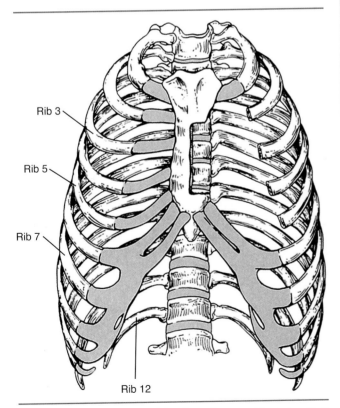

FIG. 6-2   Anterior view of the thoracic cage. A "window" has been removed (left side of thorax) to show to better advantage the relationship between the ribs and vertebrae.

compromise (Bland, 1987). The occurrence of thoracic outlet syndrome remains a matter of clinical debate, with some authorities stating that true compression of these structures is extremely rare. Others are convinced that such compression is relatively common. This section discusses the areas and structures typically associated with the thoracic outlet syndrome.

The right and left subclavian arteries and veins pass through the superior thoracic aperture. These vessels may be compromised by pathologic conditions of the lower cervical or upper thoracic viscera. Examples include lymphosarcoma affecting the lymphatics of the thoracic inlet (Moore, 1992) and tumors of the apex of the lung (Pancoast tumor), esophagus, and thyroid gland.

As the subclavian arteries and veins exit the superior thoracic aperture, they are met by the inferior structures of the brachial plexus. These neural structures include the anterior primary divisions of C8 and T1 and their union as the inferior trunk of the brachial plexus. All these vascular and neural structures pass over the first rib. The subclavian artery and inferior trunk of the brachial plexus course directly across the first rib between the insertions of the anterior and middle scalene muscles. The subclavian vein passes over the first rib in front of the anterior scalene muscle. The inferior trunk of the brachial plexus and subclavian artery are thought to be vulnerable in this region. Anomalous insertion of the scalenes or an anomalous inferior trunk of the brachial plexus that pierces either the anterior or middle scalene muscles may provide the means by which these structures can become entrapped. Extension of the neck and rotation to the same side closes the interval between the anterior and middle scalene muscles, providing another possible mechanism of compromise. An elongated TP of C7 or a cervical rib (see Chapter 5) can dramatically crowd this region, and many believe that either one is a significant contributor to "thoracic outlet syndrome" (Bland, 1987; Foreman and Crofts, 1988). Cervical ribs range considerably in size, and even the smallest cervical rib can be associated with fibrous bands that course from the cervical rib to the first rib or sternum. Any or all of these structures could restrict the subclavian vessels and inferior trunk of the brachial plexus.

The subclavian artery becomes the axillary artery at the lateral border of the first rib. Surrounding the transition region of the subclavian artery to the axillary artery are the divisions of the brachial plexus, which soon combine into the cords of the plexus. The divisions and cords accompany the axillary artery beneath the clavicle and can be compressed between the clavicle and the first rib.

The axillary artery is surrounded by the cords of the brachial plexus as the artery passes beneath the coracoid process of the scapula. The axillary vein accompanies the artery in this region. The pectoralis minor muscle passes anterior to these structures as it inserts onto the coracoid process. The axillary artery, axillary vein, and the cords of the brachial plexus may be compressed against the coracoid process and the tendon of the pectoralis minor muscle during abduction and lateral rotation of the arm.

New Terminology for Thoracic Outlet Syndrome.
Thoracic outlet syndrome is characterized generally by numbness, paresthesias, pain, or a combination of these symptoms along the posterior aspect of the shoulder, axilla, and arm regions with or without vascular compression. However, there is much confusion related to the terminology surrounding thoracic outlet syndrome. Because of this confusion, Ranney (1996) has suggested a completely different nomenclature for the condition. Figure 6-3 illustrates the anatomic structures involved and the regions used in Ranney's (1996) nomenclature.

Ranney (1996) first suggests that the term *thoracic outlet syndrome* be replaced with the term *cervicoaxillary syndrome*. Subdivisions of this syndrome would be named based on the specific anatomic region associated with the pathologic compression of neural or vascular tissues. Second, he suggests that the terms

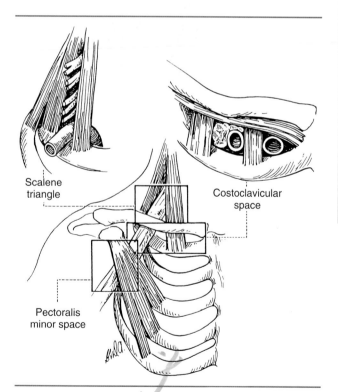

FIG. 6-3 Regions involved in cervicoaxillary syndrome. (From Berger AC & Kleiner JM. [1991]. Work related vascular injuries and diseases. In ML Kasden (Ed.). *Occupational hand and upper extremity injuries and diseases.* Philadelphia: Hunley & Belfus.)

superior thoracic aperture and *inferior thoracic aperture* should be used instead of the clinically confusing terms thoracic inlet (for the superior thoracic aperture) and thoracic outlet (for the inferior thoracic aperture). Next, he proposes that the appropriate term *scalene triangle* be used for the space bordered by the anterior scalene muscle anteriorly, the middle scalene muscle posteriorly, and the first rib inferiorly. He then suggests that the superior aspect of this triangle, housing the C5, C6, and usually the C7 cervical nerve roots, be called the *cervical outlet*. (Compression of these structures in this region sometimes is called scalenus syndrome or scalenus anterior syndrome.) The term *thoracic outlet* would be reserved for the inferior aspect of the scalene triangle for the region that normally houses the C8 and T1 nerve roots and the subclavian artery. The subclavian artery or vein or the divisions or cords of the brachial plexus can be compressed in the more distal *costoclavicular space.* This space is bounded by the clavicle superiorly and first rib inferiorly. Finally, the *pectoralis minor space* is the region bounded superiorly by the pectoralis minor muscle and coracoid process to which it inserts, as well as the thoracic cage inferiorly. The term *hyperabduction syndrome* has been used to identify compression of the axillary artery and the cords of the brachial plexus against the pectoralis minor tendon during prolonged abduction of the upper extremity. With these terms and definitions in mind, Ranney (1996) suggests that the term *cervicoaxillary syndrome* (CAS) be used for compression of neural or vascular structures anywhere along the thoracic outlet, costoclavicular space, or pectoralis minor triangle, and that the more specific subtypes of CAS to include thoracic outlet, costoclavicular, and pectoralis minor syndromes be used once the precise location of compression is identified. The term *cervical outlet syndrome* would be used to describe compression of the C5, C6, or C7 nerve roots in the upper portion of the scalene triangle and the terms *scalene syndrome* and *scalenus anticus syndrome* would be discarded.

Subclavius Posticus Muscle.
An anomalous muscle, known as the subclavius posticus muscle (also known as the chondroscapular muscle or the scapulocostalis minor muscle of Gruber) can be associated with CAS. When present, the muscle usually originates along the superior border of the scapula and the transverse scapular ligament and passes anteriorly, inferiorly, and medially to insert into the costal cartilage of the first rib. Because of its innervation from branches of the brachial plexus (e.g., the suprascapular nerve), the muscle is thought to be related to the subclavius muscle. Anatomic dissections have found the upper and middle trunks of the brachial plexus (see Fig. 5-20), as well as the subclavian artery (Forcada et al., 2001) and subclavian vein

(Akita et al., 2000), to show signs of compression by this muscle, suggesting that the muscle could cause some cases of a variant of the costoclavicular syndrome of CAS (using Ranney's terminology) and also Paget-von Schrötter syndrome (Akita et al., 2000; Forcada et al., 2001). The latter syndrome is thrombosis of the axillary vein, or its proximal continuation as the subclavian vein, that can either develop spontaneously or can be related to strenuous activity involving the upper extremity. The anomalous subclavius posticus muscle is common, being found unilaterally or bilaterally in 8.9% of cadavers (Akita et al., 2000). This anomaly should be visible on magnetic resonance imaging (MRI) (Collins et al., 1995; Akita et al., 2000).

Inferior Thoracic Aperture. The inferior thoracic aperture (thoracic outlet) is bounded by the following: T12, twelfth ribs, anterior costal margins, and xiphisternal joint. The inferior thoracic aperture contains the diaphragm, which serves as the boundary between the thorax and abdomen.

General Characteristics of the Thoracic Cage. The thoracic cage functions to protect underlying structures, support underlying structures (e.g., pericardium via sternopericardial ligaments), support overlying muscles and skin, and assist in respiration.

The adult thorax is wider from side to side than front to back. The anteroposterior diameter increases during inspiration. This is quite different than a child's thorax, which is circular in shape and therefore does not allow change to occur during inspiration. In contrast to adults, children rely almost completely on the excursions of the diaphragm for respiration.

Ribs

Certain groups of cells throughout the spine, known as the costal elements, have the ability to develop into ribs (see Chapters 2 and 12 and Fig. 12-13) and do so in the thoracic region. These thoracic costal elements push through the ventral myotomal plates, which form the intercostal muscles. The costal elements further develop to become precartilaginous ribs, which, after undergoing chondrification and then ossification, become the ribs themselves. The TPs of the thoracic vertebrae grow behind the proximal ends of the developing ribs and are united to them by mesenchyme. This mesenchyme forms the articulations and ligaments of the costocorporeal and costotransverse joints. The fully developed ribs serve to protect the underlying thoracic viscera while providing attachment sites for a wide variety of muscles (Table 6-4).

Typical Ribs. The typical ribs are ribs three through nine. Each consists of a head, neck, tubercle, and shaft (Fig. 6-4).

Table 6-4 Relationships of the Thoracic Cage

Region	Structure(s) Attached
Superiorly	Sternocleidomastoid, sternohyoid, sternothyroid, and anterior, middle, and posterior scalene muscles
Anteriorly	Pectoralis major and minor muscles, mammary glands
Posteriorly	Serratus posterior superior and inferior, and deep back muscles; trapezius, rhomboid minor and major, scapula and all muscles related to it rest against the thoracic cage
Laterally	Serratus anterior muscles
Inferiorly	Abdominal muscles attaching to thoracic cage (e.g., rectus abdominis, external and internal abdominal oblique, transversus abdominis)

The head of a typical rib articulates with two adjacent vertebral bodies (see Vertebral Bodies). Inferior and superior articular facets of the rib head articulate with the superior costal demifacet of the same-number vertebra as the rib and with the inferior costal demifacet of the vertebra above, respectively. The crest of the head is a ridge that runs between the two articular surfaces of the rib head. The crest is joined by the intraarticular ligament to the adjacent IVD. This creates the two separate components of the costocorporeal joints, one superior to the crest of the head of the rib, and one inferior to the crest (see Costocorporeal Articulations and Fig. 6-8).

The neck of a typical rib is located between its head and tubercle. The neck serves as the attachment site for the costotransverse ligament and superior costotransverse ligament.

The tubercle of a rib is a process that forms the lateral boundary of the neck and the beginning of the shaft. It possesses an articular facet (articular portion) for articulation with the transverse costal facet on the TP of a typical thoracic vertebra. The tubercle of a rib articulates with the same-number vertebra as the rib (e.g., fourth rib articulates with TP of T4). The tubercle also contains a nonarticular part lateral to the articular portion. The nonarticular region serves as an attachment site for the lateral costotransverse ligament.

The shaft of a rib begins at the articular tubercle and extends distally to the end of the rib at its articulation with the costal cartilage. The typical ribs curve inferiorly and anteriorly. Much of this anterior curve is achieved at the angle of the rib. The angle of the rib is located a few centimeters distal to the articular tubercle and is where the shaft makes the sharpest anterior bend.

A costal depression or groove, located along the inferior aspect of each rib, shelters (from superior to inferior) the intercostal vein, artery, and nerve.

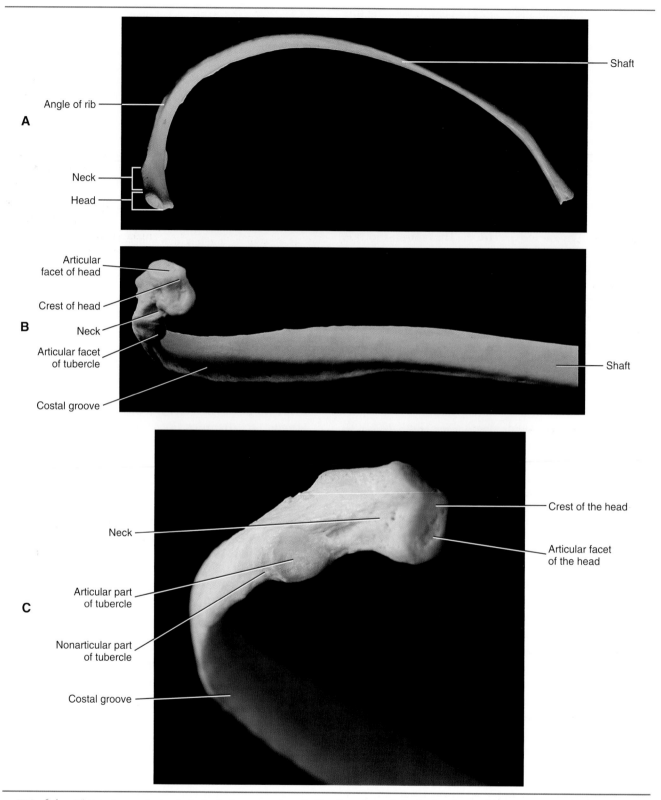

FIG. 6-4   Three views of a typical rib. **A,** Superior view. **B,** Head, angle, and shaft of a rib. **C,** Close-up of the head and neck.

Anteriorly each typical rib attaches to a costal cartilage. The costal cartilage, in turn, joins each of the first through seventh ribs with the sternum. The eighth through tenth costal cartilages articulate with the costal cartilage immediately above. The xiphoid process, seventh costal cartilage, and union of the eighth through tenth costal cartilages together form the substernal angle.

Atypical Ribs. The first, second, tenth, eleventh, and twelfth ribs all have special features (Williams et al., 1995). The first rib is short, flat, and strong. It lies almost completely in the horizontal plane and does not angle inferiorly as do typical ribs. Its superior surface is marked by a scalene tubercle (for insertion of the anterior scalene muscle). The subclavian vein passes anterior to the scalene tubercle (and the anterior scalene muscle), and the subclavian artery and inferior trunk of the brachial plexus course posterior to this tubercle. The first rib usually articulates with only one vertebra (T1). Occasionally the head also articulates with the body of C7.

The second rib is much more typical than the first and is almost twice its size. The major distinguishing characteristic of the second rib is a tuberosity on its superior surface, which serves as the partial origin of the serratus anterior muscle.

The tenth rib has only a single facet, and no crest, on its head. The head articulates with the large, single costal facet on the lateral aspect of the body (close to the pedicle) of T10. Sometimes the head of the tenth rib also articulates with the IVD between T9 and T10.

The eleventh and twelfth ribs are short, and neither possesses a neck or tubercle. They are considered free, or floating, ribs because they do not attach to costal cartilage anteriorly. As with the first and tenth ribs, the eleventh and twelfth each articulate with only one vertebra (T11 and T12, respectively).

Sternum

The sternum develops from left and right bars of mesenchyme that migrate to the midline and eventually fuse. The fully developed sternum is composed of a manubrium, body, and xiphoid process. The superior aspect of the manubrium is at the level of the T2-3 IVD. The manubrium possesses a superior concavity known as the jugular notch (see Fig. 6-2). Lateral to the jugular notch is the clavicular notch, which projects superolaterally, allowing its concavity to articulate with the clavicle. The apex of the lung extends above the sternoclavicular joint and the clavicle. The lung is vulnerable here and may be punctured from the anterior in this region. The articulation with the first costal cartilage is inferior to the clavicular notch, on the lateral aspect of the manubrium (see Fig. 6-2).

The inferior margin of the manubrium joins the body of the sternum. The manubriosternal joint is usually a symphysis, although occasionally it may develop a joint cavity, giving it characteristics of a synovial joint. The sternal angle (of Lewis) is formed by the angle between the manubrium and body of the sternum at the manubriosternal symphysis (see Fig. 6-2). This angle makes the sternum slightly convex anteriorly. The second costal cartilage articulates with the sternum at this angle. The sternal angle is located on a horizontal plane that posteriorly passes roughly through the level of the T4-5 IVD. (This level varies from the vertebral bodies of T4 to T6; see Chapter 1.) Other anatomic structures are present at the general level of this plane. These include the bifurcation of the trachea into primary (main stem) bronchi, the hilus of the lung, and the superior extent of the aortic arch.

The body of the sternum is formed by the union of four segments known as sternebrae. The lateral margin is notched for articulation with costal cartilages of ribs. The inferior process of the sternum is the xiphoid process. It is joined with the body of the sternum by a symphysis that usually ossifies by 40 years of age. The xiphoid process also articulates with the costal cartilage of the seventh rib.

The thoracic cage serves as an attachment site for a variety of structures. See Table 6-4 for structures associated with various regions of the thoracic cage.

UNIQUE THORACIC VERTEBRAE

Several thoracic vertebrae have distinct characteristics: T1, T9 (occasionally), T10, T11, and T12. They can best be considered as unique, not atypical, thoracic vertebrae.

First Thoracic Vertebra

T1 possesses two characteristics associated with cervical vertebrae but not normally found on typical thoracic vertebrae: uncinate processes and superior vertebral notches above the pedicles (Fig. 6-5). In addition, the vertebral body of T1 resembles that of a cervical vertebra, being rectangular in shape instead of heart shaped, with the transverse diameter greater than the anteroposterior diameter.

Sixteen percent of T1 vertebrae have asymmetry of greater than 10 degrees of the plane of articulation of the left and right articular processes and their facets (Boyle, Singer, and Milne, 1996).

The superior facet on the vertebral body for articulation with the head of the first rib is usually a full facet (not a demifacet). Occasionally the superior facet is a demifacet, allowing the first rib to attach to both T1 and C7 vertebral bodies and the intervening IVD. Frequently a deep depression can be found on the vertebral body of

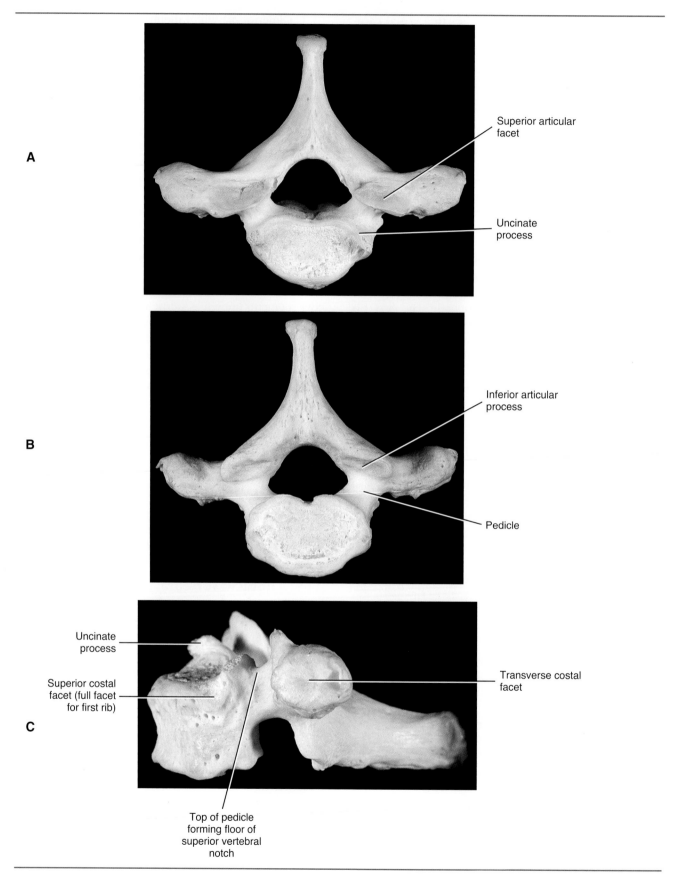

FIG. 6-5   First thoracic vertebra. **A,** Superior view. **B,** Inferior view. **C,** Lateral view.

T1 just inferior to the superior costal facet (Williams et al., 1995). The inferior demifacet of T1 is typical. The spinous process of T1 is large, projects directly posteriorly, and is often as long, and sometimes longer, than the spinous process of C7.

Ninth Thoracic Vertebra

When the tenth rib does not articulate with the T9 vertebral body, the result is the absence of the inferior demifacet on T9. The other characteristics of T9 conform to those of typical thoracic vertebrae.

Tenth Thoracic Vertebra

The vertebral body of T10 contains only a single facet on each side for articulation with the head of the left and right tenth ribs (Fig. 6-6). As stated, typical thoracic vertebrae possess two demifacets on each side for articulation with the rib of the same number and with the rib below. The single facet on T10 is usually oval or semilunar in shape. The precise shape depends on whether the tenth rib articulates with just the body of T10 or also with the body of T9 and the IVD between the two. The former results in an oval-shaped facet, and the latter results in a semilunar-shaped facet. The TP of T10 does not always have a facet for articulation with the articular tubercle of the tenth rib.

Eleventh Thoracic Vertebra

T11 also has only a single facet on each side for articulation with the head of the eleventh rib (see Fig. 6-6). However, this facet is located on the pedicle. There is also no articular facet on the TP for articulation with the articular tubercle of the rib. Therefore the eleventh rib does not articulate with the TP of T11. The vertebral body of T11 also resembles that of a lumbar vertebra. The spinous process of T11 is almost triangular in shape with a blunt apex (Williams et al., 1995).

The superior articular processes of T11 resemble those of other thoracic vertebrae. However, usually T11 represents the transition of thoracic-type articular processes to the lumbar type. Therefore the inferior articular processes usually are convex and face anteriorly and laterally. The articular processes of thoracic vertebrae allow for rotation to be the primary movement, whereas the lumbar articular processes limit rotation but encourage flexion and some extension. This transition of facet type also can occur at T12 or occasionally T10.

Asymmetry of the plane of articulation of the T11-12 articular processes and their articular facets is related to increased degenerative changes on the side of the articular process that is more closely oriented to the sagittal plane (Boyle, Singer, and Milne, 1996). The same has been found to be true at the L5-S1 articulation (Giles, 1987).

Twelfth Thoracic Vertebra

The vertebral body of T12 is large, but the TPs are small (see Fig. 6-6). In fact, each TP is actually replaced by three smaller processes (Williams et al., 1995). One process projects laterally and is the equivalent of a thoracic TP except that it is small. The largest of the three processes projects posteriorly and superiorly and is the homologue of the mamillary process of a lumbar vertebra. However, this mamillary process is not as closely related to the superior articular process as it is in the lumbar region. Finally, a small process that is homologous to the accessory process of lumbar vertebrae projects posteriorly and slightly inferiorly. T12 also has a single facet on each side for articulation with the head of the corresponding twelfth rib. The facet is circular and is located primarily on the pedicle but may extend onto the vertebral body. The small TP has no facet for articulation with the twelfth rib.

Thoracolumbar Junction

The left and right Z joints between the T12 and L1 vertebrae are unique. At this joint the L1 mamillary process (see Chapter 7) of each side overlaps the posterior aspect of the inferior articular process of T12. This usually occurs to a greater degree between these two vertebrae than at any other level. The result is that each inferior articular process of T12 fits closely into the superior articular process and overlying mamillary process of L1, much like a well-made carpenter's joint (e.g., mortise and tenon joint). This prevents almost any movement except flexion from occurring at this articulation (Singer and Giles, 1990; Singer, Giles, and Day, 1990). Singer, Giles, and Day (1990) have shown large Z joint synovial folds (see Chapter 2) protruding into this joint (Fig. 6-7). They also emphasize that normally almost no rotation occurs at this articulation.

LIGAMENTS AND JOINTS OF THE THORACIC REGION

Several ligaments found in the thoracic spine are also present in the cervical spine and are discussed in Chapter 5. These include the ligamenta flava, anterior longitudinal ligament, posterior longitudinal ligament, and interspinous ligaments. Because the interspinous ligaments in the thoracic region differ from those in the cervical region, they are discussed more fully in this section. In addition, further information is provided on the anterior longitudinal ligament, posterior longitudinal ligament, thoracic IVDs, and LF in this section. Also, the

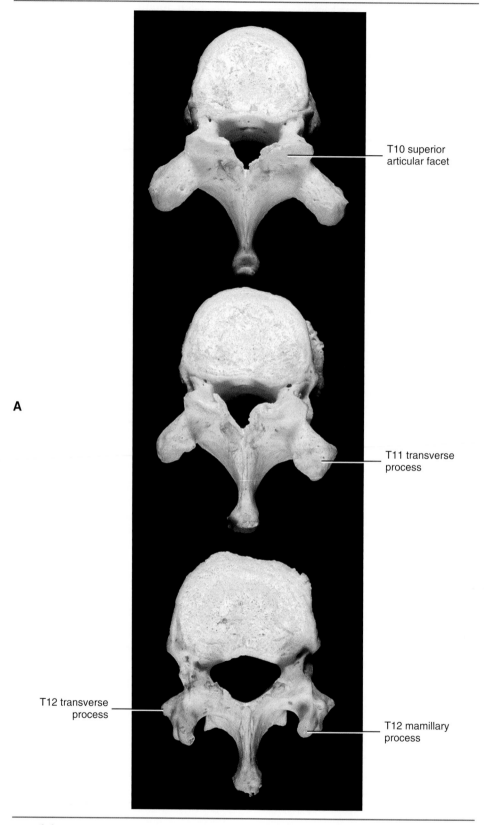

A

T10 superior
articular facet

T11 transverse
process

T12 transverse
process

T12 mamillary
process

FIG. 6-6   Tenth, eleventh, and twelfth thoracic vertebrae. **A,** Superior view.

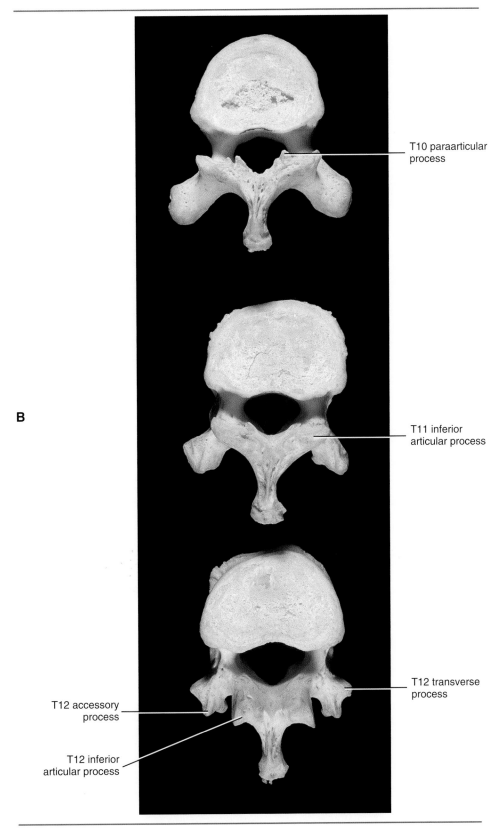

B

T10 paraarticular
process

T11 inferior
articular process

T12 transverse
process

T12 accessory
process

T12 inferior
articular process

FIG. 6-6—cont'd   Tenth, eleventh, and twelfth thoracic vertebrae. **B,** Inferior view.

Continued

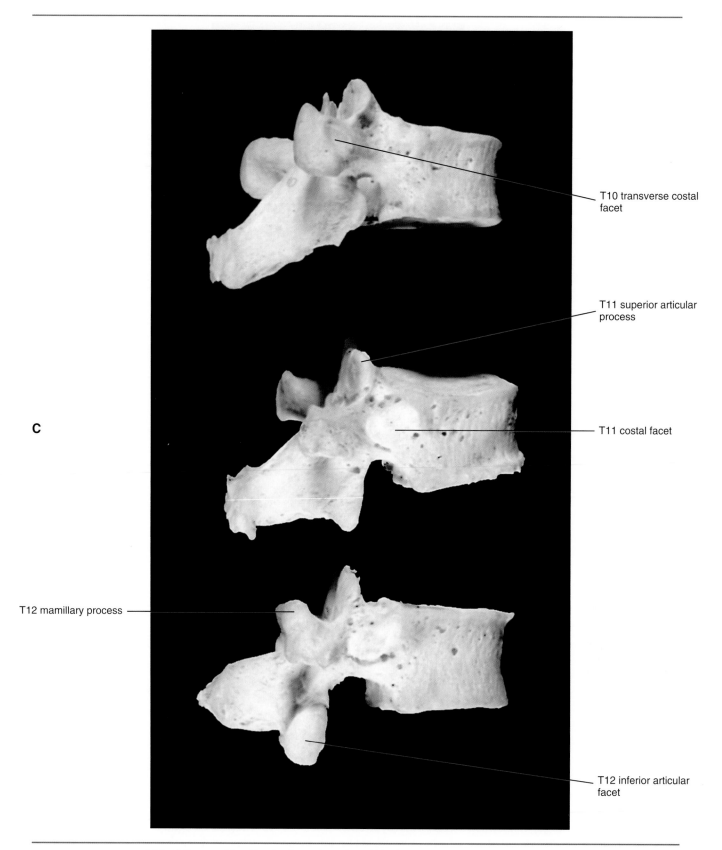

C

T10 transverse costal
facet

T11 superior articular
process

T11 costal facet

T12 mamillary process

T12 inferior articular
facet

FIG. 6-6—cont'd   Tenth, eleventh, and twelfth thoracic vertebrae. **C,** Lateral view.

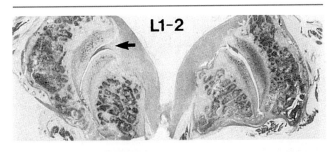

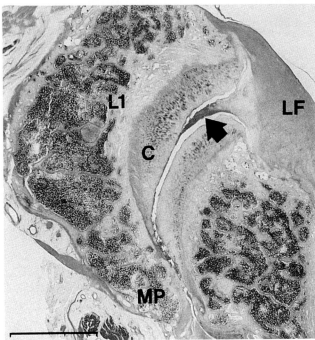

FIG. 6-7 Photomicrograph of the left Z joint at the thoracolumbar junction. L1 represents the superior articular process of L1; *C,* articular cartilage. Notice that, MP, the mamillary process of L1, protrudes medially to overlap the inferior articular process of T12. Also notice the Z joint synovial fold *(arrow)* protruding into the joint space from, *LF,* the ligamentum flavum. (From Singer KP, Giles LGF, & Day RE. [1990]. Intra-articular synovial folds of thoracolumbar junction zygapophyseal joints. *Anat Rec, 226,* 147-152.)

supraspinous ligament is discussed for the first time here. Finally, because the joints between the thoracic vertebrae and ribs are unique to the thoracic region, much of this section is devoted to these interesting and important articulations and the ligaments that support them. This section concludes with a discussion of the sternocostal and interchondral articulations.

Anterior and Posterior Longitudinal Ligaments

The anterior longitudinal ligament (ALL) in the thoracic region (see Figs. 6-10, 6-11, and 6-12, *B*) is thicker from anterior to posterior and thinner from side to side than

in either the cervical or lumbar regions. The ALL attaches firmly to the superior and inferior bony end plates of the thoracic vertebrae, but has only weak attachments to the remainder of the thoracic vertebral bodies. However, firm attachments of the ALL to the thoracic IVDs have been found in more than 50% of spines (Cramer et al., 1996). The firm attachments of the ALL to the IVDs may help prevent anterior protrusion of the IVDs in this region.

Ossification of the posterior longitudinal ligament (PLL) is much less common in the thoracic region than in the cervical region; however, when it does occur it can be severe and lead to paraplegia (Fujimura et al., 1997; Vera et al., 1997).

Ligamentum Flavum

Viejo-Fuertes et al. (1998) studied the ligamenta flava (ligamentum flavum, sing.) in the region of the thoracolumbar junction in detail. They found that each LF had two layers, superficial (posterior) and deep (anterior). The fibers of the superficial layer were oriented obliquely, and those of the deep layer were more organized and oriented in a sagittal plane. The superficial and deep layers were separated by a potential space that Viejo-Fuertes et al. (1998) called a "gliding space." Many nerve fibers were found to innervate the LF. These fibers were thought to originate from the posterior primary division of the spinal nerve, and the authors speculated that the deep layer of the LF also may receive fibers from the recurrent meningeal nerve. In addition, they found a distinct border between the superficial layers of the left and right LF and also a distinct border between the superficial layer of each LF and the more medially located interspinous ligament. They called the region between the left and right superficial layers of the LF the "zone of separation." The deep layers of the left and right LF were continuous at the midline; however, the division between the left and right sides could be identified easily by a prominent posterior midline indentation (a "cleavage separation"). The lateral aspect of each LF was crossed by the longissimus thoracis muscle, and the medial aspect was crossed by the tendons of the rotatores longus and brevis muscles. Elastic fibers dominated the fiber type of typical LF, making up 80% of the fibers in them. The remaining 20% of the fibers were collagen fibers found in densely packed arrays. When the LF was in the neutral position, the significant amount of elastin resulted in a "pretension," meaning that in the neutral position the length of the LF was increased by 15% from the length when no tension was placed on the LF. Therefore a typical ligament was stretched partially when in the neutral position. The percentage of elastin was found to be highest "at the end of fetal life and during the first years of development." With age the pretension of the LF decreased and the elastic fibers became disorganized. Also, increased numbers of chondrocytes and small regions of calcification where the LF attached to bone could be seen under magnification in aging LF. With more advanced age and degeneration, 80% of the elastic fibers were replaced with collagen and chondrocytes. In specimens that showed injury to the ligaments, only minimal replacement of elastic fibers was found and collagen fibers predominated in these regions. No elastic fibers were seen in specimens showing advanced degeneration, and the remaining collagen fibers were disorganized and an increased number of chondrocytes were seen in these specimens. In addition, the number of nerve fibers innervating the LF decreased as the degree of degeneration increased.

Viejo-Fuertes et al. (1998) described two functions of the LF, a biomechanical and neurologic function. Biomechanically the LF decreases flexion and also helps with extension of the vertebral column. Degenerative changes can cause the LF to buckle into the vertebral canal. The authors felt that the neurologic function of the LF was both proprioceptive and nociceptive in nature; the proprioceptive information received from the LF would be important in providing the central nervous system with proprioceptive information to be used for segmental muscle reflexes, and the nociceptive information would be important in relaying information related to tissue damage to the central nervous system.

The LF can ossify. The cause of such ossification is unknown and the condition is poorly understood. Although occurring infrequently, when it does occur, such ossification can increase the size of the LF dramatically, to the point of causing paraplegia secondary to compression of the spinal cord from behind. Ossification of the LF occurs most often in the thoracic region, and also can occur in the thoracolumbar junction (Hasue et al., 1983). When it is present, it usually is found at multiple levels. Some degree of compression of the spinal cord is found in 62% of cases (Yamashita et al., 1990), most of the compressions are mild (56%), and only 6% are severe. Ossification of the LF is frequently associated with ossification of the PLL, and when the two occur together they usually are found at the same level (Hasue et al., 1983; Vera et al., 1997).

Interspinous Ligaments

The interspinous ligaments pass between adjacent spinous processes, filling the gap along the anterior to posterior length of these processes. Anteriorly each interspinous ligament is continuous with the left and right ligamenta flava, and posteriorly each is continuous with the supraspinous ligament. Even though the thoracic interspinous ligaments are thin and membranous in structure, they are more fully developed in the thoracic than cervical region. Some authors dispute their existence in the cervical region altogether, stating that they are simply thin, fascial, anterior extensions of the ligamentum nuchae (Williams et al., 1995). Controversy also surrounds the precise orientation of these ligaments (Behrsin and Briggs, 1988; Williams et al., 1995). Some authors believe that the fibers of the interspinous ligament run from anterosuperior to posteroinferior, and others believe that the fibers making up this ligament run from posterosuperior to anteroinferior (Paris, 1983; Scapinelli, 1989). The latter scenario is more likely. The interspinous ligaments have been studied more fully in the lumbar region, where they are better developed (see Chapter 7).

Supraspinous Ligament

The supraspinous ligament limits flexion of the spine. It is classically described as forming a continuous band that passes from the spinous process of C7 to the sacrum (Williams et al., 1995). However, disagreement exists as to whether or not it extends all the way to the sacrum. Some investigators believe that it is almost nonexistent in the lumbar region (Behrsin and Briggs, 1988). Some authors state that it is divided into layers, with the deeper fibers running between adjacent vertebrae and the more superficial fibers spanning several (up to four) vertebrae (Williams et al., 1995). All the authors seem to agree that the deepest fibers of the thoracic supraspinous ligament become continuous with the interspinous ligaments. The supraspinous ligament seems to warrant further investigation.

Thoracic Intervertebral Discs

The thoracic IVDs have the thinnest superior-to-inferior dimension of the spine. Also, the discs of the upper thoracic region are thinner than those of the lower thoracic region. The upper thoracic region is also the least movable area of the thoracic spine. In contrast to the cervical and lumbar IVDs, which are thicker anteriorly than posteriorly, the thoracic IVDs are of more equal thickness.

Calcification of the IVD is found with greater frequency in the thoracolumbar region than in any other region of the spine. Radiographic surveys have found thoracolumbar IVD calcification in 5% to 6% of adults. Postmortem examinations have found such calcification in up to 70% of adults. Disc calcification usually is asymptomatic unless it is associated with protrusion into the vertebral canal, in which case neurologic compression symptoms result (Lipson and O'Connell, 1991).

Thoracic IVD protrusion is rather infrequent, accounting for only 0.15% to 1.8% of all disc protrusions (Alvarez, Roque, and Pampati, 1988; Bauduin et al., 1989). However, they may be more common than previously believed (Vernon, Dooley, and Acusta, 1993). When present, this condition usually affects the lower thoracic discs of individuals primarily between 30 and 60 years of age (Otani et al., 1988). Symptoms vary dramatically from none at all to motor and sensory deficits resulting from spinal cord compression (myelopathy). Pain, muscle weakness, and spinal cord dysfunction that can present with bowel and bladder dysfunction are the most common clinical symptoms. Computed tomography (CT), in conjunction with contrast enhancement of the subarachnoid space (CT myelography), and MRI are useful in the detection of these rare but significant lesions (Alvarez, Roque, and Pampati, 1988; Bauduin et al., 1989; Vernon, Dooley, and Acusta, 1993), and may allow for more frequent detection of thoracic IVD protrusion in the future.

Crean et al. (1997) found matrix metalloproteinases in degenerated IVDs and in IVDs at the peak of a scoliotic curve. The presence of these proteinases directly correlated with the degree of degeneration. These substances degrade all known extracellular matrix substances and may be associated with the "progressive nature" of IVD degeneration, including the IVD degeneration seen at the apex of scoliotic curves (Crean et al., 1997). A more thorough discussion of IVD degeneration can be found in Chapter 14.

Costovertebral Articulations

The ribs and vertebrae articulate in two locations. The first is the joint complex between the head of a rib and the adjacent vertebral bodies, known as the costocorporeal articulation. The second costovertebral articulation is between a rib and the TP, known as the costotransverse articulation. In addition to allowing the movements of the ribs so important to respiration, the costocorporeal and costotransverse articulations, along with the rib cage, provide stability to the thoracic region of the vertebral column. Whereas the articular processes of the thoracic region limit flexion and extension, the ribs and costovertebral (both costocorporeal and costotransverse) articulations limit lateral flexion and axial rotation of this region (Oda et al., 1996).

Costocorporeal Articulations. The joint between the head of a rib and the adjoining typical thoracic vertebrae consists of articulations with the two adjacent vertebral bodies and interposed IVD (Fig. 6-8). The rib head articulates with the superior demifacet of the same-number vertebra and the inferior demifacet of the vertebra above (e.g., seventh rib articulates with superior demifacet of T7 and inferior demifacet of T6). The crest of the rib head is attached to the adjacent IVD by an intraarticular ligament. This short, flat ligament creates two distinct articular compartments (upper and lower)

within the costocorporeal articulation. Both of these compartments are surrounded by a fibrous articular capsule lined with a synovial membrane. These synovial joints can best be classified as having ovoid articular surfaces, and the fibrous capsule extends around the ovoid articular surfaces of both the demifacet and adjacent articular half of the rib head (see Fig. 6-8). The capsule extends to the intraarticular ligament between the upper and lower compartments. The fibers of the fibrous capsule closest to the IVD blend with that structure, and the posterior fibers blend with the costotransverse ligament. In a fashion similar to that found in the Z joints, synovial folds, or menisci, protrude into the costocorporeal articulation, presumably to help lubricate the joint and help with the sliding and rotary motions of the joint (Meyer, 1972). The heads of the first, tenth (occasionally), eleventh, and twelfth ribs form single ovoid synovial articulations with their respective ribs.

The ligaments of this compound joint include the capsular, intraarticular (both described previously), and radiate. Each radiate ligament (see Fig. 6-8) associated with typical vertebrae attaches to the anterior aspect of the head of the articulating rib and the two vertebrae to which the head attaches. In addition, the radiate ligament attaches by horizontal fibers to the IVD between the two vertebrae. The superior fibers attach just above the superior demifacet and ascend to the vertebral body of the superior vertebra. Likewise, the inferior fibers attach just below the inferior demifacet and descend to the inferior vertebral body. The radiate ligament of the first rib has some superior fibers that attach to C7. The radiate ligaments of the tenth through twelfth ribs attach to only the vertebra with which the rib head articulates.

In addition to allowing motion of the ribs, the costocorporeal joints provide stability to the thoracic region during motions in the sagittal (flexion-extension), coronal (lateral flexion), and transverse planes (axial rotation) (Oda et al., 2002).

Confirming the work of Meyer (1972), Erwin, Jackson, and Homonko (2000) found large synovial folds protruding into the costocorporeal joints. In addition, they found that the synovial folds were innervated by free nerve endings and mechanoreceptors immunoreactive to substance P. Substance P is associated with pain transmission and functions in the perception of pain, related reflex muscle responses (flexion reflexes), and reflex responses to pain of the autonomic nervous system and endocrine system. Therefore the costocorporeal joints are similar to the Z joints with respect to being planar synovial joints with nociceptive (pain-sensitive) innervation of both the joint capsule and synovial folds. The nerve endings are most likely sensitive to tissue strain or tissue damage of mechanical origin. The authors speculated that nociception transmitted from a lesion

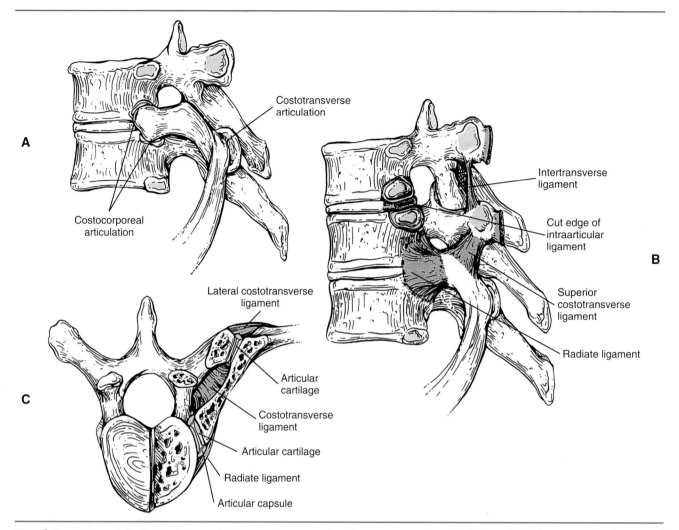

FIG. 6-8 Costovertebral articulations. **A,** Bony costocorporeal and costotransverse articulations. **B,** Ligamentous attachments of these joints. **C,** Superior view. The vertebra and rib have been horizontally sectioned on the right half of the illustration to demonstrate further the costocorporeal and costotransverse articulations.

affecting these nerve endings would probably radiate to the midline thoracic region and anteriorly along the same rib. In addition, pain from the costocorporeal joints also may be associated with atypical chest and arm pain (Erwin, Jackson, and Homonko, 2000). Others (Groen et al., 1987) have identified fibers from sympathetic chain extending to the costocorporeal joint. The fibers were found to form a dense network that surrounded the joint, and met the criteria of vasomotor fibers that would provide innervation to the vessels extending to the synovial lining of the joint capsule.

Costotransverse Articulation. This joint is composed of the costal (articular) tubercle of a rib articulating with the transverse costal facet of a TP (see Fig. 6-8). Recall that the eleventh and twelfth ribs do not articulate with the TPs of their respective vertebrae. The joint surfaces of the upper five or six costotransverse joints are curved, with the transverse costal facet being concave and the articular tubercle convex. The remaining joints are more planar in configuration (Meyer, 1972; Williams et al., 1995). A thin, fibrous capsule lined by a synovial membrane attaches to the two adjacent articular surfaces. A costotransverse foramen is found between the TP and the rib between the costotransverse and costocorporeal articulations. This foramen is filled by the costotransverse ligament. The costotransverse ligament passes from the posterior aspect of the rib neck to the anterior aspect of the adjacent TP (see Fig. 6-8). For example, the costotransverse ligament of the sixth rib attaches to the posterior aspect of that rib and to the anterior aspect of the TP of T6. Sensory nerve endings also have been found in the costotransverse ligament, indicating that it is pain sensitive (Erwin, Jackson, and Homonko, 2000). Sensory innervation to the lateral and superior costotransverse ligaments has not been investigated adequately.

The ligaments of the costotransverse articulation include the articular capsule, costotransverse ligament (both described previously), superior costotransverse ligament, and lateral costotransverse ligament (see Fig. 6-8). The strong but short lateral costotransverse ligament courses directly laterally from the lateral margin of the TP to the nonarticular region of the costal tubercle of the adjacent rib (see Fig. 6-8). This ligament is found at every thoracic segment. The ligaments of the upper thoracic vertebrae course slightly superiorly, as well as laterally, whereas the lower ones run slightly inferiorly, as well as laterally.

A superior costotransverse ligament courses between the neck of each rib, except for the first, and the TP of the vertebra above. This ligament is divided into two parts, anterior and posterior. Both parts course superiorly from a rib neck to the inferior border of the TP immediately above. The anterior layer angles slightly laterally as it ascends and blends with the posterior intercostal membrane (see Fig. 6-11, B). The posterior layer angles slightly medially. Because it is more posteriorly placed, this ligament blends laterally with the external intercostal muscle. The intercostal vein, artery, and nerve pass across the anterior surface of these ligaments. A lumbocostal ligament runs from the inferior border of the twelfth rib shaft to the superior surface of the TP of L1.

An accessory ligament is normally found medial to the superior costotransverse ligament. This accessory ligament is separated from the superior costotransverse ligament by a gap that is filled by the posterior primary division as it leaves the mixed spinal nerve to reach the more posterior structures of the spine. More specifically, the accessory ligament originates from the region of the neck of a rib medial to the attachment of the superior costotransverse ligament. It courses superiorly to reach the inferior articular process of the vertebra above, although some fibers reach the TP.

Sternocostal and Interchondral Articulations

The costal cartilages of the first through seventh ribs articulate directly with the sternum at the sternocostal joints (see Fig. 6-2). The costal cartilages of the eighth through tenth ribs attach to the costal cartilage of the rib above at articulations known as the interchondral joints.

Sternocostal Joints. A complex type of synarthrosis exists between the first costal cartilage and manubrium. A thin piece of fibrocartilage is interposed between the two surfaces and is tightly adherent to both (Williams et al., 1995). A radiate ligament also unites the two surfaces. The joint between the second costal cartilage and sternum is synovial and is separated into two compartments by an intraarticular ligament. Small synovial joints are located between the costal cartilages of the third through seventh ribs and the sternum. The costal cartilages and sternum are united by the fibrous capsules of the joints and also by the radiate ligaments that pass from the anterior and posterior surfaces of each costal cartilage to the sternum. A small amount of rotation occurs at these joints. This rotation allows the thorax to expand and contract during inspiration and expiration, respectively.

Interchondral Joints. As mentioned, the eighth through tenth costal cartilages articulate with the costal cartilage immediately above. Small synovial joints are formed at the attachment sites for the eighth and ninth ribs. The costal cartilage of the tenth rib usually is continuous with the costal cartilage of the ninth rib, and no true joint unites the two. Occasionally no attachment exists between the tenth rib and the costal cartilage of the ninth rib. Although both the sixth and seventh costal cartilages attach directly to the sternum, their most distal portions also contact one another. Small synovial joints are also located where these cartilages are in contact with one another.

RANGES OF MOTION IN THE THORACIC SPINE

Vertebral Motion

As stated, the facets of the thoracic vertebrae are oriented 60 degrees to the horizontal plane. Therefore they are more vertically oriented than the articular processes of the cervical region. This vertical orientation dramatically limits forward flexion. Extension is limited by the inferior articular processes contacting the laminae of the vertebrae below and also by contact between adjacent spinous processes. Rotation is the dominant movement in the thoracic region. However, the vertebrae are a part of the entire thoracic cage and even this motion is limited considerably. This may help to explain why the lower thoracic region, with its relation to floating ribs and ribs with only an indirect attachment to the sternum, is the most mobile part of the thoracic spine. Ranges of motion of the thoracic spine include the following:

Combined flexion and extension	34 degrees
Unilateral lateral flexion	15 degrees
Unilateral axial rotation	35 degrees

Motion of the Ribs

Motion of the ribs at the costocorporeal and costo-transverse articulations is primarily one of rotation with a slight gliding motion. Motion is limited because of the strong ligamentous attachments. Upward and downward rotation is the primary movement of the upper six ribs, accompanied by slight superior and inferior gliding. Rotation of the seventh through tenth ribs is accompanied by more gliding than in the ribs above. This is because the transverse costal facets of T7 through T10 are more flat than those of the vertebrae above and also because the facets face upward, anteriorly, and laterally. Upward rotation of these lower ribs is accompanied by posterior and medial gliding, and downward rotation is accompanied by anterior and slightly lateral gliding. These movements tend to open and close the substernal angle, respectively (Williams et al., 1995).

LATERAL CURVATURE OF THE SPINE

Lateral curvature or lateral deviation of the spine is known as scoliosis (Fig. 6-9). A slight lateral curve with the convexity on the same side as handedness (i.e., convexity to the left in left-handed individuals) is normally found in the upper thoracic region (see Chapter 2). This is a result of the pull of the stronger musculature on the side of handedness. Lateral curves other than this mild upper thoracic curve are considered to be a variation from normal spinal structure. These scolioses range from being barely perceptible and insignificant deviations to extremely dramatic and deforming curvatures.

Scoliosis can be found in any spinal region, but the thoracic region is usually the most prominently affected, partly because of its length and central location. However, the thoracic region is the most noticeably affected primarily because the attachment of the rest of the thoracic cage to the thoracic vertebrae can result in deformation of the entire thorax. In addition, curvatures of the thoracic spine are more or less "held in place" by the remainder of the thoracic cage (ribs and sternum), and proper evaluation of the ribs can be useful in the diagnosis of scoliosis. In fact, with full forward flexion of the spine, posterior elevation on one side of the thorax ("rib hump") of 6 mm or greater has been used as one of the primary indicators of scoliosis. The incidence of such posterior thoracic elevation has been reported as 4.1% in fourth-grade schoolchildren with an average age of 10.8 years (Nissinen et al., 1989).

Osteophytes of vertebral bodies frequently develop on the concave side of the curve of a scoliosis and are rarely seen on the convex side of the curve (Nathan, 1962). Occasionally scoliosis is so severe that serious compromise of lung capacity and cardiac output may result.

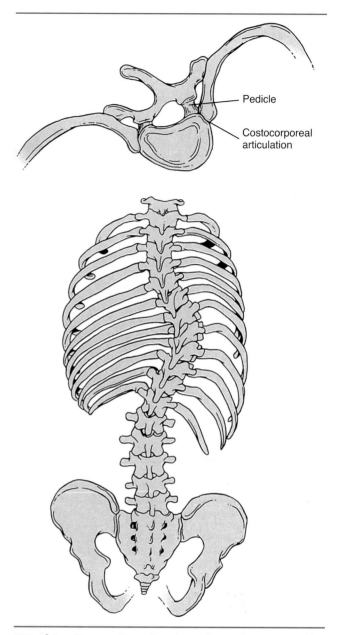

FIG. 6-9 *Bottom,* Posterior view of a scoliotic spine. *Top,* Superior view of a single vertebra and the articulating ribs. Notice the asymmetry between the left and right costocorporeal and costovertebral articulations (compare with Fig. 6-5). (Modified from Netter [1990].)

Interestingly, individuals with spines shortened as a result of pathology during childhood or early adolescence (e.g., scoliosis or tuberculosis affecting the spine) have upper and lower extremities that are statistically significantly longer (≈2 cm for each extremity) than "healthy" individuals. This increase in upper and lower extremity lengths are thought to be the result of a possible "compensatory stimulatory growth mechanism" (Upadhyay et al., 1991; Krishna and Upadhyay, 1996).

Scoliosis has many causes, ranging from developmental and anatomic, such as hemivertebra (see Chapters 2 and 12), to unknown causes (idiopathic). Idiopathic scoliosis is typically characterized by the presence of a concomitant lordosis at the apex of the lateral curve (Deacon, Archer, and Dickson, 1987).

The cause of idiopathic scoliosis remains unknown, but it is thought to be the result of many factors. There is most likely a genetic component to this disorder with both autosomal and sex-linked elements, with variable penetrance (expression) and heterogeneity (two or more genes acting independently), contributing to the genetic predisposition for idiopathic scoliosis (Kesling and Reinker, 1997; Lowe et al., 2000). This genetic predisposition is probably linked to asymmetric processing of motor and sensory information in the cerebral cortex and possibly improper processing in the paramedian pontine reticular formation (Cook et al., 1986; Wyatt et al., 1986; Goldberg et al., 1995; Carpintero et al., 1997). Secondary factors are then probably necessary for the genetic predisposition and neurologic abnormalities to be fully expressed. Such secondary factors include a decrease in melatonin production (Kanemura et al., 1997; Wang et al., 1997; Cheung et al., 2003), which leads to an increase in circulating levels of the hormone calmodulin (Lowe et al., 2000). These hormonal changes are probably related to bone growth during the pubertal growth spurt. This growth spurt has been found to begin earlier in children with idiopathic scoliosis. For this reason, the more rapid and earlier growth spurt in females compared with males may explain the higher incidence of this disorder in girls, and the fact that scoliosis tends to develop somewhat later in boys than girls (Karol et al., 1993). Changes in skeletal muscle (Carpintero et al., 1997), connective tissue (Crean et al., 1997; Duance et al., 1998), bone density, rib distortion (Lowe et al., 2000), decreased height of the posterior vertebral arch (Deane and Duthie, 1973), asymmetry of the neurocentral synchondrosis (Vital et al., 1989), and the relatively common finding (up to 26%) of syrinx formation and other neuroanatomic abnormalities in the spinal cord (Evans et al., 1996; Ghanem et al., 1997) are probably the result of the altered biomechanics of the spine and spinal cord that occur with spinal curvatures (Lowe et al., 2000).

Additional support for the involvement of high centers in the central nervous system in the cause of idiopathic scoliosis is provided by evidence that a significantly lower incidence of idiopathic scoliosis exists among hearing-impaired children (1.2% in hearing impaired children versus 4% to 10% in the general population) (Woods et al., 1995). Of note is that 80% of hearing-impaired children also have significant vestibular impairment. This vestibular impairment forces these children to shift to vision and proprioception as the primary means of detecting and establishing a vertical position in space. The vestibular system is thought to normally provide the baseline from which visual and proprioceptive information is compared when establishing the vertical posture. Woods et al. (1995) hypothesize that the central nervous system of individuals with idiopathic scoliosis may process normal vestibular information incorrectly; visual and proprioceptive information then would be compared with this consistently altered baseline information, causing the reflex efferent projections to postural muscles to be incorrect. The incorrect efferent stimulation of postural muscles then would result in the postural alterations of scoliosis. More work is still needed to verify this compelling hypothesis. Additional evidence for high central nervous system (cortical) involvement in the development of idiopathic scoliosis is that a significantly higher incidence of scoliosis is found in individuals with cerebral palsy (an incidence of 4% to 64%, dependent on the amount of muscle spasticity) (Dias et al., 1997). Possibly related to scoliosis in the cerebral palsy population is that congenital block vertebrae (lack of vertebral segmentation) in the cervical region, known as Klippel-Feil syndrome, is also more prevalent in this group of individuals (Theiss, Smith, and Winter, 1997). Much more work is still needed to unravel the cause of idiopathic scoliosis and to possibly find a way to cure this disorder.

NERVES, VESSELS, AND VISCERA RELATED TO THE THORACIC SPINE

The thoracic spine and the ribs are intimately related to many neural, vascular, and visceral structures (Figs. 6-10 and 6-11). The structures most closely related to the spine and ribs include posterior primary divisions; the intercostal arteries, veins, and nerves; azygos, hemiazygos, and accessory hemiazygos veins; thoracic duct and thoracic lymphatics; thoracic aorta; esophagus; trachea; vagus nerves; thoracic sympathetic chain; and splanchnic nerves. These structures are discussed briefly in this section. Chapter 1 and Table 1-1 relate many of the most important visceral structures to vertebral body levels to aid in the interpretation of scans presenting cross-sectional anatomy (e.g., CT, MRI). The intercostal muscles are discussed in Chapter 4.

Posterior Primary Divisions (Dorsal Rami)

The thoracic spinal nerves are formed within the IVF by the union of the thoracic dorsal and ventral roots. The roots in the upper thoracic region descend only slightly before entering the IVF, whereas the roots of the lower thoracic region may descend as much as two vertebral levels before entering the IVF. Once formed, the spinal nerves contain both sensory and motor fibers (see Fig. 3-3). Each mixed spinal nerve then divides into a

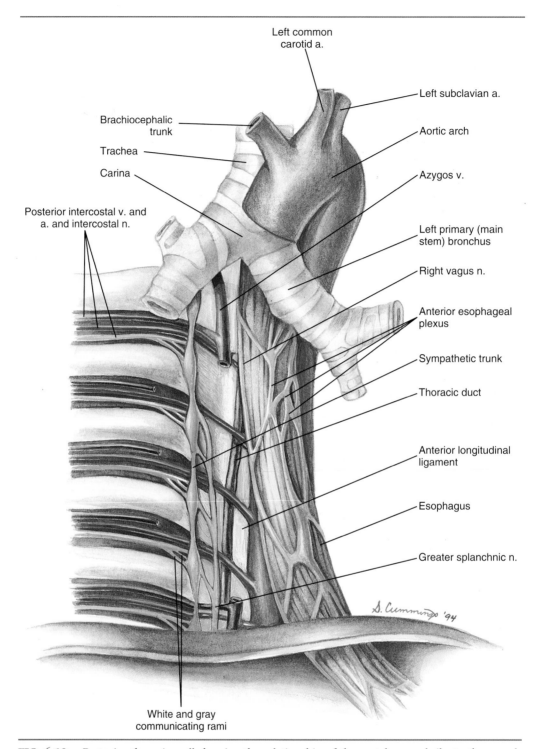

Left common
carotid a.

Left subclavian a.

Brachiocephalic
trunk

Aortic arch

Trachea

Azygos v.

Carina

Posterior intercostal v. and
a. and intercostal n.

Left primary (main
stem) bronchus

Right vagus n.

Anterior esophageal
plexus

Sympathetic trunk

Thoracic duct

Anterior longitudinal
ligament

Esophagus

Greater splanchnic n.

White and gray
communicating rami

FIG. 6-10   Posterior thoracic wall showing the relationship of the vertebrae and ribs to the vessels and nerves of the thorax. The right vagus nerve is shown sending a few branches to the anterior esophageal plexus. The more abundant and important contributions to the posterior esophageal plexus cannot be seen from this perspective.

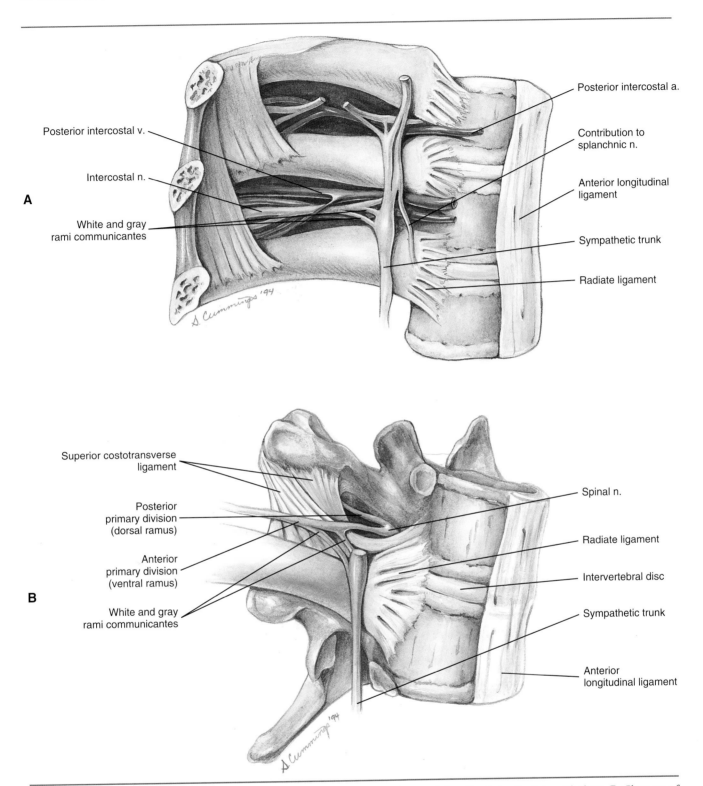

A, Posterior intercostal v.

Intercostal n.

White and gray rami communicantes

A

Posterior intercostal a.

Contribution to splanchnic n.

Anterior longitudinal ligament

Sympathetic trunk

Radiate ligament

Superior costotransverse ligament

Posterior primary division (dorsal ramus)

Anterior primary division (ventral ramus)

White and gray rami communicantes

B

Spinal n.

Radiate ligament

Intervertebral disc

Sympathetic trunk

Anterior longitudinal ligament

FIG. 6-11   A, Nerves and vessels related to three adjacent thoracic vertebrae and the ribs that articulate with them. **B,** Close-up of the nerves associated with a single thoracic motion segment (two adjacent thoracic vertebrae).

posterior primary division (dorsal ramus) and an anterior primary division (ventral ramus) as it exits the IVF (see Fig. 6-11, *B*). The anterior primary division of a thoracic nerve becomes an intercostal nerve and the subcostal nerve at the level of T12 (see the following discussion). The posterior primary division (dorsal ramus) passes posteriorly across the lateral aspect of the Z joint, to which it sends fine branches. It then passes through a small but adequate opening bounded superiorly by the TP, inferiorly by the rib of the vertebra below (e.g., T5 nerve exits between T5 and T6 vertebrae and above the sixth rib), medially by the Z joint and the accessory superior costotransverse ligament, and laterally by the superior costotransverse ligament, which attaches to the rib below. This opening is known as the *costotransverse foramen* of Cruveilhier. The dorsal ramus then divides into medial and lateral branches. The lateral branch supplies the erector spinae muscles in the region and continues to provide sensory innervation to the skin of the back.

Not all of the first six lateral branches of the posterior primary divisions reach the skin. However, the lower six lateral branches all have significant cutaneous distributions. They supply the skin superficial to the spinous processes via medial cutaneous branches (of the lateral branches of the posterior primary divisions) and supply sensory innervation to the skin several inches lateral to the midline via lateral cutaneous branches (of the lateral branches of the posterior primary divisions). The lateral cutaneous branches may descend as far as four ribs before reaching the skin. The lateral cutaneous branch of the posterior primary division of T12 reaches the upper border of the iliac crest.

A typical medial branch of a posterior primary division takes a rather tortuous course, passing between the multifidus muscle on its medial surface and the levator costarum muscle on its lateral side (Maigne, Maigne, and Guerin-Surville, 1991). It then continues posteromedially and slightly inferiorly, running medial to most of the longissimus thoracis muscle fibers. The dorsal rami of the second, third, and fourth thoracic nerves then pass through the tendon of the splenius cervicis muscle, continue through the rhomboid muscles, pierce the trapezius muscle, and then reach the skin adjacent to the spinous process of its vertebra of origin (e.g., T3 nerve innervating region of T3 spinous process). The medial branches of the fifth and sixth thoracic nerves also reach the skin of the back.

Maigne, Maigne, and Guerin-Surville (1991) found that the upper thoracic medial branches of the dorsal rami frequently appeared to be entrapped in tendons of the erector spinae or splenius cervicis muscle. They believed this helped to explain localized areas of thoracic discomfort with associated hypesthesia and paresthesia frequently seen in their clinical practice. Also, in 1 of the

16 cadavers studied, the authors found a bilateral anastomosis between the medial branch of the dorsal ramus of T2 and the accessory nerve (CN XI). They thought this might explain the occasional lack of paralysis of the trapezius muscle among certain individuals after transection of the accessory nerve during neck surgery.

Like the medial branches of the posterior primary divisions of the upper six thoracic nerves, those of the lower six pass posteriorly to innervate primarily the multifidi, rotatores, and longissimus thoracis muscles; however, they only occasionally reach the skin of the back (Williams et al., 1995).

Intercostal Nerves, Arteries, and Veins

Intercostal Nerves. The anterior primary divisions of the T1 to T11 nerves are the intercostal nerves (see Figs. 6-10 and 6-11). The ventral ramus of the T1 nerve splits, and the larger branch joins the ventral ramus of C8 to form the inferior trunk of the brachial plexus. The smaller branch of the ventral ramus of T1 forms the first intercostal nerve. The anterior primary division of the T12 nerve is the subcostal nerve.

Close to its origin, each intercostal nerve (and the subcostal and upper two lumbar nerves) sends a white ramus communicans to the sympathetic ganglion of the same level. These ganglia are located anterior to the intercostal nerves and lie along the lateral aspect of the vertebral bodies.

The intercostal nerves also receive gray rami communicantes from the neighboring sympathetic ganglia (see Fig. 6-11). This is similar to all other anterior primary divisions. The intercostal nerve then continues laterally along the subcostal groove, inferior to the intercostal vein and artery (Fig. 6-12; see also Fig. 6-10). The lateral course of the intercostal nerve, within the posterior intercostal space, is subject to a wide degree of variation. The intercostal nerve frequently runs within the middle of the intercostal space (73% of the time) and occasionally runs along the inferior aspect of the intercostal space just above the subjacent rib (Hardy, 1988).

Each intercostal nerve provides sensory, motor (somatic motor), and sympathetic (visceral motor to blood vessels and sweat glands) innervation to the thoracic or abdominal wall. This is accomplished by means of posterior, lateral, and anterior branches.

Posterior Intercostal Arteries. The third through eleventh intercostal arteries originate from the thoracic aorta and course laterally along the inferior aspect of the corresponding rib (see Figs. 6-10 and 6-12, *A*). The artery that courses below the twelfth rib is known as the subcostal artery because it lies inferior to the twelfth rib and not between two ribs. The first two intercostal arter-

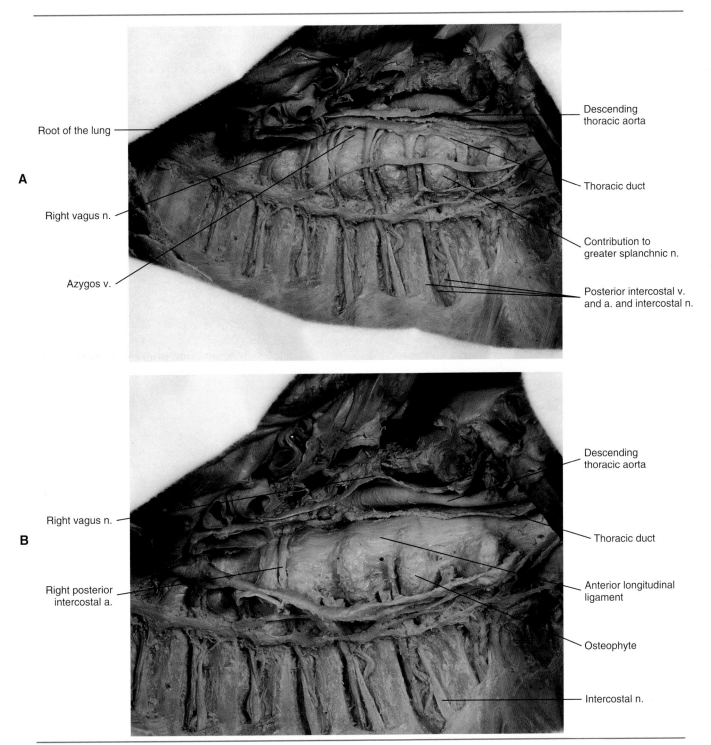

Root of the lung

Right vagus n.

Azygos v.

A

Descending thoracic aorta

Thoracic duct

Contribution to greater splanchnic n.

Posterior intercostal v. and a. and intercostal n.

Right vagus n.

Right posterior intercostal a.

B

Descending thoracic aorta

Thoracic duct

Anterior longitudinal ligament

Osteophyte

Intercostal n.

FIG. 6-12 **A,** Right side of the mediastinum and the thoracic vertebrae, ribs, and intercostal spaces associated with this region. **B,** Same specimen with the azygos vein and related intercostal veins retracted. This was done to show more clearly the anterior longitudinal ligament. Notice the large osteophytes extending from the right anterolateral aspects of the thoracic vertebrae. Typically such osteophytes are seen in dissections of this region.

ies arise from the highest intercostal artery. The highest intercostal artery is a branch of the costocervical trunk, which arises from the subclavian artery.

The intercostal arteries course between the intercostal vein superiorly and the intercostal nerve inferiorly. Because the thoracic aorta lies to the left of the thoracic spine, the right intercostal arteries must cross over the thoracic vertebral bodies to reach the right intercostal spaces. This results in the right intercostal arteries being longer than the left ones.

Each posterior intercostal artery gives rise to dorsal and lateral branches that supply the dorsal (including deep back muscles) and lateral aspects of the intercostal spaces, respectively.

Anterior Intercostal Arteries. The upper six anterior intercostal arteries arise from the internal thoracic artery (internal mammary artery). The internal thoracic artery arises from the subclavian artery, then courses inferiorly, behind and lateral to the sternocostal articulations, and divides into the superior epigastric artery and the musculophrenic artery. The musculophrenic artery, in turn, supplies the seventh, eighth, and ninth anterior intercostal arteries. The nine anterior intercostal arteries supply the intercostal muscles anteriorly, as well as the muscles of the anterior thoracic wall and breast.

Intercostal Veins and the Azygos System of Veins. Venous drainage of the thoracic cage is accomplished primarily by the intercostal veins. The intercostal venous blood generally courses in the opposite direction of the arterial supply and drains into the azygos system of veins (see Figs. 6-10 and 6-12, *A*).

The azygos vein originates from one or more of the following: inferior vena cava, right renal vein, and right ascending lumbar vein. The azygos vein passes through the diaphragm by means of the aortic hiatus. It then courses along the right anterior aspect of the thoracic vertebral bodies. Along its course this vein receives the right lower eight intercostal veins, right superior intercostal vein, and hemiazygos vein. In addition, the accessory hemiazygos vein frequently is a direct tributary of the azygos vein. The right superior intercostal vein drains the upper two to three intercostal spaces and can empty into either the azygos or right brachiocephalic vein. Other tributaries of the azygos vein include esophageal, bronchial, mediastinal, and pericardial veins. The azygos vein courses superiorly and arches (from posterior to anterior) around the superior aspect of the right primary bronchus. It then terminates by entering the superior vena cava.

The hemiazygos vein originates from the left ascending lumbar vein, left renal vein, or both. The hemiazygos vein enters the thorax through the aortic hiatus. It then continues superiorly along the left anterior aspect of the vertebral bodies. Along its path the hemiazygos vein receives the lower four or five left intercostal veins. It also frequently receives the accessory hemiazygos vein. The hemiazygos vein helps to drain the left mediastinum and left lower esophagus. The hemiazygos vein crosses from left to right at roughly the level of T9 and terminates by emptying into the azygos vein.

The accessory hemiazygos vein connects the middle three or four intercostal veins. It occasionally receives the left superior intercostal vein, which drains the upper two to three intercostal spaces. However, the left superior intercostal vein normally is a tributary of the left brachiocephalic vein. The accessory hemiazygos vein ends by either draining into the hemiazygos vein or by crossing the vertebral column from left to right, just above the hemiazygos vein, to drain into the azygos vein.

Thoracic Duct

The thoracic duct is the largest and most important lymphatic channel of the body (see Figs. 6-10 and 6-12). The thoracic duct drains the lower extremities, pelvis, abdomen, left side of the thorax, left upper extremity, and left side of the head and neck. It originates at the cisterna chyli (when present) and terminates at the junction of the left subclavian and left internal jugular veins. The cisterna chyli is a large midline lymphatic collecting structure located just inferior to the aortic hiatus of the diaphragm. It collects lymphatics from the lower extremities via left and right lateral branches and from the intestinal tract via an intestinal branch. The cisterna chyli tapers at its superior aspect and becomes the thoracic duct. Most frequently the cisterna chyli is replaced by a confluence of lymph trunks in the abdominal region. The thoracic duct subsequently enters the thorax through the aortic hiatus just to the right of the aorta. On entering the thorax, the thoracic duct continues superiorly along the anterior aspect of the thoracic vertebral bodies. Between T7 and T5 it passes to the left side of the anterior aspect of the vertebral bodies. The thoracic duct continues superiorly to empty into the junction of the left subclavian and internal jugular veins.

The right lymphatic duct drains the right side of the thorax, right upper extremity, and right side of the neck and head. It usually empties into the right subclavian vein, the internal jugular vein, or the union of the two.

The lymphatics of the thoracic cage drain into mediastinal nodes, which in turn drain into either the right lymphatic or thoracic duct. The lymphatics of the mediastinum are abundant and can be divided into four major nodes: superior mediastinal, diaphragmatic, posterior mediastinal, and tracheobronchial. These lymph nodes drain into nearby lymphatic channels. Those of the right side drain into the right lymphatic duct, and those of the left side drain into the thoracic duct.

Aortic Arch and Thoracic Aorta

Aortic Arch. The aortic arch begins at the heart as the outflow path of the left ventricle. It extends in front of the trachea, swings around the left primary bronchus, and comes to lie to the left of the midthoracic vertebrae (see Fig. 6-10). The arch then continues inferiorly as the descending thoracic aorta. There are three large branches from the aortic arch: the brachiocephalic (innominate) artery, left common carotid artery, and left subclavian artery.

Descending Thoracic Aorta. The descending thoracic aorta is the continuation of the aortic arch (see Figs. 6-10 and 6-12). It begins at approximately the T4-5 disc and continues inferiorly along the left side of the thoracic vertebrae. The thoracic aorta shifts to the midline in the lower thorax, lying on the anterior aspect of the lower thoracic vertebrae. The thoracic aorta gives off bronchial arteries (which supply the lungs) and all the intercostal arteries except the first two on each side (supplied by the highest intercostal artery of the costocervical trunk). The descending thoracic aorta also gives off the left and right subcostal arteries.

Esophagus

The esophagus (see Fig. 6-10) originates posterior to the cricoid cartilage (roughly at the level of C6) and terminates at the cardia of the stomach (at the T11 vertebral body level). Therefore the esophagus has cervical, thoracic, and abdominal regions. It is approximately 10 inches in length. The esophagus lies roughly in the midline in the upper and middle thorax, where it is located posterior to the left atrium. It curves left at the esophageal hiatus (≈T10 vertebral body level), where it lies anterior and slightly to the left of the thoracic aorta and its hiatus.

Trachea

The trachea (see Fig. 6-10) is a rigid tubular organ that lies anterior to the esophagus between the brachiocephalic artery (on the right) and the left common carotid artery (on the left). The brachiocephalic veins lie anterior to the trachea. The trachea begins at the cricoid cartilage (roughly the level of C6) and ends by bifurcating into the left and right primary bronchi at approximately the level of the T4-5 disc (see Fig. 6-10). The trachea is kept rigid and held open by 16 to 20 cartilaginous tracheal rings. These rings are C-shaped with the open end facing posteriorly. Fibroelastic tissue and smooth muscle (tracheal or trachealis muscle) span the posterior opening. The less rigid posterior surface allows the passage of food through the posteriorly located esophagus. Helping to form the tracheal bifurcation is

the carina, the inverted V-shaped inferior border of the trachea formed by the last tracheal cartilage.

The trachea receives innervation from sympathetic and parasympathetic autonomic fibers. The parasympathetics arise from the vagus nerves and their recurrent laryngeal branches. Stimulation of these nerves results in constriction of the trachea and increased secretion of the mucus cells of the tracheal epithelium. Sympathetic innervation of the trachea is derived from branches of the thoracic sympathetic trunk. Stimulation of these nerves results in dilation of the trachea and decreased mucus secretions.

Vagus Nerves

The vagus nerves (right and left) run within the carotid sheath in the neck and enter the thorax medial to the phrenic nerves (right and left). Each vagus nerve is responsible for carrying preganglionic parasympathetic fibers to all the thoracic viscera. These fibers synapse in the walls of the organs they supply. General visceral afferent fibers from these same viscera also travel within the left and right vagus nerves. The parasympathetic nervous system is described in detail in Chapter 10.

Left Vagus Nerve. The left vagus nerve enters the thorax between the left common carotid and left subclavian arteries. It continues inferiorly by crossing the aortic arch, where it gives off the large left recurrent laryngeal nerve. This nerve loops around the aortic arch from anterior to posterior just lateral to the ligamentum arteriosum. It then runs superiorly in a groove between the esophagus and trachea (tracheoesophageal groove) to supply eight of the nine laryngeal muscles on the left side. The main trunk of the vagus nerve continues inferiorly from the arch of the aorta (giving branches to the cardiac plexus) and follows the aorta posteriorly, passing behind the root of the left lung, where it participates in the pulmonary plexus. The vagus nerve then courses medially and comes to lie on the anterior aspect of the esophagus, where it helps to form the anterior esophageal plexus. The anterior esophageal plexus coalesces inferiorly to form the anterior vagal trunk. This trunk exits the thorax by traveling along the anterior aspect of the esophagus through the esophageal hiatus of the diaphragm.

Right Vagus Nerve. The right vagus nerve enters the thorax by crossing the right subclavian artery. The right recurrent laryngeal nerve is given off at this point. This nerve loops around the right subclavian artery and continues superiorly in the right tracheoesophageal groove to supply eight of the nine muscles of the larynx on the right side. The right vagus nerve continues inferiorly in the thorax, contributing to the superficial and deep cardiac plexuses, and runs posterior to the root of the right lung. Here it sends several branches to the posterior pulmonary plexus. The right vagus nerve then travels medially to the posterior aspect of the esophagus, where it forms the posterior esophageal plexus (see Figs. 6-10 and 6-12). The nerves of the posterior esophageal plexus coalesce to form the posterior vagal trunk. The posterior vagal trunk exits the thorax by traveling along the posterior aspect of the esophagus through the esophageal hiatus of the diaphragm.

Thoracic Sympathetic Chain

The sympathetic nervous system is discussed in detail in Chapter 10. Because of the close anatomic relationship between the sympathetic trunk and the thoracic verte-brae, it also is discussed briefly here.

The sympathetic trunk in the thoracic region extends from superior to inferior across the heads of the ribs and is covered by the costal pleura (see Figs. 6-10, 6-11, and 10-7, *B*). As it reaches the inferior aspect of the thorax, the trunk courses medially to be positioned along the lateral aspect of the lower thoracic vertebral bodies. The sympathetic trunk is composed of axons of neurons whose cell bodies are located in the intermediolateral cell column of the thoracic spinal cord. These axons exit the cord via a ventral root that unites with a dorsal root, forming a spinal nerve. This nerve exits the vertebral canal through the IVF. These preganglionic sympathetic fibers leave the ventral ramus close to its origin to form a white ramus communicans, which connects to the sympathetic ganglion. Once in the sympathetic ganglion, the preganglionic sympathetic fibers have several options to reach their destinations (effector organs) (see Chapter 10). One option is to help form the splanchnic nerves, which supply a large part of the abdominal viscera with sympathetic innervation.

Splanchnic Nerves

The thorax contains three splanchnic nerves: the greater, the lesser (see Figs. 6-10, 10-5, and 10-12), and the least. Each is formed from branches of the sympathetic chain. The splanchnic nerves course along the lateral aspects of the middle and lower thoracic vertebral bodies and exit the thorax by piercing the posterior aspect of the diaphragm. They then synapse in one of several pre-vertebral ganglia. The postganglionic fibers from these prevertebral ganglia provide sympathetic innervation to the vast majority of the abdominal viscera.

The three splanchnic nerves, their ganglia of origin, and the prevertebral ganglion in which they synapse are as follows:

- *Greater splanchnic nerve.* This nerve arises from thoracic ganglia five through nine (see Figs. 6-10; 6-11, *A*; and 6-12, *A*) and synapses in the celiac ganglion. Some of its fibers do not synapse here but pass

directly to the medulla of the adrenal gland, which they innervate.
- *Lesser splanchnic nerve.* The lesser splanchnic nerve arises from thoracic ganglia 9 and 10 (it may some-times arise from 10 and 11) (Williams et al., 1995). It synapses in the aorticorenal ganglion.
- *Least splanchnic nerve.* This nerve originates from the twelfth thoracic ganglion and synapses within ganglia of the renal plexus.

REFERENCES

Akita K et al. (2000). The subclavius posticus muscle: A factor in arterial, venous or brachial plexus compression? *Surg Radiol Anat, 22,* 111-115.

Alvarez O, Roque CT, & Pampati M. (1988). Multilevel thoracic disk herniations: CT and MR studies. *J Comput Assist Tomogr, 12,* 649-652.

Bailey P & Casamajor L. (1911). Osteo-arthritis of the spine as a cause of compression of the spinal cord and its roots. *J Nerv Ment Dis,* 588-609.

Bauduin E et al. (1989). Foraminal herniation of a thoracic calcified nucleus pulposus. *Neuroradiology, 31,* 287-288.

Behrsin JF & Briggs CA. (1988). Ligaments of the lumbar spine: A review. *Surg Radiol Anat, 10,* 211-219.

Bland J. (1987). *Disorders of the cervical spine.* Philadelphia: WB Saunders.

Boyle JJW, Singer KP, & Milne N. (1996). Morphological survey of the cervicothoracic junctional region. *Spine, 21,* 544-548.

Carpintero P et al. (1997). Scoliosis induced by asymmetric lordosis and rotation. *Spine, 22,* 2202-2206.

Cheung MC et al. (2003). Effect of melatonin suppression on scoliosis development in chickens by either constant light or surgical pinealec-tomy. *Spine, 28,* 1941-1944.

Collins JD et al. (1995). Compromising abnormalities of the brachial plexus as displayed by magnetic resonance imaging. *Clin Anat, 8,* 1-16.

Cook SD et al. (1986). Upper extremity proprioception in idiopathic scoliosis. *Clin Orthop, 213,* 118-123.

Cramer G et al. (1996). Identification of the anterior longitudinal ligament on cadaveric spines and comparison with appearance on MRI. *Proc 1996 Internat Conf Spinal Manipulation (ICSM),* Bournemouth, England, October 17-19, 151-152.

Crean JKG et al. (1997). Matrix metalloproteinases in the human interver-tebral disc: Role in disc degeneration and scoliosis. *Spine, 22,* 2877-2884.

Deacon P, Archer J, & Dickson RA. (1987). The anatomy of spinal deformity: A biomechanical analysis. *Orthopedics, 10,* 897-903.

Deane G & Duthie RB. (1973). A new projectional look at articulated scoliotic spines. *Acta Orthop Scand, 44,* 351-365.

Dias RC et al. (1997). Revision spine surgery in children with cerebral palsy. *J Spinal Disord, 10,* 132-144.

Duance VC et al. (1998). Changes in collagen cross linking in degenerative disc disease and scoliosis. *Spine, 23,* 2545-2551.

Dupuis PR et al. (1985). Radiologic diagnosis of degenerative lumbar spinal instability. *Spine, 10,* 262-276.

Edelson JG & Nathan H. (1988). Stages in the natural history of the vertebral end plates. *Spine, 13,* 21-26.

Erwin WM, Jackson PC, & Homonko DA. (2000). Innervation of the human costovertebral joint: Implications for clinical back pain syndromes. *J Manipulative Physiol Ther, 23(6),* 395-403.

Evans SC et al. (1996). MRI of 'idiopathic' juvenile scoliosis: A prospective study. *J Bone Joint Surg [Br], 78-B,* 314-317.

Forcada P et al. (2001). Subclavius posticus muscle: Supernumerary muscle as a potential cause for thoracic outlet syndrome. *Clin Anat, 14,* 55-57.

Foreman SM & Crofts AC. (1988). *Whiplash injuries: The cervical acceleration/deceleration syndrome.* Baltimore: Williams & Wilkins.

Fujimura Y et al. (1997). Long-term follow-up study of anterior decom-pression and fusion for thoracic myelopathy resulting from ossification of the posterior longitudinal ligament. *Spine, 22,* 305-311.

Ghanem IB et al. (1997). Chiari I malformation associated with syringo-myelia and scoliosis. *Spine, 22,* 1313-1318.

Giles LGF. (1987b). Lumbo-sacral zygapophysial joint tropism and its effect on hyaline cartilage. *Clin Biomech, 2,* 2-6.

Goldberg CJ et al. (1995). Adolescent idiopathic scoliosis and cerebral asymmetry. *Spine, 20,* 1685-1691.

Groen GJ et al. (1987). Branches of the thoracic sympathetic trunk in the human fetus. *Anat Embryol, 176*, 401-411.

Hardy PA. (1988). Anatomical variation in the position of the proximal intercostal nerve. *Br J Anaesth, 61*, 338-339.

Harrison DD et al. (2003). Do alterations in vertebral and disc dimensions affect an elliptical model of thoracic kyphosis? *Spine, 28*, 463-469.

Hasue M et al. (1983). Anatomic study of the interrelation between lumbosacral nerve roots and their surrounding tissues. *Spine, 8*, 50-58.

Humzah MD & Soames RW. (1988). Human intervertebral disc: Structure and function. *Anat Rec, 220*, 337-356.

Kanemura T et al. (1997). Natural cause of experimental scoliosis in pinealectomized chickens. *Spine, 22*, 1563-1567.

Karol LA et al. (1993). Progression of the curve in boys who have idiopathic scoliosis. *J Bone Joint Surg, 75-A*, 1804-1810.

Kesling KL & Reinker KA. (1997). Scoliosis in twins: A meta-analysis of the literature and report of six cases. *Spine, 22*, 2009-2014.

Kothe R et al. (1996). Internal architecture of the thoracic pedicle. *Spine, 21*, 264-270.

Krishna M & Upadhyay SS. (1996). Increased limb lengths in patients with shortened spine due to tuberculosis in early childhood. *Spine, 21*, 1045-1047.

Lemire JJ et al. (1996). Scheuermann's's juvenile kyphosis. *J Manipulative Physiol Ther, 19(3)*, 195-201.

Ley F. (1974). Contribution to the study of thoracic vertebral articular cavities between the articular processes. *Arch Anat Hist Embr, 57*, 61-114.

Lipson SJ & O'Connell JX. (1991). A 47-year-old woman with back pain and a lesion in a vertebral body. *N Engl J Med, 325*, 794-799.

Lowe TG et al. (2000). Current concepts review etiology of idiopathic scoliosis: Current trends in research. *J Bone Joint Surg, 82-A*, 1157-1166.

Maigne JY, Maigne R, & Guerin-Surville H. (1991). Upper thoracic dorsal rami: Anatomic study of their medial cutaneous branches. *Surg Radiol Anat, 13*, 109-112.

Marchesi D et al. (1988). Morphometric analysis of the thoracolumbar and lumbar pedicles, anatomico-radiologic study. *Surg Radiol Anat, 10*, 317-322.

McLain RF, Ferrara L, & Kabins M. (2002). Pedicle morphometry in the upper thoracic spine: Limits to safe screw placement in older patients. *Spine, 27*, 2467-2471.

McLain RF & Pickar JG. (1998). Mechanoreceptor endings in human thoracic and lumbar facet joints. *Spine, 23*, 168-173.

Meyer PR. (1972). Contribution to the study of costo-vertebral articular cavities. *Arch Anat Hist Embr, 55*, 283-360.

Moore KL. (1992). *Clinically oriented anatomy* (3rd ed.). Baltimore: Williams & Wilkins.

Nathan H. (1959). The para-articular processes of the thoracic vertebrae. *Anat Rec, 133*, 605-618.

Nathan H. (1962). Osteophytes of the vertebral column: An anatomical study of their development according to age, race, and sex with considerations as to their etiology and significance. *J Bone Joint Surg, 44-A*, 243-268.

Nissinen M et al. (1989). Trunk asymmetry and scoliosis. *Acta Paediatr Scand, 78*, 747-753.

Oda I et al. (1996). Biochemical role of the posterior elements, costovertebral joints, and rib cage in stability of the thoracic spine. *Spine, 21*, 1423-1429.

Oda I et al. (2002). An in vitro human cadaveric study investigating the biomechanical properties of the thoracic spine. *Spine, 27*, E64-E70.

Otani K et al. (1988). Thoracic disc herniation: Surgical treatment in 23 patients. *Spine, 13*, 1262-1267.

Pal GP et al. (1988). Trajectory architecture of the trabecular bone between the body and the neural arch in human vertebrae. *Anat Rec, 222*, 418-425.

Paris S. (1983). Anatomy as related to function and pain. *Orthop Clin North Am, 14*, 476-489.

Pascoe DD et al. (1997). Influence of carrying book bags on gait cycle and posture of youths. *Ergonomics, 40*, 631-641.

Ranney D. (1996). Thoracic outlet: An anatomical redefinition that makes clinical sense. *Clin Anat, 9*, 50-52.

Scapinelli R. (1989). Morphological and functional changes of the lumbar spinous processes in the elderly. *Surg Radiol Anat, 11*, 129-133.

Singer KP & Giles LGF. (1990). Manual therapy considerations at the thoracolumbar junction: An anatomical and functional perspective. *J Manipulative Physiol Ther, 13*, 83-88.

Singer KP, Giles LGF, & Day RE. (1990). Intra-articular synovial folds of thoracolumbar junction zygapophyseal joints. *Anat Rec, 226*, 147-152.

Spapen HD et al. (1990). The straight back syndrome. *Neth J Med, 36*, 29-31.

Theiss SM, Smith MD, & Winter RB. (1997). The long-term follow-up of patients with Klippel-Feil syndrome and congenital scoliosis. *Spine, 22*, 1219-1222.

Upadhyay SS et al. (1991). Disproportionate growth in girls with adolescent idiopathic scoliosis: A longitudinal study. *Spine, 8 (suppl)*, s343-s347.

Vera CL et al. (1997). Paraplegia due to ossification of ligamenta flava in x-linked hypophosphatemia. *Spine, 22*, 710-715.

Vernon L, Dooley J, & Acusta A. (1993). Upper lumbar and thoracic disc pathology: A magnetic resonance imaging analysis. *J Neuromusculo-skeletal Sys, 1*, 59-63.

Viejo-Fuertes D et al. (1998). Morphologic and histologic study of the ligamentum flavum in the thoraco-lumbar region. *Surg Radiol Anat, 20*, 171-176.

Vital J et al. (1989). The neurocentral vertebral cartilage: Anatomy, physiology and physiopathology. *Surg Radiol Anat, 11*, 323-328.

Wang X et al. (1997). Characterization of the scoliosis that develops after pinealectomy in the chicken and comparison with adolescent idiopathic scoliosis in humans. *Spine, 22*, 2626-2635.

White AW & Panjabi MM. (1990). *Clinical biomechanics of the spine.* Philadelphia: JB Lippincott.

Williams PL et al. (1995). *Gray's anatomy* (38th ed.). Edinburgh: Churchill Livingstone.

Woods LA et al. (1995). Decreased incidence of scoliosis in hearing impaired children. *Spine, 20*, 776-781.

Wyatt MP et al. (1986). Vibratory response in idiopathic scoliosis. *J Bone Joint Surg, 68*, 714-718.

Yamashita Y et al. (1990). Spinal cord compression due to ossification of ligaments: MRI imaging. *Radiology, 175*, 843-848.

CHAPTER 7

The Lumbar Region

Gregory D. Cramer

The lumbar portion of the vertebral column has the ideal structure to simultaneously optimize the functions of mobility and stability (Putz and Müller-Gerbl, 1996). This region of the spine is sturdy and is designed to carry the weight of the head, neck, trunk, and upper extremities.

However, pain in the lumbar region is one of the most common complaints of individuals, experienced by approximately 80% of the population at some time in their lives (Nachemson, 1976; Jonsson, 2000). The estimated annual cost for low back pain claims in the U.S. in 1995 was $8.8 billion (Borenstein, 2000) and is undoubtedly greater than that today. The total annual costs of treatment, loss of productivity, and resulting disability are estimated to be more than $28 billion in the United States (Rizzo, Abbott, and Berger, 1998). Low back pain is the most common complaint of patients who go to clinics that deal primarily with musculoskeletal conditions. Low back pain of mechanical origin is the most frequent subtype found in this group (Cramer et al., 1992a). The most common sources of low back pain are the lumbar zygapophysial joints (Z joints) and intervertebral discs (IVDs) (Bogduk, 1985).

Much of the reason for the high incidence of low back pain is probably related to humans being bipedal. Being able to walk on the hind limbs is accompanied by increased freedom of movement and increased ability to interact with the environment, other species, and other members of the same species. Animals that walk on the hind legs (primarily humans) can normally turn their heads with relative ease to look around to both the left and right sides. They also have the ability to use their hands for an almost infinite number of tasks without having to be concerned about using their upper extremities to help maintain balance.

However, the ability to walk on the lower extremities (the bipedal stance) has one significant drawback: Increased stress is placed on the spine. The weight of the body is concentrated on a smaller region compared with quadrupeds. The weight of the human trunk is completely supported by the lower extremities and lumbar spine during standing and it is completely absorbed by

242

the lumbar spine and sacroiliac joints during sitting. Therefore the lumbar region, sacrum, and sacroiliac joints are susceptible to more problems than are encountered by four-legged animals. These problems can be divided into three types of lumbar disorders and sacroiliac joint difficulties:

1. Problems with the lumbar region
   a. *The Z joints* (facet joints; see Figs. 7-3 through 7-6). Increased weight borne by these joints can be a direct cause of back pain. These joints also are susceptible to arthritic changes (e.g., osteoarthritis; arthritis associated with wear and tear).
   b. *The intervertebral disc.* The IVDs absorb most of the increased stress received by the low back in bipeds. The discs may bulge or protrude, and by doing so compress the spinal nerves that exit behind them (see Figs. 7-24, 7-25, 11-10, and 11-11). Such protrusion can result in back pain that also has a sharp radiation pattern into the thigh and sometimes into the leg and foot. This type of pain is frequently described as feeling like a "bolt of lightning" or a "hot poker" (see Chapter 11). The IVDs may undergo degeneration also. This narrows the space between the vertebrae, which may result in arthritic changes and additional pressure on the Z joints (see Chapters 2 and 14). The discs themselves are supplied by sensory nerves and therefore can be a direct source of back pain (i.e., they do not have to compress neural elements to cause back pain).
   c. The muscles of the low back in bipeds are called on to hold the spine erect (erector spinae muscles; see Chapter 4). Therefore when they are required to carry increased loads (this sometimes includes the added weight of a protruding abdomen), these muscles can be torn (strained).
   Note: The lumbosacral region, between L5 and the sacrum, receives the brunt of the biomechanical stress of the biped spine. The lumbosacral joints (interbody joint and left and right Z joints between L5 and the sacrum) are a prime source of low back pain. In addition to the biomechanical stresses, the opening for the spinal nerve at this level is the smallest in the lumbar region, making it particularly vulnerable to IVD protrusions and compression from other sources.
2. The sacroiliac joints are the joints between the sacrum and the left and right ilia. The weight carried in the upright posture also can result in damage to the sacroiliac joint, another source of low back pain (see Chapter 8).

The lumbar region has been the focus of extensive high-quality research because of its clinical importance. Numerous descriptive, quantitative, and experimental studies have been completed on this area of the spine.

This chapter concentrates on the unique characteristics of the lumbar vertebrae and the ligamentous, neural, and vascular elements of the lumbar region. It also includes the most pertinent results of research in an attempt to explain clearly the most important and clinically relevant idiosyncrasies of this intriguing area of the spine.

All the lumbar vertebrae are considered to be typical, although the fifth lumbar vertebra is unique. This chapter presents the typical characteristics of lumbar vertebrae, the lumbar vertebral canal, and the intervertebral foramina (IVFs). A description of the unique characteristics of L5 and the lumbosacral articulation follows. The ranges of motion of the lumbar region are included also. The chapter concludes with a discussion of the nerves, vessels, and related viscera of the lumbar region.

LUMBAR LORDOSIS AND CHARACTERISTICS OF TYPICAL LUMBAR VERTEBRAE

Developmental Considerations and the Lumbar Curve (Lordosis)

The development of lumbar vertebrae is similar to the development of typical vertebrae in other regions of the spine (see Chapter 12). Two additional secondary centers of ossification on each vertebra are unique to the lumbar region. This brings the total number of secondary centers of ossification per lumbar vertebra to seven. These additional centers are located on the posterior aspect of the superior articular processes and develop into the mamillary processes.

Between 2 and 16 years of age, the lumbar vertebrae grow twice as fast as the thoracic vertebrae. Because the anteroposterior curves of these two regions face in opposite directions (thoracic kyphosis versus lumbar lordosis), the posterior elements of thoracic vertebrae probably grow faster than their vertebral bodies; the reverse (lumbar vertebral bodies grow faster than their posterior elements) is true in the lumbar region (Clarke et al., 1985).

Normally the lumbar lordosis is more prominent than the cervical lordosis. The lumbar lordosis extends from T12 to the L5 IVD, and the greatest portion of the curve occurs between L3 and L5 (Fig. 7-1). The lumbar lordosis is created by the increased height of the anterior aspect of both the lumbar vertebral bodies and the lumbar IVDs, with the discs contributing more to the lordosis than the increased height of the vertebral bodies.

Either an increase or decrease of the lumbar lordosis may contribute to low back pain (Mosner et al., 1989). This has sparked an interest in measurement of the lumbar curve; as a result, the lumbar curve has been measured in a variety of ways. One method, developed by Mosner et al. (1989), used measurements from lateral

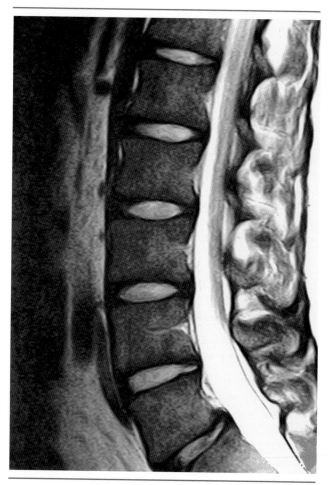

FIG. 7-1 Magnetic resonance imaging scan demonstrating the lumbar lordosis.

x-ray films taken with the patient in the supine position. A line was drawn across the superior vertebral end plate of L2 and another across the superior aspect of the sacral body. These two lines were continued posteriorly until they intersected, and the angle between them was measured. Using this method, an angle of 47 and 43 degrees was found to be normal for women and men, respectively. This is in agreement with the values given by other authors (Williams et al., 1995).

Another relatively common method of measuring the lumbar lordosis calls for passing a line across the superior aspect of the body of L1 and another such line across the body of the first sacral segment, and then measuring the angle formed by the intersection of the continuation of the two lines. However, care must be taken when making such measurements. Normally the first lumbar vertebral body is slightly taller anteriorly than posteriorly; however, a relatively frequent anomaly is for the first lumbar vertebral body to be wedge shaped, so that it is shorter anteriorly than posteriorly. Such wedging of the vertebra being used as a landmark

for measurement can cause significant variation of measurements of the lumbar lordosis (Worril and Peterson, 1997).

In the past, many clinicians incorrectly assumed that the lumbar lordosis in the black population was greater than that in the white population, but this has been found to be incorrect; the lordosis is approximately the same in both races (Mosner et al., 1989).

Clinical Considerations. Certain individuals develop a painful degenerative lumbar kyphosis that is characterized by disc and vertebral body wedging and weakness of lumbar paraspinal muscles. This condition may be related to a prolonged working posture in flexion. For example, a higher incidence of this condition has been found in Japanese dairy farmers when compared with Japanese field farmers. The working posture of the former group calls for long periods of forward flexion while squatting. This posture is maintained for the majority of each working day throughout the workers' careers, which can last for many decades (Takemitsu et al., 1988). Such prolonged flexion is thought to cause remodeling of the vertebral bodies of the lumbar region so that they are shorter anteriorly than posteriorly.

The lumbar lordosis is often significantly increased in achondroplasia. This can lead to a marked compensatory thoracic (thoracolumbar) kyphosis, which can be severe in some cases (Giglio et al., 1988).

A high incidence of scoliosis (64%) exists in the lumbar region of individuals with Marfan syndrome. Other lumbar vertebral anomalies associated with Marfan syndrome include a high incidence of transitional lumbosacral segments (18%), concavity of both the superior and inferior aspects of the vertebral bodies (biconcavity), and longer than normal transverse processes (Tallroth et al., 1995).

Vertebral Bodies

When viewed from above, the vertebral bodies of the lumbar spine are large and kidney shaped with the concavity facing posteriorly (Fig. 7-2). However, L5 is more elliptical in shape. In addition, the inferior and superior bony end plates of adjacent vertebrae sharing the same IVD are similar in size and shape. Although the lumbar vertebral bodies of males generally have greater dimensions than those of females, the shapes of the vertebral bodies are similar (Hall et al., 1998). The superior surfaces of the vertebral bodies possess small elevations along their posterior rim. These represent remnants of the uncinate processes of the cervical region. The inferior surfaces of the vertebral bodies have two small notches along their posterior rim. These notches correspond to the uncinate-like elevations of the vertebra below. These elevations and notches have been used as landmarks on x-ray films as a means for evaluating normal and abnormal movement between adjacent lumbar segments (Dupuis et al., 1985).

The vertebral bodies are wider from side to side (lateral width) than from front to back and are taller in front (anteriorly) than behind. Therefore as mentioned, the vertebral bodies are partially responsible for the creation and maintenance of the lumbar lordosis.

Normally the lateral width of the lumbar vertebrae increases from L1 to L3. L4 and L5 are somewhat variable in width (Williams et al., 1995). Ericksen (1976, 1978) found that the L1-4 vertebral bodies (he did not study L5) became wider from side to side with age. Also, he noted a decrease in height of the vertebral body's anterior aspect, corresponding with an increase in its lateral width, in both males and females. Further, the increase in lateral width in males was accompanied by a corresponding decrease in height of the vertebral body's posterior aspect (Erickson, 1976, 1978).

Up to 90% of the compressive loads received by the vertebral bodies are carried by the inner cancellous (trabecular) bone (Silva, Keaveny, and Hayes, 1997); however, this may be an overestimation (Cao, Grimm, and Yang, 2001). The remaining 10% (or more) of the compressive loads are carried by the thin outer cortical shell of the vertebral bodies (Silva, Keaveny, and Hayes, 1997). However, with the bone loss associated with osteoporosis a higher percentage of the compressive loads are carried by the outer extra cortical shell of bone (Cao, Grimm, and Yang, 2001).

Perhaps somewhat paradoxically, the bony end plates of the vertebral bodies are particularly important in resisting compressive loads placed on the spine. Oxland et al. (2003) found that removal of the bony end plates decreased the ability of the vertebral bodies to resist compression fracture by 66%. The end plates of the lumbar region are weakest in the center, and strongest posterolaterally. In addition, the inferior end plates are stronger than the superior ones, and the sacral end plate is similar in strength to the inferior lumbar bony end plates (Grant, Oxland, and Dvorak, 2001).

The blood supply to the lumbar vertebral bodies is extensive and complex (Bogduk, 1997). Each lumbar segmental artery gives off up to 20 primary periosteal arteries as it courses across the anterolateral aspect of the vertebral body. The posterior aspect is supplied by many branches of the anterior vertebral canal artery. The anterior vertebral canal artery refers to the anterior branch of the artery that passes through the IVF. The artery that passes through the IVF sometimes is known as the spinal ramus of the (lumbar) segmental artery.

The end branches of periosteal arteries form a ring around both the superior and inferior margins of the vertebral body. These rings are known as the metaphyseal anastomoses (superior and inferior). They not only help to supply the metaphyseal region of the vertebral body, but also send penetrating branches (metaphyseal arteries) to the region of the vertebral end plate (Bogduk, 1997). A dense capillary network is associated with the superior and inferior vertebral end plates. This network receives contributions from the metaphyseal and nutrient arteries.

Nutrient arteries also arise from the anterior vertebral canal arteries. The nutrient arteries enter the center of the posterior aspect of the vertebral body, pass deep within the substance of the cancellous bone of the vertebral body's center, and then give off superior (ascending) and inferior (descending) branches. In addition to giving off periosteal arteries, the lumbar segmental arteries also send branches that enter the cancellous bone of the anterior and lateral aspects of the vertebral bodies. These branches enter along the superior-to-inferior midpoint of the vertebral bodies. Known as the equatorial arteries, these vessels are similar to the nutrient arteries in that they also give rise to ascending and descending branches deep within the substance of the vertebral bodies (Bogduk, 1997). See Chapter 2 and Figure 2-3 for further details on the blood supply to and venous drainage of typical vertebrae.

The lumbar vertebral bodies serve as attachment sites for several structures. Table 7-1 lists those structures that attach to the lumbar vertebral bodies.

Clinical Considerations. Osteophytes of the lumbar vertebral bodies can be large. They are much more prominent laterally than anteriorly (the opposite of what is commonly found in the thoracic region), and usually they are completely absent anteriorly at the L3-4 and L4-5 levels. This seems to be associated with the pulsing action of the abdominal aorta and proximal portions of the common iliac arteries (Edelson and Nathan, 1988).

Fractures of the secondary centers of ossification associated with the superior and inferior vertebral end plates, the ring apophyses (sometimes known as anular apophyses; see Chapters 2 and 12), have been reported. These fractures are rare but occur most frequently during adolescence. The signs and symptoms of apophyseal ring fractures resemble those of IVD protrusions. Such fractures may go unnoticed on conventional x-ray films. Sagittally reformatted computed tomography (CT) is currently the imaging modality that shows these fractures to best advantage (Thiel, Clements, and Cassidy, 1992).

Pedicles

The pedicles of the lumbar spine are short but strong (see Fig. 7-2). They attach lower on the vertebral bodies than the pedicles of the thoracic region, but higher than those of the cervical region. Therefore each lumbar vertebra

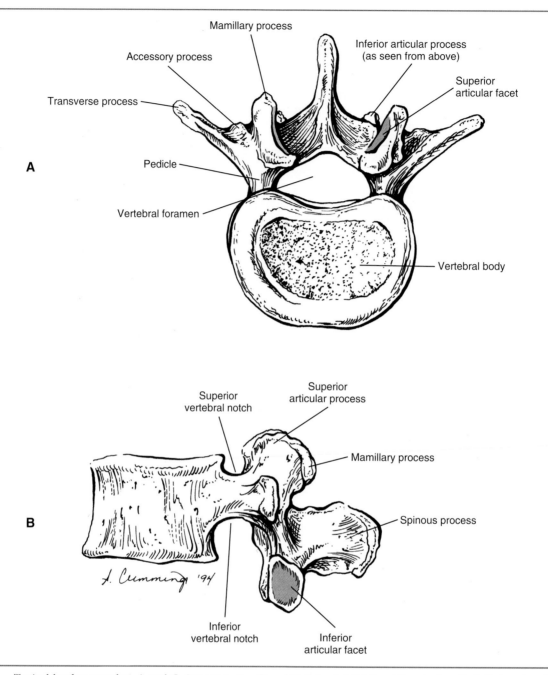

FIG. 7-2   Typical lumbar vertebra. **A** and **C**, Superior view. **B** and **E**, Lateral (slightly oblique) view. **D**, Inferior view. **F**, posterior view. Notice in **C** that the superior articular process of this typical vertebral is concave posteriorly; also notice the labeled nutrient foramen (one of many) located at the junction of the pedicle and transverse process. Notice in **E** the superior vertebral notch located above the pedicle.

has a superior vertebral notch that is less distinct than that of the cervical region. On the other hand, the inferior vertebral notch of lumbar vertebrae is prominent.

The size of the pedicles, like the size of many spinal structures, can vary among individuals of different ethnic backgrounds. Such normal ethnic variations should be kept in mind when evaluating x-ray films and CT or magnetic resonance imaging (MRI) scans. For example,

the length of the pedicles of individuals of East Indian descent is less than that of whites (Mitra, Datir, and Jadhav, 2002).

The role of the pedicles in the transfer of loads is discussed in Chapter 2. More study is needed to confirm the role played by the pedicles in the transfer of loads in the upper lumbar region (Pal et al., 1988). However, the trabecular pattern of the L4 and L5 pedicles seems to

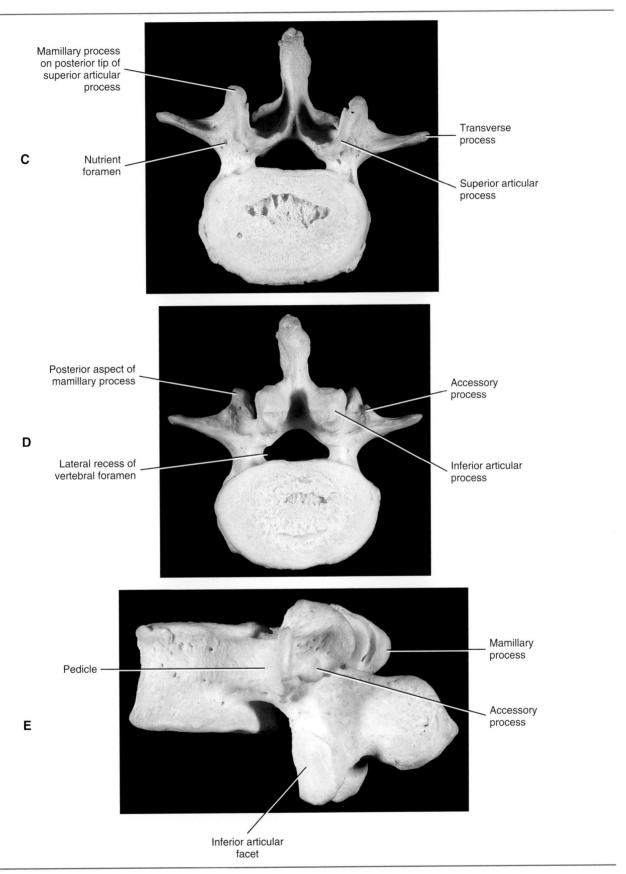

C

Mamillary process on posterior tip of superior articular process

Nutrient foramen

Transverse process

Superior articular process

D

Posterior aspect of mamillary process

Lateral recess of vertebral foramen

Accessory process

Inferior articular process

E

Pedicle

Inferior articular facet

Mamillary process

Accessory process

FIG. 7-2—cont'd

Continued

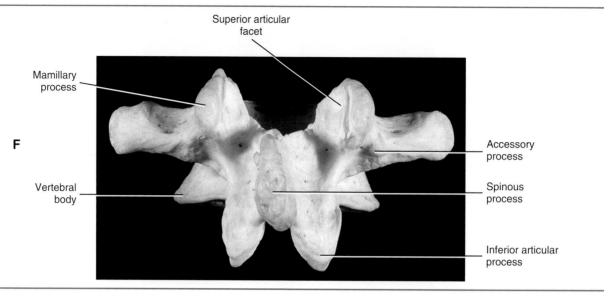

FIG. 7-2—cont'd

Table 7-1	Attachments to Lumbar Vertebral Bodies
Region	**Structure(s) Attached**
Anterior surface	Anterior longitudinal ligament on superior and inferior borders
Posterior surface	Posterior longitudinal ligament on superior and inferior borders
Lateral surface	Crura of the diaphragm (anterolateral surface of left L1 and L2 and right L1, L2, and L3)
	Origin of the psoas major muscle (posterolateral aspect of superior and inferior surface of all lumbars); a series of tendinous arches between vertebral attachments of the psoas major muscle creates concave openings between arches and vertebral bodies, allowing for passage of segmental arteries, veins, and gray communicating rami of sympathetic chain.

From Williams PL et al. (1995). *Gray's anatomy* (38th ed.). Edinburgh: Churchill Livingstone.

indicate that most loads placed on these vertebrae may be transferred from the vertebral bodies to the region of the posterior arch, specifically to the pars interarticularis (see Laminae).

Transverse Processes

Each transverse process (TP) (left and right) of a typical lumbar vertebra projects posterolaterally from the junction of the pedicle and the lamina of the same side (see Fig. 7-2). It lies in front of (anterior to) the articular processes and behind (posterior to) the lumbar IVF.

The lumbar TPs are quite long, the TPs of L3 being the longest. The distance between the apices of the left and right TPs is much greater on L1 than T12. This distance increases on L2 and is the greatest in the entire spine on L3. The intertransverse distance between the left and right L4 TPs is smaller than that of L3 and is even smaller for L5. The lumbar TPs are flat and thin from front to back. They are also narrower from superior to inferior than their thoracic counterparts. They possess neither articular facets (as do thoracic TPs) nor foramina of the transverse processes (as do cervical TPs). The anterior aspect of the lumbar TPs also are known as the costal elements, and they occasionally develop into ribs. This happens most frequently at L1.

The lateral aspect of the anterior surface of the lumbar TPs is creased by a ridge that runs from superior to inferior. This ridge is created by the anterior layer of the thoracolumbar fascia. The middle layer of the thoracolumbar fascia attaches to the apex of the TPs. Table 7-2 lists structures that attach to the lumbar TPs.

Accessory Processes. The accessory processes are unique to the lumbar spine. Each accessory process projects posteriorly from the junction of the posterior and inferior aspect of the TP with the corresponding lamina. These processes serve as attachment sites for the longissimus thoracis muscles (lumbar fibers) and the medial intertransversarii lumborum muscles (Williams et al., 1995). (See Figure 4-5, *B*, for the attachment of the medial intertransversarii lumborum muscles to the accessory processes.)

Table 7-2   Attachments to Lumbar Transverse Processes

Region	Structure(s) Attached
Anterior surface	Psoas major and quadratus lumborum muscles
	Anterior layer of thoracolumbar fascia (separates psoas major and quadratus lumborum muscles)
	Medial and lateral arcuate ligaments (lumbocostal arches) (L1)
Apex	Middle layer of thoracolumbar fascia
	Iliolumbar ligament (L5, occasionally L4)
Superior border	Lateral intertransversarius muscle
Inferior border	Lateral intertransversarius muscle
Posterior surface	Deep back muscles (longissimus thoracis)

From Williams PL et al. (1995). *Gray's anatomy* (38th ed.). Edinburgh: Churchill Livingstone.

Articular Processes

Superior Articular Processes. Left and right superior articular processes are formed on every vertebrae of the lumbar spine (see Fig. 7-2). Each superior articular process possesses a hyaline cartilage–lined superior articular facet that is oriented in a vertical plane. That is, these facets are not angled to the vertical plane like the superior articular facets of the cervical and thoracic regions.

All the lumbar superior articular facets face posteriorly and medially. The articular surface of a typical superior articular facet can be gently curved with the concavity facing medially (Figs. 7-3 and 7-4), or the articular surface can be angled abruptly. When the articular surface is angled abruptly, two relatively distinct articulating surfaces are formed. One surface faces posteriorly and forms almost a 90-degree angle with the second surface, which faces medially. As with the curved facet,

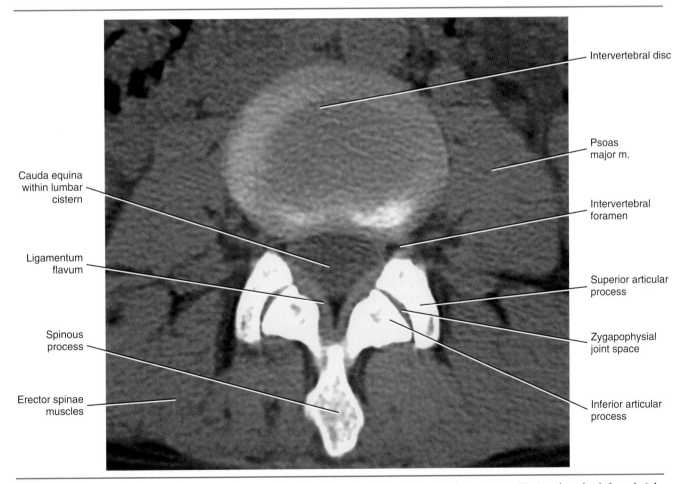

Intervertebral disc

Psoas major m.

Intervertebral foramen

Superior articular process

Zygapophysial joint space

Inferior articular process

Cauda equina within lumbar cistern

Ligamentum flavum

Spinous process

Erector spinae muscles

FIG. 7-3 Horizontal computed tomography scan showing the orientation of the lumbar Z joints. Notice that the left and right superior articular processes face posteriorly and medially. (Image courtesy Dr. Dennis Skogsbergh.)

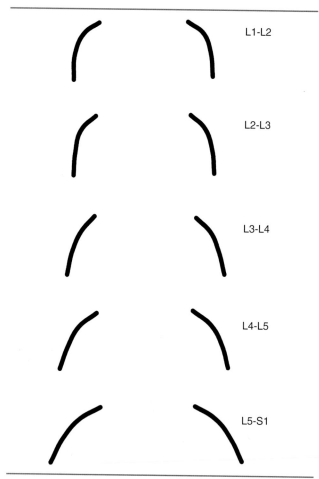

FIG. 7-4   Orientation of lumbar Z joints. Notice the changes from L1-2 to L5-S1. (From Taylor JR & Twomey LT. (1986). Age changes in lumbar zygapophyseal joints: Observations on structure and function. *Spine, 11*, 739-745.)

the concavity faces posteriorly and medially. In either case (curved or angled articular surface), the shape conforms almost perfectly to the inferior articular facet of the vertebra above. The hyaline cartilage of the central region of the superior articular facet (the area of greatest concavity) increases in thickness with age, probably because this region receives much of the load during flexion of the spine (Taylor and Twomey, 1986). Also, the articular processes may fracture as a result of age-related degeneration (Kirkaldy-Willis et al., 1978).

The orientation of the superior articular facets varies from one vertebral level to another (see Fig. 7-4). A line passed across each superior articular facet, on transverse CT scans, shows that the L4 superior facets (and therefore the L3-4 Z joints) are more sagittally oriented than the L5 facets. Also, the S1 superior facets (and therefore the L5-S1 Z joints) are more coronally oriented than the L4 and L5 facets (Van Schaik, Verbiest, and Van Schaik, 1985). (See Zygapophysial Joints for further detail

on the orientation of the superior and inferior articular facets.)

The mamillary processes (see Fig. 7-2), which project posteriorly from the superior articular processes of lumbar vertebrae, are unique to the lumbar spine. Each mamillary process is a small rounded mound of variable size. Some are almost indistinguishable, whereas others are relatively prominent. The mamillary processes serve as attachment sites for the multifidi lumborum muscles.

Mamillo-Accessory Ligament.   A mamillo-accessory ligament (Bogduk, 1981; Lippitt, 1984) is found between the mamillary and accessory processes on the left and right sides of each lumbar vertebra. Occasionally one or more of these ligaments may ossify in the lower lumbar levels (L3-5). The incidence of ossification increases in frequency from L3 to L5. Ossification of these ligaments at L5 occurs at a frequency of 10% (Bogduk, 1981) to 26% (Maigne, Maigne, and Guervin-Surville, 1991). Maigne, Maigne, and Guervin-Surville (1991) studied 203 lumbar spines and found that ossification of this ligament at L5 occurred twice as often on the left. They gave no reason why the ligament ossified more frequently on this side. However, they believed the ossification was the result of osteoarthritis, because they found no evidence of ossification on the spines of children and young adults. These authors also stated that an ossified mamillo-accessory ligament could occasionally be seen on standard lumbar x-ray films.

The mamillo-accessory ligament has been described as a tough, fibrous band that may represent tendinous fibers of origin of the lumbar multifidi muscles or fibers of insertion of the longissimus thoracis pars lumborum muscle (Bogduk, 1981). Regardless of its precise structure, the reported purpose of the mamillo-accessory "ligament" is to hold the medial branch of the dorsal ramus of the above spinal nerve (e.g., the L2 medial branch is associated with the L3 mamillo-accessory ligament) against (a) the bone between the base of the superior articular process and the base of the transverse process, and (b) the Z joint, which is slightly more medial (Fig. 7-5). The medial branch of the dorsal ramus gives off articular branches to the capsule of the Z joint as it passes deep to the mamillo-accessory ligament. The medial branch then continues medially across the vertebral lamina to reach the multifidus muscle (Bogduk, 1981). Therefore the medial branch of the dorsal ramus (posterior primary division) is held within a small osteofibrous canal along the posterior arch of a lumbar vertebra. The medial branch could possibly become irritated or even entrapped within this tunnel, which would result in low back pain. However, more investigation is necessary to determine if such irritation or entrapment occurs and, if so, its frequency (Bogduk, 1981; Maigne, Maigne, and Guerin-Surville, 1991).

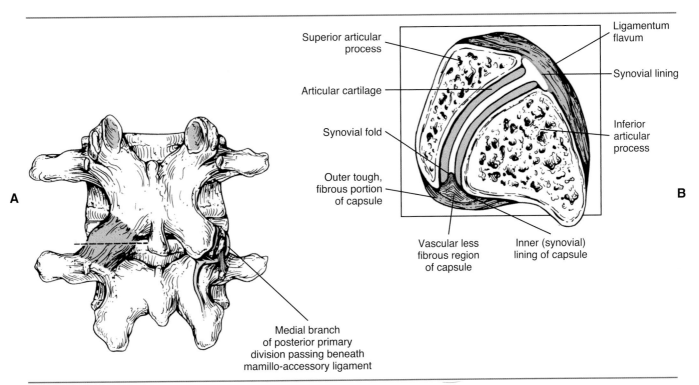

FIG. 7-5   The lumbar Z joints. **A,** Joint capsule *(left)*. Mamillo-accessory ligament and its relationship to the medial branch of the dorsal ramus of the spinal nerve *(right)*. **B,** Cross section through the left Z joint at the level of the dotted line shown in **A.** Notice the ligamentum flavum anteriorly and the Z joint capsule posteriorly. The lateral aspect of the capsule blends with the articular cartilage, and the medial aspect extends for a considerable distance along the posterior aspect of the inferior articular process. Also notice that a synovial fold can be seen extending into the joint space.

Inferior Articular Processes. The inferior articular processes of lumbar vertebrae are convex anteriorly and laterally. They possess inferior articular facets that cover their anterolateral surface. As with the superior articular facets, the inferior ones vary in shape. Even though articular processes vary from one vertebral level to another, and even from one side to another, superior and inferior articulating processes of one Z joint conform to one another. This conformation is such that each inferior articular facet usually fits remarkably well into the posterior and medial concavity of the adjoining superior articular facet.

Zygapophysial Joints

General Considerations. The Z joints have been positively identified as a source of back pain (Mooney and Robertson, 1976; Yamashita et al., 1990; Bogduk, 1992; Dreyfuss and Dreyer, 2001). In addition, Rauschning (1987) states that these joints "display typical degenerative and reparative changes which are known to cause osteoarthritic pain in peripheral synovial joints." Therefore the lumbar Z joints are highly significant clinically. Because these joints are discussed in detail in Chapter 2,

this section focuses on the unique and clinically significant aspects of the lumbar Z joints.

The lumbar Z joints are considered to be complex synovial joints oriented in the vertical plane (Williams et al., 1995). They are fashioned according to the shape of the superior and inferior articular facets (see previous discussion). Therefore the lumbar Z joints are concave posteriorly and even have been described as being biplanar in orientation (Taylor and Twomey, 1986). That is, they have a coronally oriented, posterior-facing, anteromedial component and a large, sagittally oriented, medial-facing, posterolateral component. Taylor and Twomey (1986) state that the lumbar Z joints are coronally oriented in children and that the large sagittal component develops as the individual matures. The sagittal component limits rotation, whereas the coronal component limits flexion. More specifically, the shape of the lumbar Z joints allows a large amount of flexion to occur in the lumbar region, yet the size of the lumbar Z joints is what eventually limits flexion at the end of the normal range of motion. Therefore the long contact surfaces between the coronal component of the superior articular processes and the adjacent inferior articular processes finally limit flexion by "restraining the forward translational component of flexion" (Taylor and Twomey, 1986).

Even though the size of the Z joints eventually limits flexion, approximately 60 degrees of flexion is able to occur in the lumbar region before the bony restraints of the lumbar articular processes prevent further movement. However, the size and shape of the Z joints dramatically limit rotation. By limiting rotation, the Z joints protect the IVDs from rotational injury. During rotation of the lumbar region, distraction (or gapping) occurs between adjacent lumbar articular facets (superior facet of vertebra below and inferior facet of vertebra above) on the side of rotation. For example, right rotation results in gapping of the facets on the right side. Also during rotation, the two opposing facets of the opposite side are pressed together. This causes them to act as a fulcrum for the distracting facets on the side of rotation (Paris, 1983; Cramer et al., 2003). Side posture spinal adjusting, performed by chiropractors and other health practitioners, also causes gapping of the Z joints. The gapping action produced by such adjustive procedures is thought to break-up fibrous adhesions that develop in Z joints that are moving less than normal (are hypomobile) (Cramer et al., 2000, 2002, 2003).

Extension of the lumbar region is limited by the inferior articular process on each side of a lumbar vertebra contacting the junction between the lamina and superior articular process of the vertebra below. This junction between the lamina and superior articular process is known as the pars interarticularis.

Variation of Zygapophysial Joint Size and Shape.

A considerable degree of variation exists between individual Z joints at different lumbar levels and the left and right Z joints at the same vertebral level. The shapes range from a slight and gentle curve, concave posteriorly, to a pronounced, dramatic, posteriorly concave curve, and in some cases to a joint in which the posterior and medial components face one another at an angle of nearly 90 degrees. Generally, the Z joints of the upper lumbar levels are more sagittally oriented than those of the lower lumbar levels (see Fig. 7-4). This makes the lower lumbar joints more susceptible to recurrent rotational strain (Kirkaldy-Willis et al., 1978).

Biomechanical Considerations.

The articular facets do not absorb any of the compressive forces of the spine when humans are sitting erect or standing in a slightly flexed posture. The IVD and vertebral bodies absorb almost all the compressive loads under these conditions. However, when standing erect (slight extension), the facets resist approximately 16% (range, 3% to 25%) of the compressive forces between vertebrae. Disc degeneration may lead to increased stress on the Z joints, causing them to resist up to approximately 47% of the

loads. This results in pain, not from the articular cartilage, but usually from pressure on the subchondral bone of the articular processes, soft tissue being caught between the articular facets, or added strain on the articular capsules (Dunlop, Adams, and Hutton, 1984; Yang and King, 1984; Hutton, 1990). In addition, beyond the limit of normal physiologic flexion, the inferior articular process is forced over the superior articular process, and the compressive loads carried by the facets again increase from those carried in the neutral position (Shirazi-Adl and Drouin, 1987).

The superior and inferior articular processes of the Z joints also resist anterior shear forces. The articular processes carry approximately one third of the anterior shear forces during forward flexion, whereas the IVDs carry approximately two thirds of the shear loads (when the load is applied suddenly). However, because of the viscoelasticity of the IVD, if a shear load is applied slowly, the vertebra above creeps further forward than when shear loads are applied rapidly. Thus the shear forces on the articular processes are increased with slowly applied and long-lasting loads in forward flexion (e.g., bending forward for long periods to weed a garden).

Articular Capsules.

An articular capsule covers the posterior aspect of each lumbar Z joint (see Fig. 7-5), and the ligamentum flavum covers the anteromedial aspect of the Z joint. The articular capsule is tough, possesses a rich sensory innervation, and is well vascularized (Giles and Taylor, 1987; Ashton et al., 1992).

The bundles of collagen fibers that form the thick outer fibrous layer of a typical lumbar Z joint capsule are oriented in different directions, depending on whether the fibers are located in the superior, middle, or inferior aspect of the capsule. The superior fibers attached laterally to the groove that is located between the mamillary process and posterior ridge of the superior articular process. From here the fibers of the superior capsule course medially across the superior joint recess, attaching to the medial aspect of the laminae of the superiormost vertebrae forming the Z joint. Fibers of the middle part of the Z joint capsule course more horizontally (lateral to medial), beginning from their attachment to the posterior aspect of the mamillary process (on the posterior aspect of the superior articular process) (Yamashita et al., 1996). These fibers then cross the Z joint gap and attach to the medial part of the lamina of the suprajacent vertebra. The fibers just described extend a considerable distance medially and become continuous with the lateral fibers of the interspinous ligament. Finally, the fibers of the more inferior aspect of the capsule course from superomedial to inferolateral, covering the joint space and the inferior end of the inferior Z joint recess. The superomedial fibers attach to the medial and inferior part of the lamina. The bundles of collagen fibers of this inferior aspect of the capsule are longer and thicker than those of the superior aspect of the capsule (Yamashita et al., 1996).

The orientation of the fibers within the tough outer layer of the capsule helps to limit forward flexion (Paris, 1983). The medial to lateral arrangement of the fibers in the central part of the Z joint may tend to stabilize the joint during axial rotation, while allowing movement in flexion and extension (Yamashita et al., 1996). The contribution of the lumbar Z joint capsule to stabilize and perhaps even helping to limit motion during axial rotation also has been supported by biochemical studies that show evidence of increased capsular resistance to tension in regions of the capsule that would receive the greatest stretch during this motion (Boszczyk et al., 2001). The collagen fibers of the superior and middle aspects of the Z joint are shorter than those of the inferior aspect of the capsule and are thought to be under more tensile stretch than the inferior aspect of the capsule. The posterosuperomedial-most corner of capsule (just inferior to the superior Z joint recess) is thought to be the area of the capsule that receives the highest tensile stretch (Yamashita et al., 1996). In fact, Yamashita et al. (1996) stated that the lumbar Z joint capsules undergo "extensive stretch under physiological loads."

The collagen fibers of the inferior aspect of the lumbar Z joint capsules are thicker and more heavily innervated than the superior and middle aspects of the capsules. This may be because the inferior aspects of the capsule can be compressed (therefore requiring increased thickness), and even pinched (thus resulting in pain from additional nociceptive nerve endings), during full extension of the lumbar region (Yamashita et al., 1996).

Laterally, fibers of each articular capsule frequently are continuous with the articular cartilage lining the superior articular facet. A gradual transition occurs from the fibrous tissue of the capsule to fibrocartilage and finally to the hyaline cartilage of the superior articular facet (Taylor and Twomey, 1986).

Each capsule has a relatively large superior and inferior recess that extends away from the joint. The capsular fibers (or fibers of the ligamentum flavum, anteriorly) surrounding these recesses are relatively thin and loose, and there may be openings through which neurovascular bundles enter the recesses (Taylor and Twomey, 1986). Paris (1983) states that effusion within the Z joint may enter the superior recess and as little as 0.5 ml of effusion may cause the superior recess to enter the anteriorly located IVF. Once in the IVF, this expanded superior capsular recess may compress the dorsal root ganglion or the exiting spinal nerve, resulting in radiculopathy (see Chapter 11 for a full discussion of radiculopathy). Such a distinct protrusion of the superior recess of the Z joint capsule constitutes an example of a large Z joint synovial cyst (Xu et al., 1991; Bougie, Franco, and Segil, 1996).

Xu et al. (1991), in a study of 50 pairs of lumbar Z joints from an elderly population, found that the capsules varied greatly in thickness and regularity. They found that the capsules were "irregularly thickened, amorphous, and calcified in 22 cases." In addition, they found that in most subjects the synovium of the joint space extended 1 to 2 mm outside the boundaries of the joint in one or more locations. These synovial extensions, which could be considered to be small synovial cysts, maintained communication with the joint space, and were found on both the anterior and posterior aspects of the joint. Anteriorly the spaces most often extended along the posterior border of the ligamentum flavum (64% of Z joints). Sometimes a synovial joint extension extended directly into the ligamentum flavum (8% of cases). Posteriorly the synovial cysts usually extended either laterally along the superior articular process (7% of cases) or medially along the inferior articular process (29%). Extensions were found on both the inferior and superior articular processes in 41% of the Z joints, and no synovial extensions were found in 23% (7% of individuals) of the Z joints. Xu et al. (1991) believed that the synovial joint extensions (synovial cysts) probably were more common in the older population (e.g., the specimens in their study) than in younger age groups. They stated that their findings may explain why Z joint arthrography (visualization of the Z joint after injection with radiopaque dye) could be successful even when the joint space was not entered with the injecting needle (i.e., the needle could enter a synovial extension).

In another study, Xu, Haughton, and Carrera (1990) visualized the synovial joint extensions (cysts) with MRI. Their positive identification of these synovial joint extensions was aided with the injection of paramagnetic contrast medium (gadodiamide, Winthrop Pharmaceuticals). Their imaging was performed on dissected spines using small surface coils, long acquisition times, and thin slice thicknesses. Therefore clear delineation of these extensions is probably still beyond the resolving capabilities of MRI scans obtained in a typical clinical setting. However, Xu et al. (1991) thought their results helped to explain the variable appearance of the facet joints on MRI scans. They stated that "the inhomogeneity detected at MR imaging and computerized tomography in the ligamentum flavum near the facet joint most likely represents extension of the joint capsule between the ligamentum flavum and the articular processes. . . ." (Xu et al., 1991).

The superior and inferior recesses are filled with fibrofatty pads. These pads are well vascularized and are lined with a synovial membrane. They also protrude a significant distance into the superior and inferior aspects of the Z joint. Engel and Bogduk (1982) state that adipose tissue pads probably develop from undifferentiated mesenchyme of the embryologic Z joint. Furthermore, they note that in certain instances, mechanical stress to the joint may cause an adipose tissue pad to undergo fibrous metaplasia, which results in the formation of a large fibroadipose meniscoid (an adipose tissue pad with a fibrous tip composed of dense connective tissue). The authors believed that both the adipose tissue pads and the normally found synovial folds, or meniscoids, "play some form of normal functional role" (see Fig. 7-5).

In addition, "fringes" of synovium extend from the capsule to the region between the articular facets. These fringes fill the small region in which the facets do not completely come together.

Sometimes a fatty synovial fold develops a relatively long fibrous tip that extends a considerable distance between the joint surfaces, where it may become compressed (Taylor and Twomey, 1986). Such protruding synovial folds have been associated with the early stages of degeneration (Rauschning, 1987). Rauschning (1987) typically found hemarthrosis and effusion into the Z joints when the meniscal folds of this type were torn or "nipped" between the joint surfaces.

Occasionally a piece of articular cartilage breaks from the superior or inferior articular facet as humans age. The piece usually breaks along the posterior aspect of the Z joint, parallel to the joint space. However, the attachment to the articular capsule usually is maintained. The result is the presence of a large, fibrocartilaginous meniscoid inclusion within the joint. Taylor and Twomey (1986) reported that the formation of this type of meniscoid is partially caused by the regular pulling action on the posterior articular capsule by the multifidi muscles that originate from these capsules. The attachment of the capsule to the periphery of the articular cartilage may then result in the cartilage tears found to run parallel with the joint surface. Again, the torn cartilage fragment is capable of developing into a Z joint meniscoid, which can become interposed between the two surfaces of the joint. The authors also noted that the posterior aspect of the Z joint may open when the multifidi and other deep back muscles relax, allowing the meniscoids and other joint inclusions to bow into the joint space and become entrapped. The result of this type of entrapment could be (a) loss of motion (locked back), resulting from the cartilage being lodged between two opposing joint surfaces; (b) pain, because the meniscoids remain attached and therefore might put traction on the pain-sensitive joint capsule; or (c) both decreased motion and pain.

As described in Chapter 2, the Z joint articular capsule receives sensory innervation from the medial branch of the posterior primary division of three consecutive spinal nerves. Using nerve tracing techniques in rats, Suseki et al. (1997) found that some sensory neurons innervating the lower lumbar Z joint capsules arise from the L1 and L2 dorsal root ganglia. These sensory fibers course through the lumbar sympathetic chain and then through gray communicating rami to reach the lower lumbar Z joints. These authors felt that this innervation of lower lumbar spinal tissues by sensory nerves arising from upper lumbar dorsal root ganglia might help to explain the clinical finding that pathology of lower lumbar spinal tissues sometimes can be described by patients as referring to regions innervated by higher lumbar segments (e.g., radiation into the inguinal region from a painful L5-S1 Z joint).

The pain-sensitive articular capsule and the synovial lining of the ligamentum flavum of each lumbar Z joint normally are held out of the joint by three structures. First, the multifidus lumborum muscles take part of their origin (several originate from each vertebra) from the posterior aspect of each articular capsule (Taylor and Twomey, 1986). These muscles pull the capsule out of the joint's posterior aspect. Second, the ligamentum flavum pulls the synovium out of the joint's anterior aspect. Third, when the joint surfaces are compressed, the Z joint synovial folds push the capsule out of the joint (Paris, 1983). If either of the two mechanisms associated with the articular capsule fails to function properly, the result could be painful pinching of the capsule, with subsequent acute low back pain and muscle tightness (spasm).

In addition, recall that the Z joint folds possess nociceptive fibers (Giles, 1987a, 1988; Giles and Taylor, 1987). Consequently, entrapment within a Z joint of these innervated folds may be a primary source of back pain and muscle tightness (spasm) even without traction of the capsule. Chapter 2 describes Z joint synovial folds and other Z joint inclusions in further detail.

Narrowing of the IVD space results in increased pressure on the articulating surfaces of the Z joint. This pressure is further increased with extension of the lumbar region. Disc space narrowing also causes or increases the severity of impingement of synovial folds. Therefore increased pressure on the subchondral bone of the articular processes and increased impingement of articular tissues (soft-tissue "nipped" between the facets) may be two causes of back pain in patients with decreased height of one or more IVDs (Dunlop, Adams, and Hutton, 1984).

Zygapophysial Joint Degeneration. A strong correlation has been found between increasing age and degeneration of the Z joints (Peterson, Boulton, and Wood, 2000). Kirkaldy-Willis et al. (1978) stated that such changes include inflammatory reaction of the synovial lining of the Z joint, changes of the articular cartilage, loose bodies in the Z joint, and laxity of the joint capsule.

All these result in joint instability. Changes of the Z joints (left and right) of any given vertebral level frequently are accompanied by degenerative changes in the IVD of the same level (Kirkaldy-Willis and Mierau, 1995; Peterson, Boulton, and Wood, 2000). Disc degeneration leads to increased rotational instability of the Z joints, resulting in further degeneration of these structures. This process of degenerative changes of the IVDs leading to degeneration of the Z joints also has been supported with computer models of spine function (Goel et al., 1993). The Z joint degenerative changes usually take the form of increased bone formation (e.g., arthrosis, spur formation), which can compress the exiting spinal nerve (Epstein et al., 1973; Rauschning, 1987). Much less frequently, degenerative change takes the form of erosion of the superior articular process (Kirkaldy-Willis et al., 1978). This can lead to degenerative spondylolisthesis. Figure 7-6 shows the process of Z joint and disc degeneration and the interrelation between the two.

Individuals with low back pain secondary to trauma have been found to have more advanced degeneration of the Z joints than low back pain patients who do not experience trauma, although no difference between pain and disability has been found between these two groups of patients. In addition, as low back pain increases, the number of lumbar Z joints showing signs of degeneration and the severity of the degeneration also increase (Peterson, Boulton, and Wood, 2000).

The articular cartilage lining and the lumbar Z joints usually become irregular with age (Taylor and Twomey, 1986). The cartilage of the posterior aspect of the joint frequently is worn thin or even may be completely absent. The articular cartilage of the anterior aspect of the joint usually remains thick but may show many fissures (known as cartilaginous fibrillation) that extend from the articular surface of the cartilage deep to the attachment of the cartilage to the subchondral bone. These types of articular cartilage changes often are more pronounced at the most superior and inferior aspects of the joint (Taylor and Twomey, 1986).

As mentioned, osteophytes (or bony spurs) often develop with age on the superior and inferior articular processes. Frequently this occurs along the periphery of the Z joint along the attachment sites of the ligamentum flavum or the articular capsule. The osteophytes most often develop at the attachment site of the ligamentum flavum on the anteromedial aspect of the superior articular process and extend into the posterolateral aspect of

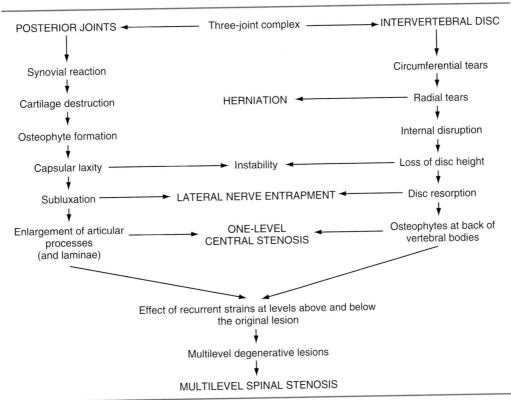

FIG. 7-6 The process of Z joint and disc degeneration and the interrelation between the two. (From Kirkaldy-Willis WH et al. [1978]. Pathology and pathogenesis of lumbar spondylosis and stenosis. *Spine, 3,* 319-328.)

the vertebral canal and also into the IVF. Taylor and Twomey (1986) found that fat-filled synovial pads developed in the region of osteophytes associated with the Z joints. These pads formed a cushion between the osteophytes and inferior articular process. The authors also occasionally found that a prominent pad had developed within the inferior recess of the Z joint. This pad was found to lie between the tip of the inferior articular process and the lamina at the base of the subjacent vertebra's superior articular process. This is where the inferior articular process contacts the lamina during extension of the lumbar spine. This fat pad often was found to become thickened and sclerotic with age, probably in response to the mechanical stimulation of the inferior articular process.

Laminae

The laminae in the lumbar region are broad and thick but do not completely overlap one another. Therefore in contrast to the thoracic region, a distinct space exists between the laminae of adjacent lumbar vertebrae in a dried preparation. This space allows relatively easy access to the spinal subarachnoid space and is used in many diagnostic and therapeutic procedures.

Each lumbar lamina can be divided into superior and inferior portions. The superior part is curved and smooth on its inner surface, whereas the inferior part has a rough inner surface for attachment of the ligamentum flavum. Also, the inferior part of the lamina forms a buttress for the inferior articular process (Van Schaik, Verbiest, and Van Schaik, 1985) (see Fig. 7-2, F).

The region of the lumbar lamina located between the superior and inferior articular processes is known as the pars interarticularis. This region can be fractured rather easily, a condition known as spondylolysis. As mentioned, at the levels of L4 and L5 loads probably are transferred from the vertebral bodies to the pars interarticularis by means of the pedicles. As the trabeculae in the L4 and L5 pedicles pass posteriorly, they are most highly concentrated where they extend into the pars interarticularis. Because trabeculae develop along the lines of greatest stress, the trabecular arrangement leading to the pars interarticularis of the L4 and L5 pedicles has been used to explain the frequency of spondylolysis at these levels.

As a result of spondylolysis, the vertebral body, pedicles, TPs, and superior articular processes can displace anteriorly. This anterior displacement is known as spondylolisthesis. Spondylolysis and spondylolisthesis are most common at L5. However, they may occur at any lumbar level. (The subsection entitled Spondylolysis and Spondylolisthesis of the section Fifth Lumbar Vertebrae found later in this chapter describes these conditions in more detail.)

Lumbar Vertebral Foramen and Vertebral Canal

General Considerations. The vertebral foramina in the lumbar region generally are triangular in shape, although they are somewhat more rounded in the upper lumbar vertebrae and more triangular, or trefoil, in the lower lumbar vertebrae. The triangular shape of the vertebral foramina of the middle and lower lumbar vertebrae is reminiscent of the shape of these openings in the cervical region; however, the lumbar foramina are smaller than those of the cervical region. On the other hand, the lumbar vertebral foramina are larger and more triangular than the rounded foramina of the thoracic region.

The maximum midsagittal diameter in the horizontal plane of the lumbar vertebral foramina is reached by the age of 4 years. Therefore if development is delayed in early childhood, "catch-up growth" does not occur for this dimension. However, the distance between the pedicles (interpedicular distance) increases until adulthood. Thus the lumbosacral vertebral canal becomes more trefoil in appearance with age, reaching its adult dimensions in the early to mid-twenties (Papp, Porter, and Aspden, 1994; Taitz, 1996).

The size of the lumbar vertebral canal ranges from 12 to 20 mm in its anteroposterior dimension at the midsagittal plane. The transverse diameter ranges from 18 to 27 mm, and averages 23.2 to 24.4 mm (Dommisse and Louw, 1990; Ebraheim et al., 1997b). Flexion of the lumbar region significantly increases the size of the vertebral canal at the level of the IVDs (both cross-sectional area and midsagittal diameter) and lumbar extension significantly decreases canal size (Inufusa et al., 1996). Stenosis has been defined as a narrowing below the lowest value of the range of normal (Dommisse and Louw, 1990). Because of the clinical significance of the vertebral canal, Table 7-3 has been included as a ready

Table 7-3	Dimensions of the Lumbar Vertebral Foramina (Vertebral Canal)*
Dimension	**Size (range)†**
Anteroposterior (in midsagittal plane)	12–20 mm
Transverse (interpedicular distance)	18–27 mm

*Dimensions below the lowest value indicate spinal (vertebral) canal stenosis (Dommisse & Louw, 1990). A typical vertebral foramen is rather triangular (trefoil) in shape. However, the upper lumbar vertebral foramina are more rounded than the lower lumbar foramina. L1 is the most rounded, and each succeeding lumbar vertebra becomes increasingly triangular, with L5 the most dramatically trefoil of all.

†Dimensions of lumbar vertebral foramina usually are smaller than those of the cervical region but larger than those of the thoracic region.

source of the dimensions of this region. However, care must be taken when using published values of morphometric measurements of anatomic structures to make clinical decisions. For example, the mid-sagittal diameter of the vertebral foramina is smaller in Asians than in Europeans or North Americans (You-Lu and Wu, 1988; Lee et al., 1995).

Lumbar epidural adipose tissue has been found to be histologically different from adipose tissue in other regions of the body (e.g., subcutaneous adipose tissue). Epidural fat is less solid than subcutaneous fat. The adipocytes are almost identical in size and shape throughout epidural adipose tissue. In addition, epidural adipose tissue has less connective tissue within it and the connective tissue present forms "gliding planes" separated by distinct "slits." The adipocytes of subcutaneous fat are irregular and varied in shape, there is much more connective tissue, and no gliding planes separated by slits are found. The epidural fat in fetuses completely surrounds the dura mater and is evenly distributed from superior to inferior in the lumbar vertebral canal. However, in the adult spine, the lumbar epidural fat is found almost exclusively along the posterior aspect of the dura mater and is most prominent at the level of the IVDs. The epidural fat is isolated into these "pads" by thin connective tissue membranes that are located on the anterior surface of the adipose tissue. These thin connective tissue membranes lie against the posterior surface of the spinal dura mater, and attach laterally to the lateral aspects of the left and right ligamenta flava and intervertebral foramina, and attach superiorly and inferiorly to the suprajacent and subjacent laminae, respectively. Each adipose tissue pad is connected by a small connective tissue pedicle to the posterior midline. Therefore in horizontal section, the pads are triangular in shape with their apex pointing posteriorly and their base resting anteriorly against the posterior spinal dura mater. The size (volume) of the pads increases from the L1-2 to the L4-5 level. These anatomic features suggest a functional role of the epidural adipose tissue, a role designed to aid in the smooth passage of the dura mater during flexion and extension movements across the bony and ligamentous structures of the posterior aspect of the vertebral canal (Beaujeux et al., 1997).

It should be recalled that the conus medullaris of the spinal cord extends to about the L1 vertebra in adults (roughly S1 in fetuses, L3 in neonates, and L1 within the first few months to 2 years of life) (Wilson and Prince, 1989; Macdonald et al., 1999; Malas et al., 2000). (See Chapter 3 for a full discussion of this topic.) Inferior to the level of L1 the vertebral canal (Figs. 7-7 and 7-8) contains the cauda equina. The cauda equina is bathed in the cerebrospinal fluid of the subarachnoid space. The subarachnoid space in the lumbar vertebral canal is large compared with that in the cervical and thoracic regions. Because of its size, the subarachnoid space below the level of the L1 vertebral foramen is known as the lumbar cistern. Also within the lumbar vertebral canal are the meninges: pia mater, attached to rootlets; arachnoid; and dura mater, which surrounds the arachnoid and to which the arachnoid is closely applied. In addition, adipose tissue, vessels, and nerves are located within the epidural space of the vertebral canal. Clinicians who specialize in diagnostic imaging frequently use the term *thecal sac* when collectively referring to the dura mater, arachnoid, and subarachnoid space within the vertebral canal. This term is not restricted to the lumbar region and is used when referring to these structures in the cervical and thoracic regions as well.

Tethered cord syndrome. The conus medullaris extends further inferiorly than normal in a condition known as "tethered cord syndrome." In the fully developed spine this condition is caused by either a thickened filum terminale or adhesions connecting the filum terminale to adjacent tissues (Marchiori and Firth, 1996; Salbacak et al., 2000). Normally the filum terminale stretches when experiencing tension, as with the tension that occurs during flexion of the cervical region (Lew, Morrow, and Lew, 1994). However, with infiltration of adipose tissue, or the formation of a lipoma within the filum terminale, the filum can lose its resilience and can even shorten. Although fat infiltration of the filum terminale is found in approximately 5% of individuals, only a small percentage of these have a tethered spinal cord. If the filum terminale becomes hardened or shortened, a traction injury (e.g., a hyperflexion injury of the cervical region) can place abnormal tensile forces on the conus medullaris and the lower lumbar spinal cord segments. Such stretching of the lower spinal cord results in low back pain accompanied by a variety of motor and sensory signs and symptoms in the lower extremities. MRI is the imaging modality of choice for tethered cord syndrome. MRI shows the conus medullaris extending further inferiorly than normal with infiltration of adipose tissue into the filum terminale, or a lipoma in the filum terminale, if tethered cord syndrome is present (Marchiori and Firth, 1996). See Chapter 3 for additional information on this very clinically relevant condition.

Dural Attachments within the Vertebral Canal. The dura mater of the lumbar spine has a series of attachments to neighboring vertebrae and ligaments. These attachments are found at each segmental level and are usually located at the level of the IVD (Rauschning, 1987). They have been called the dural attachment complex (Dupuis, 1988), meningovertebral ligaments (Bashline, Bilott, and Ellis, 1996), or Hoffmann ligaments

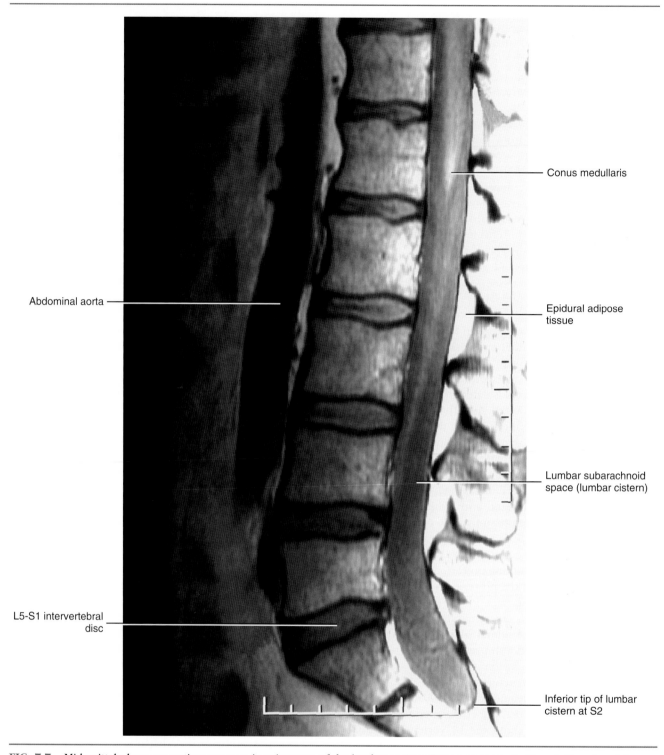

Conus medullaris

Abdominal aorta

Epidural adipose tissue

Lumbar subarachnoid space (lumbar cistern)

L5-S1 intervertebral disc

Inferior tip of lumbar cistern at S2

FIG. 7-7 Midsagittal plane magnetic resonance imaging scan of the lumbar region. (Image courtesy Dr. Dennis Skogsbergh.)

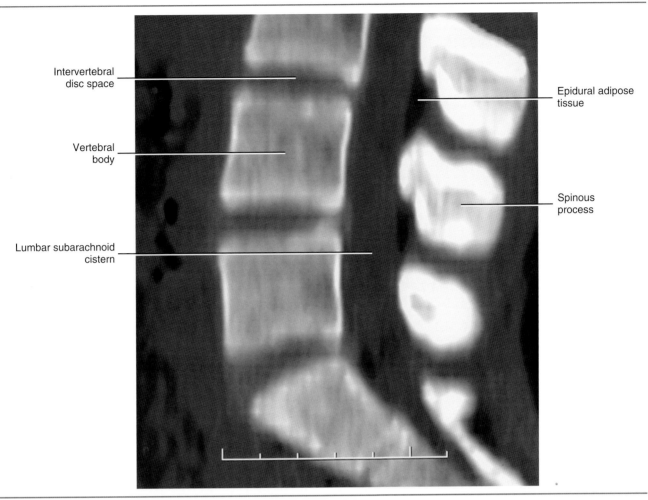

Intervertebral disc space

Vertebral body

Lumbar subarachnoid cistern

Epidural adipose tissue

Spinous process

FIG. 7-8   Horizontal computed tomography images digitally reformatted by computer to obtain this midsagittal plane image of the lumbar vertebral canal. (Image courtesy Dr. Dennis Skogsbergh.)

(Rauschning, 1987; Dupuis, 1988). A centrally placed set of connective tissue bands attaches the anterior aspect of the dura mater to the posterior aspect of the lumbar vertebral bodies and the posterior longitudinal ligament. This set of bands has been called midline Hoffmann (meningovertebral) ligaments (Dupuis, 1988). These are the most numerous and the most robust of the meningovertebral ligaments (Bashline, Bilott, and Ellis, 1996). A second set attaches the anterior and lateral aspects of the dura mater to the lateral, flared extension of the posterior longitudinal ligament, which is attached to the IVD (Fig. 7-9). These bands have been called the lateral Hoffmann (meningovertebral) ligaments (Dupuis, 1988), and are less common and less robust than the midline meningovertebral ligaments (Bashline, Bilott, and Ellis, 1996). A third set of connective tissue bands attaches the exiting dural root sleeves with the inferior pedicles forming the IVFs. These are known as the lateral root ligaments, and may act to limit medial and superior mobility

of the nerve root. These meningovertebral ligaments are the least common (i.e., not found at all lumbar vertebral levels) and least robust, but are still found in all specimens (Bashline, Bilott, and Ellis, 1996) (see Connective Tissue Attachments of the Dura to the Border of the Intervertebral Foramina). These three types of meningovertebral ligaments are variable in distribution, size, and length (varying in length from a few millimeters to as long as 2.5 cm) (Bashline, Bilott, and Ellis, 1996). Posterior Hoffmann (meningovertebral) ligaments also have been identified. They are much less common than the others and course from the posterior aspect of the dura mater to the ligamentum flavum and the posterior aspects of the neural canal (Bashline, Bilott, and Ellis, 1996). Although meningovertebral ligaments have been identified in the thoracic and cervical regions, they are much less common and substantive that those of the lumbosacral region (Scapinelli, 1990; Bashline, Bilott, and Ellis, 1996). However, sturdy attachments of the

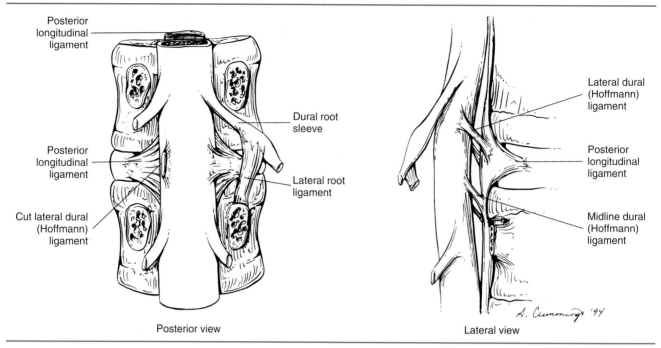

Posterior longitudinal ligament

Posterior longitudinal ligament

Cut lateral dural (Hoffmann) ligament

Dural root sleeve

Lateral root ligament

Posterior view

Lateral dural (Hoffmann) ligament

Posterior longitudinal ligament

Midline dural (Hoffmann) ligament

Lateral view

FIG. 7-9   Attachments of the dura mater to surrounding structures. (Dupuis PR. [1988]. The anatomy of the lumbosacral spine. In W. Kirkaldy-Willis (Ed.). *Managing low back pain* (2nd ed). New York: Churchill Livingstone.)

cervical dura mater to the ligamentum nuchae and rectus capitis posterior minor muscle have been found (see Chapter 5).

It should be recalled that irritation of the anterior aspect of the lumbar spinal dura mater has been found to result in pain felt in the midline, radiating into the low back and superior aspect of the buttock (Edgar and Ghadially, 1976). This pattern of referral is also seen in irritation of the posterior longitudinal ligament (see Ligaments of the Lumbar Region). Bashline, Bilott, and Ellis (1996) speculated that with bulging or protrusion of the IVD, the presence of midline and lateral meningovertebral ligaments would cause traction of the dura mater and the related nerve roots, increasing back and lower extremity pain. They later verified that a bulging IVD can cause traction of the dura mater by means of meningovertebral ligaments (Bashline, Bilott, and Ellis, 1996). They further speculated that the absence of meningovertebral ligaments at some levels in some individuals may be one reason why disc bulges of the same size in two individuals, or at two different levels in the same individual, may present with dramatically different signs and symptoms. The abundance of meningovertebral ligaments in the lumbar region, coupled with the higher incidence of disc bulging and protrusion in this region, would make the lumbar region the most susceptible to this phenomenon. Bashline, Bilott, and Ellis (1996) further speculated that the greater number of anterior meningovertebral ligaments in the lumbar

region may result from the greater volume of the lumbar vertebral canal, allowing for more ligaments of greater size. Another possible reason given was that more stabilization of the dural sac may be needed in the lumbar region than in other regions of the vertebral column. The authors also hypothesized that these ligaments would pull the dural sac anteriorly with spondylolisthesis and be a source of pain in this condition (Bashline, Bilott, and Ellis, 1996). In addition, calcification of some of these ligaments has been noted. Such calcification could potentially cause mechanical irritation of the anterior aspect of the dura mater and the underlying nerve roots (Spencer, Irwin, and Miller, 1983; Bashline, Bilott, and Ellis, 1996). In addition, Spencer, Irwin, and Miller (1983) believed that the commonly seen "cap" of bone present along the posterior aspect of lumbar vertebral bodies could result from the attachment of meningovertebral ligaments causing a type of "traction spur."

Spinal Canal Stenosis.   Narrowing of the vertebral canal (spinal canal) is most often known as spinal canal stenosis, or simply, spinal stenosis. Many variations of this condition exist in the lumbar region, several of which are discussed in the following. The possible pathologic condition that can result from spinal canal stenosis and that is common to all the variations is compression of one or more of the nerves that course through the vertebral canal. Such compression can lead to pain and dysfunction, probably caused by ischemia of the entrapped nerves (Lancourt, Glenn, and Wiltse, 1979). Lumbar spinal canal stenosis affects the nerves of the cauda equina or the dorsal and ventral roots as they leave the vertebral canal and enter IVFs.

Spinal stenosis is usually characterized by diffuse and bilateral low back pain accompanied by radicular pain (see Chapter 11) that radiates along the posterior aspect of one or both thighs and extends to or below the knees. In addition to low back and radicular pain, a patient with spinal stenosis usually experiences weakness of the lower extremities that occurs after prolonged standing with the lumbar region in extension or after walking (neurogenic claudication) (Amundsen et al., 1995). Takahashi et al. (1995) and Takahashi, Shima, and Porter (1999) measured epidural pressure by means of epidural transducers in patients with spinal stenosis. The epidural pressure was found to be low when patients were sitting or lying down and were high when patients were standing. Flexion decreased epidural pressure and extension increased it. The epidural pressure was found to be the highest during extension while standing. The increased pressures also were positively associated with neurologic symptoms of cauda equina compression.

Subdivisions of spinal stenosis include lateral recess stenosis and foraminal (intervertebral foraminal) stenosis. The exiting nerve roots travel through the narrower lateral aspect of the vertebral canal, known as the lateral recess, before entering the IVF. As the roots pass through this region of the vertebral canal, pressure may be placed on them. This is known as lateral recess stenosis. Another type of stenosis includes narrowing of the IVF. This condition is known as foraminal stenosis.

Causes. Spinal canal stenosis may be congenital in nature (Verbiest, 1954; Arnoldi et al., 1976). That is, some people are born with a "tight tube," and their vertebral canal remains narrow throughout their lives. Spinal canal stenosis also can be the result of degenerative changes. The most common causes of degenerative spinal stenosis include arthrosis (increased bone formation) of the medial aspect of the Z joint, especially of the superior articular process. Thickening (hypertrophy) of the ligamentum flavum also can be a degenerative cause of spinal canal stenosis (Arnoldi et al., 1976; Liyang et al., 1989).

Other causes of spinal canal stenosis include spondylolisthesis, Paget's disease, fluorosis, degenerative changes after trauma (Kirkaldy-Willis et al., 1978), and iatrogenic (physician-induced) causes. The latter category includes complication after laminectomy, spinal fusion, and chemonucleolysis (Arnoldi et al., 1976). Box 7-1 lists possible causes of spinal stenosis.

Any combination of congenital and degenerative causes of spinal canal stenosis may be present at one time. Because the contents of the lumbar vertebral canal

---

BOX 7-1
POSSIBLE CAUSES OF SPINAL (VERTEBRAL) CANAL STENOSIS

Congenital
Degenerative
    Facet arthrosis
    Ligamentum flavum thickening (hypertrophy)
    Subsequent to trauma
Spondylolisthesis
Paget's disease
Fluorosis
Iatrogenic
    After laminectomy, spinal fusion, or chemonucleolysis
Any of above causes in conjunction with intervertebral
    disc protrusion

---

are more frequently affected by disc protrusions than the contents of the cervical and thoracic regions (Clarke et al., 1985), a protruding or bulging IVD can increase the severity of signs and symptoms in a patient who has spinal stenosis. Arnoldi et al. (1976), who developed a classification system for this condition, have included IVD protrusion in their system of nomenclature for spinal canal stenosis (e.g., congenital stenosis with IVD protrusion, degenerative stenosis with IVD protrusion).

Also important in the development of signs and symptoms of spinal canal stenosis is the ratio between the size of the neural elements within the lumbar vertebral canal (the cauda equina) and the dimensions of the vertebral canal (Liyang et al., 1989). A person with relatively narrow vertebral foramina may be free of symptoms if the size of the roots making up the cauda equina and the surrounding meninges are proportionately small. On the other hand, if a person has a normal-sized vertebral canal and one or more enlarged nerve roots, as can occur with a schwannoma of the cauda equina (Caputo and Cusimano, 1997), compression of many or all of the nerve roots of the cauda equina can occur. Conversely, if the vertebral canal is narrow (either congenitally or secondary to pathologic conditions or degeneration) and the roots making up the cauda equina are of normal size, signs and symptoms of spinal stenosis can occur. Two possible results of a normal-sized cauda equina within a narrow vertebral canal are the conditions known as neurogenic claudication and redundant nerve roots.

Neurogenic claudication. Neurogenic claudication is pain, paresthesias, and weakness in one or both lower extremities that is aggravated by walking, and is the result of compression of cauda equina, at more than one vertebral level. Compression of the cauda equina at more than one level leads to venous pooling and stasis within the veins draining the cauda equina between the compression sites. The resulting increased venous pressure is thought to lead to a lack of sustained dilation of the arterioles to the cauda equina after exercise (walking), which in turn results in decreased motor nerve function (similar to that found in an entrapment neuropathy such as carpal tunnel syndrome) and subsequent weakness of the lower extremity muscles supplied by the affected nerves (Porter, 1996).

Men experience neurogenic claudication more often than women, and the condition is most common after the age of 50 years. Those affected often have a congenitally narrow vertebral canal that is also affected by degenerative changes (e.g., osteophytes extending from the posterior aspect of the vertebral bodies and also from the articular processes). Neurogenic claudication can be difficult to differentiate from claudication caused by peripheral vascular disease (intermittent claudication), and the two conditions frequently are found together. Standard x-rays can identify a narrow vertebral canal, and advanced imaging procedures (e.g., CT, MRI, and CT-myelography) can assess the extent of degeneration and determine the number of stenotic vertebral levels.

Redundant nerve roots. Redundant nerve roots refers to roots of the cauda equina that bend, curve frequently (undulate within the vertebral canal), or buckle during their course through the vertebral canal. The buckling can be quite severe, blocking the flow of radiopaque dye on myelography. The roots in some cases appear to form dramatic loops (redundancies) when viewed during spinal surgery (Tsuji et al., 1985). The redundancies usually occur rather high in the lumbar spinal canal. Degenerative spinal stenosis is thought to be the usual cause of this condition.

Redundant nerve roots once were considered a rare occurrence, but they may occur more frequently than previously expected. Tsuji et al. (1985) found this condition in 45% of a series of 117 consecutive cadavers without a recorded history of low back or leg pain. They also found that "22 of 56 patients (39%) had obvious redundant nerve roots, which indicates that this condition is a rather common abnormality in degenerative spinal stenosis."

Tsuji et al. (1985) presented a hypothesis of the progression of redundant nerve roots, which is summarized in Box 7-2. Their hypothesis began with the finding that the vertebral column decreases in superior-to-inferior length with age (an average of 14 mm). Shortening of the vertebral canal would force the roots of the cauda equina to become somewhat redundant, causing them to fill the subarachnoid space (thecal space) more completely. Posterior spondylosis (osteophytes) from the vertebral bodies, or other constrictions within the vertebral canal, could then more easily rub against the roots during

movement. (Their study showed that considerable movement of the roots probably occurs during flexion-extension excursions of the spine.) The pressure from spondylosis (or other compressive elements) over many years could result in a friction neuritis. The friction neuritis was thought to result in the large redundant roots seen in several specimens. During walking and standing (extension), increased pressure is placed on the nerve roots (Fig. 7-10), which would cause ischemia of the neural elements. Nerve root ischemia results in the

---

BOX 7-2
DEVELOPMENT OF REDUNDANT NERVE ROOTS AND THE CONSEQUENCES

Vertebral column decreased in length with age
↓
Redundant nerve roots
↓
Spondylosis results in friction neuritis
↓
Increased root size
↓
Nerve root ischemia
↓
Cauda equina claudication

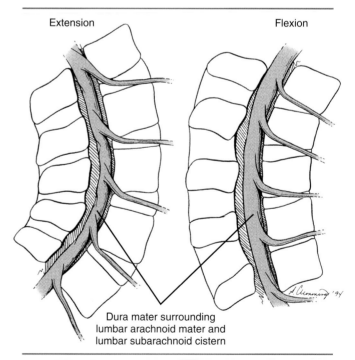

Extension   Flexion

Dura mater surrounding lumbar arachnoid mater and lumbar subarachnoid cistern

FIG. 7-10 Changes that occur within the lumbar vertebral canal during flexion and extension. Notice that the lumbar cistern enlarges during flexion and decreases in volume during extension. The lumbar vertebral canal has also been found to increase in length by almost 2 cm during flexion.

signs and symptoms of intermittent claudication (pain and weakness in the lower extremities during standing and walking), which frequently are associated with spinal stenosis and redundant nerve roots. An average conduction velocity of 50% below normal values was found in cauda equina roots of individuals with redundant nerve roots. Tsuji et al. (1985) believed that such neurologic changes were probably permanent.

Ischemia during stenosis. As mentioned, stenosis of the vertebral canal has been implicated as a possible cause of ischemia to the roots of the cauda equina (Lancourt, Glenn, and Wiltse, 1979; Tsuji et al., 1985; Dommisse and Louw, 1990). This ischemia probably occurs in the roots' "vulnerable region" of vascularity. The roots that form the cauda equina receive their blood supply (vasa nervorum) distally from radicular arteries and also proximally from the cruciate anastomosis surrounding the conus medullaris (see Chapter 3). The proximal and distal vessels form an anastomosis at about the junction of the proximal and middle thirds of the cauda equina roots. This has been called the "critical zone" of vascularity and represents a region where the roots are vulnerable to compression (Dommisse and Louw, 1990). Compression in this region results in neural ischemia causing the symptoms and signs usually associated with spinal stenosis (see the following discussion).

Symptoms. The symptoms of spinal canal stenosis usually include pain radiating from the lumbar region into the lower extremities, occasionally inferior to the knee. The symptoms usually are posture dependent and are made worse by standing or walking for variable periods of time. Flexion of the lumbar region usually relieves the pain.

It should be recalled that flexion of the lumbar region significantly increases the size of the vertebral canal (both cross-sectional area and midsagittal diameter) and extension significantly decreases canal size (Inufusa et al., 1996). In addition, Liyang et al. (1989) found that the volume of the dural sac (subarachnoid space), as studied in 10 cadavers, increased by 3.5 to 6.0 ml during excursion from full extension to full flexion. These changes were found to be highly significant ($p<0.001$). The sagittal diameter of the dural sac (subarachnoid space), as measured from myelograms of the cadaveric spines, also was found to increase significantly during flexion; the greatest increase occurred at the level of L5. Also, the length of the lumbar vertebral (spinal) canal was found to increase by an average of 19.4 mm during flexion. The epidural pressure measurements of Takahashi et al. (1995) and Takahashi, Shima, and Porter (1999) discussed previously supports all of these findings. These results help to explain the clinical findings that flexion

generally relieves the symptoms of spinal canal stenosis (see Fig. 7-10).

Because extension of the lumbar region is accompanied by broadening of the cauda equina, slackening of the ligamenta flava, bulging of the IVDs into the vertebral (spinal) canal, and narrowing of the IVF, one can understand how extension of the lumbar region can increase the symptoms of spinal canal stenosis (see Fig. 7-10). Therefore therapeutic interventions that increase flexion and reduce extension are indicated in patients with this condition (Liyang et al., 1989). Such interventions include exercises that increase tone of abdominal muscles, weight reduction if indicated, and adjustive (manipulative) procedures that promote flexion (Kirk and Lawrence, 1985; Cassidy and Kirkaldy-Willis, 1988; Cox, 1990; Bergmann, Peterson, and Lawrence, 1993). If stenosis is severe, positive effects from manipulation may be more difficult to achieve. "Nevertheless, it can be helpful in some patients and is worth a try in the early management of this syndrome" (Cassidy and Kirkaldy-Willis, 1988). Several authors have reported positive results from wearing a brace to keep the lumbar spine in flexion. Liyang et al. (1989) suggested that spinal stenosis be treated by surgical decompression (laminectomy) of the spinal (vertebral) canal, followed by fixation of the spine in flexion. Interestingly, Kikuchi et al. (1984) found that infiltration of a single nerve root with local anesthetic usually extinguished the symptoms of cauda equina claudication secondary to spinal stenosis. This seems to be contrary to the widely held belief that neurogenic claudication is the result of compression of the entire cauda equina.

Spinous Processes

The spinous processes of lumbar vertebrae are broad from superior to inferior, narrow from side to side, and project directly posteriorly. They are, more or less, flat and rectangular in shape. Their posteroinferior ridge is thickened for the attachment of ligaments and muscles.

The lumbar spinous processes have been found to undergo morphologic changes after age 40, reaching the highest incidence of change in persons over age 60 (Scapinelli, 1989). The most common change is the addition of bone along the posterior aspect of the spinous processes, which may increase their anteroposterior length by as much as 1 cm or more. The greatest increase in length is usually at L3. Frequently the added bone presents a sharp, spurlike margin, usually on the posterosuperior aspect of the spinous process. A smaller increase in the superior-to-inferior dimension usually occurs simultaneously with the anteroposterior change. Occasionally the spinous processes touch one another in the neutral position. This is known as "kissing spines," or Baastrup's syndrome, and can be a source of localized pain.

These changes in the size of the lumbar spinous processes are created by replacement of ligamentous tissue of the supraspinous and interspinous ligaments and the related fibrous tissue below L3 (the supraspinous ligament usually does not extend below L3) with fibrocartilage and eventually bone. Scapinelli (1989) believes these changes are associated with decreased movement as one ages, an increased lumbar lordosis, and traction from ligaments and tendons of muscles. The greatest increase in bone is in individuals with degenerative changes of the vertebral bodies and Z joints (degenerative spondyloarthrosis), especially those with diffuse idiopathic skeletal hyperostosis (DISH, or Forestier's disease). With the exception of DISH, the changes are believed to increase the lever arm of the erector spinae muscles, helping with the maintenance of an erect posture (Scapinelli, 1989).

Table 7-4 lists those structures that normally attach to the lumbar spinous processes.

Lumbar Intervertebral Foramina and Nerve Root Canals

General Considerations. The bony and ligamentous canals called the intervertebral foramina (sing., foramen) are described in Chapter 2. However, several features of the lumbar IVFs are unique. In addition, these regions have been the subject of extensive descriptive and clinical investigation. The relationship between the lumbosacral nerve roots and their surrounding tissues is important in the proper diagnosis of low back pain and pain radiating into the lower extremity (Hasue et al., 1983). This section therefore focuses on the unique aspects of the anatomy of the lumbar IVFs, the pertinent conclusions of previous and current studies of the IVF, and the clinical relevance of this fascinating area.

Many features of the region of the lumbar IVFs are different from those of the rest of the spine because of the unique characteristics of the lumbar and sacral spinal nerves (Fig. 7-11). Because the spinal cord ends at generally the level of L1, the lumbar and sacral dorsal and ventral roots must descend, sometimes for a considerable distance, within the subarachnoid space of the lumbar

Table 7-4	Attachments to Lumbar Spinous Processes
Type	**Structure(s) Attached**
Ligaments	Thoracolumbar fascia (posterior lamella) Supraspinous and interspinous
Muscles	Deep back muscles (spinalis thoracis, multifidus, interspinalis)

From Williams PL et al. (1995). *Gray's anatomy* (38th ed.). Edinburgh: Churchill Livingstone.

vertebral canal. This region of subarachnoid space is known as the lumbar cistern. The exiting nerves (dorsal and ventral rootlets or roots) leave the lumbar cistern by entering a sleeve of dura mater. This usually occurs slightly inferior to the level of the IVD at the level *above* the IVF that the roots eventually will occupy. For example, the L4 roots enter their dural sleeve just beneath the L3-4 disc and then course inferiorly and laterally to exit the L4-5 IVF. More specifically, on leaving the subarachnoid space of the lumbar cistern, the exiting dorsal and ventral roots pass at an oblique inferior and lateral angle while retaining a rather substantial and very distinct covering of dura mater. This covering, known as the dural root sleeve, surrounds the neural elements and their accompanying radicular arteries and veins until they leave the confines of the IVF (see Fig. 2-13).

Frequently the dorsal and ventral rootlets that arise from the spinal cord do not all unite to form dorsal and ventral roots until they are well within the dural root sleeve (Rauschning, 1987; Dupuis, 1988). In addition, the dorsal and ventral roots combine to form the spinal nerve while within the distal aspect of the funnel-shaped dural root sleeve. This latter union occurs at the level of the IVF. The exiting spinal nerve has been found to be larger than the combined size of the individual dorsal and ventral roots (dePeretti et al., 1989). On reaching the lateral edge of the IVF, the dural root sleeve becomes continuous with the epineurium of the spinal nerve.

Many authors (Vital et al., 1983; Bose and Balasubramaniam, 1984; Rauschning, 1987; Lee, Rauschning, and Glenn, 1988) have described the region beginning at the exit of the neural elements from the lumbar subarachnoid cistern and continuing to the lateral edge of the IVF as having significant clinical importance. Perhaps because of the clinical significance of this region, several terms have been used to describe it, including lumbar radicular canal (Vital et al., 1983), nerve root canal, or simply root canal (Rauschning, 1987) (Fig. 7-12). The term *nerve root canal* (NRC) is used in the following paragraphs when discussing the course of the dural root sleeve and its contents, and the term IVF is used to describe the terminal part of the NRC that lies between the pedicles of two adjacent vertebrae.

Within the dural root sleeve an interneural complex of fibrous connections (Dupuis, 1988) anchors the neural elements (rootlets and roots) to the surrounding dura mater of the NRC. More specifically, these connections course from the dura and inner arachnoid mater of the sleeve to the pia mater surrounding the rootlets and roots. Recall that farther laterally the root sleeve unites with the spinal nerve to form its epineurium.

Connective Tissue Attachments of the Dura to the Borders of the Intervertebral Foramina. The external surface of the dural root sleeve is usually

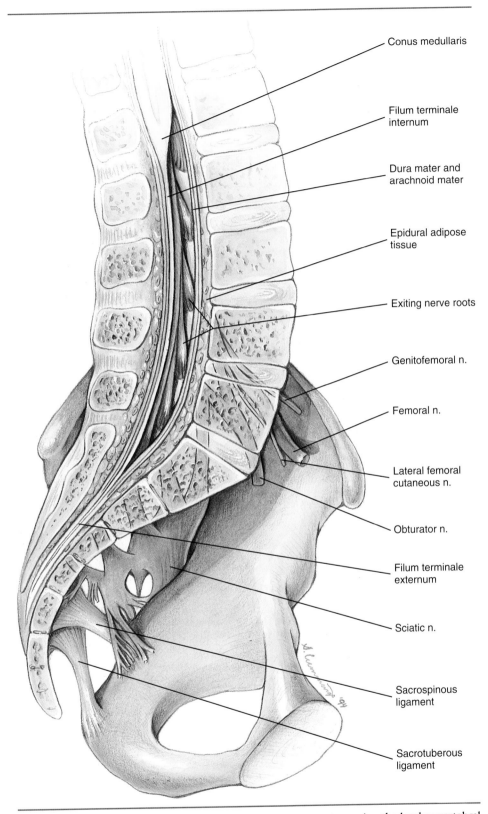

Conus medullaris

Filum terminale
internum

Dura mater and
arachnoid mater

Epidural adipose
tissue

Exiting nerve roots

Genitofemoral n.

Femoral n.

Lateral femoral
cutaneous n.

Obturator n.

Filum terminale
externum

Sciatic n.

Sacrospinous
ligament

Sacrotuberous
ligament

FIG. 7-11 Midsagittal view of the spine showing nerve roots traversing the lumbar vertebral canal, exiting the intervertebral foramina, and forming the lumbar and sacral plexuses.

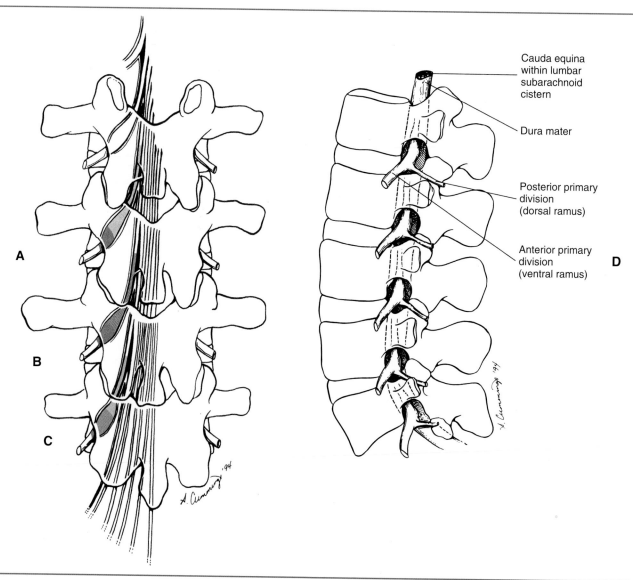

FIG. 7-12 **A–C,** Regions of the intervertebral foramen (IVF) as described by various authors. **A,** The nerve root canal (NRC) as the course of the dural root sleeve and its contents (*yellow* and *red* regions combined). Other terms used when referring to this general region are lumbar radicular canal (Vital et al., 1983) and root canal (Rauschning, 1987). The IVF is shown in red as the terminal part of the NRC, located between the pedicles of two adjacent vertebrae. This also represents the classic anatomic description of the IVF. **B,** Regions of the NRC (lumbar radicular canal) as described by Vital et al. (1983). Notice the retrodiscal portion in blue. This is the portion of the NRC that lies posterior to the intervertebral disc (IVD) superior to the level that the spinal nerve eventually exits. The parapedicular portion of the NRC (*green*) is the region medial to the pedicle. Vital et al. (1983) refer to the region occupied by the uniting dorsal and ventral roots and the exiting spinal nerve as the IVF proper (*red*). Table 7-8 describes the borders of the retrodiscal, parapedicular, and IVF proper subdivisions of the NRC. **C,** Divisions of the NRC (root canal) as described by Rauschning (1987) and Lee et al. (1988). The entrance zone (*pink*) is the region that begins as the dorsal and ventral roots enter the dural root sleeve and extends through the lateral recess. Other authors use lateral recess, lateral canal, subarticular gutter, or lateral nerve canal when referring to the entrance zone. The middle zone, or pedicle zone, (*blue*) is the region of the NRC located between the two adjacent pedicles that make up an IVF. This area was described in the preceding (**A** and **B**) as the IVF proper (Vital et al., 1983). The term exit zone, or foramen proper, is used by Rauschning (1987), and Lee et al. (1988) to refer to the almost two-dimensional opening ("doorway") formed by a parasagittal plane passed along the lateral edge of the two pedicles that help to form an IVF. The exit zone is shown in red in **C. D,** Lateral view of the lumbar IVFs. The specific dimensions of the lumbar IVFs are given in Chapter 2 (see Tables 2-6 and 2-7 and Fig. 2-21).

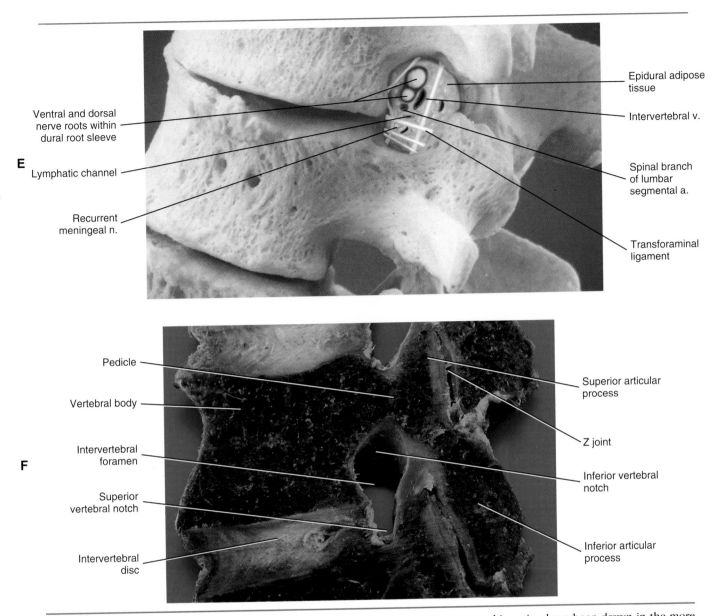

E

Epidural adipose tissue

Ventral and dorsal nerve roots within dural root sleeve

Intervertebral v.

Lymphatic channel

Recurrent meningeal n.

Spinal branch of lumbar segmental a.

Transforaminal ligament

F

Pedicle

Vertebral body

Intervertebral foramen

Superior vertebral notch

Intervertebral disc

Superior articular process

Z joint

Inferior vertebral notch

Inferior articular process

FIG. 7-12—cont'd   **E,** Lateral view of two IVFs. The structures that normally traverse this region have been drawn in the more superior IVF. The most common locations of the transforaminal ligaments also are shown traversing this IVF. **F,** Parasagittal section through the fourth lumbar IVF. A typical lumbar IVF is sometimes described as being shaped like an "inverted teardrop" or an "inverted pear" when viewed from the side. (**E** and **F,** Courtesy the National University of Health Sciences.)

attached by one or more connective tissue bands to the inferior pedicle of the IVF (see Fig. 7-9). This connective tissue attachment is called the lateral root ligament (Dupuis, 1988). It limits the medial and upward mobility of the root sleeve and its contents (Rauschning, 1987). Fibrous connections from the lateral aspect of the IVF to the exiting spinal nerve have also been identified (Hasue et al., 1983; dePeretti et al., 1989). Grimes, Massie, and Garfin (2000) found four connective tissue attachments from the dural root sleeve to the adjacent borders of the IVF at all lumbar levels. One such attachment passed posteriorly to the lateral-most aspect of the ligamentum

flavum as it blended with the joint capsule. Another connective tissue attachment was found to extend superiorly to the pedicle above, and a third formed a mirror image to the second by extending inferiorly to the pedicle below. Finally, another connective tissue attachment extended anteriorly to the posterior aspect of the IVD (Grimes, Massie, and Garfin, 2000). An appropriate term for these connective tissue attachments would seem to be "intraforaminal meningovertebral ligaments," after Bashline, Bilott, and Ellis (1996), who used the term *meningovertebral ligaments* to refer to Hoffmann's ligaments connecting the dura mater to surrounding tissues within the vertebral (spinal) canal. These structures were found to stabilize the neural structures within the IVF and to resist considerable traction applied to the spinal nerve and anterior primary division distal to the connective tissue attachments (dePeretti et al., 1989; Grimes, Massie, and Garfin, 2000). These fibrous attachments also have been found to give considerable resistance to traction of the anterior primary divisions. Therefore they serve to spare the lumbar roots from traction injuries. The dural root sleeve also provides resistance to traction. In fact, the dural root sleeve ruptures before avulsion of the rootlets from the conus medullaris occurs. These resistive forces, when combined with the fact that the rootlets and roots forming the spinal nerves are of excess length within the dura mater, indicate that the IVF seems to provide an almost insurmountable protective barrier to traction forces placed on the exiting spinal nerves (dePeretti et al., 1989).

Entrapment of the Neural Elements. Unfortunately, the exiting neural elements are not as well protected from pressure injuries as they are from traction injuries. Compression, or entrapment, of neural elements as they pass through the NRC or the IVF is of extreme clinical importance (Lancourt, Glenn, and Wiltse, 1979). Also a detailed understanding of this region is essential because treatment may differ depending on the cause of entrapment. The clinician should attempt to localize a lesion as precisely as possible to determine the structure causing the problem and to identify the specific neural elements being affected (Rauschning, 1987). These neural elements include the dorsal and ventral roots and their union as the spinal nerve. Causes of such compression include degenerative changes of the superior articular processes and posterior vertebral bodies, IVD protrusion, and pressure from the superior pedicle of the IVF (McNab, 1971; Hasue et al., 1983; Vital et al., 1983) (see Chapter 11).

Occasionally osteophytes from the Z joints and vertebral bodies can become so large that they can almost completely divide the IVF into two smaller foramina, one on top of the other (Kirkaldy-Willis et al., 1978). Such changes may result in entrapment of the exiting spinal nerve. However, osteophytes of the superior articular processes forming the Z joints cause venous obstruction of the intervertebral veins more often than compression of nerves in the IVF. This leads to "compression, congestion, and resultant dilation of foraminal veins." The venous changes are also associated with intraneural and perineural fibrosis, focal demyelination, and edema of the nerve roots. These neural changes probably result from ischemia secondary to poor venous return from the nerve roots upstream to the venous obstruction (Hoyland, Freemont, and Jayson, 1989).

Because of the clinical importance of the NRCs and the IVFs, a more accurate anatomic description is necessary.

Anatomy of the Nerve Root Canals. The sizes of the NRCs vary considerably from the upper to lower lumbar segments. They are smaller in length at the level of L1 and L2 because, after exiting the lumbar cistern, the L1 and L2 nerves course almost directly laterally to reach the IVF. This led Crock (1981) to state that the concept of a nerve root *canal* at L1 and L2 is useless, because the beginning of the dural root sleeve lies against the inferior and medial aspect of the IVF's upper pedicle. Therefore no true dural "canal" exists for these nerve roots.

Table 7-5 gives the obliquities and lengths of the lumbar NRCs. Other authors (e.g., Ebraheim et al., 1997b) have found lower values for obliquity (i.e., more obliquity) than those presented in the table (Bose and Balasubramaniam, 1984). The NRCs become progressively longer from L1 to S1 as the dural root sleeves exit at a more oblique inferior angle. Therefore the NRCs of L5 and S1 are the longest in the lumbar region and the most susceptible to damage from pathologic conditions of surrounding structures (Crock, 1981). Tables 7-6 and 7-7 describe the relationships of the L5 and S1 NRCs, respectively. Many, if not most, of the types of borders described in Table 7-6 for the L5 NRC also apply to the L3 and L4 NRCs as well.

All the exiting rootlets or roots course over an IVD either just before entering their dural root sleeve (L1 and L2) or, in the case of L3-S1, directly in the region in where they enter the dural root sleeve. However, only the S1 dural root sleeve (and contents) passes completely over an IVD (the L5 disc). The S1 NRC passes through a movable, narrow opening between the L5 disc anteriorly and the L5-S1 ligamentum flavum posteriorly. Therefore the S1 nerve is exposed to possible compression both anteriorly

Table 7-5	Obliquity and Length of the Lumbar Nerve Root Canals		
Level (degrees)	Obliquity*	Length†	Length*
L1	70	NVG	AN
L2	80	NVG	AN
L3	60	NVG	NVG
L4	60	6.7 mm	25 mm
L5	45	7.8 mm	30 mm
S1	30	8.0 mm	35 mm

AN, Almost nonexistent; *NVG,* no value given.
*According to Bose and Balasubramaniam (1984); obliquity given in degrees from a sagittal plane (low values, much inferior obliquity).
†According to Vital et al. (1983) (see Fig. 7-12).

Table 7-6	Relationships of the L5 Nerve Root Canal
Surface	**Relationship**
Origin	L4-5 Intervertebral disc (sometimes does not begin this far superiorly, in which case begins at L5 vertebral body)
Medial surface	Lateral aspect of S1 nerve root canal
Lateral surface	Medial aspect of pedicle of L5, then enters L5 intervertebral foramina
Anterior surface*	Posterior aspect of L5 vertebral body
Posterior surface†	L5-S1 Z joint and overlying ligamentum flavum
Other relationships	Surrounded by epidural adipose tissue, and small arteries, veins, and lymphatics (small)

From Bose K & Balasubramaniam P. (1984). Nerve root canals of the lumbar spine. *Spine, 9,* 16-18.
*Just distal to origin.
†Posterior relationships vary considerably depending on length of the nerve roots and orientation of the L5 lamina, which changes with a change in the angle between L5 and the sacrum (Crock, 1981).

Table 7-7	Relationships of the S1 Nerve Root Canal
Surface	**Relationship**
Origin	Medial aspect of L5 pedicle
Medial surface	Lateral aspect of dural sac
Lateral surface	L5 nerve root, then L5-S1 intervertebral foramina, then S1 pedicle, then enters S1 intervertebral foramina
Anterior surface	Posterior aspect of L5 vertebral body, then L5 intervertebral disc, then posterior aspect of the S1 vertebral body
Posterior surface*	Bony ridge of anterior aspect of L5 lamina (formed by the attachment of ligamentum flavum), then ligamentum flavum, then anteromedial aspect of S1 superior articular process
Other relationships	Surrounded by epidural adipose tissue, and small arteries, veins, and lymphatics (small)

From Crock HV. (1981). Normal and pathological anatomy of the lumbar spinal nerve root canals. *J Bone Joint Surg, 63,* 487-490 and Vital JM et al. (1983). Anatomy of the lumbar radicular canal. *Anat Clin, 5,* 141-151.
*Posterior relationships vary considerably depending on length of the nerve roots and orientation of the L5 lamina, which changes with a change in the angle between L5 and the sacrum (Crock, 1981).

(disc protrusion) and posteriorly (ligamentum flavum bulging or buckling, hypertrophy of superior articular process of sacrum) in this region (Rauschning, 1987).

Anomalies of the Neural Elements and the Dural Root Sleeves. Anomalies of the rootlets as they come off of the spinal cord are common. Such anomalies occur much more often with the dorsal rootlets than the ventral rootlets (Kikuchi et al., 1984). The anomalies take the form of rootlets of one spinal cord segment passing to the root of the nerve below or above. Such anomalies could conceivably result in the perception of radicular symptoms different from the normal pain pattern.

Anomalies of the roots making up the cauda equina while within the lumbar cistern also are quite common. These usually consist of nerve bundles from one root passing to a neighboring root. The clinical implications of this type of anomaly are the same as those just discussed for anomalous rootlets.

Congenital anomalies associated with the dural root sleeves also occur with some frequency. Hasue et al. (1983) found anomalies in 5 of the 59 cadavers (8.5%) in their study. Several types of anomalies have been identified (Hasue et al., 1983; Neidre and MacNab, 1983; Kikuchi et al., 1984; Aota et al., 1997; Bogduk, 1997) (Fig. 7-13). The first type is known as conjoined nerve roots and is the most common type of dural sleeve anomaly (see Fig. 7-13, *C*). With this anomaly, roots of adjacent spinal cord segments share the same dural root sleeve for a short distance. The roots then separate into their own

dural root sleeve and exit the appropriate IVF. Conjoined nerve roots cause one set of dorsal and ventral roots (or both sets) to take a tortuous course, possibly making them more susceptible to traction across a bulging disc or narrow NRC.

The second type of root sleeve anomaly is the most dramatic. The dorsal and ventral roots of two distinct spinal cord levels, within their appropriate root sleeves, exit the same IVF, leaving the adjacent IVF devoid of exiting roots (see Fig. 7-13, *B*). In a variation of this anomaly, an additional dorsal and ventral root and their covering dural root sleeve pass through the same IVF with the neural and dural structures that normally pass through the IVF. In this instance, all of the IVFs have roots within them, and one IVF has two pairs of roots passing through it (see Fig. 7-13, *D*). The nerves within an IVF containing more than one set of roots in these types of anomalies are more susceptible to entrapment. Entrapment of two sets of roots within one IVF might lead to radicular symptoms of more than one dermatome (see Chapters 9 and 11).

In the third type of dural root sleeve anomaly, a communicating branch, surrounded by its own dural sheath, passes from one NRC to its neighbor before

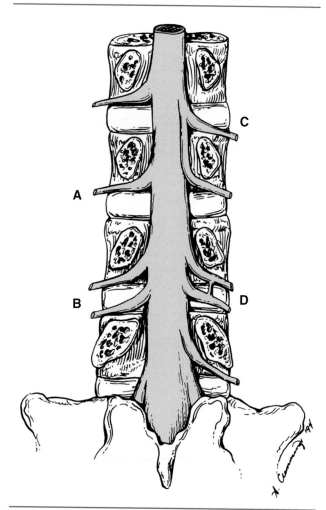

FIG. 7-13 Posterior view of the vertebral canal showing anomalies of dural root sleeves. **A,** The dural root sleeve is normal. Notice that it is exiting the upper region of the intervertebral foramen (IVF). **B,** The anomaly shows the roots of two distinct spinal cord levels, within their appropriate root sleeves, exiting the same IVF. This leaves an adjacent IVF devoid of exiting roots. **C,** The anomaly shows conjoined nerve roots. In this case the roots of adjacent spinal cord segments share the same dural root sleeve for a short distance. The roots then separate into their own dural root sleeve and exit the appropriate IVF. Conjoined nerve roots cause one of the roots (or both) to take a rather tortuous course. **D,** The anomaly is a variation of **B.** The anomaly shows an additional dorsal and ventral root, and their covering dural root sleeve, passing through the same IVF with the neural and dural structures that normally pass through that IVF. Therefore all the IVFs on the right side of the illustration have roots within them, and one IVF has two pairs of roots passing through it. Also notice that another type of anomaly is shown here. A communicating branch, surrounded by its own dural sheath is seen passing from one dural sleeve to its neighbor, before either exit the IVF. **B–D,** All these types of anomalies can have significant clinical implications (see text). (From Bogduk N & Twomey LT. [1991]. *Clinical anatomy of the lumbar spine.* London: Churchill Livingstone.)

either primary root exits its IVF. The result of this anomaly could be similar to that of roots sending connecting branches to neighboring roots, causing dispersion of radicular symptoms to include an adjacent segment (e.g., L5 compression may result in some pain or paresthesia in the distribution of L4). However, because it runs within its own dural root sleeve, the neural elements within the "bridging sleeve" are more vulnerable to compression either inside a lateral recess or as they pass behind an IVD. This type of anomaly also can occur in conjunction with the variation of the second type of anomaly mentioned. In this case a communicating branch is found between two dural root sleeves as they both exit the same IVF (see Fig. 7-13, *D*).

Anomalies of the nerve roots and dural sleeves can be a sole cause of radicular symptoms. They also can augment radicular symptoms from other causes (Hasue et al., 1983). Even though the incidence of symptoms as a result of such NRC anomalies is thought to be rare, they should be kept in mind when patients have unusual distribution patterns of radicular pain (Bogduk, 1997).

Terminology Associated with the Nerve Root Canals and the Intervertebral Foramina. Terminology with regard to the exiting roots can be confusing. Some authors (Vital et al., 1983) describe the beginning of the NRC (that portion posterior to the IVD directly above the level of the IVF of exit) as the retrodiscal portion of the NRC (see Fig. 7-12, *B*). As the nerve continues to descend more laterally in what is described by many as the lateral recess, the nerve lies medial to the pedicle that forms the upper border of the IVF, which the nerve roots eventually exit. This region is sometimes called the parapedicular portion of the NRC (Vital et al., 1983). The portion of the IVF occupied by the uniting dorsal and ventral roots and the exiting spinal nerve is called the IVF proper. Table 7-8 describes the borders of the retrodiscal, parapedicular, and IVF proper subdivisions of the NRC. This table is included to help clarify the regions where the nerve roots and (mixed) spinal nerve are most vulnerable to various types of pathologic conditions.

Moving from the upper to the lower lumbar region, the parapedicular portion (lateral recess) of the NRC widens in the transverse plane (i.e., left to right), becomes shorter from top to bottom, and becomes narrower from anterior to posterior (average, 12 mm at L2 and 8 mm at L5) (Vital et al., 1983); therefore this part of the NRC becomes more like a true lateral recess, or gutter, as one descends the lumbar spine.

The position of the entire lumbar region affects the NRC and the neural elements (Vital et al., 1983). The anteroposterior dimension of the retrodiscal space narrows in the upright posture. This is because of slight posterior bulging of the IVD and slight anterior buckling

Table 7-8 Relationships of the Various Regions of the S1 Nerve Root Canal

Region and Surface Relationships

Retrodiscal Region
Anterior	Intervertebral disc*
Posterior	Superior articular process,* ligamentum flavum*

Parapedicular Region (Lateral Recess)
Anterior	Posterior surface of vertebral body
Posterior	Ligamentum flavum,* superior articular process,* pars interarticularis (isthmus)*
Lateral	Medial surface of pedicle
Medial	Dura of lumbar cistern

Intervertebral Foramina Proper
Superior	Lower margin of upper pedicle
Anterior	Upper and lower vertebral bodies, intervertebral disc in between them*
Inferior	Upper margin of lower pedicle
Posterior	Z joint and ligamentum flavum*

*Indicates relationships that are of key clinical importance.

of the ligamentum flavum. During flexion of the lumbar region, the neural elements become stretched and pressed against the anterior walls of the retrodiscal and parapedicular spaces. Also, the IVF proper increases in height and width during flexion. Extension of the lumbar region results in slackening of the neural elements. They also move against the posterior wall of the lateral recess during extension. In addition, the IVF becomes significantly shorter from superior to inferior and anterior to posterior during extension (Mayoux-Benhamou et al., 1989).

A different set of terms was put forth by Rauschning (1987) and Lee, Rauschning, and Glenn (1988) (see Fig. 7-12, C). These authors used the term *entrance zone* when referring to the region that begins as the roots enter the dural root sleeve and continues through the lateral recess. Other authors use the terms *lateral recess, lateral canal, subarticular gutter,* or *lateral nerve canal* when referring to this region (Rauschning, 1987). This area corresponds to the combination of the retrodiscal and parapedicular regions previously described. The most common cause of stenosis in the entrance zone is hypertrophic osteoarthritis of the Z joint, usually of the superior articular process. Other causes include congenital variations of the Z joints or a congenitally short pedicle. Also, a bulging anulus fibrosus (e.g., L3 anulus compressing the L4 nerve) or osteophytic spurs from the superior vertebral end plate coursing along the anulus could compress the neural elements in the entrance zone.

Rauschning (1987) and Lee, Rauschning, and Glenn (1988) use the term *midzone* or *pedicle zone* when referring to the region of the NRC located between the

two adjacent pedicles that make up an IVF (see Fig. 7-12, C). This area was described previously as the IVF proper (Vital et al., 1983) (see Fig. 7-12, A). The dorsal root (spinal) ganglion and ventral root are located within this region and can be compressed here. Because of its large size, the dorsal root ganglion is more susceptible to minor compression than the ventral root. Osteophyte formation along the ligamentum flavum (anterior to the pars interarticularis) and hypertrophy of fibrous tissue along a fracture of the pars interarticularis was cited by Lee, Rauschning, and Glenn (1988) as being the most common causes of stenosis in the middle zone. They also believed that clinicians may overlook stenosis of this region because the middle zone is difficult to evaluate with diagnostic imaging procedures. They stated that neural entrapment of the middle zone may result in symptoms of activity-related, intermittent, neurogenic claudication. They also noted that some patients progress until they experience constant pain and diminished sensation even during times of rest. These unprovoked resting symptoms may be caused by spontaneous action potentials arising from compressed or entrapped ganglionic cells (Lee et al., 1988).

The term *exit zone,* or *foramen proper,* was used by Rauschning (1987) and Lee, Rauschning, and Glenn (1988) to refer to the almost two-dimensional opening ("doorway") formed by a parasagittal plane passed along the lateral edge of the two pedicles that help to form an IVF (see Fig. 7-12, C). The most common causes of stenosis in this region were cited as "hypertrophic osteoarthritic changes of the facet joints (Z joints) with subluxation and osteophytic ridge formation along the superior margin of the disc" (Lee, Rauschning, and Glenn 1988).

Clinical Conditions Related to the Nerve Root Canals. Narrowing of the IVD, particularly at the L5-S1 level, causes narrowing of the IVF at the same level (L5-S1 IVF in this case) and also narrowing of the NRC of the nerve exiting at the IVF below (the S1 NRC in this case). Crock (1981) stated that the remaining anulus fibrosus of the disc may bulge posteriorly, bringing the posterior longitudinal ligament along with it. The superior articular facet of the segment below (S1) moves superiorly and anteriorly, again compressing the NRC (S1). The combination of posterior anulus bulge along with anterior displacement of the superior articular facet of the vertebra below can result in dramatic narrowing of the NRC that runs between these two structures (Rauschning, 1987). Osteophyte (bony spur) formation is fairly common, both from the vertebral body along the attachment of the anulus fibrosus and the superior articular process along the attachment of the ligamentum flavum. These spurs can further compress the neural and vascular elements of the NRC (Rauschning, 1987). In addition, a bony ridge may develop along the anterior and inferior surface of the lamina. This can compress the more medial NRC (that of the nerve exiting at the IVF of the level below, S1 in this instance) and also the lateral and distal (inferior) aspect of the NRC of the nerve exiting at the same level (in this case, L5).

The L5 NRC is related to both the L4-5 (at its origin) and the L5-S1 (at its exit) IVDs. Therefore with suspected entrapment of the L5 nerve, a differentiation between compression from an L4 or L5 disc bulge or protrusion, or from another structure along the L5 NRC, must be made (Bose and Balasubramaniam, 1984).

Congenital hypertrophy of the L5-S1 articular processes and facets may cause localized obstruction of the L5-S1 IVF. Osteoarthritis of the L5-S1 facets may cause the same condition, but usually such arthritis tends to cause obstruction more medially, affecting the descending S1 NRC (Crock, 1981).

Intervertebral Foramina Proper. When viewed from the side, the lumbar IVFs face laterally. A typical lumbar IVF is sometimes described as being shaped like an inverted teardrop or an inverted pear (Fig. 7-14). The specific dimensions of the lumbar IVFs are given in Chapter 2 (see Tables 2-6 and 2-7).

The spinal nerve is located in the upper third of each lumbar IVF. As it enters the IVF, the spinal nerve is close to the medial and inferior aspect of the superior pedicle that forms the upper boundary of the IVF (Crock, 1981). Here the nerve is accompanied by a branch (or sometimes branches) of the lumbar segmental artery, the superior intervertebral (segmental, or pedicle) veins, which connect the external and internal vertebral venous plexuses, and by the sinuvertebral nerve (Rauschning, 1987). The spinal nerve occupies approximately one third of the IVF in the lumbar region. However, the spinal nerve can be as close as 0.4 mm (range, 0.4 to 0.8 mm)

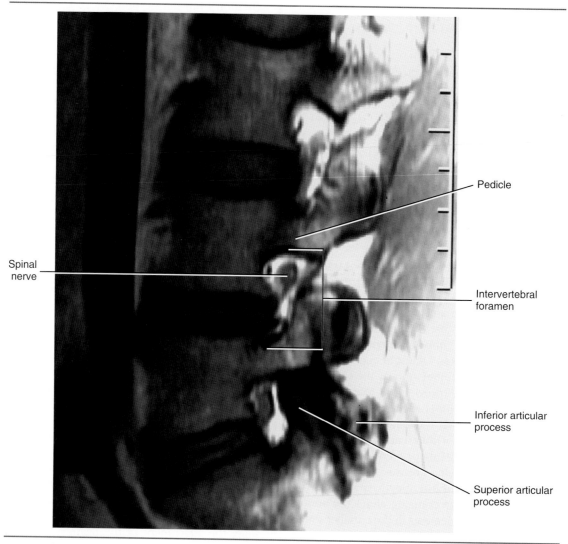

FIG. 7-14 Parasagittal plane magnetic resonance imaging scan of the lumbar region. Note the prominent intervertebral foramina. (Image courtesy Dr. Dennis Skogsbergh.)

to the bony anterior and posterior IVF borders (Giles, 1994). This allows crowding by the articular facets during extension (Bose and Balasubramaniam, 1984; Rauschning, 1987). The inferior aspect of the IVF is usually narrowed to a slit by the anulus fibrosus, which normally bulges slightly posteriorly. The inferior aspect of the IVF is also narrowed by the posteriorly located ligamentum flavum. The inferior intervertebral (segmental, discal) veins usually lie in this narrow space. As with the superior intervertebral (pedicle) veins, the inferior veins also unite the internal (epidural) vertebral venous plexus with the external vertebral venous plexus and the ascending lumbar vein.

The lateral borders of the IVFs are covered with an incomplete layer of transforaminal fascia (Paz-Fumagalli and Haughton, 1993). This fascia condenses in several locations at each IVF to form the accessory ligaments of the IVF (see Chapter 2). An exiting spinal nerve could be affected by these structures as it leaves the IVF (Bachop and Janse, 1983; Bachop and Ro, 1984; Bose and Balasubramaniam, 1984; Rauschning, 1987; Bakkum and Mestan, 1994). In addition to compression by accessory ligaments or transforaminal fascia, Rauschning (1987) states that lateral disc herniations and bony structures such as the TPs (usually of L5, but at higher lumbar levels on rare occasions) "may compress, kink, or constrict the lumbar nerves beyond the foraminal outlet." The author calls this region the extraforaminal region or the postcanal zone.

Also, the lateral borders of the L1 through L4 IVFs are associated with the origin of the psoas major muscle. In fact, because of the posterior origin of the psoas major muscle from the front of the TPs and its anterior origin from the lumbar vertebral bodies and IVDs, the psoas major almost completely surrounds the lateral opening of the first four lumbar IVFs. Therefore the anterior primary divisions (ventral rami), by necessity, run through the substance of the psoas major muscle, frequently uniting with neighboring ventral rami within the muscle to form the branches of the lumbar plexus. In addition to the protection given by the dural root sleeve and the meningovertebral (Hoffman) ligaments (see previous discussion and Fig 7-9), the psoas major muscle may provide some protection for the dorsal and ventral roots during traction of the peripheral nerves of the lumbar plexus (dePeretti et al., 1989). Such traction may occur as a result of hyperflexion or hyperextension of the lower extremity.

The boundaries of the IVF can be imaged well with both MRI and CT (Cramer et al., 1994) (Fig. 7-15; see also Fig. 7-14). Occasionally ossification of the superior attachment of the ligamentum flavum results in foraminal spurs, which can be seen on CT. These spurs are considered to be normal variants; may project well into the IVF, posterior to the dorsal root ganglion; are frequently bilateral; and are usually asymptomatic (Helms and Sims, 1986).

Changes in Dimensions of the Intervertebral Foramina.

Flexion of the lumbar region has been shown to significantly increase the height and width of the IVFs by separating the pedicles (increases height), decreasing the normal bulging of the anulus fibrosus of the IVD (increases IVF width), and by decreasing the thickness of the ligamentum flavum (increases IVF width) (Fujiwara et al., 2001). Extension significantly decreases the height and width of the IVFs by having the opposite effects as flexion (Fujiwara et al., 2001). Flexion increases the cross-sectional sagittal area of the IVF from the neutral position by 12%, whereas extension decreases the area of the IVF from the neutral position by 15% (Inufusa et al., 1996). Distraction (traction) has been found to increase IVF size in cadavers (Schlegel et al., 1994), and compression decreases the height of the IVFs (Nowicki et al., 1990). Titanium cages (BAK Interbody Fusion System) implanted in the IVDs during interbody fusion spine surgery also have been shown to increase IVF volume at L4-5 and L5-S1 (Chen et al., 1995). Many of the pathologic conditions described as affecting the NRC, such as anterior osteophytes on the superior articular processes of the Z joints, also can diminish the dimensions of the IVF proper (Bailey and Casamajor, 1911; Giles, 1994). In addition, recall that the IVD forms a part of the anterior border of the IVF. Because of this, a far lateral IVD prolapse can cause a significant decrease in the anterior to posterior dimension of the IVF, resulting in a dramatic change of shape of the spinal nerve in the IVF and the development of fibrotic adhesions in and around the spinal nerve (Hadley, 1948). In addition, a decrease in disc height also results in a decrease of the vertical dimension of the IVF (Crock, 1981; Cinotti et al., 2002). However, a decrease in IVF height of only 4 mm, when combined with lumbar extension, can cause compression of the dorsal root ganglion or the spinal nerve within the IVF (Revel et al., 1988). This is most likely because the dorsal root ganglion and spinal nerve normally can be as close as 0.4 mm to the bony anterior and posterior borders of the IVFs (Giles, 1994). Cinotti et al. (2002) found that a decrease in the sagittal diameter of the vertebral (spinal) canal was related to a decreased width of the IVF at the same level (usually resulting from decreased length of the pedicles). This relationship of decreased spinal canal size with decreased IVF size, along with the close relationship of disc degeneration and acquired spinal canal and foraminal stenosis and decreased IVF height, led Cinotti et al. (2002) to conclude that IVF stenosis should be suspected whenever spinal canal stenosis is present. For these reasons, having access to the normal size of the lumbar IVFs as they appear on MRI scans can be clinically useful. (These

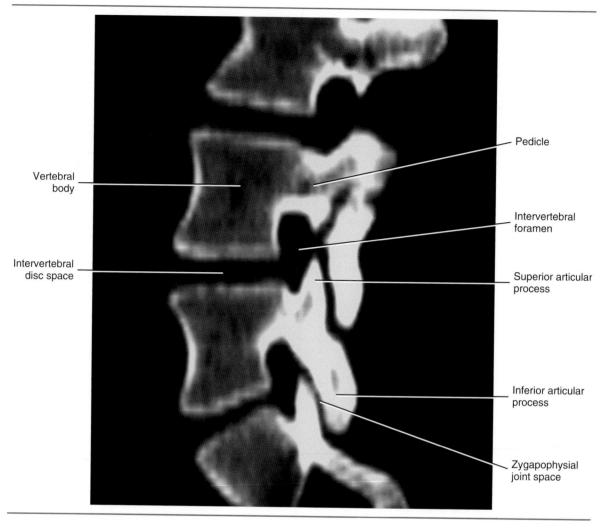

Vertebral body

Intervertebral disc space

Pedicle

Intervertebral foramen

Superior articular process

Inferior articular process

Zygapophysial joint space

FIG. 7-15   Digitally reformatted parasagittal plane computed tomography image showing the region of the Z joints and IVFs. (Image courtesy Dr. Dennis Skogsbergh.)

values are presented in Chapter 2 in the section Intervertebral Foramen, Tables 2-6 and 2-7.)

L5 Nerve Root Canal and L5 Intervertebral Foramina. The anatomy of the L5 NRC is unique, and because of this the L5 roots and nerve are susceptible to compression in many different locations. This canal is longer and runs at a more oblique anterior angle than the rest of the lumbar NRCs. Also, the lateral recess of the L5 vertebra is the deepest laterally and often the narrowest from anterior to posterior of the entire spine. This narrow lateral recess may lead to compression of the L5 nerve in some instances (Rauschning, 1987). Hasue et al. (1983) found histologic evidence of compression (intraneural fibrosis) of the L5 dorsal root. Compression occurred between the superior articular process of S1 and the posterior aspect of the vertebral body of L5 (Hasue et al., 1983).

After leaving the lateral recess, the L5 roots and their dural root sleeve continue along the L5 NRC by wrapping around the posterior and lateral aspect of the L5 vertebral body. The roots continue around the posterolateral aspect of the L5 IVD and unite to form the spinal nerve. The L5 nerve, which is the *largest* of the lumbar nerves, exits the lateral border of the L5 NRC (the IVF proper), which is the *smallest* IVF of the lumbar spine (Olsewski et al., 1991; Cramer et al., 2003). This makes the L5 nerve particularly susceptible to compression within its IVF.

The anterior primary division (APD) of L5 is given off at the most lateral aspect of the IVF and then passes along a depression on the front of the sacral ala. The APD frequently is bounded anterosuperiorly in this region by the corporotransverse ligament (Bachop and Janse, 1983; Bachop and Ro, 1984; Rauschning, 1987). The corporotransverse ligament passes from the vertebral body and IVD of L5 to the TP of L5. Several investigators (Nathan, Weizenbluth, and Halperin, 1982; Olsewski et al., 1991; Briggs and Chandraraj, 1995) report that the inferior band of the iliolumbar ligament, known as the lumbosacral ligament (LSL), consistently courses from the vertebral body and TP of L5 to the ala of the sacrum (see Fig. 7-22). The descriptions of the corporotransverse ligament by Bachop and Janse (1983) and Bachop and Ro (1984) are consistent with what Nathan, Weizenbluth, and Halperin (1982) consider to be the fibers of origin of the LSL. This indicates that the fibers of origin of the LSL are much more substantial than those fibers found more inferiorly and laterally, and that frequently a distinct tough, fibrous band, the corporotransverse ligament, is formed in the region of origin of the LSL.

After passing beneath the corporotransverse ligament and the LSL, the APD of L5 continues inferiorly (Nathan, Weizenbluth, and Halperin, 1982; Bachop and Janse, 1983; Bachop and Ro, 1984; Olsewski et al., 1991). Therefore the corporotransverse ligament of Bachop and the LSL significantly extend the osteoligamentous canal of the L5 NRC, and the most inferior aspect of the LSL forms the anterior and inferior boundary of the L5 osteoligamentous canal. Nathan, Weizenbluth, and Halperin (1982) state that the gray communicating ramus from the sympathetic chain to the APD of L5 pierces the LSL. Previous studies had shown that, throughout the spine, osteophytes from vertebral bodies frequently exert pressure on the sympathetic trunk, rami communicantes, and spinal nerves. This was found to be particularly true with the neural elements of L5 (Nathan, Weizenbluth, and Halperin, 1982). Finally, just inferior to the LSL, a branch of the APD of L4 joins the APD of L5 to form the lumbosacral trunk.

The unique characteristics of the L5-S1 NRC, IVF proper, and the lateral osteoligamentous canal of the L5 APD make the L5 nerve "extremely vulnerable to compression by any of the structures forming the tunnel. A tight LSL, osteophytes on the border of the L5-S1 disc or a combination of the two may impinge on the nerve and compress it against the ala of the sacrum" (Nathan, Weizenbluth, and Halperin, 1982). Olsewski et al. (1991) reported that the APD of L5 was observed to be compressed by the LSL in 11% of the 102 cadaveric specimens they studied by gross dissection. Histologic evidence of compression (e.g., perineurial and endoneurial fibrosis, peripheral thinning of myelin sheaths, and shift to a smaller fiber diameter) was shown in 3% of L5 APD specimens studied by Olsewski et al. (1991), and in 9% of the specimens studied by Briggs and Chandraraj (1995). Osteophytes extending posterolaterally from both the inferior surface of the L5 body and the upper border of the body of the sacrum were found to narrow the L5 osteoligamentous canal further in 1 of 59 spines (2%) studied by Olsewski et al. (1991). This was found to contribute to compression of the APD of L5. Nathan, Weizenbluth, and Halperin (1982) found such osteophytes "frequently" and also noted that the L5 nerve was "very often" entrapped or compressed to some degree by osteophytes or the LSL while passing through the

osteoligamentous tunnel. Briggs and Chandraraj (1995) found that IVD narrowing also contributed to compression of the L5 APD; they felt that the reason for this may be that additional fibers were added to the LSL to help stabilize the region after IVD degeneration.

Compression of the L5 APD by the corporotransverse ligament or the LSL could result in pain along the distribution of L5 nerves to include the L5 dermatome (lateral aspect of the leg distally to the great toe [Floman and Mirovsky, 1990]) and possible loss of motor function of the muscles primarily innervated by the L5 APD (motor paresis of the extensor hallucis longus muscle is found in 5% to 11% of patients with L5 nerve root compression [Jönsson and Stromqvist, 1995]). Referred pain may be experienced in the lumbar region (see Chapter 11), although this has not been fully documented. Myelography, discography, standard CT scans, and transverse plane MRI scans would all be negative (Olsewski et al., 1991). Far lateral parasagittal MRI scans (farther lateral than standard MRI protocols) may show the relationship between the L5 nerve and the corporotransverse ligament and the LSL (Nowicki and Haughton, 1992). Perhaps far lateral parasagittal MRI would be a useful diagnostic procedure for patients exhibiting L5 dermatomal and motor symptoms and signs when other imaging modalities do not reveal a possible cause of entrapment (see Fig. 2-24). Further investigation in this region is warranted. In the meantime, "in the patient presenting with L5 root signs, if the myelogram, discogram, and CT scan do not reveal any defect, then the possibility of extraforaminal compression must be considered as a possible source of the clinical signs" (Olsewski et al., 1991).

Because of the unique anatomy of this region, several distinct conditions, besides those already described, can affect the L5 nerve roots, the L5 spinal nerve, or the APD of L5. For example, because the neural elements of L5 are related to the L5 IVD for a relatively long distance, far lateral L5 IVD protrusion (lateral to the IVF) may affect the L5 spinal nerve or the APD of L5. Another example of the unique vulnerability of the L5 neural elements is spondylolisthesis after spondylolysis (see Fig. 7-17). This condition may result in compression of the L5 nerve along its course from behind the L5 disc to the nerve's lateral relation with the corporotransverse ligament and the L5 TP, both of which lie above the nerve (Bachop and Janse, 1983; Bachop and Ro, 1984; Rauschning, 1987).

A 20% or greater anterior shift of a spondylolisthetic L5 vertebra may result in compression of the APD of L5 between the TP of L5 and the sacral ala (Wiltse et al., 1984). Such compression is usually unilateral but occasionally may be bilateral. Also, both asymmetric degeneration of the L5 IVD and degenerative lumbar scoliosis result in lateral tilting and rotation of L5. As with spondylolisthesis, this also can result in compression of the L5 nerve between the TP of L5 and the sacral ala. Such far lateral compressions of the L5 nerve have been called the "far-out syndrome (Wiltse et al., 1984) of Wiltse" (Dommisse and Louw, 1990). Wiltse et al. (1984) stated that the lateral entrapment caused by either degenerative scoliosis or asymmetric disc degeneration probably was most common in elderly patients, whereas lateral entrapment as a result of spondylolisthesis was found most frequently in a somewhat younger group of adult patients. The authors also stated that far lateral entrapment occasionally could occur at levels higher than L5 and may be accompanied by the radiographic findings of marked scoliosis with closely approximated TPs of two adjacent vertebrae. CT was found to be the imaging modality of choice to view the region of entrapment. A "wide window" setting for the CT scan was necessary to view the laterally placed TPs. CT images reformatted in the coronal plane were particularly useful in evaluating the relationship between the L5 TPs and the sacral ala (Wiltse et al., 1984).

Nathan, Weizenbluth, and Halperin (1982) found that branches of the iliolumbar artery and relatively large veins always accompanied the APD of L5 beneath the LSL. Using examples of neuralgias and pareses of cranial nerves caused by compression of these nerves by adjacent arteries, they hypothesized that likewise the APD of L5 could become entrapped within its osteoligamentous tunnel by branches of the iliolumbar artery and accompanying veins. This would be particularly feasible when the APD of L5 already was partially compressed within a narrow tunnel or by osteophytes extending posterolaterally from the inferior border of the L5 body.

UNIQUE ASPECTS OF THE LUMBAR VERTEBRAE

Fifth Lumbar Vertebra

The L5 vertebra, its relationship with the sacrum, and soft tissue elements in between are some of the most clinically relevant anatomic structures of the spine. Pain in this region is extremely common (Cramer et al., 1992a); therefore an accurate working knowledge of the L5-S1 region is essential for those treating patients with low back and leg pain. The anatomy of this region is subject to much variation. Nathan, Weizenbluth, and Halperin (1982) stated that "such skeletal variations are accompanied by changes and adjustments of the related soft tissues, including the nerves and vessels." Therefore clinically relevant variations frequently accompany the normal anatomy of this area.

The L5 vertebral body is the largest of the entire spine (Fig. 7-16). It is taller anteriorly than posteriorly, which contributes to the increase in the lower lumbar lordosis (the lower lumbar lordosis is frequently called the lumbosacral angle). The spinous process of L5 is the

smallest of all those of the lumbar vertebrae. It projects inferiorly, and its posterior aspect is more rounded in appearance than the rest of the lumbar spinous processes (see Fig. 7-16). The TPs of L5 are much wider from anterior to posterior and from superior to inferior than those of the rest of the lumbar spine. They originate from the entire lateral aspect of the pedicles, and their origin continues posteriorly to the adjacent lamina (see Fig. 7-16). However, the TPs do not extend as far laterally as other lumbar TPs (see Transverse Processes). The lateral aspect of the TPs of L5 also angle slightly superiorly, with the angulation beginning at about the midpoint of each of the two (left and right) processes.

Spondylolysis and Spondylolisthesis. Spondylolysis is a defect of the lamina (Fig. 7-17) between the superior and inferior articular processes. This region is known as the pars interarticularis. Controversy exists as to whether this defect is most frequently caused by trauma or if it is hereditary (Schwab, Farcy, and Roye, 1997). Causes of pars (isthmic) defects include lytic or stress fractures of the pars interarticularis (probably the most common cause), elongated but intact pars (not spondylolysis), and acute fracture of the pars (Day, 1991). The fifth lumbar vertebra is the segment most vulnerable to acute pars fracture (Ebraheim et al., 1997a). Athletes whose sport requires them to rapidly alternate between flexion and extension of the lumbar region are commonly afflicted with acute fractures of the pars interarticularis (McGill, 1997). Bilateral spondylolysis may result in forward slippage of that portion of the vertebra located anterior to the laminar defect (i.e., vertebral body, pedicles, TPs, superior articular processes). This leaves the inferior articular processes, a portion of the laminae, and the spinous process behind. Such forward displacement is known as spondylolisthesis and is found in 5% of lumbar spines (Williams et al., 1995) (see Fig. 7-17). Although most common at L5, spondylolisthesis occurs with some frequency at L4 and may be seen at any level of the lumbar spine. Other causes of spondylolisthesis include (a) improper formation of the posterior vertebral arch, known as the dysplastic type of spondylolisthesis; (b) degeneration and subsequent erosion of the superior articular process; (c) fracture of part of the posterior arch other than the pars interarticularis (e.g., pedicle fracture); and (d) pathologic conditions of the bone forming the posterior arch (e.g., Paget's disease).

Sometimes the pars defect fills with connective tissue. The connective tissue attachment has been termed the spondylolysis ligament (Wiltse, 1962) and contains several zones of fibrous and cartilaginous tissues (Nordström et al., 1994). Einstein et al. (1994) found that this "ligament" was innervated by nerves that met the criteria of pain-sensitive (nociceptive) fibers (e.g.,

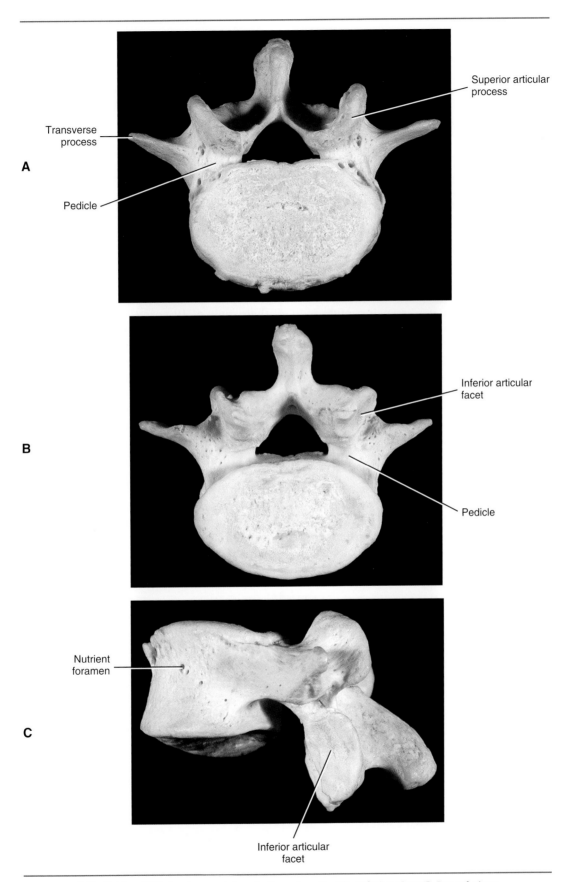

FIG. 7-16   Fifth lumbar vertebra. **A,** Superior view. **B,** Inferior view. **C,** Lateral view.

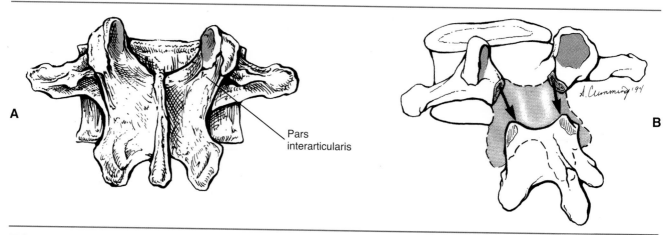

FIG. 7-17 **A,** Posterior view of a typical lumbar vertebra. **B,** Bilateral fracture of the pars interarticularis (spondylolysis) and a separation (spondylolisthesis) of the region anterior to the pars interarticularis from the remainder of the posterior arch.

immunoreactivity to calcitonin gene-related peptide and vasoactive intestinal peptide), indicating that deformation of the ligament during spondylolisthesis could result in low back pain. Of course, several other tissues (e.g., IVD, muscles, ligaments) that are stretched because of spondylolisthesis also could generate pain as well (Einstein et al., 1994).

Standard x-ray films and CT remain the imaging modalities of choice for visualizing spondylolysis. However, parasagittal MRI does help to reveal a defect of the pars, which appears as a decrease in signal intensity perpendicular to the plane of the articular facets on these images (Grenier et al., 1989a). Occasionally, rather than the development of a spondylolisthesis, the *posterior* segment created by bilateral spondylolysis moves further posteriorly. When such posterior displacement occurs, it can frequently be identified on sagittal plane MRI scans (Ulmer et al., 1995).

Spondylolisthesis is graded by the degree to which the affected vertebral body is anteriorly displaced in relation to the vertebral (or sacral) body located immediately inferior to it. For example, a 25% spondylolisthesis represents forward displacement of a vertebral body (measured at the posterior and inferior border of the vertebral body) along one fourth of the length of the vertebral body (or sacral body) directly inferior to it. Spondylolisthesis also can be graded on a scale of 1 to 4, with each grade representing an additional 25% of anterior slippage. A grade 4 describes a vertebral body that has been displaced completely off of the vertebra (or usually, the sacrum) directly beneath it.

Although spondylolysis with spondylolisthesis has been implicated as a cause of spinal canal (specifically, lateral recess) stenosis at the level of the pars interarticularis defect, Liyang et al. (1989) reported an increase in vertebral canal dimensions at the level of spondylolisthesis in one cadaveric spine, which was included in

their study of 10 normal spines. Spondylolisthesis at L5 also may result in entrapment of the L5 nerve as it passes laterally, in front of the pars interarticularis, to exit the L5 IVF. The entrapment is caused by the portion of the pars located above the fracture site. This is the part of the pars that is displaced anteriorly with the vertebral body and pedicles. By moving anteriorly, it can compress the L5 nerve (Kirkaldy-Willis et al., 1978).

Degenerative spondylolisthesis is a condition in which the superior articular processes undergo erosion with age rather than the usual increase in bone formation that frequently occurs in these processes with age. This erosion results in the vertebrae above (usually L4, the next most common is L3) moving anteriorly, bringing its posterior arch with it. The amount of anterior slippage (olisthesis) with degenerative spondylolisthesis ranges from 8% to 43% (Postacchini and Perugia, 1991). The consequence of this anterior slippage of the entire vertebra, including the posterior arch, is spinal canal stenosis with possible compromise of the cauda equina (Kirkaldy-Willis et al., 1978). As mentioned, most frequently L4 moves anteriorly on L5, and the inferior articular processes of L4 entrap the L5 and S1 nerve roots against the posterior aspect of the vertebral body of L5 (Dommise and Louw, 1990).

At the opposite end of the clinical spectrum for the pars interarticularis: the pars can occasionally enlarge as a result of degeneration. This is significant at the level of L5 because it can lead to entrapment of the S1 nerve as it courses along the lateral aspect of the vertebral canal (lateral recess).

Lumbosacral Articulation

The lumbosacral articulation is actually composed of several articulations between L5 and the sacrum. It consists of two components: the joining, by the fifth lumbar IVD, of the inferior aspect of the L5 body with the body of the S1 segment; and the joints between the left and right inferior articular processes of L5 and the superior articular processes of the sacrum. These latter joints are not nearly as curved as are the Z joints of the rest of the lumbar spine. The plane of articulation of the lumbosacral Z joints is subject to much variation, ranging 20 to 90 degrees to the sagittal plane (average, 40 to 60 degrees). Frequently asymmetry, known as tropism, exists between the left and right L5-S1 Z joints. Tropism may be a cause of premature degeneration and pain (Farfan, Huberdeau, and Dubow, 1972; Lippitt, 1984), with increased degenerative changes of the articular cartilage having been found on the side of the superior and inferior articular processes that are more closely oriented along the sagittal plane (Giles, 1987). However, the clinical significance of tropism remains a matter of controversy. For example, no association has been found between asymmetric facets and prolapsed IVD (Vanharanta et al., 1993; Boden et al., 1996) or degenerative spondylolisthesis (Boden et al., 1996); however, an association has been found between both of those clinical entities and bilateral sagittally oriented facets. This positive association holds true for sagittally oriented facets at both L4-L5 and L5-S1 (Boden et al., 1996).

The L5-S1 IVD is typically narrower than the IVDs of the rest of the lumbar region (Nicholson, Roberts, and Williams, 1988). This may contribute to the IVF at this level being smaller than those of the rest of the lumbar spine. It should be recalled that the spinal nerve at this level is the largest lumbar spinal nerve. Therefore more than one third of the L5-S1 IVF is filled by the spinal nerve. Even though the IVD and IVF are smaller in this region, the L5-S1 articulation is by far the most movable of all the lumbar joints (5 degrees of unilateral rotation, 3 degrees of lateral bending, 10 degrees of flexion, 10 degrees of extension). These factors, along with the others discussed in the previous section devoted to the L5 NRC, make the L5 roots and spinal nerve vulnerable to compression as they traverse the L5 NRC.

The intraarticular space of the left and right lumbosacral Z joints usually is wider than those of the remainder of the lumbar region. A recess normally exists along the inferomedial edge of the lumbosacral Z joints. This recess has been shown to be filled with a large intraarticular synovial fold, which is primarily composed of adipose tissue. Another intraarticular synovial protrusion usually projects into the superomedial aspect of the L5-S1 Z joint (Giles and Taylor, 1987). These synovial folds are susceptible to entrapment between the apposing L5-S1 articular facets and are a likely source of low back pain and subsequent muscle tightness. Gentle, well-controlled spinal manipulation to open the facets and allow an entrapped synovial fold to be pulled out of the joint by its attachment to the joint capsule has been suggested as the treatment of choice for this condition (Giles and Taylor, 1987).

A transitional segment between the lumbar spine and sacrum is found in 5% of the population (Nicholson, Roberts, and Williams, 1988). This takes the form of either a lumbarization of the S1 segment or, more frequently, a sacralization of the L5 vertebra. Sacralization refers to elongation of the TPs of L5 with varying degrees of fusion or articulation with either the sacral ala or the iliac crest. The union between L5 and the sacrum may be bilateral, but usually it is only unilateral (see Figs. 12-14, G and H). The L5-S1 IVD in cases of sacralization is normally significantly thinner than that of typical L5-S1 segments (Nicholson, Roberts, and Williams, 1988; Hsieh et al., 2000). It is also usually devoid of nuclear material, and therefore usually does not undergo pathologic change or degeneration to the degree seen in discs above the sacralized segment (Nicholson, Roberts, and Williams, 1988).

LIGAMENTS AND INTERVERTEBRAL DISCS OF THE LUMBAR REGION

Most of the ligaments associated with the lumbar region have been discussed in previous chapters. The articular capsules of the Z joints, ligamenta flava, supraspinous ligament, interspinous ligaments, intertransverse ligaments, and anterior and posterior longitudinal ligaments are discussed in Chapters 5 and 6, and the IVDs are discussed in Chapter 2. The mamillo-accessory ligament is discussed in this chapter (see Articular Processes). This section is devoted to characteristics of the mentioned ligaments that are unique to the lumbar region. The iliolumbar ligaments (left and right), which are found only in the lower lumbar region, also are covered in this section.

Lumbar Anterior Longitudinal Ligament

The anterior longitudinal ligament (ALL) is wider from side to side in the lumbar than in the thoracic region. It has also been found to be thicker than the posterior longitudinal ligament (PLL) (Grenier et al., 1989b). The lumbar ALL extends across the anterior aspect of the vertebral bodies and IVDs to attach inferiorly to the sacrum (Fig. 7-18). Like the ALL throughout the vertebral column, the lumbar ALL is firmly attached to a significant portion of the superior and inferior bony end plates of the vertebral bodies, but is only lightly attached to the center of the vertebral bodies or IVDs (Cramer et al., 1996, 1998a). Table 7-9 demonstrates the percentage of the width of the spine taken up by the ALL at the center of the vertebral bodies and at the center of the IVD. Figure 7-18, A, shows the lumbar ALL drawn to scale. Notice that the ALL bows out slightly at the level of the lumbar IVDs. This flaring of the ALL at the IVDs is unique

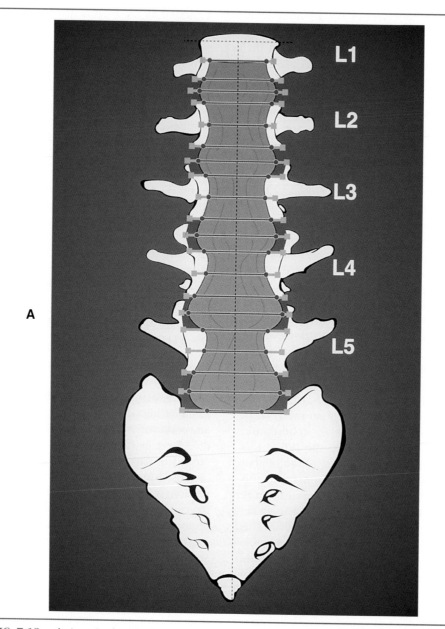

FIG. 7-18   **A,** Anterior longitudinal ligament (ALL) in the lumbar region. The ALL is illustrated to scale using the data of Table 7-9 and shows the lateral extensions of the ALL.

to the lumbar region of the vertebral column (Cramer et al., 1996, 1998).

The ALL functions to limit extension, and it may be torn during extension injuries of the spine. It receives sensory (nociceptive and proprioceptive) innervation from branches of the gray communicating rami of the lumbar sympathetic trunk; therefore damage to the ALL during extension injuries can be a direct source of pain.

The ALL and PLL have been collectively termed the intercentral ligaments because they connect the anterior and posterior surfaces of adjacent vertebral bodies (centra), respectively (Grenier et al., 1989b). They also

help attach the vertebral bodies to the IVDs and are important in stabilizing the spine during flexion (PLL) and extension (ALL). They also function to *limit* flexion (PLL) and extension (ALL) of the spine.

Lumbar Posterior Longitudinal Ligament

The PLL in the lumbar region is denticulated in appearance (Figs. 7-19 and 7-20). That is, it is narrow over the posterior aspect of the vertebral bodies and flares laterally at each IVD, where it attaches to the posterior aspect of the anulus fibrosus. The lumbar PLL is

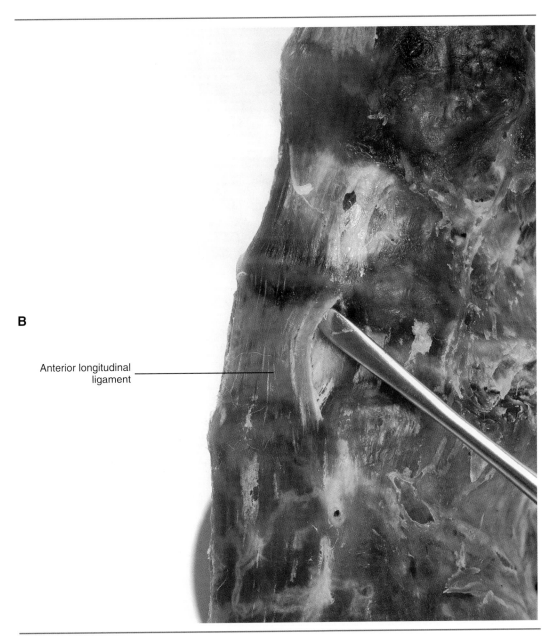

B

Anterior longitudinal ligament

FIG. 7-18—cont'd   B, Dissection of the lumbar ALL. Notice the probe passing posterior to the ligament, demonstrating its firm superior attachment to the bony end plate of the vertebral body.

Continued

composed of two strata of fibers, superficial and deep. The superficial fibers form a distinct midline band that spans several vertebral levels. The deep fibers are much shorter, and they converge on the IVD and extend laterally to the wide attachment sites of the PLL to the anulus fibrosus of the IVD (Parke and Schiff, 1993).

The width of the central attachment of the PLL to the lumbar vertebral bodies narrows as one moves down the spine, whereas the discal attachments remain relatively constant in width (Table 7-10 and Fig. 7-20). The PLL firmly attaches to the superior and inferior bony end plates of all lumbar vertebrae, and also firmly attaches to the superior aspect of the S1 segment. However, the PLL does not attach to the central regions of the L1-S1 vertebral bodies. The PLL is also firmly attached to the IVD along the peripheral margins of the PLL, but does not firmly attach to the IVD centrally to these peripheral attachments. This creates a rhomboid-shaped fascial cleft deep to the PLL in the center of the IVD. This fascial cleft may be important in helping to contain IVD extrusions (Oshima et al., 1993; Parke and Schiff, 1993; Yu et al., 1996; Cramer et al., 1998b).

The PLL receives sensory innervation from the recurrent meningeal nerve (sinuvertebral nerve). Substance P,

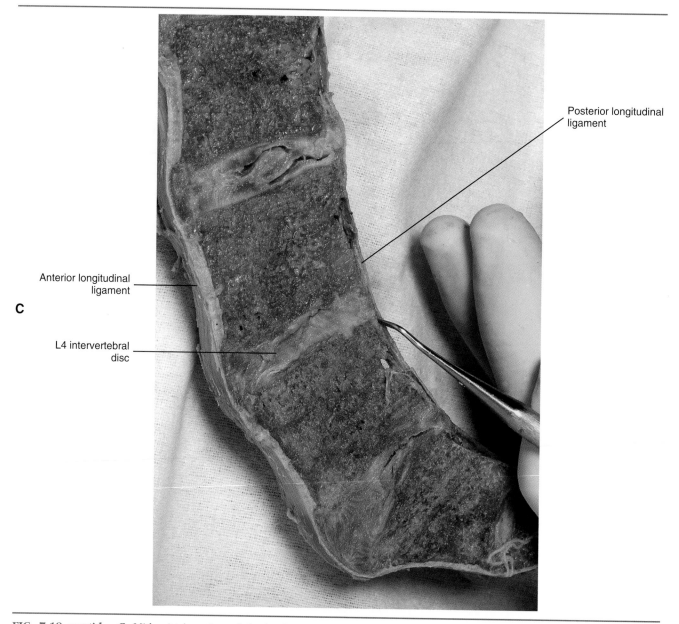

Posterior longitudinal ligament

Anterior longitudinal ligament

C

L4 intervertebral disc

FIG. 7-18–cont'd **C,** Midsagittal section of the lumbar region showing the anterior and posterior longitudinal ligaments. The probe is passing in front of (anterior to) the posterior longitudinal ligament.

a known sensory neurotransmitter that is usually associated with pain sensation, has been found in the terminal fibers of the sinuvertebral nerve innervating the lumbar PLL. Korkala et al. (1985) also found enkephalins, a known neuromodulator, in the PLL. Together these findings substantiate previous suppositions that the PLL is pain sensitive and may indicate that the PLL (at least in the lumbar region) is *highly* sensitive to pain. The pain sensitivity of the PLL has been demonstrated by mechanical irritation of the ligament in patients with only local anesthesia of the overlying skin. The pain was felt in the midline and radiated into the low back and

superior aspect of the buttock (Edgar and Ghadially, 1976).

In some instances, posterior and posterolateral IVD extrusions may penetrate the PLL. This is a strong sign that the extrusion is not contained within the anulus fibrosis (see Intervertebral Disc in Chapter 11 and later discussion). This may be an indication for surgical removal of the disc. The penetrated PLL is able to be distinguished from a bulging anulus fibrosus on parasagittal MRI scans. The PLL appears as an area of low signal intensity on these images. Using MRI, Grenier et al. (1989b) were able to determine when the PLL was *not*

Table 7-9 Width Measurements* of the Anterior Longitudinal Ligament and Spine at Seven Locations

Level	ALL	Spine	Percent ALL/Spine†
L2 Body	31.7 (3.5)	40.7 (3.4)	78.1% (±9.1%)
L2 Disc	42.9 (5.4)	55.1 (4.8)	77.9% (±7.7%)
L4 Body	32.6 (4.3)	46.2 (3.3)	70.5% (±8.9%)
L4 Disc	50.9 (4.5)	60.5 (5.5)	84.4% (±7.9%)
L5 Body	33.7 (4.4)	51.9 (4.4)	65.2% (±9.8%)
L5 Disc	50.5 (6.1)	59.8 (7.7)	85.5% (±8.8%)
S1 Superior margin	29.8 (5.0)	58.4 (6.9)	51.1% (±8.8%)

These data allowed for the development of the composite diagram of the lumbar spine and the ALL shown in Figure 7-18, A.

ALL, Anterior longitudinal ligament.

*Measurements are in millimeters with standard deviations in parentheses.

†These are the actual averages of the percentages obtained for each specimen (30 specimens), not results obtained from values of column two divided by those of column three. These values represent the percent of the width of the spine occupied by the ALL at the specified level.

disrupted (not penetrated by the anulus fibrosus or nucleus pulposus) 100% of the time and were able to determine when the PLL *was* disrupted 78% of the time. The authors concluded that MRI was useful in the detection of PLL disruption.

Lumbar Ligamenta Flava

The paired ligamenta flava of the lumbar region are the thickest of the entire spine. They extend between the laminae of adjacent vertebrae throughout the lumbar region, including the junction between the laminae of L5 and those of the S1 segment. Each ligamentum flavum is thickest medially. Laterally the ligament passes more anteriorly to form the anterior joint capsule of the Z joint, attaching to the superior and inferior articular processes that form this joint. The most lateral fibers attach to the pedicle of the vertebra below (Fig. 7-21).

Olszewski, Yaszemski, and White (1996) evaluated the ligamenta flava in the lumbar region. They found that rather than a left and right ligament being found at each level, the two sides actually were continuous with one another in the midline. However, a deep midline recess of several millimeters was found extending posteriorly in the midline. The authors were convinced that previous investigators had mistaken this midline recess for a separation of the two sides of the ligamentum flavum. The authors also found that each ligamentum flavum of the lumbar region had a superficial (posterior) and a deep (anterior) component. The two components adhered tightly to one another, except at their inferior attachment

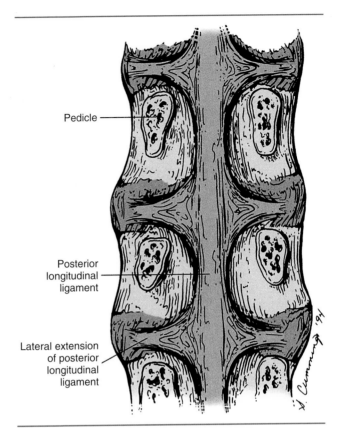

Pedicle

Posterior longitudinal ligament

Lateral extension of posterior longitudinal ligament

FIG. 7-19 Posterior longitudinal ligament is shown coursing along the anterior aspect of the lumbar vertebral canal.

Table 7-10 Width Measurements* of the Posterior Longitudinal Ligament and Spine at Six Locations

Level	PLL	Spine	Percent PLL/Spine†
L2 Body	7.84 (2.07)	40.74 (3.58)	19.5% (±5.5%)
L2 Disc	28.18 (3.87)	55.18 (4.96)	47.8% (±12.4%)
L4 Body	4.67 (1.70)	46.39 (3.47)	12.4% (±7.2%)
L4 Disc	28.68 (4.12)	60.29 (5.45)	44.3% (±11.3%)
L5 Body	2.50 (1.05)	52.36 (4.47)	7.6% (±7.1%)
L5 Disc	25.81 (5.03)	59.46 (7.60)	45.4% (±11.0%)

These data allowed for the development of the composite diagram of the lumbar spine and the PLL shown in Figure 7-20, A.

PLL, Posterior longitudinal ligament.

*Measurements are in millimeters with standard deviations in parentheses.

†These are the actual averages of the percentages obtained for each specimen (33 specimens), not results obtained from values of column two divided by those of column three. These values represent the percent of the width of the spine occupied by the PLL at the specified level.

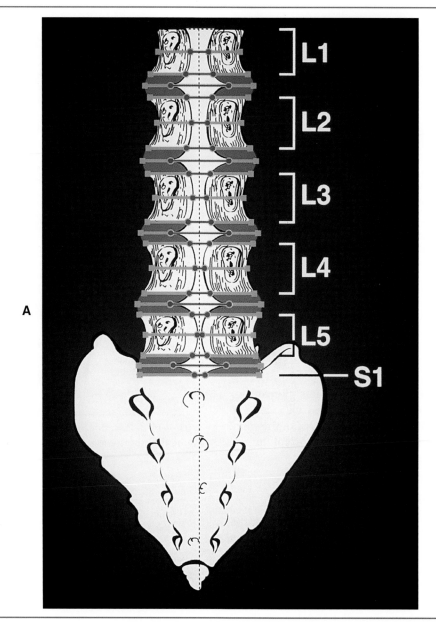

FIG. 7-20   **A,** Posterior longitudinal ligament (PLL) in the lumbar region. The PLL is illustrated to scale from the data presented in Table 7-10.

sites. Superiorly the adherent superficial and deep components attached to the anteroinferior aspect of the laminae above. The amount of the anterior surface of the laminae that was covered by the fibers extending superiorly increased from the upper to lower lumbar regions (a little less than 60% at L1 to approximately 70% at L5). Inferiorly the attachments of the superficial and deep components of the ligamentum flavum differed. The superficial component was found to attach to the posterosuperior aspect of the lamina below, as classically taught; however, the deep component attached to the anterosuperior aspect of the lamina below. Again, a much

greater portion of the anterior surface of the lamina was covered by the deep component of the ligamentum flavum as one descended the lumbar region, with the combination of the superior attachment of the ligament below and the inferior attachment of the ligament above covering a little more than 60% of the lamina at L1 (the inferior aspect of the T12-L1 ligamentum flavum covered little of the anterior surface of L1), 75% to 80% at L3 and L4, and 100% of the lamina at L5 (Olszewski, Yaszemski, and White, 1996).

The exiting dorsal and ventral nerve roots of the lumbar region come in direct contact with the anterior

B

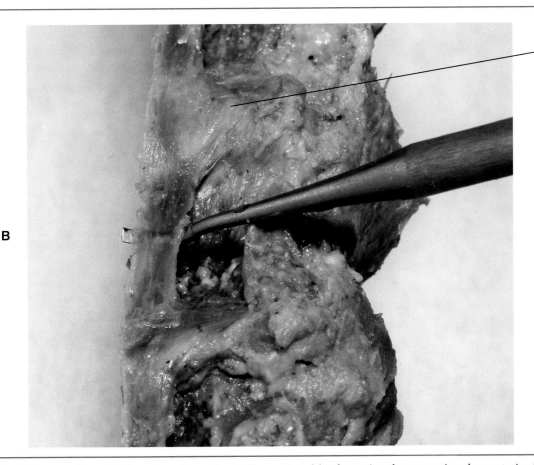

Lateral attachment
of posterior
longitudinal
ligament to
intervertebral
disc

FIG. 7-20—cont'd   B, Dissection of a midsagittally sectioned lumbar spine demonstrating the posterior longitudinal ligament. Notice how narrow the ligament is in the region of the vertebral body, where the probe is passing anterior to it, and how the ligament flares laterally as it firmly attaches to the intervertebral discs.

aspect of the ligamentum flavum as the ligament forms the anterior capsule of the Z joint within the IVF (Hasue et al., 1983). A recess has been found in the lateral, articular portion of the ligament. Paris (1983) states that this recess may allow the synovium of the facet joint to pass through the ligamentum flavum. Under certain circumstances the synovium could then extend into the IVF, where it could conceivably compress the spinal nerve.

Sensory fibers, probably arising from the medial branch of the posterior primary division (Bogduk, 1983), have been found innervating the ligamenta flava (Edgar and Ghadially, 1976). Therefore damage to these ligaments may result in back pain. The sensory receptors within the ligamenta flava have been found to be both mechanoreceptors (i.e., Ruffini corpuscles, Ruffini end organs, Pacinian corpuscles), for proprioception, and free nerve endings for nociception (Yahia, Newman, and Rivard, 1988; Yahia, St-Georges, and Newman, 1988). In fact, tissue samples of the ligamenta flava taken from low back pain patients at surgery have been found to contain a significant number of nociceptive fibers, similar in number to the Z joint capsule and significantly more than the IVD (Bucknill et al., 2002). Therefore tissue damage and inflammation of the ligamentum flavum may stimulate an additional ingrowth of sensory neurons, as has been found in other tissues (e.g., the IVD). However, as the ligamentum flavum undergoes aging and degeneration the number of nerve fibers decreases (Viejo-Fuertes et al., 1998). In addition, the role of the ligamenta flava as a secondary source of back pain in spinal stenosis (by compressing the nerve roots) is also well documented (see Lumbar Vertebral Foramen and the Vertebral Canal; Lumbar Intervertebral Foramina and the Nerve Root Canals). Hypertrophy of the ligamenta flava can contribute to spinal canal stenosis. The ligamenta flava have been found to undergo hypertrophy in some individuals during simple aging of the spine. More frequently, hypertrophy of the ligamenta flava occur as other spinal tissues, such as the IVDs and Z joints, undergo degenerative changes and decrease the stability of the motion segments. These hypertrophic changes of the ligamenta flava may result from an increase in the growth factor, transforming growth factor-beta 1

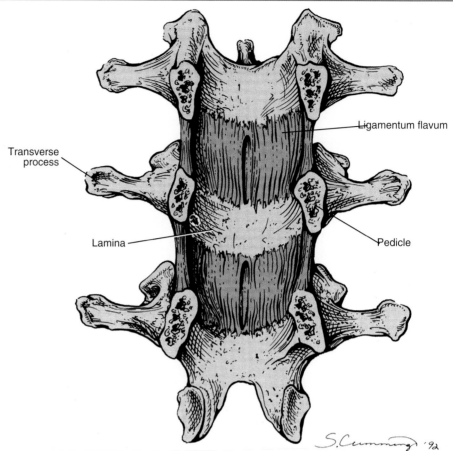

A

Ligamentum flavum

Transverse process

Lamina

Pedicle

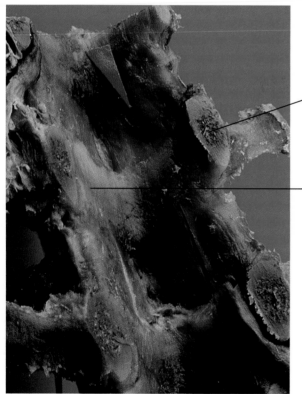

B

Pedicle

Lamina

FIG. 7-21   Pedicles have been sectioned in a coronal plane to reveal the posterior aspect of the vertebral canal. **A,** Artist's rendering. **B,** Cadaveric specimen. Notice the ligamenta flava (*red arrow*) passing between the adjacent laminae. (**B,** Courtesy the National University of Health Sciences.)

(TGF-β1) in ligamentum flavum fibroblasts (Park, Chang, and Lee, 2001). In addition, calcium pyrophosphate deposition disease (pseudogout) is also associated with hypertrophy of the ligamenta flava (Markiewitz et al., 1996).

Lumbar Interspinous Ligaments

The results of descriptive studies of these ligaments in the lumbar region have led to elaboration on their structure in this particular area of the spine. Therefore a brief discussion of the unique aspects of these ligaments is included here, even though the interspinous ligaments were described with the thoracic region (see Chapter 6).

Several authors have described the structure of a typical lumbar interspinous ligament as being composed of three parts: anterior, middle, and posterior (Behrsin and Briggs, 1988; Bogduk, 1997). These three parts run between adjacent spinous processes, filling the gap along the length of these processes.

The anterior portion of the interspinous ligament is paired (left and right) anteriorly, with each part attaching to the ligamentum flavum of the same side. A thin layer of adipose tissue separates the two halves. Posteriorly the two sides of this part of the interspinous ligament unite to form a single ligament. The fibers of this part of the interspinous ligament pass posteriorly and superiorly from their origin (ligamentum flavum) to attach to the anterior half of the inferior aspect of the spinous process of the vertebra above.

The middle portion of the interspinous ligament is the most substantial region. It originates from the anterior half of the upper surface of a spinous process and passes posteriorly and superiorly to insert onto the posterior half of the lower surface of the spinous process of the vertebra above. Although this orientation of fibers in the interspinous ligament would not seem to limit flexion of the lumbar region, the collagen fibers of this ligament have a complex interaction that increases stiffness of the ligament, helping it to limit flexion (Dickey, Bednar, and Dumas, 1996).

The posterior aspect of the interspinous ligament attaches to the posterior half of the upper surface of a spinous process and continues superiorly to pass behind (posterior to) the vertebra above, becoming continuous with the supraspinous ligament (see following discussion). Bogduk (1997) does not consider this posterior portion to be a true part of the interspinous ligament because it does not attach to two adjacent bones.

The interspinous ligament appears to be quite capable of being torn. One investigator found its fibers to be ruptured in 21% of cadavers examined. The middle fibers were found to be torn most frequently (Behrsin and Briggs, 1988). Because this ligament is supplied with sensory innervation containing both mechanoreceptive and nociceptive nerve endings (Yahia, Newman, and St-Georges, 1988), tearing of the ligament is likely a source of low back pain.

The interspinous ligaments and supraspinous ligament limit the end stage of lumbar flexion, and they are the first to sprain during hyperflexion of the lumbar region (Hutton, 1990).

Lumbar Supraspinous Ligament

The supraspinous ligament is strongest in the lumbar region. It is classically described as extending to the sacrum. However, Behrsin and Briggs, (1988) believe that the supraspinous ligament ends at L5 and does not extend to the sacrum, and Paris (1983) states that it usually ends at L4 and rarely at L5, never extending to the sacrum. Paris (1983) has found that the strong fibers of origin of the lumbar erector spinae muscles and the thoracolumbar fascia take the place of this ligament inferior to the spinous process of L4. This fascia continues inferiorly to the median sacral crest. Bogduk (1997) states that the supraspinous ligament is not a true ligament in the lumbar region. He believes it is primarily made up of strong tendinous fibers of the longissimus thoracis and multifidus muscles, and crisscrossing fibers of the thoracolumbar fascia. In addition, a condensation of the membranous (deep) layer of the superficial fascia of the back forms the superficial layer of the supraspinous ligament (Bogduk, 1997). In spite of this, the term *supraspinous ligament* continues to be used quite frequently by clinicians and researchers alike. In such instances, they are probably referring to the tough combination of midline tendons of the longissimus thoracis muscle, intersecting fibers of the thoracolumbar fascia, and membranous layer of superficial fascia. The term *lumbar supraspinous restraints* would seem to reflect more accurately the true nature of the fibrous band of tissue that is found along the posterior aspect of the lumbar spinous processes and interspinous spaces. Regardless of the true origin of the tissue forming these supraspinous restraints, they do receive sensory innervation that consists of both mechanoreceptive and nociceptive nerve endings (Yahia, Newman, and St-Georges, 1988); therefore damage to these restraints is likely to cause low back pain.

Lumbar Intertransverse Ligaments

The general characteristics of the intertransverse ligaments are described in Chapter 5. Some authors describe the lumbar intertransverse ligaments as being thin membranous bands that connect two adjacent TPs (Behrsin and Briggs, 1988). Others consider the intertransverse ligaments to be rather discrete and well-defined bands; still other authors consider them to consist of two lamellae (Behrsin and Briggs, 1988). The latter view appears to be gaining acceptance (Bogduk, 1997).

The posterior lamella of the intertransverse ligament passes medially to the posterior aspect of the Z joint. It is pierced by the posterior primary division and continues medially to help reinforce the Z joint capsule from behind. Laterally the membranous intertransverse ligament also has a posterior layer. The posterior layer of the lateral aspect of the intertransverse ligament becomes continuous with the aponeurosis of the transversus abdominis muscle and then becomes continuous with the middle layer of the thoracolumbar fascia (Bogduk, 1997).

The anterior lamella of the intertransverse ligament passes medially to form a layer of fascia over the IVF, where it is pierced by the APD and the spinal branches of lumbar segmental arteries and veins. The anterior lamella then continues anteriorly and medially to become continuous with the ALL. The accessory (transforaminal) ligaments that span the IVF (see Chapter 2 and previous discussion on corporotransverse ligament under L5 NRC) are probably condensations of the anterior lamella of the intertransverse ligament (Bogduk, 1997). It should be recalled that laterally the membranous intertransverse ligament also has anterior and posterior layers. The anterior layer becomes continuous with the anterior layer of the thoracolumbar fascia and covers the anterior aspect of the quadratus lumborum muscle.

A V-shaped groove (with the apex of the V facing laterally) is formed by the medially located anterior and posterior lamellae of the intertransverse ligament. The region between the two lamellae is filled with a small amount of adipose tissue that is continuous with the adipose tissue within the Z joint. This V-shaped region is known as the superior articular recess (see Zygapophysial Joints). It aids the Z joint by allowing for its adipose contents to be displaced during extension of the spine (Bogduk, 1997).

Iliolumbar Ligaments

The left and right iliolumbar ligaments (ILLs) course from the left and right TPs of L5 (and rarely L4) to the sacrum and iliac crest of the same side. Each is composed of as many as five parts (Bogduk, 1997). The most prominent part consists of an inferior and superior band (Olsewski et al., 1991; Williams et al., 1995). The inferior band is present 97% of the time and is also known as the lumbosacral ligament (LSL). The LSL extends from the inferior aspect of the L5 TP and the body of L5 to the anterosuperior aspect of the sacral ala, where it blends with the ventral sacroiliac ligament (Fig. 7-22). The LSL extends from the TP and body of L5 to the sacral promontory at least 3% of the time (Olsewski et al., 1991).

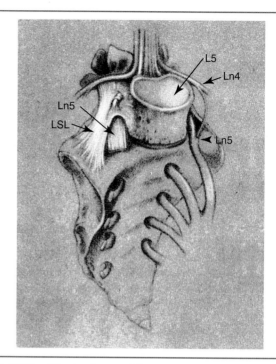

FIG. 7-22   The lumbosacral ligament (LSL). Notice the relationship between the LSL and the ventral ramus of L5 (Ln5). (From Olsewski JM et al. [1991]. Evidence from cadavers suggestive of entrapment of fifth lumbar spinal nerves by lumbosacral ligaments. *Spine, 16,* 336-347.)

The superior band of the ILL courses farther laterally than the LSL and attaches to the iliac tuberosity in front of the superior aspect of the sacroiliac joint. This band is continuous with the attachment of the quadratus lumborum muscle to the TP of L5, and usually consists of two distinct bands, anterior and posterior (Fig. 7-23), although one of the bands can be absent in some individuals. The anterior band is flat and fan shaped, narrow medially and wide laterally. Its dimensions average 30 to 40 mm long, 8 to 10 mm wide, and 2 to 3 mm thick. The medial attachment of the anterior band is to the anterior, inferior, and lateral aspect of the TP of L5. From here the anterior band passes laterally, within the horizontal plane, to reach its lateral attachment to the medial aspect of the ilium, inferior to the iliac crest (specifically, to the upper and anterior-most aspect of the iliac tuberosity). The posterior band is more rod shaped. The medial attachment of this band is to the lateral tip of the L5 TP. From here the posterior band courses laterally, posteriorly (at a 45- to 55-degree angle to a horizontal line passing through the TP of L5), and superiorly, reaching its lateral attachment to the superior and anterior aspects of the iliac tuberosity, just above and behind the anterior band (Hanson and Sonesson, 1994; Basadonna, Gasparini, and Rucco, 1996; Rucco, Basadonna, and Gasparini, 1996).

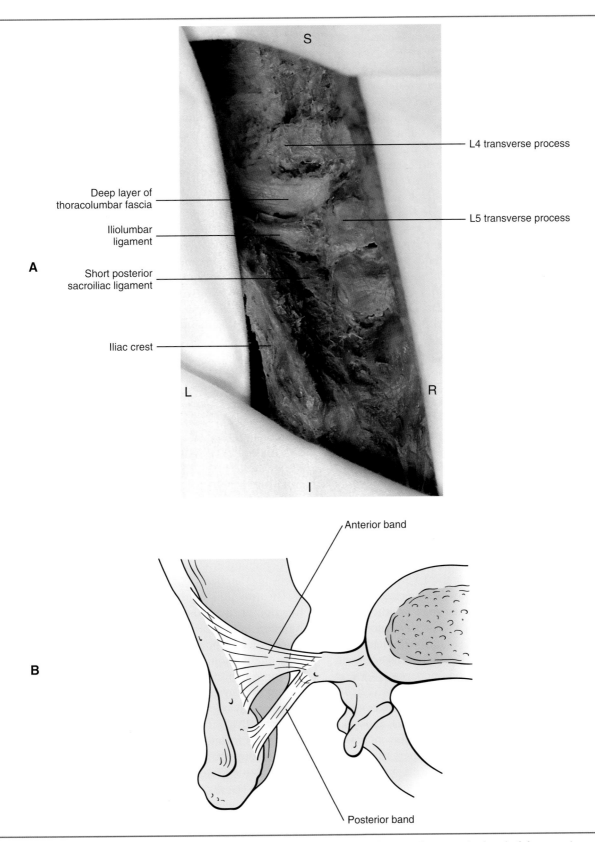

L4 transverse process

Deep layer of
thoracolumbar fascia

Iliolumbar
ligament

L5 transverse process

Short posterior
sacroiliac ligament

Iliac crest

A

Anterior band

B

Posterior band

FIG. 7-23   The iliolumbar ligament (ILL). **A,** Posterior view of a dissection showing the posterior band of the superior component of this ligament. *S,* Superior; *I,* inferior; *L,* left; and, *R,* right. **B,** Illustration (superior view) demonstrating the anterior and posterior bands of the superior component (band) of the ILL. (**B,** Based on Rucco V, Basadonna PT & Gasparini D. [1996] Anatomy of the Iliolumbar ligament: A review of its anatomy and a magnetic resonance study. *Am J Phys Med Rehabil* 75: 451-455.)

This is the band that is most commonly seen during typical dissections of the lower lumbar region using the standard posterior approach. When L5 is located more inferiorly in the pelvis, the anterior and posterior bands of the ILLs pass more obliquely superiorly, and when L5 is more superiorly positioned with respect to the pelvis, the anterior and posterior bands are shorter and have a more horizontal orientation (Rucco, Basadonna, and Gasparini, 1996). Other, less significant, portions of the ILL include inferior (not the LSL) and vertical parts. These are both said to originate from the TP of L5 and attach to the ilium (Bogduk, 1997); however, not all authors agree about their existence (Hanson and Sonesson, 1994).

Previously the ILL was thought to develop as a result of metaplasia of epimysium (outer covering) of the inferior fibers of the quadratus lumborum muscle. However, Uhthoff (1993) found this ligament to be well developed in 12 of 12 fetuses beyond 11.5 weeks of gestational age. Further, he found that the direction of the collagen fibers was 90 degrees to the muscle fibers of the quadratus lumborum muscle. He concluded that the ILL develops in a fashion similar to most of the other ligaments of the body and is not formed by metaplasia of the inferior fibers of the quadratus lumborum muscle. The findings of Hanson and Sonesson (1994), who fully dissected the ILLs in 100 spines, 50 of them in cadavers between birth and 10 years of age, confirm the results of Uhthoff (1993).

The ILLs probably function to stabilize the L5-S1 junction, helping to maintain the proper relationship of L5 on S1 (Olsewski et al., 1991), and also to prevent disc degeneration at this level (Aihara et al., 2002). Shorter posterior bands of the superior ILL, as measured in cadavers, are associated with less IVD degeneration at the L5-S1 level and greater disc degeneration at the L4-5 level. The greater degeneration at the L4-5 level is presumably the result of increased loads being transmitted there, secondary to decreased motion at the L5-S1 motion segment in specimens with a short posterior band of the superior ILL (Aihara et al., 2002). In addition to stabilizing the L5 vertebra on the first sacral segment, the ILL limits flexion (L5 motion increases 77.5% in flexion when ILL is experimentally cut), extension (20.4% increase when cut), lateral flexion (141.7% increase in contralateral lateral flexion when ILL is cut), and axial rotation of L5 on S1 (surprisingly, L5 motion increases only 5.3% in unilateral axial rotation when the ILL is experimentally cut) (Basadonna, Gasparini, and Rucco, 1996; Sims and Moorman, 1996).

The ILL is innervated by posterior primary divisions of the neighboring spinal nerves and consequently may be a primary source of back pain. Therefore sprain of the ILL can be painful, and enthesopathy of the posterior band of the superior ILL can develop. Enthesopathy refers to inflammation at the attachment site of a liga-ment to bone that frequently results in calcification of the ligament at the site of attachment (in this case, the illium). The narrower attachment sites of the posterior aspect of this ligament may explain the development of such enthesopathy. Such a narrow attachment causes the loads to be more focused, placing more stress on the ligamentous attachment site (Basadonna, Gasparini, and Rucco, 1996; Sims and Moorman, 1996).

Lumbar Intervertebral Discs

Because of their tremendous clinical significance, much has been written in this chapter about the lumbar IVDs. In addition, Chapter 2 describes the make-up of the IVDs and much of the clinical significance associated with their unique morphology, Chapter 11 discusses disc bulge and protrusion and their biologic consequences, and Chapter 14 discusses the microscopic anatomy of the IVDs and IVD aging and degeneration. This chapter focuses on the unique characteristics of the lumbar IVDs with an emphasis on their clinical significance.

In general, IVDs of the lumbar region are the thickest (tallest) of the spine. As discussed in Chapter 2, they are made up of a central nucleus pulposus, an outer anulus fibrosus composed of 15 to 25 lamellae (Marchand and Ahmed, 1990; Twomey and Taylor, 1990), and the vertebral (cartilaginous) end plates that line the superior and inferior IVD borders. The thickness of the lamellae of the anulus fibrosus of lumbar IVDs varies considerably from one lamella to the next and also varies within the same lamella. In addition, the thickness of the lamellae also increases with age. Often lamellae are incomplete and do not continue all the way around the anulus fibrosus. Consequently, some lamellae are ending and some are beginning in any given 20-degree sector of the anulus fibrosus (Marchand and Ahmed, 1990).

The function of the lumbar IVDs is similar to the function of the IVDs throughout the spine. That is, they function with the vertebral bodies to absorb loads placed on the spine from above (axial loading) and allow for some motion to occur (Hutton, 1990) while restricting too much motion. The lumbar discs become shorter during the day because they carry the load of the torso. They usually regain their shape within 5 hours of sleep. During active hours the discs require movement to maintain proper hydration. Decreased movement and decreased axial loading have been strongly associated with disc degeneration (Twomey and Taylor, 1990).

The IVDs do not always become narrower from superior to inferior with age (Twomey and Taylor, 1990). Their central region can become more convex with age and push into the central region of the adjacent vertebral bodies. The central aspects of the vertebral bodies lose transverse trabeculae with age and become somewhat shorter from superior to inferior. The peripheral margins of the bodies lose much less height, causing the bony end plates to become concave.

The lumbar IVDs are normally thicker (taller) anteriorly than posteriorly. This helps in the formation of the lumbar lordosis. Liyang et al. (1989) found that the shapes of the lumbar IVDs change significantly during flexion and extension of the lumbar region. Flexion was found to narrow the anterior aspect of the disc by approximately 1 to 5 mm and to increase the height of the posterior aspect of the disc by between approximately 1.5 to 3 mm. Consequently, lumbar flexion significantly increases tension on the posterior fibers of the anulus fibrosus (Hedman and Fernie, 1997). In addition, the nucleus pulposus tends to move posteriorly during flexion and anteriorly during extension (Fennell, Jones, and Hukins, 1996). Interestingly, IVDs with greater height and a smaller area (i.e., tall IVDs with small vertebral bodies) are the most susceptible to protrusion (Natarajan and Andersson, 1999).

Rather than considering IVD injury as the result of a single event, McGill (1997) and others (Yang et al., 1988; Gordon et al., 1991) describe lumbar IVD injury as usually occurring over a long period of time as a consequence of cumulative trauma (or "loading") with the spine in a forward flexed position. Disc protrusion has been found to be rare when the spine is loaded in axial compression in the neutral position; under these circumstances the bony end plates of the vertebral bodies usually fracture (McGill, 1997).

The IVDs usually are protected from anterior displacement, or shear stress, by the Z joints and the lumbar extensor muscles (Hutton, 1990). However, fracture of the pars interarticularis allows anterior displacement of the IVDs to occur.

Pain Originating from the Intervertebral Disc.
Because each lumbar disc is in direct contact with two or three pairs of dorsal roots (Taylor, 1990), bulging, or protrusion, of the IVD is considered by most authors to be a major cause of radicular pain (Fig. 7-24). However, clinicians should keep in mind that each IVD is innervated by sensory nerve endings and, as a result, can be a primary source of back pain. The IVD receives both nociceptive and proprioceptive fibers (McCarthy, 1993) (see Chapter 2). The posterior aspect of the disc receives innervation from the recurrent meningeal nerve (sinuvertebral nerve), and the lateral and anterior aspect of the disc is supplied by branches of the gray communicating rami of the lumbar sympathetic trunk (Edgar and Ghadially, 1976; Bogduk, Tynan, and Wilson, 1981).

Nociceptive fibers from that part of the IVD innervated by branches of the gray communicating rami (left and right at each level) probably course through the gray rami to the anterior primary divisions and then enter the dorsal horn of the spinal cord in a fashion similar to other nociceptive fibers of the somatic nervous system (Bogduk, 1983). However, some fibers innervating the anterior and lateral aspects of the discs, and to a lesser extent even the posterior aspect of the IVDs (Ohtori et al., 1999) have been found in animal models (rats) to ascend several segments in the sympathetic chain before passing through a gray communicating ramus, anterior primary division, and dorsal root and ganglion to enter the dorsal horn of the spinal cord several segments higher than the level of innervation. This is thought to explain the broad referral patterns (e.g., pain referred into the inguinal region from IVD pathology as low as L5-S1) seen in various presentations of low back pain of primary discal origin (Morinaga et al., 1996; Ohtori et al., 1999, 2001). For example, Yukawa et al. (1997) have reported that approximately 4.1% of patients with protrusion of the IVD at L4-5 or L5-S1 experience groin pain. (Chapters 9 and 11 discuss the central connections of fibers conducting nociception.) Bogduk (1990) has described a series of events that explain the mechanisms by which the IVD can be a primary source of pain without IVD herniation. He states that there are two mechanisms by which the disc causes pain without herniation: torsional injuries to the disc and compression of the IVD.

Torsional injury to the IVD refers to a sprain of the outer layers of the anulus fibrosus after excessive axial rotation. Normally tearing of the anulus does not occur because the collagen fibers of the 15 to 25 anular lamellae of a lumbar IVD are able to withstand more than 3 degrees of axial rotation without being stretched beyond their capacity. In fact, 22.6 degrees of unilateral axial rotation are needed to cause failure of the anular fibers. This amount of segmental rotation of a single lumbar motion segment only can occur under experimental conditions after complete removal of the Z joints (facetectomy) in unembalmed cadaveric spines (Farfan, 1973). Therefore rotation of the lumbar spine does not normally cause damage to the IVD (Hutton, 1990), because axial rotation between two adjacent segments is primarily limited by the Z joints and usually does not exceed 3 degrees (see Range of Motion in the Lumbar Spine). However, flexion significantly increases tension on the posterior aspect of the anulus fibrosus (Hedman and Fernie, 1997), and if flexion is added to axial rotation, the collagen fibers of the anulus fibrosus can be stretched beyond their limits, resulting in circumferential tears of the anulus (Fig. 7-25). Because of the nociceptive innervation of the outer third of the IVD, these tears can result in pain of discal origin. However, even though these injuries have been produced experimentally, have been identified in cadavers, and match the signs and symptoms expressed by many patients who have back pain after injuries involving rotation combined with flexion, no definitive studies irrevocably link isolated

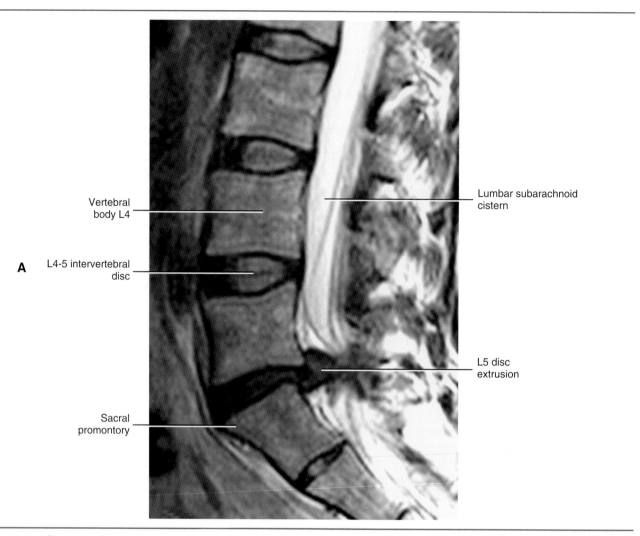

A

Vertebral body L4

L4-5 intervertebral disc

Sacral promontory

Lumbar subarachnoid cistern

L5 disc extrusion

FIG. 7-24   Magnetic resonance imaging scans demonstrating a protrusion of the L5-S1 intervertebral disc. **A,** Sagittal view.

circumferential tears of the IVD with low back pain (Bogduk, 1990).

If several episodes of excessive loading of the disc during flexion and axial rotation occur, the result may be circumferential tears of several adjacent lamellae of the anulus fibrosus. If enough anular lamellae tear in this way, the anulus fibrosus may be weakened to the point that the nucleus pulposus may be allowed to tear a path created by the circumferential tears of weakened adjacent anular lamellae. Such a path courses from the centrally located nucleus pulposus to the periphery through successive layers of the anulus fibrosus, and is known as a radial tear (see Fig. 7-25). A radial tear can result in protrusion and extrusion of nuclear contents into the vertebral canal. Once in the canal, entrapment or stretching of the neural elements can occur. As discussed, a protruding or extruding disc can affect the neural elements as they course within the vertebral canal, pass through the IVF, or both.

MRI is gaining wide acceptance in the evaluation of disc protrusion. However, a significant number of false-positive findings have been found with MRI. Therefore close correlation of MRI findings with other clinical findings is essential before a diagnosis of disc protrusion can be made with certainty (Boden et al., 1990).

The second type of injury that can result in pain originating from the IVD itself results from excessive compression of the IVD. Compression injuries can result in pain of discal origin by two mechanisms, chemical and mechanical (Bogduk, 1990). Bogduk (1990) has described a series of events that may occur after excessive compression of a lumbar IVD. These events are summarized in Box 7-3. Note that fracture of the cartilaginous and bony end plate is a key feature in this sequence of events. During compressive loading of the spine (forces being placed on the spine from directly above), the vertebral (cartilaginous) and bony end plates have been shown to fracture before tearing of the anulus

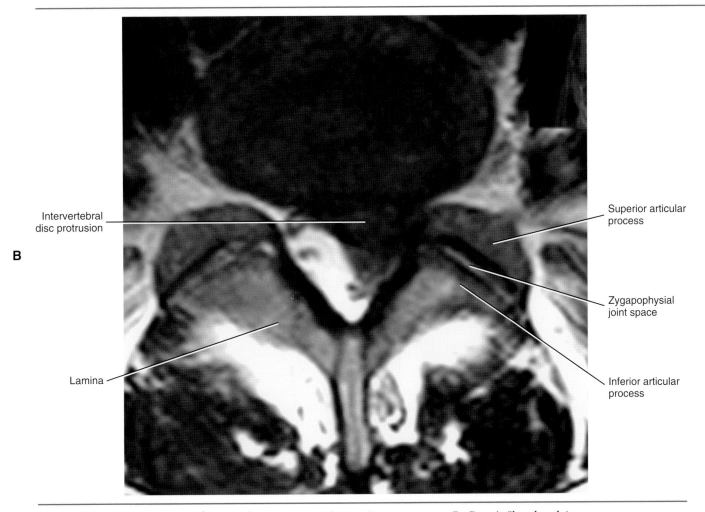

Intervertebral disc protrusion

B

Lamina

Superior articular process

Zygapophysial joint space

Inferior articular process

FIG. 7-24—cont'd   **B,** Horizontal view. (Images courtesy Dr. Dennis Skogsbergh.)

fibrosus or protrusion of the nucleus pulposus occurs. Such fractures may heal completely and go unnoticed. However, a dramatic repair response may occur if the fracture extends into the cancellous bone of the vertebral body and the IVD comes in contact with the vascular supply of the vertebral body. This response is characterized by the nucleus pulposus being treated as if it were foreign to the body. The result has been described as an autoimmune type of response (Bogduk, 1990). This response leads to destruction of the proteoglycan aggregates and proteoglycan monomers that make up the disc. The result of this destruction is a condition known as internal disc disruption (Kirkaldy-Willis et al., 1978).

Internal disc disruption can result in spinal stenosis (including foraminal stenosis), protrusion of the nucleus pulposus, or both. The processes by which these two entities develop are summarized in Boxes 7-4 and 7-5.

Internal disc disruption also can result in resorption, or loss, of IVD material. The loss of discal material, over time, may make extrusion of the nucleus pulposus less

likely. Kirkaldy-Willis et al. (1978) state that discography has shown a marked correlation between loss of disc height, the presence of traction spurs (osteophytes), and disruption of the disc. Therefore even if patients escape nuclear bulge or extrusion (see Box 7-5), they remain vulnerable to lateral recess stenosis (see Box 7-4).

In addition, as disruption continues toward the outer layers of the anulus fibrosus, pain of purely discal origin also can result. Bogduk (1990) has reviewed two mechanisms by which this can occur. These mechanisms are summarized in Boxes 7-6 and 7-7. The first mechanism that produces pain of discal origin is chemical in nature. Progression of the inflammatory process of internal disc disruption results in the direct stimulation of nociceptors in the outer third of the anulus fibrosus. The second process causes pain from the anulus as a result of its decreased ability to handle mechanical stress adequately. As the process of disruption progresses, the inner lamellae of the anulus break down, causing the outer layers to absorb all the loads placed on the disc. The anulus

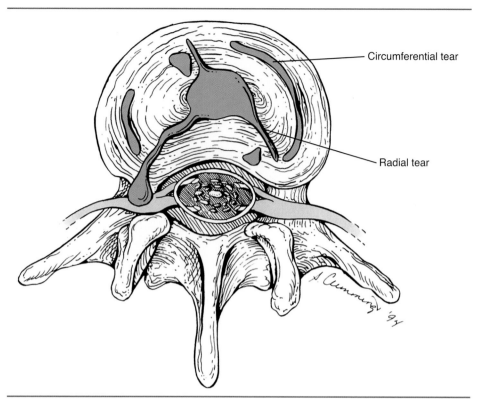

FIG. 7-25   Circumferential and radial tears of the intervertebral disc. Notice that one of the radial tears is allowing the nucleus pulposus to extrude posterolaterally on the left side.

BOX 7-3
EFFECTS OF COMPRESSIVE LOADING

Fall or excessive compressive load
↓
Fracture of vertebral end plate
↓
Nuclear material exposed to blood supply of vertebral body
↓
Unrestrained inflammatory repair response
↓
Degradation of IVD proteoglycans
↓
Internal disc disruption

Modified from Bogduk N. (1990). Pathology of lumbar disc pain. *Manual Med, 5,* 72-79.

BOX 7-4
SCENARIO ONE

Internal disc disruption
↓
Circumferential bulging of the anulus fibrosus
↓
Osteophyte formation
↓
Isolated disc resorption
↓
Foraminal or spinal stenosis

Modified from Bogduk N. (1990). Pathology of lumbar disc pain. *Manual Med, 5,* 72-79.

---

is rendered more susceptible to circumferential tears, which are likely to produce pain. Therefore this type of pain, secondary to internal disc disruption, is the result of mechanical forces. The two mechanisms just described (pain of chemical and mechanical origin) can occur simultaneously (Bogduk, 1990).

Finally, Box 7-8 summarizes the clinical findings in a patient with early internal disc disruption. The neurologic findings are negative because the disc remains contained, especially in the early stages. Pain from internal disc disruption has characteristics similar to those of other somatic causes of low back pain (e.g., Z joint pathology), making the diagnosis more challenging. If the pain is prolonged or becomes severe, injection of

---

BOX 7-5
SCENARIO TWO

Rapid internal disc disruption
↓
Centrifugal erosion of the anulus fibrosus
↓
Radial fissures
↓
Fissure track (path)
↓
Nuclear protrusion

BOX 7-8
CLINICAL FINDINGS WITH INTERNAL DISC DISRUPTION

1. Pain restricted to back or referred to lower limb
2. Pain aggravated by movements or compression of disc
3. Muscle guarding could be present
4. Neurologic examination normal
5. Standard x-ray examination, myelography, and computed tomography scan normal
6. Computed tomography discography with pain provocation positive

---

BOX 7-6
PAIN FROM INTERNAL DISC DISRUPTION: ONE

Degradation of nucleus reaches outer third of anulus fibrosus
↓
Stimulation of nociceptors of outer anulus fibrosus
↓
Chemically induced pain

BOX 7-7
PAIN FROM INTERNAL DISC DISRUPTION: TWO

Disruption of anular collagen
↓
Decrease in number of collagen fibers
↓
Application of loads results in increased stress to outer anulus fibrosus
↓
Anular sprain
↓
Mechanically induced pain

Intervertebral Disc Degeneration and Its Consequences. Decreased disc height and osteophyte formation are the best indicators of IVD degeneration on x-ray. A low signal in the IVD on MRI is also an indication of disc degeneration (Marchiori et al., 1994). It should be recalled that the IVD and the two Z joints between two adjacent vertebrae make up a three-joint complex. Pathologic conditions or dysfunction of one component can adversely affect the others (Kirkaldy-Willis et al., 1978; Haher et al., 1992) (see Fig. 7-6). As disc degeneration increases, segmental motion, particularly in axial rotation, also increases; however, in the final stages of degeneration, intersegmental motion decreases (Fujiwara et al., 2000; Krismer et al., 2000). The increased motion during the initial stages of IVD degeneration results in decreased IVD stiffness; however, during the later stages of IVD degeneration, stiffness increases as intersegmental motion decreases (Brown, Holmes, and Heiner, 2002). In addition, loss of disc height as a result of disc degeneration, protrusion, internal disc disruption, resorption of the disc, chemonucleolysis, and discectomy may lead to added loads being placed on the Z joint capsules and the articular processes, resulting in degenerative changes of the articular processes. Disc deterioration at one level also can lead to increased strain and possible degeneration of the discs immediately above or below the level of primary involvement (Kirkaldy-Willis et al., 1978).

Loss of disc height also can result in subluxation of the Z joints and upward and forward displacement of the superior articular processes (Kirkaldy-Willis et al., 1978). This in turn results in narrowing of the lateral recesses of the vertebral canal. Narrowing of the lateral recess may result in entrapment of the exiting nerve roots as they proceed to the medial aspect of the IVF proper. Therefore loss of disc height from any cause can result in abnormal joint position and abnormal motion. Such abnormal joint position and abnormal motion of both the interbody joint and the Z joints of two adjacent vertebrae has been termed instability (Dupuis et al.,

radiopaque dye into the disc followed by CT (CT discography) usually shows disruption into the anulus fibrosus when internal disc disruption is present. In addition, CT discography reproduces the patient's symptoms. Extrusion of dye into the anulus combined with provocation of the patient's symptoms confirms the condition of internal disc disruption (Schwarzer et al., 1995). In addition, a disc affected by internal disc disruption may be identified as an area of reduced signal intensity when viewed on sagittal MRI scans.

1985). Instability, in turn, can lead to repeated entrapment of the spinal nerve exiting between the two adjacent segments.

RANGES OF MOTION IN THE LUMBAR SPINE

Several factors help to limit specific movements of the lumbar region. These include the unique configuration of the lumbar articular facets and the restraints of the Z joint capsules, ligaments of the lumbar region, deep back muscles, and lumbar IVDs. For example, flexion of the lumbar region is primarily limited by the Z joint capsules (Hutton, 1990) and the articular processes themselves (Taylor and Twomey, 1986). The ligamenta flava, IVDs, and interspinous and supraspinous ligaments also help to limit flexion. Hutton (1990) found that the interspinous and supraspinous ligaments (supraspinous restraints) were the first to tear during hyperflexion of the lumbar region.

A few items about lumbar flexion are worth noting. First, all of the lumbar vertebrae do not move simultaneously during flexion. In fact, lumbar flexion occurs in a stepwise fashion, beginning at L1-L2, and continuing through L5-S1 (Kanayama et al., 1996). Second, advancing age also can affect lumbar flexion. That is, lumbar flexion decreases with age, with the most marked change beginning in the sixth decade of life (McGregor, McCarthy, and Hughes, 1995).

Extension is limited by the ALL, the Z joint capsular ligaments (Dupuis et al., 1985), and the bony "stop" of the inferior articular processes coming against the pars interarticularis of the subjacent vertebra.

The tightly interlocking facets of this region dramatically limit axial rotation. However, the reciprocal concave and convex surfaces of the respective superior and inferior articular processes allow for a very small amount of axial rotation to occur. Gapping of the Z joint occurs on the same side of vertebral body rotation (i.e., gapping of right Z joint with right rotation) (Boszczyk et al., 2001; Cramer et al., 2002). Axial rotation is finally stopped by the impact of articular processes that make up the Z joint of the side opposite that to which the vertebral body is rotating. This limitation usually occurs at 1 to 2 degrees of axial rotation between adjacent vertebrae from L1 to L4 (Hutton, 1990). The L5-S1 segment is able to attain more axial rotation than the other lumbar segments (see values at the end of this section).

Lateral flexion in the lumbar region is limited primarily by the contralateral intertransverse ligaments. The contralateral capsular ligaments and ligamenta flava are also important in the limitation of lateral flexion. In addition, the configuration of the articular processes helps to limit this motion (Dupuis et al., 1985). Lateral

flexion in the lumbar region usually is coupled with axial rotation such that left lateral flexion results in right rotation of the vertebral bodies (left rotation of the spinous processes), and vice versa (i.e., right lateral flexion is coupled with left rotation of the vertebral bodies). Probably this is caused by the sagittal orientation of the lumbar Z joints, combined with the effect of the relatively strong lumbar interspinous and supraspinous restraints. The latter restraints tend to hold the spinous processes together during lateral flexion. Abnormally loose posterior stabilizers (e.g., interspinous ligaments, supraspinous restraints, deep back muscles, Z joints) can result in abnormal coupling during lateral flexion so that left lateral flexion is coupled with left rotation of the vertebral body and right rotation of the spinous process (the opposite of the normal coupling pattern). This abnormal coupling pattern, which can be detected on standard x-ray films, is an indication of lumbar instability (Dupuis et al., 1985).

Lumbar instability (abnormally high intersegmental motion) may result in low back pain if abnormal stress is placed on the unstable segments. A patient with lumbar instability may have centralized low back pain without leg pain or central and lateral low back pain combined with radiation into the buttock and thigh. Some patients with lumbar instability have signs of nerve root entrapment. Differentiation between pain caused by lumbar instability and that caused by primary IVD or Z joint pathology may be challenging, because the latter structures may be receiving increased mechanical loading and thus may be generating pain themselves. Examination of dynamic x-ray films taken in flexion, extension, and lateral flexion that demonstrate increased motion have been found to aid in this differentiation (Dupuis et al., 1985).

Table 7-11 lists the total ranges of motion for the lumbar region as reported by several different authors.

The following is a list of ranges of motion (in degrees) for each lumbar segmental level (White and Panjabi, 1990).
Combined flexion and extension
   L1-2: 12 degrees
   L2-3: 14 degrees
   L3-4: 15 degrees
   L4-5: 17 degrees
Unilateral lateral flexion
   L1-2: 6 degrees
   L2-3: 6 degrees
   L3-4: 8 degrees
   L4-5: 6 degrees
Unilateral axial rotation
   L1-2: 2 degrees
   L2-3: 2 degrees
   L3-4: 2 degrees
   L4-5: 2 degrees

Table 7-11	Total Ranges of Motion for the Lumbar Region
Direction	Motions and ranges reported in the literature
Flexion	60°
	39-55° (average: 45.95° ± 4.28,[*]
	52° ± 18)[†]
L4-5 segment	14.5-19.0° (average: 15.95° ± 1.38)[*]
Extension	20°
	16° ± 10[†]
Lateral flexion[‡]	25-30°
Axial rotation[‡]	10-15°
	5°[†]

[*]Data from Liyang D et al. (1989). The effect of flexion-extension motion of the lumbar spine on the capacity of the spinal canal, an experimental study. *Spine, 14,* 523-525.
[†]Data from Bogduk N. (1997). *Clinical anatomy of the lumbar spine* (3rd ed.). London: Churchill Livingstone.
[‡]Unilateral motion.

Plamondon, Gagnon, and Maurais (1988) used stereometry (method of measurement using sets of x-ray films taken at 90 degrees to one another) to determine the motion of individual lumbar vertebrae. The following list represents the amount of motion they found, *per segment,* for the L1 to L4 vertebrae:

Flexion: 10 degrees
Extension: 4 degrees
Axial rotation: 1 degree
Lateral flexion: 4 degrees

It should be recalled that the L5-S1 articulation is the most movable segment in flexion, extension, and axial rotation in this region. The following is a list of the ranges of motion at this level (White and Panjabi, 1990):

Combined flexion and extension: 20 degrees
Unilateral lateral flexion: 3 degrees
Unilateral axial rotation: 2.5 degrees

However, some texts present data that show less motion at the L5-S1 region (Bogduk, 1997).

SOFT TISSUES OF THE LUMBAR REGION: NERVES AND VESSELS

The muscles associated with the lumbar region are discussed in Chapter 4. This includes a discussion of the diaphragm and the muscles of the anterior and posterior abdominal walls, including the abdominal obliques, transversus abdominis, rectus abdominis, quadratus lumborum, and psoas major and minor muscles. Consequently, this section on soft tissue structures of the lumbar region focuses on vessels and nerves related to the lumbar spine.

Nerves of the Lumbar Region

The innervation of the lumbar portion of the vertebral column and the soft-tissue structures of the lumbar region is a topic of supreme clinical importance. Having knowledge of the innervation of the spine gives the clinician a better understanding of the source of the patient's pain. Perhaps Bogduk (1983) stated it best, "The distribution of the intrinsic nerves of the lumbar vertebral column systematically identifies those structures that are potential sources of primary low back pain."

Because the basic neural elements associated with the spine are covered in Chapters 2, 3, 5, and 6, this chapter concentrates on those aspects of innervation unique to the lumbar region. However, many key features of the basic neural elements also are included here to maintain continuity and minimize the need to refer to previous chapters.

The cauda equina and exiting roots and spinal nerves have been discussed (see Lumbar Vertebral Foramen and Lumbar Intervertebral Foramina and the Nerve Root Canals, respectively). This section briefly covers the dorsal and ventral roots and the spinal nerve. It concentrates on the neural elements once they have left the confines of the IVF. Because the vast majority of spinal structures are innervated by either the recurrent meningeal nerves or posterior primary divisions (PPDs), these nerves and the structures they innervate are covered in more detail. This is followed by a discussion of the anterior primary divisions (APDs) and the lumbar plexus. It should be recalled that the lateral and anterior aspects of the IVDs and the ALLs are innervated by direct branches of the lumbar sympathetic trunk and also by branches from the lumbar gray rami communicantes. The specific innervation of the IVD has been discussed in greater detail earlier (see Pain Originating from the Intervertebral Disc).

General Considerations. Three types of nerve endings have been found in almost all the innervated structures of the lumbar vertebral column: free nerve endings, other nonencapsulated endings, and encapsulated endings. This seems to indicate that most innervated structures of the spine are sensitive to pain, pressure, and proprioception (Jackson et al., 1966).

Of particular interest, and sometimes of particular frustration to clinicians and researchers alike, is that innervation overlaps throughout the spine. This has been particularly well documented in the lumbar region. Most spinal structures seem to be innervated by nerves from at least two adjacent vertebral levels. This led Edgar and Ghadially (1976) to state, "The poor localization of much low back pain and its tendency to radiate may be related to this neurological pattern." This can at times make the task of identifying the cause of low back pain particularly challenging.

Dorsal and Ventral Roots and Spinal Nerves.
The dorsal and ventral roots of the lumbar spine travel inferiorly as the cauda equina. They then course through the NRC before exiting the IVF (see previous material). The nerve roots can be irritated by many structures and pathologic processes (see previous discussions and Chapter 11). These include disc protrusion or other space-occupying lesions, structural lesions of the vertebral canal, chemical irritation, and intrinsic radiculitis (Bogduk, 1976). The dorsal and ventral roots unite to form a spinal nerve before exiting the IVF. Each lumbar spinal nerve emerges from a lumbar IVF and immediately divides into an APD (ventral ramus) and PPD (dorsal ramus).

Dorsal Root Ganglia.
Each dorsal root has a marked enlargement, known as the dorsal root (spinal) ganglion (DRG), that is located immediately proximal to the union of the dorsal and ventral roots to form the spinal nerve. DRGs increase in diameter from L1 to S1. Because the dural root sleeve of S1 is relatively short, the S1 DRG is frequently (77.3% to 79%) within the superior aspect of the sacral canal, rather than within the first sacral IVF. However, the locations of the lumbar and sacral DRGs are variable, and can even be asymmetric from left to right. The positions of the DRGs are clinically relevant. Kikuchi et al. (1994) studied the locations of the L4, L5, and S1 DRGs, and Hasegawa et al. (1996) studied the location of the L1-5 DRGs. They categorized the ganglia as being intraspinal (within the vertebral canal), intraforaminal (within the IVF), or extraforaminal (lateral to the IVF). The following is a breakdown of the percentage of DRGs found in each category (the values of Hasegawa et al., 1996, are in parentheses):

Intraspinal: L4-9.3%; L5-19.2%; S1-77.3%
Intraforaminal: (L1-92%, L2-98%, L3-100%) L4-86.1% (100%); L5-72.8% (95%); S1-22.7%
Extraforaminal: L4-4.6%; L5-8.0%; S1-0.0%

In addition, Hamanishi and Tanaka (1993) found values similar to those of Kikuchi et al. (1994) (i.e., more intraforaminal and extraforaminal DRGs).

When a lumbar DRG is located within the IVF, it generally occupies 23% to 30% of the area of the IVF within a parasagittal plane passing through the DRG. The more superior DRGs (L1 and L2) have a tendency to be more laterally placed within the IVF, or are located lateral to their IVF altogether (extraforaminal location), whereas the more inferior DRGs (L5 and S1) generally are located in the medial aspect of the IVF, or can be within the vertebral (spinal) canal (intraspinal location), or in the case of S1 within the superior-most aspect of the sacral canal. Intraspinal L5 or S1 DRGs have an increased incidence of DRG compression with associated radiculopathy. The DRG compressions in these instances usually are secondary to bulging of an IVD, Z joint articular facet arthropathy, or a combination of both conditions (Hasegawa et al., 1996). Compression of intraspinal DRGs (indentation seen at postmortem examination) has been found to be more frequent with advancing age (Kikuchi et al., 1994).

Recurrent Meningeal (Sinuvertebral) Nerves.
The recurrent meningeal nerves (RMNs) at each level innervate many structures located within the IVF and the vertebral canal. Because they have been found to carry fibers that conduct nociception (pain), structures innervated by RMNs are considered to be capable of producing back pain. However, in addition to nociceptive input, the RMNs also probably carry thermal sensation and proprioception (Edgar and Ghadially, 1976). Even though the RMNs are discussed in Chapters 5 and 6, they are included here because of their clinical importance.

The RMNs are found at each IVF of the vertebral column. They each originate from the most proximal portion of the APD just distal to the IVF that they eventually reenter. They receive a branch from the closest gray communicating ramus and then enter the anterior aspect of the IVF close to the pedicle that forms the roof of this opening. Usually, more than one RMN enters each IVF, and up to six have been found at one level. Consequently, compression of the RMNs within the confines of the IVF may be a cause of back pain (Edgar and Ghadially, 1976).

The RMNs ramify extensively on entering the IVF. Great variation is associated with their distribution within the vertebral canal (Groen, Baljet, and Drukker, 1990). Usually each gives off a large ascending branch and smaller descending and transverse branches, although the transverse branch is not always present. The ascending branch usually extends superiorly for at least one vertebral level above its level of entrance. The branches of the RMNs anastomose with those of adjacent vertebral segments, including those of the opposite side of the spine (Bogduk, 1976; Edgar and Ghadially, 1976; Groen, Baljet, and Drukker, 1990). They innervate the posterior aspect of the IVD, PLL, periosteum of the posterior aspect of the vertebral bodies, epidural venous plexus, and anterior aspect of the spinal dura mater (see Chapter 11). Therefore all these structures have been implicated as possible sources of back pain. In addition, compression of the RMNs in the vertebral canal may be a component of spinal stenosis (Edgar and Ghadially, 1976). However, because of the great variability in the distribution of the RMNs, the pattern of pain referral as a result of nociceptive input received from them also may be inconsistent.

Less frequently cited possible causes of back pain that receive innervation by the RMNs include venous congestion within the vertebral bodies (intravertebral venous congestion) and varicosities of the epidural veins (Edgar and Ghadially, 1976) and basivertebral veins (Bogduk, 1976). Edgar and Ghadially (1976) stated that, in addition to relieving pressure on nerve roots, decompression of the vertebral canal via laminectomy may reduce back pain by relieving venous congestion in the epidural and intravertebral veins.

Posterior Primary Divisions. Whereas the recurrent meningeal nerves innervate the structures located on the anterior aspect of the vertebral canal, the posterior primary rami innervate those structures of the posterior aspect of the vertebral canal (vertebral arch structures). This difference of innervation may be significant; the RMNs may be responsible for information related to potential or real harm to the neural elements of the vertebral canal, and the PPDs may be responsible for relaying information related to the structural integrity of the spine (Edgar and Ghadially, 1976).

Each PPD of the lumbar region leaves the spinal nerve at the lateral border of the IVF and passes over the TP of the lower vertebra participating in the formation of the IVF (e.g., the L3 nerve passes over the L4 TP). The PPD then passes through a small osteoligamentous canal. This canal, which is unique to the lumbar region, lies between the base of the anterior surface of the superior articular process medially and the posterior lamella of the intertransverse ligament laterally. The nerve then sends a twig to the intertransversarius medialis muscle and continues posteriorly, where it divides into a medial and lateral branch. The medial branch passes deep to the mamillo-accessory ligament (see Articular Processes) and supplies sensory innervation to the Z joint and then motor innervation to the multifidi. This innervation to the lumbar multifidi has been found to be specific (Bogduk, Wilson, and Tynan, 1982). The medial branch of a PPD innervates those fibers that insert onto the spinous process "of the same segmental number as the nerve" (Bogduk, Wilson, and Tynan, 1982). For example, the medial branch of the L3 PPD innervates the multifidi muscles that insert onto the L3 spinous process. The medial branch then continues further medially to innervate the rotatores and interspinalis muscles and provide sensory innervation to the interspinous ligament, supraspinous "ligament" (restraints), ligamentum flavum, and periosteum of the posterior arch, including the spinous process (Box 7-9 and Fig. 7-26). Along its course, the medial branch anastomoses with medial branches of adjacent levels and sends an inferior branch to the Z joint of the level below and an ascending branch to the level above (Bogduk, 1976; Edgar and Ghadially, 1976). Therefore each Z joint typically is innervated by medial branches of three PPDs (Bogduk et al., 1982; Jeffries, 1988).

The lateral branch of the PPD supplies motor innervation to the erector spinae muscles. Bogduk (1983)

BOX 7-9
STRUCTURES INNERVATED BY THE MEDIAL BRANCH OF A LUMBAR POSTERIOR PRIMARY DIVISION (STRUCTURES CAPABLE OF PRODUCING PAIN)

Z joint
Interspinous ligament
Supraspinous restraints
Ligamentum flavum
Periosteum of posterior arch and posterior aspect of spinous process
Muscles, including intertransversarius mediales, multifidi, rotatores, and interspinous muscles (motor and sensory innervation to these)

---

found that the lateral branch supplies the iliocostalis lumborum muscle while an intermediate branch stems from the lumbar PPDs to supply the longissimus thoracis muscle. After innervating the longissimus thoracis muscle, the intermediate branches form an anastomosis with the intermediate branches of adjacent levels. The PPD of L5 has only two branches, a medial branch with a typical distribution and a more lateral branch that corresponds with the intermediate branches of higher levels because it innervates the longissimus thoracis muscle. Because the muscle fibers of the iliocostalis lumborum do not extend inferiorly to the level of the L5 nerve, the absence of a nerve corresponding to a typical lateral branch of higher levels is understandable (Bogduk, 1983). Neither the medial branches of the PPDs nor any branches of the L4 and L5 PPDs supply the skin of the back.

The (T11) T12, L1, L2, and L3 lateral branches are sometimes known as the superior clunial nerves. They supply sensory innervation to the skin over the upper buttocks. The medial superior cluneal nerve can become entrapped, resulting in pain localized to the iliac crest and radiating into the buttock (Maigne and Doursounian, 1997). The medial superior cluneal (MSC) nerve originates from L1 60% of the time, L2 40% of the time, and occasionally receives a contributing branch from L3. The MSC courses over the iliac crest approximately 7 cm lateral of the midline. As it rests on the iliac crest, the MSC passes under a bridge of fibrous tissue formed by the thoracolumbar fascia. Occasionally the fibrous tissue wraps too tightly around the nerve at this location, causing constriction and the signs and symptoms of the entrapment neuropathy described in the preceding. Superior cluneal nerve injury also has been implicated as a cause of postoperative pain after iliac crest harvesting for spine fusion surgery (Maigne and Doursounian, 1997).

Anterior Primary Divisions and the Lumbar Plexus. The APDs, or ventral rami, branch from the

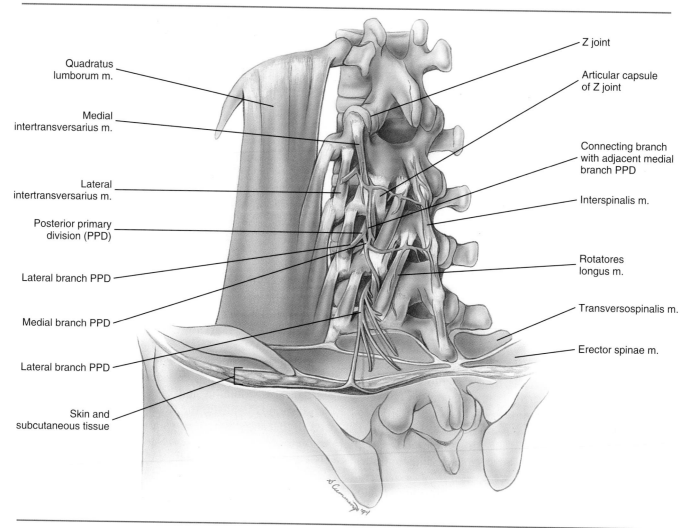

Quadratus
lumborum m.

Medial
intertransversarius m.

Lateral
intertransversarius m.

Posterior primary
division (PPD)

Lateral branch PPD

Medial branch PPD

Lateral branch PPD

Skin and
subcutaneous tissue

Z joint

Articular capsule
of Z joint

Connecting branch
with adjacent medial
branch PPD

Interspinalis m.

Rotatores
longus m.

Transversospinalis m.

Erector spinae m.

FIG. 7-26   Structures innervated by the posterior primary divisions of typical lumbar spinal nerves. The quadratus lumborum muscle, which is innervated by the anterior primary divisions, also is shown.

spinal nerves at the lateral border of the IVF and immediately enter the psoas major muscle. The ventral rami of the first four lumbar nerves then branch within the substance of the psoas major muscle to form the lumbar plexus. As mentioned in this chapter, the psoas major muscle may provide some protection for the dorsal and ventral roots from traction forces placed on the peripheral nerves of the lumbar plexus (dePeretti et al., 1989).

The lumbar plexus is derived from the ventral rami of only the first four lumbar nerves. The ventral ramus of L5 unites with a branch of the ventral ramus of L4 to form the lumbosacral trunk. The lumbosacral trunk then enters the pelvis to unite with the APDs of the sacral spinal nerves and in doing so helps to form the sacral plexus. Frequently the twelfth thoracic (subcostal) nerve also participates in the lumbar plexus.

The branches of the lumbar plexus are listed next, along with the closely related subcostal nerve and lumbosacral trunk.

- *Subcostal nerve (T12).* The subcostal nerve is sensory to the region under the umbilicus and is also motor to the pyramidalis and quadratus lumborum muscles.
- *Iliohypogastric nerve (L1).* This nerve is sensory to the gluteal, inguinal, and suprapubic regions. It also provides some motor innervation to the muscles of the anterior abdominal wall.
- *Ilioinguinal nerve (L1).* This nerve is motor to the muscles of the anterior abdominal wall.
- *Genitofemoral nerve (L1 and L2).* The femoral branch is sensory to the region of the femoral triangle, and the genital branch is motor to the dartos and cremaster muscles of the male (no important innervation by this branch in the female).

♦ *Lateral femoral cutaneous nerve (L2 and L3)*. This nerve is sensory to the lateral aspect of the thigh.

♦ *Femoral nerve (L2, L3, and L4)*. The femoral nerve provides motor innervation to the psoas and iliacus muscles before leaving the abdominopelvic cavity posterior to the inguinal ligament. Distal to the inguinal ligament, this nerve innervates the quadratus femoris and pectineus muscles and supplies sensory innervation to the anterior thigh and medial leg. Spratt, Logan, and Abrahams (1996) found that aberrant slips of the psoas major or iliacus muscle pierced the femoral nerve unilaterally in 4 of 68 cadavers. In one case a slip of iliacus muscle originated from the iliolumbar ligament and pierced the femoral nerve before inserting onto the lesser trochanter. The authors felt that such anomalies could traction the femoral nerve, possibly leading to referred pain to the hip or knee or along the L2-4 dermatomes.

♦ *Obturator nerve (L2, L3, and L4)*. The obturator nerve is motor to the adductor muscles of the thigh and supplies sensory innervation to the medial aspect of the thigh.

♦ *Lumbosacral trunk (L4 and L5)*. The lumbosacral trunk is not officially a part of the lumbar plexus. This nerve passes inferiorly to participate in the sacral plexus. It therefore serves as a connection between the lumbar and sacral plexuses.

Autonomic Nerves of the Lumbar Region.

The abdominal and pelvic viscera receive their motor innervation from autonomics derived from both the sympathetic and parasympathetic nervous systems. Sensory nerves originating from the same visceral structures also travel along the sympathetic and parasympathetic nerve fibers. The diffuse nature of the sympathetic and parasympathetic systems is responsible for the equally diffuse nature of the sensory innervation that travels along with them. This is one reason pain from an abdominal or pelvic viscus may "refer" to a region some distance from the affected organ.

Sympathetic innervation of the abdominal viscera is derived from two sources, the thoracic and lumbar splanchnic nerves. The parasympathetics are supplied by either the left and right vagus nerves or pelvic splanchnic nerves. The clinical relevance and specific nerves that comprise both the sympathetic and parasympathetic divisions of the autonomic nervous system are discussed in detail in Chapter 10.

Vessels of the Abdomen Related to the Spine

This synopsis of the arteries and veins of the abdomen is included because of the close relationship of the abdominal vessels to the anterior and anterolateral aspects of the lumbar vertebral bodies and lumbar IVDs. This section is by no means complete; it is meant to provide a ready reference for the student and clinician.

Abdominal Aorta and Its Branches.

The abdominal aorta receives its name as the continuation of the thoracic aorta, after passing through the aortic hiatus, which is about in the midline at the level of the twelfth lumbar vertebral body. The abdominal aorta continues along the anterior aspect of the lumbar vertebral bodies and IVDs (which are covered anteriorly by the ALL) and subtly deviates to just left of center before bifurcating into the left and right common iliac arteries. Each of these latter arteries supplies the structures of the pelvis (via the internal iliac artery) and lower extremity (via the external iliac artery) of the same side. The bifurcation of the aorta occurs at the level of the vertebral body of L4 67% of the time, with variations extending from L3 to L5 in the remainder of cases (more often higher than lower). No variation in an individual's age or sex has been found with respect to the location of the aortic bifurcation; however, the frequency of transitional lumbar segments makes for additional variation of the aortic bifurcation. When lumbarization of the first sacral segment is present, the aortic bifurcation occurs at L4 40% of the time, at the L4-5 IVD 33% of the time, and below this level in the remainder of the cases. When sacralization of the L5 vertebra is present, the aortic bifurcation occurs at L3 59% of the time, and below that level in the remainder of the cases (Chithriki, Jaibaji, and Steele, 2002).

Three large, unpaired branches of the aorta—the celiac trunk, the superior mesenteric artery, and the inferior mesenteric artery—exit the anterior aspect of the abdominal aorta and supply the gastrointestinal tract from the stomach to the superior aspect of the rectum. In addition, the celiac trunk supplies the spleen, liver, gallbladder, and a large part of the pancreas. Paired branches of the abdominal aorta also are present throughout its length and are closely related to the posterior abdominal wall. For this reason, they are more relevant to the current discussion (Fig. 7-27). The paired branches of the abdominal aorta are listed and briefly discussed next.

♦ *Inferior phrenic artery*. The left and right inferior phrenic arteries branch from the aorta as it enters the abdominal cavity through the aortic hiatus. Each courses superiorly to supply the posteroinferior aspect of the diaphragm and, along its way, gives many superior suprarenal (adrenal) arteries.

♦ *Middle suprarenal (adrenal) arteries*. These are several paired branches that course directly to the adrenal gland.

♦ *Renal artery*. The large left and right renal arteries course behind the renal veins to enter the hilus of the left and right kidneys. At the hilus, each divides into

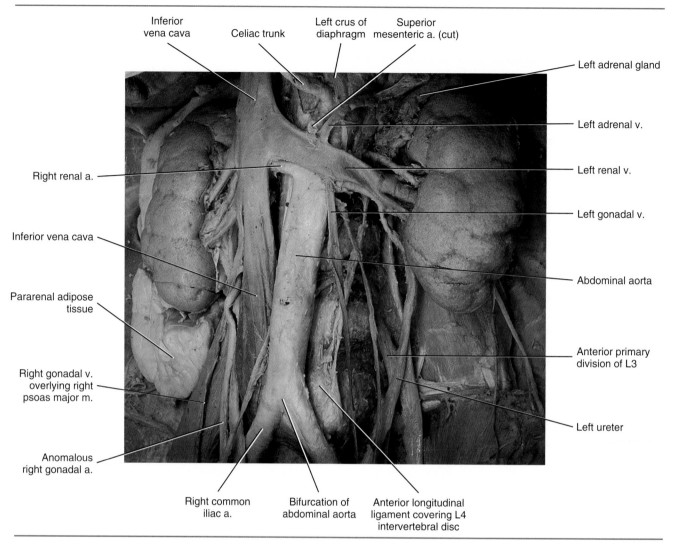

Inferior
vena cava

Celiac trunk

Left crus of
diaphragm

Superior
mesenteric a. (cut)

Left adrenal gland

Left adrenal v.

Right renal a.

Left renal v.

Left gonadal v.

Inferior vena cava

Abdominal aorta

Pararenal adipose
tissue

Anterior primary
division of L3

Right gonadal v.
overlying right
psoas major m.

Left ureter

Anomalous
right gonadal a.

Right common
iliac a.

Bifurcation of
abdominal aorta

Anterior longitudinal
ligament covering L4
intervertebral disc

FIG. 7-27   Important vessels of the abdomen related to the lumbar vertebral column.

five branches (four anterior and one posterior) that supply the five renal arterial segments.

◆ *Gonadal artery (testicular artery in males and ovarian artery in females).* The left and right gonadal arteries arise from the anterior aspect of the abdominal aorta in a staggered fashion. That is, one of the arteries (usually the left) originates up to several centimeters superior to the other. The gonadal vessels have a long inferolateral course within the abdomen and pelvis. The testicular artery of each side enters the deep inguinal ring on its way to the testes. The left and right ovarian vessels enter the pelvis by crossing the external iliac artery of the same side before supplying the ovary.

◆ *Lumbar arteries and the blood supply to the lumbar region of the spine.* These are four (occasionally five) paired segmental arteries that arise from the posterolateral aspect of the aorta. The left and right lumbar

arteries (LAs) arise only a few millimeters apart from one another. Each course laterally along the center of the anterior and lateral aspects of the vertebral bodies, sending branches to the psoas major muscle, the ALL, and the vertebral bodies themselves. They also give off many small branches to retroperitoneal tissues and the posterior peritoneum. In addition, each LA gives off short centrum branches that immediately enter the center of the vertebral body. Each LA also gives off ascending and descending branches that proceed toward the superior and inferior aspects of the vertebral body. These ascending and descending arteries give branches that enter the vertebral body along the way.

As a LA reaches the intervertebral foramen, it gives off three main sets of branches: (a) to the abdominal wall (sometimes called the anterior branches, these arteries pass behind the psoas major muscle, then course along the quadratus lumborum muscle, pierce the transversus abdominis muscle, and course between that muscle and the internal abdominal oblique muscle); (b) spinal canal branches (or "spinal branches" or "spinal rami"); and (c) to the posterior spinal elements (sometimes called posterior branches). Each spinal ramus of a LA divides into three branches: an anterior branch that courses to the vertebral body, a posterior branch that supplies the posterior arch structures, and a neural branch that courses along the spinal nerve and then divides into anterior and posterior radicular arteries, supplying these neural structures (see Chapters 2 and 3 and Fig. 2-4 for further details). The anterior branch to the vertebral body gives off large branches that enter the center of the posterolateral aspect of the body. Once within the vertebral body these branches send smaller branches that either pass superiorly or inferiorly within the body. Before sending these branches to the vertebral body, the anterior branch divides into an ascending and descending branch. These branches course along the external surface of the vertebral body. The ascending branch crosses the IVD above to unite with the descending branch from the level above. The descending branch passes near the pedicle, supplying it, before anastomosing with the ascending branch from the level below. Both ascending and descending branches send twigs into the posterior aspect of the vertebral body, and also supply the PLL (Crock and Yoshizawa, 1976) (Fig. 2-4, B).

The posterior branch of the LA courses to the inner surface of the lamina and ligamentum flavum, and then usually continues as a large branch that pierces the base of the spinous process and continues posteriorly within this process until it reaches the posterior tip of the spinous process. Along its course, the posterior branch sends some twigs to the extradural adipose tissue and others to the posterior aspect of the spinal dura mater. A large laminar branch enters the lamina very close to the union of the lamina with the pedicle. Once within the bone an ascending branch and descending branch (the longer of the two) course through the superior and inferior articular processes, respectively, sending smaller branches that reach the subchondral bone of the articular facets (Fig. 2-4). The posterior branch of the LA also has a branch that courses posterior to the neural arch. This branch supplies the transversospinalis and erector spinae muscles (Crock and Yoshizawa, 1976).

Therefore a series of relatively large arteries pierce the center of the vertebral bodies (VBs) along their entire circumference. On entering the VB, these arteries form a dense plexus of arteries within the central horizontal plane of the VB. From this central plexus many small branches ascend and descend to reach the superior and inferior margins of the VBs; these margins are adjacent to the cartilaginous end plates (Crock and Yoshizawa, 1976) (Fig. 2-4).

- ◆ *Median (middle) sacral artery.* This is a small, unpaired artery that arises from the posterior aspect of the abdominal aorta just before its bifurcation into right and left common iliac arteries. The median sacral artery passes inferiorly along the midline of the anterior sacrum. Although the median sacral artery is almost always present, it is rather variable with respect to its location, typically lying more than 5 mm to the left or right of the midline of the sacrum (Tribus and Belanger, 2001).

Interestingly, a much higher incidence of blocked lumbar segmental arteries and blockage of the middle sacral artery has been found in subjects with low back pain than in age-matched controls (Kauppila and Tallroth, 1993).

Veins of the Abdomen. The two large veins of the abdomen are the portal vein and inferior vena cava (IVC). The portal vein receives the blood from the entire gastrointestinal tract and spleen and pancreas. The IVC receives blood from the remainder of the abdominal and pelvic viscera and the lower extremities. The IVC begins as the union of the left and right common iliac veins. These latter vessels course posteriorly and slightly to the right of the arteries of the same name. The common iliac arteries and veins form an inverted V over the vertebral body of L5. Tribus and Belanger (2001) found that the left common iliac vein and right common iliac artery were separated by an average of 33.5 mm at the level of the L5-S1 IVD, and that the left common iliac vein generally was found approximately 12 mm to the left of the midline at this level. In general the venous return to the IVC follows a similar course to that of the arterial supply from the abdominal aorta. Some unique features of the abdominal venous system are listed next.

- ◆ *Venous drainage of spinal structures.* Large veins accompany each LA and drain into either the IVC or the left common iliac vein. These large veins are connected by vertical channels, known as the ascending lumbar veins. The relationship of the ascending lumbar veins to the azygos system of veins is described in Chapter 2. Intervertebral veins exit the IVFs and drain blood from the internal vertebral venous plexus to join this drainage system (i.e., entering lumbar veins and ascending lumbar veins). Veins also accompany the posterior branches of the LA. These veins also drain into the large veins that accompany the LA themselves (Crock and Yoshizawa, 1976). The external vertebral venous plexus also drains into the ascending lumbar veins.
- ◆ *Hepatic veins.* These veins drain the liver and empty into the IVC as it passes through the fossa for the IVC on the posteroinferior surface of the liver.
- ◆ *Renal veins.* These tributaries of the IVC drain the kidneys. The right renal vein communicates with the

azygos vein, whereas the left renal vein communicates with the hemiazygos vein. The azygos and hemiazygos veins course along the right and left sides of the upper lumbar vertebral bodies, respectively.

♦ *Ascending lumbar veins.* As described, the right and left ascending lumbar veins course superiorly along the posterior and lateral aspects of the lumbar vertebral bodies. They receive tributaries from both the internal and external vertebral venous plexuses. Superiorly the right and left ascending lumbar veins communicate with the azygos and hemiazygos veins, respectively. The drainage of the azygos and hemiazygos veins and their specific relationship to the venous drainage of the vertebral column are described in Chapter 2, and a full discussion of the azygos system of veins is found in Chapter 6.

REFERENCES

Aihara T et al. (2002). Does the morphology of the iliolumbar ligament affect lumbosacral disc degeneration? *Spine, 27,* 1499-1503.

Amundsen T et al. (1995). Lumbar spinal stenosis. *Spine, 20,* 1178-1186.

Antoniou J et al. (1996). The human lumbar end plate. *Spine, 21,* 1153-1161.

Aota Y et al. (1997). Presurgical identification of extradural nerve root anomalies by coronal fat-suppressed magnetic resonance imaging: A report of six cases and a review of the literature. *J Spinal Disord, 10,* 167-175.

Arnoldi CC et al. (1976). Lumbar spinal stenosis and nerve root entrapment syndromes. *Clin Orthop, 115,* 4-5.

Ashton IK et al. (1992). Morphological basis for back pain: The demonstration of nerve fibers and neuropeptides in the lumbar facet joint capsule but not in ligamentum flavum. *J Orthop Res,10,* 72-78.

Bachop W & Janse J. (1983). The corporotransverse ligament at the L5 intervertebral foramen. *Anat Rec, 205* (abstract).

Bachop WE & Ro CS. (1984). A ligament separating the nerve from the blood vessels at the L5 intervertebral foramen. *J Bone Joint Surg, 8,* 437.

Bailey P & Casamajor L. (1911). Osteo-arthritis of the spine as a cause of compression of the spinal cord and its roots. *J Nerv Ment Dis, 38,* 588-609.

Bakkum B & Mestan M. (1994). The effects of transforaminal ligaments on the sizes of T11 to L5 human intervertebral foramina. *J Manipulative Physiol Ther, 17,* 517-522.

Basadonna PT, Gasparini D, & Rucco V. (1996). Iliolumbar ligament insertions. *Spine, 21,* 2313-2316.

Bashline SD, Bilott JR, & Ellis JP. (1996). Meningovertebral ligaments and their putative significance in low back pain. *J Manipulative Physiol Ther, 19,* 592-596.

Beaujeux R et al. (1997). Posterior lumbar epidural fat as a functional structure? *Spine, 22,* 1264-1269.

Behrsin JF & Briggs CA. (1988). Ligaments of the lumbar spine: A review. *Surg Radiol Anat, 10,* 211-219.

Bergmann TF, Peterson DH, & Lawrence DJ. (1993). *Chiropractic technique: Principles and procedures.* New York: Churchill Livingstone.

Boden SC et al. (1996). Orientation of the lumbar facet joints: Association with degenerative disc disease. *J Bone Joint Surg, 78-A,* 403-411.

Boden SD et al. (1990). Abnormal magnetic-resonance scans of the lumbar spine in asymptomatic subjects. *J Bone Joint Surg, 72,* 401-408.

Bogduk N. (1976). The anatomy of the lumbar intervertebral disc syndrome. *Med J Aust, 1,* 878-881.

Bogduk N. (1981). The lumbar mamillo-accessory ligament: Its anatomical and neurosurgical significance. *Spine, 6,* 162-167.

Bogduk N. (1983). The innervation of the lumbar spine. *Spine, 8,* 286-293.

Bogduk N. (1985). Low back pain. *Aust Fam Physician, 14,* 1168-1171.

Bogduk N. (1990). Pathology of lumbar disc pain. *Manual Med, 5,* 72-79.

Bogduk N. (1992). The causes of low back pain. *Med J Aust, 156,* 151-153.

Bogduk N. (1997). *Clinical anatomy of the lumbar spine* (3rd ed.). London: Churchill Livingstone.

Bogduk N, Tynan W, & Wilson A. (1981). The nerve supply to the human lumbar intervertebral discs. *J Anat, 132,* 39-56.

Bogduk N, Wilson A, & Tynan W. (1982). The human lumbar dorsal rami. *J Anat, 134,* 383-397.

Borenstein DG. (2000). Epidemiology, etiology, diagnostic evaluation, and treatment of low back pain. *Curr Opin Rheumatol, 12(2),* 143-149.

Bose K & Balasubramaniam P. (1984). Nerve root canals of the lumbar spine. *Spine, 9,* 16-18.

Boszczyk BM et al. (2001). Related an immunohistochemical study of the dorsal capsule of the lumbar and thoracic facet joints. *Spine, 26(15),* e338-e343.

Bougie JD, Franco D, & Segil CM. (1996). An unusual cause for lumbar radiculopathy: A synovial facet joint cyst of the right L5 joint. *J Manipulative Physiol Ther, 19,* 48-51.

Briggs CA & Chandraraj S. (1995). Variations in the lumbosacral ligament and associated changes in the lumbosacral region resulting in compression of the fifth dorsal root ganglion and spinal nerve. *Clin Anat, 8,* 339-346.

Brown MD, Holmes DC, & Heiner AD. (2002). Measurement of cadaver lumbar spine motion segment stiffness. *Spine, 27,* 918-922.

Bucknill AT et al. (2002). Nerve fibers in lumbar spine structures and injured spinal roots express the sensory neuron-specific sodium channels SNS/PN3 and NaN/SNS2. *Spine, 27,* 135-140.

Butterman GR. (1998). Lumbar fusion results related to diagnosis. *Spine, 23,* 116-127.

Cao KD, Grimm MJ, & Yang KH. (2001). Load sharing within a human lumbar vertebral body using the finite element method. *Spine, 26,* E253-E260.

Caputo LA & Cusimano MD. (1997). Schwannoma of the cauda equina. *J Manipulative Physiol Ther, 20,* 124-129.

Cassidy J & Kirkaldy-Willis W. (1988). Manipulation. In W Kirkaldy-Willis (Ed.). *Managing low back pain* (2nd ed.). New York: Churchill Livingstone.

Chen D et al. (1995). Increasing neuroforaminal volume by anterior interbody distraction in degenerative lumbar spine. *Spine, 20,* 74-79.

Chithriki M, Jaibaji M, & Steele RD. (2002). The anatomical relationship of the aortic bifurcation to the lumbar vertebrae: A MRI study. *Surg Radiol Anat, 24,* 308-312.

Cinotti G et al. (2002). Stenosis of lumbar intervertebral foramen. *Spine, 27,* 223-229.

Clarke GA et al. (1985). Can infant malnutrition cause adult vertebral stenosis? *Spine, 10,* 165-170.

Cox J. (1990). *Low back pain: Mechanism, diagnosis, and treatment* (5th ed.). Baltimore: Williams & Wilkins.

Cramer GD et al. (1992a). Generalizability of patient profiles from a feasibility study. *J Can Chiropractic Assoc, 36,* 84-90.

Cramer GD et al. (1992b). Lumbar intervertebral foramen dimensions from thirty-seven human subjects as determined by magnetic resonance imaging. *Proc 1992 Intern Conf of Spinal Manipulation, 1,* 3-5.

Cramer GD et al. (1994). Comparison of computed tomography to magnetic resonance imaging in the evaluation of the lumbar intervertebral foramina. *Clin Anat, 7,* 173-180.

Cramer GD et al. (1996). Identification of the anterior longitudinal ligament on cadaveric spines and comparison with appearance on MRI. *Proc 1996 Intern Conf Spinal Manipulation (ICSM),* Bournemouth, England, October 17-19, 151-152.

Cramer GD et al. (1998a). Morphometric evaluation of the anterior longitudinal ligament on cadaveric spines by means of magnetic resonance imaging. *J Chiropract Educ, 11,* 141.

Cramer GD et al. (1998b) Morphometric evaluation of the posterior longitudinal ligament on cadaveric spines by means of magnetic resonance imaging. *Proc Intern Conf Spinal Manipulation,* Vancouver, BC, July 16-19, 24-26.

Cramer GD et al. (2000). Effects of side-posture positioning and side posture adjusting on the lumbar zygapophysial joints as evaluated by magnetic resonance imaging: A before and after study with randomization. *J Manipulative Physiol Ther, 23,* 380-394.

Cramer GD et al. (2002). The effects of side posture positioning and spinal adjusting on the lumbar Z joints: A randomized controlled trial of 64 subjects. *Spine, 27,* 2459-2466.

Cramer GD et al. (2003). Dimensions of the lumbar intervertebral foramina as determined from the sagittal plane magnetic resonance imaging scans of 95 normal subjects. *J Manipulative Physiol Ther, 26,* 160-170.

Crock HV. (1981). Normal and pathological anatomy of the lumbar spinal nerve root canals. *J Bone Joint Surg, 63,* 487-490.

Crock HV & Yoshizawa H. (1976). The blood supply of the lumbar vertebral column. *Clin Orthop, 115,* 6-21.

Day MO. (1991). Spondylolytic spondylolisthesis in an elite athlete. *Chiro Sports Med, 5,* 91-97.

dePeretti F et al. (1989). Biomechanics of the lumbar spinal nerve roots and the first sacral root within the intervertebral foramina. *Surg Radiol Anat, 11,* 221-225.

Dickey JP, Bednar DA, & Dumas GA. (1996). New insight into the mechanics of the lumbar interspinous ligament. *Spine, 21,* 2720-2727.

Dommisse GF & Louw JA. (1990). Anatomy of the lumbar spine. In Y Floman (Ed.). *Disorders of the lumbar spine.* Rockville, Md, and Tel Aviv: Aspen and Freund.

Dreyfuss PH & Dreyer SJ. (2001). Lumbar zygapophysial (facet) joint injections. North American Spine Society. *Contemp Concepts Spine Care,* 1-16.

Dunlop RB, Adams MA, & Hutton WC. (1984). Disc space narrowing and the lumbar facet joints. *J Bone Joint Surg, 66,* 706-710.

Dupuis PR. (1988). The anatomy of the lumbosacral spine. In W Kirkaldy-Willis (Ed.). *Managing low back pain* (2nd ed). New York: Churchill Livingstone.

Dupuis PR et al. (1985). Radiologic diagnosis of degenerative lumbar spinal instability. *Spine, 10,* 262-276.

Ebraheim NA et al. (1997a). Anatomic considerations of the lumbar isthmus. *Spine, 22,* 941-945.

Ebraheim NA et al. (1997b). Anatomic relations between the lumbar pedicle and the adjacent neural structures. *Spine, 22,* 2338-2341.

Edelson JG & Nathan H. (1988). Stages in the natural history of the vertebral end plates. *Spine, 13,* 21-26.

Edgar M & Ghadially J. (1976). Innervation of the lumbar spine. *Clin Orthop, 115,* 35-41.

Einstein SM et al. (1994). Innervation of the spondylolysis "ligament." *Spine, 19,* 912-916.

Engel R & Bogduk N. (1982). The menisci of the lumbar zygapophysial joints. *J Anat, 135,* 795-809.

Epstein JA et al. (1973). Lumbar nerve root compression at the intervertebral foramina caused by arthritis of the posterior facets. *J Neurosurg, 39,* 362-369.

Ericksen MF. (1976). Some aspects of aging in the lumbar spine. *Am J Phys Anthropol, 45,* 575-580.

Ericksen MF. (1978). Aging in the lumbar spine. *Am J Phys Anthropol, 48,* 241-245.

Farfan HF. (1973). *Mechanical disorders of the low back.* Philadelphia: Lea & Febiger.

Farfan HF, Huberdeau RM, & Dubow HI. (1972). Lumbar intervertebral disc degeneration. *J Bone Joint Surg, 54-A,* 492-510.

Fennell AJ, Jones AP, & Hukins DWL. (1996). Migration of the nucleus pulposus within the intervertebral disc during flexion and extension of the spine. *Spine, 21,* 2753-2757.

Floman Y & Mirovsky Y. (1990). The physical examination of the lumbosacral spine. In Y Floman (Ed.). *Disorders of the lumbar spine.* Rockville, Md, and Tel Aviv: Aspen and Freund.

Fujiwara A et al. (2000). The effect of disc degeneration and facet joint osteoarthritis on the segmental flexibility of the lumbar spine. *Spine, 25,* 3036-3044.

Fujiwara A et al. (2001). Morphologic changes in the lumbar intervertebral foramen due to flexion-extension, lateral bending, and axial rotation an in vitro anatomic and biochemical study. *Spine, 26,* 876-882.

Giglio GC et al. (1988). Anatomy of the lumbar spine in achondroplasia. *Basic Life Sci, 48,* 227-239.

Giles LG. (1987) Lumbo-sacral zygapophysial joint tropism and its effect on hyaline cartilage. *Clin Biomech, 2,* 2-6.

Giles LG. (1988). Human zygapophyseal joint inferior recess synovial folds: A light microscopic examination. *Anat Rec, 220,* 117-124.

Giles LG & Taylor JR. (1987). Human zygapophyseal joint capsule and synovial fold innervation. *Br J Rheumatol, 26,* 93-98.

Goel VK et al. (1993). A combined finite element and optimization investigation of lumbar spine mechanics with and without muscles. *Spine, 18,* 1531-1541.

Gordon SJ et al. (1991). Mechanism of disc rupture: A preliminary report. *Spine, 16,* 450-456.

Grant JP, Oxland TR, & Dvorak MF. (2001). Mapping the structural properties of lumbosacral vertebral end plates. *Spine, 26,* 889-896.

Grenier N et al. (1989a). Isthmic spondylolisthesis of the lumbar spine: MR imaging at 1.5T. *Radiology, 170,* 489-493.

Grenier N et al. (1989b). Normal and disrupted lumbar longitudinal ligaments: Correlative MR and anatomic study. *Radiology, 171,* 197-205.

Grimes PF, Massie JB, & Garfin SR. (2000). Anatomic and biomechanical analysis of the lower lumbar foraminal ligaments. *Spine, 25,* 2009-2014.

Groen G, Baljet B, & Drukker J. (1990). Nerves and nerve plexuses of the human vertebral column. *Am J Anat, 188,* 282-296.

Hadley LA. (1948). Apophysial subluxation. *J Bone Joint Surg,* 428-433.

Haher TR et al. (1992). Instantaneous axis of rotation as a function of the three columns of the spine. *Spine, 17,* s149-s154.

Hall LT et al. (1998). Morphology of the lumbar vertebral end plates. *Spine, 23,* 1517-1522.

Hamanishi C & Tanaka S. (1993). Dorsal root ganglia in the lumbosacral region observed from the axial views of MRI. *Spine, 18(13),* 1753-1756.

Hanson P & Sonesson B. (1994). The anatomy of the iliolumbar ligament. *Arch Phys Med Rehabil, 75,* 1245-1246.

Hasegawa T et al. (1996). Morphometric analysis of the lumbosacral nerve roots and dorsal root ganglia by magnetic resonance imaging. *Spine, 21,* 1005-1009.

Hasue M et al. (1983). Anatomic study of the interrelation between lumbosacral nerve roots and their surrounding tissues. *Spine, 8,* 50-58.

Hedman TP & Fernie GR. (1997). Mechanical response of the lumbar spine to seated postural loads. *Spine, 22,* 734-743.

Helms CA & Sims R. (1986). Foraminal spurs: A normal variant in the lumbar spine. *Radiology, 160,* 153-154.

Hoyland JA, Freemont AJ, & Jayson MIV. (1989). Intervertebral foramen venous obstruction: A cause of perridicular fibrosis. *Spine, 14,* 558-568.

Hsieh C et al. (2000). Lumbosacral transitional segments: Classification, prevalence, and effect on disc height. *J Manipulative Physiol Ther, 23,* 483-489.

Hutton WC. (1990). The forces acting on a lumbar intervertebral joint. *J Manual Med, 5,* 66-67.

Inufusa A et al. (1996). Anatomic changes of the spinal canal and intervertebral foramen associated with flexion-extension movement. *Spine, 21,* 2412-2420.

Jackson HC et al. (1966). Nerve endings in the human lumbar spinal column and related structures. *J Bone Joint Surg, 48,* 1272-1281.

Jeffries B. (1988). Facet joint injections. *Spine: State of the art reviews, 2,* 409-417.

Jerusalem G et al. (2003). PET scan imaging in oncology. *Eur J Cancer, 39,* 1525-1534.

Jönsson B & Stromqvist B. (1995). Motor affliction of the L5 nerve root in lumbar nerve root compression syndromes. *Spine, 20,* 2012-2015.

Jonsson E. (2000). Back pain, neck pain. SBU Project Group 2000, Summary & Conclusions, *Report, 145.*

Kanayama M et al. (1996). Phase lag of the intersegmental motion in flexion-extension of the lumbar and lumbosacral spine. *Spine, 21,* 1416-1422.

Kauppila LI & Tallroth K. (1993). Postmortem angiographic findings for arteries supplying the lumbar spine: Their relationship to low-back symptoms. *J Spinal Disord, 6,* 124-129.

Kikuchi S et al. (1984). Anatomic and clinical studies of radicular symptoms. *Spine, 9,* 23-30.

Kikuchi S et al. (1994). Anatomic and radiographic study of dorsal root ganglia. *Spine, 19,* 6-11.

Kirk CR & Lawrence DJ. (1985). *States manual of spinal, pelvic, and extravertebral techniques* (2nd ed.). Baltimore: Waverly Press.

Kirkaldy-Willis WH et al. (1978). Pathology and pathogenesis of lumbar spondylosis and stenosis. *Spine, 3,* 319-328.

Korkala O et al. (1985). Immunohistochemical demonstration of nociceptors in the ligamentous structures of the lumbar spine. *Spine, 10,* 156-157.

Krismer M et al. (2000). Motion in lumbar functional spine units during side bending and axial rotation moments depending on the degree of degeneration. *Spine, 25,* 2020-2027.

Lancourt JE, Glenn WV, & Wiltse LL. (1979). Multiplanar computerized tomography in the normal spine and in the diagnosis of spinal stenosis. A gross anatomic-computerized tomographic correlation. *Spine, 4,* 379-390.

Lee CK, Rauschning W, & Glenn W. (1988). Lateral lumbar spinal canal stenosis: Classification, pathologic anatomy and surgical decompression. *Spine, 13,* 313-320.

Lee H et al. (1995). Morphometric study of the lumbar spinal canal in the Korean population. *Spine, 20,* 1679-1684.

Lew PC, Morrow CJ, & Lew AM. (1994). The effect of neck and leg flexion and their sequence on the lumbar spinal cord. *Spine, 19,* 2421-2425.

Lippitt AB. (1984). The facet joint and its role in spine pain: Management with facet joint injections. *Spine, 9,* 746-750.

Liyang D et al. (1989). The effect of flexion-extension motion of the lumbar spine on the capacity of the spinal canal, an experimental study. *Spine, 14,* 523-525.

Macdonald A et al. (1999). Level of termination of the spinal cord and the dural sac: A magnetic resonance study. *Clin Anat, 12,* 149-152.

Maigne JY & Doursounian L. (1997). Entrapment neuropathy of the medial superior cluneal nerve. *Spine, 22,* 1156-1159.

Maigne JY, Maigne R, & Guerin-Surville H. (1991). The lumbar mamillo-accessory foramen: A study of 203 lumbosacral spines. *Surg Radiol Anat, 13,* 29-32.

Malas MA et al. (2000). The relationship between the lumbosacral enlargement and the conus medullaris during the period of fetal development and adulthood. *Surg Radiol Anat, 22,* 163-168.

Marchand F & Ahmed A. (1990). Investigation of the laminate structure of lumbar disc anulus fibrosus. *Spine, 15,* 402-410.

Marchiori DM & Firth R. (1996). Tethered cord syndrome. *J Manipulative Physiol Ther, 19,* 265-267.

Marchiori DM et al. (1994). A comparison of radiographic signs of degeneration to corresponding MRI signal intensities in the lumbar spine. *J Manipulative Physiol Ther, 17,* 238-245.

Markiewitz AD et al. (1996). Calcium pyrophosphate dehydrate crystal deposition disease as a cause of lumbar canal stenosis. *Spine, 21,* 506-511.

Mayoux-Benhamou MA et al. (1989). A morphometric study of the lumbar spine, influence of flexion-extension movements and of isolated disc collapse. *Surg Radiol Anat, 11,* 97-102.

McCarthy PW. (1993). The innervation of lumbar intervertebral discs: An update. *Eur J Chiropract, 41,* 21-29.

McGill SM. (1997). The biomechanics of low back injury: Implications on current practice in industry and the clinic. *J Biomechanics, 30,* 465-475.

McGregor AH, McCarthy ID, & Hughes SP. (1995). Motion characteristics of the lumbar spine in the normal population. *Spine, 20,* 2421-2428.

McNab I. (1971). Negative disc exploration: An analysis of the causes of nerve-root involvement in sixty-eight patients. *J Bone Joint Surg, 53A,* 891-903.

Mitra SR, Datir SP, & Jadhav SO. (2002). Morphometric study of the lumbar pedicle in the Indian population as related to pedicular screw fixation. *Spine, 27,* 453-459.

Mooney V & Robertson J. (1976). The facet syndrome. *Clin Orthop, 115,* 149-156.

Morinaga T et al. (1996). Sensory innervation to the anterior portion of the lumbar intervertebral disc. *Spine, 21,* 1848-1851.

Mosner EA et al. (1989). A comparison of actual and apparent lumbar lordosis in black and white adult females. *Spine, 14,* 310-314.

Nachemson AL. (1976). The lumbar spine, and orthopedic challenge. *Spine, 1,* 59-71.

Natarajan RN & Andersson GBJ. (1999). The influence of lumbar disc height and cross-sectional area on the mechanical response of the disc to physiological loading. *Spine, 24,* 1873.

Nathan H, Weizenbluth M, & Halperin N. (1982). The lumbosacral ligament (LSL), with special emphasis on the "lumbosacral tunnel" and the entrapment of the 5th lumbar nerve. *Int Orthop, 6,* 197-202.

Neidre A & MacNab I. (1983). Anomalies of the lumbosacral nerve roots: Review of 16 cases and classification. *Spine, 8,* 294-299.

Nicholson AA, Roberts GM, & Williams LA. (1988). The measured height of the lumbosacral disc in patients with and without transitional vertebrae. *Br J Radiol, 61,* 454-455.

Nordström D et al. (1994). Symptomatic lumbar spondylolysis. *Spine, 19,* 2752-2758.

Nowicki BH et al. (1990). Effect of axial loading on neural foramina and nerve roots in the lumbar spine. *Radiology, 176,* 433-437.

Nowicki BH & Haughton VM. (1992). Ligaments of the lumbar neural foramina: A sectional anatomic study. *Clin Anat, 5,* 126-135.

Ohtori S et al. (1999). Sensory innervation of the dorsal portion of the lumbar intervertebral disc in rats. *Spine, 24,* 2295.

Ohtori S et al. (2001). Neurones in the dorsal root ganglia of T13, L1 and L2 innervate the dorsal portion of lower lumbar discs in rats. A study using diI, an anterograde neurotracer. *J Bone Joint Surg [Br], 83(8),* 1191-1194.

Olsewski JM et al. (1991). Evidence from cadavers suggestive of entrapment of fifth lumbar spinal nerves by lumbosacral ligaments. *Spine, 16,* 336-347.

Olszewski AD, Yaszemski MJ, & White AA. (1996). The anatomy of the human lumbar ligamentum flavum: New observations and their surgical importance. *Spine, 21,* 2307-2312.

Oshima H et al. (1993). Morphologic variation of lumbar posterior longitudinal ligament and the modality of disc herniation. *Spine, 18,* 2408-2411.

Oxland TR et al. (2003). Effects of end plate removal on the structural properties of the lower lumbar vertebral bodies. *Spine, 28,* 771-777.

Pal GP et al. (1988). Trajectory architecture of the trabecular bone between the body and the neural arch in human vertebrae. *Anat Rec, 222,* 418-425.

Papp T, Porter RW, & Aspden R. (1994). The growth of the lumbar vertebral canal. *Spine, 19,* 2270-2273.

Paris S. (1983). Anatomy as related to function and pain. *Symposium on Evaluation and Care of Lumbar Spine Problems,* 475-489.

Park JB, Chang H, & Lee JK. (2001). Quantitative analysis of transforming growth factor-beta 1 in ligamentum flavum of lumbar spinal stenosis and disc herniation. *Spine, 26,* E492-E495.

Parke WW & Schiff DC. (1993). The applied anatomy of the intervertebral disc. *Orthop Clin North Am, 2,* 309-324.

Paz-Fumagalli R & Haughton VM. (1993). Lumbar cribriform fascia: Appearance at freezing microtomy and MR imaging. *Radiology, 187,* 241-243.

Peterson CK, Boulton JE, & Wood AR. (2000). A cross-sectional study correlating lumbar spine degeneration with disability and pain. *Spine, 25,* 218-223.

Plamondon A, Gagnon M, & Maurais G. (1988). Application of stereo-radiographic method for the study of intervertebral motion. *Spine, 13,* 1027-1032.

Porter R. (1996). Spinal stenosis and neurogenic claudication. *Spine, 21,* 2046-2052.

Postacchini F & Perugia D. (1991). Degenerative lumbar spondylolisthesis. *It J Orthop Traumatol, 17,* 165-173.

Putz RL & Müller-Gerbl M. (1996). The vertebral column: A phylogenetic failure? A theory explaining the function and vulnerability of the human spine. *Clin Anat, 9,* 205-212.

Rauschning W. (1987). Normal and pathologic anatomy of the lumbar root canals. *Spine, 12,* 1008-1019.

Revel M et al. (1988). Morphological variations of the lumbar intervertebral foramina during flexion-extension and disc collapse. *Revue du Rhumatisme, 55,* 361-366.

Rizzo JA, Abbott TA III, & Berger ML. (1998). The labor productivity effects of chronic backache in the US. *Medical Care, 36(10),* 1471-1488.

Rucco V, Basadonna PT, & Gasparini D. (1996). Anatomy of the iliolumbar ligament. *Am J Phys Med Rehabil, 75,* 451-455.

Salbacak A et al. (2000). An investigation of the conus medullaris and filum terminale variations in human fetuses. *Surg Radiol Anat, 22,* 89-92.

Scapinelli R. (1989). Morphological and functional changes of the lumbar spinous processes in the elderly. *Surg Radiol Anat, 11,* 129-133.

Scapinelli R. (1990). Anatomical and radiologic studios on the lumbosacral meningovertebral ligaments of humans. *J Spinal Disord, 3,* 6-15.

Schlegel JD et al. (1994). The role of distraction in improving the space available in the lumbar stenotic canal and foramen. *Spine, 19(18),* 2041-2047.

Schwab FJ, Farcy JC, & Roye DP Jr. (1997). The sagittal pelvic tilt index as a criterion in the evaluation of spondylolisthesis. *Spine, 22,* 1661-1667.

Schwarzer AC et al. (1995). The prevalence and clinical features of internal disc disruption in patients with chronic low back pain. *Spine, 20,* 1878-1883.

Shirazi-Adl A & Drouin G. (1987). Load-bearing role of facets in a lumbar segment under sagittal plane loadings. *J Biomech, 20(6),* 601-613.

Silcox DH et al. (1995). The effect of nicotine on spinal fusion. *Spine, 20,* 1549-1553.

Silva MJ, Keaveny TM, & Hayes WC. (1997). Load sharing between the shell and centrum in the lumbar vertebral body. *Spine, 22,* 140-150.

Sims JA & Moorman SJ. (1996). The role of the iliolumbar ligament in low back pain. *Med Hypoth, 46,* 511-515.

Spencer DL, Irwin GS, & Miller JAA. (1983). Anatomy and significance of fixation of the lumbosacral nerve roots in sciatica. *Spine, 8,* 672-679.

Spratt JD, Logan BM, & Abrahams PH. (1996). Variant slips of psoas and iliacus muscles, with splitting of the femoral nerve. *Clin Anat, 9,* 401-404.

Suseki K et al. (1997). Innervation of the lumbar facet joints. *Spine, 22,* 477-485.

Takahashi K et al. (1995). Epidural pressure measurements. *Spine, 20,* 650-653.

Takahashi K, Shima I, & Porter RW. (1999). Nerve root pressure in lumbar disc herniation. *Spine, 24,* 2003.

Takemitsu Y et al. (1988). Lumbar degenerative kyphosis. *Spine, 13,* 1317-1326.

Tallroth K et al. (1995). Lumbar spine in Marfan syndrome. *Skeletal Radiol, 24,* 337-340.

Taylor JR. (1990). The development and adult structure of lumbar intervertebral discs. *J Manual Med, 5,* 43-47.

Taylor JR & Twomey LT. (1986). Age changes in lumbar zygapophyseal joints: Observations on structure and function. *Spine, 11,* 739-745.

Theil HW, Clements DS, & Cassidy JD. (1992). Lumbar apophyseal ring fractures in adolescents. *J Manipulative Physiol Ther, 15,* 250-254.

Tribus CB & Belanger T. (2001). The vascular anatomy anterior to the L5-S1 disk space. *Spine, 26,* 1205-1208.

Tsuji H et al. (1985). Redundant nerve roots in patients with degenerative lumbar spinal stenosis. *Spine, 10,* 72-82.

Twomey L & Taylor JR. (1990). Structural and mechanical disc changes with age. *J Manual Med, 5,* 58-61.

Uhthoff H. (1993). Prenatal development of the iliolumbar ligament. *J Bone Joint Surg, 75,* 93-95.

Ulmer JL et al. (1995). Lumbar spondylolysis without spondylolisthesis: Recognition of isolated posterior element subluxation on sagittal MR. *Am J Neuroradiol, 16,* 1393-1398.

Van Schaik J, Verbiest H, & Van Schaik F. (1985). The orientation of laminae and facet joints in the lower lumbar spine. *Spine, 10,* 59-63.

Vanharanta H et al. (1993). The relationship of facet tropism to degenerative disc disease. *Spine, 18,* 1000-1005.

Verbiest H. (1954). A radicular syndrome from developmental narrowing of the lumbar vertebral canal. *J Bone Joint Surg, 36-B,* 230-237.

Viejo-Fuertes D et al. (1998). Morphologic and histologic study of the ligamentum flavum in the thoraco-lumbar region. *Surg Radiol Anat, 20(3),* 171-176.

Vital JM et al. (1983). Anatomy of the lumbar radicular canal. *Anat Clin, 5,* 141-151.

Vleeming A et al. (1996). The function of the long dorsal sacroiliac ligament. *Spine, 21,* 556-562.

White AW & Panjabi MM. (1990). *Clinical biomechanics of the spine.* Philadelphia: JB Lippincott.

Williams PL et al. (1995). *Gray's anatomy* (38th ed.). Edinburgh: Churchill Livingstone.

Wilson DA & Prince JR. (1989). John Caffey award. MR imaging determination of the location of the normal conus medullaris throughout childhood. *AJR Am J Roentgenol, 152(5),* 1029-32.

Wiltse LL et al. (1984). Alar transverse process impingement of the L5 spinal nerve: The far-out syndrome. *Spine, 9,* 31-41.

Worril NA & Peterson CK. (1997). Effect of anterior wedging of LI on the measurement of lumbar lordosis: Comparison of two roentgenological methods. *J Manipulative Physiol Ther, 20,* 459-467.

Xu GL et al. (1991). Normal variations of the lumbar facet joint capsules. *Clin Anat, 4,* 117-122.

Xu GL, Haughton VM, & Carrera GF. (1990). Lumbar facet joint capsule: Appearance at MR imaging and CT. *Radiology, 177,* 415-420.

Yahia H, Newman N, & St-Georges M. (1988). Sensory nerve endings in the posterior ligaments of the lumbar spine. *Electrophysiol Kinesiol,* 455-458.

Yahia LH, Newman N, & Rivard C. (1988). Neurohistology of lumbar spine ligament. *Acta Orthop Scand, 59,* 508-512.

Yamashita T et al. (1990). Mechanosensitive afferent units in the lumbar facet joint. *J Bone Joint Surg, 72-A,* 865-870.

Yamashita T et al. (1996). A morphological study of the fibrous capsule of the human lumbar facet joint. *Spine, 21,* 538-543.

Yang KH & King AI. (1984). Mechanism of facet load transmission as a hypothesis for low-back pain. *Spine, 9,* 557-565.

Yang KH et al. (1988). Annulus fibrosus tears. An experimental model. *Orthop Trans, 12,* 86-87.

You-Lu Z & Wu W. (1988). CT measurement of the normal cervical and lumbar spinal canal in Chinese. *Chin Med J, 101,* 898-900.

Yu SW et al. (1996) Identification of the posterior longitudinal ligament on magnetic resonance imaging scans: Comparison between MRI and a cadaveric specimen. *Proc 1996 Intern Conf Spinal Manipulation (ICSM),* Bournemouth, England, October 17-19, 153-154.

Yukawa Y et al. (1997). Groin pain associated with lower lumbar disc herniation. *Spine, 22,* 1736-1740.

CHAPTER 8

The Sacrum, Sacroiliac Joint, and Coccyx

Gregory D. Cramer
Chae-Song Ro

This chapter begins with a discussion of the bony sacrum. Then, because of its clinical significance, the sacroiliac joint is covered in detail. This is followed by a discussion of the anatomy of the coccyx.

THE SACRUM

The sacrum is composed of five fused vertebral segments. The sacral segments decrease in size from the first to the fifth, making the sacrum triangular in shape. Consequently, the wider superior surface of the sacrum is known as the sacral base, and the smaller inferior surface is known as the apex (Figs. 8-1 and 8-2). The sacrum is concave anteriorly (kyphotic), and as with the other primary kyphosis (the thoracic region), its curvature helps to increase the size of a bony body cavity, in this case the pelvis. The sacrum is normally positioned so that its base is located anterior to its apex. Therefore the sacral curve faces anteriorly and inferiorly (Williams et al., 1995). The sacral curve is more pronounced in humans than in other mammals, including monkeys and apes. In addition, the human sacral curve is almost nonexistent in infants but becomes more pronounced with age (Abitbol, 1989). The combination of upright posture, supine sleeping posture, and a well-developed levator ani muscle are responsible for the increased sacral curve in humans. Abitbol (1989) also found that the frequency of sleeping in the supine posture, and the younger the age when this posture was first assumed for sleeping, were positively associated with the size of the sacral curve.

The sacrum ossifies much like any other vertebra, with one primary center located in the anterior and centrally located primitive vertebral body and one primary center in each posterior arch. Unique to the sacrum is that the costal elements develop separately and then fuse with the remainder of the posterior arch to form the solid mass of bone lateral to the pelvic sacral foramina. Secondary centers of ossification are complex,

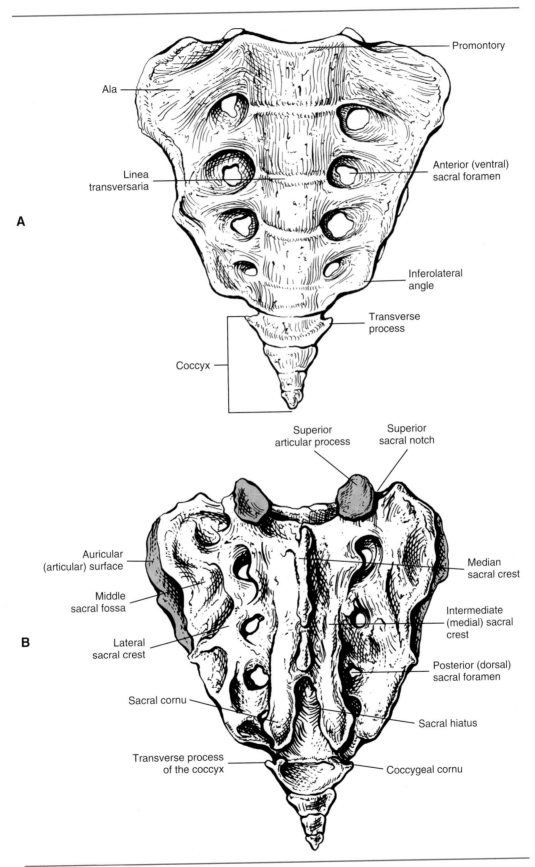

FIG. 8-1   The sacrum. **A,** Anterior view. **B,** Posterior view.

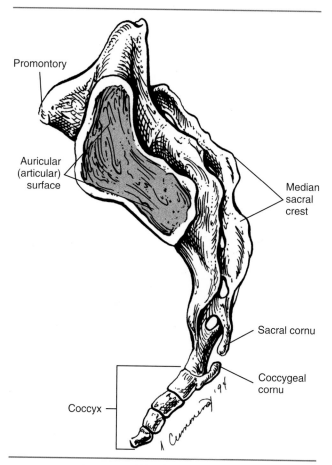

Promontory

Auricular
(articular)
surface

Median
sacral
crest

Sacral cornu

Coccygeal
cornu

Coccyx

FIG. 8-2   Lateral view of the sacrum.

with centers developing on the superior and inferior aspects of each sacral vertebral body, the lateral and the anterior aspects of each costal element, the spinous tubercles, and the lateral (auricular) surface of the sacrum. Most centers fuse by approximately the twenty-fifth year of life, but ossification and fusion of individual segments continue until later in life. Early in development, fibrocartilage forms between sacral bodies. These represent rudimentary intervertebral discs (IVDs) and usually become surrounded by bone as the sacral bodies fuse with one another. However, the central region of these "discs" usually remains unossified throughout life.

Sacral Base

The sacral base is composed of the first sacral segment. It has a large body that is the homologue of the vertebral bodies (see Figs. 8-1 and 8-2). This body is wider from left to right than from front to back. The anterior lip of the sacral body is known as the promontory. The vertebral foramen of the first sacral segment is triangular in shape and forms the beginning of the sacral canal. This canal extends the length of the sacrum. The pedicles of the

first sacral segment are small and extend to the left and right laminae. The laminae of the first segment meet posteriorly to form the spinous tubercle. The transverse processes (TPs) extend laterally and fuse with the costal elements to form the large left and right sacral alae, which are also known as the lateral sacral masses. The bony trabeculae of the inner cancellous bone of the sacral ala are significantly less dense than those in the sacral bodies (Peretz, Hipp, and Heggeness, 1998). Each lateral sacral mass is concave on its anterior surface, allowing it to accommodate the psoas major muscle. The psoas major passes across the sacrum before inserting onto the lesser trochanter of the femur.

Extending superiorly from the posterior surface of the sacral base are the left and right articular processes. These processes generally face posteriorly and slightly medially. However, the plane in which these processes lie varies considerably (Dommisse and Louw, 1990). Their orientation ranges from nearly a coronal plane to almost a sagittal one. These processes also frequently are asymmetric in orientation, with one process more coronally oriented and the other more sagittally oriented. Such asymmetry is known as tropism and usually can be detected on standard anterior-posterior x-ray films. The superior articular processes possess articular facets on their posterior surfaces that articulate with the inferior articular facets of the L5 vertebra. The zygapophysial (Z) joints formed by these articulations are more planar than those between two adjacent lumbar vertebrae, and they usually are much more coronally oriented than the lumbar Z joints (see Chapter 7). However, because of the wide variation of the plane in which the superior articular processes lie, the orientation of the lumbosacral Z joints also varies in corresponding fashion.

The left and right superior sacral notches are just lateral to the superior articular facets. These notches allow for passage of the left and right posterior primary divisions of the L5 spinal nerve.

The muscular and ligamentous attachments to the sacral base and the anterior and posterior surfaces of the sacrum are listed in Table 8-1. This table also provides the key anatomic relationships between these regions of the sacrum, and the neural, muscular, and visceral structures that contact them.

Lateral Surface

The lateral surface of the sacrum (see Fig. 8-2) is composed of the TPs of the five sacral segments, fused with the costal elements of the same segments. This surface contains the auricular surface. The auricular surface of the sacrum articulates with the auricular surface of the ilium. The sacral auricular surface is concave posteriorly and extends across the lateral aspects of three of the five sacral segments. Within the region surrounded by the

Table 8-1	Attachments and Relationships to the Sacrum
Surface	**Attachments or Relationships**
Base	
Anterior	Ligaments: anterior longitudinal, iliolumbar, ventral sacroiliac
	Muscles: psoas major and iliacus (cover the base)
	Nerves: lumbosacral trunk (crosses over the base)
Posterior	Ligaments: posterior longitudinal, ligamentum flavum (to lamina of S1), posterior sacroiliac, interosseous sacroiliac
Ventral	Muscle: piriformis
	Ligament: sacrospinous
	Nerves: S1-4 ventral rami (S1-3 are anterior to piriformis), sympathetic trunks (left and right)
	Arteries: median sacral, lateral sacral (left and right), superior rectal
	Viscera: parietal peritoneum (S1-3 bodies), sigmoid mesocolon (S1-3 bodies), rectum (S3-5 bodies)
Dorsal	Muscles: erector spinae, multifidus (between median and lateral sacral crests)
	Ligament: sacrotuberous

From Williams PL et al. (1995). *Gray's anatomy* (38th ed.). Edinburgh: Churchill Livingstone.

concavity of the auricular surface are several elevations and depressions that serve as attachment sites for the ligaments that support the sacroiliac joint posteriorly. These ligaments and the sacroiliac joint are discussed in detail later in this chapter. Inferior to the auricular surface, the lateral surface of the sacrum curves medially and becomes thinner from anterior to posterior. The inferior and lateral angle of the sacrum is located at roughly the level of the junction of the fourth and fifth sacral segments. Below this angle the sacrum rapidly tapers to the sacral apex. The apex of the sacrum has an oval-shaped facet on its inferior surface for articulation with a small disc between the sacrum and coccyx.

Sacral Canal and Sacral Foramina

The sacral canal is composed of the vertebral foramina of the five fused sacral segments. The left and right lateral walls of the canal each contain four intervertebral foramina (IVFs). Each IVF is continuous laterally with a ventral (pelvic) and dorsal sacral foramen. The sacral canal ends inferiorly as the sacral hiatus (see the following discussion).

The cauda equina extends inferiorly through the beginning of the sacral canal and within the subarach-

noid space. The arachnoid mater and dura mater end at roughly the level of the S2 spinous tubercle. The sacral roots exiting below this level must pierce the inferior aspect of the arachnoid and dura to continue inferiorly through the sacral canal. In the process, these roots receive a dural root sleeve. Dorsal and ventral roots unite within their dural sleeve to form a spinal nerve and then exit a sacral IVF.

Structures Exiting the Sacral Hiatus. Both the left and the right S5 nerves and the coccygeal nerve of each side exit the sacral hiatus just medial to the sacral cornua of the same side. They proceed inferiorly and laterally, wrapping around the inferior tip of the sacral cornua (see Dorsal Surface). The posterior primary divisions (PPDs) of these nerves pass posteriorly and inferiorly to supply sensory innervation to the skin over the coccyx. The S5 and coccygeal anterior primary divisions pass anteriorly to pierce the coccygeus muscle and enter the inferior aspect of the pelvis. Here they are joined by the ventral ramus of the S4 nerve to form the coccygeal plexus. This small plexus gives off the anococcygeal nerves that help to supply the skin adjacent to the sacrotuberous ligament.

The end of the filum terminale also passes through the sacral hiatus. The filum terminale originates from the most inferior aspect of the spinal cord, where it is known as the filum terminale internum. It passes through the lumbar cistern of cerebrospinal fluid (CSF), pierces the inferior aspect of the arachnoid and dura (at generally the level of the S2 segment), and then becomes known as the filum terminale externum. After exiting the sacral hiatus, the filum terminale externum attaches to the posterior surface of the first coccygeal vertebral segment.

Ventral Surface

The junctions of the five fused sacral segments form lines that can be seen running across the central aspect of the anterior, or pelvic, surface of the sacrum. These junctions are known as the linea transversaria (also known as transverse lines, or transverse ridges). Remnants of the IVDs are located just deep to the transverse lines. These "discs" frequently remain throughout life and can be seen on standard x-ray films and magnetic resonance imaging (MRI) scans. The vertebral bodies of the five fused sacral segments lie between the transverse lines and medial to the pelvic sacral foramina (see Fig. 8-1).

The ventral surface of the sacrum displays four pairs of ventral (pelvic or anterior) sacral foramina. These foramina are continuous posteriorly and medially with the sacral IVFs. The sacral IVFs, in turn, are continuous with the more medially located sacral canal. The anterior primary divisions (APDs) of the S1 through S4 sacral nerves exit the pelvic sacral foramina. The APDs are accompanied within these openings by branches of the lateral and median sacral arteries and by segmental veins. Located between the pelvic sacral foramina of the same side are the costal elements. The cortical bone in these regions between the ventral sacral foramina is sturdy (dense), and the cortical bone between the S1 and S2 ventral sacral foramina is the most dense bone of the entire sacrum (Ebraheim et al., 2000). The costal elements fuse posteriorly with the TPs of the sacral segments.

The muscular and ligamentous attachments to the anterior surface of the sacrum are listed in Table 8-1. Also, Figures 8-20 and 8-21 demonstrate the major arteries and nerves associated with the anterior surface of the sacrum.

Dorsal Surface

The dorsal surface of the sacrum is irregular in shape (see Fig. 8-1). The superior articular processes extend from the superior aspect of the sacral base (see Sacral Base).

Four pair of dorsal (posterior) sacral foramina are located among the five fused sacral segments. These openings are continuous anteriorly with the IVFs of the sacral segments. The PPDs of the S1 through S4 spinal nerves exit through these openings. The PPDs are accompanied by small segmental arteries and veins.

The posterior surface of the sacrum contains five longitudinal (vertical) ridges known as the median, intermediate (left and right), and lateral (left and right) sacral crests (see Fig. 8-1). These crests are homologous to the spinous processes, articular processes, and the TPs of the rest of the spine, respectively.

The median sacral crest is composed of four spinous tubercles that are fused with one another and form the posterior boundary of the sacral canal. Each sacral tubercle is formed by the union of the left and right laminae of the sacral vertebral segments. The median sacral crest ends as the only normally occurring spina bifida of the vertebral column because the left and right laminae of the fifth sacral segment normally do not fuse, forming an opening at the inferior end of the sacral canal known as the sacral hiatus.

The left and right intermediate, or medial, sacral crests are located just medial to the posterior (dorsal) sacral foramina. They are formed by four fused articular tubercles on each side of the sacrum (S2-5 tubercles; the S1 articular process is distinct). The left and right fifth articular tubercles extend inferiorly as the sacral cornua. The sacral cornua come to blunted tips inferiorly. They form the left and right inferior boundaries of the sacral hiatus (Fig. 8-1).

Finally, the left and right lateral sacral crests lie lateral to the dorsal sacral foramina. These crests are formed by the fused transverse tubercles of the five sacral segments.

The muscular and ligamentous attachments to the posterior surface of the sacrum are listed in Table 8-1.

Several differences exist between male and female sacra, although sometimes these changes may be subtle. Generally, the male sacrum is narrower from left to right and longer from superior to inferior than that of the female. The wider sacrum of the female results in a larger pelvic inlet (i.e., region bounded by the pecten of the pubis, arcuate line of the ilium, sacral ala, and sacral promontory). A larger pelvic inlet results in more room for the passage of the fetal head during delivery. The sacrum in the female is also oriented slightly more horizontally than that of the male. This results in an increase of the lumbosacral angle. The ventral surface of the female sacrum is more concave than that of the male. This concavity provides more space in the pelvic cavity proper than would otherwise be the case, and it also results in a more prominent S2 spinous tubercle on the posterior surface of the female sacrum.

Fusion of the L5 vertebra with the sacrum (sacralization) is discussed in Chapter 7 and shown in Figures 12-14, *G* and *H*. The first sacral segment also may separate from the sacrum, known as lumbarization. The separation may be complete but usually is unilateral, and a joint may develop between the TP of the lumbarized segment and the remainder of the sacrum. Also, the first coccygeal segment may fuse with the sacrum.

Sacrococcygeal Joint

A fibrocartilaginous disc typically exists between the apex of the sacrum and the coccyx, making this joint a symphysis. However, occasionally a synovial joint develops here. At the other extreme, this region may completely fuse in older individuals (Williams et al., 1995).

Table 8-2 lists all the ligaments of the sacrococcygeal joint by their coccygeal attachments, as well as the muscles attaching to the coccyx.

Clinical Implications. Sacral fractures are present in as many as 45% of pelvic fractures (Gibbons, Soloniuk, and Razack, 1990). These fractures may go undetected if caudal, cephalic, and oblique x-ray examinations of the pelvis are not performed. Fractures of the sacrum can damage the APDs of the lumbosacral plexus, and fractures involving the sacral canal may affect the sacral roots before they are able to exit the sacrum.

Gibbons, Soloniuk, and Razack (1990) found neurologic deficits in 34% of patients with sacral fractures. They also noted that the neurologic deficits usually improved with time. The presence and type of nerve injury correlated with the type of sacral fracture. Patients with injuries that involved only the sacral ala had the

Table 8-2	Attachments and Relationships to the Coccyx
Surface	**Attachments or Relationships**
Anterior	Pubococcygeus, iliococcygeus, and ischiococcygeus (coccygeus) muscles, ventral sacrococcygeal ligament (similar to anterior longitudinal ligament)
Posterior	Gluteus maximus and sphincter ani externus (to tip of apex) muscles, intercornual ligaments, deep and superficial dorsal sacrococcygeal ligament,* filum terminale externum
Lateral	Lateral sacrococcygeal ligament (from transverse process of coccyx to inferolateral angle of sacrum)

From Williams PL et al. (1995). *Gray's anatomy* (38th ed.). Edinburgh: Churchill Livingstone.

*The superficial part runs between the sacral cornua (it closes the inferior aspect of the sacral canal at the sacral hiatus). The deep part is similar in location (and function) to the posterior longitudinal ligament. The filum terminale externum passes between the two parts of this ligament before attaching to the coccyx.

lowest incidence of neurologic deficit, although L5 or S1 radiculopathy was found in 24% of these patients. The mechanism of L5 radiculopathy was thought to be caused by entrapment of the APD of L5 between the fractured, superiorly displaced ala and the TP of L5.

Gibbons, Soloniuk, and Razack (1990) also found that fractures involving the pelvic sacral foramina usually were vertical fractures that passed through all four foramina of one side. These injuries always were associated with other pelvic fractures and had a 29% incidence (two of seven fractures) of unilateral L5 or S1 nerve root involvement. However, bowel and bladder functions were maintained; a bilateral lesion is necessary to affect these functions.

Fractures involving the sacral canal can be either transverse (horizontal) or vertical and have the greatest chance of causing nerve damage (57% with horizontal and 60% with vertical). Vertical fractures usually are associated with other pelvic fractures and can result in bladder and bowel dysfunction (Gibbons, Soloniuk, and Razack, 1990; Ebraheim, Biyani, and Salpietro, 1996).

Horizontal fractures of the sacrum affecting the sacral canal are not necessarily associated with other pelvic fractures. They can be isolated injuries caused by a direct blow, as might occur from a long fall. The inferior fragment sometimes is considerably displaced, and severe neurologic deficits, involving bladder and bowel functions, can occur if the fracture is above the S4 segment (Gibbons, Soloniuk, and Razack, 1990).

SACROILIAC JOINT

General Considerations

The degree to which low back pain is caused by pathologic conditions or dysfunction of the sacroiliac joint (SIJ) has been discussed for many decades. The SIJ is now gaining added attention as a primary source of low back pain (Cassidy and Mierau, 1992; Daum, 1995; Schwarzer, Aprill, and Bogduk, 1995; Dreyfuss et al., 1996). One reason for this is that protrusion of the IVD is now considered to be a relatively infrequent cause of low back pain, accounting for less than 10% of the pain in this region (Cassidy and Mierau, 1992). On the other hand, pain arising from the SIJ is reported to account for more than 20% of low back pain (Kirkaldy-Willis, 1988) and may be implicated to some extent in more than 50% of patients with low back pain (Cassidy and Mierau, 1992). This makes the SIJ an area of significant clinical importance. An understanding of the unique and interesting anatomy of this joint is essential before a clinician can properly diagnose and treat pain arising from this articulation.

The pelvic ring possesses five distinctly different types of joints: the lumbosacral Z joints, the anterior lumbosacral (L5-S1 IVD), coxal (hip), SIJ, and symphysis pubis. The dynamic interactions between these joints are not well understood. Because the pelvic ring is complex and actually involves a total of eight joints (left and right Z joints, coxals, and SIJs; plus the single lumbosacral joint and the pubic symphysis), any change in the trunk or lower extremity is compensated in some way by the complicated dynamic mechanism of the pelvic ring (Lichtblau, 1962; Winterstein, 1972; LaBan et al., 1978; Sandoz, 1978; Grieve, 1981; Fidler and Plasmans, 1983; Wallheim, Olerud, and Ribbe, 1984; Drerup and Hierholzer, 1987). In fact, a survey of the pelvic rings of asymptomatic schoolchildren 7 to 8 years of age revealed distortion (asymmetry) in 40% of them. Surgical removal of graft material from the pelvic bone (iliac crest) also causes distortion of the pelvic ring (Grieve, 1975; Beal, 1982; Diakow, Cassidy, and DeKorompay, 1983).

The SIJ and symphysis pubis move a small amount. At first inspection, what little motion they have may seem enigmatic at best. Some authors have stated that the sole function of these two joints simply is to widen the pelvic ring during pregnancy and parturition. The joints are aided in this action by the hormone relaxin (Simkins, 1952; Bellamy, Park, and Rodney, 1983). Others believe the SIJs move during many activities. An incomplete list of activities thought to enlist the movement of the SIJ includes the following: locomotion, spinal and thigh movement, and changes of position (from lying to standing, standing to sitting, etc.).

The SIJ is thought to move a minimum of 2 mm and 2 degrees, but this small amount of movement is complex (Pitkin and Pheasant, 1936b; Weisl, 1955; Colachis et al., 1963; Wood, 1985; Sturesson, 1989; Brunner, Kissling, and Jacob, 1991; Barakatt et al., 1996; Smidt et al., 1997). Janse (1978) stated that the function of movement in the SIJ is to convert the pelvis into a resilient, accommodating receptacle essential to the ease of locomotion, weight bearing, and shock absorption. This is in agreement with other authors (DonTigny, 1990; King, 1991) who state that the function of SIJ is to buffer, absorb, direct, and compensate for forces generated from above (gravity, carrying the torso, and muscle action) and below (forces received during standing and locomotion).

Unique Characteristics

Differences between humans and quadrupeds.
The pelvis tilts anteriorly and inferiorly in the bipedal human, and the SIJ is aligned in parallel fashion with the vertebral column, whereas the pelvis of quadrupedal animals is tilted more posteriorly. The SIJ of the bipedal human has other differences associated with a two-legged stance. These include the articulating surfaces of the SIJ that are shaped like an inverted L, the interosseous ligaments that are more substantial and stronger posteriorly, and the many bony interlockings between the sacrum and the ilium that develop with age (Walker, 1986).

Differences among humans. The plane of articulation of SIJs can vary from one individual to another; and the left and right SIJs of one individual can even lie in different planes (Ebraheim et al., 1997b). The weight of the human trunk is transmitted by gravity through the lumbosacral joint and is then divided onto the right and left SIJs. In addition, the ground reaction, or bouncing force, is transmitted through the hip joints and also acts on the SIJs. Adapting to the bipedal requirements of mobility and stability may account for the tremendous amount of variation and asymmetry found in the human SIJ. The joint structure and the surface contours of the SIJ have changes associated with age, sex, and the mechanical loads that are placed on them (Walker, 1986). Therefore the functional requirements of the SIJ, to a great extent, may influence the structural changes found in them (Weisl, 1954a). For example, one may speculate that more mobility is necessary in the SIJ in younger persons, females around the time of parturition, and athletes. On the other hand, more stability is necessary in older persons, males (generally larger body weight), and those who frequently carry heavy weights. This stability may be provided by the development of stronger interosseous ligaments and a more prominent series of bony interlockings (Table 8-3). Also, the osteophytes and ankylosis frequently seen in the SIJs of older individuals may develop to increase stability.

Table 8-3 "Tongue and Groove" Relationships (Bony Interlockings) between the Sacrum and Ilium*

Sacral E or D	Iliac E or D
Sacral groove (D)	Iliac ridge (E)
Middle sacral fossa (see text) (D)	Iliac tuberosity (E)
Sacral tuberosity (E)	Sulcus between iliac ridge and iliac tuberosity (iliac sulcus) (D)
Additional elevation on posterior and superior surface of sacral ala (alar tuberosity) (E)	Depression anterior and superior to iliac tuberosity (D)

E, Elevation; *D*, depression.
*Compare with Fig. 8-9.

Structure

General Relationships. The SIJ is an articulation between the auricular surface of the lateral aspect of the sacrum and the auricular surface of the medial aspect of the ilium (see Figs. 8-6 and 8-7). Previously this joint was classified as an amphiarthrosis. However, the SIJ is now classified as an atypical synovial joint with a well-defined joint space and two opposing articular surfaces (Cassidy and Mierau, 1992). Each auricular surface is shaped like an inverted L (Williams et al., 1995). Other authors have described it as being C shaped (Cassidy and Mierau, 1992). The superior limb of this surface is oriented posteriorly and superiorly, and the inferior limb is oriented posteriorly and inferiorly (Figs. 8-2 to 8-9). Consequently, the upper, middle, and lower regions of the SIJ have distinctly different appearances when viewed in the horizontal plane, as is done with MRI and computed tomography (CT) scans (Fig. 8-10). An articular capsule lines the SIJ's anterior aspect, whereas the SIJ's posterior aspect is covered by the interosseous sacroiliac (S-I) ligament. No articular capsule has been found along the posterior joint surface.

The sacral auricular surface has a longitudinal groove, known as the sacral groove, along its center that extends from the upper end to the lower end. The posterior rim of this groove is thick and is known as the sacral tuberosity. The iliac auricular surface has a longitudinal ridge, known as the iliac ridge, which corresponds to the sacral groove. The inferior end of this iliac ridge ends as the posterior inferior iliac spine (PIIS). The sacral groove and iliac ridge interlock for stability and help to guide movement of the SIJ (see Table 8-3 and Figs. 8-8 and 8-9).

The region of the sacrum within the posterior concavity of the SIJ is covered by the interosseous sacroiliac ligament and consists of three fossae (see Fig. 8-9). The

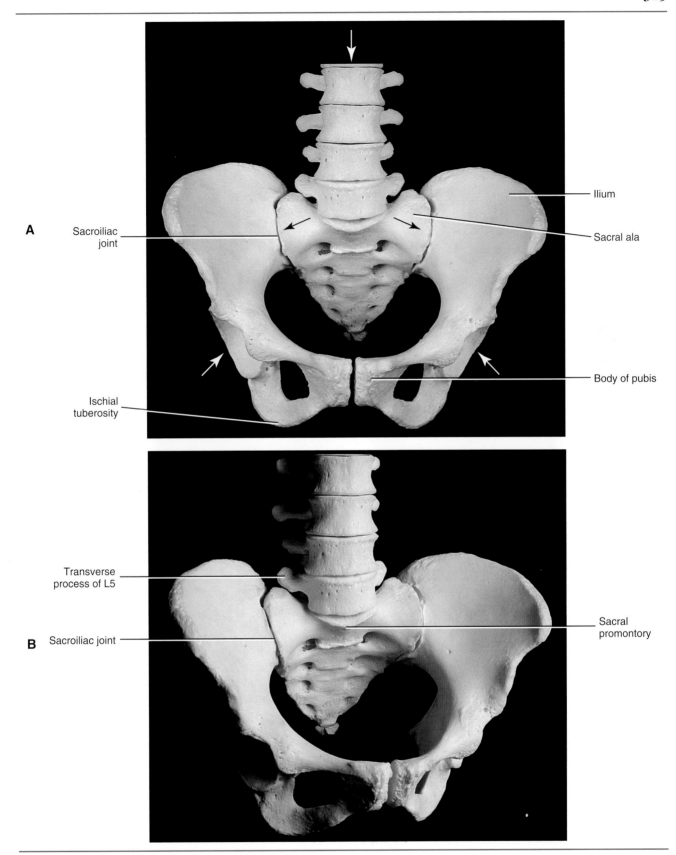

FIG. 8-3 **A,** Anterior, and, **B,** anterior oblique views of the bony pelvis. The anterior aspect of the left and right sacroiliac joints (SIJs) can be seen. The large arrows in **A** indicate the forces transmitted to the SIJs. Notice that the SIJs receive forces from above and below. Those from above are generated primarily from carrying the weight of the trunk, other weight lifted by the upper extremities, and forces generated during pushing or bending. Forces from below are generated primarily from the lower extremities during walking, running, and so on and are transmitted through the acetabula. Forces from below also can be transmitted through the ischial tuberosities during sitting.

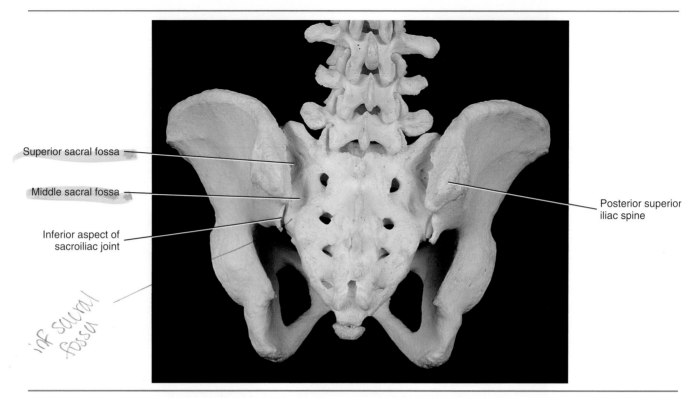

FIG. 8-4 Posterior view of the pelvis. Several sacral fossae associated with the sacroiliac joint are visible from this perspective.

middle fossa is the estimated location of the axis of SIJ rotation. It is in the region of this fossa that the iliac ridge moves circularly in the sacral groove. The iliac tuberosity is posterior to the auricular surface of the ilium. The anterior aspect of the iliac tuberosity inserts into the middle sacral fossa, creating a pivot around which the iliac ridge turns within the sacral groove (Bakland and Hanse, 1984) (see Table 8-3). There is a sulcus between the iliac tuberosity and iliac ridge. The sulcus promotes stability by interlocking with the sacral tuberosity (see the following discussion). Finally, anterior and superior to the iliac tuberosity is a depression that interlocks with an additional elevation on the posterior and superior surface of the sacral ala (alar tuberosity). Therefore stability of the SIJ is promoted by a series of "tongues and grooves." Figures 8-8 and 8-9 show this series of interlocking elevations and depressions that aid the stability of the SIJ, and Table 8-3 summarizes the tongue and groove relationships between these "hills and valleys." This series of interlocking prominences and depressions becomes more enhanced and irregular with age.

Ligaments

Articular capsule. The fibrous articular capsule of the SIJ is only located along the anterior surface of the joint (Fig. 8-11). Its outer portion is thick and tough, and

its inner portion is lined internally with a synovial membrane (Jaovisidha et al., 1996). The articular capsule is innervated with nociceptive and proprioceptive (mechanoreceptive) nerve endings. No articular capsule is located along the posterior border of the SIJ.

Interosseous sacroiliac ligament. The interosseous ligament of each SIJ connects the three sacral fossae (see previous section) to the iliac tuberosity and the area around the tuberosity (Figs. 8-12 to 8-16; see also Figs. 8-8 to 8-11). The interosseous ligament consists of superficial and deep layers. Furthermore, the deep layer has a cranial band and a caudal band. The cranial band is oriented transversely, and the caudal band is oriented more vertically. The superficial layer is membranous and is covered by the posterior S-I ligaments (long and short). Nerves and blood vessels pass between the posterior sacroiliac ligament and the superficial layer of the interosseous ligament. Because there is no posterior joint capsule of the SIJ, the interosseous S-I ligament is what limits the SIJ posteriorly.

A small band, known as the superior intracapsular ligament, or Illi's ligament (Illi, 1951; Janse, 1976), has been found to extend between the superior aspects of the sacral and iliac auricular surfaces in 75% of 31 cadavers studied (Freeman, Fox, and Richards, 1990). This

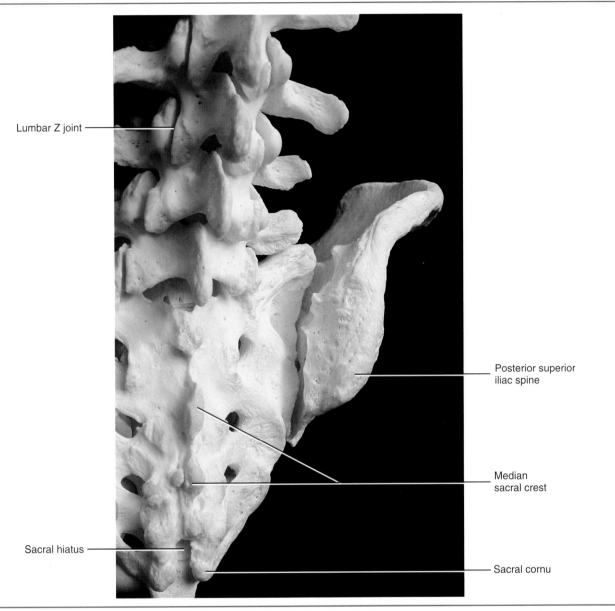

Labels on figure:
- Lumbar Z joint
- Posterior superior iliac spine
- Median sacral crest
- Sacral hiatus
- Sacral cornu

FIG. 8-5 Close-up of the posterior aspect of the sacroiliac joint, showing the normal anatomic relationships of the sacrum and the ilium.

ligament may be an anterior and superior extension of the interosseous S-I ligament, but Freeman, Fox, and Richards (1990) found that it was quite distinct. The superior intracapsular ligament may have relatively little biomechanical value.

Anterior sacroiliac ligament. The pelvic surface and articular capsule of each SIJ is covered by the anterior, or ventral, S-I ligament (see Fig. 8-12). The fibers of the superior part of the ventral S-I ligament course in a slight superolateral direction from the sacrum to the ilium, the fibers in the middle of the ligament are horizontally oriented, and those of the inferior aspect of the ligament course inferolaterally (Jaovisidha et al., 1996). The ventral S-I ligament does not provide as much support to the SIJ as either the interosseous or posterior S-I ligaments. The ventral S-I ligament blends with the anterior joint capsule of the SIJ. These two structures cannot be distinguished from each other during gross dissection, but can be distinguished from one another histologically by evaluating the different direction taken by the collagen fibers of each structure. The ventral S-I

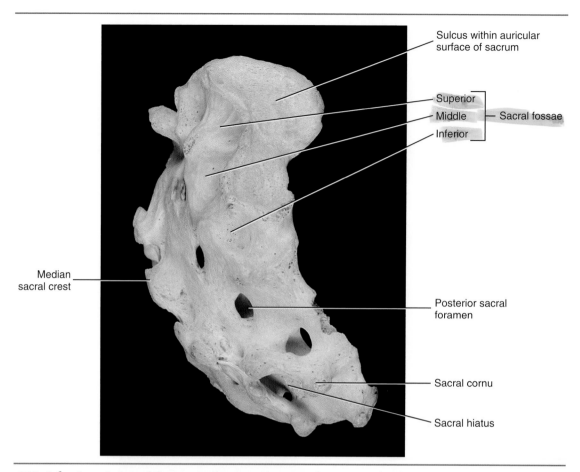

Sulcus within auricular surface of sacrum

Superior
Middle — Sacral fossae
Inferior

Median sacral crest

Posterior sacral foramen

Sacral cornu

Sacral hiatus

FIG. 8-6   Lateral view of the sacrum demonstrating several structures that help to form the sacroiliac joint.

ligament and articular capsule combined are approximately 2 mm thick (Jaovisidha et al., 1996). The ligament–articular capsule complex is thicker inferiorly, near the region of the posterior inferior iliac spine, than superiorly (Weisl, 1954b; Freeman, Fox, and Richards, 1990; Jaovisidha et al., 1996). The APD of L5 supplies sensory innervation to the superior aspect of this ligament, and the APD of S2 (occasionally with additional fibers from the sacral plexus) supplies the lower part of the ventral S-I ligament (Jaovisidha et al., 1996).

Posterior sacroiliac ligament. The posterior (dorsal) sacroiliac (S-I) ligament is made up of two distinct parts (see Figs. 8-12 and 8-13):

♦ *Long posterior sacroiliac ligament.* The long posterior S-I ligament (LPSIL) consists of two distinct bands that originate from the posterior superior iliac spine (PSIS), and the sacral tubercles of S3 and S4, respectively. These bands course vertically along the posterior aspect of the SIJ and then end by blending inferiorly with the sacrotuberous ligament. The LPSIL

can be palpated immediately inferior to the PSIS. The ligament is tough at this location and throughout its course from the PSIS to the sacrotuberous ligament. Many important structures attach to this ligament, including the deep fascia of the gluteus maximus muscle, the deep fibers of the posterior layer of the thoracolumbar fascia (attaching to the medial aspect of the LPSIL), and the aponeurotic attachments of the common origin of the erector spinae muscle. The LPSIL is under tension during the transmission of forces from the lower extremities to the trunk and vice versa. Vleeming et al. (1996) found that the ligament is tensed during counternutation of the sacrum (posterior rocking of the sacral base) and is slackened during sacral nutation (anterior rocking of the sacral base; see Sacroiliac Joint Motion).

♦ *Short posterior sacroiliac ligament.* This ligament originates from the sacral tubercles of S1 and S2. It runs in the horizontal plane covering the SIJ posteriorly, and attaches to the medial aspect of the posterior surface of the iliac crest and the iliac tuberosity.

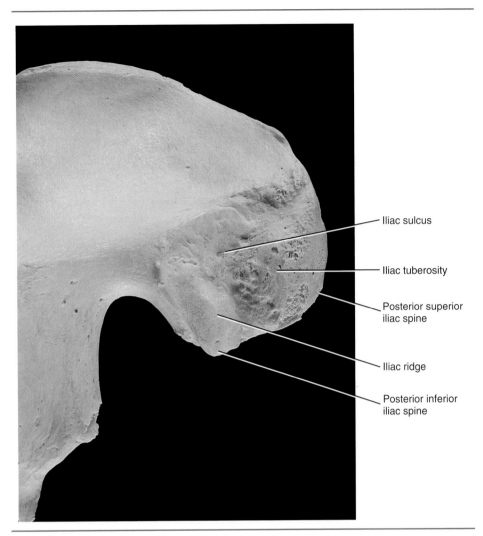

Iliac sulcus

Iliac tuberosity

Posterior superior
iliac spine

Iliac ridge

Posterior inferior
iliac spine

FIG. 8-7   Medial surface of the posterior ilium of a dried skeletal specimen. Several structures that participate in the formation of the sacroiliac joint are demonstrated.

Accessory sacroiliac ligaments. The stability of the SIJ is enhanced by two accessory S-I ligaments (see Fig. 8-12). A third ligament, the iliolumbar ligament (see Chapter 7 and Fig. 8-13), also provides stability to the region.

- ◆ *Sacrotuberous ligament.* This ligament passes inferiorly and laterally from the posterior and inferior aspects of the sacrum to the ischial tuberosity. The lesser sciatic foramen is formed between this ligament and the sacrospinous ligament.
- ◆ *Sacrospinous ligament.* The sacrospinous ligament courses from the anterior surface of the sacrum (fused second, third, and fourth segments) to the spine of the ischium (see Fig. 8-12). The greater sciatic foramen is located superior to this ligament.

The sacrotuberous and sacrospinous ligaments help to limit the small amount of anterior and inferior nodding (nutational) motion of the sacrum at the SIJ. This is accomplished by restricting the amount the sacral apex can move posteriorly and superiorly when the promontory of the sacrum moves anteriorly and inferiorly. These ligaments also help to stabilize the inferior aspect of the SIJ.

- ◆ *Iliolumbar ligament.* The iliolumbar ligament connects the iliac crest with the adjacent TP of the L5 vertebra. Part of the iliolumbar ligament (lumbosacral ligament, see Fig. 8-20) attaches to the anterior and superior part of the sacrum (see Chapter 7). The iliolumbar ligament helps to limit lateral tilting of the pelvis and gapping of the superior aspect of the SIJ.

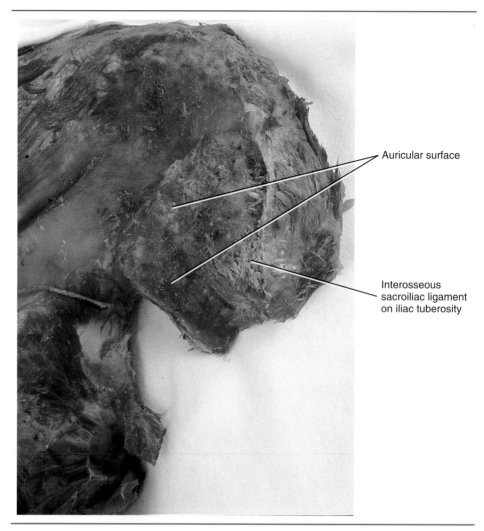

Auricular surface

Interosseous sacroiliac ligament on iliac tuberosity

FIG. 8-8 View similar to that seen in Figure 8-7, only with more soft tissue visible on this cadaveric specimen. The auricular surface can be identified readily on this medial surface of the posterior ilium. Also notice the cut fibers of the interosseous sacroiliac ligament.

Arterial Supply and Venous Drainage

Both the anterior and posterior aspects of the SIJ are served by the superior branch of the lateral sacral artery and vein, which are branches of the internal iliac artery and vein, respectively. These vessels anastomose with the superficial branch of the superior gluteal artery and vein (Williams et al., 1995). Figures 8-20 and 8-21 demonstrate the major arteries and nerves associated with the anterior surface of the SIJ.

Innervation

The SIJ receives sensory innervation, and the joint capsule and sacroiliac ligaments possesses both nociceptors (pain receptors) and mechanoreceptors (for joint position sense, i.e., proprioception). This may indicate that the sensory receptors of the SIJ relay information related to movement and joint position and in doing so may help to keep the body upright and balanced. However, the complete innervation of the SIJ has not been fully characterized, and Sakamoto et al. (2001) found many more nociceptive nerve endings in the SIJ than mechanoreceptive endings. The most pain-sensitive structures in this region are the posterior inferior iliac spine and superior portion of the sacroiliac fissure (Pitkin and Pheasant, 1936a; Norman and May, 1956). The specific innervation of the SIJ is variable, even between the left and right sides of the same individual.

The anterior (pelvic) part of the SIJ is innervated by the APDs of L2 through S2 (Bernard and Cassidy, 1993), with L4 and L5 being the most frequent source of innervation (Cassidy and Mierau, 1992). The posterior

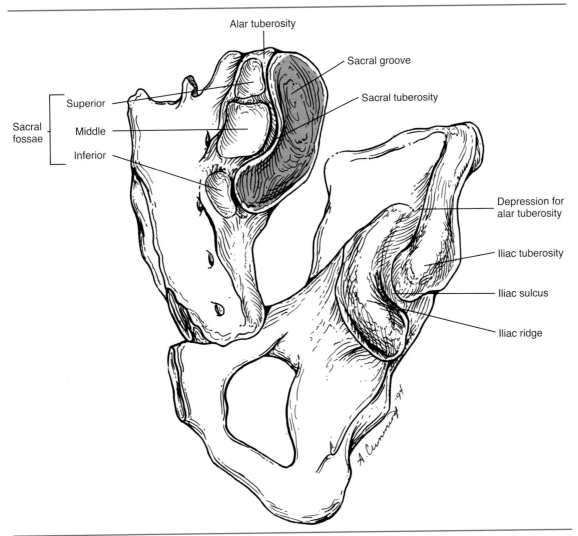

FIG. 8-9   Medial surfaces of the right side of the sacrum and right ilium showing the series of elevations and depressions associated with the sacroiliac joint (SIJ). These elevations and depressions are thought to help increase stability of the SIJ. Table 8-3 lists the important elevations and depressions of the SIJ.

part of the SIJ, according to most authors, is innervated by PPDs of S1 and S2. However, the innervation of this part of the joint is probably more extensive than just the upper sacral segments. Bernard and Cassidy (1993) state that the posterior part of the SIJ is innervated by the lateral branches of the PPDs of L4 to S3. Ro (1990) has demonstrated that the lateral branch of the L5 PPD can extend inferiorly and pass between the superficial layer of the interosseous and posterior S-I ligaments.

The variable innervation of the SIJ from person to person and even from the left to the right side of the same person may be one reason for the wide range of pain referral patterns described by patients experiencing discomfort of SIJ origin (Bernard and Cassidy, 1993). Furthermore, the wide variation of referral patterns may help to explain the difficulty researchers and clinicians

have had in identifying the incidence with which SIJ dysfunction occurs.

A portion of the sacral plexus is formed along the anterior surface of the SIJ. Figures 8-20 and 8-21 demonstrate the relationship of the sacral plexus to the anterior aspect of the SIJ.

Microscopic Anatomy

The histologic makeup of the cartilage lining the auricular surface of the sacrum differs from that lining the auricular surface of the ilium. The sacral surface is lined by hyaline cartilage, and the iliac surface is lined by what is best described as fibrocartilage. The hyaline cartilage of the adult sacral surface is three times thicker than the cartilage of the iliac surface. Large, round, paired

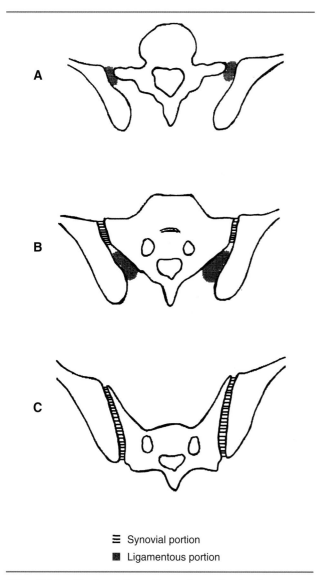

≡ Synovial portion

■ Ligamentous portion

FIG. 8-10 Horizontal sections through, **A,** the upper, **B,** middle, and **C,** lower portions of the sacroiliac joint (SIJ). The diagram also demonstrates the synovial versus fibrous (ligamentous) portions of the SIJ. (From Prassopoulos PK et al. [1999]. Sacroiliac joints: Anatomic variants on CT. *J CAT, 23,* 323-327.)

chondrocytes are distributed throughout the hyaline matrix of the sacral auricular surface and are arranged in columns parallel to the articulating surface. The hyaline cartilage is homogeneous with a small amount of fibrous tissue. Its smooth surface aids the gliding motion of the joint.

The iliac cartilage is thin (≈1 mm) and contains smaller spindle-shaped chondrocytes clumped in a fibrous matrix. The cell columns are oriented at right angles to the surface. Postpartum the iliac cartilage degenerates early, and the amount of fibrous tissue increases. The sacral cartilage degenerates throughout life, and in later

adult life it may appear fibrous as well (Sashin, 1929; Bowen and Cassidy, 1981; Paquin et al., 1983). These changes cause the synovial portion of the SIJ to narrow with age. Sometime this narrowing can be seen on standard x-rays that include the SIJ (Sgambati et al., 1997).

Development

The SIJ begins development during the seventh week of fetal life with the ilia moving superiorly and also posterior to the sacrum. During the eighth week of development, the mesenchyme between the two bones becomes arranged into three layers. At the tenth week, multiple cavities develop in the mesenchyme. These cavities are separated by septa, which disappear by the time the fetus reaches term. The sacral hyaline cartilage develops first, followed by the development of the iliac surface. At birth the sacral hyaline cartilage is thick and almost fully developed, whereas the iliac cartilage is thin and irregular. The iliac surface has the appearance of fibrocartilage by the time of infancy (Cassidy and Mierau, 1992).

Before puberty, both sacral and iliac auricular surfaces are flat, straight, and vertically oriented (Beal, 1982). The joint can conceivably have a gliding movement in any direction, being restricted only by ligaments. After puberty the auricular surfaces change shape to form a horizontal and vertical limb. The horizontal limb, which can be longer than the vertical limb, is possibly formed to aid stability (Otter, 1985). Also during this time the longitudinal groove is formed in the sacral auricular surface. This groove runs from top to bottom, down the center of this surface. The corresponding iliac ridge develops simultaneously on the iliac auricular surface. The interlocking groove and ridge limit the direction of motion, but increase stability.

The interosseous ligaments are strengthened during the third decade of life. The many bony tuberosities and corresponding grooves and fossae develop and probably increase the stability of the SIJ by their interlocking relationships (see Table 8-3 and Fig. 8-9). The differences in depth and height of the interlocking system of grooves and crests among different individuals cause a wide variation of normal appearances of the SIJ on CT scans (Prassopoulos et al., 1999). This led Prassopoulos et al. (1999) to conclude that all SIJs have a distinct appearance on CT (at least subtly).

Beginning in the fourth decade of life, marginal osteophytes frequently begin to develop, particularly on the anterior and superior portions of the SIJ along the articular capsule. These degenerative changes develop earlier in the male. They probably increase stability of the joint, at the expense of decreased joint mobility. In later life the cartilage undergoes degeneration and further marginal ankylosis develops. Total fibrous ankylosis eventually

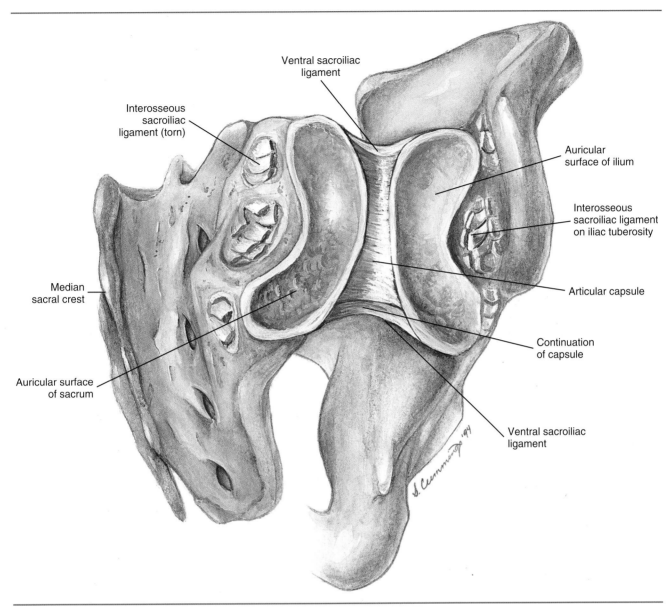

Interosseous
sacroiliac
ligament (torn)

Ventral sacroiliac
ligament

Auricular
surface of ilium

Interosseous
sacroiliac ligament
on iliac tuberosity

Median
sacral crest

Articular capsule

Auricular surface
of sacrum

Continuation
of capsule

Ventral sacroiliac
ligament

FIG. 8-11 Posterior view of an opened right sacroiliac joint demonstrating some of the important bony and soft tissue components. Notice that the articular capsule is found only anteriorly. Posteriorly the interosseous sacroiliac ligament supports the joint. This ligament is shown torn to illustrate the deeper structures of the opened joint.

may occur. During the eighth decade of life, SIJ mobility usually is lost completely, making body movement stiff (Walker, 1986).

Sacroiliac Joint Motion

The SIJ provides substantial, yet resilient, stability to the region between the spine and the lower extremities while also allowing for slight mobility to occur between the sacrum and ilium. The SIJ has a small amount of movement (Solonen, 1957; Frigerio, Stowe, and Howe, 1974; Egund et al., 1978), but the movement is difficult to

evaluate because of its location deep to the origin of the erector spinae muscle group, the posterior S-I ligament, and the interosseous S-I ligament. SIJ movement is three dimensional and contains several elements. The primary movements appear to be anteroinferior and posterosuperior nodding (called nutation and counternutation, respectively) of the sacral base in relation to the ilium (Fig. 8-17, *B*). This represents rotation along the sacral groove, with the center of rotation located in the middle sacral fossa of the SIJ. The full range of motion of the SIJ is not expressed until the extremes of hip motion are reached.

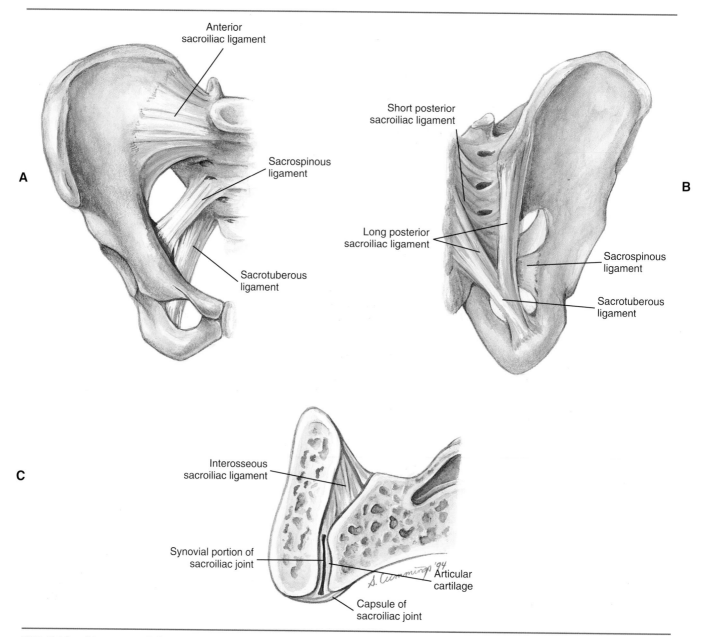

FIG. 8-12   Ligaments of the sacroiliac joint (SIJ.) **A,** Anterior view. **B,** Posterior view. **C,** SIJ in horizontal section. Notice that the capsule of the SIJ joint is only present anteriorly.

Smidt et al. (1997) found in a study evaluating SIJ motion in five unembalmed cadavers (age range 52 to 68) that each SIJ moved an average of 7.5 degrees (range, 3 to 17 degrees) in the sagittal plane during full flexion and extension of the hips. In addition, SIJ ranges of motion of 22 to 36 degrees have been reported in young gymnasts and nongymnasts (Barakatt et al., 1996).

Another type of movement is rotatory movement along an axis that passes longitudinally through the iliac ridge of the SIJ (Fig. 8-17, *C*). The movement of the posterior aspect of the ilium in this case is superomedial

and inferolateral. Although the iliac ridge may move only 2 mm during this type of movement, the distance between the two anterosuperior iliac spines increases or decreases by as much as 10 mm (Hadley, 1952; Wilder, Pope, and Frymoyer, 1980; Ehara, El-Khoury, and Bergman, 1988).

Gapping of the superior and inferior aspects of the SIJ has also been described. This could be interpreted as a third type of SIJ motion (Fig. 8-17, *A*).

Initiation of SIJ movements is made by the vertebral column and lower extremities. The forces inducing

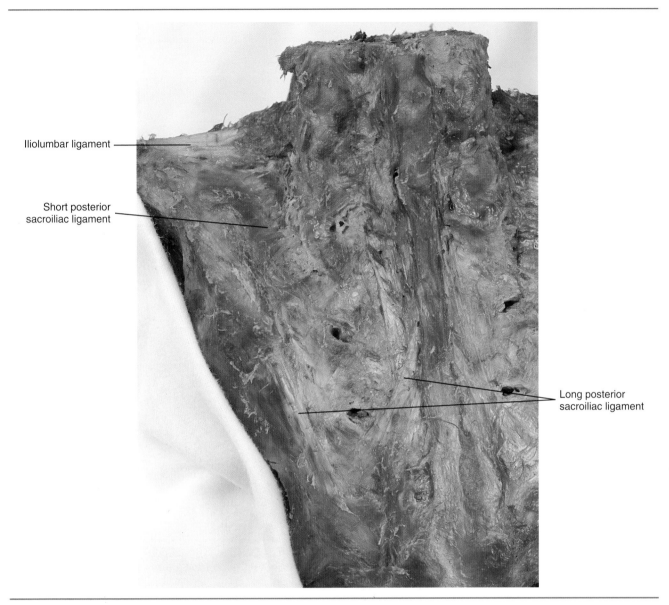

FIG. 8-13   Posterior view of the sacrum and the left posterior ilium, showing the iliolumbar ligament and the posterior sacroiliac ligament. The posterior sacroiliac ligament has long fibers, which are vertically oriented, and short fibers, which are horizontally oriented.

SIJ motion are gravity (trunk weight), ground reaction (bouncing) force, and muscle contraction. Postural changes of the vertebral column (e.g., during lying, sitting, standing) and motion of the vertebral column (e.g., flexion, extension, rotation) cause the sacrum to move relative to the ilium. Change of thigh position (e.g., during sitting, standing, standing on one leg) and active motion of the thigh during flexion, extension, abduction, adduction, and rotation cause the iliac surface of the SIJ to move relative to the sacral surface of the SIJ. In addition, abduction and adduction of the thigh causes a certain amount of gapping motion. The mechanism of walking is

extremely complex, thereby causing movements of the SIJ to be complicated.

Even though there appears to be no muscle specifically designed for movement of the SIJ, approximately 40 muscles can influence this joint. Some of the most important are the erector spinae, quadratus lumborum, multifidus lumborum, iliopsoas, rectus abdominis, gluteus maximus, and piriformis muscles (Fligg, 1986).

As mentioned, stability is increased and mobility is decreased with age. Until puberty, stability is maintained primarily by ligaments. After puberty, the bony interlockings that enhance stability begin to form (see Table

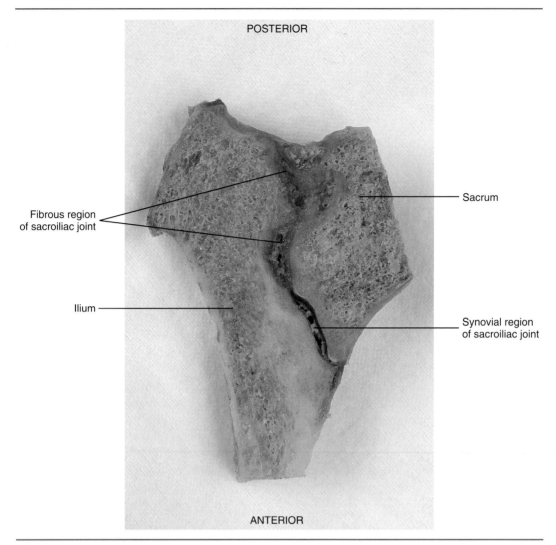

FIG. 8-14   Horizontal section through the right sacroiliac joint. Notice the synovial portion of the joint anteriorly and the fibrous portion posteriorly. The posterior fibrous portion of the joint is filled with the interosseous sacroiliac ligament.

8-3 and Fig. 8-9). Recall that after the fourth decade of life, osteophytes are formed and ankylosis may begin to occur, increasing stability. Near the eighth decade of life, total fibrous degeneration develops for stability; consequently, SIJ movement usually completely stops at approximately this age.

Clinical Considerations

Disorders of the Sacroiliac Joint. Because of its role in weight bearing and perhaps also because of its unique anatomy, the SIJ can become a source of pain (Daum, 1995; Schwarzer, Aprill, and Bogduk, 1995; Dreyfuss et al., 1996). This section briefly highlights some of the most common causes of pain arising from this clinically important articulation. Brief mention also

is made of the most important factors involved in the clinical evaluation of the SIJ. Also, some of the most common methods currently used to treat SIJ dysfunction are mentioned. However, a complete consideration of the pathologic conditions, diagnosis, and treatment of SIJ disorders is beyond the scope of this book.

Trauma and repeated minor forces can cause SIJ disorders. Examples of minor forces include those received while driving for long periods over rough terrain or while driving on poorly maintained roads in a vehicle with inadequate suspension (Abel, 1950). The SIJ receives its greatest stresses from below during sitting. This is because the ground reaction (bouncing) force reaches the SIJ directly without going through any other joint (Johnson, 1964; Schuchman and Cannon, 1986; Bermis and Daniel, 1987).

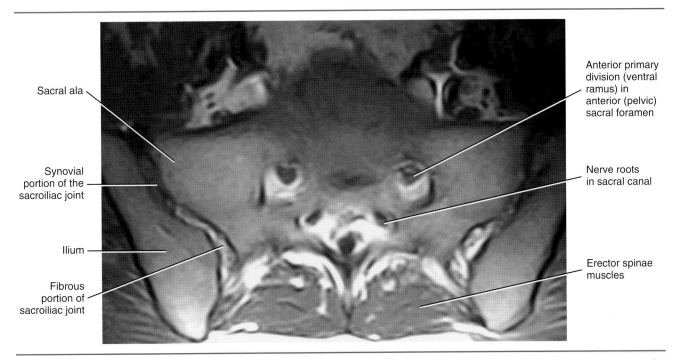

FIG. 8-15 Magnetic resonance imaging scan performed in a horizontal plane that shows the sacroiliac joint. (Image courtesy Dr. Dennis Skogsbergh.)

An accessory SIJ frequently forms within the posterior (fibrous) portion of the joint (Fig. 8-18). Such accessory joints are more common in obese individuals than in individuals of normal weight. Accessory SIJs also are more common in older than younger individuals, and are also associated with other signs of degeneration (e.g., sclerosis and roughening of the articular surfaces). Therefore accessory SIJs are most likely acquired rather than congenital in nature (Prassopoulos et al., 1999). Prassopoulos et al. (1999) found an accessory SIJ in 19.1% of the patients in their series of pelvic CT scans that excluded frank SIJ disease. This anomaly was more frequently associated with periodic low back pain than other lumbosacral and pelvic anomalies.

Low back pain during pregnancy is common and may have a different etiology than low back pain unrelated to pregnancy (Kristiansson, Svärdsudd, and von Schoultz, 1996). Women appear to be more susceptible to SIJ syndrome (pain as a result of mechanical irritation) than men. This is probably caused by the actions of the hormone relaxin during menstruation and pregnancy, and for a short time after childbirth (Cassidy and Mierau, 1992). Relaxin decreases the tension of the S-I ligaments, allowing them to become more pliable (or lax). The best known SIJ disease is osteitis condensans ilii, which occurs secondary to pregnancy and parturition (Nykoliation, Cassidy, and Dupuis, 1984; Olivieri et al., 1990).

A partial list of disorders of the SIJ includes joint space widening or narrowing, cystic or erosive change, osteosclerosis, osteophytosis, and idiopathic hyperosto-sis. Some causes of SIJ dysfunction include trauma, disease of bone, infection, and arthropathy (Fryette, 1936; Romanus, 1955; Blumel, Evans, and Eggers, 1959; Resnik, Dwosh, and Niwayama, 1975; Dunn et al., 1976; DeCavalho and Graudal, 1980; Bose, 1982; Cone and Resnick, 1983; Blower and Griffin, 1984; Vogler et al., 1984; Resnik and Resnick, 1985; Jajic and Jajic, 1987; Burns, Mireau, and Howlett, 1995). Bacterial infection of the SIJ is a rare cause of low back pain. However, when the source of SIJ pathology is bacterial infection, immediate treatment with antibiotics is essential to prevent permanent destruction of adjacent bone (Burns, Mireau, and Howlett, 1995). Table 8-4 provides a more complete list of some of the causes of SIJ dysfunction.

Evaluation and Treatment. Examination of the SIJ is challenging for many reasons. First, the SIJ is subject to a wide range of normal anatomic variation (Prassopoulos et al., 1999). Second, its unusual location and oblique position make direct palpation almost impossible. Also, evaluation is made more challenging because spinal radiography does not always correspond well with symptoms. In addition, pain patterns associated with SIJ disorders can be diverse (Dreyfuss et al., 1996). Outside of diagnostic anesthetic blocks of the SIJ, differentiating SIJ pain from pain arising from structures of the lumbar spine can be difficult. However, one potential clue is that pain arising from the SIJ *usually* does not radiate superiorly to the L5 level of the lumbar region (low back) (Dreyfuss et al., 1996).

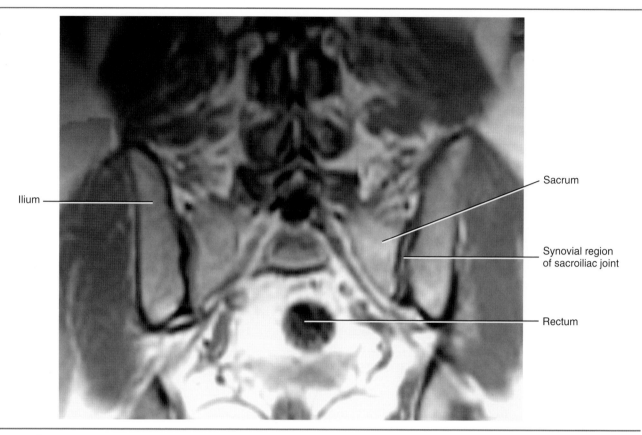

Ilium

Sacrum

Synovial region of sacroiliac joint

Rectum

FIG. 8-16   Magnetic resonance imaging scan taken in a coronal plane that shows the sacroiliac joint. (Image courtesy Dr. Dennis Skogsbergh.)

As always, the patient's history can be extremely revealing. The patient may complain of pain over the PSIS that radiates into the buttock and less frequently to the groin and lower extremity (Cassidy and Mierau, 1992). Neurologic signs are negative, and the pain is not of dermatomal distribution.

Useful methods of palpatory examination for the SIJ include the palpation of neighboring prominences (PSIS and the S2 spinous tubercle) during thigh flexion (motion palpation). In addition, several orthopedic tests for SIJ dysfunction exist (Lawrence, 1990). Potter and Rothstein (1985) investigated the reliability of many physical tests for SIJ dysfunction and found the most reliable test to be a measurable widening of the distance between the left and right anterior superior iliac spines from a standing to a supine position. Using this method, a 94% agreement was found between multiple observers. A measured narrowing of the distance between the left and right anterior superior iliac spines after compression in the side-lying posture was the second most reliable method, with a 76% agreement found among observers. Also, certain orthopedic tests may be helpful in evaluating disorders of the SIJ. Using bone scans, Cassidy and Mierau (1992) found SIJ dysfunction to be particularly correlated with orthopedic testing when at least two out of three of the following orthopedic tests for SIJ sprain were positive: Patrick-Faber (pathologic conditions of the hip previously ruled out), Gaenslen's test (forced thigh flexion), and Yeoman's test (forced thigh extension). However, other investigators have found much lower reliability of orthopedic tests for SIJ dysfunction (Dreyfuss et al., 1996).

Differentiation between enteric disorders, pelvic disorders, and inflammatory arthritides from SIJ dysfunction can be challenging, and two of these disorders may coexist. Such conditions include Crohn's disease, psoriasis, Reiter's syndrome, Behçet's syndrome, and other inflammatory bowel disorders. Differential diagnosis may be aided by anesthetic injection into the SIJ, with relief of pain after anesthetic injection being an indication of SIJ dysfunction (McEwen et al., 1971; Russell et al., 1977; Davis, Thomson, and Lentle, 1978; Dekker-Saeys et al., 1978; Yazici, Tuzlaci, and Yurdakul, 1981; Olivieri et al., 1990; Ro, 1990).

Fortunately SIJ syndrome usually is self-limiting and responds well to rest. However, in some individuals the condition becomes chronic and disabling. Chiropractic manipulation has been used to treat SIJ disorders. More

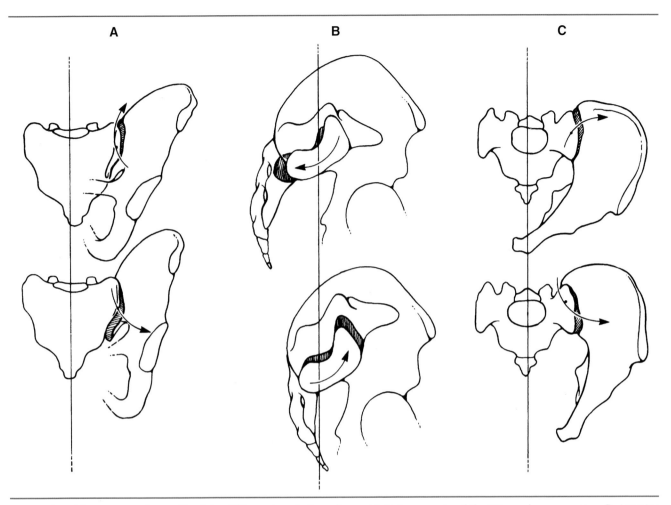

FIG. 8-17   Three types of sacroiliac joint (SIJ) motion. **A,** Superior and inferior aspects of the SIJ are shown gapping. **B,** Anterior and posterior rocking of the sacral base. This is sometimes known as nutation and counternutation, respectively. **C,** Movement of the ilium on the sacrum that takes place in the horizontal plane. **A** and **C,** Arrows show motion of the ilium. **B,** Arrows show sacral motion. These movements are accentuated for demonstrative purposes in this illustration.

than 90% of patients presenting to a university hospital disabled with chronic SIJ syndrome responded favorably to a regimen of sacroiliac manipulation (Cassidy and Mierau, 1992). Some believe examination and treatment of the soft tissues surrounding the SIJ is the best way to manage spinal and SIJ problems (Lavignolle et al., 1983; Maltezopoulos and Armitage, 1984). Injection of local anesthetic not only may prove useful in the diagnosis of these disorders, but also may provide long-term relief in some patients who do not respond to other treatments (Cassidy and Mierau, 1992). The use of belts to stabilize the SIJ, injections of proliferant (to decrease mobility), exercises, and fusion also have been used to treat SIJ disorders (Cassidy, 1993).

Increased stiffness of the SIJ can potentially protect against sprains of the SIJ ligaments. Richardson et al. (2002) assessed stiffness of the SIJ by measuring vibrations of the sacrum and ilium adjacent to the SIJ, after the

application of vibrations with a frequency of 200 Hz to the anterior superior iliac spine. Through use of these methods, contraction of the left and right transversus abdominis muscles was found to increase stiffness of the sacroiliac joint.

THE COCCYX

The coccyx (Fig. 8-19) is formed by three to five fused segments (usually four), and each develops from one primary center of ossification. The coccygeal segments develop between the ages of 1 (first segment) and 20 (fourth segment) years, although the time when coccygeal ossification centers develop varies. Fusion of the coccygeal segments usually occurs in the late twenties but may be delayed considerably (Williams et al., 1995). Sometimes the first coccygeal segment does not fuse with the remainder of the coccyx at all. The first

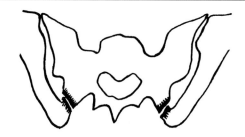

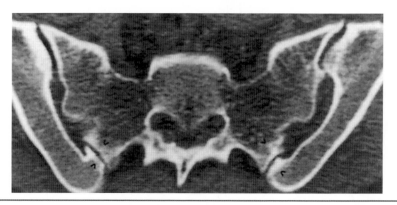

FIG. 8-18 Accessory sacroiliac joints (darkened region in upper illustration and arrowheads in the CT scan). (From Prassopoulos PK et al. [1999]. Sacroiliac joints: Anatomic variants on CT. *J CAT, 23,* 323-327.)

Table 8-4	Causes of Sacroiliac Joint Dysfunction
Type	**Possible Causes**
Trauma	Direct trauma, falls, locus minoris resistentiae
Disease of bone	Osteitis condensans ilii, infection
Arthropathies	Ankylosing spondylitis, enteropathic arthropathies, gouty arthritis
Other causes	Hyperparathyroidism, paraplegia, lower extremity disorders, activity related (e.g., athletic activity), after hip surgery, neoplasm

coccygeal segment has several prominences (see the following discussion), whereas the second through fifth coccygeal segments are rather simple and are homologous to vertebral bodies of typical vertebrae.

As with the sacrum, the coccyx is triangular in shape; with the superior surface the base and the inferior surface the apex (see Fig. 8-19). The base of the coccyx is formed by the first coccygeal segment. The top of the base has an articular facet for articulation with a small disc that intervenes between it and the apex of the

sacrum. Also, a TP extends from the left and right lateral surfaces of the coccygeal base. Posteriorly the coccygeal cornua are in register with the sacral cornua. Intercornual ligaments connect the cornua of the sacrum with those of the coccyx. The S5 and coccygeal nerves of each side exit the sacral hiatus (see The Sacrum) and pass between the apex of the sacrum and intercornual ligament (i.e., the nerves pass deep to this ligament). They then give off the dorsal rami, which pass posterior to the TP of the coccyx.

A series of fibrocartilaginous discs develop, before and after birth, between the individual coccygeal segments. These discs eventually are replaced by bone as the segments fuse during the second or third decades of life.

Structures That Attach to the Coccyx and the Borders of the Pelvic Outlet

Table 8-2 lists the muscles and ligaments that attach to the coccyx. The apex of the coccyx helps to form the boundaries of the pelvic outlet. The boundaries of this outlet follow:

Anterior: pubic symphysis
Posterior: tip of coccyx
Lateral: ischial tuberosities

NERVES AND VESSELS ASSOCIATED WITH THE SACRUM AND COCCYX

Location of Sacral Dorsal Root Ganglia

Ebraheim and Lu (1998) evaluated the locations of the first through the fourth sacral dorsal root ganglia (DRGs) within the sacral canal and sacral foramina. They found that the S1 DRG was intraforaminal (defined as lateral to the medial border of the sacral pedicle) 55% to 60% of the time and "intracanalar" (defined as medial to medial aspect of the sacral pedicles) 40% to 45% of the time. The S2 DRG was intraforaminal 15% to 50% of the time and intracanalar 50% to 85% of the time. The S3 and S4 DRGs always were intracanalar, and no DRGs were found to be extraforaminal. The S1 DRGs were the largest, and the DRGs became smaller from S1 to S4, and the S1 and S2 DRGs were significantly larger than the S3 and S4 DRGs. Ebraheim and Lu (1998) were convinced that intracanalar S1 and S2 DRGs were more susceptible than intraforaminal DRGs to compression from L5-S1 IVD protrusions and other space-occupying lesions causing stenosis of the sacral canal. Kikuchi et al. (1994) found an even higher incidence (77.3%) of intraspinal "intracanalar" S1 DRGs than did Ebraheim and Lu (1998).

Sacral Plexus

The sacral plexus is formed by the anterior primary divisions (ventral rami) of L4 and L5 (lumbosacral trunk), S1-3, and part of S4. Of note is that the lumbosacral trunk is approximately 30 mm in length. It crosses the SIJ approximately 2 cm inferior to the pelvic brim (i.e., 2 cm below the internal arcuate line of the ilium) and is fixed to the sacral ala by fibrous connective tissue. In addition, the APD of S1 is the widest APD (9.0 mm) contributing to the lumbosacral plexus (Ebraheim et al., 1997a). The anterior primary division of S4 also contributes to the coccygeal plexus.

The sacral plexus is located on the posterior pelvic wall, specifically, anterior to the piriformis muscle (Figs. 8-20 and 8-21). The branches of the sacral plexus follow (contributing spinal cord segments appear in parentheses):
- Posterior cutaneous nerve of the thigh (S1-3)
- Pudendal nerve (S2-4)
- Sciatic nerve (L4, L5, S1-3)
- Superior gluteal nerve (L4, L5, S1)
- Inferior gluteal nerve (L5, S1, S2)
- Nerve to the obturator internus (and superior gemellus) (L5, S1, S2)
- Nerve to the quadratus femoris (and inferior gemellus) (L4, L5, S1)

Chapters 9 and 10 provide further information on the nerves of the sacral plexus. Chapter 10 also discusses the relationship between the nerves of the sacral plexus and pelvic autonomic fibers.

Pelvic Autonomic Nerves

The S2 to S4 segments provide parasympathetic innervation to the pelvic viscera via nerves of the sacral plexus. In addition, each sympathetic trunk has five sacral ganglia that are located along the anterior surface of the sacrum. These ganglia supply sympathetic innervation to the pelvic viscera via gray rami. The two sympathetic chains join inferiorly on the anterior surface of the coccyx at a single ganglion, which is called the ganglion impar. The inferior hypogastric autonomic plexus, which receives contributions from the lumbar splanchnic nerves (sympathetic), sacral sympathetics, and pelvic splanchnic nerves (parasympathetic), helps to supply the pelvic viscera with autonomic fibers. Chapter 10 thoroughly discusses the pelvic autonomics.

Arteries Associated with the Sacrum and Coccyx

The aorta bifurcates at roughly the body of L4 into left and right common iliac arteries. Each common iliac artery, in turn, bifurcates into an internal and external iliac artery. The external iliac artery courses toward the inguinal ligament, giving off the inferior epigastric and deep circumflex iliac arteries before crossing under the inguinal ligament to become the femoral artery. The left and right internal iliac arteries supply the pelvic viscera, inferior aspect of the posterior abdominal wall, pelvic wall, gluteal region, ischioanal (ischiorectal) fossa, perineum, and adductor region of the thigh. Each internal iliac artery can be described as having an anterior, or visceral, division and a posterior, or somatic, division. The branches of each division of the internal iliac artery are listed in the following section.

Posterior Division of the Internal Iliac Artery

1. *Iliolumbar artery.* This is the first branch of the internal iliac artery. The iliolumbar artery further divides into two branches:
   a. An iliac branch that passes along the superior border of the iliac crest to supply the iliacus and quadratus lumborum muscles.
   b. A lumbar branch courses superiorly to help supply the psoas muscle.
2. *Lateral sacral artery.*
   This artery has been mentioned previously and is shown in Figure 8-21. It courses along the anterior and lateral surface of the sacrum, sending branches into the anterior sacral foramina. It serves as a major source of blood to the sacrum and sacral nerve roots.

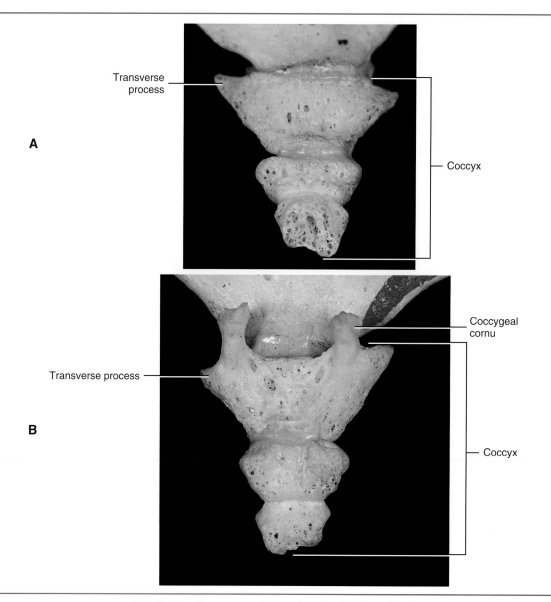

A

Transverse process

Coccyx

B

Transverse process

Coccygeal cornu

Coccyx

FIG. 8-19   The coccyx. **A,** Anterior view. **B,** Posterior view.

3. *Superior gluteal artery.* This artery usually passes between the lumbosacral trunk and S1 ventral ramus to exit the pelvis. (In some cases it exits between the S1 and S2 ventral rami.) The superior gluteal artery helps to supply the gluteal region.

Anterior Division of the Internal Iliac Artery

1. *Inferior gluteal artery.* This artery usually exits the pelvis by passing between the S1 and S2, or the S2 and S3, ventral rami. As with the superior gluteal artery, this artery also helps to supply the buttock and thigh.

2. *Internal pudendal artery.* This artery usually exits the pelvis between the S2 and S3 ventral rami. It then passes around the posterior surface of the sacrospinous ligament to enter the ischioanal (ischiorectal)

fossa, where it continues anteriorly within the pudendal (Alcock's) canal. It terminates near the symphysis pubis by dividing into the deep and dorsal arteries of the penis.

3. *Inferior vesical artery.* This artery is only found in the male. In the female its place is taken by the vaginal artery. The inferior vesical (or a branch of the vaginal artery in the female) supplies the inferior aspect of the bladder.

4. *Middle rectal artery.* This artery usually is small and may arise from the inferior vesical artery or the internal pudendal artery. It helps to supply the rectum.

5. *Obturator artery.* The obturator artery has a rather long intrapelvic course before exiting the pelvis at the obturator foramen. It then supplies the adductor

region of the thigh. Before exiting the pelvis, this artery gives a branch that anastomoses with the pubic branch of the inferior epigastric artery. This anastomosis frequently is called the accessory obturator artery. Occasionally the pubic branch of the inferior epigastric artery replaces the obturator artery.

6. *Umbilical artery.* This artery is the direct continuation of the internal iliac artery. It courses from the superior aspect of the bladder to the anterior abdominal wall, where its continuation forms the medial umbilical ligament. The superior vesical arteries are branches of the proximal portion of the umbilical artery. As the name implies, these arteries pass inferiorly from the umbilical artery to supply the superior aspect of the bladder.

Branches Found Only in the Female.

1. *Uterine artery.* This artery courses beneath (inferior to) the ureter to reach the lateral aspect of the uterus, which it supplies.

2. *Vaginal artery.* This artery not only supplies the vagina, but also takes the place of the male inferior

vesical artery. Therefore it also supplies the inferior aspect of the bladder.

Median sacral artery. The median sacral artery is another vessel associated with the anterior surface of the sacrum. The median (middle) sacral artery (see Chapter 7) is a tiny unpaired artery that arises from the posterior surface of the abdominal aorta just before the aorta bifurcates into right and left common iliac arteries. It then passes inferiorly along the midline of the anterior sacrum, sending branches into the anterior sacral foramina. These foraminal branches are accompanied by branches of the lateral sacral artery.

Veins Associated with the Sacrum and Coccyx

The venous drainage of the sacrum, coccyx, and pelvic viscera generally flows in the opposite direction as the arterial supply and drains into the internal iliac veins (left and right). Each internal iliac vein drains into the common iliac vein of the same side, and the common

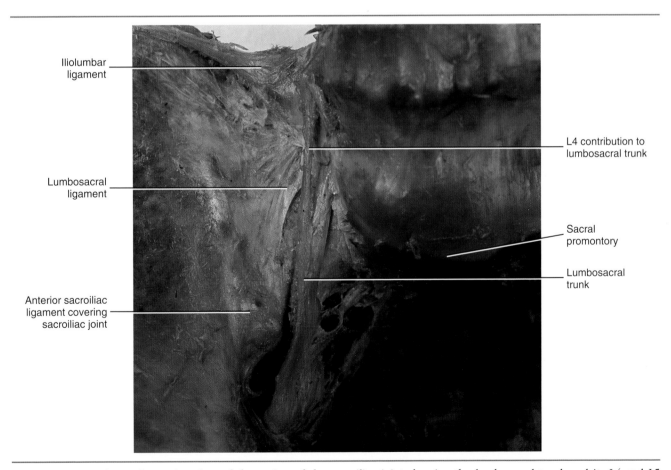

FIG. 8-20 Anterior and superior view of the region of the sacroiliac joint showing the lumbosacral trunk and its L4 and L5 contributions.

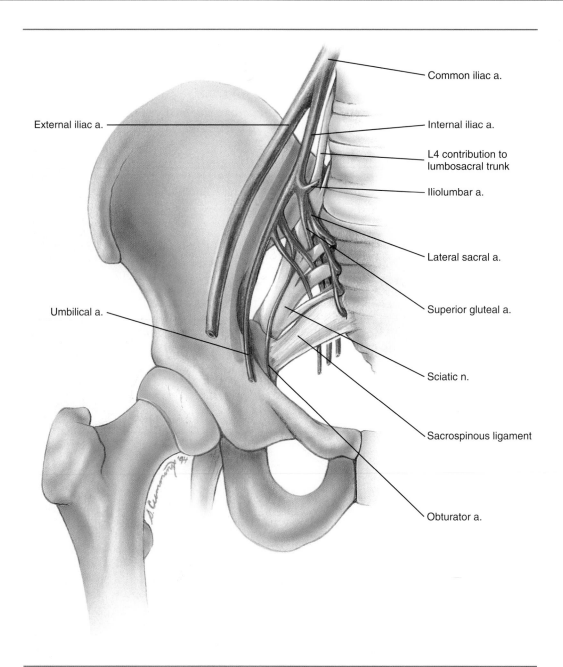

External iliac a.

Umbilical a.

Common iliac a.

Internal iliac a.

L4 contribution to lumbosacral trunk

Iliolumbar a.

Lateral sacral a.

Superior gluteal a.

Sciatic n.

Sacrospinous ligament

Obturator a.

FIG. 8-21   Arteries and nerves associated with the anterior aspect of the sacrum and sacroiliac joint.

iliac vein drains into the inferior vena cava. One exception to this is the superior rectal vein, which helps to form the inferior mesenteric vein. The inferior mesenteric vein, in turn, drains into either the splenic or superior mesenteric veins. The latter two veins combine to form the portal vein. Blood from the inferior rectal vein eventually drains into the inferior vena cava. The anastomosis between the superior rectal veins and the inferior and middle rectal veins forms an important portal-caval anastomosis.

The internal and external vertebral venous plexuses also help to drain the sacrum. These venous plexuses are discussed with the vertebral canal in Chapter 2.

REFERENCES
Abel MS. (1950). Sacroiliac joint changes in traumatic paraplegics. *Radiology, 55,* 235-239.
Abitbol M. (1989). Sacral curvature and supine posture. *Am J Phys Anthropol, 80,* 379-389.
Bakland O & Hanse J. (1984). The axial sacroiliac joint. *Anat Clin, 6,* 29-36.
Barakatt E et al. (1996) Interinnominate motion and symmetry: comparison

between gymnasts and nongymnasts. *J Orthop Sports Phys Ther, 23,* 309-319.

Beal MC. (1982). The sacroiliac problem: Review of anatomy, mechanics and diagnosis. *J Am Osteopath Assoc, June,* 667-673.

Bellamy N, Park W, & Rodney PJ. (1983). What do we know about the sacroiliac joint? *Arthritis Rheum, 12(3),* 282-309.

Bermis T & Daniel M. (1987). Validation of the long sitting test on subjects with sacroiliac dysfunction. *J Orthop Sports Phys Ther, 8,* 336-343.

Bernard T & Cassidy D. (1993). As quoted from: The sacroiliac joints revisited: Report from the San Diego congress on the sacroiliac joint. *Chiro Rep, 7(2),* 1-6.

Blower PW & Griffin AJ. (1984). Clinical sacroiliac joint test in ankylosing spondylitis and other causes of low back pain: 2 studies. *Ann Rheum Dis, 43,* 192-195.

Blumel J, Evans EB, & Eggers GWN. (1959). Partial and complete agenesis or malformation of the sacrum with associated anomalies. *J Bone Joint Surg, 41A,* 497-518.

Bose RN. (1982). Ankylosing spondylitis: Treatment. *Am Chiro, June,* 50.

Bowen V & Cassidy JD. (1981). Macroscopic and microscopic anatomy of sacroiliac joint from embryonic life until the eighth decade. *Spine, 6(6),* 620-628.

Brunner C, Kissling R, & Jacob HAC. (1991). The effects of morphology and histopathologic findings on the mobility of the sacroiliac joint. *Spine, 16(9),* 1111-1117.

Burns SH, Mireau DR, & Howlett E. (1995). Sacroiliac joint pain due to bacterial infection: A report of two cases. *J Can Chiro Assoc, 39,* 139-146.

Cassidy D. (1993). As quoted from: The sacroiliac joints revisited: Report from the San Diego congress on the sacroiliac joint. *Chiro Rep, 7(2),* 1-6.

Cassidy JD & Mierau DR. (1992). Pathophysiology of the sacroiliac joint. In S Haldeman (Ed.). *Principles and practice of chiropractic* (2nd ed.). East Norwalk, Conn: Appleton & Lange.

Colachis SC et al. (1963). Movement of sacroiliac joint in adult male: A preliminary report. *Arch Phys Med Rehabil, 44,* 490-497.

Cone RO & Resnick D. (1983). Roentgenographic evaluation of the sacroiliac joints. *Orthop Rev, 12(1),* 95-105.

Daum WJ. (1995). The sacroiliac joint: An underappreciated pain generator. *Am J Orthop, June,* 475-478.

Davis P, Thomson ABR, & Lentle BC. (1978). Quantitative sacroiliac scintigraphy in patients with Crohn's disease. *Arthritis Rheum, 21(2),* 234-237.

DeCavalho A & Graudal H. (1980). Sacroiliac joint involvement in classical or definite rheumatoid arthritis. *Acta Radiol Diagn, 21,* 417-423.

Dekker-Saeys BJ et al. (1978). Prevalence of peripheral arthritis, sacroiliitis and ankylosing spondylitis in patients suffering from inflammatory bowel disease. *Ann Rheum Dis, 37,* 33-35.

Diakow P, Cassidy JD, & DeKorompay VL. (1983). Post-surgical sacroiliac syndrome: A case study. *J Can Chiro Assoc, 27(1),* 19-21.

Dommisse GF & Louw JA. (1990). Anatomy of the lumbar spine. In Y Floman (Ed.). *Disorders of the lumbar spine.* Rockville, Md, and Tel Aviv: Aspen and Freund.

DonTigny RL. (1990). Anterior dysfunction of sacroiliac joint as a major factor in the etiology of idiopathic low back pain syndrome. *Phys Ther, 70(4),* 250-265.

Drerup B & Hierholzer E. (1987). Movement of human pelvis and displacement of related anatomical landmarks on body surface. *J Biomech (Br), 20(19),* 971-977.

Dreyfuss P et al. (1996). The value of medical history and physical examination in diagnosing sacroiliac joint pain. *Spine, 21,* 2594-2602.

Dunn EJ et al. (1976). Pyogenic infections of the sacroiliac joint. *Clin Orthop, 118,* 113-117.

Ebraheim NA & Lu J. (1998). Morphometric evaluation of the sacral dorsal root ganglia. *Surg Radiol Anat, 20,* 105-108.

Ebraheim NA et al. (1997a). Radiology of the sacroiliac joint. *Spine, 22,* 869-876.

Ebraheim NA et al. (1997b). The relationship of lumbosacral plexus to the sacrum and the sacroiliac joint. *Am J Orthop, Feb,* 105-110.

Ebraheim NA et al. (2000). Internal architecture of the sacrum in the elderly. *Spine, 25,* 292-297.

Ebraheim NA, Biyani A, & Salpietro B. (1996). Zone III fractures of the sacrum: A case report. *Spine, 21,* 2390-2396.

Egund N et al. (1978). Movement of sacroiliac joint, demonstrated with roentgen stereophotogrammetry. *Acta Radiol Diagn, 19,* 833-846.

Ehara S, El-Khoury GY, & Bergman RA. (1988). The accessory sacroiliac joint, a common anatomic variant. *AJR, Am J Roentgenol, 150,* 857-859.

Fidler MW & Plasmans CMT. (1983). The effect of four types of support on segmental mobility of the lumbosacral spine. *J Bone Joint Surg, 65A,* 943-947.

Fligg DB. (1986). Piriformis technique. *J Can Chiro Assoc, 30(2),* 87-88.

Freeman MD, Fox D, & Richards T. (1990). The superior intracapsular ligament of the sacroiliac joint: Confirmation of Illi's ligament. *J Manipulative Physiol Ther, 13(7),* 374-390.

Frigerio NA, Stowe RR, & Howe JW. (1974). Movement of sacroiliac joint. *Acta J Chiro, 8,* 161-166.

Fryette HH. (1936). Some reasons why sacroiliac lesions recur. *J Am Osteopath Assoc, 36(3),* 119-122.

Gibbons K, Soloniuk D, & Razack N. (1990). Neurological injury and patterns of sacral fractures. *J Neurosurg, 72,* 889-893.

Grieve E. (1981). Lumbopelvic rhythm and mechanical dysfunction of the sacroiliac joint. *Physiotherapy, 67(6),* 171-173.

Grieve GP. (1975). The sacroiliac joint. *Norfolk Norwich Hosp,* 384-401.

Hadley LA. (1952). Accessory sacroiliac articulations. *J Bone Joint Surg, 34A(1),* 149-155.

Illi FW. (1951). *The vertebral column: Lifeline of the body.* Chicago: National College of Chiropractic.

Jajic I & Jajic Z. (1987). The prevalence of osteoarthrosis. *Clin Rheum, 6,* 39-41.

Janse J. (1976). *Principles and practice of chiropractic: An anthology.* Lombard, Ill: National College of Chiropractic.

Janse J. (1978). The clinical biomechanics of sacroiliac mechanism. *ACA J Chiro, 12,* s1-s8.

Jaovisidha S et al. (1996). Ventral sacroiliac ligament: Anatomic and pathologic considerations. *Invest Radiol, 31,* 532-541.

Johnson JW. (1964). Sacroiliac strain. *J Am Osteopath Assoc, 63,* 1132-1148.

Kikuchi S et al. (1994). Anatomic and radiographic study of dorsal root ganglia. *Spine, 19,* 6-11.

King L. (1991). Incidence of sacroiliac joint dysfunction and low back pain in fit college students. *J Manipulative Physiol Ther, 14(5),* 333-334.

Kirkaldy-Willis W. (1988). The pathology and pathogenesis of low back pain. In W Kirkaldy-Willis (Ed.). *Managing low back pain* (2nd ed.). New York: Churchill Livingstone.

Kristiansson P, Svärdsud K, & von Schoultz B. (1996). Back pain during pregnancy. *Spine, 21,* 702-709.

LaBan MM et al. (1978). Symphyseal and sacroiliac joint pain associated with pubic symphysis instability. *Arch Phys Med Rehabil, 59,* 470-472.

Lavignolle B et al. (1983). An approach to functional anatomy of sacroiliac joint in vivo. *Anat Clin, 5,* 169-176.

Lawrence DJ. (1990). Sacroiliac joint. Part two. Clinical considerations. In JM Cox (Ed.). *Low back pain: Mechanism, diagnosis and treatment* (5th ed.). Baltimore: Williams & Wilkins.

Lichtblau S. (1962). Dislocation of sacroiliac joint. *J Bone Joint Surg, 44A,* 193-198.

Maltezopoulos V & Armitage N. (1984). A comparison of four chiropractic systems in the diagnosis of sacroiliac malfunction. *Eur J Chiro, 32,* 4-42.

McEwen C et al. (1971). Ankylosing spondylitis and spondylitis accompanying ulcerative colitis, regional enteritis, psoriasis and Reiter's disease. *Arthritis Rheum, 14(3),* 291-318.

Norman GP & May A. (1956). Sacroiliac condition simulating intervertebral disc syndrome. *WJSO & G, (August),* 401-402.

Nykoliation JW, Cassidy JD, & Dupuis P. (1984). Osteitis condensans ilii, a stress phenomenon. *J Can Chiro Assoc, 28(1),* 21-24.

Olivieri I et al. (1990). Differential diagnosis between osteitis condensans ilii and sacroiliitis. *J Rheum, 17(1),* 1504-1512.

Otter R. (1985). A review study of differing opinions expressed in the literature about the anatomy of the sacroiliac joint. *Eur J Chiro, 33,* 221-242.

Paquin JD et al. (1983). Biomechanical and morphological study of cartilage from adult human sacroiliac joint. *Arthritis Rheum, 26(6),* 887-895.

Peretz AM, Hipp JA, & Heggeness MH. (1998). The internal bony architecture of the sacrum. *Spine, 23,* 971-974.

Pitkin HC & Pheasant HC. (1936a). Sacroarthrogenic telalgia. *J Bone Joint Surg, 18A(1),* 111-133.

Pitkin HC & Pheasant HC. (1936b). A study of sacral mobility. *J Bone Joint Surg, 18A,* 365-374.

Potter NA & Rothstein JM. (1985). Intertester reliability for selected clinical tests of the sacroiliac joint. *Phys Ther, 65(11),* 1671-1675.

Prassopoulos PK et al. (1999). Sacroiliac joints: Anatomical variants on CT. *J CAT, 23,* 323-327.

Resnik CS & Resnick D. (1985). Radiology of disorders of sacroiliac joints. *JAMA, 253(19),* 2863-2866.

Resnik D, Dwosh IL, & Niwayama G. (1975). Sacroiliac joint in renal osteodystrophy: Roentgenographic-pathologic correlation. *J Rheum, 2(3),* 287-295.

Richardson CA et al. (2002). The relation between the transverses abdominis muscles, sacroiliac joint mechanics, and low back pain. *Spine, 27,* 399-405.

Ro CS. (1990). Sacroiliac joint. In JM Cox (Ed.). *Low back pain: Mechanism, diagnosis and treatment* (5th ed.). Baltimore: Williams & Wilkins.

Romanus R. (1955). *Pelvo-spondylitis ossificans.* Chicago: Year Book.

Russell AS et al. (1977). The sacroiliitis of acute Reiter's syndrome. *J Rheum, 4(3),* 293-296.

Sakamoto N et al. (2001). An electrophysiologic study of mechanoreceptors in the sacroiliac joint and adjacent tissues. *Spine, 26,* E468-E471.

Sandoz RW. (1978). Structural and functional pathologies of the pelvic ring. *Ann Swiss Chiro Assoc,* 101-155.

Sashin D. (1929). A critical analysis of the anatomy and the pathologic changes of the sacroiliac joints. *Bull Hosp Joint Dis,* 891-910.

Schuchman JA & Cannon CL. (1986). Sacroiliac strain syndrome, diagnosis and treatment. *Tex Med, 82,* 33-36.

Schwarzer AC, Aprill CN, & Bogduk N. (1995). The sacroiliac joint in chronic low back pain. *Spine, 20,* 31-37.

Sgambati E et al. (1997). Morphometric analysis of the sacroiliac joint. *It J Anat Embryol, 102,* 33-38.

Simkins CS. (1952). Anatomy and significance of the sacroiliac joint. *AAO Yearbook,* 64-69.

Smidt GL et al. (1997). Sacroiliac motion for extreme hip positions. *Spine, 22,* 2073-2082.

Solonen KA. (1957). The sacroiliac joint in the light of anatomical, roentgenographical and clinical studies. *Acta Orthop Scand, 27,* 160-162.

Vleeming A et al. (1996). The function of the long dorsal sacroiliac ligament. *Spine, 21,* 556-562.

Vogler JB et al. (1984). Normal sacroiliac joint: A CT study of asymptomatic patients. *Radiology, 151(2),* 433-437.

Walker JM. (1986). Age-related differences in the human sacroiliac joint: A histological study; implications for therapy. *J Orthop Sports Phys Ther, 7(6),* 325-334.

Wallheim GG, Olerud S, & Ribbe T. (1984). Motion of symphysis in pelvic instability. *Scand J Rehabil Med, 16,* 163-169.

Weisl H. (1954a). The articular surface of sacroiliac joint and their relation to the movement of the sacrum. *Acta Anat, 22,* 1-14.

Weisl H. (1954b). The ligaments of sacroiliac joint examined with particular reference to their function. *Acta Anat, 20(30),* 201-213.

Weisl H. (1955). The movement of the sacroiliac joint. *Acta Anat, 23,* 80-91.

Wilder DG, Pope MH, & Frymoyer JW. (1980). The functional topography of sacroiliac joint. *Spine, 5(6),* 575-579.

Williams PL et al. (1995). *Gray's anatomy* (38th ed.). Edinburgh: Churchill Livingstone.

Winterstein JF. (1972). *Spinographic evaluation of pelvic and lumbar spine.* Lombard, Ill: National College of Chiropractic.

Wood J. (1985). Motion of the sacroiliac joint. *Palmer Coll Res Forum, Spring,* 1-16.

Yazici H, Tuzlaci M, & Yurdakul S. (1981). A controlled survey of sacroiliitis in Behçet's disease. *Ann Rheum Dis, 40,* 558-559.

PART II

NEUROANATOMY OF THE SPINAL CORD, AUTONOMIC NERVOUS SYSTEM, AND PAIN OF SPINAL ORIGIN

C H A P T E R 9

Neuroanatomy of the Spinal Cord

Susan A. Darby
Robert J. Frysztak

The vertebral column and its adjacent musculature are discussed in detail in the previous chapters. Because of the intimate anatomic and functional relationship between the vertebral column and spinal cord (which is protected by the vertebral column), knowledge of both is equally important. Chapter 3 describes the meninges, external surface, and vasculature of the spinal cord. In addition, it provides a cursory description of the cord's internal organization. The purpose of this chapter is to elaborate on this internal organization by discussing the neurons, which form the circuitry of the spinal cord, and the ascending and descending tracts, which provide a connection among the spinal cord, the peripheral nerves, and the higher centers of the central nervous system. This information forms the basis of important neuroanatomic concepts that are necessary for an understanding of clinical neuroscience. The knowledge of these concepts is imperative for diagnosing pathologic conditions of the cord, some of which may be caused by vertebral column dysfunction. Examples demonstrating the application of these neuroanatomic principles to pathologic conditions are presented at the end of the chapter.

PERIPHERAL NERVOUS SYSTEM

Peripheral Receptors

Peripheral receptors are sensory endings of peripheral nerves; they are scattered throughout the body. They are found in great numbers along the vertebral column and within the ligaments, muscles, and skin that surround the spine. These receptors and the sensory systems that transmit their input provide information concerning one's environment. Each receptor is sensitive to a particular form of physical energy, or stimulus, and transduces the stimulus into electrochemical energy or action potentials, which is the "language" the central nervous system (CNS) can understand.

Receptors may be divided into two types, rapidly adapting and slowly adapting. A slowly adapting receptor, such as a Merkel's disc, responds continuously to a sustained stimulus, whereas a rapidly adapting receptor does not. A rapidly adapting receptor, such as a pacinian corpuscle, responds to any dynamic change in the receptor. For example, if the pressure onto a pacinian corpuscle is continuously increased, the corpuscle will continue to produce action potentials until the stimulus strength becomes constant. A stimulus furnishes a receptor with four basic characteristics: modality (type of stimulus), intensity (strength of stimulus), duration (perceived time that the stimulus is present), and location (where on the body the stimulus is being perceived). When a receptor is adequately stimulated, a generator potential occurs across its membrane and may lead to an action potential. The action potential propagates along the sensory neuron into the CNS. The CNS then is able to combine the four characteristics of the stimulus into a perceived sensation.

The sensory neurons of the peripheral nervous system (PNS) are pseudounipolar neurons. Their cell bodies are located in the dorsal root ganglia. The peripheral process, which may be myelinated or unmyelinated, is the part of the fiber continuous with the receptor. It is the sensory component of a peripheral nerve. The other part of the fiber, the central process, enters the CNS. A bundle of central processes form a dorsal root. The peripheral processes are classified according to their conduction velocity, and conduction velocity is related to the axon diameter. Fibers with large diameters conduct the fastest. Based on the relationship between velocity and diameter, cutaneous fibers are classified alphabetically as A-beta, A-delta, and C fibers. Similarly, afferents from muscle tissue usually are classified numerically from heavily myelinated to unmyelinated as I, II, III, and IV. Type I also has subgroups of Ia and Ib. Afferents from visceral interoceptors often are classified as A-delta and C fibers. Motor (efferent) fibers also are classified according to the alphabetic listing. Large somatic motor neurons correspond to the A-alpha and A-gamma group, and autonomic efferent fibers correspond to the B and C groups. Table 9-1 summarizes the classifications of the afferent and efferent fibers.

Peripheral receptors can be classified by their morphology, location, and the type of stimulus to which they respond. Morphologically, receptors may be encapsulated by connective tissue and nonneural cells, or they may simply be nonencapsulated, bare arborizing endings. Receptors classified by their location of distribution are called exteroceptors, proprioceptors, or interoceptors. Exteroceptors are superficial and located in the skin. Modalities such as nociception (pain), temperature, and touch (and the submodalities of pressure and vibration) are conveyed by these receptors. Proprioceptors are located in the muscles, tendons, and joints of the body and provide information concerning limb position, while the limbs are either stationary (static) or moving (dynamic or kinesthetic) (Williams et al., 1995; Kiernan, 1998; Pearson and Gordon, 2000a; Nolte, 2002). Interoceptors are located in the viscera, glands, and vessels and convey poorly localized information from such systems as the digestive and urinary. Examples of the types of information conveyed by interoceptors include distention or fullness and ischemic pain.

Receptors classified by the type of stimulus to which they respond are called mechanoreceptors, thermoreceptors, chemoreceptors, or nociceptors. Mechanoreceptors respond to deformation or displacement of self or adjacent cells. Thermoreceptors respond to changes in temperature. Chemoreceptors respond to chemical stimuli and are important in the special senses of taste and olfaction. Nociceptors respond to stimuli that damage tissue cells, and their stimulation results in the sensation of pain. The classification of receptors by location overlaps with the classification by stimulus type, such that nociceptors also can be exteroceptors, and mechanoreceptors also can be proprioceptors.

Cutaneous Receptors. Cutaneous receptors (exteroceptors) include mechanoreceptors, thermoreceptors, and nociceptors and subserve such modalities as touch,

---

Table 9-1   Summary of the Classification of Peripheral Fibers

Fiber Diameter (Microns)	Efferent Fibers	Afferent Fibers (From Cutaneous Receptors)*	Afferent Fibers (From Skeletal Muscle and Articular Receptors)	Myelination
12–20[†,‡]	A-alpha (skeletomotor)	A-alpha (from mechanoreceptors) (rapidly adapting)	Type I (from mechanoreceptors)	Heavily myelinated
6–12[‡]		A-beta (from mechano-receptors) (slowly adapting)	Type II (from mechanoreceptors)	Myelinated
3–8[†]	A-gamma (fusimotor)			Myelinated
1–6[‡]		A-delta (from nociceptors and thermoreceptors)	Type III (from mechanoreceptors and nociceptors)	Thinly myelinated
1–3[†]	B[†,§] (preganglionic autonomic fibers)			Myelinated
0.2–1.5[†,‡]	C[†,§] (postganglionic autonomic fibers)	C (from nociceptors and thermoreceptors)	Type IV (from nociceptors)	Unmyelinated

*Afferent fibers from visceral receptors are classified as A-delta and C fibers.
[†]Kiernan JA. (1998). *The human nervous system* (7th ed.). Philadelphia: JB Lippincott.
[‡]Gardner EP, Martin JH, & Jessell TM. (2000). The bodily senses. In ER Kandel, JH Schwartz, & TM Jessell (Eds.). *Principles of neural science* (4th ed.). New York: McGraw-Hill.
[§]Williams PL et al. (1995). *Gray's anatomy* (38th ed.). Edinburgh: Churchill Livingstone.

pressure, vibration, temperature, and nociception (pain) (Fig. 9-1). Mechanoreceptors include the nonencapsulated Merkel's discs, nonencapsulated endings surrounding hair follicles (peritrichial), and encapsulated endings such as Ruffini endings, pacinian corpuscles, and Meissner's corpuscles. The fibers supplying these receptors are primarily A-beta. Thermoreceptors are nonencapsulated, free nerve endings that occupy areas approximately 1 mm in diameter. Cold thermoreceptors respond in the range of 5° C (41° F) to 40° C (104° F) relative to the normal skin temperature of 34° C (93.2° F) and fire most frequently at 25° C (77° F). Warm thermoreceptors are stimulated in the temperature range 29° C (84.2° F) to 45° C (113° F) and are most active at 45° C (Gardner, Martin, and Jessell, 2000). Cold receptors are supplied by A-delta or C fibers, but warm receptors are supplied by C fibers alone.

An understanding of nociceptors is helpful in the comprehension of pain of spinal origin. Nociceptors are free nerve endings, and they respond to stimuli that may threaten or actually damage adjacent tissue cells. The damage to cells causes the release of chemical mediators that may sensitize (e.g., prostaglandins, leukotrienes, substance P) previously unresponsive free nerve endings by lowering their threshold for activation or activate (e.g., histamine, bradykinin, potassium, serotonin) the free nerve endings. In some instances, activated free nerve endings release substance P and calcitonin gene-related peptide into the surrounding area, causing vasodilation, extravasation of fluid, and release of histamine from tissue cells. These changes in turn lead to lowering the threshold for activation of more nociceptors. The inflammatory process that results from the activity of these nociceptors is termed neurogenic inflammation (Basbaum and Jessell, 2000). Three types of nociceptors appear to exist: (a) mechanical, which are stimulated by mechanical damage such as by a sharp object; (b) thermal, which are stimulated by temperatures higher than 45° C (113° F) or lower than 20° C (68° F); and (c) polymodal, which respond to damaging mechanical, thermal, or chemical stimuli. Mechanical and thermal nociceptors send their information via A-delta fibers, whereas polymodal receptors use C fibers. The three types of nociceptors often are activated simultaneously and thus work together. For example, if a person stubs a toe, initially there is sharp (fast) pain resulting from stimulating mechanical nociceptors followed by an achy prolonged pain resulting from stimulating polymodal nociceptors that use slower C fibers.

The cutaneous fibers of these receptors form overlapping horizontal plexuses in the dermis and subcutaneous layers of the skin. The density and variety of receptors vary in different regions. For example, in hairy skin the peritrichial endings are most common, but Merkel's discs and free nerve endings are also present. In glabrous (hairless) skin, free nerve endings are present, as are Merkel's discs and Meissner's corpuscles. The latter two receptors have small receptive fields and help to discriminate the spatial relationship of stimuli. This ability to discriminate is well developed on the fingertips. In fact, Meissner's corpuscles have been located only in primate animals (Kiernan, 1998). The subcutaneous tissues of both types of skin are provided with pacinian corpuscles and Ruffini endings, both of which have large receptive fields and therefore are less discriminatory (Gardner, Martin, and Jessell, 2000).

Cutaneous modalities that may be easily tested during a neurologic examination include vibration, temperature, pain (nociception), and tactile sensation. Tactile sensation can be described as simple touch (which includes light touch, touch pressure, and crude localization) and tactile discrimination (which includes deeper pressure and spatial localization), which is sometimes called two-point discriminatory touch. On the fingertips, for example, tactile discrimination is precise enough to localize two points of stimulation applied simultaneously 2 mm apart. Such tactile discrimination is necessary for further analysis of objects concerning their size, shape, texture, and movement pattern. This analysis is completed in sensory integrative areas of the cerebral cortex. Identifying common objects held in the hand and letters drawn on the back of the hand without visual cues are called stereognosis and graphesthesia, respectively. These are further examples that demonstrate tactile discrimination. The clinical relevance of these cutaneous modalities is discussed at the end of this chapter.

Muscle, Tendon, and Joint Receptors. The majority of the receptors located in muscles, tendons, and joints are involved with the sense of proprioception. The receptors are classified as proprioceptors based on their location. They are classified as mechanoreceptors based on the type of stimulus to which they respond. These receptors convey proprioception, the term used to describe the sensory information that contributes to the sense of movement and position of one's own limbs and body without visual input. The mechanoreceptors involved with providing proprioception (excluding the vestibular system of the inner ear) are the joint receptors, neuromuscular spindles, and Golgi tendon organs (neurotendinous spindles). They function in the coordination and control of movements and the maintenance of upright posture by monitoring both the stationary position and movement (kinesthesia) of body parts, and then relaying that information into the CNS. This information, often called joint position sense, may be perceived consciously. In addition, cutaneous mechanoreceptors also

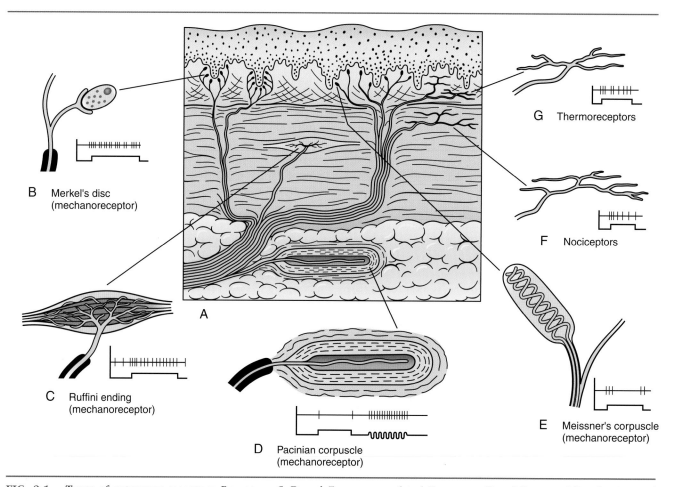

FIG. 9-1 Types of cutaneous receptors. Receptors *C, D,* and *E* are encapsulated. Receptors *D* and *E* are rapidly adapting and receptors *B, C, F,* and *G* are slowly adapting. The tracings illustrate that the slowly adapting receptors fire continuously throughout the stimulus and the rapidly adapting receptors fire at the onset and offset of the stimulus.

may function in the overall assessment of proprioception. For example, they may aid other proprioceptors in the task of discriminating different thicknesses of objects held between the thumb and finger and in the manipulation of objects of different shapes and sizes (McCloskey, 1994; Gardner, Martin, and Jessell, 2000).

Joint receptors are located in the superficial and deep layers of the joint capsules and in the ligaments. Four types of receptors exist, classified as I, II, III, and IV. The first three types are encapsulated mechanoreceptors that have a proprioceptive function. The fourth type consists of unmyelinated free nerve endings. The receptors classified as I, II, or III provide information about such activities as the direction, velocity, and initiation of joint movements. They do this by responding to tension applied to the connective tissue surrounding them. The group IV free nerve endings, which mediate nociception and normally are silent, respond to potentially injurious mechanical or inflammatory processes (Wyke, 1985).

Neuromuscular spindles are complex encapsulated proprioceptors that monitor muscle fiber length. They

are located within a skeletal muscle close to the tendon and are surrounded by muscle fibers. They provide the sensory arc of the stretch, or myotatic, reflex. Each spindle consists of a connective tissue capsule that is fixed at each end to adjacent muscle fibers. The capsule encloses specialized muscle fibers called intrafusal fibers, which are either nuclear bag fibers or nuclear chain fibers. The total and individual numbers of nuclear bag and chain fibers vary among spindles. The innervation of the nuclear bag and chain fibers of the spindle is provided by group Ia and II sensory fibers. In addition, the spindle is a unique peripheral receptor in that it also has a motor innervation furnished by gamma motor neurons. The motor innervation of the intrafusal fibers allows the spindle to remain sensitive to muscle fiber length during muscle contraction. The section Spinal Motor Neurons and Motor Coordination describes the function of the muscle spindle and stretch reflex.

Golgi tendon organs (GTOs), or neurotendinous spindles, respond to tension that is applied to a tendon. They consist of tendon collagen fibers surrounded by connective tissue, with group Ib afferent fibers twisted among the collagen fibers in such a way that they may become "squeezed" under the appropriate amount of tension. On stimulation, the group Ib afferent fiber stimulates a Ib interneuron. This interneuron then inhibits the alpha motor neuron that supplies the skeletal muscle associated with that stimulated GTO. This action is opposite to that of a stimulated neuromuscular spindle, which produces excitation of the alpha motor neuron supplying the skeletal muscle associated with that spindle. The GTOs and spindles not only function at the spinal level, but also send input to higher centers (see Ascending Tracts). The section Spinal Motor Neurons and Motor Coordination describes the functional relationship between muscle spindles and GTOs.

Visceral Receptors. These receptors also may be classified as interoceptors because of their location. They include mechanoreceptors that respond to movement or distention of the viscera. These are found in locations such as the mesentery, connective tissue enclosing the organs, and along blood vessels. Nociceptors are found in the viscera, as well. These are capable of responding to noxious mechanical, thermal, and chemical stimuli (Willis Jr. and Coggeshall, 1991). Chapter 10 discusses the relationship of these receptors and their afferent fibers to somatic and autonomic efferents.

Peripheral Nerves

The spinal cord receives impulses from receptors and sends output to effectors via the PNS. Because the PNS transmits this essential information, its components are considered in this section.

Thirty-one pairs of spinal nerves exist, and each is formed by the convergence of a dorsal root and a ventral root usually within the intervertebral foramen (IVF). Just distal to this union, each spinal nerve divides into a dorsal ramus (posterior primary division, PPD) and a ventral ramus (anterior primary division, APD) (see Fig. 3-3). The dorsal rami of spinal nerves innervate the zygapophysial joints, skin over the back, and deepest muscles of the neck and back. The ventral rami innervate the extremities and the ventrolateral aspect of the trunk. Successive thoracic ventral rami retain a clear segmental distribution along the thoracic region. However, the back of the head, the anterior and lateral neck, shoulder, and upper and lower extremities are innervated by plexuses. Each plexus is formed by a regrouping of adjacent ventral rami. The plexuses are called the cervical, brachial, and lumbosacral plexuses, and each is briefly described here.

The cervical plexus is formed by ventral rami of the C1 through C4 cervical nerves. It supplies cutaneous innervation to the dorsolateral part of the head, neck, and shoulder. Motor fibers in this plexus course to the deep cervical muscles, hyoid muscles, diaphragm, and sternocleidomastoid and trapezius muscles (see Chapter 5).

The brachial plexus is formed by ventral rami of the C5 through T1 spinal nerves (often with a contribution from C4 and T2). This plexus supplies the upper extremity. Subsequent to the mixing of the ventral rami in the plexus, numerous branches are formed, including five large terminal branches: the axillary, musculocutaneous, radial, ulnar, and median nerves. The axillary nerve (C5 to C6) supplies cutaneous branches to the deltoid region and muscular branches to the deltoid and teres minor muscles. The musculocutaneous nerve (C5 to C7) is sensory to the anterolateral and posterolateral aspect of the forearm. It supplies motor innervation to the flexors of the arm, which includes the biceps brachii. The radial nerve (C5 to C8, possibly T1) has an extensive area of distribution in both the arm and forearm. Its cutaneous branches innervate the posterior aspect of the arm and forearm. The superficial radial nerve supplies the skin of the lateral half of the dorsum of the hand and the first three and a half digits, excluding the nails. The radial nerve also innervates the extensor muscles of the upper extremity. The ulnar nerve (C8 and T1, sometimes C7) courses through the arm to supply structures in the forearm and hand. Its motor distribution includes one and a half forearm flexors (ulnar side) and intrinsic hand muscles, including the hypothenar and all interossei muscles and some thenar muscles. Its cutaneous distribution is present only in the hand and encompasses the ulnar half of the hand, including the fifth and medial one half of the fourth digits. The median nerve (C6 to C8 and T1, sometimes C5) supplies motor fibers to the forearm flexors (excluding those with ulnar innervation) and some intrinsic hand muscles, including most of the thenar muscles. As with the ulnar nerve, its sensory area is only in the hand and includes the lateral palmar surface and first three and a half digits, including the nails (Williams et al., 1995) (Figs. 9-2 and 9-3 and Table 9-2). (See Chapter 5 for a full description of the brachial plexus and its proximal branches.)

The lumbosacral plexus is the third plexus, which is composed of ventral rami L2 through S2 (with contributions from L1 and S3). The major branches of this network are the femoral, obturator, gluteal, sciatic, common fibular (peroneal) (and its branches), and tibial nerves. Cutaneous nerves with large areas of distribution include, but are not limited to, the lateral femoral cutaneous, saphenous, posterior femoral cutaneous, and sural nerves. (Chapters 7 and 8 describe the lumbar plexus and its smaller branches [iliohypogastric and ilioinguinal] and the sacral plexus and its branches.)

The obturator nerve (L2 to L4) supplies motor branches to the adductor muscles of the thigh and gracilis muscle.

Also it is cutaneous to the inner thigh. The femoral nerve (L2 to L4) sends motor branches to the anterior thigh muscles (e.g., quadriceps), which extend the leg. Cutaneous innervation by the femoral nerve supplies the anterior and anteromedial thigh and, via the saphenous nerve (L3 and L4), the medial leg and foot. The thigh's lateral side is innervated by cutaneous branches of the lateral femoral cutaneous nerve (L2 and L3). The sciatic nerve (L4 to S3) is the body's largest nerve. This nerve actually is composed of two parts (tibial and common fibular) but usually is ensheathed to form one nerve in the posterior thigh. Motor branches in the posterior thigh innervate the hamstring muscles (biceps femoris, semitendinosus, semimembranosus), which flex the leg. The cutaneous innervation of the posterior thigh is furnished by the posterior femoral cutaneous nerve (S1 to S3). The sciatic nerve divides into the common fibular (peroneal) and tibial nerves at varying levels proximal to the knee.

The common fibular (peroneal) nerve (L4, L5, S1, and S2) courses laterally around the neck of the fibula and divides into two major branches: superficial fibular (peroneal) and deep fibular (peroneal). The superficial fibular (peroneal) nerve supplies muscular branches to the fibularis (peronei) muscles, which are responsible for eversion of the foot, and cutaneous branches to the distal and anterolateral third of the leg and dorsum of the foot (excluding the first digital interspace). The deep fibular (peroneal) nerve sends motor fibers to the anterior leg muscles, which provide dorsiflexion of the foot and extension of the toes. Cutaneous branches supply the skin between the first two toes. The other branch of the sciatic nerve is the tibial nerve (L4, L5, S1, S2, and S3). This nerve provides motor innervation to posterior leg muscles (including the gastrocnemius muscle), which are responsible for plantar flexion of the foot. A branch of the tibial nerve and contributing fibers from the common fibular (peroneal) nerve form the sural nerve. This supplies sensory innervation to the posterior and lateral surfaces of the leg. The tibial nerve divides into medial and lateral plantar nerves at the region of the medial malleolus. These nerves supply motor and sensory innervation to the plantar aspect of the foot (see Figs. 9-2 and 9-3 and Table 9-2).

The inferior and superior gluteal nerves innervate muscles moving the hip joint. The inferior gluteal nerve (L5, S1, and S2) is responsible for the motor innervation of the strongest hip extensor, the gluteus maximus. The superior gluteal nerve (L4, L5, and S1) innervates the gluteus medius and minimus muscles and the tensor fascia latae muscle, which are responsible for hip abduction (see Table 9-2).

This has been a cursory description of the innervation of major individual muscles and muscle groups and the cutaneous distribution of the major nerves. Because of developmental events, one muscle is innervated by multiple cord segments, and one cord segment may be involved with the innervation of more than one muscle. The intermingling of dorsal root fibers in the plexuses produces a peripheral nerve with an area of distribution that is different from a dermatomal pattern. However, the origin (cord segments) of a peripheral nerve innervating a particular cutaneous region includes the same cord segments as those supplying the dermatomes of that same area. For example, the lateral femoral cutaneous nerve is formed from cord segments L2 and L3, and its peripheral nerve pattern includes parts of the L2 and L3 dermatomal regions.

Realize the differences between peripheral nerve and dermatomal patterns (and remember there is much variation in dermatomal maps) (see Figs. 9-2 and 9-3). Know both the segmental and peripheral innervation of major skeletal muscles. This knowledge of peripheral innervation of muscles and skin is imperative, because a neurologic examination includes the assessment of a patient's motor functions (reflexes and muscle strength; Table 9-3) and sensory functions. The information gained from this assessment is useful for distinguishing if the lesion is in the CNS or PNS and subsequently for determining the specific location of the lesion along one of these two systems.

INTERNAL ORGANIZATION OF THE SPINAL CORD

Gray Matter

The gray matter of the spinal cord appears in cross section as an H- or butterfly-shaped region. Each of the two symmetric halves consists of a dorsal horn, which includes a head, neck, and base; an intermediate region; and a ventral horn. An additional lateral horn is present in cord segments T1 through L2 or L3. In general, the dorsal horn is a receptacle for sensory afferent input, and the ventral horn is involved in motor functions, including housing the cell bodies of motor neurons. Microscopically the gray matter is a dense region of neuron cell bodies, cell processes and their synapses, neuroglia cells, and capillaries.

The neurons that compose the gray matter are subdivided into four groups: motor neurons, the axons of which leave the spinal cord and innervate the effector tissues (skeletal, smooth, and cardiac muscles, and glands); tract neurons, the axons of which ascend in the white matter to higher centers; interneurons, which have short processes; and propriospinal neurons, the axons of which provide communication between cord segments. Propriospinal neurons are classified as long, intermediate, or short. Long propriospinal neurons extend the length of the cord in the ventral funiculus and ventral part of the lateral funiculus (see White

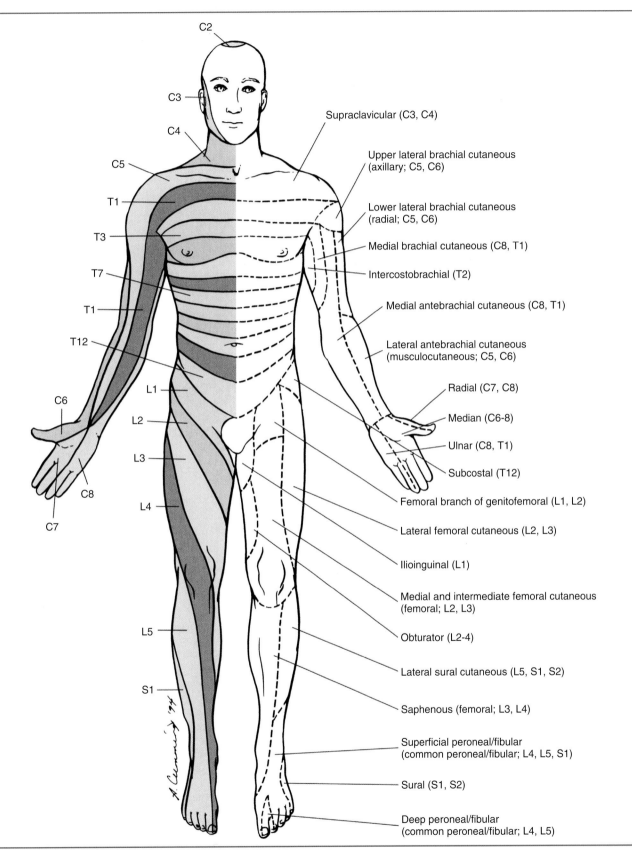

FIG. 9-2 Anterior view of the body showing its cutaneous innervation. *Left*, Dermatomal pattern, which may vary according to different authors. This dermatomal mapping is based on studies by JG Keegan and FV Garrett (1948). *Right*, Areas of cutaneous peripheral nerve distributions. Note the similarity of cord segment origins between the two sides.

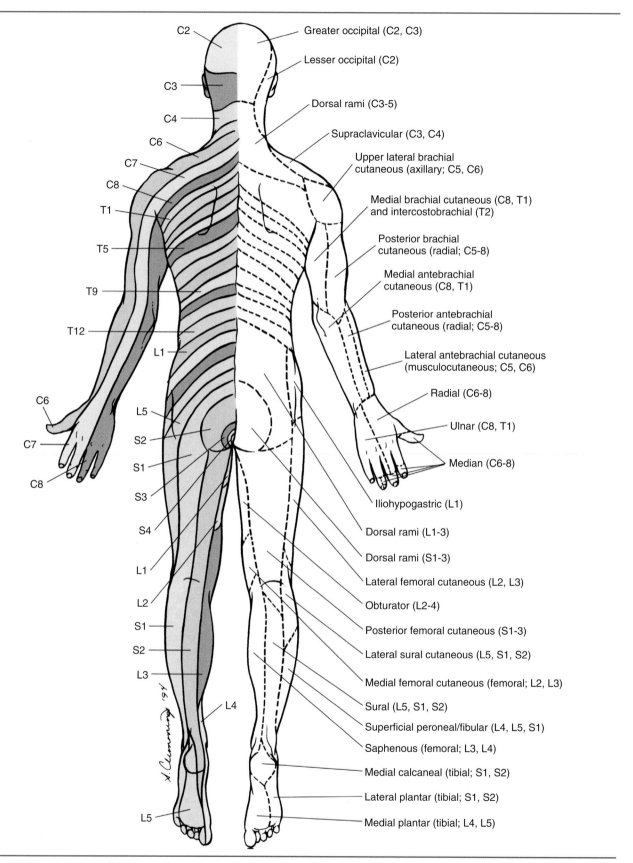

FIG. 9-3 Posterior view of the body showing its cutaneous innervation. *Left,* Dermatomal pattern, which may vary according to different authors. This dermatomal mapping is based on studies by JG Keegan and FV Garrett (1948). *Right,* Areas of cutaneous peripheral nerve distributions. Note the similarity of cord segment origins between the two sides.

Table 9-2	Muscles Supplied by Terminal Branches of the Brachial Plexus and the Lumbosacral Plexus	
Muscle(s) Supplied	**Peripheral Nerve**	**Cord Segments**
Deltoid, teres minor	Axillary	C5, C6
Anterior arm	Musculocutaneous	C5-7
Extensors of upper extremity	Radial	C5-8 (T1)*
Flexor carpi ulnaris, flexor digitorum profundus (medial half), hypothenar eminence, interossei, adductor pollicis, lumbricals (3rd and 4th)	Ulnar	(C7)*, C8-T1
Anterior forearm (except above), thenar eminence (except above), lumbricals (1st and 2nd)	Median	(C5)*, C6-T1
Medial thigh	Obturator	L2-4
Anterior thigh	Femoral	L2-4 (mostly L3 and L4)
Posterior thigh	Sciatic	L4-S3
	Common fibular (peroneal)	L4-S2
Lateral leg	Superficial	(mostly S1)
Anterior leg	Deep	
Posterior leg	Tibial	L4-S3 (mostly S1)
Gluteus maximus	Inferior gluteal	L5-S2 (mostly S1)
Gluteus medius and minimus	Superior gluteal	L4-S1 (mostly L5)

*This level represents clinically significant contributions in a small portion of the population.

Matter). Descending propriospinal fibers (axons) course bilaterally and the ascending axons project mostly contralaterally. Short propriospinal neurons extend six to eight segments in the ipsilateral lateral funiculus, and intermediate propriospinal neurons course primarily ipsilaterally more than eight segments but less than the cord's entire length. Most of the propriospinal fibers are located immediately adjacent to the gray matter in the fasciculus proprius, but some travel more laterally in the funiculi. The axons of medial propriospinal neurons are long and include extensive branches. For example, some extend the length of the cord to coordinate the movements of neck and pelvic axial musculature for postural corrections. Laterally placed propriospinal fibers influence neurons innervating more distal muscles, communicate with a smaller number of segments, and branch

less extensively. Because the distal musculature is less connected to other muscle groups, these muscles function more independently. This independence permits more diverse somatic motor activities (Williams et al., 1995; Ghez and Krakauer, 2000). Through their communication with neurons in other cord segments, propriospinal neurons are involved not only with the coordination of somatic motor activity, but also with the autonomic innervation of sweat glands, smooth muscle of the vasculature, and viscera such as the bladder and bowel (Williams et al., 1995).

In the early 1950s, Rexed (1952) studied feline spinal cords and proposed that the organization of the gray matter formed 10 layers, or laminae. He described lamina I as being located at the tip of the dorsal horn, followed sequentially into the ventral horn by laminae II through IX. Lamina X formed the connecting crossbar of the gray matter, that is, the gray commissure. This organization has been accepted for the human spinal cord as well (Fig. 9-4). Each lamina includes at least one of the four general types of neurons: motor, tract, interneuron, or propriospinal. Each lamina also may be the site of the termination of primary afferents, descending tracts, propriospinal neurons, and interneurons of neighboring laminae. The laminae may vary in size throughout regions of the spinal cord and even may be absent in some regions. Also within each lamina, neurons may be organized into smaller groups, called nuclei or cell columns, based on commonalities such as cell morphology and function. The following is a brief description of each of these laminae.

Laminae I through VI (Dorsal Horn). The dorsal horn consists of laminae I through VI. Laminae I through IV form the head, lamina V the neck, and lamina VI the base of the dorsal horn. Laminae I and II are collectively known as the superficial dorsal horn and are heavily involved with the processing of nociception. The majority of A-delta and C fibers terminate here. Lamina I is also known as the marginal zone of Waldeyer. Most of the primary afferent input into lamina I originates from cutaneous nociceptors and thermoreceptors via A-delta fibers. Additional input is conveyed by C fibers (from nociceptors, thermoreceptors, and histamine-sensitive receptors conveying the sensation of "itch" [Schmelz et al., 1997; Andrew and Craig, 2001; Craig, Zhang, and Blomqvist, 2002]) and a small group of thinly myelinated muscle, joint, and visceral afferent fibers (Willis and Coggeshall, 1991; Williams et al., 1995). Many neurons within lamina I are considered to be nociceptive specific, whereas others are classified as wide-dynamic-range neurons that respond to both noxious and innocuous stimuli. Thermoreceptive-specific neurons also terminate in lamina I (Han, Zhang, and Craig, 1998) along with numerous interneurons. Tract neurons originate in lamina I as

Table 9-3   Muscle Testing and Deep Tendon (Muscle Stretch) Reflexes

Muscle Action	Cord Segments	Peripheral Nerve(s)	Reflex
Shoulder abduction (deltoid)	C5	Axillary	
Elbow flexion (biceps brachii, brachialis, brachioradialis)	C5	Musculocutaneus	Biceps
	C6	Radial brachioradialis	
Elbow extension (triceps brachii)	C7	Radial triceps	
Wrist extension (posterior forearm muscles)	C6 (C7)*	Radial	
Wrist flexion (anterior forearm muscles)	C7	Median, ulnar	
Finger extension (extensor digitorum)	C7	Radial	
Finger flexion (flexor digitorum)	C8	Median, ulnar	
Finger abduction (interossei)	T1	Ulnar	
Hip flexion (iliopsoas)	T12-L3	Lumbar plexus (L2-4), femoral	
Hip extension (gluteus maximus)	S1	Inferior gluteal	
Hip adduction (adductors)	L2-L4	Obturator	
Hip abduction (gluteus medius and minimus)	L5	Superior gluteal	
Knee extension (quadriceps femoris)	L2-L4	Femoral	Patellar (L4)
Foot inversion and dorsiflexion (tibialis anterior)	L4	Deep fibular (peroneal)	
Foot eversion, with plantar flexion (peronei)	S1	Superficial fibular (peroneal)	
Foot eversion, with dorsiflexion (extensor digitorum longus, peroneus tertius)	L5	Deep fibular (peroneal)	
Foot plantar flexion (gastrocnemius, soleus)	S1 (S2)*	Tibial	Achilles
Toe extension (hallux) (extensor hallucis longus)	L5	Deep fibular (peroneal)	
Toe extension, except above (extensor digitorum brevis)	S1, S2	Deep fibular (peroneal)	

*This level represents clinically significant contributions in a small portion of the population.

well, and provide the major output for the superficial dorsal horn.

Lamina II is known as the substantia gelatinosa of Rolando. The many processes, the presence of small neurons, and the absence of myelinated axons gives this layer a gelatinous appearance on close inspection. The primary afferent input into lamina II enters by C afferent fibers from cutaneous nociceptors, thermoreceptors, and mechanoreceptors. A few A-delta fibers also terminate here. The neurons of lamina II are almost entirely interneurons (both excitatory and inhibitory), the dendrites of which arborize within the lamina and also project into other laminae. Some interneurons respond to noxious stimuli, whereas others respond to both noxious and innocuous stimuli (Basbaum and Jessell, 2000).

Laminae III and IV are similar and are described together. These laminae (and sometimes the upper part of lamina V) often are called the nucleus proprius. The majority of the primary afferent input arrives via A-beta fibers, which transmit innocuous input from mechanoreceptors such as pacinian corpuscles, peritrichial endings surrounding hair follicles, and Meissner's corpuscles. Although direct afferent input synapses on the interneurons within laminae III and IV, the dendrites of these interneurons also project dorsally into lamina II. Some lamina II neurons also project axons ventrally into these laminae and thus influence laminae III and IV neurons and their sensory input. Thus considerable inter-

laminar communication occurs. The types of neurons present in these laminae include interneurons and some tract neurons.

Lamina V forms the neck of the dorsal horn. Primary afferent input comes via A-delta fibers from cutaneous mechanical nociceptors and group III and IV muscle and joint afferents, and nociceptive visceral afferents (Willis and Coggeshall, 1991; Basbaum and Jessell, 2000). Additional input to this lamina (such as input from C fibers) is most likely received via the dendritic projections located within more dorsal laminae. Many neurons within this lamina are wide-dynamic-range tract neurons that are the site of viscerosomatic convergence for visceral referred pain (Benarroch et al., 1999), whereas others are interneurons and propriospinal neurons.

Lamina VI is the base of the dorsal horn and is anatomically close to motor regions in the ventral horn, suggesting it is involved with regulation of movement. This lamina is diminished and sometimes absent in segments other than those forming the cervical and lumbosacral enlargements. Proprioceptive information enters via large-diameter afferent fibers such as the group Ia and A-beta fibers. These fibers form the primary afferent input to this lamina. In addition, many descending tracts terminate in this area. Numerous interneurons and propriospinal neurons are present in this lamina also.

In summary, the first six laminae that comprise the dorsal horn are the major receiving areas for sensory

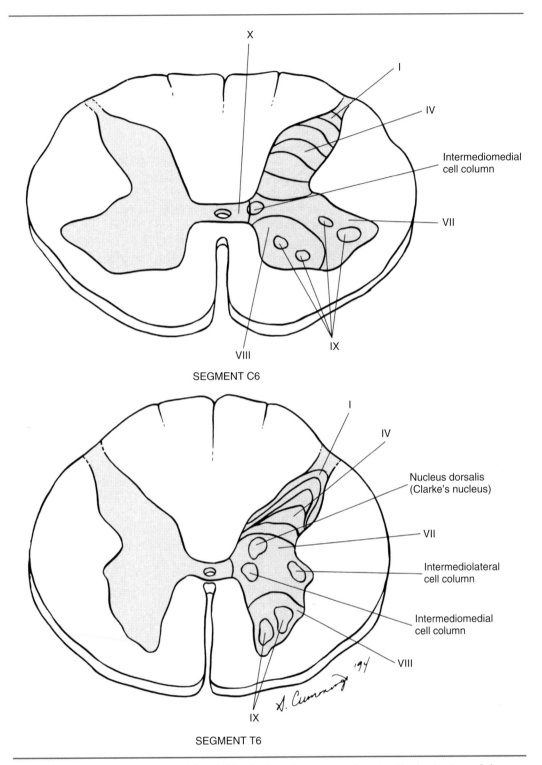

FIG. 9-4 Cross sections of the C6 and T6 spinal cord segments showing the lamination of the gray matter. Examples of nuclei located within the laminae are shown.

information. Pain and temperature input appears to terminate primarily in superficial layers; mechanical types of stimuli terminate in the middle region; and proprioceptive input ends in the base of the dorsal horn near the motor regions. Each primary afferent fiber has many collateral branches that synapse in the circuitry of more than one lamina and feed into more than one ascending pathway. For example, one Ia afferent fiber from a neuromuscular spindle may have 500 or more branches terminating within the gray matter of the cord (Nolte, 2002). Many of the laminae communicate with each other via profuse dendritic branching and the axonal projections of their interneurons. This provides a mechanism by which incoming sensory signals may be processed and modified (modulated) before ascending to higher centers. This modulation occurs at the level of the synapse between presynaptic and postsynaptic neurons and involves not only the release of neurotransmitters and neuromodulators but also the different receptors with which these chemicals bind. This is exemplified by studies of the nociceptive interneurons in lamina II that show that numerous chemicals can modulate synaptic transmission.

Dorsal horn interneurons. Interneurons in the dorsal horn play a key role in modifying sensory information and ongoing movements, as well as controlling all reflexive movements. The extensive branching of the afferent inputs to the spinal cord results in simultaneous activation of many types of interneurons. The activity of these interneurons and their subsequent synapses on cells in the ventral horn (motor systems), ascending tracts (sensory perception of stimuli), descending tracts (sensitivity of motor and sensory pools), and other interneurons in the spinal cord controls the overall sensitivity and general responsiveness of all neurons in the spinal cord. In addition to the input from afferent fibers, the spinal interneurons also receive input from the descending systems, ventral horn alpha motor neurons, local (at the level) interneurons, short propriospinal interneurons (from one or two levels above or below), and long propriospinal interneurons (ascending and descending between all levels of the cord). This vast array of interconnections among and between the various interneurons also contributes to the general responsiveness of the spinal cord to both afferent (sensory or reflexive) and efferent (motor or voluntary) stimuli. The interconnections between the interneurons are mutually inhibitory, meaning that only one set of pathways can be active at any time. When one particular response pathway and its corresponding interneurons are activated, all other interneuronal pathways typically are inhibited. This allows the spinal cord to respond selectively to any input, either afferent or efferent, without inappropriately activating other antagonistic pathways that might hinder

the appropriate response. In addition, interneurons can modulate or alter the normal output of higher-order neurons. One example of this is related to the gate control theory of pain (see Fig. 11-6), in which nonnociceptive afferents reduce the output of second-order pain fibers via inhibitory interneurons in the dorsal horn. Therefore interneurons are the key building blocks of all spinal reflexes, and can control or modulate most afferent and efferent information at the level of the spinal cord (see the Spinal Motor Neurons and Motor Coordination section later in this chapter).

Relationship between the dorsal horn and trigeminal nerve. The dorsal horn of the upper three or four cervical cord segments has an interesting relationship with the trigeminal nerve. The trigeminal nerve (cranial nerve V) provides sensory innervation to the skin of the face and other structures, including the paranasal sinuses, cornea, temporomandibular joint, and oral and nasal mucosae. Cranial nerve V (CN V) also supplies motor fibers to the muscles of mastication and several other small muscles of the head. The afferent fibers of CN V enter the brain stem at the level of the pons and synapse in a nuclear column that extends from the midbrain through the pons and medulla and into the upper cervical cord segments. The portion of the nuclear column located in the medulla and upper cervical cord segments is known as the spinal trigeminal nucleus (Fig. 9-5). Afferent fibers conveying pain and temperature (and some touch) that enter the brain stem within CN V (and also in the facial and glossopharyngeal nerves) descend as the spinal trigeminal tract and synapse in this nucleus. The most inferior portion of the spinal trigeminal nucleus is the nucleus caudalis. This nuclear region continues from the caudal medulla into the upper three or four cervical cord segments and blends with laminae I through IV, and possibly V and VI, of the dorsal horn of those segments (Carpenter, 1991; Williams et al., 1995). This area of gray matter that is the site of convergence of trigeminal and cervical afferents is also called the trigeminocervical (Bogduk, 1992; Biondi, 2001) or trigeminospinal nucleus. The descending spinal trigeminal tract fibers also continue into the dorsolateral tract of Lissauer in the upper cervical segments. Afferent fibers conveying similar information and traveling in dorsal roots of the upper three or four cervical nerves also synapse in these same laminae. In fact, some of these cervical dorsal root afferents may ascend into the rostral medulla and synapse in the spinal trigeminal nucleus (Abrahams, 1989).

The relationship between the dorsal horn and trigeminal system is clinically significant (Pollman, Keidel, and Pfaffenrath, 1997; Biondi, 2000, 2001; Bogduk, 2001). The upper three cervical spinal nerves innervate the muscles (including the trapezius and sternocleidomastoid muscles), ligaments, and joints in the region of the upper three cervical vertebral segments, C2-3 intervertebral discs, vertebral and internal carotid arteries, and dura mater of the upper spinal cord and posterior cranial fossa of the skull. Second-order neurons in the dorsal horn, which project to the brain, receive afferents from pain generators in these structures and potentially from pain generators innervated by lower cervical nerves whose central processes have ascended in the dorsolateral tract of Lissauer. In addition, these second-order neurons receive input from pain generators innervated by CN V primary afferents. When the brain receives this nociceptive information from these spinal pain generators, it can misinterpret the input as coming from the more familiar source, resulting in the perception that the origin is in the territory of CN V. Thus this region of convergence becomes the anatomic basis for pain referral

from the neck to regions innervated by CN V (typically the forehead or orbital region), and vice versa (sometimes called the trigemino-cervical reflex (Lance, 1989; Pollmann, Keidel, and Pfaffenrath, 1997; Browne et al., 1998; Sessle, 1998; Milanov and Bogdanova, 2003). Head pain or headache that is the result of stimulation of pain generators located in the cervical spine is called cervicogenic headache.

Laminae VII through X. Lamina VII composes most of the intermediate region of the gray matter and also extends into the ventral horn (see Fig. 9-4). The shape of lamina VII varies in different regions. For example, in the T1 to L2 or L3 segments, lamina VII includes the lateral horn. Most primary afferent input into this lamina (excluding the lateral horn) and the remaining ventral horn concerns proprioception, although some

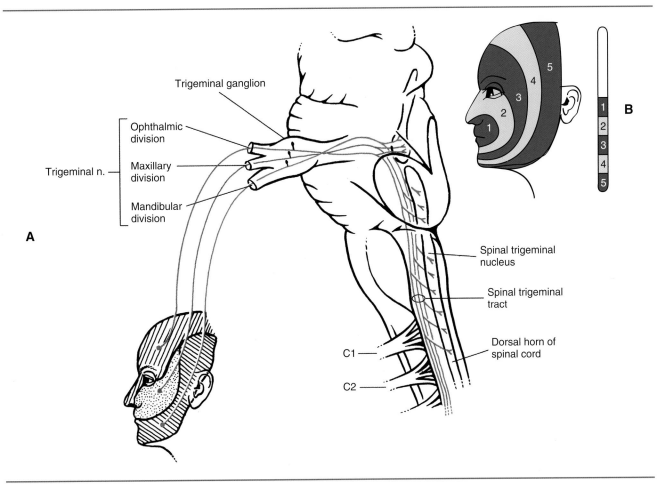

FIG. 9-5 Trigeminal system. **A,** The trigeminal nerve fibers conducting pain and temperature enter the pons of the brain stem and descend in the medulla (as the spinal trigeminal tract) and into the upper three or four cervical cord segments. They synapse in the adjacent spinal trigeminal nucleus of the medulla and dorsal horn of the upper cervical cord segments. This provides the anatomical substrate for pain referral (see text). Note that the descending fibers are arranged within the medulla such that the ophthalmic fibers are ventral, the mandibular fibers are dorsal, and the maxillary fibers are in between. **B,** Representation of trigeminal afferents in the nucleus caudalis of the spinal trigeminal nucleus. Note the "onion skin" pattern created by the five zones and that, 5, the most posterior zone is represented in the most caudal part of the nucleus (approximately at the C3 cord level). The white area in the nucleus receives afferents from the oral cavity and teeth.

neurons receive noxious stimuli via polysynaptic connections (Basbaum and Jessell, 2000). The lateral part of lamina VII (excluding the lateral horn) is involved with the regulation of posture and movement. These neurons, including tract neurons, have numerous ascending (tract neurons) and descending connections with the cerebellum and midbrain. The medial part of lamina VII includes interneurons and propriospinal neurons that connect adjacent laminae and cord segments for reflexes concerned with movement and autonomic activities. In the ventral part of the lamina, inhibitory interneurons, such as Renshaw cells and Ia inhibitory interneurons, have been identified (Williams et al., 1995). Clearly defined nuclei and cell columns also are within lamina VII. One of these is the nucleus dorsalis of Clarke (nucleus thoracicus). This oval nucleus consists of tract neurons and is located in the medial part of lamina VII in segments C8 through L3. It is best defined in the T10 to L2 segments (Carpenter and Sutin, 1983). The axons of these neurons ascend ipsilaterally in the spinal cord white matter to the cerebellum as the dorsal spinocerebellar tract (see Ascending Tracts). A cluster of four nuclei that is associated with the innervation of autonomic effectors also is located in lamina VII (see Chapter 10). The largest of the four is the intermediolateral cell column, which is located in the lateral horn in cord segments T1 to L2 or L3 and consists of autonomic motor neuron cell bodies. The axons of these motor neurons are preganglionic sympathetic fibers that exit in the ventral root and synapse in autonomic sympathetic ganglia. They are involved with the innervation of smooth and cardiac muscles and glands. The sacral autonomic nucleus is found in cord segments S2 to S4, and although there is no lateral horn at that level, this nucleus is located in a similar position to that of the intermediolateral cell column. The sacral autonomic nucleus contains cell bodies, the axons of which form preganglionic parasympathetic fibers. These fibers exit via the S2 to S4 ventral roots, synapse in autonomic ganglia, and innervate the smooth muscle and glands of the pelvic and lower abdominal regions. An additional group of neurons forms the intermediomedial nucleus of lamina VII. This is found in the medial aspect of this lamina and is considered by some authors to be the termination site of visceral afferent fibers (Carpenter and Sutin, 1983). Chapter 10 provides a thorough description of the autonomic nervous system. From this description, it is apparent that lamina VII is composed of all four neuron types: interneurons, tract, propriospinal, and motor neurons.

Lamina VIII is also located in the ventral horn. In spinal cord segments of the cervical and lumbar enlargements, it is found in the medial aspect of the ventral horn. In thoracic segments, lamina VIII is located in the base of the ventral horn. Input to the interneurons and propriospinal neurons of this lamina originates from descending tracts and some proprioceptive afferents. Interneurons from adjacent laminae and the contralateral lamina VIII project here as well.

Lamina IX is found in the ventral horn and consists of well-defined medial and lateral longitudinal nuclear columns, and a central nuclear group of motor neurons (anterior horn cells) (see Fig. 9-4) (Williams et al., 1995). The position and presence of the groups vary at different spinal regions. The medial group (subdivided into dorsal and ventral parts) is found in all cord segments and provides the axons that innervate the axial musculature. The lateral group (subdivided into dorsal, ventral, and retrodorsal groups) is responsible for innervating the muscles of the extremities. These clusters of neurons are organized so that the more lateral the motor neurons, the more distal the muscles they innervate. Also, the dorsal motor neuronal groups innervate the flexor muscles, and the ventral motor neuronal groups innervate the extensor muscles. In addition, one specific group of ventrolateral neurons located in the S1 and S2 segments forms Onuf's nucleus. The axons from this nucleus innervate the perineal musculature (Williams et al., 1995). The addition of these lateral motor neuronal groups in cord segments supplying the extremity muscles creates a distinctive lateral enlargement in the ventral horn.

The third nuclear group of lamina IX is the central group. This group includes three nuclei located in specific cord segments. One of these is the lumbosacral nucleus, which is located in the L2-S1 cord segments. The projections from this nucleus are unknown (Williams et al., 1995). Another nuclear column forms the phrenic nucleus, which is found in the C3 to C5 segments. The axons of these segments, and in particular C4, form the phrenic nerve, which provides innervation to the diaphragm. Based on cadaveric studies, Routal and Pal (1999) suggest that the phrenic nucleus is not part of a central column but instead actually is a subdivision of the medial column. The diaphragm develops as an axial muscle and therefore the phrenic nucleus is located near the other motor neurons that innervate the axial musculature (i.e., the medial motor column). The location of the nucleus in the C3-5 segments and the location of the nucleus' efferent fibers also may have clinical significance. As exemplified by two case studies, severe cases of cervical spondylotic myelopathy could traumatize the phrenic nucleus or its efferent fibers, resulting in phrenic paresis (Parke and Whalen, 2001). The other nucleus is the accessory nucleus, which extends from the lower medulla into the C5 cord segment (Routal and Pal, 1999). Axons from this nucleus form the spinal root of the spinal accessory nerve (CN XI). They ascend in the vertebral canal dorsal to the denticulate ligament and travel through the foramen magnum to enter the cranial cavity and briefly join the cranial root of CN XI. Subsequently this nerve exits the cranial cavity, and the spinal root fibers branch away to innervate the sternocleidomastoid and trapezius muscles. This nucleus may be somatotopically organized in a craniocaudal direction and subdivided into two parts, with the upper part of the nucleus projecting to the sternocleidomastoid muscle, and the lower part projecting to the trapezius muscle (Routal and Pal, 1999).

Each of these three major groups of lamina IX includes alpha motor neurons, which project to extrafusal skeletal muscle fibers and are subdivided into tonic (to slow muscle fibers) and phasic (to clusters of fast muscle fibers) neurons; beta motor neurons, which course to extrafusal and intrafusal fibers; and gamma motor neurons, which innervate the contractile portion of the neuromuscular spindles located within skeletal muscles and are subdivided into static and dynamic types (Williams et al., 1995; FitzGerald and Folan-Curran, 2002). The alpha and gamma motor neurons are tightly packed into pools responsible for the innervation of a particular skeletal muscle. Both types of motor neurons receive excitatory and inhibitory input from neighboring interneurons that have formed local reflex circuits, propriospinal neurons, and some descending tract fibers. These connections modulate the activity of the motor neurons. Alpha motor neurons also receive the primary afferent fibers from neuromuscular spindles that form the sensory arc of the stretch (myotatic) reflex (see Spinal Motor Neurons and Motor Coordination). The cell bodies of the alpha motor neurons, which are large and range from 30 to 70 μm in size, receive a tremendous amount of synaptic input. An estimated 10,000 excitatory boutons of descending fibers from the brain and propriospinal neurons may synapse on the extensive dendritic tree of a typical alpha motor neuron, and some 5000 inhibitory propriospinal boutons synapse on the cell bodies of alpha motor neurons (FitzGerald and Folan-Curran, 2002). These connections indicate the extensive level of neuronal integration occurring at this cell. Gamma motor neurons are smaller (10 to 30 μm) and have a lower threshold to stimuli than alpha motor neurons (Davidoff and Hackman, 1991; Williams et al., 1995). In addition to the motor neurons, lamina IX includes some interneurons and propriospinal neurons (Carpenter and Sutin, 1983; Williams et al., 1995; Kiernan, 1998).

The last lamina to be mentioned is lamina X. This region forms the commissural area between the two halves of the gray matter and surrounds the central canal. It consists of interneurons and some decussating axons. Lamina X receives input from A-delta fibers transmitting information from mechanical nociceptors and group C visceral afferents (Willis and Coggeshall, 1991).

In summary, the gray matter is divided into 10 laminae, each of which may vary in size and shape within the different cord segments (Fig. 9-6). This variation results in a notable difference in the overall amount and shape of gray matter present in the various regions of the spinal cord. Also, there is a difference in the appearance and amount of white matter throughout the cord because of the presence or absence of certain tracts at different levels. For example, the amount of white matter is greater in the cervical cord than in other areas because all ascending and descending tracts to and from the brain traverse this region (Fig. 9-6). Table 9-4 summarizes the types of neuron cell bodies found in each lamina, the primary afferent fiber types terminating in each lamina, and the laminae in which descending (motor) fibers from higher centers synapse.

Dorsal Root Entry Zone

Peripheral receptors and the spinal gray matter are linked together through sensory afferent fibers. Stimulated receptors transmit their information to the CNS via peripheral processes. These processes may be classified according to their velocity of conduction as a group A or group C cutaneous or visceral fiber or as a group I, II, III, or IV fiber from muscle or joint receptors. Peripheral processes course with efferent motor fibers in peripheral nerves, dorsal and ventral rami, and spinal nerves. They are processes of pseudounipolar neurons, the cell bodies of which form a dorsal root ganglion. This ganglion is located in the IVF. The pseudounipolar neuron also has a central process, which, with many other central processes, forms a dorsal root. Because each peripheral and central process is a component of one neuron, this sensory or afferent neuron does not synapse until it reaches the CNS. As the dorsal root approaches the spinal cord within the vertebral canal, it branches into numerous rootlets. Each rootlet becomes a myriad of fibers conveying various types of sensory information.

As the rootlet fibers enter the dorsal root entry zone, they become arranged into lateral and medial divisions (Fig. 9-7). The lateral division contains thinly myelinated and unmyelinated fibers, which include the nociceptive (pain) and temperature, or A-delta and C fibers. These fibers first enter an area of white matter located at the tip of the dorsal horn called the dorsolateral tract of Lissauer and then continue into the gray matter of the cord. The dorsolateral tract of Lissauer is found in all cord segments, but it is most developed in the upper cervical segments. Collateral branches of the entering fibers are given off within the dorsolateral tract of Lissauer, some of which ascend or descend a few segments before also synapsing in the gray matter. It has been suggested that visceral afferent fibers may give off collateral branches that span as many as five segments (Chandler, Zhang, and Foreman, 1996; Jänig, 1996). In addition to the ascending and descending branches, the dorsolateral tract of Lissauer also contains fibers from the substantia

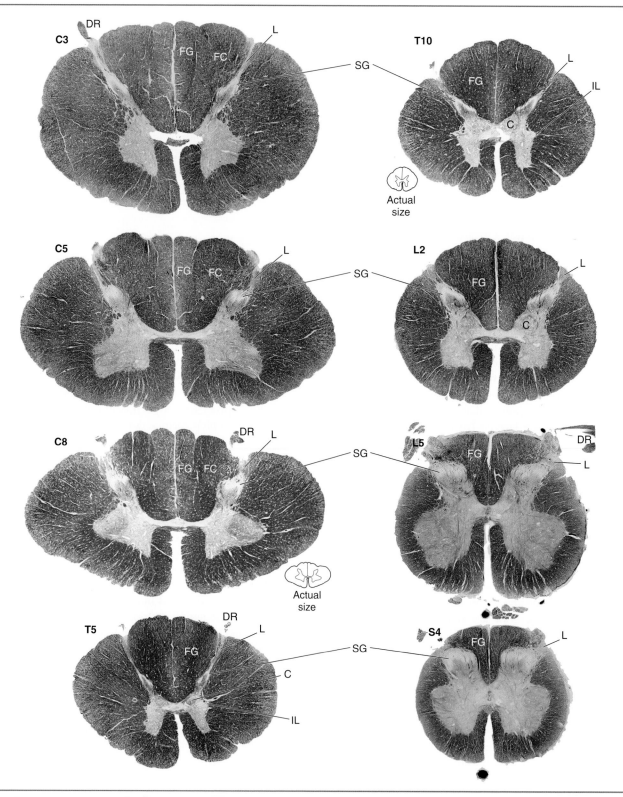

FIG. 9-6   Cross sections of the spinal cord. Note the variation in the overall shapes and the different amounts and appearances of gray matter and white matter present in the various regions of the spinal cord. *FG,* Fasciculus gracilis; *FC,* fasciculus cuneatus; *L,* Lissauer's tract; *DR,* dorsal root; *SG,* substantia gelatinosa; *C,* Clarke's nucleus; and, *IL,* intermediolateral cell column. (From Nolte J. [2002]. The human brain [5th ed.]. St Louis: Mosby.)

Table 9-4   General Summary of Input to and Neurons in the Laminae of Rexed

Lamina	Tract	Motor	Interneuron	Propriospinal	Primary Afferent Fiber Type	Termination of Descending Motor Fibers
	Types of Neurons Present					
I	X		X		A-delta, (C)	
II			X		C, (A-delta)	
III	(X)*		X		A-beta	
IV	(X)		X		A-beta	(X)
V	X		X	X	A-delta, III, IV	X
VI	(X)		X	X	I, II	X
VII	X	X	X	X	I, II	X
VIII	(X)		X	X	(I, II)	X
IX		X	X	X	I, (II)	(X)
X			X		A-delta	

*All parentheses indicate minor contribution.

gelatinosa (lamina II) that interconnect with laminae II of other levels. Other propriospinal fibers also have been identified in the dorsolateral tract (Williams et al., 1995). At all levels, the lateral division primary afferent fibers may synapse on tract neurons in the dorsal horn and intermediate gray, interneurons in the dorsal horn, and interneurons involved with somatic and visceral reflex responses.

The medial division of the dorsal root entry zone contains large- and intermediate-diameter fibers from such receptors as proprioceptors (e.g., neuromuscular spindles) and mechanoreceptors (e.g., Meissner's and pacinian corpuscles). These fibers enter medial to Lissauer's tract. Branches of these fibers may ascend directly in the dorsal white column of the spinal cord to the medulla of the brain stem, or give off collateral branches to the dorsal horn and then ascend. In addition, branches may synapse on tract neurons in the intermediate gray (e.g., Clarke's nucleus in lamina VII) or on interneurons and motor neurons involved with segmental reflexes (e.g., lamina IX and the stretch reflex), or synapse on dorsal horn interneurons involved with pain modulation.

As stated, after entering the cord each of these primary afferent fibers is the origin of many branches that synapse with numerous neurons in various laminae and in cord segments at multiple levels. Consequently, one primary afferent fiber may be involved with many local neuronal circuits and pathways and thus have an impact on a variety of neuronal activities.

When the primary afferents enter the dorsal horn, they synapse in the gray matter and release neurotransmitters. These neurotransmitters include excitatory amino acids and neuropeptides. Many primary afferents appear to release glutamate (or aspartate or both) as their primary neurotransmitter. Glutamate has been localized in peripheral nerves, dorsal root ganglia, dorsal

roots, and the dorsal horn. Excitatory neuropeptides found in the presynaptic terminals of small-diameter primary afferent fibers include substance P and calcitonin gene-related peptide (CGRP). Substance P is synthesized in the cell bodies found in the dorsal root ganglia and is transported (via fast axonal transport) to the terminals of small-diameter nociceptive fibers in the dorsal horn. The fibers' terminals are prevalent in laminae I and II. CGRP has been identified in the cell bodies found in the dorsal root ganglia (often co-localized along with substance P), in group A-delta and C dorsal root fibers, Lissauer's tract, and the presynaptic terminals of afferent fibers that synapse in dorsal horn laminae. Additional excitatory neuropeptides released by small-diameter afferent fibers, which are less well known, include somatostatin, cholecystokinin, thyrotropin-releasing hormone, and vasoactive intestinal polypeptide (Willis and Coggeshall, 1991).

In summary, the pathway for sensory information generally can be described as beginning in a peripheral receptor and continuing through peripheral nerves, dorsal or ventral rami, spinal nerves, dorsal roots, and dorsal rootlets. Within each rootlet a fiber travels in either the medial or the lateral division. Once in the spinal cord, the fiber's future course depends on the type of information it is conveying. Most fibers terminate in various laminae of the gray matter. The next section describes the white matter of the spinal cord and the continuation of sensory information to higher centers.

White Matter

The white matter of the spinal cord is seen in cross section to be a distinct region located peripheral to the gray matter. It contains myelinated and unmyelinated axons, glial cells, and capillaries. The white matter consists of three regions: a dorsal funiculus (column)

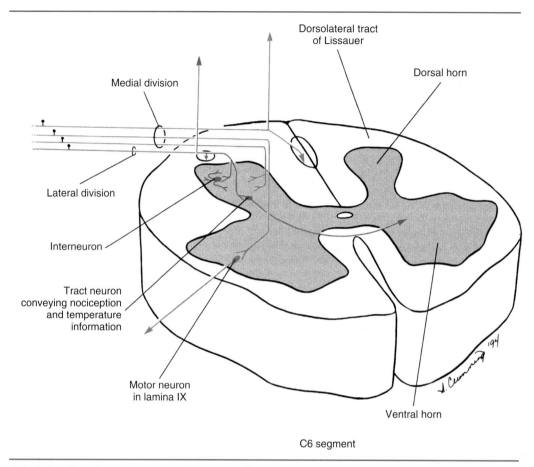

C6 segment

FIG. 9-7 Dorsal root entry zone illustrating fibers in one rootlet. The lateral division fibers use the dorsolateral tract of Lissauer to enter the laminae associated with nociception (pain) and temperature. Collateral branches of these fibers ascend and descend in Lissauer's tract before they enter the dorsal horn of nearby segments. The medial division fibers, which include large-diameter fibers, enter the cord medial to Lissauer's tract, where many ascend and descend. Others enter the medial aspect of the gray matter to synapse in various laminae, such as lamina IX of the ventral horn, the location of alpha motor neurons.

between the dorsal horns, a lateral funiculus (column) between each dorsal horn and ventral horn, and a ventral funiculus (column) between the ventral horns. Tracts, or fasciculi, are present within each of these regions (Fig. 9-8). These may be ascending tracts, which convey sensory information to higher centers, or descending tracts, which originate in higher centers and send descending signals to the cord. These descending signals are involved primarily with some type of motor information. Other axons are confined to the spinal cord and interconnect cord segments at various levels. These form the fasciculus proprius, which is an area of white matter located immediately adjacent to the gray matter. It consists of descending and ascending axons of propriospinal neurons. Concerning the ascending and descending tracts associated with higher centers, each tract contains axons that have a common origin, destination, and function. During a neurologic examination, the integrity of

certain tracts is tested. Therefore familiarity of the location of these tracts aids the clinician in localizing lesions within the CNS.

Ascending Tracts. In general, an ascending tract can be classified into one of three groups based on the three different functions that are provided by the somatosensory system. One group contains tracts that transmit information concerning the type, location, and intensity of a stimulus. These are considered to be direct or discriminatory tracts. A second group consists of tracts that transmit information about the initiation of reflexes that may be concerned with arousal, affective, and motivational responses to a stimulus. The third group of tracts includes those that transmit information concerning the unconscious monitoring and control of motor activity, such as posture and movement (Benarroch et al., 1999). Ascending tracts convey information that has originated from a stimulated peripheral receptor located in the skin, muscles, tendons, joints, or viscera. When a receptor is stimulated, it transmits an action potential via the peripheral and central processes of sensory (afferent) neurons to the CNS. The sensory fibers that convey the action potential from the peripheral receptors are sometimes called first-order neurons, because they are the first neuron in a chain of neurons that proceeds to a higher center such as the cerebral cortex for conscious awareness of the stimulus, or the cerebellar cortex for regulation of motor patterns (Fig. 9-9). On entering the cord, numerous first-order neurons synapse on neurons in the gray matter of the spinal cord, whereas others, after contributing collateral branches to the gray matter, ascend and synapse in nuclear gray matter in the caudal medulla of the brain stem. The next neuron of the chain that leaves the gray matter of the cord or medulla to ascend to higher centers is known as the second-order neuron. Along with many others, this neuron makes up a specific tract. If sensory information is perceived consciously, the second-order neuron decussates and subsequently synapses with a third-order neuron in the thalamus, which is located in the diencephalon of the brain. The thalamus is an oval-shaped area of gray matter that consists of numerous nuclear subgroups (Fig. 9-10). All sensory information traveling to the cerebral cortex (except olfaction) synapses in one of these thalamic nuclei. From here, the third-order thalamic neuron fibers course in a

thick bundle of axons called the internal capsule (which also includes efferent fibers from the cerebral cortex) and terminate in the cortex, thus completing the chain. The thalamus is not simply a relay station through which sensory information is routed to reach its cortical destination. In fact, there is a crude awareness of pain and temperature sensations at this level. In reality, the thalamus functions more like a complex processing center, or gatekeeper. Through the processing within a thalamic nucleus, and in conjunction with excitatory and inhibitory input from other centers (e.g., brain stem nuclei, reticular formation, and cerebral cortex), the thalamus is able to modulate its sensory output to the cerebral cortex based on the immediate needs of the individual (Amaral, 2000).

Certain important characteristics should be identified when considering the tracts of the CNS. These include the direction of the tract (i.e., ascending or descending, which usually is indicated by the name), the specific type of information the tract is conveying, if the tract crosses, and the location of crossing. This information is summarized in Tables 9-5 and 9-6. The ascending tracts are discussed first, beginning with the most clinically and anatomically relevant. These major tracts are well defined, and much information has been gathered about them. Secondary tracts are then discussed, about which limited information is available. They appear to supplement the major tracts by conveying similar types of information.

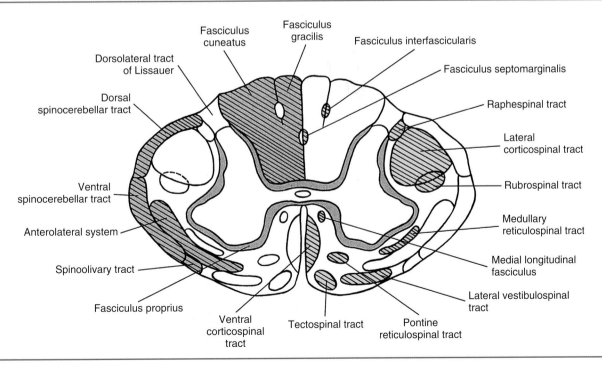

FIG. 9-8   Cross section of the spinal cord illustrating the organization of white matter into fasciculi and tracts. Boundaries usually overlap but are well defined here for illustrative purposes. Ascending tracts are indicated on the left side (*green*). Descending tracts are indicated on the right side (*yellow*); the fasciculus proprius also is shown (*blue*).

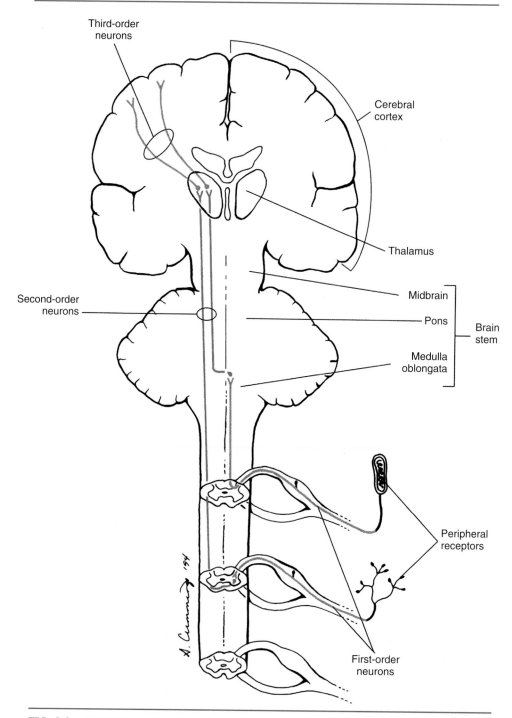

FIG. 9-9 Neuronal organization of ascending information to the cerebral cortex. Note that there are three neurons involved. The first-order neuron (*blue*) cell body is in the dorsal root ganglion. The second-order neuron cell body is located in either the gray matter of the spinal cord or medulla of the brain stem. Its axon (*red*) ascends contralaterally and terminates in the thalamus. The third-order neuron (*green*) courses to the cerebral cortex.

Dorsal column-medial lemniscal system. The first system of ascending fibers to be discussed is the dorsal column-medial lemniscus (DC-ML). Dorsal column refers to the first-order fibers located ipsilaterally (in reference to the side of fiber entry) in the dorsal white column of the spinal cord. Medial lemniscus refers to the second-order fibers located contralaterally in the brain stem. The DC-ML system conveys discriminatory (two-point) touch, some light (crude) touch, pressure, vibration, and joint position sense (conscious proprioception). This input provides temporal and spatial discriminatory qualities that allow for the conscious awareness of body part position at rest and during movements, and the conscious appreciation of the intensity and localization of touch, pressure, and vibration.

The peripheral receptors, which are mechanoreceptors (e.g., neuromuscular spindles, joint receptors, GTOs), have been discussed. The afferent fibers of these mechanoreceptors are large diameter; therefore they are located in the medial division of the dorsal root entry zone and subsequently enter the cord just medial to the dorsolateral tract of Lissauer. As these first-order neurons enter, they bifurcate into long ascending and short descending branches. The descending branches descend as the fasciculus interfascicularis in the upper half of the cord and as the fasciculus septomarginalis in the lower cord segments (see Fig. 9-8). These synapse in spinal gray matter and are involved in mediating reflex responses. The longer fibers contribute collateral branches to the spinal gray matter to participate in intersegmental

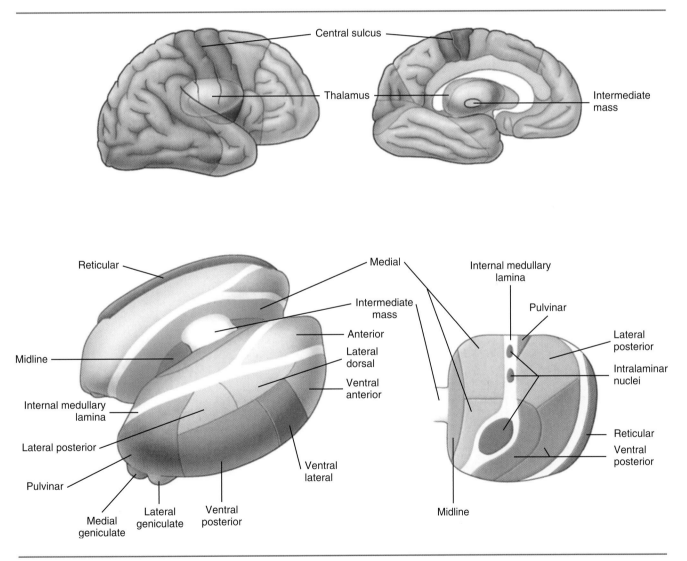

FIG. 9-10   Thalamus. This area of gray matter is located approximately in the center of the brain and is divided into nuclear subgroups. Note the ventral posterior nucleus and intralaminar nuclei, which are the synaptic locations for tract axons conveying general sensory information from the body. (From Tortora GJ, & Grabowski SR. [2003]. *Principles of Anatomy and Physiology* [10th ed.]. New York: John Wiley & Sons, Inc.)

Table 9-5 Ascending Tracts

Tract	Information Conveyed	First-Order Cell Bodies	Second-Order Cell Bodies	Crossed	Third-Order Cell Bodies	Termination
Dorsal column-medial lemniscus	Two-point touch, light touch, joint position sense, vibration, pressure, stereognosis, graphesthesia	Dorsal root ganglia (DRG)	Gracilis and cuneate nuclei	Yes; internal arcuate fibers (in medulla)	Ventral posterior (lateral) nucleus of thalamus (VPL)	Postcentral gyrus and paracentral lobule (posterior part)
Spinothalamic: neo and paleo	Pain, temperature, light touch	DRG	Dorsal horn laminae	Yes; in ventral white commissure	VPL (neo) and intralaminar (paleo) thalamic nuclei	Postcentral gyrus and paracentral lobule (posterior part) (neo) and widespread cortex/limbic system (paleo)
Spinoreticular	Pain and temperature	DRG	Intermediate gray laminae	Majority; in ventral white commissure	—	Pontine and medullary reticular formation
Spinomesencephalic (spinotectal)	Pain (and temperature)	DRG	Dorsal horn laminae	Yes; in ventral white commissure	—	Midbrain: superior colliculus and periaqueductal gray
Dorsal spinocerebellar	Lower limb position sense	DRG	Clarke's nucleus (nucleus dorsalis)	No	—	Cerebellum via inferior cerebellar peduncle
Cuneocerebellar	Upper limb position sense	DRG	Lateral cuneate nucleus	No	—	Cerebellum via inferior cerebellar peduncle
Ventral spinocerebellar	Lower limb position sense	DRG	Lamina VII	Yes; in cord and recrosses in cerebellum	—	Cerebellum via superior cerebellar peduncle
Spino-olivary	Limb position sense	DRG	Spinal gray	Yes; in medulla	—	Inferior olivary nucleus

Table 9-6   Descending Tracts

Tract	Function	Origin	Crossed	Termination
Corticospinal	Voluntary (skilled) movement	Motor (some sensory) cerebral cortex	Majority cross (lateral corticospinal tract) as pyramidal decussation (in medulla)	Intermediate gray and ventral horn
Rubrospinal	Facilitates flexor and inhibits extensor muscle groups	Red nucleus	Yes; ventral tegmental decussation (in midbrain)	Intermediate gray and ventral horn
Medullary reticulospinal	Facilitates/inhibits muscle groups	Medullary reticular formation	Some cross (others remain uncrossed)	Intermediate gray and ventral horn
Pontine reticulospinal	Facilitates/inhibits muscle groups	Pontine reticular formation	No	Ventral horn
Lateral vestibulospinal	Facilitates antigravity muscles	Lateral vestibular nucleus	No	Ventral horn
Tectospinal	Reflex postural movements in response to visual, auditory, and somatic sensory stimuli	Superior colliculus	Yes; dorsal tegmental decussation (in midbrain)	Ventral horn of cervical segments
Medial vestibulospinal (in MLF)	Coordinates head and eye movements	Medial vestibular nucleus	Some crosse (others remain uncrossed)	Ventral horn of cervical segments
Raphespinal	Pain inhibition	Raphe nuclei	No	Dorsal horn
Descending autonomic fibers	Modulates autonomic nervous system functions	Hypothalamus and brain stem nuclei	No	Spinal gray matter

MLF, Medial longitudinal fasciculus.

reflexes and ascend ipsilaterally in the dorsal (white) column of the cord and continue into the medulla of the brain stem (Fig. 9-11). The first synapse occurs here in the nuclei gracilis and cuneatus, which are deep to the tubercles of the same name (Fig. 9-12). As the first-order neurons enter the dorsal white column, each neuron comes to lie more laterally to the fibers that entered more inferiorly. For example, information entering via a lumbar nerve ascends in the dorsal column in axons located lateral to the axons conveying information entering via a sacral nerve. In a cross section of the C3 spinal cord, first-order neurons conveying information (specific for the DC-ML system) from areas of the body innervated by sacral nerves are found most medial, followed in a lateral sequence by axons conveying information from areas innervated by lumbar, thoracic, and cervical nerves (see Fig. 9-11).

At the midthoracic level of the cord and above, the dorsal column is divided by the dorsal intermediate sulcus into a medial fasciculus gracilis and lateral fasciculus cuneatus. The dorsal intermediate sulcus extends ventrally from the cord's periphery to approximately one half of the way into the dorsal column. This sulcus acts as a mechanical barrier preventing medial migration of the cuneate fibers (Smith and Deacon, 1984). Thus the

fasciculus gracilis, which is found in all cord segments, includes axons of middle and lower thoracic, lumbar, and sacral nerves and therefore generally conveys information from the ipsilateral lower extremity. Smith and Deacon (1984) investigated the dorsal columns of human spinal cords and found that the orientation of the fasciculus gracilis fibers varied. In the most caudal part of the fasciculus, the fibers were oriented parallel to the medial side of the dorsal horn, whereas the upper lumbar and lower thoracic fibers were parallel to the dorsal median septum. However, the fibers in the fasciculus gracilis located in the remaining cord segments were oriented obliquely in a ventromedial-to-dorsolateral fashion. The authors also found that some overlapping of fibers occurred within the fasciculus gracilis but little if any occurred between the fasciculus gracilis and fasciculus cuneatus.

The fasciculus cuneatus includes axons of upper and middle thoracic and cervical nerves and, in general, conveys information from the ipsilateral upper extremity (see Fig. 9-11).

In addition to the mediolateral arrangement of fibers in the dorsal column, the type of modality is organized during the fibers' ascent such that input from hair receptors is superficial, whereas tactile and vibratory information ascends via deeper fibers (Williams et al.,

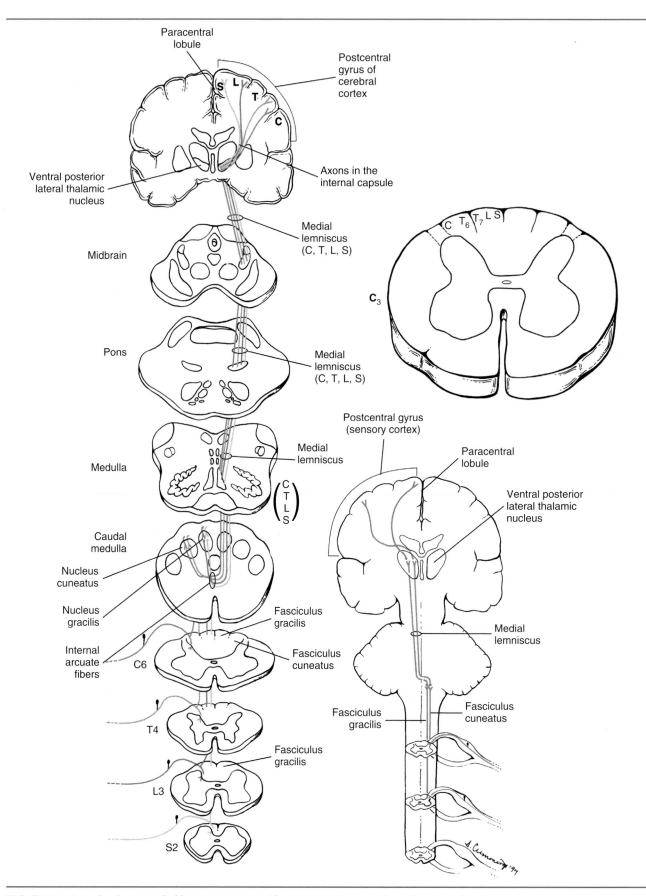

FIG. 9-11   Dorsal column-medial lemniscus system. The cross sections are through various locations of the central nervous system and show the location of the ascending fibers. The ascending fibers are color coded (*yellow*, sacral; *red*, lumbar; *blue*, thoracic; *green*, cervical) to correspond to their cord level of entry. Note the somatotopic organization of these fibers in the spinal cord and brain stem as they ascend to the cerebral cortex.

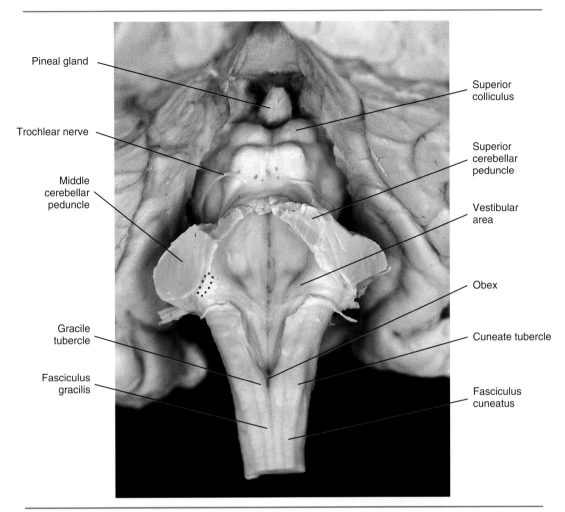

FIG. 9-12   Dorsal view of the brain stem. The cerebellum has been removed to expose the floor of the fourth ventricle. Red stippled area indicates the inferior cerebellar peduncle.

1995). Smith and Deacon (1984) demonstrated that the cross-sectional shape of each fasciculus (both gracilis and cuneatus) is different in each of the upper thoracic and cervical segments, and thus characteristic of that particular segment. The authors also believe that the fasciculi gracilis and cuneatus should be regarded as separate anatomic entities.

As mentioned, the first-order neurons of the fasciculi gracilis and cuneatus synapse with second-order neurons in the nuclei of the same name in the caudal medulla. The axons of the second-order neurons decussate (cross) in the caudal medulla (in a region called the sensory or lemniscal decussation); as they do so, they form a bundle of fibers known as the internal arcuate fibers (see Fig. 9-11). These second-order neurons then ascend through the brain stem as a fiber bundle known as the medial lemniscus. The lemniscal fibers are organized in the medulla such that information originating from the lower extremity and transmitted to the spinal cord in

lumbar and sacral nerves is conveyed by fibers that are ventral to fibers conveying information originating from the upper extremity and transmitted to the cord in (primarily) cervical nerves. In the pons the fibers shift so that the lower extremity information is conveyed by fibers located lateral to the fibers conveying information from the upper extremity. In the midbrain of the brain stem, the lower extremity fibers become located dorsolateral to the upper extremity fibers. Clinically, it is imperative to recognize that the decussation of fibers occurs in the medulla. A unilateral lesion (e.g., trauma, vascular insufficiency, tumor) in the medial lemniscus of the brain stem produces contralateral deficits (e.g., loss of vibration, loss of joint position sense), whereas a lesion in the dorsal column of the spinal cord produces ipsilateral deficits.

The medial lemniscus ascends to the ventral posterior (lateral part) nucleus of the thalamus and synapses on third-order neurons (see Figs. 9-10, 9-11, and 9-14). The axons of the third-order neurons travel in the internal capsule (a mass of axons going to and coming from the cerebral cortex) by way of the corona radiata to the primary sensory area of the cerebral cortex, which is located in the postcentral gyrus and paracentral lobule (posterior part) of the parietal lobe (Figs. 9-13 and 9-14; see also Fig. 9-11). From here, neurons project to adjacent cortical areas for further higher-level processing. This includes the integration of the information that is useful for the execution of movements and the same for the appreciation of the significance of the sensory input. For example, through the sense of touch and without visual input, one is able to recognize an object placed in the hand (stereognosis) or identify numbers or letters traced on the skin (graphesthesia). The DC-ML system maintains the spatial relationships of all parts of the body throughout its course in the CNS and allows the surface and underlying body structures to be mapped onto the primary sensory area of the cerebral cortex. This arrangement is called somatotopic organization. This organiza-

tion is illustrated by a mapping of the entire body surface on the somatosensory cortex that depicts the location and amount of cortex dedicated to the processing of sensory information from a particular part of the body. The map, called the homunculus, represents the density of the innervation, rather than the size, of that particular body part (Fig. 9-15).

Anterolateral system. The remaining tracts discussed in this chapter follow a basic plan in which first-order neurons terminate in the spinal cord gray matter. One group of tracts conveys nociception (pain) and temperature and some light touch. The tracts of this group ascend in the anterolateral quadrant of the spinal cord white matter and are collectively called the anterolateral system (ALS). This system consists of the spinothalamic, spinoreticular, and spinomesencephalic tracts (Young, 1986; Willis and Coggeshall, 1991; Basbaum and Jessell, 2000; Nolte, 2002). Nociception is conveyed by fast-conducting A-delta fibers (6 to 30 m/s) and slow-

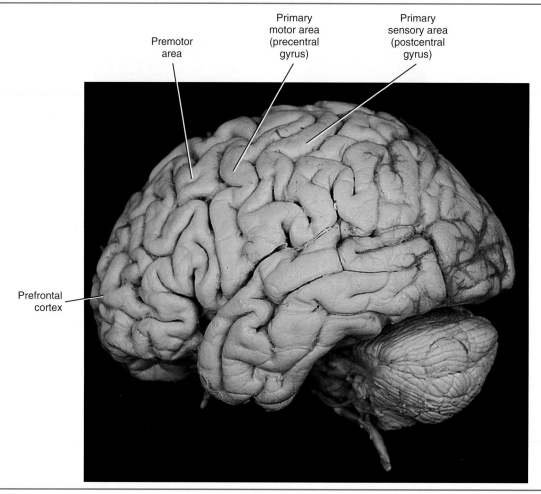

FIG. 9-13   Lateral view of the brain showing the primary motor (precentral gyrus), premotor, and primary sensory (postcentral gyrus) areas of the cerebral cortex. Prefrontal cortex is also indicated.

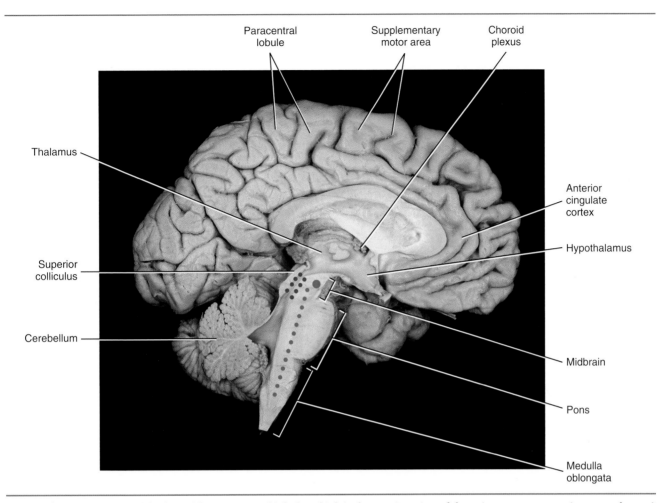

Paracentral
lobule

Supplementary
motor area

Choroid
plexus

Thalamus

Anterior
cingulate
cortex

Hypothalamus

Superior
colliculus

Cerebellum

Midbrain

Pons

Medulla
oblongata

FIG. 9-14   Medial view of the brain. The paracentral lobule, which is the continuation of the primary motor area (precentral gyrus) and primary sensory area (postcentral gyrus) of the cerebral cortex, is indicated. Purple stippled area outlines the periaqueductal gray. Solid red area indicates the location of the red nucleus. Green stippled area indicates the reticular formation.

conducting C fibers (0.5 to 2 m/s) and is divided into two main types of pain. The A-delta fibers convey nociceptive information that is precisely localized and is perceived as being sharp, acute, or pinpricklike pain. It is perceived approximately 0.1 seconds after the stimulus has occurred and acts to alert the individual to potential tissue damage. It is typically confined to the skin. Slow-conducting C fibers convey nociceptive information that is described as burning, aching, or throbbing pain and is felt 1 second or later after the stimulus has occurred. This pain is appreciated secondarily to the fast pain, lasts much longer, and is poorly localized. It can occur from damage in any tissue (Snell, 2001). Temperature sense is also conveyed by A-delta and C fibers.

The first-order neurons of all of the ALS tracts enter the cord via the lateral division of the dorsal root entry zone and pass into the dorsolateral tract of Lissauer. Here, collateral branches ascend and descend, as well

as enter and then synapse, in spinal cord laminae (Fig. 9-16). The spinothalamic tract originates primarily in laminae I, IV to VI, and even from laminae VII and VIII (Young, 1986; Hodge and Apkarian, 1990; Noback, Strominger, and Demarest, 1991; Willis and Coggeshall, 1991; Williams et al., 1995; Willis and Westlund, 1997). The second-order fibers decussate in the cord's ventral white commissure within one or two segments of entry, although recent studies suggest that the fibers cross transversely rather than diagonally (Nathan, Smith, and Deacon, 2001). The fibers then ascend in the anterolateral white matter of the cord and brain stem to terminate in the thalamus. As they travel through the brain stem, collateral branches are given off to the reticular formation. Fibers from the thalamus course through the internal capsule to terminate in the cerebral cortex.

The spinothalamic and spinoreticular tracts are sometimes differentiated based on the order of their appearance during vertebrate evolution. The spinoreticular

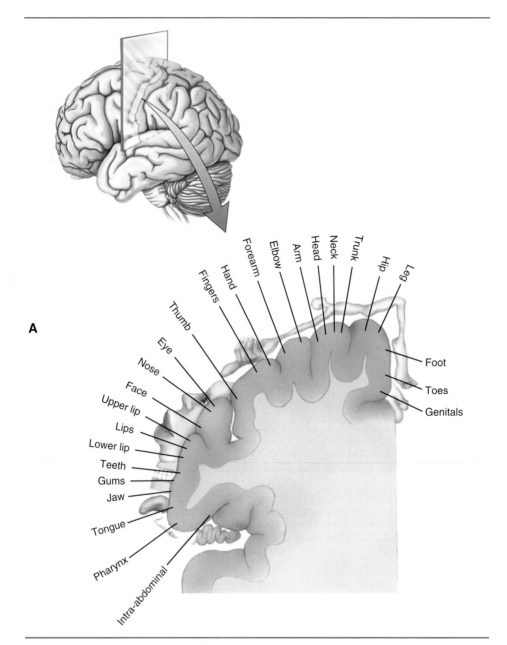

FIG. 9-15   The homunculus. **A,** The sensory homunculus is a somatotopic mapping of the body surface on the cortex (postcentral gyrus and posterior part of the paracentral lobule) indicating the location and amount of cortex assigned to the processing of sensory information from a particular part of the body. (From Bear, Connors, & Paradiso. [2001]. *Neuroscience: Exploring the brain* [2nd ed.]. Baltimore: Lippincott Williams & Wilkins.)

tract appeared first (i.e., is present in lower vertebrate animals), terminating in the reticular formation. Third-order neurons then project to the medial thalamic nuclear group. When mammals evolved, a group of fibers developed that coursed directly to the medial thalamic nuclear group but included collateral branches to the reticular formation. These fibers are called the paleo-spinothalamic tract or spinoreticulothalamic tract. This tract is similar to the spinoreticular tract. Lastly, a tract evolved that coursed directly to the lateral thalamic nuclear group and became the most developed in primates. This is called the neospinothalamic tract (Basbaum and Jessell, 2000; FitzGerald and Folan-Curran, 2002). The neospinothalamic tract originates from tract neurons

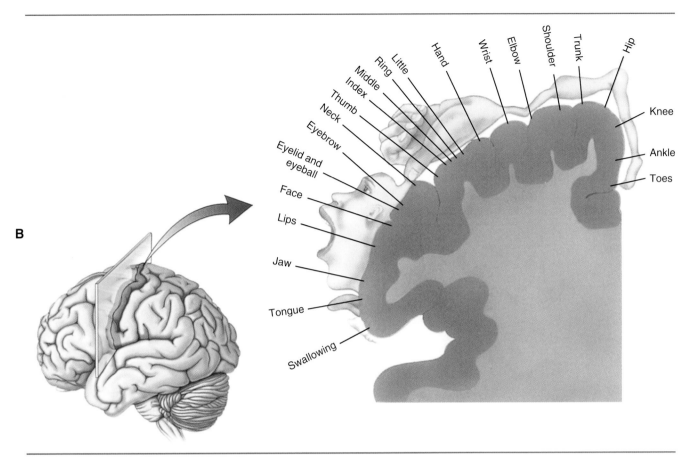

B

FIG. 9-15—cont'd **B,** The motor homunculus is a somatotopic mapping indicating the location and amount of cortex (precentral gyrus and anterior part of the paracentral lobule) associated with a specific motor neuron pool, which controls muscles of a particular part of the body. (From Bear, Connors, & Paradiso. [2001]. *Neuroscience: Exploring the brain* [2nd ed.]. Baltimore: Lippincott Williams & Wilkins.)

primarily in laminae I and V to VII (Basbaum and Jessell, 2000) and conveys sharp or A-delta fiber nociception (pain), temperature, light (crude) touch, and pressure.

In addition, many of the neospinothalamic tract neurons in thoracic cord segments also receive convergent input from visceral afferent fibers and thus are called viscerosomatic neurons. This intersection of visceral input and somatic input on the same tract neuron may explain the phenomenon of visceral referred pain (Williams et al., 1995; Basbaum and Jessell, 2000) (see Chapter 10). The fibers of the neospinothalamic tract then ascend contralaterally through the brain stem to the ventral posterior (lateral part) nucleus (see Fig. 9-10) and possibly the posterior nucleus of the thalamus, where they synapse on third-order neurons (see Fig. 9-16, *A*). The third-order neurons ascend to the sensory part of the cerebral cortex, which is the postcentral gyrus and paracentral lobule (posterior part) of the parietal lobe (see Figs. 9-13 and 9-14). The type of pain information ascending in this tract, exemplified by a pinprick, is well localized and discriminatory. The fibers ascend in the spinal cord in a dorsolateral-to-ventromedial somatotopic pattern, with the axons conveying information from sacral nerves found dorsolaterally and axons conveying information from cervical nerves located mostly ventromedially (see Fig. 9-16, *A*). There is also evidence that pain and temperature fibers are segregated within the tract such that nociceptive fibers are located ventral to fibers conducting temperature (Friehs, Schrottner, and Pendi, 1995; Williams et al., 1995; Snell, 2001).

The paleospinothalamic tract conveys dull, achy, or slow C-fiber nociception (pain) and temperature. The cell bodies of second-order neurons are located in laminae VII and VIII, and their axons decussate in the ventral white commissure to ascend in the brain stem (see Fig. 9-16, *A*). Their dendrites extend into laminae I through IV, and numerous interneurons are involved in the neurotransmission between first- and second-order neurons. The tract sends some collateral branches to the reticular formation of the brain stem on its course to the thalamus (Kiernan, 1998; Snell, 2001) (see Fig. 9-16, *A*). When reaching the thalamus, the second-order neurons

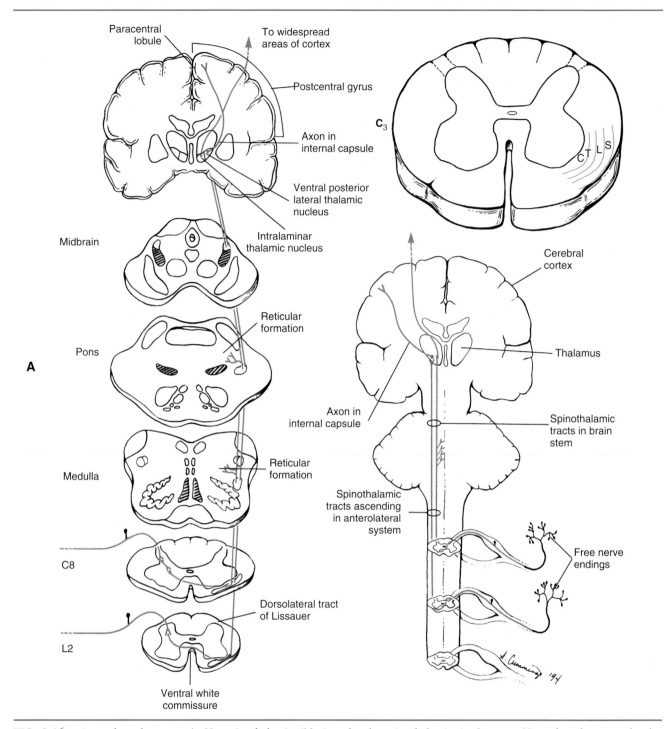

FIG. 9-16 Anterolateral system. **A,** Neospinothalamic (*blue*) and paleospinothalamic (*red*) tracts. Note that the second-order neurons cross in the ventral white commissure of the spinal cord. The somatotopic organization of the neospinothalamic tract is illustrated in the C3 cross section. The medial lemniscus is shaded to show its anatomic relationship to the spinothalamic tracts within the brain stem.

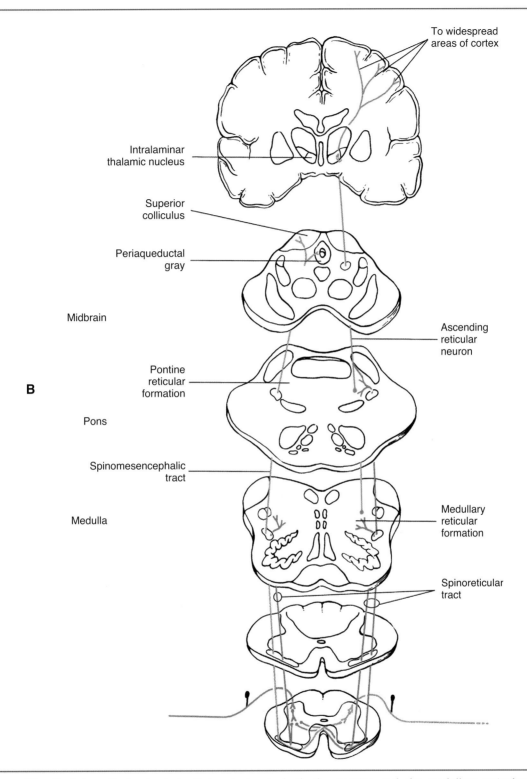

FIG. 9-16—cont'd   **B,** Spinoreticular tract (*red*) terminates in both the pontine and the medullary reticular formations. Information from the reticular formation (represented by the neuron [*green*]) continues to the thalamus and then to the cortex. Spinomesencephalic tract is also shown (*blue*).

of the paleospinothalamic tract synapse in the intralaminar nucleus (see Fig. 9-10). From this nucleus, third-order neurons travel to the same cortical areas as the spino-reticular tract (see the following) where the information relative to the affective and motivational aspect of pain is processed. Sometimes, perhaps unnecessarily (Williams et al., 1995; Kiernan, 1998; Snell, 2001; Nolte, 2002), the spinothalamic tract is divided into a lateral spinothalamic tract, which is thought to convey nociception and temperature, and an anterior (ventral) spinothalamic tract conveying light (crude) touch and pressure. However, physiologic studies indicate that all of these fibers are extensively intermingled and they should be considered as one entity (Williams et al., 1995).

The spinoreticular tract originates from second-order neurons located primarily in laminae VII and VIII (Young, 1986; Willis and Westlund, 1997; Basbaum and Jessell, 2000) but also in lamina V (Williams et al., 1995). The second-order fibers ascend to synapse in various nuclei in the medullary and pontine reticular formation. The majority of these axons ascend contralaterally, although some ascend ipsilaterally (Williams et al., 1995; Willis and Westlund, 1997; Basbaum and Jessell, 2000) (see Fig. 9-16, B). The reticular formation is a network of neurons located in the core of the brain stem (see Fig. 9-14), which is similar to the intermediate gray matter of the spinal cord. It consists of highly organized and differentiated neuronal populations that receive input from fibers of sensory systems ascending through the cord and brain stem. The reticular formation has numerous functions, including mediating cranial nerve reflexes, modulating somatic motor activity, influencing autonomic functions and the endogenous pain system (see Chapters 10 and 11), and regulating the level of consciousness. From the reticular formation, neurons project to the intralaminar and midline thalamic nuclei (see Fig. 9-10) and then, after synapsing, these neurons project to widespread areas of the cerebrum via the anterior cingulate (see Fig. 9-14) and insular cortices. These areas are important components of the limbic system, which consists of areas of the brain that are involved with the emotions and behaviors necessary for survival. The spinoreticular tract is thought to convey cutaneous information associated with alertness and consciousness and also dull, achy pain. Unlike the spinothalamic tract, which transmits information pertaining to the discriminatory qualities of painful stimuli (i.e., location and intensity), the spinoreticular tract is involved with transmitting information that is part of the affective and motivational aspects of pain (i.e., the unpleasantness of the pain and desire to eliminate or reduce it). These latter aspects of pain result in autonomic, behavioral, and emotional responses to the painful stimuli. The brain stem reticular formation also is part of a group of structures comprising the ascending reticular activating system (ARAS). This system functions in arousal of the cortex to maintain alertness and attentiveness and, relative to the spino-reticular tract, the nature of the painful stimuli and subsequent responses.

The third tract found in the anterolateral quadrant consists of a group of fibers, called the spinomesencephalic tract, which terminates in the midbrain (see Fig. 9-16, B) (Young, 1986; Williams et al., 1995; Willis and Westlund, 1997; Basbaum and Jessell, 2000; Nolte, 2002). The spinomesencephalic tract also is likely to be involved with the motivational-affective component of pain. In addition, it is associated with the activation of a descending analgesic system. This crossed tract originates primarily in laminae I and V and conveys nociceptive information to midbrain nuclei, such as the superior colliculus (the fibers to this nucleus are called the spinotectal tract [Williams et al., 1995; Snell, 2001; FitzGerald and Folan-Curran, 2002]), the mesencephalic reticular formation, and the periaqueductal gray (PAG) of the midbrain (see Figs. 9-12, 9-14, and 9-16, B). The superior colliculus is thought to be concerned with spinovisual reflexes; for example, turning the head and eyes toward a stimulus. The PAG has been implicated as being part of an endogenous pain control system. The PAG is capable of modulating pain circuitry in the dorsal horn of the spinal cord via the descending raphe-spinal tract (see Other Descending Fibers).

Remember that most conscious pain and temperature information ascends contralaterally in the anterolateral region and that the decussation of the second-order fibers occurs within the ventral white commissure within one or two segments of entry. Therefore a lesion in the spinal cord or brain stem produces a contralateral loss of pain and temperature below the level of the lesion (injury).

Spinocervicothalamic tract. The spinocervicothalamic tract is involved with conveying tactile and nociceptive information (Williams et al., 1995; Willis and Westlund, 1997; Basbaum and Jessell, 2000; Nolte, 2002). First-order neurons terminate in the gray matter of the dorsal horn. Axons of tract neurons in laminae III and IV ascend ipsilaterally in the dorsolateral funiculus as the spinocervical tract to synapse in the lateral cervical nucleus. This nucleus is located in the white matter lateral to the tip of the dorsal horn in the first two cervical cord segments. Axons of this nucleus decussate and ascend with the medial lemniscus to the thalamus, where they synapse. Axons from the thalamic nuclei subsequently project to the cerebral cortex. Although the lateral cervical nucleus is prominent in many mammals, especially carnivores, and is likely part of an important somatosensory pathway, its presence and importance in humans is unclear.

Spinohypothalamic tract. This tract originates in various laminae of the spinal cord gray matter (e.g., laminae VII and VIII) (Sewards and Sewards, 2002), laminae I, VII, and X (Willis and Westlund, 1997), and laminae I, V, and VIII (Basbaum and Jessell, 2000) and ascends bilaterally to the hypothalamus (see Fig. 9-14). The tract may be involved with the motivational aspect of pain and the resulting emotional and autonomic responses.

Postsynaptic dorsal column pathway. This pathway originates from neurons located around the central canal in lamina X. It ascends in the dorsal column and synapses in the dorsal column nuclei of the caudal medulla. From here fibers travel to visceroceptive neurons in the VPL nucleus of the thalamus. This tract is a visceral nociceptive pathway and is viscerotopically organized such that fibers conveying information from pelvic viscera travel in the midline of the dorsal column and nociception from upper abdominal organs travel in fibers located more laterally (Nauta et al., 1997; Willis and Westlund, 1997, 2001).

The previous description of ascending tracts has emphasized the fact that these tracts terminate in specific CNS targets. Neuroanatomic and neurophysiologic evidence collected through the use of more advanced techniques in tract-tracing methods and low threshold point antidromic mapping methods indicates that there are spinal dorsal horn neurons that project to double or multiple targets (Lu and Willis, 1999). This is not unexpected, because axons are known to display extensive branching and collateralization. Identified systems that appear to have double or multiple projecting systems include subpopulations that are related to the spinothalamic tract system, dorsal column postsynaptic tract system, and spinohypothalamic tract system. When compared with the anatomic description of the more classically defined multisynaptic and direct projecting systems, these pathways appear to be a phylogenetically intermediate group of tracts. Also, these pathways may function to transmit afferent information that has converged and been processed in the dorsal horn to multiple sites. These multiple sites may influence autonomic, affective, and motivational responses, as well as modulate descending control systems.

Spinocerebellar tracts. The next group of ascending tracts terminates in the cerebellum and conveys unconscious proprioception. Numerous spinocerebellar tracts have been implicated, although all their origins are not well known (Ekerot, Larson, and Oscarsson, 1979; Grant and Xu, 1988; Xu and Grant, 1988). The best known of these are the dorsal spinocerebellar tract, cuneocerebellar tract, and ventral spinocerebellar tract.

DORSAL SPINOCEREBELLAR TRACT. The dorsal spinocerebellar tract (DSCT) is located on the periphery of the lateral funiculus ventral to the dorsolateral tract of Lissauer and lateral to the lateral corticospinal tract (see Fig. 9-8). It begins in the L2 or L3 segments and ascends (Fig. 9-17). The cell bodies of these tract fibers are located in the nucleus dorsalis (thoracicus), also known as Clarke's nucleus. This nucleus is located in lamina VII in cord segments C8 or T1 through L3 and is best developed in the upper lumbar and lower thoracic segments (Nolte, 2002). Recent evidence suggests that axons of neurons located within the intermediate and dorsal laminae of similar segments also contribute to the DSCT (Bosco and Poppele, 2001). The DSCT is believed to carry proprioceptive and cutaneous touch and pressure information from the trunk and lower extremities. The vast majority of first-order neurons, along with collaterals of dorsal column primary afferents (Williams et al., 1995; Nolte, 2002), enter at the levels of C8 or T1 to L3 and synapse in Clarke's nucleus. However, first-order neurons entering in dorsal roots L4 and inferiorly first ascend in the fasciculus gracilis to reach Clarke's nucleus in the lower thoracic and upper lumbar segments, where they then synapse. Because the second-order neurons originating from Clarke's nucleus and adjacent laminae ascend in the lateral white column as the DSCT, the tract itself is only present at the levels in which Clarke's nucleus is found and superiorly (i.e., L3 and above). The DSCT ascends into the medulla of the brain stem and then exits the medulla via the inferior cerebellar peduncle (see Fig. 9-12) to terminate in the vermal and paravermal region (spinocerebellum) of the cerebellum (Figs. 9-17 and 9-18).

CUNEOCEREBELLAR TRACT. The upper limb equivalent to the DSCT is the cuneocerebellar tract. Its first-order fibers enter the spinal cord and ascend in the fasciculus cuneatus into the caudal medulla (see Fig. 9-17). Here they synapse in the lateral or accessory cuneate nucleus, which is lateral to the nucleus cuneatus of the DC-ML system. Axons from the lateral cuneate nucleus form the cuneocerebellar tract and course with the DSCT, leaving the brain stem via the inferior cerebellar peduncle and terminating in the vermal and paravermal regions of the cerebellum.

VENTRAL SPINOCEREBELLAR TRACT. A third tract, which like the DSCT is involved with lower extremity unconscious proprioception, is the ventral spinocerebellar tract (VSCT) (see Fig. 9-17). This tract does not originate in Clarke's nucleus but instead originates from spinal border cells located in the periphery of the ventral horn (Grant and Xu, 1988; Xu and Grant, 1988) and from other neurons located in laminae V through VII in cord

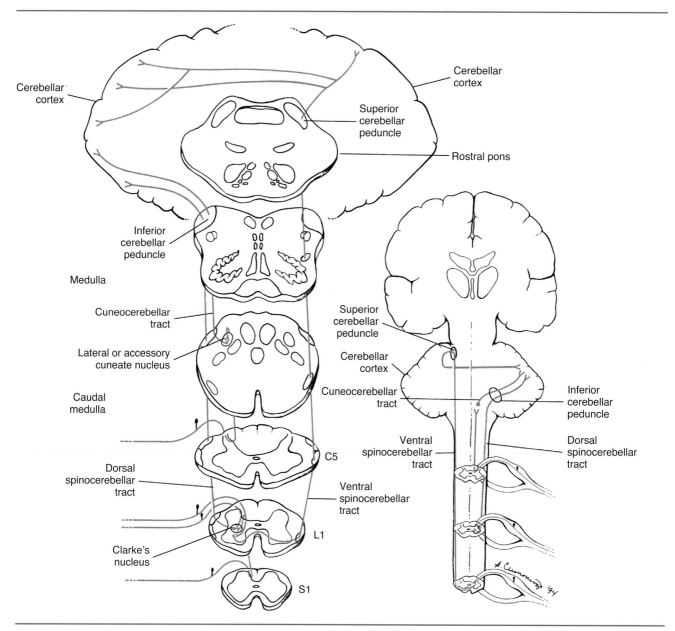

FIG. 9-17   Spinocerebellar tracts as they ascend through the spinal cord, medulla, and rostral pons: the dorsal spinocerebellar tract (and its first-order neuron) (*blue*), ventral spinocerebellar tract (and its first-order neuron) (*red*), and cuneocerebellar tract (and its first-order neuron) (*green*). The second crossing of the ventral spinocerebellar tract is within the white matter of the cerebellum. Note that the side of the cerebellum that receives the input is ipsilateral to the side of the body where the input originated.

segments L1 and below (Carpenter and Sutin, 1983; Noback, Strominger, and Demarest, 1991). The majority of the tract fibers decussate in the ventral white commissure and are first observed in the lower lumbar cord segments (Carpenter and Sutin, 1983). They ascend in the lateral white column just ventral to the DSCT. The VSCT ascends through the medulla and into the rostral pons and then exits the brain stem via the superior cerebellar peduncle (see Fig. 9-12). Before terminating in the vermal and paravermal regions of the cerebellum

(see Fig. 9-18), the majority of the tract fibers decussate again within the cerebellum and thus terminate in the cerebellar hemisphere ipsilateral to the side of the body, where the primary afferent fibers originated. The upper extremity equivalent to the VSCT, called the rostral spinocerebellar tract, rarely is seen in humans and is not described here.

The tracts just discussed are components of the mossy fiber system of the cerebellum. Their termination in the cerebellum is functionally highly organized and is

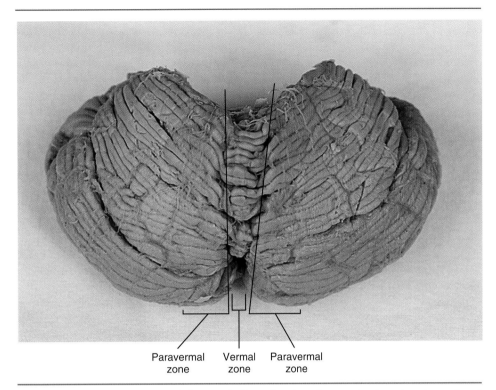

FIG. 9-18 Superior surface of the cerebellum showing the termination sites (vermal and paravermal zones) of the dorsal and ventral spinocerebellar and cuneocerebellar tracts.

Paravermal zone   Vermal zone   Paravermal zone

somatotopically arranged. The DSCT and VSCT terminate in the region of the cerebellar cortex for the lower limbs, and the cuneocerebellar tract ends in the upper limb area of the cerebellum. These tracts are involved with muscle coordination during movements and maintenance of posture (Carpenter and Sutin, 1983). The DSCT and cuneocerebellar tract neurons receive input monosynaptically from neuromuscular spindles and GTOs from individual limb muscles, joint receptors, and also from cutaneous (touch and pressure) receptors (Ekerot, Larson, and Oscarsson, 1979; Carpenter and Sutin, 1983; Williams et al., 1995). The classical view of the function of the DSCT was that it transmits information that is used for the precise coordination of individual limb muscles during posture and limb movements. However, several investigators recently have proposed that the DSCT neurons process sensory input about global limb parameters, such as the position of the limb endpoint and its direction of movement. Although there are well-defined ipsilateral monosynaptic connections with DSCT neurons, there is also a bilateral polysynaptic afferent input via interneurons to DSCT neurons. This allows the DSCT to convey information about the status of the coordination of both lower limbs (Bosco and Poppele, 2001; Poppele, Rankin, and Eian, 2003). Studies of the step cycle in decerebrate cats with cut dorsal roots indicate that the sensory feedback to the cerebellum via the

DSCT occurs only during ongoing movements (Ghez and Thach, 2000). The other major spinal input to the cerebellum is the ventral spinocerebellar tract. The VSCT neurons receive a complex array of input from type I afferents (mainly GTOs) and cutaneous afferents and also from segmental motor centers that may be excitatory or inhibitory (Ekerot, Larson, and Oscarsson, 1979). The motor centers are complex interneuronal pools that receive input from primary afferents and descending tracts and then synapse on local motor neurons. Some of the centers are pattern generator areas for automatic movements such as stepping. Studies show that the VSCT functions to transmit information concerning the activity of this central locomotor rhythmic area and interneuronal pools, as well as the activity of primary afferent fibers (Ghez and Thach, 2000). Unlike the DSCT, it is strongly modulated by the descending tracts, especially during locomotion; in response, it may relay information back to the cerebellum. In doing so, the VSCT may aid in monitoring the activity of the descending pathways (Noback, Strominger, and Demarest, 1991).

SPINO-OLIVARY TRACT. In addition to the spinocerebellar and cuneocerebellar tracts, which project to the cerebellum with few synapses, the less direct spino-olivary tract also conveys proprioceptive and exteroceptive information to the cerebellum by way of brain stem nuclei. Second-order neurons from deep laminae of the spinal gray matter decussate in the cord and ascend to the inferior olivary nucleus, which is located deep to the olive of the medulla (see Fig. 9-20). From the inferior olivary nucleus, the axons project through the inferior cerebellar peduncle to the contralateral side of the cerebellum. This tract may transmit information about motor learning occurring at the level of the cerebellum, as well as input to alter olivocerebellar connections concerning the correction of a moving body part meeting an obstacle (FitzGerald and Folan-Curran, 2002).

In summary, unconscious proprioception to the cerebellum is conveyed in the DSCT, cuneocerebellar tract, and VSCT, which use the fewest synapses and are thus the fastest, and also in the spino-olivary tract. Pain and temperature sensations are conveyed in the anterolateral quadrant in the spinothalamic, spinoreticular, and spinomesencephalic tracts, which cross in the spinal cord. Discriminative qualities of sensation (e.g., two-point touch) ascend in the DC-ML system, which decussates in the lower medulla. Light (crude) touch ascends in both the spinothalamic tract and DC-ML system. Descending pathways from the cerebral cortex and brain stem nuclei also play an important role in the ascending systems. These descending pathways modulate (inhibit or facilitate) the transmission of the ascending tract neurons of the spinal cord.

Clinically, the most important ascending tracts are the DC-ML and spinothalamic. These tracts convey information that can be tested during a neurologic examination, such as vibration, joint position sense, stereognosis, light touch, pain, and temperature. Because lesions may disrupt these tracts, it is crucial that their functions, locations within the CNS, and points of decussation be remembered in order to localize the lesion site.

Descending Tracts. As discussed in the previous section, ascending tracts convey sensory information to higher centers. Some of this processed information is integrated to enable the human brain to form a conscious perception of the environment. Sensory input also is used by autonomic centers to help maintain homeostasis and by motor centers to allow for efficient control of somatic movement. Continuous sensory input such as visual, auditory, cutaneous, and proprioceptive input keeps higher centers informed about such facts as an object's location in space relative to body position, and body position (stationary or moving) in space. This information is integrated and assessed, and is used for programming and adjusting movements (Ghez and Krakauer, 2000).

Three major motor areas receive this input and are involved with controlling movements. They are arranged in a hierarchy; the first is the spinal cord. Neurons in the spinal cord involved with motor activity supply muscles (via alpha and gamma motor neurons) either directly or they form local circuits that mediate reflexes and automatic movements such as locomotion. Although some reflexes are monosynaptic, most reflex circuitry is complex and includes polysynaptic interneuronal pools. Descending inputs from higher centers terminate on motor neurons and interneurons, thus coordinating motor activity by influencing, through excitation or inhibition, the output of the interneuronal pools on the motor neurons. The second motor area is the brain stem, which includes nuclear regions that receive input from ascending tracts and also information from the eyes, inner ear, and even higher centers. The brain stem in turn sends information back to spinal cord neurons to modulate circuitry and thus influence the alpha and gamma motor neurons involved with postural adjustments, purposeful movements, and the control of coordinated head and eye movements. The third motor area is the cerebral cortex. The frontal lobe of the cerebral cortex includes three specific motor areas: (a) primary (located in the precentral gyrus and anterior part of the paracentral lobule); (b) premotor (located in the region anterior to the precentral gyrus); and (c) supplementary (located in the medial frontal gyrus anterior to the paracentral lobule) (see Figs. 9-13 and 9-14). These areas project directly to the spinal cord and brain stem nuclei, which in turn project to the spinal cord. The premotor and supplementary areas receive input from the sensory cortex and prefrontal cortex, project to the adjacent primary motor area, and, in general, are involved with coordinating and planning complex motor activities (Ghez and Krakauer, 2000). Two additional higher centers, the basal ganglia and cerebellum, through their projections to the cortex and brain stem nuclei, are also involved with planning, coordinating, and correcting motor activities.

All these motor areas provide control over such activities as maintaining balance and posture and performing purposeful, skilled movements. In general, three classes of movements can be described. These classes, which may function separately or be combined, are reflex movements, which, although coordinated and elicited by somatosensory input, are the simplest and are involuntary; automatic rhythmic movements (e.g., chewing, swallowing, and locomotion), which typically are initiated by somatosensory input to motor circuits located in the cord and brain stem and are voluntary at their initiation and cessation; and voluntary movements, which are performed for a purpose and may be learned and subsequently improved. Voluntary movements vary in complexity from turning a doorknob to playing the piano (Ghez and Krakauer, 2000).

All three types of movements are influenced by the brain stem and cerebral cortex. These areas produce two sets of parallel descending pathways, through which they can control somatic motor activity by indirectly (via interneurons) and directly influencing the alpha and gamma motor neurons that innervate the muscles that produce movements. Although most descending tracts are involved with somatic motor control, some influence primary sensory afferents and autonomic functions. The descending pathways (tracts) are described in the subsections that follow, beginning with pathways that descend from the cerebral cortex, and followed by those that descend from the brain stem. The locations of the tracts within the spinal cord are described in general terms because their boundaries often overlap.

Corticospinal tract. The largest descending tract is the corticospinal tract (CST), which is often called the pyramidal tract (Fig. 9-19). This tract transmits information concerning voluntary (especially skillful) motor activity. The majority (approximately two thirds) of the fibers originate in the motor cortex (precentral or primary motor and premotor cortices) of the frontal lobe (Davidoff, 1990; Schoenen, 1991; Williams et al., 1995; Nolte, 2002), whereas other cell bodies are located in the adjacent sensory cortex of the parietal lobe. The CST courses through the posterior limb of the internal capsule and continues to descend within the ventral (basal) portion of the brain stem (see Fig. 9-19). The fibers in the medulla become very compact and form two elevations called the medullary pyramids (Fig. 9-20). At the caudal level of the medulla, 80% to 90% of the fibers cross at the pyramidal decussation (hence the name). The crossed fibers become the lateral CST and descend in the lateral white column (funiculus) of the spinal cord between the fasciculus proprius and the DSCT. When the DSCT is not present (below the L2 or L3 spinal cord segments), the lateral CST may extend to the periphery of the cord.

The CST is relatively new phylogenetically and found only in mammals. It is best developed in humans and becomes fully myelinated by the end of the second year of life. In each human medullary pyramid, there are approximately 1 million axons, and the vast majority are myelinated (DeMyer, 1959; Williams et al., 1995). (However, a recent study using a more discriminating staining technique suggests that there actually are less than 100,000 axons in the human medullary pyramid [Wada et al., 2001]). Axons with a diameter of 1 to 4 μm make up approximately 90% of the tract fibers, whereas less than 2% of the axons range from 11 to 22 μm in diameter (Carpenter and Sutin, 1983; Williams et al., 1995). As the tract descends in the white matter, the size of the tract becomes progressively smaller. In the cervical cord segments, 55% of the fibers leave the tract and synapse on neurons in the gray matter. (It is understandable that such a large percentage of fibers terminate in these segments, because this is the location of the neurons that supply the muscles of the upper extremity,

including the hand, which can perform highly skilled movements.) The gray matter in the thoracic cord segments receives 20% of the descending fibers, and the gray matter of the lumbar and sacral segments receives the remaining 25% of the tract axons. Like the somatosensory cortex, the motor cortex also is associated with a mapping of the body (motor homunculus) relative to the density of cortical neurons associated with a specific motor neuron pool (see Fig. 9-15). In addition, the lateral CST, as with the spinothalamic and DC-ML tracts, is somatotopically organized. The fibers that synapse in the cervical segments are located most medial, followed laterally by the fibers that synapse in the thoracic, lumbar, and sacral segments, respectively (see Fig. 9-19, *A*). The lateral CST fibers terminate in laminae IV to VIII. Some also synapse directly on motor neurons in lamina IX.

A small number (approximately 2%) of the fibers that do not decussate descend ipsilaterally just ventral to the lateral CST. These thin fibers synapse in lamina VII and in the base of the dorsal horn (Carpenter, 1991). The larger remaining group of uncrossed fibers forms the ventral CST (see Fig. 9-19). This tract descends in the ventral white funiculus and is best seen in cervical segments. Before terminating in the intermediate gray and ventral horn (primarily lamina VII), most fibers cross in the ventral white commissure; therefore approximately 98% of all corticospinal fibers terminate contralaterally.

CST fibers terminate on various neurons in the spinal cord, including Renshaw cells (see Spinal Motor Neurons and Motor Coordination), excitatory and Ia inhibitory interneurons, and primary afferent fibers (FitzGerald and Folan-Curran, 2002). Studies suggest that the axon terminals release the excitatory neurotransmitters glutamate or aspartate (Carpenter, 1991; Williams et al., 1995). In addition, fibers terminate on and coactivate both the alpha and gamma motor neurons that innervate the same muscle, facilitating flexors and inhibiting extensors. Various laminae are the recipients of human CST fibers. These include laminae IV to VI (lateral portion), VII, VIII, and IX (dorsolateral group and the lateral aspects of the central and ventrolateral groups of nuclei [Williams et al., 1995]). Although it is accepted that CST fibers terminate almost exclusively via polysynaptic connections in lower mammals, there is evidence to support the theory that CST fibers project directly (monosynaptically) on upper limb motor neuronal pools in humans and primates (Pierrot-Deseilligny, 1996; Maertens de Noordhout et al., 1999; Nicolas et al., 2001). Studies also show that the descending excitatory cortical fibers can influence upper limb motor neuronal pools indirectly via propriospinal premotoneurons. These are neurons located at the superior (C3-4) edge of the cervical enlargement that receive direct input from CST fibers, input from low threshold upper limb peripheral afferents, and input from both "feed forward" inhibitory interneurons

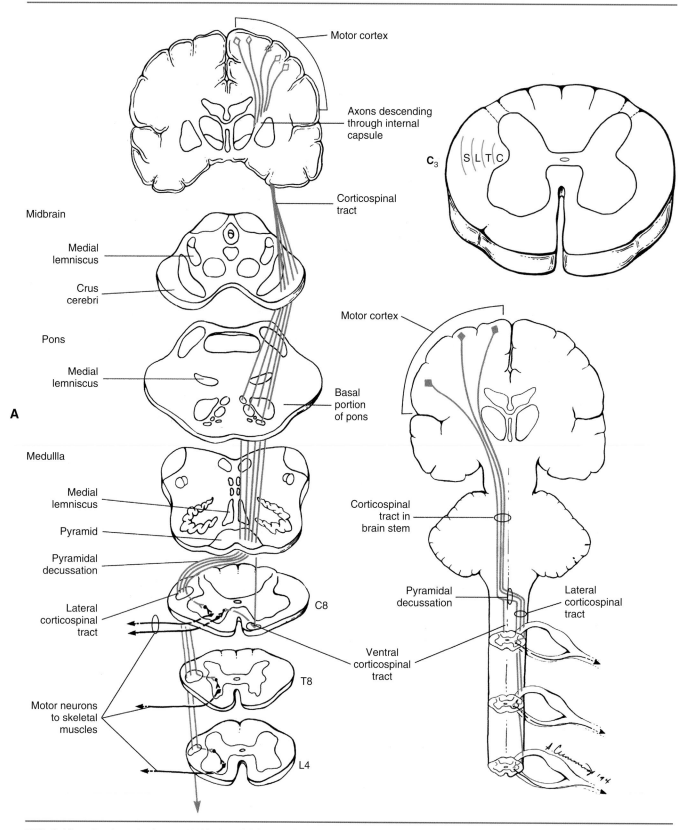

FIG. 9-19 Corticospinal tract (CST). **A,** CST descends within the basal (ventral) region of the brain stem. Most fibers cross in the caudal medulla and descend in the lateral funiculus of the cord as the lateral CST. Note the somatotopic organization of the lateral CST at the level of C3. The uncrossed fibers descend in the ventral funiculus as the ventral CST. These fibers cross before terminating in the gray matter.

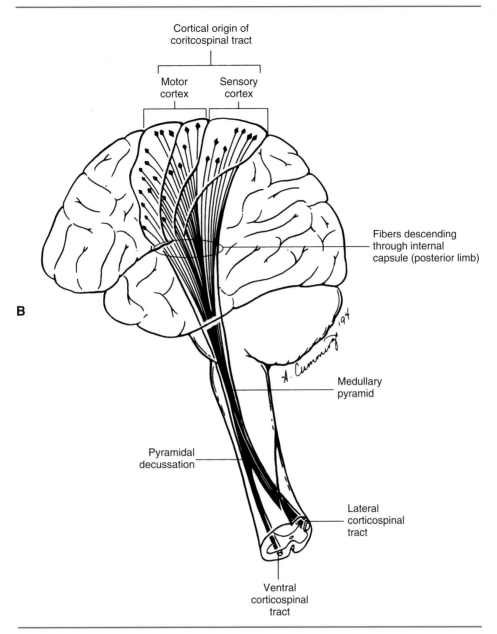

Cortical origin of
coritcospinal tract

Motor
cortex

Sensory
cortex

Fibers descending
through internal
capsule (posterior limb)

B

A. Cummings '94

Medullary
pyramid

Pyramidal
decussation

Lateral
corticospinal
tract

Ventral
corticospinal
tract

FIG. 9-19—cont'd   B, Origin of the CST, its course through the internal capsule, and its continuation into the brain stem and spinal cord.

and feedback inhibitory interneurons. The projections of the propriospinal premotoneurons to motor neurons are excitatory. This intervening pool of premotoneurons neurons may integrate cortical commands for movement with sensory feedback from the moving upper limb, and help regulate and adjust the activation of the selected motor neuronal pool (Pierrot-Deseilligny, 1996; Nicolas et al., 2001).

Studies by Nathan, Smith, and Deacon (1990) have resulted in more information concerning adult human spinal cord CSTs. They found that the extent of the area occupied by the lateral CST varied as a result of the size of the dorsal and ventral horns, the width of the fasciculus proprius that surrounds the gray matter, and the shape of the cord. In some cases the CST extended throughout a wide area of the dorsolateral white column, reaching the cord's periphery, and even extending ventral to a coronal plane through the central canal. In cervical regions the lateral CST varied from segment to segment, whereas in thoracic segments it became more constant.

This variability is important clinically because surgical procedures, such as percutaneous cordotomy and dorsal root entry zone coagulation, may damage these fibers

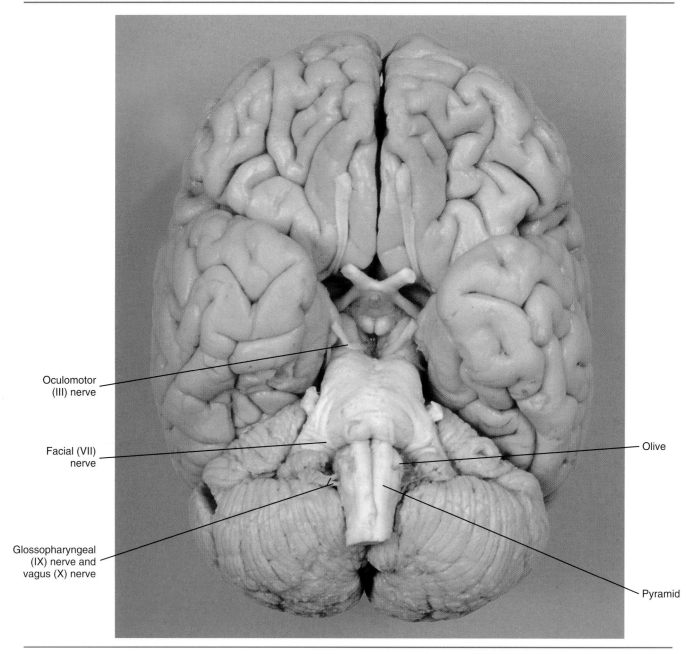

Oculomotor
(III) nerve

Facial (VII)
nerve

Glossopharyngeal
(IX) nerve and
vagus (X) nerve

Olive

Pyramid

FIG. 9-20   View of the ventral surface of the brain stem. Notice the olive immediately lateral to the pyramid on the medulla and cranial nerves III (oculomotor), VII (facial), IX (glossopharyngeal), and X (vagus). (From Lundy-Ekman L. [2002]. *Neuroscience: Fundamentals for rehabilitation* [2nd ed.]. Philadelphia: Saunders.)

because of the tract's proximity (although the denticulate ligament provides a landmark) to the anterolateral system and entering dorsal roots, respectively. The ventral CST also was described by Nathan, Smith, and Deacon (1990) as being located in the ventral white funiculus adjacent to the ventral median fissure. Although some authors believe it is found primarily in cervical and upper to mid-thoracic levels (Davidoff, 1990; Carpenter, 1991; Williams et al., 1995; Snell, 2001; FitzGerald and

Folan-Curran, 2002; Nolte, 2002), Nathan, Smith, and Deacon (1990) found that it was a distinct tract, and in some cases it extended into sacral segments. Curiously, but of related interest, they also found that cord asymmetry was a common characteristic. In the 50 normal spinal cords studied, 74% were asymmetric, and in spinal cords of 22 patients with amyotrophic lateral sclerosis, 73% were unequal. Of the total asymmetric cords, 75% were found to be larger on the right side. This asymmetry appears to be caused by the size of the CSTs. In cases in which the right side was larger than the left, it was observed that a larger number of CST fibers were located in the right side. This was because more CST fibers crossed from the left pyramid into the cord's right side than CST fibers crossing from the right pyramid into the left side. Also, more ventral CST fibers were found on the right side of the cord, because a reciprocal relationship exists between the number of ventral CST fibers and the number of contralateral lateral CST fibers. Therefore the larger (right) half included the larger lateral CST and also the larger ventral CST. A disproportionately large number of uncrossed fibers in some spinal cords (not the ventral CST fibers) that cross in the spinal cord before terminating may explain why lesions in the internal capsule may produce ipsilateral hemiplegia. Although this asymmetry is quite interesting, it does not appear to be related to handedness, and handedness does not appear to be related to the fact that fibers decussating from left to right do so at a higher level than those that decussate from right to left (Nathan, Smith, and Deacon, 1990).

The CST functions to augment the brain stem's control of motor activity and also to provide voluntary, skilled (purposeful) movements. The CST allows movements of manual dexterity and manipulative movements to be performed, primarily by control of the distal musculature of the extremities, through the independent use of individual muscles of the hand and fingers. This type of fine motor activity is called fractionation, and the integrity of the motor cortex is essential for it to occur. Buttoning a shirt and tying a shoelace are examples of this type of motor activity. In addition, the CST adds precision and speed to fractionation and other basic voluntary movements (Wise and Evarts, 1981). However, the CST is not necessary for the production of voluntary movements. This is demonstrated by lesions specific to the CST, which result in loss of independent finger and hand movements and not paralysis. Although the basic features of voluntary movements are generated by other descending tracts (see the following), a functioning CST is necessary for providing the skill, precision, fractionation, speed, and agility used during voluntary motor activity. As stated, the CST takes its origin in part from the sensory cortex (parietal lobe). These CST fibers descend and provide feedback to sensory relay areas such as the dorsal horn (lateral part of laminae IV to VI and VII [Williams et al., 1995]) and gracile and cuneate nuclei (of the DC-ML system). The corticocuneate fibers have been implicated in the primate to function as a means of regulating and adjusting (modulating) spatial and temporal input to this nucleus before and during hand movements (Bentivoglio and Rustioni, 1986). The descending fibers also are likely to modulate sensory input to motor areas. The variability of the CST in mammalian species may indicate its functional importance in various

species. In the rat the CST synapses in the dorsal horn and intermediate zone, indicating that it may be part of that animal's sensory system (Miyabayashi and Shirai, 1988). In species in which manual dexterity is nonexistent, such as the pig, the CST is not evident in the spinal cord (Palmieri et al., 1986). It is best developed in humans, providing feedback to sensory systems and also controlling voluntary skilled movements.

Other descending tracts: general considerations. The remaining descending tracts that influence motor activity originate in the brain stem and can be divided into two groups based on their location in the cord's white matter, their termination in the gray matter, and their general functions. The ventromedial group fibers course in the ventral funiculus and ventrolateral aspect of the white matter and include the vestibulospinal tracts, the reticulospinal tracts, and tectospinal tract (see Fig. 9-8). The fibers of the lateral group travel in the lateral funiculus and include the rubrospinal tract. Although the tracts are assigned to one of the two groups, the groups are not completely isolated from each other. There is communication between the two groups at the supraspinal level, and the termination of the two groups of tracts is on shared interneuronal pools. Also, there is a functional relationship between the two groups such that postural muscles frequently are caused to contract by one group as a stabilizing force during the simultaneous activation of distal musculature for purposeful movements by another group (Kuypers, 1981; Williams et al., 1995; Canedo, 1997).

The tracts of the ventromedial group, in addition to their location, also have the following functional characteristics in common: They give off many collateral fibers (collateralization), which become involved with maintaining posture; they integrate axial and limb movements and provide input associated with movements of an entire limb; and they govern head and body position in response to visual and proprioceptive stimuli. Also, they terminate in the ventromedial gray (e.g., laminae VII and VIII) on long and intermediate propriospinal neurons (which in turn project bilaterally in the fasciculus proprius) and on interneurons associated with the motor neurons supplying the axial muscles and proximal muscles of the extremities.

The fibers located in the lateral group are located near the lateral corticospinal tract. They have little collateralization and enhance the functions of the ventral group by providing independent flexion-based movements of the extremities, especially through their influence on the neurons that innervate the distal muscles of the upper extremity. These tracts terminate in laminae V, VI, and VII (dorsal part) on short propriospinal neurons (which in turn project ipsilaterally in the fasciculus proprius), numerous interneurons, and some motor neurons (Kuypers,

1981; Carpenter and Sutin, 1983; Schoenen, 1991; Williams et al., 1995). Each of the tracts in these two groups are discussed in detail in the following paragraphs.

Reticulospinal tracts. These tracts originate from the reticular formation (RF), which, as stated, is a phylogenetically old group of neurons and processes that has a network appearance in cross section. The RF consists of various nuclei located within the core of the brain stem (see Fig. 9-14). Through extensive neuronal processes, the nuclei directly and indirectly connect with all areas of the CNS and are involved in numerous activities, including the sleep-arousal cycle, regulating visceral responses such as cardiovascular and respiratory functions, modulating pain perception, and controlling somatic motor function. This chapter discusses the fibers involved with somatic muscle control. The reticulospinal tracts (ReSTs) consist of the medullary and pontine tracts (Fig. 9-21, *A*). These tracts originate in the medullary and pontine reticular formation, respectively, and show little if any somatotopic organization. The medullary ReST arises from neurons in the medial two thirds of the medullary reticular formation and descends bilaterally in the ventral and ventrolateral white columns of the cord. The pontine ReST originates in the reticular formation of the medial pontine tegmentum (core of the pons) and descends ipsilaterally in the ventral white column. These tracts are difficult to evaluate in humans, and most data have been compiled from feline studies. However, Nathan, Smith, and Deacon (1996) studied human spinal cords and looked at characteristics of reticulospinal fibers. The fibers, which did not form well-defined tracts, were located in the ventral, ventrolateral, and lateral white columns, and descended primarily ipsilaterally, although some were bilateral. They were intermingled with other ascending and descending tracts in the white matter. Many fibers shifted their position from the ventral white into the lateral white matter as they descended in the cord. In general, during movements these tracts adjust and regulate reflex actions. Either facilitation or inhibition can be produced depending on the area of stimulation in the reticular formation.

The pontine ReST facilitates motor neurons supplying axial muscles and limb extensors. The medullary ReST may inhibit or excite motor neurons innervating cervical muscles and excites motor neurons supplying back muscles in the thoracic and lumbosacral regions. Both alpha and gamma motor neurons are influenced by these tracts via monosynaptic and polysynaptic connections (Williams et al., 1995). The reticular formation integrates large amounts of information from the motor areas of the cerebral cortex (corticoreticular fibers) and other systems involved with motor control (e.g., cerebellum and brain stem nuclei). It functions to control and coordinate automatic movements such as locomotion (rhyth-mical actions such as walking and running) and posture (see Spinal Motor Neurons and Motor Coordination). Locomotion is regulated by networks of spinal interneurons known as pattern generators that activate flexor and extensor motor neurons in a rhythmic and reciprocal manner. However, the initiation of locomotion, as well as the control of speed, is a function of the mesencephalic locomotor region of the brain stem. Neurons from the mesencephalic locomotor region project to the medullary RF, which in turn sends fibers in the ventrolateral white region of the cord to the locomotor cord pattern generators, thus modulating their activity. To fine tune locomotor activity (e.g., controlling balance, refining and coordinating movements for actions such as avoiding an obstacle), afferent input about the terrain from the skin, muscles, tendons, visual system, and inner ear (vestibular apparatus), which projects to segmental neurons, cerebellum, and the motor cortex, is also necessary (Pearson and Gordon, 2000a). Posture, simply defined either as the position of body parts held between movements (standing or sitting) or the stabilization of proximal limb joints so voluntary movement of distal limbs can occur, is also influenced by the RF through ReSTs. For example, when a standing cat lifts its front paw off the ground (corticospinal input), its body weight shifts to other paws to ensure balance while the movement is occurring. However, if the medullary reticular formation is inoperative, the postural correction does not occur although the limb movement is attempted (Ghez, 1991). In general, the ReSTs influence stereotypical movements (i.e., nonskillful movements) concerned with posture, crude stereotypical limb movements, and steering head and trunk movements in response to external stimuli (Williams et al., 1995).

Vestibulospinal tracts. Two tracts originate from the vestibular nuclei of the brain stem. These nuclei (lateral, medial, inferior, and superior) are located in the vestibular area in the floor of the brain stem's fourth ventricle (see Fig. 9-12). The nuclei receive proprioceptive input from the inner ear and cerebellum. They project to brain stem nuclei for coordinating conjugate eye movements and to gray matter in the spinal cord. One of these tracts is the lateral vestibulospinal tract, which originates in the lateral vestibular (Deiter's) nucleus. The tract fibers descend the length of the cord ipsilaterally. Initially they are in the peripheral part of the ventrolateral white column of the cord, but move medially into the ventral white column at lower cord levels. The fibers synapse in lamina VIII and the medial part of lamina VII of the ventral horn (Fig. 9-21, *B*). The tract effects antigravity muscles by facilitating (polysynaptically and monosynaptically) the motor neurons supplying the extensor muscles of the neck, back, and limbs, and inhibiting the motor neurons (via

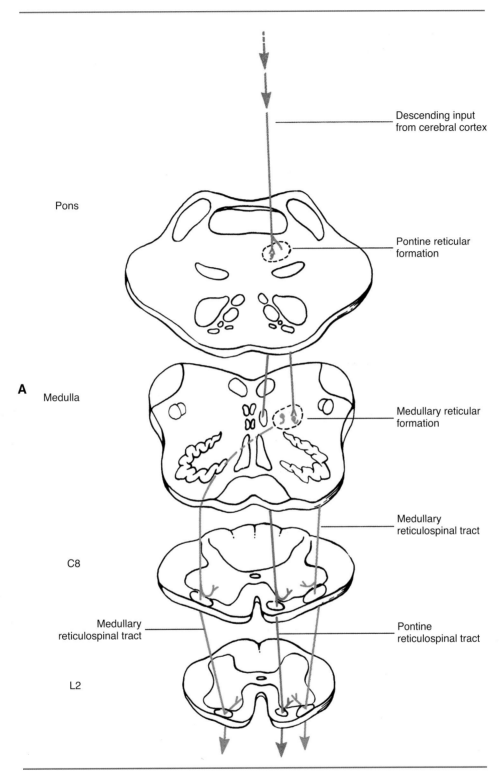

FIG. 9-21   Descending tracts that originate in the brain stem. **A,** Reticulospinal tracts: medullary (*green*) and pontine (*red*). Descending input from the cerebral cortex is represented by arrows and the neuron (*blue*).

Continued

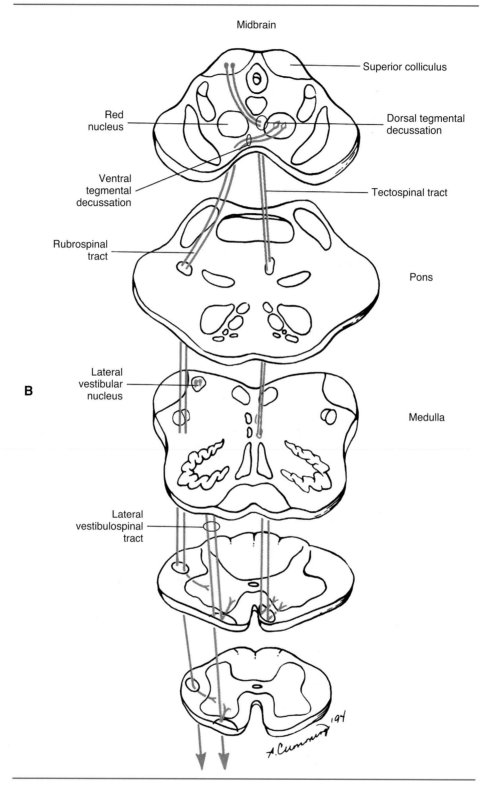

FIG. 9-21—cont'd B, Lateral vestibulospinal tract (*green*), rubrospinal tract (*red*), and tectospinal tract (*blue*).

Ia inhibitory interneurons) supplying the limb flexor muscles (Williams et al., 1995). Its function is to maintain balance and upright posture by compensating for unanticipated movements made by the body while standing or during locomotion.

The other vestibulospinal tract is the medial vestibulospinal tract, which originates primarily from the medial vestibular nucleus. These fibers descend bilaterally near the midline in the ventral white column of the cord within the medial longitudinal fasciculus (MLF), and synapse in laminae VII and VIII in the cervical and upper thoracic cord segments. The tract is responsible for stabilizing head position and accurately maintaining head position in relation to eye movements in response to vestibular stimuli.

Tectospinal tract and medial longitudinal fasciculus. The tract fibers that have just been discussed are located throughout the spinal cord and most likely influence somatic motor activity in the trunk and all four extremities. The tectospinal tract and MLF are two additional descending tracts located in the ventral funiculus that also influence skeletal muscle activity, but they are not found in all cord segments.

The tectospinal tract originates in the superior colliculus of the midbrain (see Figs. 9-12 and 9-14). The fibers cross in the midbrain as the dorsal tegmental decussation and descend through the brain stem and into the medial part of the ventral white column of the cord (see Fig. 9-21, *B*). The majority of fibers terminate in the upper four cervical cord segments in laminae VI through VIII (Carpenter, 1991; Williams et al., 1995), although in lower mammals (e.g., rat, cat, monkey) fibers also terminate in the segments of the cervical enlargement (Coulter et al., 1979). This tract is involved with orienting an animal toward stimuli in the environment (e.g., visual, auditory, cutaneous) by reflex turning of the head (and eyes via tectal fibers to cranial nerve nuclei) toward the stimulus. It is also involved with the head and eye movements used in tracking a moving visual stimulus (e.g., watching a tennis match from seats at midcourt).

The MLF (descending component of the MLF) is located in the cord's ventral white column and terminates in the cervical cord segments. (Ascending fibers of the MLF are involved with eye movements and course to brain stem motor nuclei of the oculomotor, trochlear, and abducens nerves.) This pathway includes (houses) the medial vestibulospinal tract and possibly the tectospinal, ventral corticospinal, and the cervical portions of reticulospinal tracts (Williams et al., 1995; Kiernan, 1998; FitzGerald and Folan-Curran, 2002; Nolte, 2002). The tract is responsible for accurately maintaining head position relative to eye movements in response to vestibular stimuli.

Rubrospinal tract. The rubrospinal tract is part of (with the lateral corticospinal tract) the lateral group of tracts. The rubrospinal tract originates in the red nucleus of the midbrain (see Fig. 9-14). The tract crosses in the midbrain as the ventral tegmental decussation and descends somatotopically in the lateral white column just ventral to the lateral CST (see Fig. 9-21, *B*). The fibers synapse in the dorsal part of lamina VII and in laminae V and VI. Although the rubrospinal tract is well established in the cat and monkey and extends the length of the spinal cord, its localization, termination, and function in the human cord is still unclear. Nathan and Smith (1982) studied the human rubrospinal tract from the brains of nine patients and found that the tract was small, and when it could be traced into the cord, it extended only into the upper cervical segments. The red nucleus receives input from the cerebellum and motor cortex and may be an indirect route to the motor neurons of the spinal cord. Stimulation of the red nucleus produces facilitation of the contralateral motor neurons supplying flexor muscles and inhibition of the contralateral motor neurons supplying extensors. Although it is well developed in lower mammals, its importance probably diminished phylogenetically as the CST became more developed.

Other Descending Fibers. Three other groups of descending fibers are located in the spinal cord white matter, although they are not well defined. One of these is a group of fibers comprising central autonomic pathways. Animal studies indicate that these fibers originate in various hypothalamic and brain stem nuclei. These fibers descend in the lateral funiculus to synapse on preganglionic autonomic neurons located in cord segments T1 to L2 (L3) and S2 to S4 and modulate such functions as blood pressure, heart rate, respiration rate, sweating, vasomotor tone, and bladder and bowel functions (see Chapter 10). Human studies show that there is a compact bundle of descending (central sympathetic) reticulospinal fibers surrounding and terminating in the lateral horn. These fibers are seen best in the upper seven or eight thoracic segments and rarely descend into the L1 segment. They most likely originate in the ipsilateral pons and provide input for sympathetic innervation to blood vessels and sweat glands (Nathan, Smith, and Deacon, 1996).

The second group of fibers comprise an aminergic pathway (FitzGerald and Folan-Curran, 2002; Nolte, 2002). These fibers, which primarily use the neurotransmitters norepinephrine and serotonin, include the raphespinal tract and are part of the ceruleospinal system. They originate in the brain stem, descend in the ventral and lateral white columns, and synapse mainly in the dorsal horn. They are involved with the endogenous analgesic system (see Chapter 11).

The third small group of fibers comprises the solitariospinal tract that originates in the solitary nucleus of the medulla and the medullary reticular formation. The fibers of this tract descend mostly contralaterally in the ventral and ventrolateral white columns and terminate in the phrenic motor nucleus and on motor neurons supplying intercostal muscles. The solitariospinal tract is involved with the rhythmic muscle actions associated with respiration and possibly other autonomic functions (Williams et al., 1995; Kiernan, 1998).

In summary (see Tables 9-5 and 9-6), ascending fibers conveying input from peripheral receptors and descending axons from higher centers (e.g., motor areas of cerebral cortex and brain stem nuclei) are organized into fairly well-defined, although often overlapping, bundles in the spinal cord white matter. Ascending sensory input is ultimately integrated within the cerebral cortex, and along with visual, auditory, and olfactory information, it allows the human brain to form an overall perception of the environment.

The major descending tracts influencing somatic motor activity can be classified as ventromedial or lateral depending on their spinal cord location, function, and site of termination; or they may be classified as those that terminate in cervical cord segments (e.g., tectospinal and medial vestibulospinal) and all cord segments (e.g., corticospinal or pyramidal tract, lateral vestibulospinal tract, rubrospinal tract, reticulospinal tracts). Most descending tracts are involved with motor control of posture and equilibrium, automatic movements, and voluntary purposeful movements. These tracts act primarily through interactions with interneurons that in turn synapse on the motor neurons that innervate the musculature. Although these tracts obviously are of major importance in providing normal motor activity, neuronal interactions at the segmental level of the spinal cord form connections essential for normal motor activity. These segmental connections are influenced by descending tracts that allow for an increase in the complexity of movements. The next section discusses spinal cord motor neurons and their functions in coordinating muscle contractions for reflex responses, posture, locomotion, and voluntary movements.

SPINAL MOTOR NEURONS AND MOTOR COORDINATION

Motor coordination is the process of linking the contractions of many independent muscles so that they can act synergistically and be controlled as a single unit. This is typically accomplished via the spinal reflexes, which act to coordinate most actions of groups of muscles. Most reflexes at the level of the spinal cord are polysynaptic, which allows for modification of responses by higher centers within the CNS and by local circuits in the spinal cord. Movement of a skeletal muscle is a direct result of stimulation of that muscle by specific controlling elements called the motor units. A *motor unit* is defined as an alpha motor neuron (spinal motor neuron) and all of the muscle fibers it innervates (Loeb and Ghez, 2000). It is the smallest controllable element of the CNS (Fig. 9-22). Each muscle fiber is innervated by only one alpha motor neuron. However, each motor neuron innervates many muscle fibers. The number of muscle fibers a motor neuron innervates determines that motor neuron's *innervation ratio*. All of the muscle fibers innervated by a single motor neuron (a motor unit) respond in an identical manner. The innervation ratio varies between muscles, but is roughly proportional to the size of the muscle and the size of the alpha motor neuron. For example, the gastrocnemius muscle has an innervation ratio of approximately 2000:1 and is innervated by large motor neurons, whereas the small muscles of the hand generally have an innervation ratio of approximately 10:1 and are innervated by relatively small motor neurons. A low innervation ratio indicates finely graded control of muscle force.

Three types of motor neurons can be found in the ventral horn of the spinal cord. One type is the alpha motor neurons (skeletomotor efferents), which are the largest and exclusively innervate skeletal muscle. The alpha motor neurons can be further segregated into three groups based on the size of the alpha motor neuron and the biochemical properties of the muscle fiber they innervate. However, the alpha motor neuron determines the biochemical properties of the muscle tissue. The largest alpha motor neurons have the highest innervation ratios, and innervate muscle tissue that can contract and relax rapidly, but also fatigue rapidly (<1 min). These are known as *fast glycolytic* or *fast fatigable* motor units (Rhoades and Tanner, 2003) (see Fig. 9-22, *B*). The muscle tissue they innervate has few mitochondria, low myoglobin content, high glycogen and glycolytic enzyme content, high adenosine triphosphatase (ATPase) activity, can develop the largest forces of muscle tension (up to 80 g), and generally has the greatest cross-sectional area. These muscle fibers can actually function anaerobically for short periods of time because of their glycolytic metabolic pathways. Moderate-size motor units have intermediate innervation ratios, and innervate muscle tissue that has slightly slower contraction times and are resistant to fatigue, meaning they can maintain their force of contraction for many minutes. These are known as the *fast oxidative* or *fast fatigue-resistant* motor units (Loeb and Ghez, 2000; Rhoades and Tanner, 2003). The muscle tissue they innervate has many mitochondria, high myoglobin content, oxidative and glycolytic enzymes, a powerful myosin ATPase, and intermediate force development (20 to 40 g). The smallest alpha motor neurons have the smallest innervation ratios and

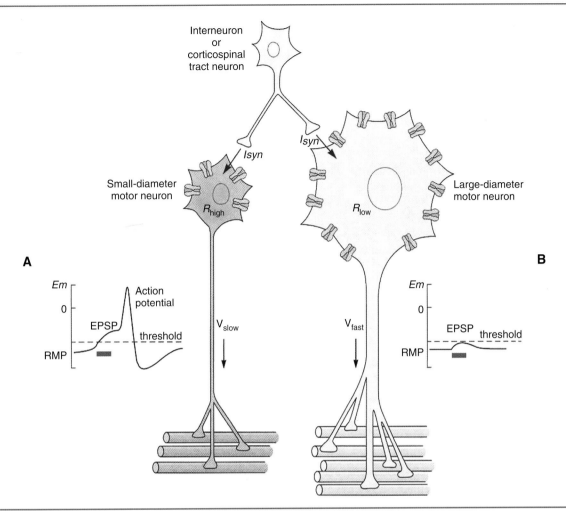

FIG. 9-22   The Motor unit. The motor unit consists of the alpha motor neuron and all of the muscle fibers it innervates. **A,** Small motor neurons generally have a small innervation ratio and are recruited first in the motor neuron pool. After stimulation, the small surface area and relatively high membrane resistance (due to fewer leak channels; R_{high}) results in a large synaptic potential that can more readily reach threshold, resulting in an action potential in this case. This action potential then stimulates the small number of muscle fibers to contract. The force generated by these fibers is relatively low, but can usually be maintained indefinitely. **B,** Large motor neurons generally have a high innervation ratio and are recruited last in the motor neuron pool. After stimulation, the large surface area and low membrane resistance (R_{low}) results in a smaller synaptic potential that is usually subthreshold. Therefore summation must occur before this neuron can create an action potential and cause contraction of its muscle fibers. Once recruited, the force generated by the large number of muscle fibers is quite large, but relatively short-lived. (Modified from Loeb GE, & Ghez C. [2000]. The Motor unit and muscle action. In ER Kandel, JH Schwartz & TM Jessell [Eds.]. *Principles of neural science* [4th ed.]. New York: McGraw-Hill.)

innervate muscles that contract slowly and precisely, and can maintain their contraction for many hours without fatigue. They are known as *oxidative* or *slow* motor units (Loeb and Ghez, 2000; Rhoades and Tanner, 2003) (see Fig. 9-22, *A*). The muscle tissue these fibers innervate has many mitochondria, many oxidative enzymes, high myoglobin content (which is an O_2 chelator), and has the smallest force development (<20 g). In addition, the firing rate of these slow motor units generally is low, and the motor units have a large hyperpolarizing after-

potential. This afterpotential aids in the summation of action potentials in the muscle, and helps prevent the occurrence of additional action potentials (self-limiting). Individual muscles contain varying proportions of all three sizes of motor units. Their muscle fibers are distributed within the muscle tissue based on their selective metabolic needs. Slow-type fibers typically are more numerous and require the greatest metabolic support, and therefore are located deep in the muscle tissue closest to the blood supply. Fast-type fibers can use glycolysis and function anaerobically, and therefore usually are located peripherally in muscle. The proportion of motor unit types within a muscle corresponds to its functional needs. Postural muscles (e.g., the soleus muscle) have a larger percentage of slow-type compared with fast fatigable-type fibers, whereas strength muscles (e.g., the biceps and gastrocnemius muscles) have a larger proportion of fast-type fibers.

The second and smallest type of motor neuron found in the spinal cord is the gamma motor neuron or fusimotor neuron (Leksell, 1945). The gamma motor neuron exclusively innervates the polar regions of the muscle spindles (see Receptors in the Motor System) and can control their level of sensitivity.

The third type is the beta motor neuron, which is known to innervate both skeletal muscle and the muscle spindles and is known as the *skeletofusimotor* neuron (Bessou, Emonet-Demand, and Laporte, 1965).

These three types of motor neurons are not segregated within the spinal cord, but rather are mixed together in the ventral horn into groupings called pools. A given motor neuron pool generally innervates one particular muscle. The various motor neuron pools are segregated into longitudinal columns normally extending two to four spinal segments. This arrangement of using motor neuron pools rather than having to stimulate each individual alpha motor neuron simplifies the task of the CNS in controlling movements of muscles. Two major strategies are employed by the CNS to control the force and velocity of contractions in skeletal muscle. First, motor units are recruited or stimulated in a fixed order from weakest (slow-type) to strongest (fast fatigable-type). In this fashion, larger motor neurons are only recruited after a significant increase in the stimulus strength. This phenomenon is called the *size principle* (Loeb and Ghez, 2000) (see Fig. 9-22). Weak inputs to a motor neuron pool in the ventral horn recruit only the smallest neurons first—those of the slow motor units— which can generate a small but consistent force that can be maintained almost indefinitely. As the input to the motor neuron pool increases, the fast fatigue-resistant motor neurons also are recruited and thereby increase the force of the contraction. Finally, if a large force or rapid contraction is necessary, the input to the motor neuron pool again increases, and the largest motor neurons— those belonging to the fast fatigable motor units—are recruited in addition to all of the other motor units, and the force of the contraction increases to its maximum. Based on the constraints of the size principle, the most numerous motor units (typically the slow fibers) are used first and most often, and are provided with the greatest metabolic support.

The second major strategy employed by the CNS to modulate muscle force or velocity is by altering the frequency of firing of the motor units. This process is known as *rate modulation* (Loeb and Ghez, 2000). As the CNS increases the firing rate of the motor neuron pool, successive twitches can summate more effectively. This summation results in the muscle contracting and moving the joint to a new position. There is a physiologic range for stimulation of muscle, because of the "low-pass filtering" properties of muscle (action potential generation in muscle is inherently slower than in the CNS). That physiologic range is 8 to 25 Hz. During normal firing of an alpha motor neuron, there is insufficient time for the calcium ions to be completely pumped back into the sarcoplasmic reticulum of the muscle before the next stimulus occurs. This results in a sustained saturation of calcium in the cytoplasm of the muscle, which results in a sustained contraction (tetanus). Stimulation rates below 8 Hz tend to produce "jerky" types of movements, whereas those above 25 Hz simply are ignored by the muscle. Regardless of the frequency of stimuli sent to the muscle, most movements are executed "smoothly" because of the asynchronous firing of the various motor units making up a muscle and the individual response properties of the individual sarcomeres within a motor unit.

Therefore muscle force, velocity of contraction, and length are *not* determined by higher centers of the CNS, but rather by the motor neuron pool in the ventral horn of the spinal cord. Muscles simply act like springs, and stimulation of the motor units controls the "stiffness" of the spring and the overall set point around a joint. In the simplest design, the CNS would increase activity to the desired motor unit, which would result in shortening of the contractile element (muscle), which in turn resets the tension and a new equilibrium is reached. Unfortunately, joints are *not* simple, unopposed hinges. The agonist muscle group is opposed by tendons and antagonist muscles, as well as ligaments around the joint, the joint capsule, skin, clothing, and any pathology associated with a joint or the muscles that move it. To correctly position the joint, an accurate assessment of both the static (steady-state) and dynamic (actively contracting) properties of the muscle are essential. This is the responsibility of the muscle receptors.

Receptors in the Motor System

Force and changes in muscle length are dependent on three properties: the initial length of the muscle, velocity of length change, and effect of external loads opposing movement. All of these are determined by specialized receptors in muscle tissue known as *muscle spindles* and *Golgi tendon organs* (Fig. 9-23, *A*). The muscle spindles are encapsulated organs, ranging from 4 to 10 mm in length. The spindles are fusiform-shaped and contain two to twelve specialized muscle fibers known as *intrafusal fibers*. They are found *within* the extrafusal

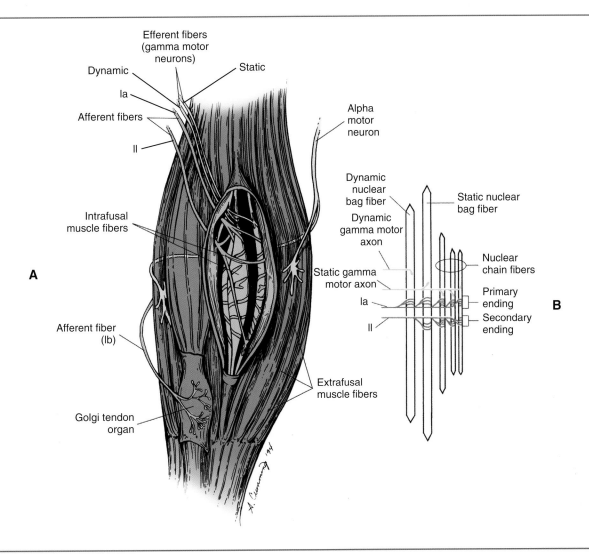

FIG. 9-23   Receptors in the motor system. **A,** Golgi tendon organs (GTOs) and muscle spindles are two types of specialized receptors associated with skeletal muscle. Extrafusal muscle fibers make up most of the muscle and are innervated by alpha motor neurons. The GTOs are positioned at the junction between extrafusal muscle fibers and the tendon (in series) and are innervated by only one afferent fiber, the type Ib afferent. Located within the fleshy part of skeletal muscle (in parallel) are the muscle spindles. The spindles are composed of intrafusal fibers innervated by both afferent (type Ia and II) and efferent (gamma motor neuron) fibers. **B,** Each muscle spindle is composed of three types of intrafusal muscle fibers. The average muscle spindle contains one dynamic nuclear bag fiber, one static nuclear bag fiber, and three or more nuclear chain fibers. A group Ia (dynamic) fiber innervates every intrafusal fiber regardless of the number. A group II (static) afferent fiber innervates the static nuclear bag fibers and all nuclear chain fibers. Each intrafusal fiber also receives motor innervation to the distal (contractile) regions to control is overall length and sensitivity. The dynamic nuclear bag fiber is innervated by dynamic gamma motor axons, whereas the static nuclear bag fiber and the all of the nuclear chain fibers are innervated by static gamma motor axons. (Modified from Gordon J & Ghez C. [1991]. Muscle receptors and spinal reflexes: The stretch reflex. In ER Kandel, JH Schwartz & TM Jessell [Eds.]. *Principles of neural science* [3rd ed.]. New York: Appleton & Lange.)

(skeletal) muscle fibers in parallel with (surrounded by) the skeletal muscle fibers. The spindles are surrounded by a connective tissue sheath (Hunt, 1990) and are innervated by both sensory and motor neurons.

Two separate classifications of sensory intrafusal muscle fibers have been identified. They are known as the nuclear chain and nuclear bag fibers (Fig. 9-23, *B*). The

nuclear chain fibers are the smaller of the two, and their nuclei are arranged in a column or row. They are innervated by both the type Ia and II afferent fibers. The *nuclear bag muscle fibers* are thicker, and their nuclei are clumped together near the center of the fiber. These fibers can be subdivided into two types, based on their physiologic properties. The *dynamic nuclear bag fiber* is most sensitive to the rate of change of the intrafusal fiber, and is a rapidly adapting type of receptor. It is innervated by only a type Ia afferent fiber. The *static nuclear bag fiber* is most sensitive to the overall position of the fiber and is innervated by both type Ia and II afferent fibers (Boyd, 1980).

The physiologic response patterns of the two afferent nerve fibers innervating the muscle spindle differ considerably, and send different types of information back to the spinal cord. The primary afferent fiber is the type Ia, or annulospiral, afferent. These fibers originate from both spindle types (bag and chain). This type of afferent fiber encodes information about the dynamic, or actively changing, state of the receptor. These are rapidly adapting types of receptors that are most sensitive to taps, vibration, and small changes in the overall length of the muscle (Fig. 9-24, *A*). They encode information about the speed (velocity) and position of the muscle during any type of movement (voluntary or involuntary) of the muscle. The secondary fiber is the type II, or flower-spray, afferent. These fibers originate only from the static bag and chain fibers. This type of afferent fiber encodes information about the steady-state position of the receptor. These are slowly adapting types of receptors that send continuous information about overall muscle position (length) back to the spinal cord (see Fig. 9-24, *A*). Both types of nerve fibers can indirectly alter their sensitivity independently via the gamma motor neurons. The dynamic nuclear bag fiber is innervated by a dynamic gamma motor neuron, whereas the static bag and static chain fibers are innervated by a static gamma motor neuron. This innervation pattern allows the different sensory components to have different levels of sensitivity, based on the predicted outcomes of the current motor task assigned to the extrafusal muscle fibers (Pearson and Gordon, 2000b). For activities that require speed or large forces, the dynamic gamma motor neuron has a relatively greater output compared with the static motor neuron. For tasks that require precise movements or postural adjustments only, the static gamma motor neuron has a relatively greater output than the dynamic motor neuron. This independent control of sensitivity to the static and dynamic sensory components allows the CNS to *preset* the level of sensitivity for specific types of tasks, and is termed the *fusimotor set* (Fig. 9-24, *B*). This mechanism of control also allows the greatest flexibility for a wide range of tasks. In addition to the gamma motor neurons, beta motor neurons (Bessou, Emonet-Demand, and LaPorte, 1965) and sympathetic efferents (Hubbard and Berkoff, 1993) also have been shown to innervate intrafusal fibers. The extent, nature, and clinical relevance of these connections to the muscle spindles are not yet well understood.

GTOs are found at the junction of the muscle fibers and the tendon (in series with muscle), and not in the tendon proper (Jami, 1992) (see Fig. 9-23, *A*). The GTOs are encapsulated organs approximately 0.5 mm in length and 0.1 mm in diameter that interface with a discrete number of muscle fibers. The GTO is innervated by a single large afferent fiber (the Ib afferent), which is entwined in the weave of collagen fibers that compose the receptor (see Fig. 9-23, *A*). The entire GTO is surrounded by a thick lamellar sheath that is continuous with the perineural sheath of the Ib afferent. As weight or tension is placed on the muscle and tendon, the weave of collagen fibers within the GTO compresses the afferent fiber and allows depolarization of the receptor. This allows the GTO fiber to function as a monitor of muscle tension, regardless of whether the extrafusal fibers are being stretched or not, and provides the CNS with crucial information about muscle tension in the face of fatigue or changing workloads.

Comparison of the output of both the spindles and GTOs during passive stretch and active contraction highlights the differences in the information these receptors convey to the spinal cord. Passive stretch applied to a muscle results in increased stretch of the intrafusal and extrafusal fibers, and therefore an increase in the output of the receptors (type Ia and II) found in the muscle spindles. In addition, passive stretch increases the tension on the muscle and tendon, and therefore causes an increase in the output of the GTO receptors (type Ib). In contrast, during active contraction of a muscle, the muscle begins to shorten and "unloads" the muscle spindle, resulting in a decrease in the amount of stretch being applied to the receptors (spindles) and a decrease in the output of those receptors. However, the GTO senses a greater tension on the tendon and muscle because of the combined forces of the load and the force of contraction, which results in a further increase in the output of the GTO receptor (type Ib). Because the GTO is in series with the muscle (between the muscle and its tendon), it is incapable of sensing muscle length, but is highly efficient at sensing changes in muscle tension. During passive stretch, much of the force is absorbed by the extrafusal fibers, and the GTO senses only a minimal increase in muscle tension. However, during active contraction both the load and contractile force of contraction are sensed by the GTO, and combine to dramatically increase the output of this receptor. The intrafusal fibers of the muscle spindle, being in parallel with the extrafusal fibers, can accurately detect changes in muscle length, but not tension. During passive stretch, both the intrafusal and extrafusal fibers are stretched by the applied load, and the spindles increase their afferent input into the CNS in direct relation to the amount of force needed to stretch the muscle. However, during active contraction the muscle shortens, and the forces applied to the spindle afferents decrease, resulting in a decreased afferent input into the CNS.

Without a resetting of the sensitivity of the muscle spindle, shortening of the extrafusal fibers could result in the muscle spindle being unable to sense further changes in the length of the muscle, resulting in a loss of position sense (proprioception) (see Fig. 9-24, *C*). To prevent this loss of proprioceptive information from occurring, the gamma motor neuron system (fusimotor system) functions to keep tension on the muscle spindles during active (voluntary) contraction of muscles. During active contraction of muscle, both the alpha and gamma motor neurons fire simultaneously. The alpha motor neuron functions to contract the extrafusal fibers, whereas the gamma motor neurons function to contract the intrafusal (muscle spindle) fibers at the same rate or velocity as the extrafusal fibers. This serves to "fill in" the signal that normally would be lost from the muscle spindle and allows it to continue to sense changes in the muscle length that might occur (see Fig. 9-24, *C*). This process of stimulating both the alpha and gamma motor neurons is known as *alpha-gamma coactivation*. In a sense, the gamma motor neuron forces the spindle to "keep pace" with the contraction of the muscle (and the alpha motor neuron), and prevents the loss of proprioception from the muscle receptor.

Based on prior experiences, the gamma motor system controls both the static and dynamic components of the fusimotor system. These components can be controlled independently of one another, depending on the type of motor function activated (Prochazka et al., 1988). If the movement is a slow, deliberate, or postural type of movement, the output of the *static* gamma motor neurons is increased by the CNS before and during the movement to ensure good overall position. Because there is little need to increase the dynamic sensitivity during these slow or postural types of movements, the output of the dynamic gamma motor neuron generally is kept low by the CNS. In contrast, if the desired movement requires either great force or velocity, the *dynamic* gamma motor neuron output is increased by the CNS, and the static component is kept low. For movements that require both postural adjustments and great force or velocity, both components can be increased by the CNS. This variability in the output to the gamma motor neurons, which is based on the expected movement, is called the fusimotor set (see Fig. 9-24, *B*). The functional role of the gamma efferents is to preserve muscle spindle sensitivity over the wide range of muscle lengths that occur during normal voluntary contractions. In general, the sensitivity is kept quite low to prevent errors in signaling to the muscles. If the sensitivity is too high, corrections occur as the muscle overshoots the expected endpoint. If too low, the muscle "lags behind" the pace of the expected movement. Therefore the sensitivity of the muscle spindle afferents plays a key role in regulating the responsiveness of the muscles based on the planned

voluntary movements (Pearson and Gordon, 2000b). These proprioceptive afferent fibers, along with all of the other sensory afferents, help modulate most of the motor actions of the muscles.

Spinal Reflexes

Spinal interneurons, the small excitatory and inhibitory connections within the spinal cord, are the building blocks of all spinal reflexes. The *spinal reflexes* act to coordinate most actions of groups of muscles, typically across joints, and most spinal reflexes are polysynaptic, which allows modifications of these connections. Most of the spinal reflexes are relatively simple neural circuits. These circuits also are used by descending influences (pathways) to generate and modify more complex motor actions. The actions of the interneurons are restricted to the spinal cord. The types of connections they control are numerous and include divergence of sensory afferents in the dorsal horn, convergence of multiple inputs onto the motor neurons and other interneurons, direct gating of neural circuits (such as the pain pathways; see Chapter 11), indirect gating through presynaptic facilitation and inhibition, activation of reverberating (repeating) circuits, and control of rhythmic pattern generators responsible for complicated motor tasks such as walking. The inhibitory interneurons coordinate muscle actions around a joint so that agonists, synergists, and antagonists act together as a *myotatic unit*. The myotatic unit regulates the stiffness of the entire joint (Pearson and Gordon, 2000b). The myotatic or muscle stretch reflex is a useful clinical and physiologic tool to understand how the spinal reflexes are controlled by interneurons. The Ia inhibitory interneuron is used to control this reflex.

The central connections involved in a stretch reflex are relatively simple and well known. A tendon is tapped, which stretches the intrafusal and extrafusal muscle fibers. The dynamic component of the spindle activates the Ia afferent fibers, which make a direct connection onto the alpha motor neurons that innervate that same muscle. The alpha motor neuron fires, causing that same muscle to contract to "reset" the muscle back to its original position. The spindle afferent often has monosynaptic connections with alpha motor neurons innervating synergistic muscles as well. In addition to the direct connection to the alpha motor neuron (agonist) and synergistic muscles, the spindle afferent also makes direct connections with inhibitory interneurons (Ia inhibitory interneurons) that inhibit the alpha motor neurons of the antagonistic or opposing muscle group (Fig. 9-25, *A*). This allows the agonist group to contract more freely (with less resistance). Stimulation of the agonist while simultaneously inhibiting the antagonist via the Ia inhibitory interneuron is called *reciprocal*

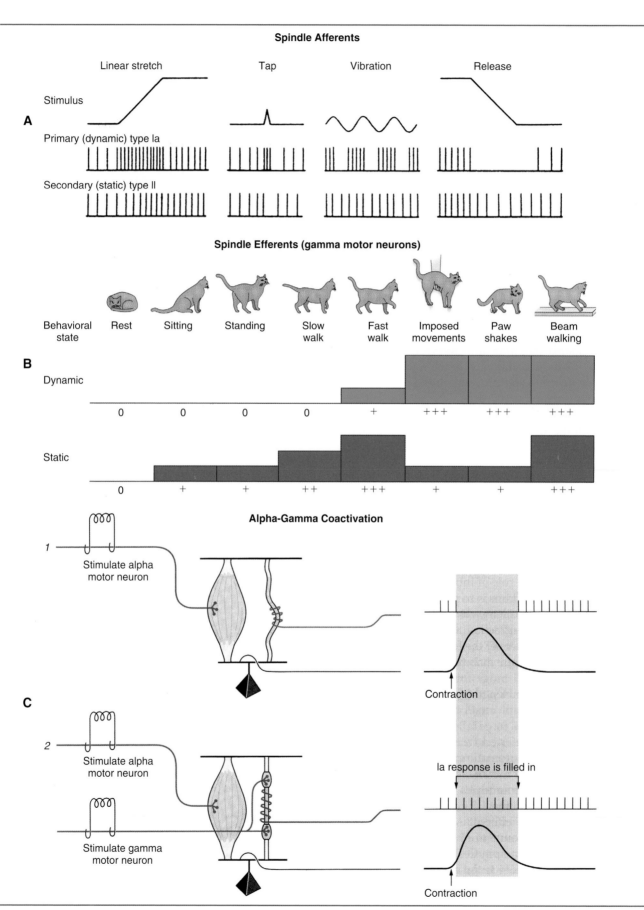

FIG. 9-24

For legend see opposite page.

FIG. 9-24   Muscle spindle afferent and efferent functions. **A,** Comparison of responses from the primary and secondary muscle spindle afferents to various stimuli. The primary receptor (type Ia) is a rapidly adapting receptor that responds to transient stretch of muscle fibers with a burst of action potentials, and release (shortening) of muscle fibers with a dramatic decrease in firing. The secondary receptor (type II) is a slowly adapting receptor that reaches a steady-state firing of action potentials that reflects the overall length of the muscle, but does not respond well to transient changes in muscle length. **B,** Fusimotor set, or gamma motor neuron activity, can be independently set at different levels, based on different types of behaviors. During activities where muscle length changes occur slowly or predictably (standing, sitting, or walking), only the static gamma motor neurons are activated. During activities in which rapid or unpredictable responses occur (imposed movements, rapid coordinated movements), the dynamic gamma motor neurons are activated. **C,** During a muscle contraction, *1,* where only the alpha motor neuron is activated, the muscle shortens, thereby unloading the muscle spindle and resulting in a decrease in its output. Any further reduction in length would be undetectable by the spindle. To prevent this loss of signal, *2,* both the alpha and gamma motor neurons fire during voluntary contractions. The spindle therefore shortens at the same rate as the extrafusal fibers, and the spindle is not unloaded during the contraction. This allows the spindle to "fill in" the missing action potentials and maintain sensitivity during voluntary contractions. This is termed "alpha-gamma coactivation." (Modified from Gordon J & Ghez C. [1991]. Muscle receptors and spinal reflexes: The stretch reflex. In ER Kandel, JH Schwartz & TM Jessell [Eds.]. *Principles of neural science* [3rd ed.]. New York: Appleton & Lange.)

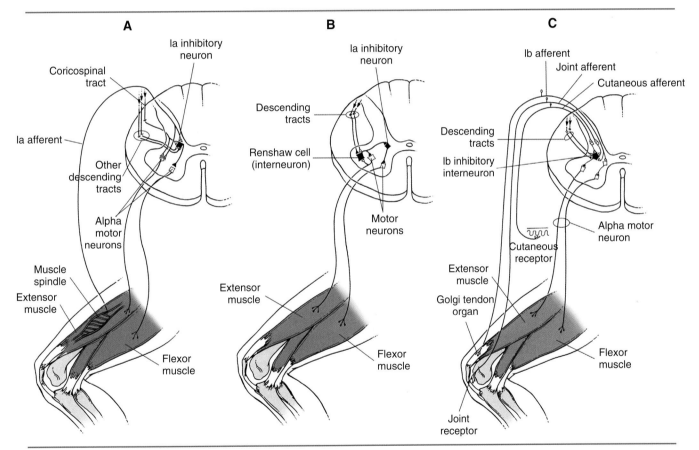

FIG. 9-25   Reflex circuitry in the spinal cord. Inhibitory interneurons that control voluntary and reflexive movements in the ventral horn of the spinal cord. **A,** The Ia afferent fiber from the spindle enters the dorsal horn and makes direct synaptic connection with an alpha motor neuron that directly innervates that muscle. The Ia afferent also makes a direct synaptic connection with a Ia inhibitory interneuron that inhibits the alpha motor neuron innervating the antagonist. This inhibition allows unopposed movement of the agonist and is called reciprocal inhibition. **B,** The Renshaw cell is another type of inhibitory interneuron that is stimulated directly from higher cortical areas and/or by a collateral branch of an alpha motor neuron. When stimulated, the Renshaw cell inhibits the agonist (and synergistic) motor neuron pool, thus shortening or reducing the motor neuron's response. In addition, the Renshaw cell simultaneously inhibits the Ia inhibitory interneuron of the antagonist group, thus disinhibiting (releasing) the antagonist muscle group and initiating cocontraction. Cocontraction serves to stabilize the joint during strenuous activity. **C,** The Ib inhibitory interneuron is activated polysynaptically by the Ib afferent (GTO), joint receptors, cutaneous receptors, and by descending pathways. The Ib inhibitory interneuron serves to inhibit the motor neuron(s) to the homonymous muscle. It also allows disinhibition of the antagonistic motor neuron pool. The inhibition of the agonist motor neuron pool and indirect stimulation of the antagonist pool allow the affected joint to be released from the tension affecting it. (Δ, Excitatory; ▲, inhibitory).

innervation or *reciprocal inhibition*. This type of contraction is used also by the CNS for voluntary movements whenever it can accurately gauge the load opposing the movement, such as during isotonic contractions (change in muscle position without change in force or tension) (Fig. 9-26, *A*). The Ia inhibitory interneuron also receives descending information from the cerebral cortex for voluntary movements, brain stem and cerebellar efferents, as well as information from other spinal interneurons.

The Renshaw cell is a second type of inhibitory interneuron found prominently in the spinal cord. The Renshaw cell is excited primarily by collateral branches from alpha motor neurons in the ventral horn. They function to inhibit the alpha motor neuron that activated the Renshaw cell, as well as other neighboring motor neurons in the motor pool (Fig. 9-25, *B*). This type of inhibition is termed *recurrent* or *feedback inhibition*, and tends to decrease or limit the output of the myotatic unit. In addition, the Renshaw cells also inhibit the Ia inhibitory interneuron, which normally inhibits the antagonistic muscle group. By decreasing or removing the inhibition (also termed *disinhibition*) of the opposing muscle group, the Renshaw cell allows all the muscles around a joint to be activated simultaneously. This concurrent activation of both agonists and antagonists is termed cocontraction, and acts to stabilize the firing rate and counteract large transient changes in joint position during movement (Fig. 9-26, *B*). The Renshaw cells also receive significant descending input (Davidoff and Hackman, 1991), which modulates the excitability of the Renshaw cells and adjusts the myotatic unit as a whole around a joint. These connections are important in ongoing postural adjustments, minor changes in muscle length (Brooks, 1986), and cases in which the precise value of the load affecting the motor pool is unknown or unpredictable.

The Ib inhibitory interneuron is a third type of inhibitory interneuron affecting the motor neurons in the ventral horn. The Ib inhibitory interneurons receive input from GTOs, joint receptors, pain receptors, and general somatic afferents from around the joint affected by the motor neuron pool. All of these afferent fibers converge either directly (monosynaptic) or indirectly (polysynaptic) onto the Ib inhibitory interneuron. The Ib interneuron has a powerful inhibitory connection to the agonist and synergistic muscles of the pool (Fig. 9-25, *C*). This connection often is called the inverse myotatic reflex, although it is not clinically testable because of the polysynaptic nature of the connections involved. A similar function of this reflex can be observed in the crossed-cord reflex called Phillipson's reflex, where flexion of one limb causes extrusion of the contralateral limb. In addition to the numerous somatic connections, the Ib

inhibitory interneuron also receives significant connections from higher centers (Jami, 1992) and other local interneurons. The significant number of convergent connections onto the Ib inhibitory interneuron represents a spinal mechanism that acts to mediate control of movements when integration of different sensory modalities is important, as in guiding limb and hand movements during exploration, allowing precise adjustments of muscle tension once an object is encountered, and preventing damage to the joint during strenuous activity by limiting or terminating agonist activity during maximum contraction.

Preprogrammed Movements. Groups of interneurons function together to build most of the preprogrammed or stereotyped movements used in everyday activities. One such circuit is the *flexion withdrawal reflex*. This reflex is triggered by noxious (damaging) stimuli, and consists of contralateral extension followed by ipsilateral flexion of muscle groups in an attempt to relieve or reduce the noxious stimulus. It involves coordinated contractions of multiple joints using reciprocal innervation and the opposite response in the opposing limb (crossed extension reflex), which provides postural support (typically extension) during withdrawal (typically flexion) of the affected limb. The flexion withdrawal reflex also is involved in coordinating some voluntary movements. This is accomplished by descending control. The descending control sends collateral connections to spinal interneurons known as *flexor reflex afferents*.

Highly stereotyped movements such as those just described involve many interneurons, and, like most reflexes, are dependent on stimulus intensity (Pearson and Gordon, 2000b). Cutaneous stimuli elicit complex protective and postural functions. Contraction of specific muscle groups in response to a stimulus at a precise location on the body is termed a "local sign." Most cutaneous stimuli have a subthreshold effect on motor neuron excitability, and the effects are spatially specific and reciprocal. The type of response elicited depends on the type of stimulus perceived. For example, a stimulus applied to the base of the foot can trigger different circuits and responses based on the strength and pattern of the afferent input into the spinal cord. Stroking the bottom of the foot with a blunt object simulates "slipping" of the foot and elicits plantar flexion, as the toes attempt to "grip" the ground. Light pressure applied to the entire plantar surface of the foot elicits the extensor thrust response (postural adjustment), which allows us to stand. Painful stimuli to the bottom of the foot activate the flexion withdrawal response, which acts to remove the foot from the painful stimulus. Most primary sensory afferent connections and all central connections involve polysynaptic pathways, and modification occurs at local

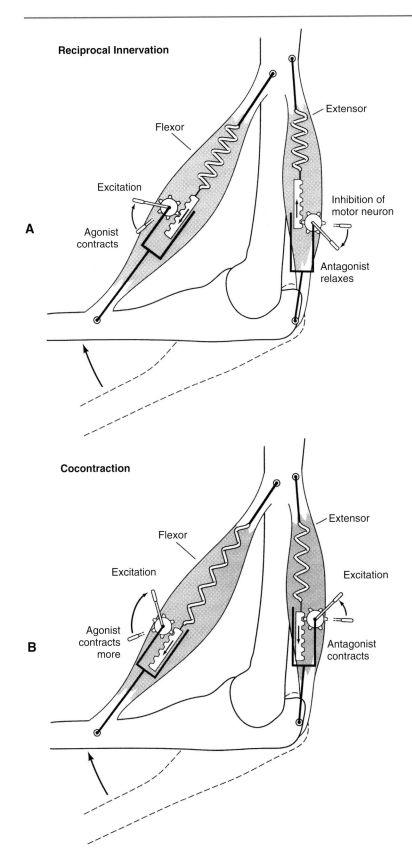

Reciprocal Innervation

Flexor

Extensor

Excitation

Inhibition of
motor neuron

A

Agonist
contracts

Antagonist
relaxes

Cocontraction

Flexor

Extensor

Excitation

Excitation

B

Agonist
contracts
more

Antagonist
contracts

FIG. 9-26 Mechanisms of muscle contraction. Movement around a joint employs one of two strategies: reciprocal innervation or cocontraction. **A,** During reciprocal innervation, the motor neurons to the agonist group (flexor) are stimulated, while the motor neurons to the antagonist group (extensor) are inhibited. This results in contraction of the flexor and relaxation of the extensor, and the joint flexes. This form of movement is extremely efficient as long as the loads placed on the muscle groups are known precisely. **B,** During cocontraction, the motor neurons to both the agonist and antagonist groups are stimulated simultaneously. Whichever group receives the greater amount of stimulation (in this case the flexor group) is the direction in which the joint will move. The overall effect is an increase in joint stiffness and stability, and allows the nervous system to control both the angle and the overall stiffness of the joint independently. (Modified from Gordon J & Ghez C. [1991]. Muscle receptors and spinal reflexes: The stretch reflex. In ER Kandel, JH Schwartz & TM Jessell [Eds.]. *Principles of neural science* [3rd ed.]. New York: Appleton & Lange.)

spinal cord connections only. To prevent the various sensory afferents and descending modulatory connections from simultaneously activating multiple or conflicting responses, most pathways are *mutually inhibitory*. Only one pathway is active at a time, and all other pathways are inhibited or prevented from responding when one circuit is active. In this fashion, the CNS can control most movements and reflexes via differential activation of selected, prewired circuits at the level of the spinal cord.

Muscle Tone and Postural Control Mechanisms

Muscle Tone. Muscle tone is the resistance of a muscle to active or passive stretch, or the overall stiffness of the muscle. Skeletal muscle has an intrinsic resistance to stretch resulting from the elastic properties of the tendons, connective tissue, and the muscle tissue itself. Therefore muscle behaves much like a spring. Reflexes also function to counteract the active or passive stretch of the muscle tissue via the monosynaptic connections from the spindles to the alpha motor neurons, and work with the elastic components of muscle to resist stretch. Normal muscle tone serves three important functions. First, it assists in maintaining posture, or the resistance of the muscle to the forces of gravity. Muscle tone helps to ensure that the center of gravity is aligned over the base of support. Secondly, because of a muscle's inherent ability to act as a spring, it can store energy and release it at a later time. This is particularly important for movements such as walking. When a leg pushes off, some of the stored energy is released and helps propel the leg and body forward, thereby assisting the muscles that normally pull the leg forward. Lastly, because muscles act like springs, they help dampen out jerky movements and allow for more "fluidlike" movements of most muscles (Ghez, 1991).

Control of muscle tone is achieved largely through feedback mechanisms. Negative feedback helps to counteract deviations from the desired muscle position. Overall muscle length is chosen by the CNS and regulated by descending connections to the motor neuron pool in the spinal cord. Deviations in the intended position are detected by the muscle spindles and relayed back to the motor neuron pool. Increases in the length of the muscle result in an increased output from the muscle spindle and increased stimulation of the motor neuron pool, which result in an increase in the force of contraction of that muscle to counteract the increase in length. Decreases in muscle length have the opposite effect. Therefore the stretch reflex functions continuously to keep the muscle position as close as possible to the length chosen by the CNS. Two crucial elements of the feedback system are the *gain* of the system and the

loop delay (Gordon and Ghez, 1991). Gain of the system is largely determined by the fusimotor set discussed earlier, and relates to the overall sensitivity of the muscle spindles. The higher the gain (greater sensitivity of spindles), the larger is the reflexive force of contraction by a muscle to counteract a given change in length. Gain can be adjusted by the overall level of fusimotor (intrafusal) activity, presynaptic modulation by excitatory and inhibitory interneurons (activated by various sensory input), and by direct connections to the motor neuron pool by descending input. The loop delay is the time between the detection of a disturbance or error and the actual compensatory response by the muscle to counteract that error. The loop delay is a sum of the conduction times from the sensory afferents, the motor neurons leading back to the muscle, and the mechanical response from the muscle. The loop delay usually is insignificant when movements are slow. During rapid or extremely precise movements, the loop delay can play a significant role in accurately regulating movement around a joint. Muscle tone also plays a substantial role in most postural control mechanisms.

Postural Control Mechanisms. Posture represents the overall position of the body and limbs relative to one another and their orientation in space. Adjustments to posture should be integrated with voluntary movements to keep the head and body aligned and to "prepare" the body for specific types of voluntary movements. There are three fundamental functions of adjustments to body posture. The first is to support the head and body against gravity and other external forces. The second is to maintain center of body mass aligned and balanced over the base of support. The third is to stabilize the supporting parts of the body while others are being moved. These three functions are achieved by two principal mechanisms: *anticipatory feed-forward mechanisms* and *compensatory feedback mechanisms*. Anticipatory feed-forward mechanisms help to *predict* disturbances by activating preprogrammed (prewired) responses. These responses are modified by experience and their effectiveness improves with practice. These postural adjustments generally occur before voluntary movements are activated. Compensatory feedback mechanisms occur after loss of balance (increased body sway). These responses are automatic and extremely rapid (reflexive in nature), are scaleable (size of response depends on size of stimulus), and use stereotyped spatiotemporal organization (muscles closest to loss of balance are activated first) to achieve stable posture. These responses also are continuously refined by experience. Sensory input from visceral, cutaneous, and proprioceptive receptors trigger anticipatory or compensatory responses that typically are automatic, and maintain posture without one's awareness. Postural control is monitored by three primary neural systems: the proprioceptive system (spindles, GTOs, joint receptors, and general sensory afferents), the vestibular system (both static and dynamic components located in the inner ear) and the visual system. Visual, vestibular, or proprioceptive information alone is not sufficient to trigger an adjustment to posture; there must be a combination of these stimuli to elicit an adjustment (Nashner, 1976). Responses that stabilize posture become *facilitated* (enhanced) with repeated trials, whereas responses that destabilize posture become *adapted* (weakened). Responses to sway are shaped by experience and continually adjusted to maintain balance. Most postural adjustments that occur to maintain equilibrium and stabilize the body are activated before the voluntary movements that may destabilize the body are initiated. *Postural set* is the preparatory state when a specific postural response is selected in advance of a stimulus so the adjustment is executed automatically either before or along with a voluntary movement (Ghez, 1991). Descending influences generated by postural set generally act via spinal interneurons to gate (control) and modulate overall tone and posture at the level of the spinal cord.

Locomotion and Voluntary Movements

Locomotion. Locomotion is a rhythmic behavior that functions to move an animal through space, and is relatively automatic. Most locomotor movements, such as walking or the scratch reflex in dogs, are controlled by groups of spinal interneurons, and these responses can outlast the initiating stimulus (Sherrington, 1947). The spinal interneurons controlling locomotion form complex circuits consisting of excitatory and inhibitory interneurons, and alpha and gamma motor neurons, which can be modulated or modified by higher CNS centers by means of descending pathways. These complicated circuits form the basis of the "rhythmic pattern generators" found in the spinal cord. Spinal animals (experimental animals having a transection of the spinal cord above C2) are actually capable of "walking" (rhythmic stepping), because of the activation of the still intact rhythmic pattern generators found within the spinal cord (Brown, 1911; Grillner and Wallen, 1985). The overall pattern consists of an alternation between contractions of the flexor and extensor muscle groups. The alternating pattern is controlled by a unique combination of excitatory and inhibitory interneurons. These interneurons act synergistically to ensure that only one group of motor neurons (flexors or extensors) is activated at a time in a given limb, and also ensure that the opposing muscle groups are activated in the opposite limb. Walking consists of two distinct phases: the swing phase (foot off of the ground and flexing forward) and the stance phase (foot planted, extended, and bear-

ing weight). The movements controlled by these circuits are timed differentially, and a spatially distributed synergy of muscular contractions exists. These elegantly timed series of muscular contractions are controlled almost exclusively by the interneurons and motor neurons that form the rhythmic pattern generators (Engberg and Lundberg, 1969; Calancie et al., 1994; Belanger et al., 1996; Pearson and Gordon, 2000a). In fact, there are separate pattern generators for each limb (Grillner and Wallen, 1985). The separate pattern generators are interconnected by other local interneurons, and both pattern generators send general information to the postural control systems of the spinal cord via long and short propriospinal interneurons.

More specifically, in normal locomotion (walking), the pattern generators for the left and right limbs are coupled to one another via a complex network of excitatory and inhibitory interneurons. These interneurons can be influenced by other networks, such as sensory afferent information (proprioception [Pearson, 1995], pain, and general somesthetic afferents), which can modify the output of the network to accommodate changing sensory inputs. The neuronal network that links the pattern generators of each limb forms a central pattern generator. This central pattern generator also can function independently, without the need for sensory feedback to maintain its pattern. Both alpha and gamma motor neurons are coactivated during locomotion; therefore the spindle afferents increase their output during locomotion because of the increased gain in the fusimotor set (Severin, Orlovsky, and Shik, 1967). In addition, tonic descending signals from the brain stem can activate the spinal circuits responsible for locomotion. However, this signal is unrelated to the rhythm of locomotion (Shik and Orlovsky, 1976). Thus a relatively simple control signal from the brain stem (mesencephalic locomotor region), modulated in intensity only, can activate locomotion and facilitate changes in speed. However, the pattern itself is controlled by circuits found in the spinal cord.

Normal locomotion requires multiple levels of neural control to support the body against gravity, maintain normal balance during ongoing movements, and propel it forward. These movements are coordinated by spinal circuits that are influenced by both sensory afferent information and descending control systems, such as the corticospinal, reticulospinal, vestibulospinal, and rubrospinal pathways.

Voluntary Movements. Although a spinal animal can reflexively "walk" (produce rhythmic, alternating movements of the limbs) if supported on a treadmill, it is not capable of balance or goal-directed voluntary movements. These purposeful movements require that an intact motor cortex, basal ganglia, cerebellum, and vestibular system be connected to the spinal cord to initiate the purposeful movements and modulate them. Most daily movements are voluntary in nature, and require that *all* levels of the CNS, from cerebral cortex to spinal cord, be intact.

There are several key differences between reflexive and voluntary movements. First, with voluntary movements motor systems can use different strategies in different situations to achieve the same result, a concept termed *motor equivalence* (Krakauer and Ghez, 2000). Secondly, the effectiveness of voluntary movements improves with experience and learning; precision increases while variability decreases. Finally, external stimuli need not be present to initiate a voluntary movement. The voluntary system can dissociate the content of the movement (what and how) from the initiation of the movement (when).

Several events must take place before a voluntary movement can be performed. First, there must be identification of an action that is to be performed. Second, a plan of action must be formulated in the cerebral cortex. After these two initial steps have been performed, there must finally be a "GO" signal that results in execution of the planned response. These three steps (identification, planning, and execution) are controlled by distinct regions of the cerebral cortex: the posterior parietal cortex, premotor regions of the frontal cortex (supplementary motor cortex and premotor cortex), and primary motor cortex, respectively. Each of these cortical areas, which controls a different aspect of the overall voluntary movement, is discussed below. In addition, other subcortical areas also can influence motor activity. These include the thalamus, cerebellum and basal ganglia, but their scope of influence is not discussed here.

The *posterior parietal cortex* is essentially a sensory integration area that helps develop the plan of action and may contribute to the identification of the task to be performed. This region is critical for integrating visual information on targeted movements and helps to focus attention on salient stimuli. The posterior parietal cortex has a strong motivational component and strong hemispheric specialization. It also receives input from the primary sensory cortex, sensory association areas, and the vestibular system and limbic (motivational) areas of the brain. It is also modulated by states of attention. This area provides the motor regions of the cortex with information about overall body position and sensory inputs and also reflects the subject's intentions for a specific action.

The *premotor areas* of the frontal cortex receive strong projections from the posterior parietal cortex, and prepare the motor system for movement. Under optimal conditions, a person can respond (reflexively) to a stimulus in 120 to 150 ms, with proprioceptive responses being the quickest. However, voluntary tasks can take hundreds of milliseconds to initiate. The time it takes to plan or initiate a voluntary response increases linearly with the complexity of the task or number of choices involved. Premotor areas control these more complex actions and also control movements that require a specific sequence of activation for execution (Krakauer and Ghez, 2000). The supplementary motor area of the premotor cortex is important for programming sequences (e.g., orienting the body before executing voluntary movements) and coordination of bilateral movements (such as clapping). The supplementary motor area is also important for mentally rehearsing specific movements and tasks before execution, controlling proximal limb and axial muscles and the initial orientation of body and limbs to a target (coordinating posture and voluntary movement), and responding to instructions for execution of specific actions. Understanding of instructions or cues is normally independent of the time frame for actual execution or initiation of the planned response. Neurons from premotor areas do not control the fine detail of actions to be executed, but rather they are concerned primarily with the global aspects (overall sequence of action) of a motor task and the initiation of the execution command to the primary motor cortex.

Individual neurons in the *primary motor cortex* code for the force exerted by the muscle, not direction of movement (Krakauer and Ghez, 2000). Distal muscles (fine control) are represented at more than one site in the primary motor cortex, but this is the cerebral cortex's *only* output to these muscles. Small muscles in the hands and the muscles of facial expression do not have concomitant neurons in the other motor areas of the cerebral cortex. The axons of most neurons in the primary motor cortex diverge to influence several motor neuron pools in the spinal cord, with the greatest number of connections being associated with proximal (postural or axial) muscles. In addition, most neurons in the primary motor cortex typically are activated before actual muscle contraction, and they may contribute to the initiation of movement. Direction is encoded by stimulating populations of neurons in the primary motor cortex, rather than stimulating a single neuron (Krakauer and Ghez, 2000). Individual neurons of this cortical region have a preferred direction or orientation (greatest output), and most respond over a wide range of directions, but with reduced output. Therefore groups of neurons determine the final direction of movement (*population vector*), whereas individual neurons code for the force or velocity exerted by a particular motor neuron pool in the spinal cord. Output of the primary motor cortex is variable, depending on the task and level of motivation. Input about limb position and speed of movement is updated continuously by means of direct connections from the primary sensory cortex, and indirectly from sensory afferents from the proprioceptive system by way of the thalamus, cerebellum, and basal ganglia. In this way, the primary motor cortex can adjust the output to motor neuron pools in the spinal cord to compensate for changes or disturbances in the planned movement, or to refine the voluntary movement.

By analyzing a relatively simple movement, such as throwing a ball, one can begin to understand how all of the afferent and efferent information being processed by the spinal cord and higher-order systems (e.g., brain stem nuclei, cerebellum, basal ganglia, and cerebral cortex) work together to complete this task (Fig. 9-27). First, the "idea" of throwing the ball has to be formulated somewhere in the cerebral cortex. This idea is relayed, along with all current proprioceptive information (originating primarily from the DC-ML pathways) to the premotor regions of the cortex, where a plan is developed, based on the body's current position in space. The basal ganglia also aid the premotor regions in developing the appropriate timing and initiation of movements, because of their extensive connections with virtually all areas of the cerebral cortex. The premotor and supplementary motor cortices then relay this plan for coordi-

nated movements of the legs, arms, trunk, head, and neck to the primary motor cortex. The primary motor cortex encodes force, velocity, and direction to the appropriate motor neurons via the corticospinal pathways to the ventral horn of the appropriate spinal cord segments. In addition, a copy of the planned movements is relayed to the cerebellum by the descending corticospinal tract (termed *corollary discharge*) (see Fig. 9-27). In the spinal cord, pools of alpha and gamma motor neurons are stimulated by the descending corticospinal tract (primarily lateral corticospinal tract) and cause the appropriate muscles to begin to contract. In addition, the reticulospinal and vestibulospinal pathways relay information for postural adjustments to the spinal cord to compensate for any deviations associated with the ongoing voluntary movement. Continuous assessment of these voluntary (throwing the ball) and involuntary (postural adjustments) movements are monitored by the muscle spindles, GTOs, and joint and skin receptors. The afferent fibers associated with these receptors, in addition to sending information back to the sensory and motor areas of the cortex via ascending tracts, also can modify the interneurons at the level of the spinal cord (Ia inhibitory interneurons, Renshaw cells, and Ib inhibitory interneurons) to ensure that the intended movement

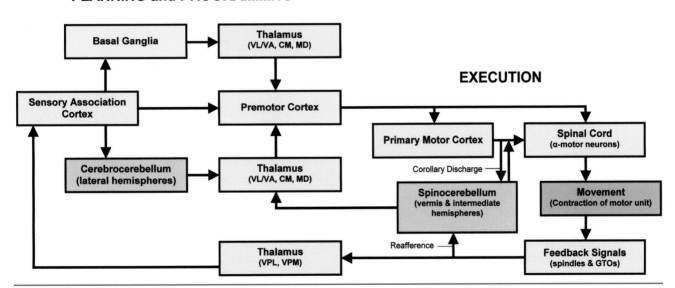

PLANNING and PROGRAMMING

FIG. 9-27 Flowchart of motor system components. This flow diagram shows the extensive integration and levels of control associated with motor function. The motor system is organized both hierarchically and in parallel. All levels of the motor system receive sensory information concerning muscle and joint position via the thalamus (*yellow*). Motor areas of the cortex (*tan*) can influence motor neurons in the spinal cord (*green*) directly and indirectly via the brain stem. The motor system is also influenced by two independent subcortical systems: the basal ganglia (*blue*) and the cerebellum (*purple*). The basal ganglia influences only motor planning, whereas the cerebellum influences both planning (cerebrocerebellum) and execution (spinocerebellum) of movements. Both the basal ganglia and cerebellum act on the cortex via the thalamus.

proceeds as planned. The primary afferent fibers also relay information to the long and short propriospinal neurons (interneurons) within the spinal cord. The short propriospinal interneurons assess and modify information across multiple joints in either the upper or lower extremity, whereas the long propriospinal interneurons assess and modify postural (axial) muscles throughout the entire length of the vertebral column and spinal cord to maintain normal balance and posture during the movement. These propriospinal interneurons can directly and indirectly modify the output of the motor neuron pools to alter the ongoing movement. All ascending proprioceptive information traveling in the DC-ML on its way to the thalamus and cortex sends collaterals to the cerebellum (termed *reafference*) and reticular formation (see Fig. 9-27). The cerebellum acts as a comparator, comparing the planned movement (via corollary discharge) with the actual ongoing movements (via reafference). If the ongoing movements do not match the intended movement, the cerebellum can modify the output of the descending corticospinal pathways via interneurons at the level of the spinal cord, thus helping to guide the movement and correct the error (termed *coordination*). The cerebellum also can correct the error by sending a signal via the thalamus to the cerebral cortex to alter the plan. Further modification of these control pathways occurs by other afferents and spinal interneurons, such as pain pathways, which can alter or modify movements after injury or in response to acute pain. The other interneuronal circuits in the spinal cord, such as gating neurons, reverberating circuits, and rhythmic pattern generators, also can work to modify or control specific types of movements based on specific afferent patterns. Therefore ascending and descending tracts, along with extensive influence and modification by the spinal interneurons, work together to produce the movements that a person relies on for most daily activities (Fig. 9-28).

CLINICAL APPLICATIONS

Neuroanatomy is the foundation on which clinical neurology is based. A clinician makes a neurologic assessment of a patient with back and extremity pain based on his or her knowledge of spinal cord anatomy and the results of the neurologic examination. The examination typically includes testing motor functions influenced by the descending tracts and sensory functions conveyed primarily by the spinothalamic tract and DC-ML system. The derivation of an anatomic diagnosis of a disorder affecting the nervous system is essential to the development of an accurate pathologic or etiologic diagnosis (Adams and Victor, 1989). The purpose of this section is to highlight the application of neuroanatomy to the localization of pathologic conditions causing signs and symptoms in particular patients. Clinical neurology is a subject unto itself; therefore the following paragraphs are intended to exemplify briefly the clinical application of only portions of the material discussed in this chapter.

Damage to areas of the body resulting in loss or alteration of function is called a lesion. Lesions of the spinal cord can occur in many ways. One means is by trauma. Spinal cord trauma occurs in approximately 10,000 individuals per year in the United States (Pearson and Gordon, 2000b). The most common cause is automobile accidents, followed by falls, gunshot wounds, and recreational activities such as diving accidents. Direct injury to the cord (e.g., by knife or bullet), compression by vertebral fragments, compression secondary to hemorrhage and coagulation, damage to vessels, or stretching of the cord can be caused by trauma. Regions most often affected are the cervical and thoracolumbar junction, followed by the thoracic and lumbar segments (Meyer et al., 1991).

Other nontraumatic examples that can cause lesions are vascular insufficiency, tumor, infections, demyelinating diseases (e.g., multiple sclerosis), or degenerative diseases (e.g., amyotrophic lateral sclerosis, Friedreich's ataxia). Patients with lesions of the spinal cord or related nerves may have strictly motor deficits, strictly sensory deficits, or a combination of the two. Disorders also may be either acute or chronic. In the following section the examples are presented in a fairly "cut and dried" manner. However, in a clinician's office a lesion may not always present as a "textbook" case.

Motor Assessment

Lower Motor Neurons. This section discusses the motor aspect of lesions, that is, lesions affecting descending tracts and the somatic motor neurons of the CNS. Two types of motor neurons are referred to clinically. One type is called the lower motor neuron (LMN) and includes the alpha and gamma motor neurons. As noted in the section on gray matter, the cell bodies of LMNs reside in lamina IX of the cord's ventral horn. Because of their location, LMNs also are called anterior horn cells. Their axons leave the cord in the ventral root, enter a spinal nerve, and continue in peripheral nerves to skeletal muscles. In general, LMNs can be defined as the only neurons that innervate skeletal muscle and are thus the final common pathway to the muscle. Without intact LMNs and intact neurons influencing them, the skeletal muscle cannot work properly, or even at all. These neurons are found in spinal nerves originating from the spinal cord and also in those cranial nerves emerging from the brain stem that innervate skeletal muscles located in the head region. Notice that

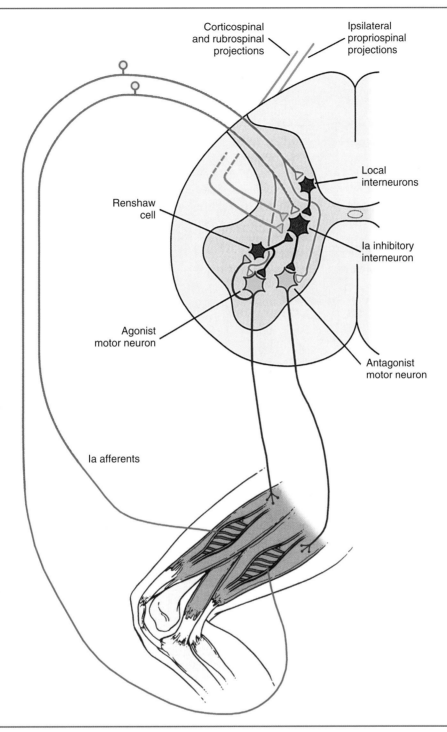

FIG. 9-28 Control of voluntary movements. The control of voluntary movements requires the integration of many different synaptic inputs as the level of the alpha motor neurons in the ventral horn of the spinal cord. By combining information from both ascending (sensory afferent information) and descending tracts (corticospinal, rubrospinal), along with extensive influence and modification by the spinal interneurons and reflex pathways "hardwired" at the level of the spinal cord, a multitude of responses can be generated that work together to produce the movements that we rely on for most of the daily activities we perform. Once a particular pathway in initiated, other competing pathways are mutually inhibited by the spinal interneurons, which results in only one set of instruction being sent to the alpha motor neurons at any one point in time to control movement. This allows the motor neurons to function as a single "myotatic unit" to produce the desired movement.

LMNs are found in both the CNS (i.e., cell bodies in the ventral horn of the cord or motor nuclei of the brain stem) and in the PNS (i.e., axons in peripheral nerves). Therefore a lesion of an LMN can occur anywhere along the entire neuron: at the level of the CNS and its cell body and more distally in the PNS, affecting the axon. Lesions of LMNs produce various signs and symptoms based on the fact that the LMN is responsible for the contraction of muscle. Because of its developmental origin, a skeletal muscle becomes innervated by more than one cord segment, and any one cord segment can innervate more than one muscle. Therefore to completely eliminate a muscle's innervation at the CNS level, a lesion must encompass all cord segments involved in the innervation of that muscle. However, a lesion of only one peripheral nerve distal to the brachial or lumbosacral plexuses may be all that is necessary to eliminate the innervation of a muscle of the extremities.

A lesion of LMNs produces characteristic signs, including the following:

- Muscle weakness
- Absent or diminished muscle tone. Tone is the amount of a muscle's resistance to stretch and is tested by passively flexing or extending a patient's joint. In LMN lesions there is a decreased resistance to passive movement called flaccid paralysis.
- Spontaneous contraction of muscle fascicles (fasciculations). This is caused by spontaneous discharging of the dying motor neurons with activation of motor units, and is visible as muscle twitching under the skin (spontaneous contractions of muscle fibers also occur but are evident only through electromyographic [EMG] recordings). The contractions peak approximately 2 or 3 weeks after denervation (Noback, Strominger, and Demarest, 1991).
- Severe neurogenic atrophy caused by denervation of the muscle and a subsequent loss of trophic (nourishing) factors normally produced by the motor neuron.
- Absent or decreased myotatic (stretch or deep tendon) reflexes (areflexia or hyporeflexia, respectively). The severity of this finding depends on the number of LMNs that remain intact to an individual muscle. One means of testing the health of a skeletal muscle, its sensory and motor fibers, and the general excitability of the CNS at a segmental level is through the muscle stretch reflex. Tapping a tendon elicits a stretch reflex that may be nonexistent, diminished, normal, or exaggerated. If a LMN lesion involves the nerve fibers innervating the muscle being tested, the reflex response of that particular muscle is nonexistent (areflexic) or diminished depending on how much of the muscle's innervation (by LMNs) is affected. For example, a lesion of an entire peripheral nerve or all the cord segments and roots forming that peripheral nerve results in areflexia, whereas a lesion of just some of the cord segments and roots results in hyporeflexia.

Upper Motor Neurons. The other type of motor neuron is the upper motor neuron (UMN). UMNs are clinically called neurons that influence LMNs. Often UMNs are considered to be the descending corticospinal fibers. In the context of this chapter, UMNs also include the vestibulospinal, rubrospinal, and reticulospinal tracts. Because UMNs are descending tracts, it is apparent that UMNs, unlike LMNs, remain in the CNS and extend from the location of their cell bodies to the termination of their axons. Therefore they are located in the cerebral cortex, internal capsule, brain stem, and white matter of the spinal cord.

Lesions of the spinal cord probably interrupt a number of descending tracts (UMNs) and produce characteristic signs that are evident after the acute effects are gone. These include the following:

- Muscle weakness
- Slow disuse atrophy
- Diminished or absent superficial (cutaneous) reflexes. These reflexes are elicited by applying an uncomfortable stimulus to the skin. An example of this type of reflex is the abdominal reflex. Stroking lateral to medial in a diamond-shaped pattern around the umbilicus normally causes the umbilicus to move toward the stimulus. This is mediated by the T8 to T12 nerves to the abdominal musculature. Another superficial reflex is the cremasteric reflex, which is tested by stroking the inner thigh. This results in elevation of the ipsilateral testicle and is mediated by the L1 and L2 nerves. This reflex is elicited best in infants. A third reflex is the plantar reflex. Stroking the lateral sole of the foot and under the toes produces a curling under of the toes and is mediated by the S1 and S2 nerves. These reflexes are under the influence of the corticospinal tract, which provides a tonic excitatory influence on segmental interneurons.
- Pathologic reflex. The most common pathologic reflex is the Babinski sign (extensor toe sign), which is a withdrawal response normally suppressed by the CST. Although any part of the leg can be stimulated producing "Babinski-like responses" (e.g., Chaddock's sign, Gordon's sign), the best technique is to stimulate the lateral sole of the foot and continue under the toes, which produces dorsiflexion of the big toe, with or without fanning of the other digits if the Babinski sign is present. Kumar and Ramasubramanian (2000) state that interpretation of a pathologic Babinski sign may be based on the following criteria:
  a. Upward movement of the great toe is pathologic only if caused by contraction of the extensor hallucis longus (EHL) muscle.

b. Contraction of the EHL muscle is pathologic only if it is occurring synchronously with reflex activity in other flexor muscles.

c. A Babinski sign does not necessarily imply that the concurrent activity of the other flexor muscles should be brisk and vice versa.

d. The true Babinski sign is reproducible, unlike voluntary withdrawal of the toes.

◆ Spasticity. Spasticity is characterized by an increase in resistance to rapid muscle stretch (hypertonia) that is especially evident in the antigravity muscles (i.e., upper extremity flexors and lower extremity extensors in humans). The resistance suddenly disappears during passive movement of an extremity. This action is similar to the opening of a pocket knife and is called the "clasp-knife" phenomenon.

It is speculated that afferents from the GTOs (proprioceptors located in muscle tendons) are stimulated, causing inhibition and release of the muscle. In addition to hypertonia, myotatic (stretch) reflexes are exaggerated (hyperreflexia). Lesioning UMNs eliminates descending excitatory input to inhibitory interneurons that synapse on LMNs. These inhibitory interneurons include Ia and Ib inhibitory interneurons, as well as presynaptic axoaxonic inhibitory interneurons (Benarroch et al., 1999). However, the components of the stretch reflex (Ia afferents and alpha motor neurons) and gamma motor neurons still are intact. This allows the gamma motor neurons to discharge at a higher rate. Although overactive gamma motor neurons may be involved in causing this phenomenon, changes in background activity of alpha motor neurons and interneurons have been implicated recently as important factors in the pathophysiology as well (Pearson and Gordon, 2000b). The spasticity produced by UMN lesions is caused by lesions in descending tracts, such as the reticulospinal tract (Bucy, Keplinger, and Siqueira, 1964; deGroot and Chusid, 1988; Snell, 2001; Nolte, 2002) rather than the corticospinal fibers. In addition, lesions of the cortical fibers projecting to the reticular formation (e.g., within the internal capsule) can cause dysfunction of the reticulospinal tract (Lance, 1980; deGroot and Chusid, 1988; Snell, 2001; Nolte, 2002).

The lack of involvement of the CST in producing spasticity is supported by experimental evidence. Selective lesions placed in the medullary pyramids of monkeys resulted in weakness of distal musculature and impairment of skilled movements of the hands but did not result in spasticity (Kuypers, 1981; Kiernan, 1998; Nolte, 2002). However, isolated case studies report that lesions in the pyramidal tract of humans cause increased tone. This may be because the lesions included reticulospinal fibers that lie close to the pyramidal fibers (Lance, 1980; Paulson, Yates, and Paltan-Ortiz, 1986).

◆ Clonus. This is another abnormal muscle activity sometimes seen as a common manifestation of hyperreflexia. Clonus occurs when muscle stretch reflexes take place in series and relaxation of one muscle triggers the contraction in another muscle, resulting in the rapid alternating contraction and relaxation of antagonistic muscles. For example, forceful and maintained dorsiflexion of the ankle joint results in continued rapid flexion and extension of the foot.

Certain components of motor activity should be evaluated when assessing the motor system. These include reflexes, muscle strength, muscle tone, muscle bulk, movements, and posture. Whenever possible, sides of the body should be compared, and proximal muscle groups should be compared with distal muscle groups. LMN lesions may be restricted to individual muscle groups, whereas UMN lesions may affect entire limbs. Both result in voluntary paralysis for different reasons. Paralysis of all four extremities is known as quadriplegia, paralysis in both lower extremities is paraplegia, one-sided paralysis is hemiplegia, and paralysis of one extremity is monoplegia. The presence of UMN lesion signs localizes the lesion to the CNS. However, LMN lesion signs may result from a lesion in the PNS or CNS. Knowledge of the peripheral nerve and cord segment innervation of muscles is imperative in determining the location of the lesion (see Table 9-3 and Peripheral Nerves).

Sensory Assessment

Evaluating the sensory systems involves testing the integrity of the DC-ML system and spinothalamic tract. Sensory modalities that may be tested include pain, temperature, touch, vibration, and conscious proprioception. Pain (nociception), which ascends contralaterally in the spinothalamic tract, is tested by pinpricking the skin in a dermatomal pattern. Light (crude) touch, which can be evaluated by brushing a wisp of cotton across the skin, ascends in both the spinothalamic tract and the DC-ML system. Testing for its presence gives general information about CNS integrity. Vibration is tested by placing a vibrating tuning fork over various bony prominences, such as the malleoli or olecranon process. This information ascends ipsilaterally in the cord's dorsal column. Conscious proprioception is evaluated by the clinician flexing or extending the patient's big toe or finger and asking the patient to identify if the digit is up or down. The patient's eyes are closed during each part of the examination. More discriminative sensations, including two-point touch, stereognosis, and graphesthesia, also ascend in the DC-ML system. These are complexly integrated in the parietal lobe association cortex located posterior to the postcentral gyrus of the cerebral cortex. The analysis by the cortex produces discriminatory capabilities that are important in the daily activities of human existence.

Two-point touch is tested on the patient's fingertips by stimulating two points on the skin simultaneously. The two points should be recognized within 2 to 3 mm of each other. Graphesthesia is tested by tracing numbers or letters on the skin of the back of the patient's hand and having the patient identify them. Stereognosis is tested by placing a common object in the hand and asking for its identification. The patient's eyes should be closed during these tests. Whenever possible, symmetry must be considered while evaluating these systems. Testing stereognosis and graphesthesia allows the clinician to assess higher cortical functioning.

As with motor assessment, knowledge of the innervation of the area tested, as well as knowledge of the ascending tracts involved, is imperative when assessing sensory functions. Peripheral nerve and dermatomal patterns of innervation (see Figs. 9-2 and 9-3) differ and must be distinguished.

Lesions

Discussing the pathologic conditions of the CNS is beyond the scope of this chapter. Therefore the following discussion generally describes specific lesions with the sole intent of emphasizing the key concepts in this chapter.

Lesions of the Dorsal and Ventral Roots. Various symptoms are present depending on the extent of injury to a dorsal root. Cutaneous afferents in the dorsal root are destined to innervate a specific strip of skin (dermatome). Therefore a lesion at this site produces symptoms that are localized in a dermatomal distribution rather than a peripheral nerve distribution (see Figs. 9-2 and 9-3). Because dermatomes overlap each other, sectioning (rhizotomy) one dorsal root produces different symptoms than sectioning many dorsal roots. For example, sectioning one dorsal root produces hypesthesia (slightly diminished sensation) or paresthesia (abnormal spontaneous sensation such as "tingling" or "pins and needles" typically experienced as when the foot "falls asleep"). Cutting several consecutive dorsal roots produces anesthesia except in the outermost dermatomes; that is, lesioning the L2 to L4 dorsal roots causes loss of all sensation only in the L3 dermatome. Some injuries may not be as severe, and lesions instead may cause pressure or irritation to the root (radix). Pressure may produce paresthesia and hypesthesia in a dermatomal pattern, whereas irritation and subsequent inflammation (or pressure resulting in ischemia) may

result in radicular (root) pain located in a dermatomal area. Because of the innervation of other (deeper) tissues by the involved nerves, radicular pain and paresthesias also may be experienced in patterns reflecting myotomal (dermomyotomal) and sclerotomal derivation as well (see Chapters 7 and 11).

In addition to the cutaneous effects seen, lesioning dorsal roots also disturb motor function, producing observable motor deficits. The destruction of all dorsal roots involved with the innervation of an extremity, for example, results in hypotonia and areflexia, even though the LMNs are intact. This occurs because the afferents of the stretch reflex are destroyed. Sensory afferents, such as from touch receptors and proprioceptors, also provide feedback about motor activity, which is essential for movements to occur properly. In fact, the extremity frequently is regarded by the individual as useless without this input, although it can be voluntarily moved. Experimental lesions of this nature on primates show that the animal does not use the extremity for climbing, walking, or grasping (Carpenter, 1991).

Tabes dorsalis, a form of neurosyphilis, affects the dorsal roots and also causes degeneration of the dorsal white columns. Initially radicular pain and paresthesias are present, followed later by impairment of sensation and reflexes, hypotonia, and loss of proprioception. Loss of proprioception results in sensory ataxia and an ataxic gait, described as being broad based with the feet slapping the ground. Visual cues are important in maintaining balance. This loss of proprioception is evidenced by the patient's inability to stand with the feet together and eyes closed without swaying or falling. This is called a Romberg sign and is indicative of damage to the dorsal column.

Ventral root lesion signs reflect the loss or disruption of the innervation to effectors. Destroying LMN fibers produces LMN lesion signs, whereas destroying autonomic efferents in the T1 to L2 (L3) and S2 to S4 roots affects visceral function (see Chapter 10). Pressure applied to the roots results in diminished reflexes and muscle weakness.

Cord Transection. An anatomic or physiologic transection of the spinal cord isolates the spinal cord from higher centers and other cord segments. Such a transection may produce a paraplegic or quadriplegic patient depending on the lesion's location. Initially and lasting days to weeks, a phenomenon called spinal shock ensues in which all or most spinal reflex activity below the level of the lesion is temporarily lost or depressed. This is thought to occur as a result of the sudden withdrawal of tonic facilitatory input (or some sort of trophic influence) from descending tracts to cord neurons leading to synaptic transmission alterations and impaired interneuronal conduction. Clinical signs manifested by spinal shock are muscle paralysis, flaccid muscle tone, and loss of stretch reflexes seen below the level of the lesion. Autonomic functions, including reflexes involved with blood pressure regulation and thermoregulation and control of colon and bladder activity, are variably affected depending on the level of the lesion. In general, reflex activity associated with the isolated segments closest to the transection are most severely affected, whereas reflex functions of distal segments may show little functional loss. For example, patients with lesions in lower cervical cord segments may still retain the sacral reflexes such as the bulbocavernosus reflex (contraction of the anal sphincter in response to compression of the penile shaft) and the anal wink (contraction of the anus in response to stroking of the perianal skin) (Atkinson and Atkinson, 1996; Chiles and Cooper, 1996; Hiersemenzel, Curt, and Dietz, 2000).

Recovery from spinal shock is heralded by an increase in excitability of muscle stretch reflexes, an increase in muscle tone, and frequent muscle spasms. At first, bilateral flexor muscle spasms predominate. In the lower extremity the flexors of the hip, knee, and foot may contract, producing the "triple-flexor response of Sherrington." In some severe cases the neurons become so hyperexcitable that the flexor response may occur in response to minimal cutaneous stimuli (e.g., pulling the bed sheet over the lower extremities of a patient) or even without any obvious stimulus (Carpenter, 1991; Noback, Strominger, and Demarest, 1991). This phase then transitions into the spastic state (spastic syndrome), which is characterized by exaggerated muscle stretch reflexes, increased muscle tone, and involuntary muscle contractions. Recovery of activity, although abnormal, may be attributed to increased numbers of postsynaptic receptors, denervation supersensitivity, a reorganization (upregulation) of membrane receptors, and sprouting of collateral branches of dorsal root axons producing new connections with cord neurons (Atkinson and Atkinson, 1996; Pearson and Gordon, 2000b). These abnormal reflex activities (UMN lesion signs) appear first in caudal segments and travel in a rostral direction up to the transected level. At this point, reflex activity is most often permanently lost (Atkinson and Atkinson, 1996; Hiersemenzel, Curt, and Dietz, 2000).

A hemisection of the left or right side of the spinal cord destroys several clinically important areas and produces a Brown-Séquard syndrome. Although most often a lesion is partial or incomplete, this syndrome is very instructive for applying concepts of neuroanatomy. In destroying a left or right half of the cord, numerous structures that are tested during a neurologic examination are involved. These are UMNs (located in the white matter), LMNs (located in the ventral horn), the clinically important ascending tracts (the dorsal column of the DC-ML and the spinothalamic tract), and the entry zone of afferent fibers and the dorsal horn (Fig. 9-29). Thus the following signs and symptoms (some of which are ipsilateral to and some contralateral to the side of the lesion) are seen at and below the level of the lesion (Fig. 9-30).

Motor assessment of cord hemisection

- Lower motor neuron lesion signs (e.g., fasciculations and flaccidity) are seen in the ipsilateral muscles innervated by the nerves originating in the lesioned cord segments.
- Upper motor neuron lesion signs (e.g., hyperreflexia, Babinski sign) are seen in the ipsilateral muscles innervated by the nerves originating from cord segments below the level of the lesion. Note that for UMN lesion signs to occur, the LMNs must be functioning.

Sensory assessment of cord hemisection

- Signs resulting from the loss of DC-ML functions are present ipsilaterally and below the level of the lesion. This includes loss of discriminating abilities (e.g., two-point touch, stereognosis, graphesthesia) and impaired joint position sense and vibratory sense. Some patients with dorsal column lesions also experience increased sensitivity to pain, temperature, and even tickling (Nathan, Smith, and Cook, 1986).
- Because of the interruption of the spinothalamic tract in the anterolateral quadrant, pain and temperature sense is lost on the contralateral side from approximately one or two segments below the level of the lesion.
- On the ipsilateral side and at the level of the lesion, anesthesia is present in a dermatomal pattern. In addition, because of the overlapping of adjacent dermatomes, hypesthesia and paresthesia are present ipsilaterally in dermatomal areas adjacent to the lesioned segments. Also, at the level of the lesion and depending on the number of cord segments involved, there usually is some contralateral impairment of pain and temperature because of the interruption of the decussating fibers that originate from the contralateral side.
- Little or no impairment of light (crude) touch exists, because this modality ascends in both the spinothalamic and the DC-ML tracts.

In localizing the site of the pathologic conditions, the UMN lesion signs are indicative of a CNS lesion, and the characteristic features of ipsilateral loss of discriminatory touch, vibration, and joint position sense and contralateral loss of pain and temperature suggest a hemisection of the spinal cord.

Syringomyelia. Syringomyelia is the progressive destruction of the central parts of the spinal cord as a

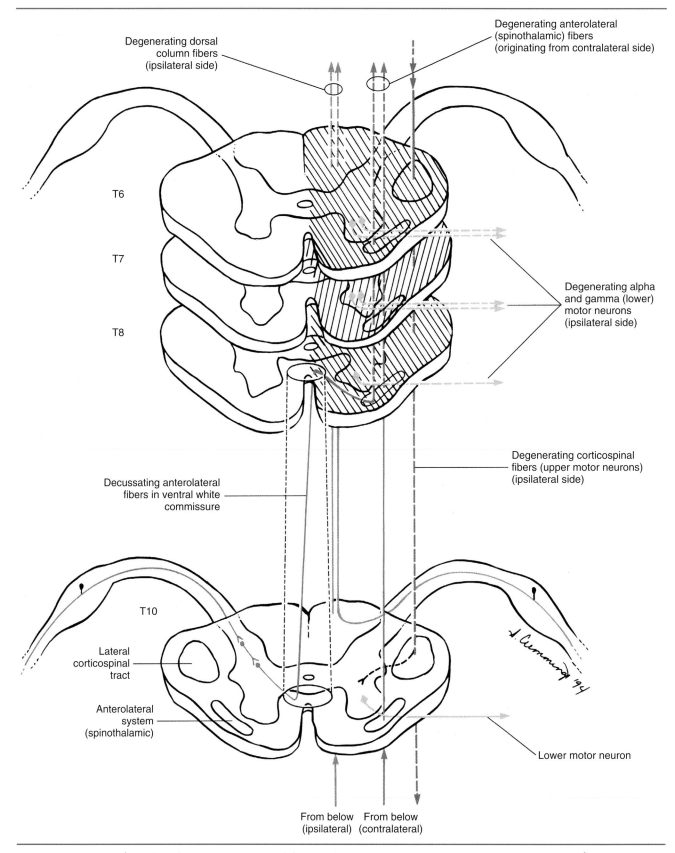

FIG. 9-29 Brown-Séquard syndrome. Hemisection of the spinal cord (*diagonal lines*) located in cord segments T6 through T8. The corticospinal tract (*green*), spinothalamic tract (*red*), dorsal column fibers (*blue*), and lower motor neurons (*yellow*) have been lesioned in those cord segments. The degenerating fibers are shown (*dashed lines*).

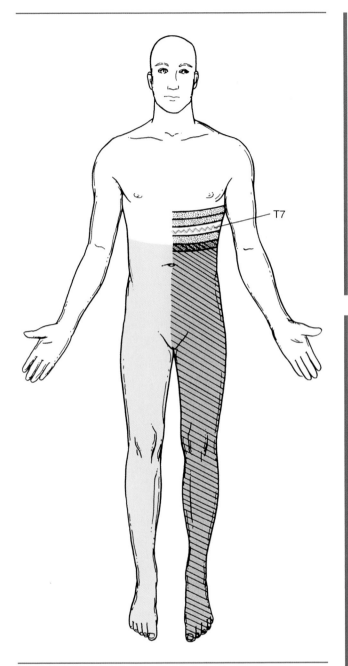

FIG. 9-30   Regions of the body affected by a hemisection (Brown-Séquard syndrome) of cord segments T6 through T8 as illustrated in Figure 9-29. The T7 dermatome (*red*) is a zone of anesthesia. Because of the overlapping between adjacent dermatomes, an area of hypesthesia and paresthesia exists (*stippled area*) on both sides of the T7 dermatome. Loss of pain and temperature sense (*blue*) occurs contralaterally below the level of the lesion. Impaired joint position sense and vibratory sense and loss of discriminatory abilities occur ipsilaterally below the level of the lesion (*light green*). Upper motor neuron lesions signs (*diagonal lines*) are present in muscles innervated by neurons originating in cord segments ipsilateral to and below the level of the lesion. Lower motor neuron signs are present in muscles innervated by neurons originating in the lesioned cord segments.

result of the formation of a cavity (syrinx) in the region of the central canal (Figs. 9-31 and 9-32). As the cavity enlarges ventrally (into the ventral white commissure), it disrupts the decussating spinothalamic fibers (see Fig. 9-32). This results in bilateral segmental loss of pain and temperature, with other sensory modalities spared. This condition is called sensory dissociation. The lesion may extend into the ventral horn, at which time it affects LMNs, producing atrophy, impaired reflexes, and weakness. The syrinx even may extend into adjacent white matter, affecting descending tracts. The lesion may not be symmetric and may vary in size from one segment to the next. Syringomyelia occurring in cervical segments and affecting the upper extremities is most common, and half of patients affected also have associated Arnold-Chiari malformation (inferior displacement of the cerebellar tonsils) (Adams and Salam-Adams, 1991).

Anterior Spinal Artery Syndrome.   The anterior spinal artery syndrome occurs as a result of the occlusion of the anterior spinal artery itself or of the arteries that reinforce it (see Chapter 3). The onset of signs and symptoms is abrupt, and the functional losses correspond to the territory of distribution that the artery supplies (i.e., the anterior two thirds of the spinal cord) (Fig. 9-33). Because the artery is unpaired, the signs are noted bilaterally. After the period of spinal shock, lower motor neuron (alpha and gamma motor neuron cell bodies in the ventral horn) lesion signs are observed in muscles innervated by the ischemic cord segments. Upper motor neuron (descending tracts in the white matter) lesion signs are seen in muscles innervated by segments caudal to the lesion. Pain and temperature sensations (conveyed in the anterolateral system) are lost bilaterally below the level of the lesion, whereas joint position sense, vibration, and discriminative touch are preserved (conveyed in the dorsal white column). The sparing of dorsal column function while losing anterolateral system (pain and temperature) function is also called a dissociated sensory loss (see Syringomyelia). Bladder and bowel function also may be impaired as well.

Amyotrophic Lateral Sclerosis.   Amyotrophic lateral sclerosis (ALS or Lou Gehrig's disease) is a progressive and degenerative motor neuron disease (see Fig. 9-33). It affects LMNs in the ventral horn, producing LMN signs in the affected muscles (e.g., atrophy, fasciculations, weakness). It also causes degeneration of upper motor neurons, and a Babinski sign may be present, as well as hyperreflexia and paralysis. Both types of motor neurons may be affected bilaterally. In addition to affecting skeletal muscles of the extremities and trunk, ALS causes degeneration of LMNs of the cranial nerves

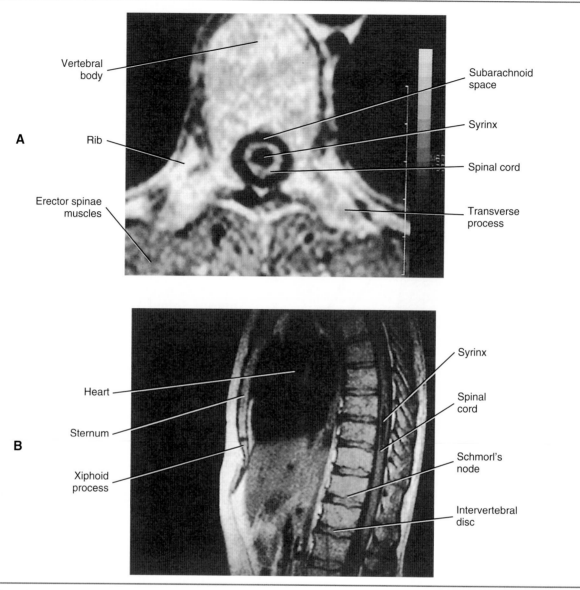

FIG. 9-31 Magnetic resonance images showing cavitation of the spinal cord resulting in syringomyelia. **A,** Horizontal section. **B,** Midsagittal section.

that innervate muscles of the face, pharynx, larynx, and tongue and may lead to serious problems of swallowing and breathing. A distinctive characteristic of this disease is that sensory functions are not impaired.

Combined Systems Disease. Combined systems disease is the combined bilateral degeneration of the dorsal white columns and the lateral white columns of the spinal cord (see Fig. 9-33). It is relatively rare and usually is associated with pernicious anemia (subacute combined degeneration). Pernicious anemia is caused by the inability to absorb vitamin B_{12} because of a lack of intrinsic factor. Combined systems disease begins with paresthesias in the hands and arms, followed by sensory ataxia as the dorsal columns of the lumbosacral cord become involved. As the disease progresses, UMN lesion signs appear, such as the Babinski sign and hyperreflexia. Peripheral nerves also may be involved; however, the symptoms are masked by those produced by the CNS lesions. Combined systems disease is treatable by the administration of weekly doses of vitamin B_{12} (cobalamin) (Adams and Salam-Adams, 1991).

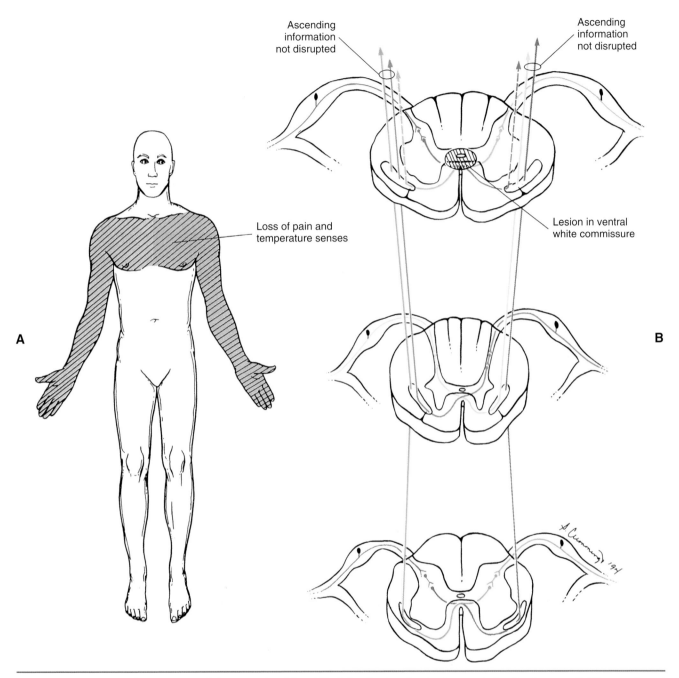

FIG. 9-32   A, Pain and temperature deficit seen in a "shawl-like" distribution that is characteristic of syringomyelia. The purple and orange areas correspond to the lesioned fibers illustrated in **B. B,** Three spinal cord cross sections. The top cross section represents spinal cord segments in which cavitation has resulted in syringomyelia. The diagonal lines indicate the lesioned area, which includes the ventral white commissure, where pain and temperature fibers from both sides of the body decussate. These lesioned fibers (*dashed lines*) are colored purple and orange. Ascending information entering the spinal cord below the lesion ascends in axons (*red, green, yellow, blue*) that are not disrupted.

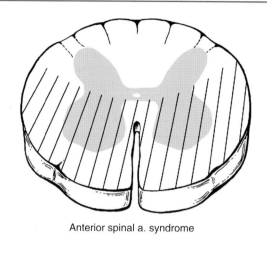

Anterior spinal a. syndrome

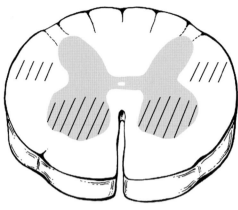

Amyotrophic lateral sclerosis

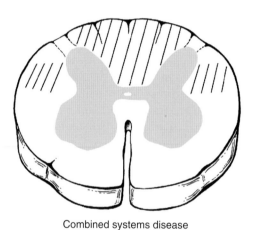

Combined systems disease

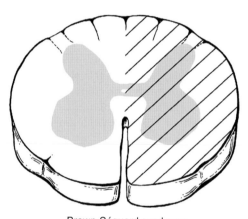

Brown-Séquard syndrome

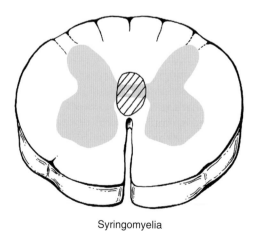

Syringomyelia

FIG. 9-33   Spinal cord lesions showing affected areas (see text for discussion).

REFERENCES

Abrahams VC. (1989).The distribution of muscle and cutaneous projections to the dorsal horn of the upper cervical cord of the cat. In F Cervero, GJ Bennett, & PM Headley (Eds.). *Processing of sensory information in the superficial dorsal horn of the spinal cord.* New York: Plenum Press.

Adams RD & Salam-Adams M. (1991). Chronic nontraumatic diseases of the spinal cord. *Neurol Clin, 9(3),* 605-623.

Adams RD & Victor M. (1989). *Principles of neurology* (4th ed.). New York: McGraw-Hill.

Amaral DG. The functional organization of perception and movement. In ER Kandel, JH Schwartz, & TM Jessell (Eds.). *Principles of neural science* (4th ed.). New York: McGraw-Hill.

Andrew D & Craig AD. (2001). Spinothalamic lamina I neurons selectively sensitive to histamine: A central neural pathway for itch. *Nat Neurosci, 4(1),* 72-77.

Atkinson PP & Atkinson JLD. (1996). Spinal shock. *Mayo Clin Proc, 71,* 384-389.

Basbaum AI & Jessell TM. (2000). The perception of pain. In ER Kandel, JH Schwartz, & TM Jessell (Eds.). *Principles of neural science* (4th ed.). New York: McGraw-Hill.

Belanger M et al. (1996).A comparison of treadmill locomotion in adult cats after spinal transaction.*J Neurophysiol, 7,* 471-491.

Benarroch EE et al. (1999). *Medical neurosciences* (4th ed.). New York: Lippincott Williams & Wilkins.

Bentivoglio M & Rustioni A. (1986). Corticospinal neurons with branching axons to the dorsal column nuclei in the monkey. *J Comp Neurol, 253,* 260-276.

Bessou P, Emonet-Demand F, & Laporte Y. (1965). Motor fibers innervating extrafusal and intrafusal muscle fibers in the cat. *J Physiol Lond, 180,* 649-672.

Biondi DM. (2000). Cervicogenic headache: Mechanisms, evaluation, and treatment strategies.*JAOA, 100(9),* S7-S13.

Biondi DM. (2001). Cervicogenic headache: Diagnostic evaluation and treatment strategies. *Curr Pain Headache Rep, 5,* 361-368.

Bogduk N. (1992). The anatomical basis for cervicogenic headache. *JMPT, 15(1),* 67-70.

Bogduk N. (2001). Cervicogenic headache: Anatomic basis and patho-physiologic mechanisms. *Curr Pain Headache Rep, 5,* 382-386.

Bosco G & Poppele RE. (2001). Proprioception from a spinocerebellar perspective. *Physiol Rev, 81,* 539-568.

Boyd IA. (1980).The isolated mammalian muscle spindle. *Trends Neurosci, 3,* 258-265.

Brooks VB. (1986). *The neural basis of motor control.* New York: Oxford University Press.

Brown TG. (1911). The intrinsic factors in the act of progression in the mammal. *Proc R Soc Lond [Biol], 84,* 308-319.

Browne PA et al. (1998). Concurrent cervical and craniofacial pain. *Oral Surg Oral Med Oral Path, 86(6),* 633-640.

Bucy PC, Keplinger JE, & Siqueira EB. (1964). Destruction of the "pyramidal tract" in man.*J Neurol, 21,* 385-398.

Calancie B et al. (1994). Involuntary stepping after chronic spinal cord injury: Evidence for a central pattern generator for locomotion in man. *Brain, 117,* 1143-1159.

Canedo A. (1997). Primary motor cortex influences on the descending and ascending systems. *Prog Neurobiol, 51,* 287-335.

Carpenter MB. (1991). *Core text of neuroanatomy* (4th ed.). Baltimore: Williams & Wilkins.

Carpenter MB & Sutin J. (1983). *Human neuroanatomy* (8th ed.). Baltimore:Williams & Wilkins.

Chandler MJ, Zhang J, & Foreman RD. (1996).Vagal, sympathetic and somatic sensory inputs to upper cervical (C1-C3) spinothalamic tract neurons in monkeys.*J Neurophysiology, 76(4),* 2555-2567.

Chiles III BW & Cooper PR. (1996). Acute spinal injury. *N Engl J Med, 334(8),* 514-520.

Coulter JD et al. (1979). Cortical, tectal and medullary descending pathways to the cervical spinal cord. *Prog Brain Res, 50,* 263-279.

Craig AD, Zhang ET, & Blomqvist A. (2002). Association of spinothalamic lamina I neurons and their ascending axons with calbindin-immuno-reactivity in monkey and human. *Pain, 97,* 105-115.

Davidoff RA. (1990).The pyramidal tract. *Neurology, 40,* 332-339.

Davidoff RA & Hackman JC. (1991). Aspects of spinal cord structure and reflex function. *Neurol Clin, 9(3),* 533-550.

deGroot J & Chusid JG. (1988). *Correlative neuroanatomy* (20th ed.). Norwalk, Conn:Appleton & Lange.

DeMyer W. (1959). Number of axons and myelin sheaths in adult human medullary pyramids. *Neurology, 9,* 42-47.

Ekerot CF, Larson B, & Oscarsson O. (1979). Information carried by the spinocerebellar paths. *Prog Brain Res, 50,* 79-90.

Engberg I & Lundberg A. (1969). An electromyographic analysis of muscular activity in the hindlimb of the cat during unrestrained locomotion. *Acta Physiol Scand, 75,* 614-630.

FitzGerald MJT & Folan-Curran J. (2002). *Clinical neuroanatomy and related neuroscience* (4th ed.). Edinburgh:WB Saunders.

Friehs GM, Schrottner O, & Pendl G. (1995). Evidence for segregated pain and temperature conduction within the spinothalamic tract.*J Neurosurg, 83,* 8-12.

Gardner EP, Martin JH, & Jessell TM. (2000).The bodily senses. In ER Kandel, JH Schwartz, & TM Jessell (Eds.). *Principles of neural science* (4th ed.). New York: McGraw-Hill.

Ghez C & Krakauer J. (2000).The organization of movement. In ER Kandel, JH Schwartz, & TM Jessell (Eds.). *Principles of neural science* (4th ed.). New York: McGraw-Hill.

Ghez C. (1991). Posture. In ER Kandel, JH Schwartz, & TM Jessell (Eds.). *Principles of neural science* (3rd ed.). Norwalk, Conn: Appleton & Lange.

Ghez C & Thach WT. (2000).The cerebellum. In ER Kandel, JH Schwartz, & TM Jessell (Eds.). *Principles of neural science* (4th ed.). New York: McGraw-Hill.

Gordon J & Ghez C. (1991). Muscle receptors and spinal reflexes: The stretch reflex. In ER Kandel, JH Schwartz, & TM Jessell (Eds.). *Principles of neural science* (3rd ed.). Norwalk, Conn:Appleton & Lange.

Grant G & Xu Q. (1988). Routes of entry into the cerebellum of spinocerebellar axons from the lower part of the spinal cord. *Exp Brain Res, 72,* 543-561.

Grillner S & Wallen P. (1985). Central pattern generators for locomotion, with special reference to vertebrates.*Ann Rev Neuroscience, 8,* 233-261.

Han ZS, Zhang ET, & Craig AD. (1998). Nociceptive and thermoreceptive lamina I neurons are anatomically distinct. *Nat Neurosci, 1(3),* 218-225.

Hiersemenzel L, Curt A, & Dietz V. (2000). From spinal shock to spasticity: Neuronal adaptations to a spinal cord injury. *Neurology, 54,* 1574-1582.

Hodge Jr CJ & Apkarian AV. (1990). The spinothalamic tract. *Crit Rev Neurobiol, 5(4),* 363-397.

Hubbard DR & Berkoff GM. (1993). Myofascial trigger points show spontaneous needle EMG activity. *Spine, 18(13),* 1803-1807.

Hunt CC. (1990). Mammalian muscle spindles: Peripheral mechanism. *Physiol Rev, 70,* 643-663.

Jami L. (1992). Golgi tendon organs in mammalian skeletal muscle: Functional properties and central actions. *Physiol Rev, 72,* 623-666.

Jänig W. (1996). Neurobiology of visceral afferent neurons: Neuroanatomy, functions, organ regulations and sensations. *Biol Psychol, 42,* 29-51.

Keegan JG & Garrett FV. (1948).The segmental distribution of the cutaneous nerves in the limbs of man. *Anat Rec, 102,* 409-437.

Kiernan JA. (1998). *The human nervous system* (7th ed.). Philadelphia: JB Lippincott.

Krakauer J & Ghez C (2000). Voluntary movement. In ER Kandel, JH Schwartz, &TM Jessell (Eds.). *Principles of neural science* (4th ed.). New York: McGraw-Hill.

Kumar SP & Ramasubramanian D. (2000). The Babinski sign: A reappraisal. *Neurol India, 48,* 314-318.

Kuypers HG. (1981). Anatomy of the descending pathways. In VB Brooks (Ed.). *Handbook of physiology.* Bethesda, Md: American Physiological Society.

Lance JW. (1980). The control of muscle tone, reflexes, and movement: Robert Wartenberg lecture. *Neurology, 30,* 1303-1313.

Lance JW. (1989). Headache: Classification, mechanism and principles of therapy, with particular reference to migraine. *Rec Prog Med, 80(12),* 673-680.

Leksell L. (1945).The action potential and excitatory effects of the small ventral root fibers to skeletal muscle.*Acta Physiol Scand, 10(suppl 31),* 1-84.

Loeb GE & Ghez C. (2000).Voluntary movement. In ER Kandel, JH Schwartz, & TM Jessell (Eds.). *Principles of neural science* (4th ed.). New York: McGraw-Hill.

Lu GW & Willis WD. (1999). Branching or collateral projections of spinal dorsal horn neurons. *Brain Res Rev, 29,* 50-82.

Maertens de Noordhout A et al. (1999). Corticomotoneuronal synaptic connections in normal man. *Brain, 122,* 1327-1340.

McCloskey DI. (1994). Human proprioceptive sensation. *J Clin Neurosci, 1(3)*, 173-177.

Meyer Jr PR et al. (1991). Spinal cord injury. *Neurol Clin, 9(3)*, 625-661.

Milanov I & Bogdanova D. (2003). Trigemino-cervical reflex in patients with headache. *Cephalalgia, 23*, 35-38.

Miyabayashi T & Shirai T. (1988). Synaptic formation of the corticospinal tract in the rat spinal cord. *Okajimas Folia Anat Jpn, 65(2-3)*, 117-140.

Nashner LM. (1976). Adapting reflexes controlling the human posture. *Exp Brain Res, 26*, 59-72.

Nathan PW & Smith MC. (1982). The rubrospinal and central tegmental tracts in man. *Brain, 105*, 223-269.

Nathan PW, Smith MC, & Cook AW. (1986). Sensory effects in man of lesions of the posterior columns and of some other afferent pathways. *Brain, 109*, 1003-1041.

Nathan PW, Smith MC, & Deacon P. (1990). The corticospinal tracts in man. *Brain, 113*, 303-324.

Nathan PW, Smith M, & Deacon P. (1996). Vestibulospinal, reticulospinal and descending propriospinal nerve fibers in man. *Brain, 119*, 1809-1833.

Nathan PW, Smith M, & Deacon P. (2001). The crossing of the spinothalamic tract. *Brain, 124*, 793-803.

Nauta HJW et al. (1997). Surgical interruption of a midline dorsal column visceral pain pathway. *J Neurosurg, 86*, 538-542.

Nicolas G et al. (2001). Corticospinal excitation of presumed cervical propriospinal neurones and its reversal to inhibition in humans. *J Physiol, 533, (3)*, 903-919.

Noback CR, Strominger NL, & Demarest RJ. (1991). *The human nervous system* (4th ed.). Philadelphia: Lea & Febiger.

Nolte J. (2002). *The human brain* (4th ed.). St Louis: Mosby.

Palmieri G et al. (1986). Course and termination of the pyramidal tract in the pig. *Arch d'Anat Micro, 75*, 167-176.

Parke WW & Whalen JL. (2001). Phrenic paresis: A possible additional spinal cord dysfunction induced by neck manipulation in cervical spondylotic myelopathy (CSM). A report of two cases with anatomical and clinical considerations. *Clin Anat, 14*, 173-178.

Paulson GW, Yates AJ, & Paltan-Ortiz JD. (1986). Does infarction of the medullary pyramid lead to spasticity? *Arch Neurol, 43*, 93-95.

Pearson K. (1995). Proprioceptive regulation of locomotion. *Curr Opin Neurobiol, 5*, 785-791

Pearson K & Gordon J. (2000a). Locomotion. In ER Kandel, JH Schwartz, & TM Jessell (Eds.). *Principles of neural science* (4th ed.). New York: McGraw-Hill.

Pearson K & Gordon J. (2000b). Spinal reflexes. In ER Kandel, JH Schwartz, & TM Jessell (Eds.). *Principles of neural science* (4th ed.). New York: McGraw-Hill.

Pierrot-Deseilligny E. (1996). Transmission of the cortical command for human voluntary movement through cervical propriospinal premoto-neurons. *Prog Neurobiol, 48*, 489-517.

Pollmann W, Keidel M, & Pfaffenrath V. (1997). Headache and the cervical spine: A critical review. *Cephalalgia, 17*, 801-816.

Poppele RE, Rankin A, & Eian J. (2003). Dorsal spinocerebellar tract neurons respond to contralateral limb stepping. *Exp Brain Res, 149*, 361-370.

Prochazka A et al. (1988). Dynamic and static fusimotor set in various behavioural contexts. In P Hnik et al. (Eds.). *Mechanoreceptors: Development, structure and function*. New York: Plenum Press.

Rexed B. (1952). The cytoarchitectonic organization of the spinal cord in the cat. *J Comp Neurol, 96*, 415-495.

Rhoades RA & Tanner GA. (2003). *Medical physiology* (2nd ed.). Philadelphia: Lippincott Williams & Wilkins.

Routal RV & Pal GP. (1999). Location of the phrenic nucleus in the human spinal cord. *J Anat, 195*, 617-621.

Schmelz M et al. (1997). Specific C-receptors for itch in human skin. *J Neurosci, 17(20)*, 8003-8008.

Schoenen J. (1991). Clinical anatomy of the spinal cord. *Neurol Clin, 9(3)*, 503-532.

Sessle B. (1998). Neurophysiological mechanisms related to craniofacial and cervical pain. *Top Clin Chiropract, 5(1)*, 36-38.

Severin FV, Orlovsky GN, & Shik ML. (1967). Work of the muscle receptors during controlled locomotion. *Biofizika, 12*, 575-586.

Sewards TV & Sewards MA. (2002). The medial pain system: Neural representations of the motivational aspect of pain. *Brain Res Bull, 59*, 163-180.

Sherrington C. (1947). *The integrative action of the nervous system* (2nd ed.). New Haven, Conn: Yale University Press.

Shik ML & Orlovsky GN. (1976). Neurophysiology of locomotor automatism. *Physiol Rev, 56*, 465-501.

Smith MC & Deacon P. (1984). Topographical anatomy of the posterior columns of the spinal cord in man. *Brain, 107*, 671-698.

Snell RS. (2001). *Clinical neuroanatomy for medical students* (5th ed.). Philadelphia: Lippincott Williams & Wilkins.

Wada A et al. (2001). Are there one million nerve fibres in the human medullary pyramid? *Okajimas Folia Anat Jpn, 77(6)*, 221-224.

Williams PL et al. (1995). *Gray's anatomy* (38th ed.). Edinburgh: Churchill Livingstone.

Willis Jr WD & Coggeshall RE. (1991). *Sensory mechanisms of the spinal cord* (2nd ed.). New York: Plenum Press.

Willis Jr WD & Westlund KN. (2001). The role of the dorsal column pathway in visceral nociception. *Curr Pain Headache Rep, 5(1)*, 20-26.

Willis Jr WD & Westlund KN. (1997). Neuroanatomy of the pain system and of the pathways that modulate pain. *J Clin Neurophysiol, 14(1)*, 2-31.

Wise SP & Evarts EV. (1981). The role of the cerebral cortex in movement. *TINS, Dec*, 297-300.

Wyke BD. (1985). Articular neurology and manipulative therapy. In EF Glasgow et al. (Eds.). *Aspects of manipulative therapy* (2nd ed.). New York: Churchill Livingstone.

Xu Q & Grant G. (1988). Collateral projections of neurons from the lower part of the spinal cord to anterior and posterior cerebellar termination areas. *Exp Brain Res, 72*, 562-576.

Young PA. (1986). The anatomy of the spinal cord pain paths: A review. *J Am Paraplegia Soc, 9*, 28-38.

CHAPTER 10

Neuroanatomy of the Autonomic Nervous System

Susan A. Darby

The autonomic nervous system (ANS) functions to maintain homeostasis by providing the optimal internal environment for the cellular components of the organism during normal and stressful periods. The ANS accomplishes this task through its control of visceral function, and generally it is considered to be a motor system consisting of fibers that innervate the smooth muscle, cardiac muscle, and glands of the body. However, sophisticated neuroanatomic techniques, such as immunocytochemistry and axonal tracing methods, have produced data indicating that visceral control involves much more than the efferents of the sympathetic and parasympathetic divisions of the ANS. Information suggests that other structures and regions are intimately associated with these efferents. These include visceral afferent fibers and the reflexes they may initiate, the widespread influence and variety of chemical mediators, and the central autonomic circuitry, which is involved with the integration and dissemination of visceral input. Therefore each of these topics generally is described along with the origin and course of the sympathetic and parasympathetic efferent fibers to present a composite picture of the ANS. The chapter concludes with examples of pathologies that affect the ANS.

AUTONOMIC EFFERENTS: SYMPATHETIC, PARASYMPATHETIC, AND ENTERIC DIVISIONS

The ANS is composed of a sympathetic and parasympathetic division. These two divisions are discussed here, followed by a description of a third division of the ANS. This third division is the enteric nervous system, which is a complex network of neurons located within the wall of the gut. Typically the anatomy and functions of the parasympathetic and sympathetic divisions are described separately. However, remember that fibers of both divisions are tonically active, and in most cases do not function as either "on" or "off." Although some tissues are predominantly or exclusively innervated by one division (e.g., sympathetic peripheral effector tissues), many tissues have a dual innervation. A balance of activity exists between the division fibers in these cases, such that when one division increases its activity, the other division decreases its activity. The central nervous system (CNS) has the ability to alter the balance of activity between these divisions. In addition, the sympathetic and parasympathetic divisions interact with the somatic nervous system and different hormonal systems to sta-

bilize the internal environment and maintain homeostasis during normal conditions or emergency situations.

The ANS can be described best after certain characteristics common to both the sympathetic and parasympathetic divisions have been reviewed. The parasympathetic and sympathetic innervation of autonomic effectors (i.e., organs, vessels, glands) is organized differently than the innervation of skeletal muscle (Fig. 10-1). Although the axons of alpha and gamma motor neurons course directly to skeletal muscles, the innervation of ANS effectors requires a chain of two neurons (see Fig. 10-1), called the preganglionic and postganglionic neurons. The cell body of the preganglionic neuron always is located

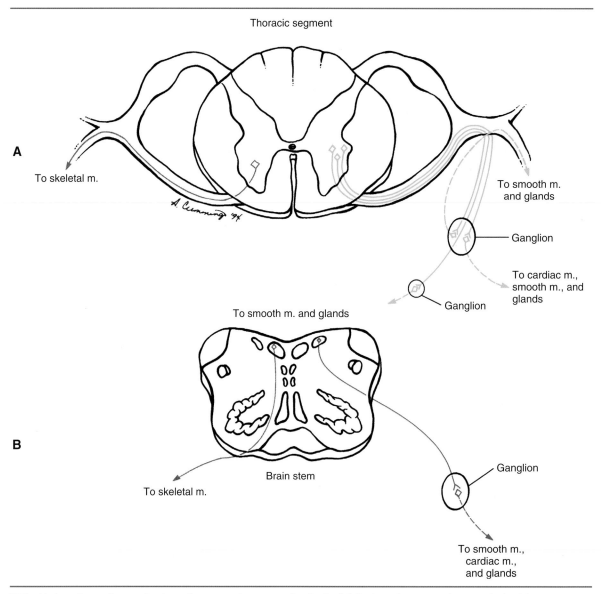

FIG. 10-1 General organization of autonomic preganglionic (*solid line*) and postganglionic (*dashed line*) neurons (*right*) compared with somatic efferent neurons (*left*). **A,** Sympathetic output and somatic output from the spinal cord. **B,** Parasympathetic output and somatic output from the brain stem.

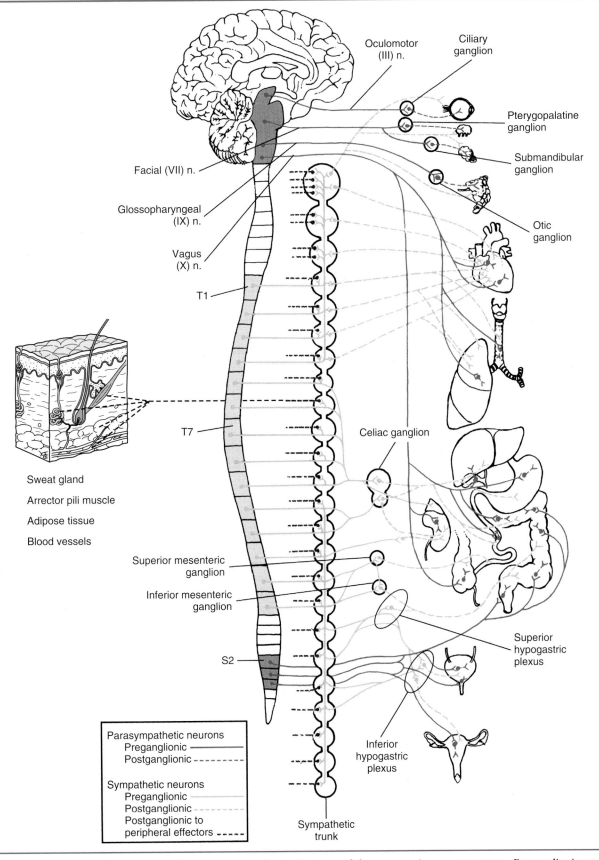

Oculomotor (III) n.

Ciliary ganglion

Pterygopalatine ganglion

Submandibular ganglion

Facial (VII) n.

Glossopharyngeal (IX) n.

Vagus (X) n.

T1

Otic ganglion

Sweat gland

Arrector pili muscle

Adipose tissue

Blood vessels

T7

Celiac ganglion

Superior mesenteric ganglion

Inferior mesenteric ganglion

S2

Superior hypogastric plexus

Parasympathetic neurons
Preganglionic ————
Postganglionic -------

Sympathetic neurons
Preganglionic ————
Postganglionic --------
Postganglionic to peripheral effectors - - - - -

Inferior hypogastric plexus

Sympathetic trunk

FIG. 10-2 Overview of the parasympathetic and sympathetic divisions of the autonomic nervous system. Preganglionic neuron cell bodies are located in the brain stem and sacral cord segments (parasympathetic or "cranio-sacral" division) and thoracic and upper lumbar cord segments (sympathetic or "thoraco-lumbar" division). The axons of these neurons synapse with postganglionic neurons, which course to the smooth muscle, cardiac muscle, and glands of the body. The postganglionic neuron cell bodies may be located in distinct autonomic ganglia, or in or very near the wall of the innervated visceral organ. Note that sympathetic fibers provide the only innervation to peripheral effectors (sweat glands, arrector pili muscles, adipose tissue, and blood vessels).

in the CNS; either in the spinal cord or brain stem (Fig. 10-2). The axon is thinly myelinated and immediately leaves the CNS within a specific ventral root of the spinal cord or within certain cranial nerves exiting the brain stem. The cell body of the postganglionic neuron is located in an autonomic ganglion that may be found in numerous places outside the CNS (see Fig. 10-2). The preganglionic neuron synapses with the postganglionic neuron within this ganglion. The axon of the postganglionic neuron is unmyelinated and innervates the effector. Both the preganglionic and postganglionic neurons frequently travel in components of the peripheral nervous system (PNS) (i.e., spinal nerves, cranial nerves) and are intermingled with afferents and somatic motor neurons of peripheral nerves. As stated, most effectors are innervated by both sympathetic and parasympathetic fibers (Table 10-1; see also Fig. 10-2). These fibers produce antagonistic but coordinated responses in the effectors. Descending input from higher integrative centers such as the hypothalamus and areas of the brain stem reaches the cell bodies of preganglionic fibers to regulate and adjust their activity. This descending input is a part of several specific visceral reflex pathways and also is used by higher centers to institute widespread bodily changes.

Sympathetic Division

The general function of the sympathetic nervous system (SNS) is to help the body cope with stressful situations. The response usually is the rapid release, and subsequent use, of energy. This is best exemplified by the reaction of the body to a dangerous situation. In this instance, sympathetic involuntary responses occur, including increased heart and respiratory rates, cold and clammy hands, wide-eyed stare, and dilated pupils. Blood is redistributed by means of vasoconstriction and vasodilation from such areas as the abdominal and pelvic organs and skin, to more important tissues such as the brain, heart, and skeletal muscles. The level of blood glucose increases, as does blood pressure. Activity of the gastrointestinal (GI) and urinary systems is less important during this stressful situation; therefore the smooth muscle of these organs is inhibited. The sympathetic division often is called the fight-or-flight division of the ANS because of this overall response.

Preganglionic Sympathetic Neurons. The cell bodies of the preganglionic sympathetic neurons are located in the spinal cord in all thoracic segments and in the upper two or three lumbar segments (see Fig. 10-2). Because of the distribution of these preganglionic cell bodies, the sympathetic division of the ANS often is called the thoracolumbar division. These preganglionic neurons comprise a heterogeneous population within the spinal cord. The dendritic arrangement of these neu-

rons ranges from simple to complex arborizations. The cell bodies are of different shapes, and their size falls in a range between the size of smaller dorsal horn neurons and larger somatic motor neurons. Of the total membranous surface area of these neurons, the cell body of each composes a maximum of 15%, which likely indicates the importance of the dendritic surface area of that neuron (Cabot, 1990).

The cell bodies of the preganglionic neurons are found in four nuclei within the intermediate gray matter of the spinal cord (Fig. 10-3) (Cabot, 1990). The largest group of these cell bodies is the intermediolateral (IML) cell column that forms the lateral horn. Throughout this column are clusters of 20 to 100 neurons that are separated by distances ranging from 200 to 500 μm in the thoracic region and 100 to 300 μm in the lumbar region. The cell bodies are approximately 12 to 13 μm in diameter and histologically are similar to motor neurons (Harati, 1993). The diameters of the axons range from 2 to 5 μm, and their speed of conduction is approximately 3 to 15 m/sec. These fibers often are classified in the B group (see Chapter 9). At the T6 and T7 levels, the mean number of these cells is approximately 5000, but it has been shown that the number decreases with age at the rate of approximately 8% per decade (Harati, 1993).

The other three nuclear groups of preganglionic neurons have been described by Cabot (1990) and are the lateral funicular area (located lateral and dorsal to the intermediolateral group), the intercalated cell group (located medial to the IML column and possibly the same cluster of neurons typically called the intermediomedial group), and the central autonomic nucleus (located lateral and dorsal to the central canal). The combination of these groups forms a ladderlike structure in longitudinal sections in which the paired IML cell columns form the sides of the ladder and the interconnected central autonomic nucleus and intercalated cell group form the rungs (Fig. 10-3). The IML cell column is the origin of the vast majority of preganglionic fibers, but the other three nuclei also give rise to some preganglionic fibers. The four nuclei are the recipients of extensive input from higher centers such as the hypothalamus and brain stem nuclei. These sources release various neurotransmitters that have been identified as monoamines, neuropeptides, and amino acids. Although the anatomic characteristics of these four nuclei have been described, the exact functions of each specific nucleus still remain unclear.

Postganglionic Sympathetic Neurons. According to the general rule of organization of the ANS, two neurons are necessary for the impulse to reach the effector. One is the preganglionic neuron, just discussed. The second neuron in the pathway to an autonomic effector is the postganglionic neuron. This neuron's axon is

Table 10-1 Functions of the Sympathetic and Parasympathetic Divisions

Structure	Sympathetic Function (Adrenergic Receptors)	Parasympathetic Function
Eye		
Sphincter muscle	—	Contraction → Constricts
Dilator muscle	Contraction → Dilates (α_1)	
Ciliary muscle	Relaxes (slightly; far vision) (β_2)	Contracts (near vision)
Heart		
Rate and force of atrial and ventricular contractions	Increases (β_1 and some β_2)	Decreases
Lungs		
Bronchial muscle	Relaxation → Dilates airway (β_2)	Contraction → Constricts airway
Glands	—	Stimulates secretion
Skin		
Sweat glands	Increases secretion (cholinergic)[1]	—
Arrector pili muscle	Contracts (α_1)	—
Glands of Head		
Lacrimal	Vasoconstriction → Reduces secretion (α)	Increases secretion
Salivary	Vasoconstriction → Secretion reduced and viscid (α); amylase secretion (β_2)	Secretion increased and watery
Blood Vessels		
Arterioles: coronary, skeletal muscle, pulmonary, abdominal viscera, renal	Contraction → Vasoconstriction (α_1) Relaxation → Vasodilation (β_2)	Vasodilation
Skin, cerebral	Contraction → Vasoconstriction (α_1)	—
Systemic veins	Contraction → Vasoconstriction (α_1) Relaxation → Vasodilation (β_2)	— —
Gastrointestinal Tract		
Motility/tone	Inhibits (α_1, β_2)	Stimulates
Sphincters	Constricts (α_1)	Relaxes
Secretion	Vasoconstriction → Inhibits secretion (α_1)	Stimulates
Liver	Breaks down glycogen (glycogenolysis), gluconeogenesis, decreased bile secretion (α, β_2)	Glycogen synthesis; increases bile secretion
Gallbladder	Relaxes (β_2)	Contracts
Pancreas	Inhibits secretion of digestive enzymes, glucagon, and insulin (α_2); increases secretion of insulin and glucagon (β_2)	Secretion of digestive enzymes, insulin, and glucagon
Spleen Capsule	Contraction (α_1) Relaxation (β_2)	— —
Adipose	Lipolysis (β_1); release of fatty acids into blood (β_1, β_3; β_3 in brown adipose tissue)	—
Kidney (juxtaglomerular cells)	Secretion of renin (β_1)	—
Urinary Bladder		
Detrusor muscle	Relaxes (minimal role) (β_2)	Contracts
Sphincter (nonstriated)	Contracts (α_1)	Relaxes
Sex Organs	Contracts smooth muscle of vas deferens, seminal vesicle, prostate → Ejaculation (α_1)	Vasodilation → Erection of clitoris (females) and penis (males)

Continued

Table 10-1 Functions of the Sympathetic and Parasympathetic Divisions—cont'd

Structure	Sympathetic Function (Adrenergic Receptors)	Parasympathetic Function
Uterus	Variable (depends on hormonal status, pregnancy, and other factors) (α_1, β_2)	Minimal effect
Adrenal Medulla	Stimulates secretion of epinephrine and norepinephrine (nicotinic ACh receptors) via preganglionic fibers	—
Pineal	Increases melatonin synthesis and secretion (β)	—

From Benarroch EE et al. (1999). *Medical neurosciences* (4th ed.). New York: Lippincott Williams & Wilkins; Bray JJ et al. (1994). *Lecture notes on human physiology* (3rd ed.). Cambridge, UK: Blackwell Science; FitzGerald MJT & Folan-Curran J. (2002). *Clinical neuroanatomy and related neuroscience* (4th ed.). Philadelphia: WB Saunders; Tortora GJ & Grabowski SR. (2003). *Principles of anatomy and physiology* (10th ed.). New York: John Wiley & Sons, Inc.; Waxman SG. (2003). *Clinical neuroanatomy* (25th ed.). Chicago: McGraw-Hill.
[1]Sweat glands are an exception; their sympathetic fibers release ACh, which binds to cholinergic receptors.

classified as a group C fiber (see Chapter 9). Generally it is described as unmyelinated, with a diameter ranging from 0.3 to 1.3 μm and a slow conduction speed ranging from 0.7 to 2.3 m/sec (Carpenter and Sutin, 1983). The cell body is located outside the CNS in an autonomic ganglion. Unlike a sensory ganglion of cranial nerves and a dorsal root ganglion of spinal nerves, in which no synapses occur, an autonomic ganglion is the location of the synapse between the preganglionic and postganglionic neurons. Preganglionic fibers disseminate their information by diverging and synapsing on numerous postganglionic fibers. This principle of divergence is based on studies of the superior cervical ganglion of mammals. Results of different studies show preganglionic

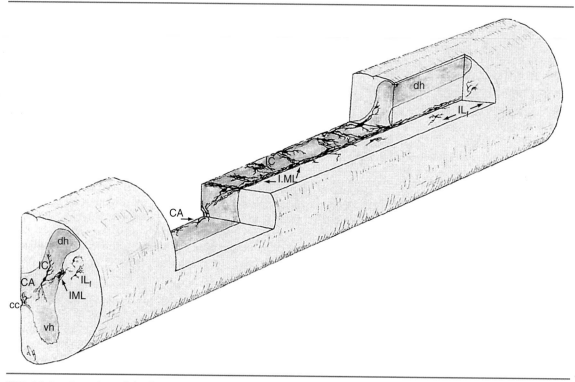

FIG. 10-3 Location of the four groups of sympathetic preganglionic neurons within the spinal cord gray matter. In the middle of the spinal cord, the horizontal plane shows the "ladderlike" arrangement of these neurons. *CA,* central autonomic nucleus; *cc,* central canal; *dh,* dorsal horn; *IC,* intercalated nucleus; *IL_f,* lateral funicular nucleus; *IML,* intermediolateral nucleus; *vh,* ventral horn. (From Cabot JB. [1990]. Sympathetic preganglionic neurons: Cytoarchitecture, ultrastructure, and biophysical properties. In AD Loewy & KM Spyer [Eds.]. *Central regulation of autonomic functions.* New York: Oxford University Press.)

to postganglionic ratios of 1:4 (Loewy, 1990a), 1:15 to 1:20, and 1:196 in a human superior cervical ganglion (Williams et al., 1995). (The parasympathetic division also has been found to exhibit divergence, but to a lesser degree.) This divergence may allow the effects of sympathetic stimulation to be more widespread throughout the body and to be of greater magnitude.

The autonomic ganglion in which the synapse occurs may be one of a chain of ganglia (called the sympathetic chain, sympathetic trunk, or paravertebral ganglia) located near the vertebral bodies of the spinal column, or it may be a prevertebral ganglion, such as the celiac ganglion (see Fig. 10-2), found within one of the autonomic nerve plexuses.

These plexuses surround the large arteries in the abdominal and pelvic cavities. The ganglion, regardless of location, is encapsulated by connective tissue. The connective tissue capsule is continuous with the epineurium of the bundle of entering preganglionic neurons and the bundle of exiting postganglionic neurons. Within the capsule are predominantly multipolar, spheroidal-shaped postganglionic neurons (Fig. 10-4). These neurons consist of cell bodies that have diameters ranging from 25 to 50 μm and dendrites that branch in a complex pattern. These dendrites are the location where preganglionic neuron axons commonly synapse. Satellite cells (neuroglial cells) that are similar to those found in the dorsal root

ganglia surround the cell bodies and dendrites. These cells provide support and help maintain the chemical environment. Interneurons are also located in the ganglion. One type, called small (cell bodies ranging in diameter from 15 to 20 μm) intensely fluorescent cells (SIFs), are present singly or in clusters. These cells contain the neurotransmitters epinephrine, serotonin, and dopamine (Hamill, 1996). When released, dopamine binds to postganglionic neurons, causing hyperpolarization. Another type of interneuron found in the ganglion is the small chromaffin cell, which also contains catecholamines. The exact difference between the chromaffin cell and SIF is unclear (Carpenter and Sutin, 1983; Harati, 1993; Williams et al., 1995).

Sympathetic Trunk. Two sympathetic trunks are located in the body, each of which lies on the anterolateral side of the vertebral column (Fig. 10-5). They both extend from the base of the skull to the coccyx. The ganglia of the sympathetic trunks are also called the paravertebral ganglia because they lie next to the vertebral column. Inferiorly the two trunks join in the midline and terminate on the anterior surface of the coccyx as the ganglion impar.

Each sympathetic trunk shares important anatomic relationships with surrounding structures. In the neck it lies between the carotid sheath and prevertebral

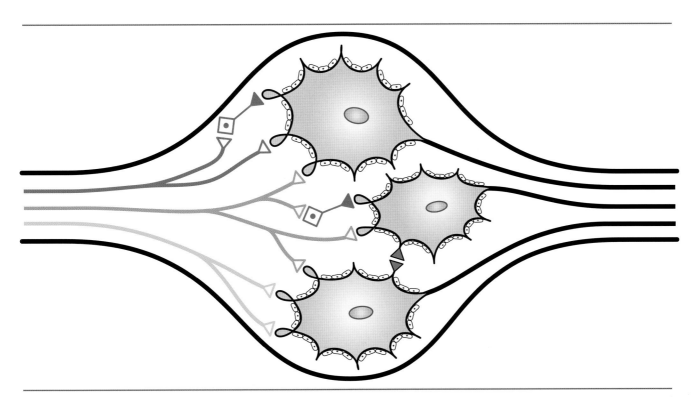

FIG. 10-4   An autonomic ganglion showing the synaptic connections between preganglionic (*green, blue,* and *yellow*) and postganglionic neurons. Note the interneurons (*red*), the dendro-dendritic synapse (*teal*), and the satellite cells surrounding the postganglionic cell bodies. Δ excitatory; ▲ inhibitory.

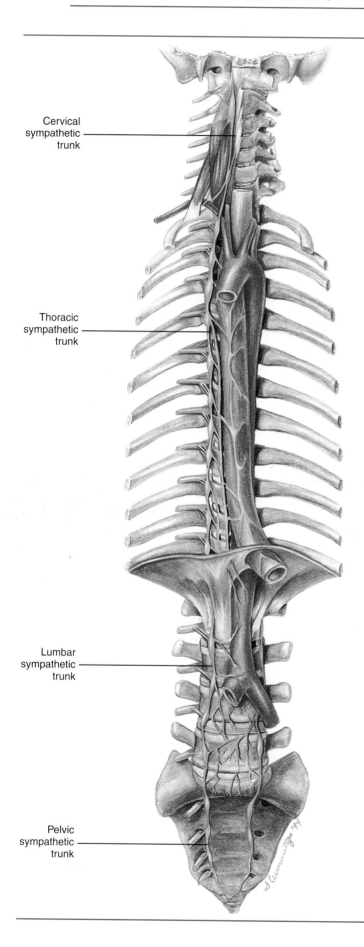

Cervical
sympathetic
trunk

Thoracic
sympathetic
trunk

Lumbar
sympathetic
trunk

Pelvic
sympathetic
trunk

FIG. 10-5   Sympathetic chain ganglia (trunk) and its anatomic location in the cervical region and the thoracic, abdominal, and pelvic cavities. (The left sympathetic trunk in the cervical and thoracic regions has been omitted for the sake of clarity.)

muscles, which cover the transverse processes (TPs) of the cervical vertebrae. It is found anterior to the heads of the ribs in the thorax, anterolateral to the bodies of the lumbar vertebrae in the abdomen, and medial to the anterior sacral foramina in the pelvis (Williams et al., 1995). As the name sympathetic chain ganglia implies, this structure consists of approximately 22 ganglia that are linked together by connective tissue surrounding ascending and descending fibers. The total number of ganglia does not correspond exactly to the number of spinal nerves because some of the ganglia have fused with one another. This fusion is most evident in the cervical region, where there are only three cervical ganglia. The thoracic portion of the sympathetic trunk includes 10 to 12 ganglia (70% of the time there are 11), the lumbar region exhibits 4 ganglia (although this number may vary), and 4 or 5 ganglia appear in the sacral region of the trunk. The union of the two sympathetic trunks forms the one coccygeal ganglion.

The preganglionic fibers exit the spinal cord in the ventral roots of cord segments T1 to L2 or L3 to reach the postganglionic neurons. Therefore at these particular levels, the ventral roots include both preganglionic sympathetic fibers and fibers to skeletal muscle (i.e., alpha and gamma motor neurons). The preganglionic fibers continue into the spinal nerve, and at the division of the spinal nerve into its dorsal and ventral rami (posterior and anterior primary divisions, respectively), the myelinated preganglionic fibers exit, forming the white (myelin is a white substance) ramus communicans, and then continue into the sympathetic trunk. (There are only 14 or 15 white rami on each side because there are only 14 or 15 spinal cord segments [T1 to L2-3] that provide preganglionic sympathetic fibers.)

The sympathetic system innervates autonomic effectors throughout the entire body. In general, cord segments T1 through T6 are involved with sympathetic innervation of autonomic effectors in the head, neck, upper extremities, and thorax. The cord segments from approximately T7 through L2 or L3 innervate the effectors in the lower extremities, abdominal cavity, and pelvic cavity. Recall that the sympathetic trunk is where synapses occur between preganglionic and postganglionic sympathetic fibers. Because the sympathetic trunk extends rostrally, adjacent to cervical vertebrae to reach the base of the skull, and caudally, adjacent to the sacrum to reach the coccyx, this trunk provides the means by which preganglionic fibers may ascend or descend to reach spinal nerves formed above or below the levels of T1 through L2 or L3. The preganglionic fibers may proceed in different directions once they pass through the white rami communicantes and enter the sympathetic trunk.

Autonomic fibers innervating peripheral blood vessels (including those in the skeletal muscles and skin), sweat glands, and arrector pili muscles of hair follicles travel in spinal nerves and subsequently peripheral nerves to innervate the appropriate effectors. These effectors are located in the area of distribution of each of the peripheral nerves. After entering the sympathetic trunk, preganglionic fibers associated with these effectors do one of three things (Fig. 10-6): ascend to synapse with postganglionic neurons in ganglia above T1 (for cervical nerves); synapse with postganglionic neurons at the level of entry into the trunk (i.e., T1 to L2 or L3 for those corresponding nerves); or descend to synapse with postganglionic neurons in ganglia below L2-3 (for lumbar and sacral nerves). From the sympathetic trunk the postganglionic fibers course through gray (these are unmyelinated fibers) rami communicantes (usually located proximal to the white rami), enter the spinal nerve at the location of its division into dorsal and ventral rami, and continue to the ANS effectors. Therefore the dorsal and ventral rami and subsequently formed peripheral nerves include sensory afferent fibers, motor neurons to skeletal muscle, and postganglionic sympathetic fibers. The ventral roots of T1 to L2-3 cord segments are unique in that they contain motor neurons to skeletal muscle and also preganglionic sympathetic fibers.

Sympathetic Preganglionic and Postganglionic Fibers. Sympathetic preganglionic fibers sending nerve impulses to effectors in the head enter the sympathetic trunk, ascend to the superior cervical ganglion, and synapse with postganglionic neurons. The postganglionic fibers course with large blood vessels to reach effectors located in the head region (Fig. 10-7, *A*). Such effectors include glands, the smooth muscle of blood vessels, and the smooth muscle of the eye. Some preganglionic fibers sending impulses to smooth muscle, cardiac muscle, and glands of the thorax also ascend on entering the trunk and synapse at rostral levels, whereas others synapse with postganglionic fibers at the level of entry. These postganglionic fibers leave the chain as branches that merge with other nerve fibers, including parasympathetic vagal fibers, to form plexuses innervating the heart and lungs. Abdominal and pelvic effectors are innervated in a different manner than the effectors of the head, thorax, and cutaneous regions. Preganglionic fibers enter the sympathetic trunk via white rami communicantes but do not synapse in the chain ganglia. Instead they pass through the chain ganglia and emerge as a collection of fibers called sympathetic splanchnic (referring to the viscera) nerves. These nerves course inferiorly in an anteromedial direction, pass through the diaphragm, and end in various prevertebral ganglia. Here they synapse on postganglionic neurons that then continue to the effectors of the abdominal and pelvic cavities (Fig. 10-7, *B*). The sympathetic prevertebral ganglia are enmeshed in plexuses of sympathetic and parasympathetic fibers

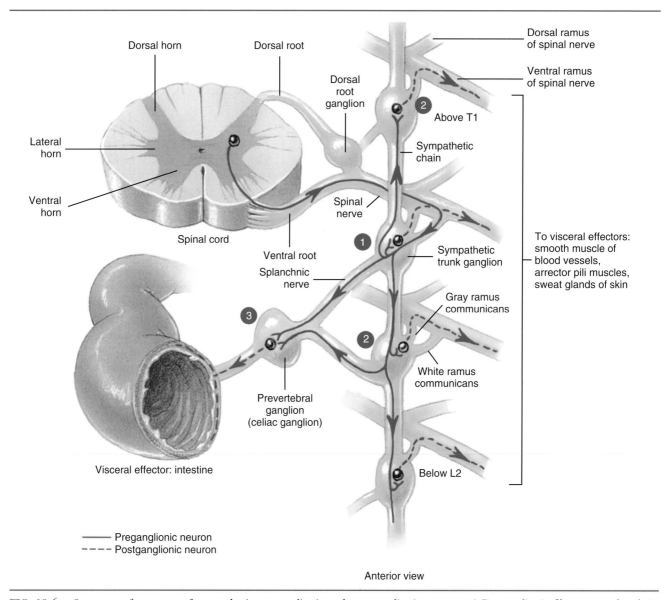

FIG. 10-6   Summary of synapses of sympathetic preganglionic and postganglionic neurons. *1,* Preganglionic fibers enter the chain via the white ramus communicans and may synapse at that level, ascend to a more superior ganglion and synapse, descend to a more inferior ganglion and synapse, or pass through the chain. *2,* Postganglionic fibers, destined to innervate peripheral effectors, exit the sympathetic chain via the gray ramus communicans (at least one for every spinal nerve) and enter into a ventral (anterior) ramus (they may enter a dorsal [posterior] ramus). *3,* Preganglionic fibers, destined to innervate viscera in the abdominal and pelvic cavities, exit the sympathetic chain without synapsing and travel to a prevertebral ganglion and synapse on postganglionic neurons. (From Tortora GJ & Grabowski SR. [2003]. *Principles of anatomy and physiology* [10th ed.]. New York: John Wiley & Sons, Inc.]

and are located near large arteries found in the abdominal cavity. Examples are the celiac, superior mesenteric, aorticorenal, and inferior mesenteric ganglia.

On entering the sympathetic trunk, a preganglionic neuron may either ascend or descend and, in each case, subsequently synapse in more than one ganglion. A preganglionic neuron also may synapse at the entry level and send collateral branches up or down to other ganglia. However, less than 2% of the neurons send a branch both up and down (Cabot, 1990). In all cases

described thus far, a preganglionic neuron has synapsed with a postganglionic neuron. However, a notable exception is the innervation of the medulla of the adrenal gland. The adrenal medulla develops from the same embryonic neural crest as postganglionic neurons. Although the medullary chromaffin cells do not resemble postganglionic neurons in appearance, they do function in a similar manner. Preganglionic neurons innervate the medulla directly, which in turn releases epinephrine and some norepinephrine into the blood-

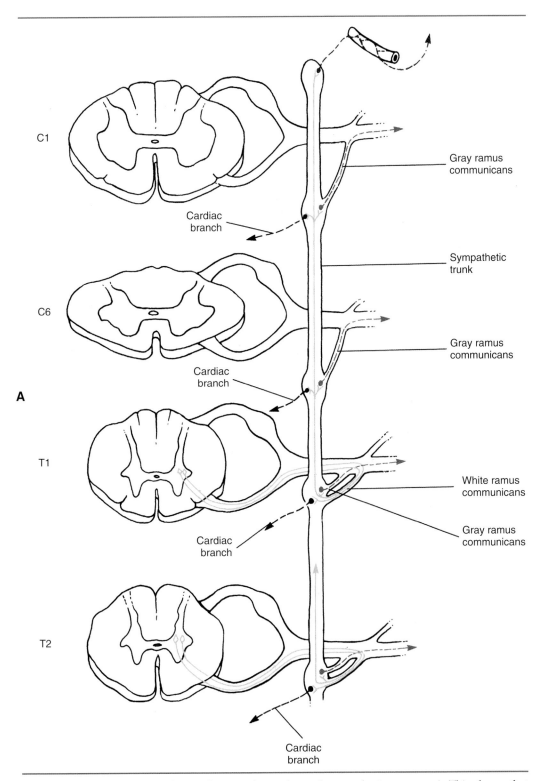

C1

Gray ramus
communicans

Cardiac
branch

Sympathetic
trunk

C6

Gray ramus
communicans

Cardiac
branch

A

T1

White ramus
communicans

Gray ramus
communicans

Cardiac
branch

T2

Cardiac
branch

FIG. 10-7 Diagrammatic scheme showing the options of sympathetic neurons. **A,** This shows that once preganglionic fibers (*yellow*) have entered the chain, they may ascend to higher levels and synapse with postganglionic fibers that may enter gray rami (*blue*) or travel on blood vessels (*green*); synapse in numerous ganglia with postganglionic neurons that leave the chain as cardiac branches (*black*); or synapse at the level of entry with postganglionic neurons that enter gray rami (*blue*).

Continued

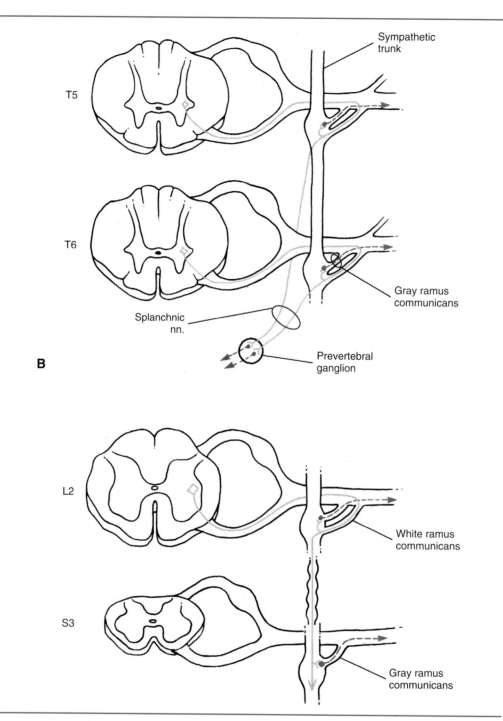

FIG. 10-7—cont'd   B, This shows that once preganglionic fibers (*yellow*) have entered the chain they may synapse at the level of entry with postganglionic neurons that enter gray rami (*blue*); descend to lower ganglia and synapse on postganglionic neurons that enter gray rami (*blue*); or pass through the chain (*purple*) without synapsing and travel to prevertebral ganglia, where they synapse with postganglionic neurons, the axons of which course to effectors in the abdominal and pelvic cavities.

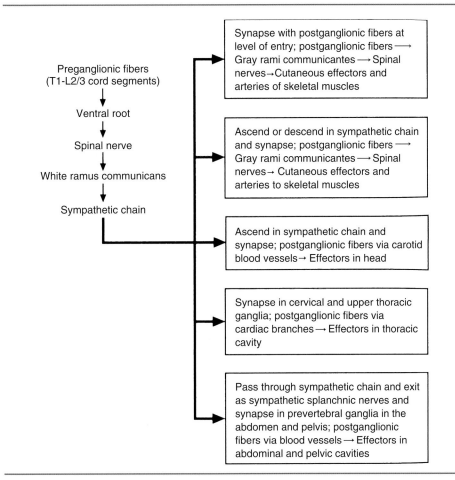

FIG. 10-8   Flowchart of pathways of the preganglionic and postganglionic sympathetic neurons.

stream. These neurotransmitters circulate throughout the body, stimulating effectors and assisting in the overall sympathetic response.

A summary of the various sympathetic nerve pathways is provided in Figures 10-6 and 10-8.

Specific Regions of the Sympathetic Trunk

Cervical sympathetic trunk. The fusion of the eight cervical ganglia results in three distinct ganglia in the region of the neck (Figs. 10-9, *A* and 10-10; see also Fig. 10-5). These are known as the superior, middle, and cervicothoracic (stellate) ganglia. (Twenty percent of the time the T1 ganglion is separate, in which case the cervicothoracic ganglion is called the inferior cervical ganglion [Harati, 1993].) The superior ganglion (Fig. 10-11, *A*; see also Figs. 10-9, *A* and 10-10) is the largest of the three and lies high in the neck adjacent to vertebrae C2 and C3, anterior to the longus capitis muscle and posterior to the cervical part of the internal carotid artery. It is also in the vicinity of the internal jugular vein

and the glossopharyngeal, vagus, spinal accessory, and hypoglossal cranial nerves (Williams et al., 1995). The proximity of the ganglion to these nerves may account for the autonomic effects seen when these nerves are lesioned in this location (Cross, 1993b). The ganglion is formed by the fusion of the first four cervical ganglia, is 2.5 to 3.0 cm long, and includes more than 1 million neurons (Carpenter and Sutin, 1983; Harati, 1993; Williams et al., 1995). Postganglionic fibers leaving this ganglion course to various regions. Some ascend as perivascular plexuses on the internal and external carotid arteries. A large branch (internal carotid nerve) from the superior cervical ganglion ascends with the internal carotid artery and divides into branches that form the internal carotid plexus (see Fig. 10-9, *A*) (Williams et al., 1995). This plexus, which surrounds the artery and innervates its wall, continues to travel with that artery, and within the cranial cavity the fibers innervate the autonomic effectors. Examples of these effectors are the dilator pupillae muscle of the eye, the

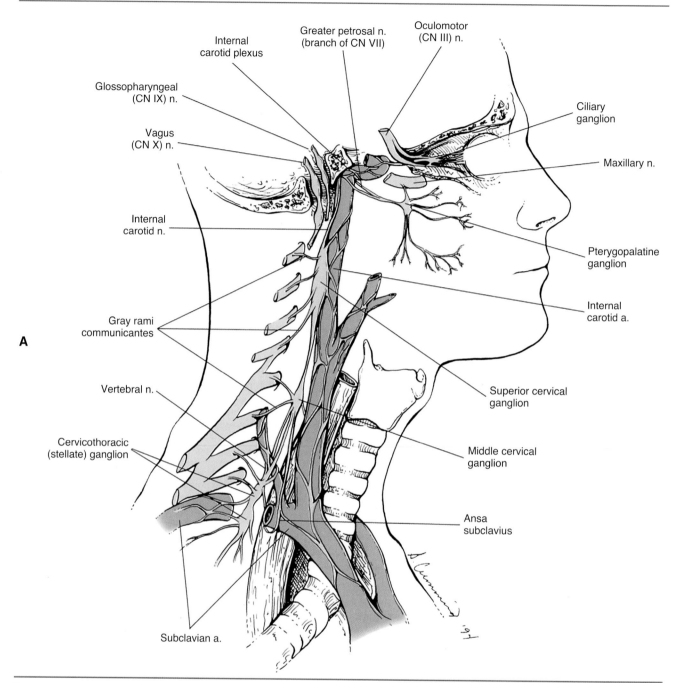

FIG. 10-9   A, Cervical sympathetic trunk and the continuation of autonomic fibers to effectors in the head. Note the relationship of the superior cervical ganglion to the vagus and glossopharyngeal cranial nerves and the internal carotid artery. Gray (not white) rami communicantes course from the cervical chain to the cervical spinal nerves. Leaving the cervicothoracic ganglion is the vertebral nerve and plexus that travel with the vertebral artery. Fibers of some postganglionic neuron cell bodies located in the superior cervical ganglion initially form the internal carotid nerve, which travels with the internal carotid artery, and subsequently branches to form the internal carotid plexus. Fibers of other postganglionic neuron cell bodies located in the superior cervical ganglion course with branches of the external carotid artery. Note that postganglionic fibers leave the blood vessels and travel with branches of cranial nerves. On the way to their destination, the sympathetic fibers may pass through, but do not synapse in, parasympathetic ganglia (e.g., ciliary and pterygopalatine).

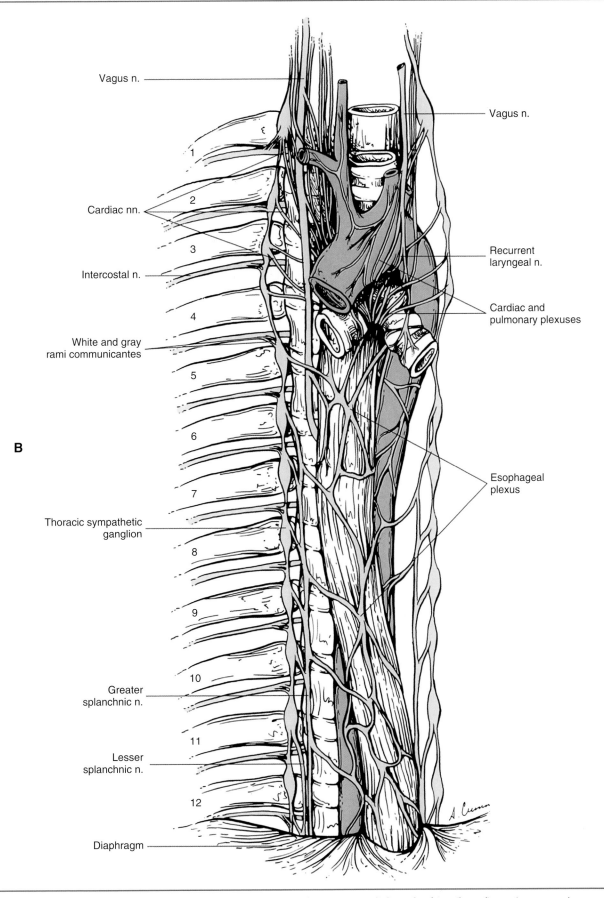

Vagus n.

Cardiac nn.

Intercostal n.

White and gray
rami communicantes

Thoracic sympathetic
ganglion

Greater
splanchnic n.

Lesser
splanchnic n.

Diaphragm

1
2
3
4
5
6
7
8
9
10
11
12

B

Vagus n.

Recurrent
laryngeal n.

Cardiac and
pulmonary plexuses

Esophageal
plexus

FIG. 10-9—cont'd **B,** The thoracic sympathetic trunk shows that gray (medial) and white (lateral) rami communicantes are present. Thoracic autonomic plexuses (e.g., cardiac, pulmonary, and esophageal), which are formed by postganglionic sympathetic fibers and vagal preganglionic fibers, are shown. Cardiac nerves and greater and lesser splanchnic nerves are also illustrated.

Continued

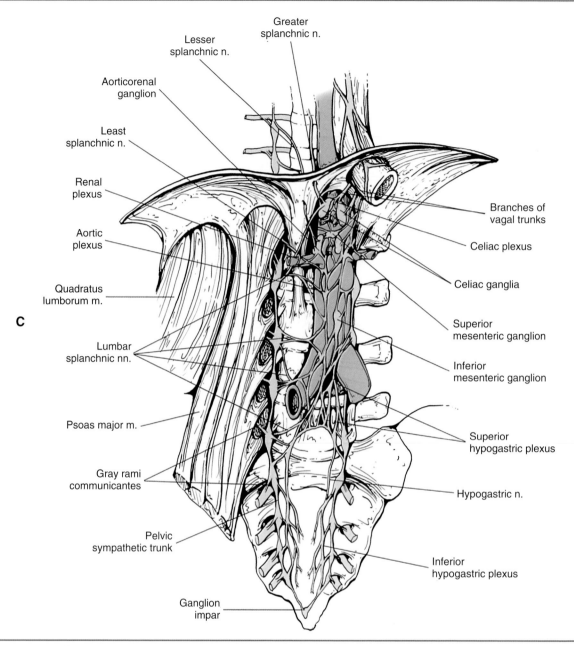

FIG. 10-9—cont'd **C,** Lumbar and pelvic sympathetic trunks and autonomic plexuses. The psoas major muscle has been reflected laterally to show the lumbar chain more clearly. The left and right pelvic sympathetic trunks can be seen uniting on the anterior surface of the coccyx to form the ganglion impar. Gray rami communicantes connecting the sympathetic trunk with spinal nerves are present at all levels. Also notice the major autonomic plexuses found in the abdominal and pelvic cavities. Sympathetic prevertebral ganglia located in the abdominal cavity (such as the celiac, superior mesenteric, and inferior mesenteric) also are shown. In the pelvic cavity the superior hypogastric plexus continues as the left and right hypogastric nerves that, with parasympathetic fibers, form the left and right inferior hypogastric (pelvic) plexuses.

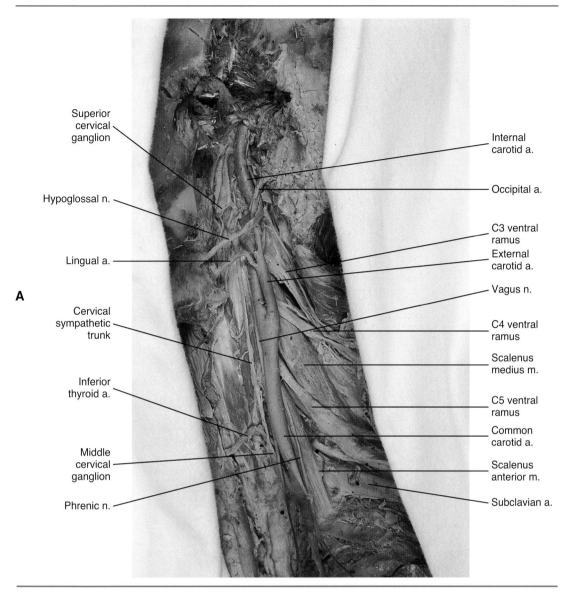

Superior
cervical
ganglion

Hypoglossal n.

Lingual a.

A

Cervical
sympathetic
trunk

Inferior
thyroid a.

Middle
cervical
ganglion

Phrenic n.

Internal
carotid a.

Occipital a.

C3 ventral
ramus

External
carotid a.

Vagus n.

C4 ventral
ramus

Scalenus
medius m.

C5 ventral
ramus

Common
carotid a.

Scalenus
anterior m.

Subclavian a.

FIG. 10-10   **A,** Left side of the neck showing the cervical sympathetic trunk. The veins and superior portion of the external carotid artery have been resected.   *Continued*

superior tarsal muscle (Müller's muscle) of the eyelid, and sweat glands in the lateral part of the forehead (Watson and Vijayan, 1995; Salvesen, 2001). In addition, some are sympathetic vasoconstrictor fibers and innervate cerebral branches of the internal carotid artery. Other postganglionic fibers leave the ganglion as medial, lateral, and anterior branches and course directly to effectors. The lateral branches include slender filaments that communicate with the glossopharyngeal, vagus, and hypoglossal nerves; and gray rami that join the first four cervical spinal nerves. The latter travel with those spinal

nerves to effectors in the areas of distribution of the nerves. The medial branches include laryngopharyngeal and cardiac (efferent) branches. The anterior branches travel with the common and external carotid arteries. Fibers continue with branches of the external carotid artery to innervate such structures as the facial sweat glands by traveling with terminal branches of the trigeminal nerve (cranial nerve [CN] V) (Williams et al., 1995).

The middle cervical ganglion (see Figs. 10-9, *A* and 10-10), formed by the fusion of the C5 and C6 ganglia, is the smallest (0.7 to 0.8 cm), and sometimes is absent.

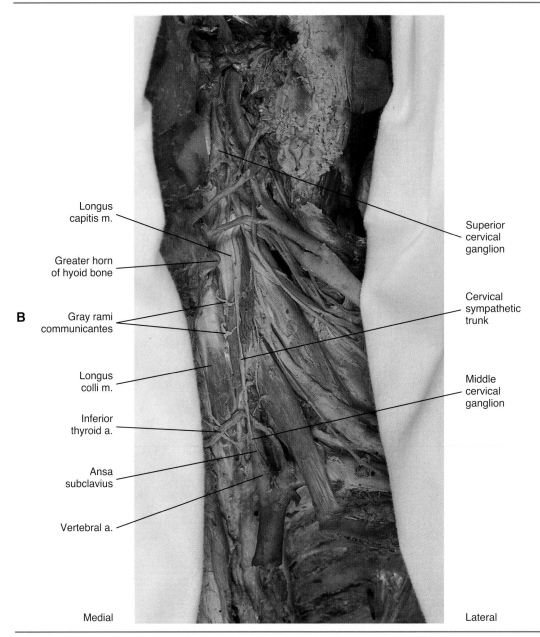

Longus
capitis m.

Greater horn
of hyoid bone

B

Gray rami
communicantes

Longus
colli m.

Inferior
thyroid a.

Ansa
subclavius

Vertebral a.

Superior
cervical
ganglion

Cervical
sympathetic
trunk

Middle
cervical
ganglion

Medial

Lateral

FIG. 10-10—cont'd **B,** The common carotid artery has been reflected laterally to expose the vertebral artery. Notice the relationship of the sympathetic trunk to the longus colli and capitis muscles and note the gray rami coursing between the two muscles.

It lies adjacent to the C6 vertebra and near the inferior thyroid artery, which is a branch of the thyrocervical trunk. Postganglionic fibers include gray rami that enter the C5 and C6 spinal nerves (sometimes the fourth and seventh), thyroid branches, and the largest sympathetic cardiac branch. The ganglion is continuous with the cervicothoracic ganglion by anterior and posterior branches. Although there is variation to this connection, typically the posterior branch splits around the vertebral artery as it descends to the cervicothoracic ganglion; the

anterior component descends and loops around the first part of the subclavian artery before connecting with the cervicothoracic ganglion. This loop is called the ansa subclavia (see Fig. 10-11, *B*).

The cervicothoracic (stellate) ganglion (see Figs. 10-9, *A* and 10-11, *B*) is formed by the fusion of the seventh, eighth, and first thoracic ganglia (and sometimes even the second, third, and fourth thoracic ganglia). It is approximately 2.8 cm long and is located between the base of the TP of C7 and the neck of the first rib lying

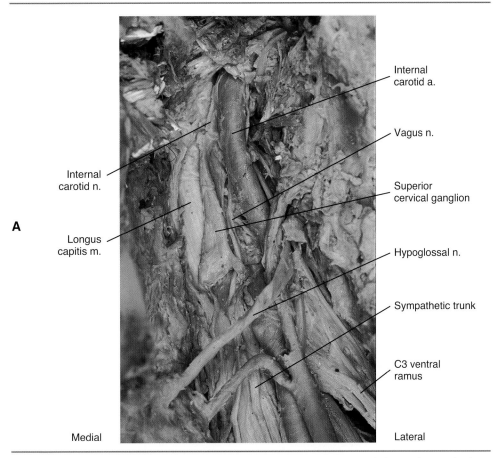

Internal carotid a.

Vagus n.

Superior cervical ganglion

Hypoglossal n.

Sympathetic trunk

C3 ventral ramus

Internal carotid n.

Longus capitis m.

A

Medial

Lateral

FIG. 10-11   A, Lateral view of the superior aspect of the deep region of the neck near the base of the skull showing the superior cervical ganglion. The internal carotid nerve (postganglionic fibers) is coursing with the internal carotid artery into the carotid canal.

Continued

on or just lateral to the longus colli muscle. A small detached portion of the stellate ganglion (or middle cervical ganglion), called the vertebral ganglion, may be present on the sympathetic trunk near the origin of the vertebral artery.

Some postganglionic fibers of the stellate (cervicothoracic) ganglion travel in gray rami communicantes to enter the C7, C8, and T1 spinal nerves, whereas others form a cardiac branch. Some other fibers form branches that course on the subclavian artery and its branches. One of these is large, and because it ascends with the vertebral artery (see Figs. 10-9,*A* and 10-11,*B*), frequently it is called the vertebral nerve (see Chapter 5 and Fig. 5-22). This nerve is joined by other branches and forms the vertebral plexus. Deep rami communicantes branch from the vertebral plexus and travel with ventral rami of the first five or six cervical spinal nerves. This plexus travels into the cranial cavity on the vertebral artery and continues on the basilar artery (and its branches) as far as the posterior cerebral artery, where it continues anteriorly to join the internal carotid artery plexus. Some

consider the vertebral plexus to be the major continuation of the sympathetic system into the cranium (Williams et al., 1995).

Although the cervical sympathetic chain has no white rami communicantes associated with it, numerous gray rami may be associated with each spinal nerve. For example, as many as five gray rami may connect with the C7 spinal nerve and the C8 spinal nerve may receive as many as three to six gray rami (Carpenter and Sutin, 1983). Also, cervical gray rami may pierce the longus capitis and scalenus anterior muscles as they course to the cervical spinal nerves (Williams et al., 1995).

Thoracic sympathetic trunk. Eleven small ganglia usually (70% of the time) are found in the thoracic sympathetic chain (Fig. 10-12; see also Fig. 10-9,*B*). (Note that 80% of the time the T1 ganglion is fused with the inferior cervical ganglion, in which case the succeeding ganglion is still named the second.) Each ganglion includes 90,000 to 100,000 neurons (Harati, 1993). The thoracic chain lies adjacent to the heads of the ribs and

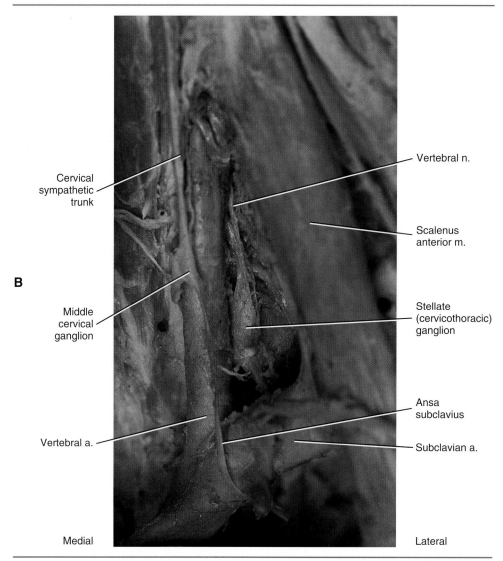

Cervical sympathetic trunk

Middle cervical ganglion

Vertebral a.

B

Vertebral n.

Scalenus anterior m.

Stellate (cervicothoracic) ganglion

Ansa subclavius

Subclavian a.

Medial

Lateral

FIG. 10-11—cont'd   **B,** Stellate ganglion, middle cervical ganglion, and ansa subclavius. The inferior thyroid artery has been resected. The vertebral nerve, which travels with the vertebral artery, courses from the superior aspect of the stellate ganglion.

posterior to the costal pleura. In this region of the chain, white rami communicantes, as well as the gray rami communicantes, are clearly evident (see Fig. 10-12, *B*). The white rami lay more distal (lateral) than the gray rami, and two or more rami may be connected to one spinal nerve. A mixed ramus formed by the fusion of the gray and white rami sometimes may be present. Postganglionic fibers originating from all thoracic ganglia enter the thoracic spinal nerves and travel with them to effectors. Some postganglionic fibers from the T1 to T5 ganglia form direct branches to the thoracic aortic, cardiac, and pulmonary plexuses of the thorax. Other large branches of the T5 to T12 ganglia supply the aorta and are associated with the three splanchnic nerves

involved with the sympathetic innervation of the abdominal and pelvic viscera. These splanchnic nerves consist of preganglionic fibers that synapse in prevertebral ganglia located in the abdominal cavity.

The greater splanchnic nerve (see Figs. 10-9, *B* and 10-12, *A*) contains preganglionic fibers exiting from the T5 to T9 or T10 ganglia. As it descends obliquely on the vertebral bodies, it sends branches to the descending thoracic aorta and then pierces the diaphragm. It courses to the medulla of the adrenal gland, the celiac ganglion, and sometimes the aorticorenal ganglion. In the ganglia, the preganglionic fibers of the greater splanchnic nerve synapse on postganglionic neurons. The lesser splanchnic nerve consists of preganglionic fibers from the T9

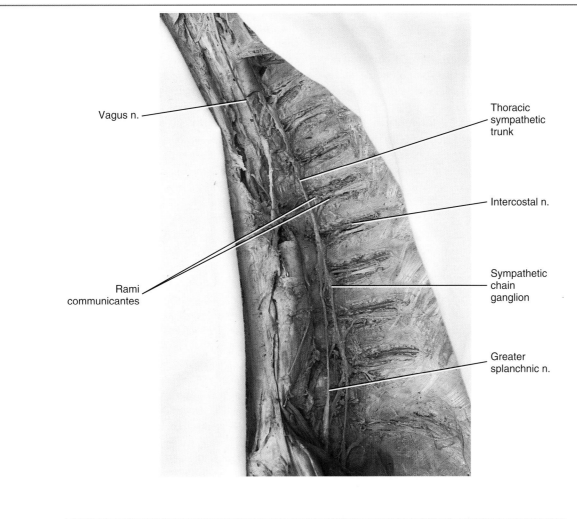

A

Vagus n.

Thoracic sympathetic trunk

Intercostal n.

Rami communicantes

Sympathetic chain ganglion

Greater splanchnic n.

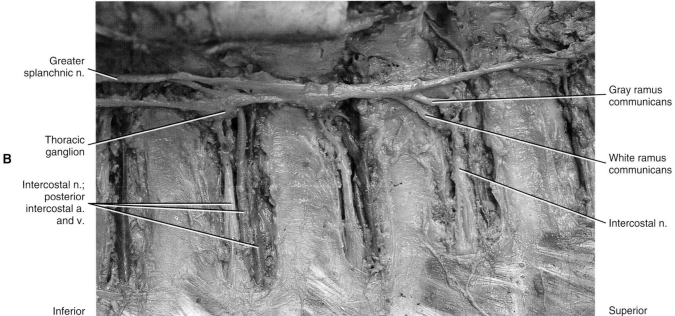

B

Greater splanchnic n.

Thoracic ganglion

Intercostal n.; posterior intercostal a. and v.

Gray ramus communicans

White ramus communicans

Intercostal n.

Inferior

Superior

FIG. 10-12 **A,** Thoracic sympathetic trunk. **B,** Closer view of the left thoracic sympathetic trunk. Both white and gray rami communicantes are shown in relationship to the intercostal nerve, artery, and vein. The greater splanchnic nerve (preganglionic fibers) is coursing inferiorly and medially from the sympathetic trunk into the abdominal cavity.

and T10 or T10 and T11 ganglia and is present 94% of the time. It traverses the diaphragm with the greater splanchnic nerve and enters the abdominal cavity to synapse in the aorticorenal ganglion (the detached lower part of the celiac ganglion). The third splanchnic nerve is the lowest or least splanchnic nerve and is present 56% of the time. Sometimes this nerve is called the renal nerve and emerges from the T12 (or lowest) ganglion to terminate in many small ganglia located in the renal plexus (Harati, 1993; Williams et al., 1995). From these prevertebral ganglia, postganglionic fibers participate in the formation of the various perivascular plexuses as they travel to abdominal effectors.

Lumbar sympathetic trunk. The thoracic sympathetic trunk passes posterior to the medial arcuate ligament (or sometimes through the crura of the diaphragm) to become continuous with the lumbar sympathetic trunk found within the abdominal cavity. The trunk has been described as consisting of four interconnected lumbar ganglia (each of which contains 60,000 to 85,000 neurons) (Harati, 1993; Williams et al., 1995). However, other data indicate that the number of ganglia varies (Mitchell, 1953; Rocco, Palombi, and Raeke, 1995). Murata et al. (2003) studied cadaveric specimens and looked at the anatomic variations of the ganglia and associated rami. They found that the number of ganglia on one side ranged from 2 to 6 (mean, 3.9) and that the majority of ganglia were located on the L2 and L3 vertebrae. Typically no ganglia were found on the L1 and L4 vertebrae. Approximately 40% of the cadavers showed the same number of ganglia on both sides, and those were asymmetrically located. In addition, Murata et al. (2003) found 5 to 12 rami communicantes per side (mean of 7.2) and noted that more than one rami communicantes could connect to a lumbar ventral ramus and that a lumbar ventral ramus often received rami communicantes from more than one ganglion. In fact, one third of the ganglia associated with the L2 and L3 vertebrae included rami that traveled to three spinal nerves. Rami associated with the L1-5 spinal nerves were measured, and it was found that the ramus of the L4 spinal nerve was significantly similar in length to the L2 and L3 rami. Although this is contrary to what would be expected because the sympathetic chain lies closer to the intervertebral foramina (IVFs) at the L4-5 vertebral levels, it may be due to the fact that there are fewer ganglia at the L4 level and the rami have farther to travel to reach a more superiorly located ganglion. The L1 rami also were significantly longer than the other lumbar rami, most likely for the same reason. The rami of L5 were significantly shorter than those of L1-4. The presence of anatomic variations in the rami and ganglia in this region may be of importance relative to the nociceptive path-

way for lower lumbar structures. Based on studies in rats that may apply to humans as well, it has been suggested that nociceptive input from low back structures is carried in two different pathways. Some nociceptive fibers from low back pain generators travel in a segmental fashion, directly within spinal nerves, and terminate in local cord segments. Other nociceptive fibers terminate centrally in a nonsegmental fashion. These course in lower lumbar spinal nerves, enter the sympathetic chain and ascend, and then exit the chain through more superiorly located rami connected to the L2 spinal nerve. These fibers terminate in the lower region of the thoracolumbar cord segments associated with the sympathetic division (Murata et al., 2003). If this pathway is present in humans it may contribute to the wide referral pattern seen in lower lumbar intervertebral discs, lower lumbar zygopophysial (Z) joints, and sacroiliac joint pain conditions (Murata et al., 2000) (see Chapters 7 and 11 for further information).

The lumbar trunk lies adjacent to the anterolateral aspect of the upper lumbar vertebrae and becomes more posterior relative to lower lumbar vertebrae (Murata et al., 2003). It also lies adjacent to the medial margin of the psoas major muscle (Fig. 10-13; see also Fig. 10-9, *C*). The inferior vena cava, right ureter, and lumbar lymph nodes lie anterior to the right sympathetic trunk. The left sympathetic trunk lies posterior to the aortic lymph nodes and lateral to the aorta. These relationships are important surgically because lumbar ganglia may have to be removed (lumbar sympathectomy) to treat certain arterial diseases of the lower extremities (Moore, 1980).

White rami communicantes are associated with the upper two or three ganglia. The gray rami are long (see previous section) as they course with lumbar arteries along the sides of the vertebral bodies to join each lumbar spinal nerve (see Fig. 10-13). The majority of these postganglionic fibers are thought to use the femoral nerve, obturator nerve, and their muscular and cutaneous branches to reach the adjoining blood vessels and cutaneous effectors. In a manner similar to the lower thoracic ganglia, some preganglionic fibers pass through the lumbar ganglia to form lumbar splanchnic nerves. In general, each lumbar splanchnic nerve corresponds to its ganglion of the same number, although the second lumbar splanchnic nerve receives additional fibers from the third ganglion, and the third lumbar splanchnic nerve also receives a contribution from the fourth ganglion. The four splanchnic nerves course into the abdomen and become part of the abdominal plexuses: the first splanchnic nerve courses within the celiac, abdominal aortic (intermesenteric), and renal plexuses; the second splanchnic nerve contributes to the inferior part of the abdominal aortic (intermesenteric) plexus; the third splanchnic nerve travels within the superior hypogastric

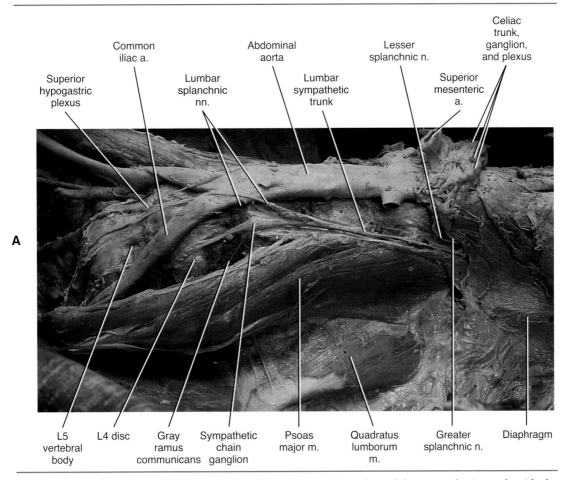

FIG. 10-13   Left lumbar sympathetic trunk. **A,** Notice the relationship of the sympathetic trunk with the psoas major muscle and vertebral bodies and discs. Lumbar splanchnic nerves are coursing from the sympathetic trunk to the superior hypogastric plexus. The greater and lesser splanchnic nerves pass through the diaphragm to synapse in the celiac ganglion and aorticorenal ganglion. The celiac trunk, superior and inferior mesenteric, and renal arteries have been resected. The inferior vena cava also has been resected.

Continued

plexus (see Figs. 10-9, *C* and 10-13); the fourth splanchnic nerve contributes to the lowest portion of the superior hypogastric plexus (or hypogastric nerve) (Williams et al., 1995). The lumbar portion of the sympathetic trunk passes inferiorly, posterior to the common iliac vessels, and becomes continuous with the pelvic portion of the trunk.

Pelvic sympathetic trunk. The pelvic chain consists of four or five ganglia that lie on the anterior aspect of the sacrum. Each side unites to form the ganglion impar on the anterior aspect of the coccyx (Fig. 10-14; see also Fig. 10-9, *C*). Postganglionic fibers leave the chain in gray rami to enter the sacral spinal nerves and coccygeal nerve. Fibers destined for blood vessels in the leg and foot course primarily with the tibial nerve to connect subsequently with (and supply) the popliteal artery

and its branches in the leg and foot. Other fibers travel with the pudendal and gluteal nerves to the internal pudendal artery and gluteal arteries. In addition, some fibers from the first two sacral ganglia send postganglionic branches into the inferior hypogastric plexus (or hypogastric nerve).

Plexuses of the Autonomic Nervous System. The autonomic plexuses that have been mentioned are a network of autonomic fibers (both sympathetic and parasympathetic) and ganglia found in the thoracic, abdominal, and pelvic cavities. They surround, and usually are named after, the large blood vessels with which they travel. The plexuses supply the autonomic effectors within the thorax, abdomen, and pelvis. The effectors and their specific innervation are discussed later in this chapter.

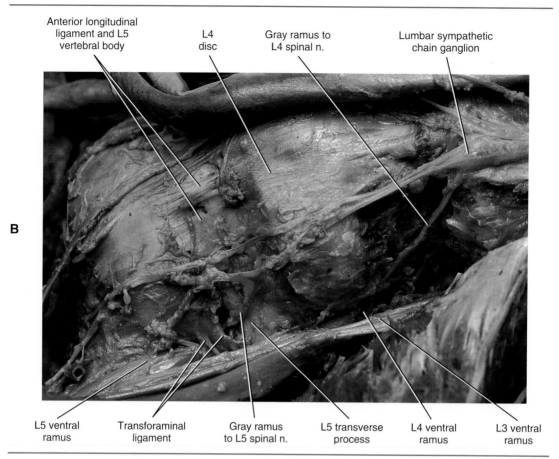

FIG. 10-13—cont'd **B,** Lumbar sympathetic trunk at the level of the L4 and L5 vertebrae. The left common iliac artery has been reflected. The psoas major muscle also has been reflected. Notice the long gray rami communicantes. A transforaminal ligament spanning the intervertebral foramen is present in this specimen. Note the relationship of the L5 ventral ramus and gray ramus communicans to this ligament.

The cardiac, pulmonary, celiac, and hypogastric plexuses are the major plexuses (Williams et al., 1995), although secondary plexuses may emanate from each one. The cardiac plexus, which is divided into deep and superficial parts, consists of cardiac branches from cervical and upper thoracic ganglia mixed with cardiac branches of the vagus nerve (see Fig. 10-9, *B*). A continuation of the cardiac plexus forms secondary coronary and atrial plexuses. The pulmonary plexus is an extension of fibers of the cardiac plexus that course with the pulmonary arteries to the lungs. Therefore the cardiac and pulmonary plexuses consist of the same sympathetic and vagal branches.

The celiac plexus is the largest autonomic plexus (see Fig. 10-9, *C*). It is located at the level of the T12 and L1 vertebrae and surrounds the celiac artery and the base of the superior mesenteric artery. This plexus is a dense fibrous network that interconnects the paired celiac ganglia. Mingling with the celiac plexus and ganglia are the greater and lesser splanchnic nerves and also branches of the vagus and phrenic nerves (Williams et

al., 1995). Numerous subsidiary ganglia and fibers extend from the celiac plexus and course along abdominal blood vessels to autonomic effectors. These fibers and ganglia form (in some cases with the help of the lesser and least splanchnic nerves) plexuses that include the phrenic, hepatic, gastric, splenic, testicular, ovarian, superior mesenteric (to small and large intestines), renal, inferior mesenteric (to lower GI tract), and abdominal aortic (intermesenteric). The latter three plexuses also include lumbar splanchnic nerves. The hepatic plexus is the largest of these smaller plexuses and supplies innervation to the liver, gallbladder, bile ducts, stomach, duodenum, and pancreas. It contains afferent and efferent sympathetic branches and parasympathetic fibers. Consequently the celiac plexus and its secondary plexuses are responsible for the innervation of the abdominal viscera. Anterior to the bifurcation of the aorta at the level of the L4 to L5 vertebral bodies, the superior hypogastric plexus (Fig. 10-13, *A,* and see Fig. 10-9, *C*) is formed by the third and fourth lumbar splanchnic nerves and fibers of the aortic plexus. This plexus sends branches

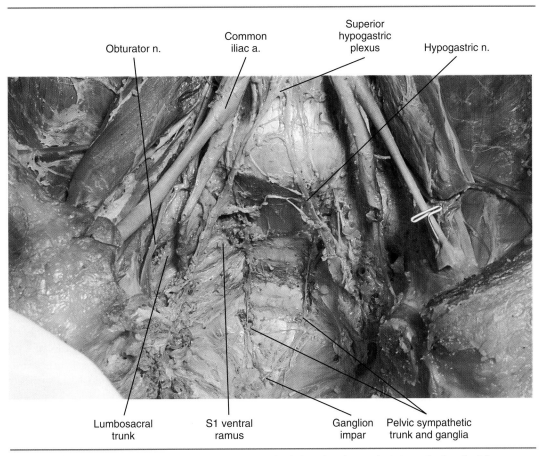

FIG. 10-14   Pelvic sympathetic trunk and ganglia. The left and right trunks join at the level of the coccyx to form the ganglion impar. The superior hypogastric plexus and hypogastric nerves also are present.

to the testicular, ureteric, ovarian, and common iliac plexuses. As the superior hypogastric plexus descends into the pelvic cavity, it divides into left and right hypogastric nerves that continue caudally to form the inferior hypogastric (pelvic) plexuses (see Fig. 10-9, *C*). Within the pelvis, pelvic splanchnic parasympathetic fibers (originating from the S2-4 cord segments) join each inferior hypogastric plexus. Preganglionic sympathetic fibers in the plexus originate in the T10-L2 cord segments and travel as lumbar splanchnics or postganglionic fibers of the lumbar and sacral chain ganglia. Extensions of the inferior hypogastric plexus, which include the middle rectal, prostatic, uterovaginal, and vesical plexuses, continue along the branches of the internal iliac artery to innervate autonomic effectors of the pelvis. The ANS innervation of the most clinically important effectors of the pelvis is discussed later in this chapter.

Parasympathetic Division

The parasympathetic division generally is concerned with conserving and restoring energy. It is coordinated with the sympathetic division in the dual and antag-

onistic innervation of autonomic effectors (see Table 10-1). However, there is no parasympathetic innervation of autonomic effectors located in the extremities and body wall (i.e., sweat glands, arrector pili muscles, peripheral blood vessels). Because the sympathetic division has been nicknamed the fight-or-flight division, the parasympathetic division could appropriately be named the rest-and-digest division, because in general, parasympathetic activation results in decreased heart rate and increased GI glandular secretion and peristalsis. In contrast to the widespread control by the sympathetic system, the parasympathetic division controls effectors at a more local level. This relates to the overall pattern of organization of the parasympathetic division of the ANS. Compared with the sympathetic division, each parasympathetic preganglionic neuron synapses with fewer postganglionic neurons, and the location of the parasympathetic ganglia is near, or frequently within, the wall of the effector organ. Although the ganglia are the site of synapses between preganglionic and postganglionic neurons, afferent fibers, postganglionic sympathetic fibers, and even branchial arch efferent fibers can course through them.

The parasympathetic division also is called the cranio-sacral division. As with the thoracolumbar (sympathetic) division, this name refers to the location of the cell bodies of preganglionic neurons (see Fig. 10-2). These cell bodies are located in autonomic nuclei of the brain stem (*cranio*) and in the second, third, and fourth sacral cord segments (*sacral*). The parasympathetic efferents of the sacral cord course within the ventral roots and subsequently form pelvic splanchnic nerves. These nerves do not use the sympathetic trunk. Axons of the cell bodies located in the brain stem leave the brain stem in the oculomotor, facial, glossopharyngeal, and vagus cranial nerves. Although numerous branches of various cranial nerves include these parasympathetic efferents, only the major branches are described. The somatic functions of the four cranial nerves are not discussed because this chapter is devoted to autonomic effectors.

Cranial Portion of the Parasympathetic Division

Oculomotor nerve. The oculomotor nerve (CN III) emerges from the ventral surface of the midbrain of the brain stem (see Chapter 9, Fig. 9-20). The origin of the autonomic efferents is in the Edinger-Westphal nucleus, which is located in the midbrain ventral to the cerebral aqueduct of Sylvius. These preganglionic fibers course within the oculomotor nerve to the ciliary ganglion, where they synapse with postganglionic neurons (Fig. 10-15). This ganglion is less than 2 mm long and contains 3000 multipolar neurons (Harati, 1993). It is located in the orbit just anterior to the superior orbital fissure. Postganglionic fibers course in the short ciliary nerves to the eye and travel between the choroid and sclera of the eye wall. Here the fibers innervate the smooth muscle of the iris (sphincter pupillae) and ciliary body (ciliary muscle). The sphincter muscle of the iris functions to constrict the pupil during the pupillary light reflex and during the accommodation-convergence reflex. Contraction of the ciliary muscle occurs during the accommodation-convergence reflex. The result of this contraction is a thickening of the lens, which improves near vision.

Facial nerve. The facial nerve (CN VII) also contains preganglionic fibers. The cell bodies of these fibers are located in the superior salivatory nucleus. This nucleus is located in the caudal part of the pons near the facial motor nucleus. The fibers emerge from the ponto-medullary junction in the nervus intermedius portion of CN VII (see Chapter 9, Fig. 9-20). Some of the fibers travel in the chorda tympani nerve, which in turn joins the lingual branch of the mandibular division of the trigeminal nerve (CN V). These preganglionic fibers continue to the submandibular (sublingual) ganglion, where they synapse with postganglionic neurons (see Fig. 10-15).

The postganglionic fibers are secretomotor and course to minor salivary glands, as well as to the larger submandibular and sublingual salivary glands. (It has been reported also that stimulation of the chorda tympani nerve results in vasodilation in the salivary glands [Williams et al., 1995].) In addition to the preganglionic fibers en route to the submandibular ganglion, other secretomotor preganglionic fibers from the lacrimal portion of the superior salivatory nucleus course in the greater petrosal nerve to the pterygopalatine ganglion (see Fig. 10-15). This ganglion is approximately 3 mm long and contains 56,500 compactly arranged neurons (Harati, 1993). It is located in the pterygopalatine fossa behind and below the orbit. Postganglionic fibers exit from here and travel in the zygomatic nerve (a branch of the maxillary division of the trigeminal nerve) and terminate in the lacrimal gland. Other secretomotor branches of the pterygopalatine ganglion course to the glands and mucous membranes of the palate and nasal mucosa.

Glossopharyngeal nerve. The glossopharyngeal nerve is CN IX. Preganglionic neurons that course in this nerve originate in the inferior salivatory nucleus, which is located caudal to the superior salivatory nucleus. CN IX emerges as three to five rootlets from the dorso-olivary sulcus on the lateral side of the medulla of the brain stem (see Chapter 9, Fig. 9-20). The preganglionic fibers travel in the lesser petrosal nerve to the otic ganglion, where they synapse with postganglionic neurons (Fig. 10-16, *A*). The postganglionic fibers are secretomotor, and the axons of these neurons travel in the auriculotemporal nerve (a branch of the mandibular division of the trigeminal nerve) to reach the parotid gland that they innervate. Evidence shows that stimulation of the lesser petrosal nerve results in vasodilation in the parotid gland, as well as serous secretion (Williams et al., 1995).

Regarding these three cranial nerves and their ganglia, it is of interest to note that sympathetic postganglionic fibers coursing to their effectors may pass through (but not synapse in) the parasympathetic ganglia. They also may travel along with branches of various cranial nerves. Parasympathetic fibers also may "hitch a ride" with cranial nerves other than III, VII, and IX.

Vagus nerve. The vagus nerve (CN X) also conveys parasympathetic fibers. In fact 75% of the total parasympathetic efferents are carried by the vagus nerve. This nerve is closely related to the glossopharyngeal nerve both anatomically and functionally. Just caudal to the glossopharyngeal nerve the vagus nerve emerges as 8 to 10 rootlets from the dorso-olivary sulcus of the medulla (see Chapter 9, Fig. 9-20). Most preganglionic fibers (some of which are extremely long) arise from the dorsal motor nucleus, which is a column of cell bodies located in the medulla of the brain stem. Some (possibly the

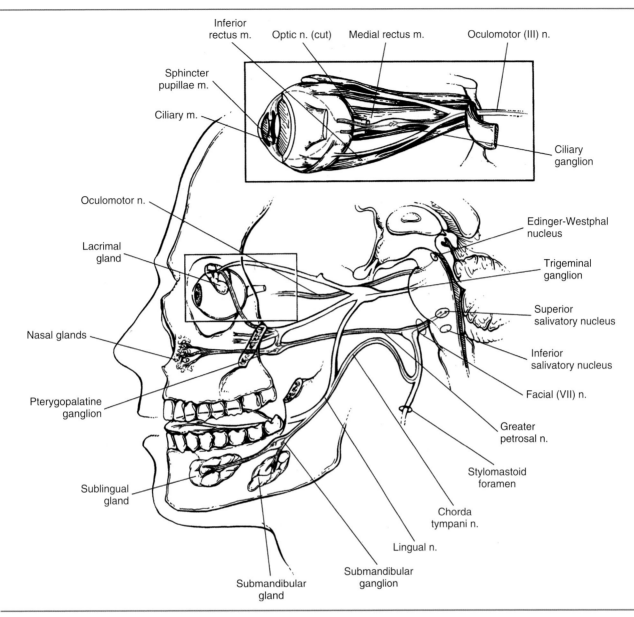

FIG. 10-15 Course of parasympathetic fibers in the oculomotor (*red*) (cranial nerve III) and facial nerves (*forest green*) (cranial nerve VII). Oculomotor preganglionic neuron cell bodies are found in the midbrain in the Edinger-Westphal nucleus. Their axons (*solid line*) synapse with postganglionic neurons in the ciliary ganglion located in the orbit. Postganglionic axons (*dashed line*) travel to the smooth muscles of the eye (sphincter pupillae and ciliary). Facial nerve preganglionic neuron cell bodies are found in the caudal pons in the superior salivatory nucleus. Their axons (*solid line*) synapse with postganglionic neurons in the pterygopalatine ganglion and submandibular ganglion. From these ganglia, postganglionic axons (*dashed line*) travel to the lacrimal gland, nasal mucosal, and sublingual and submandibular salivary glands.

majority) of preganglionic fibers destined for cardiac muscle originate in or near the nucleus ambiguus (Loewy and Spyer, 1990; Noback, Strominger, and Demarest, 1991; Wang, Holst, and Powley, 1995; Williams et al., 1995; Kiernan, 1998; Iversen, Iversen, and Saper, 2000; Nolte, 2002), which is located in the medulla ventral to the dorsal motor nucleus. However, the nucleus ambiguus is involved primarily with supplying skeletal muscles via

CNs IX, X, and XI. All the preganglionic fibers travel in the vagus nerve and its numerous branches (see Fig. 10-16, *B*). Some mingle with sympathetic fibers to form the extensive autonomic plexuses of the thoracic and abdominal cavities. The long preganglionic fibers are destined to synapse in small ganglia located within plexuses near the effector organ or ganglia within the wall of the organ itself. Some of the specific branches

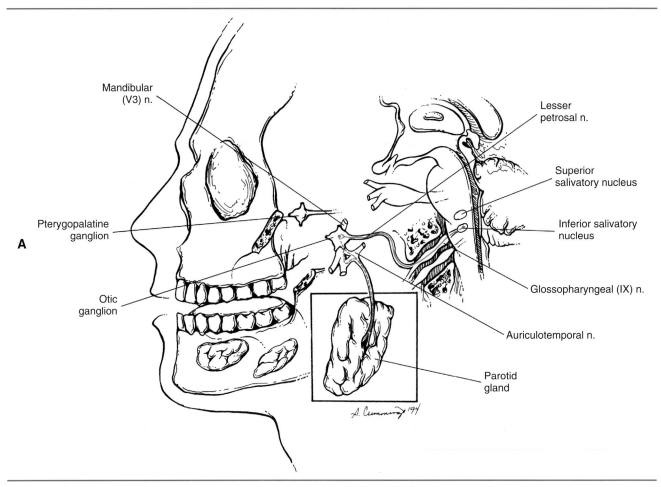

FIG. 10-16   A, Course of parasympathetic fibers within the glossopharyngeal nerve (cranial nerve IX) to the parotid gland. Preganglionic neuron cell bodies are found in the inferior salivatory nucleus in the rostral medulla. Their axons (*solid line*) synapse with postganglionic neurons (*dashed line*) in the otic ganglion.

that conduct preganglionic parasympathetic fibers are the following: in the thorax-cardiac, pulmonary, and esophageal branches that join the plexuses of the same name; and in the abdomen-gastric and intestinal branches that join in the celiac plexus (and its subsidiary plexuses) en route to the stomach, small intestine, ascending colon and most of the transverse colon, accessory glands, and kidneys.

The vagus nerve has an extensive area of distribution as can be seen in Figure 10-16, *B*. However, note that the vagus nerve does not supply autonomic effectors of the head. These are innervated by CNs III, VII, and IX. Although vagal efferents are important, the afferent fibers conveying sensory information in the vagus nerve outnumber the efferent fibers (Williams et al., 1995).

Sacral Portion of the Parasympathetic Division. Most effectors innervated by parasympathetic fibers are served by cranial nerves as can be noted from the previous discussion. The remaining effectors (e.g., the smooth muscle and glands of the pelvis) not inner-

vated by the vagus nerve are innervated by the sacral portion of the craniosacral parasympathetic division. The origin of these preganglionic fibers is in the sacral autonomic nucleus of lamina VII of sacral cord segments two, three, and four (Fig. 10-17). The preganglionic fibers exit the cord in the ventral roots of these cord segments and leave the ventral rami as pelvic splanchnic nerves. These fibers course through the hypogastric plexuses, which are formed by both parasympathetic and sympathetic fibers. They synapse in ganglia within those plexuses or in ganglia within the wall of the effector organ. Generally, these fibers supply motor innervation to part of the transverse colon, descending colon, sigmoid colon, rectum, bladder, and reproductive organs. Also, some are vasodilatory to the penis and clitoris (erectile tissue), testes, ovaries, uterine tubes, and uterus. In addition, these parasympathetic fibers convey important sensory information (Williams et al., 1995; Kiernan, 1998) that provides reflex control of normal bladder, colon, and sexual organ function.

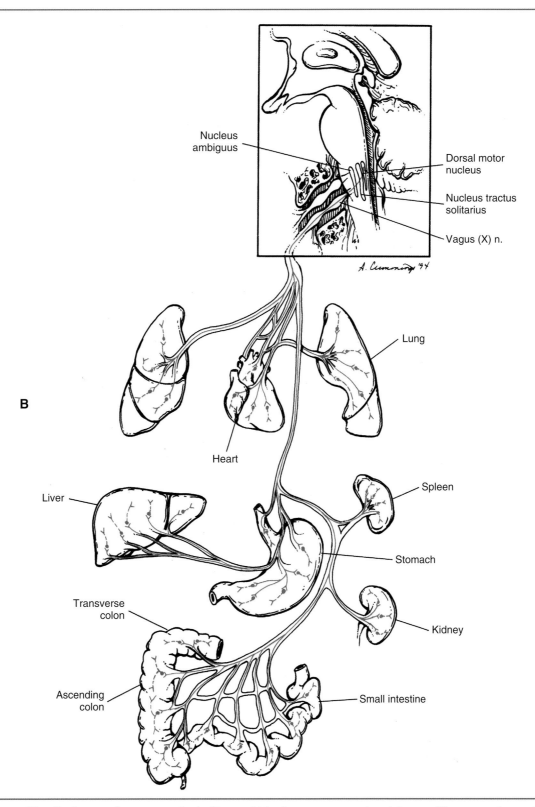

FIG. 10-16—cont'd   **B,** Course of parasympathetic fibers within the vagus nerve (cranial nerve X) to smooth muscle, cardiac muscle, and glands. Preganglionic neuron cell bodies are found in the dorsal motor nucleus located in the medulla. Their axons (*solid line*) synapse with postganglionic neurons (*dashed line*) that are in or very near the wall of innervated thoracic and abdominal visceral organs.

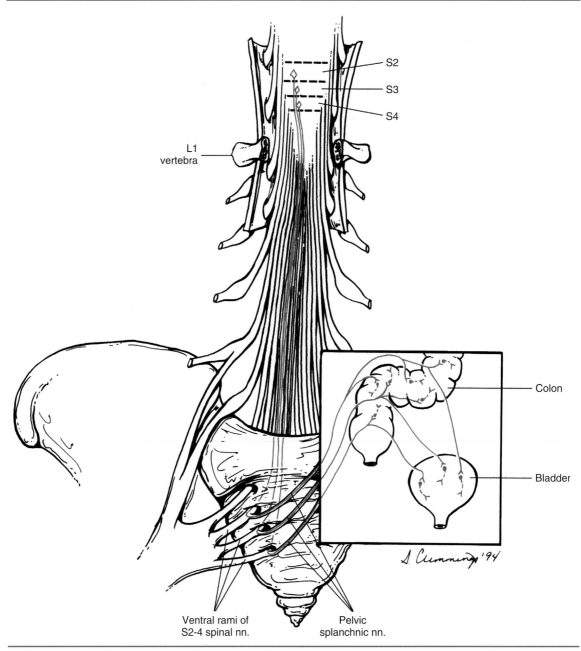

FIG. 10-17 Parasympathetic fibers originating from the spinal cord. The lumbar vertebral bodies have been removed to expose the sacral cord segments and cauda equina. The preganglionic neurons originate in the S2-4 cord segments, course within ventral roots of the cauda equina, and exit through their corresponding intervertebral foramina. They branch from ventral rami of S2-4 spinal nerves, form pelvic splanchnic nerves, and travel to ganglia (where they synapse) near or within the walls of the pelvic viscera. From the ganglia, postganglionic neurons travel to the smooth muscle and glands of the pelvic viscera.

Enteric Nervous System

The third division of the ANS is the enteric nervous system, which was first recognized as such by Langley in 1921 (Gershon, 1981). In 1899 it was first acknowledged that motility of the GI system was under autonomous control by an intrinsic nervous system, when well-coordinated and purposeful motility still occurred independently after severing nerves to the GI system (Gershon, 1981). Since that time the concept that an intrinsic group of neurons exists in the wall of the gut, pancreas, and gall bladder has been fully accepted (Williams et al., 1995). This group of neurons extends from the esophagus to the rectum; it regulates GI vaso-motor tone and motility and helps to regulate secretion and reabsorption. All of these activities are necessary for maintaining homeostasis. However, extrinsic postganglionic sympathetic fibers from prevertebral ganglia (splanchnic nerves) and preganglionic parasympathetic fibers via the vagus and pelvic splanchnic nerves provide input into these enteric neurons. This input can adjust, regulate, and (in some emergency situations) override this intrinsic system (Loewy, 1990a; Dodd and Role, 1991).

The enteric nervous system is found within the four layers of the wall of the GI tract and is considered to contain as many neurons as the spinal cord itself, approximately 100 million (Noback, Strominger, and Demarest, 1991; Camilleri, 1993; Kiernan, 1998). The enteric system consists of two major interconnected plexuses of neuron cell bodies (ganglia) and their processes (Fig. 10-18). One of these is the myenteric plexus of Auerbach, which is located between the inner circular and outer longitudinal smooth muscle layers of the muscularis externa. This plexus extends from the esophagus to the internal anal sphincter and regulates the motility of the GI tract. The second plexus is the submucosal plexus of Meissner, which is found in the submucosa of the GI tract. The submucosal plexus, which consists of deep and superficial plexuses, extends from the stomach to the internal anal sphincter and mediates the epithelial functions of secretion and absorption (Jänig, 1988; Taylor and Bywater, 1988; Loewy, 1990a; Williams et al., 1995). Nonganglionated nerve plexuses also are located in and supply various layers of the wall of the gut (Williams et al., 1995).

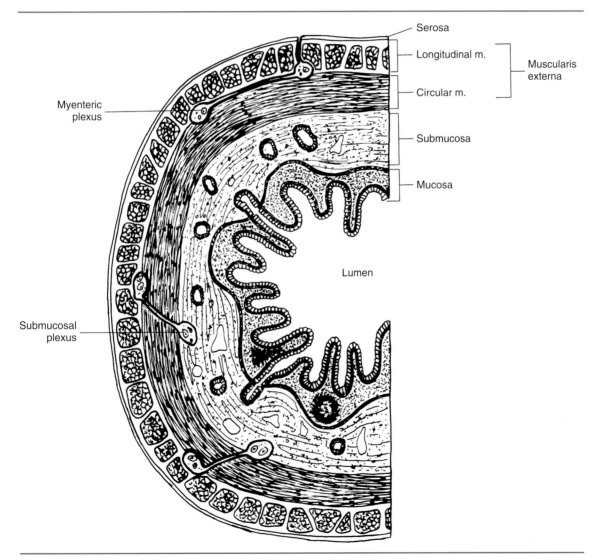

FIG. 10-18 Cross section through the wall of the gut showing the myenteric plexus (located between the two layers of smooth muscle) and the submucosal plexus (located within the submucosa layer) of the enteric nervous system. Each plexus consists of small ganglia that are interconnected.

These plexuses are more than just large, extensive parasympathetic ganglia, as previously thought. A closer look at these areas reveals that they also receive input from sympathetic postganglionic fibers, as well as preganglionic parasympathetic fibers (Fig. 10-19). In addition, they consist of cell populations different from and more complex than other autonomic ganglia. Each plexus contains clusters of neurons that are interconnected, and each cluster is made up of a heterogeneous population of neurons (Loewy, 1990a; Camilleri, 1993; Kiernan, 1998). These neurons can be classified according to their morphology, electrical properties, chemical

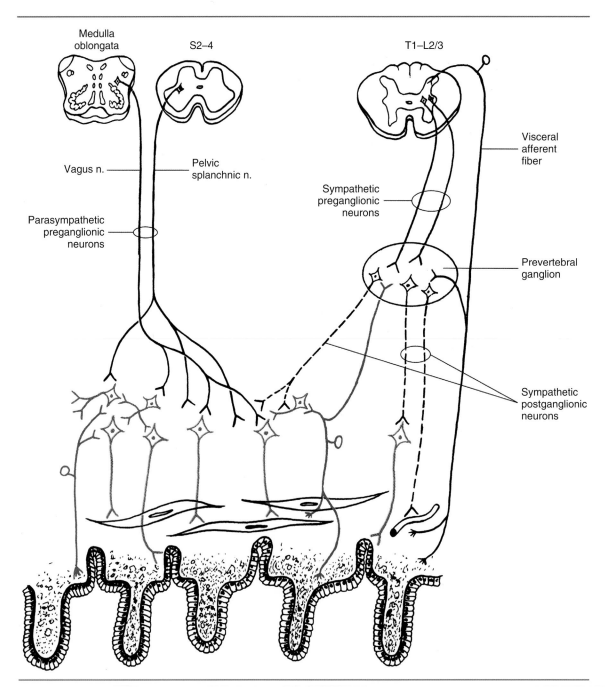

FIG. 10-19 Simplified illustration showing the sensory (*blue*), motor (*green*), and interneurons (*purple*) that compose a plexus of the enteric nervous system. Input into this group of neurons is from preganglionic parasympathetic neurons and postganglionic sympathetic neurons, both of which may modulate the function of the enteric neurons. Notice that the prevertebral sympathetic ganglion integrates input from collateral branches of primary visceral afferent fibers destined for the spinal cord, and sensory enteric neurons, thus establishing a reflex arc with postganglionic sympathetic neurons.

coding, and function (Williams et al., 1995; Furness, 2000; Hansen, 2003a). Based on size and branching patterns of the processes, seven types of neurons have been classified, although the majority are classified into three of those seven types. The neurons form multiple kinds of synapses, such as axosomatic, axoaxonal, and axodendritic. Evidence indicates that more than 30 neurotransmitters are involved in the synaptic neurotransmission. These are small molecules, peptides, or gases. The two most common chemicals are acetylcholine (ACh) and norepinephrine (NE) (Hansen, 2003a). Moreover it is suggested that one neuron may have as many as six different neuropeptides that function as neuromodulators. These modulate the release or action of the primary neurotransmitter or provide a trophic influence (Williams et al., 1995). Based on function, three types of neurons, which form complex circuits, have been classified. These are motor neurons, interneurons, and sensory neurons (see Fig. 10-19). Motor neurons are classified as one of three different types: muscle, secretomotor (some of which are vasodilators), and neurons supplying enteroendocrine cells. Muscle motor neurons innervate the smooth muscle of the GI system and are excitatory or inhibitory. The excitatory neurons use the neurotransmitters acetylcholine, substance P, and neurokinin A. The inhibitory neurons fire continuously, and thus their activity determines the amount of contraction that occurs. These neurons use numerous neurotransmitters such as nitric oxide, vasoactive intestinal polypeptide (VIP), adenosine triphosphate (ATP), gamma-aminobutyric acid (GABA), neuropeptide Y, and carbon monoxide.

Secretomotor and vasomotor (dilator) neurons of the enteric nervous system regulate secretions and blood flow. They are directly controlled by the enteric sensory neurons (intrinsic primary afferent neurons [IPANs]), which are activated by local chemical mediators released as a result of luminal stimuli. The cell bodies of both are located in the submucosa. Some of these neurons release ACh, which acts on the secretory epithelial cells. The other neurons release VIP and adjust and regulate most of the local reflex responses. These local reflexes, which maintain a balance between secretory activity and blood flow of the GI tracts, can be modulated by primarily sympathetic fibers.

A population of motor neurons also innervates enteroendocrine cells. These specialized cells are located in the mucosa and function to "taste" or detect the contents of the lumen of the gut. In response to specific stimuli (e.g., hyperosmolarity, mechanical distortion of the mucosa, bacterial products) in the lumen, they release chemical mediators, such as secretin, somatostatin, cholecystokinin (CCK), and 5 hydroxytryptamine (5-HT), that stimulate nearby afferent fibers that in turn synapse on inhibitory and excitatory neurons. The

enteroendocrine cells also activate sensory neurons and extrinsic neurons (vagal and spinal afferents). The motor innervation to these cells is extensive, although the specific motor function to *all* enteroendocrine cells is unknown. However, research has shown that there is a direct cholinergic innervation to one population of cells, the enterochromaffin cells, and this innervation controls the release of 5-HT into the lumen of the gut (Hansen, 2003a).

Interneurons aid in forming the circuitry necessary for processing sensory input. Three types of interneurons have axons that are descending (aborally directed) and are involved in local motility and secretomotor reflexes. These neurons release numerous kinds of neurotransmitters (e.g., ACh, nitric oxide, VIP, somatostatin). The other type of interneuron has an ascending orally directed axon and uses ACh as its neurotransmitter.

The sensory neurons of the enteric nervous system have dendrites that project into the mucosal layer (near the lumen), where they may play a role in epithelial functions (e.g., secretion and absorption). This allows them to act as mechanoreceptors, thermoreceptors, and chemoreceptors (e.g., detecting pH and glucose concentration) (Jänig, 1988; Dodd and Role, 1991; Camilleri, 1993). Mechanoreceptors are stimulated by distention and reflexively cause tonic muscle contractions. Peristaltic contractions are produced if the distention is maintained. Chemoreceptors and mechanoreceptors also can be stimulated by nutrients such as glucose that are located in the lumen. This produces a reflex response by stimulating secretomotor fibers that results in secretion. This response is not only local but also can be widespread throughout the GI tract by means of the integrated circuitry of the plexuses that activates secretomotor neurons at different levels. The local reflex responses are mediated by neurons primarily using substance P and VIP. However, secondary neurotransmitters such as ATP, 5-HT, ACh, and VIP also are involved in the secretory process (Hansen, 2003a,b). The axonal process of the sensory neurons synapses with interneurons and motor neurons (to smooth muscle). The peristalsis reflex is an example of the interaction of these neurons. Stretching or chemical stimuli activate the sensory neurons that project to interneurons. The interneurons in turn synapse with orally directed excitatory motor neurons and anally directed inhibitory motor neurons (Williams et al., 1995), thus creating peristalsis.

The extrinsic afferent neurons are other sensory neurons located in the GI system. These neurons send input to the CNS about the GI environment with regard to normal physiologic processes and the feelings of discomfort and pain. They become the sensory arc for sympathetic and parasympathetic reflex responses. These afferents course in the vagus nerve, pelvic splanchnic nerves, and spinal afferent nerves, and encode activity within physiologic levels. However, the spinal afferents are also activated by pathophysiologic stimuli and mediate the sensation of pain. The peripheral receptors of the spinal afferents are found in the mucosal layers, muscle, serosal membrane, and mesentery (Grundy, 2002). Spinal afferent fibers use calcitonin gene-related peptide (CGRP) and substance P as their neurotransmitters. These are known to be chemical mediators involved in the neurogenic inflammatory process and GI inflammation. Two types of vagal afferent endings are mechanosensory. One type is associated with branches that are interspersed among the circular and longitudinal muscle cell layers. These have been called "in series tension receptor endings," and they respond to muscle tension. The second type consists of endings that surround the myenteric ganglia. These monitor the stress and strains produced by muscle stretch or contraction. Also, there is evidence to show that some terminal endings of gut afferent fibers function as "efferent" sensorimotor fibers. These have collateral branches coursing to blood vessels and to the enteric ganglia where blood flow and reflexes can be modulated. Studies also indicate that some afferent fibers supplying the mucosa and coursing in the vagus nerve are sensitive to specific mediators released from the mucosal enteroendocrine cells in response to luminal nutrients. These chemical mediators are thought to initiate the neurotransmission events originating in the gut. This process is called "nutrient tasting" (Raybould, 1999; Grundy, 2002). One of these mediators is CCK, which is secreted in response to the presence of fats and protein in the intestine. In response to CCK stimulation, vagal afferent fibers become the sensory reflex limb for reflex responses controlling GI motility, secretion, and the regulation of food intake. Serotonin, in response to bacterial toxins, also functions as a mediator that stimulates vagal afferent fibers. The resulting reflex response stimulates motility and secretion and functions to protect the gut by removing the potentially harmful agent (Grundy, 2002).

The enteric sensory neurons also appear to have a broader function that involves the sympathetic system. These neurons are involved with reflexes mediated by postganglionic sympathetic fibers. Postganglionic sympathetic neurons project to numerous effectors in the GI system, including blood vessels, smooth muscle of the sphincters, myenteric plexus (concerning motility), submucosal plexus (regulating secretion and absorption), and even the organized lymphatic tissue of the GI wall (Jänig, 1988). The axons of the sensory (enteric) afferent neurons project from the myenteric plexus to sympathetic prevertebral ganglia (see Fig. 10-19). Animal studies of the prevertebral celiac ganglion show that three populations of noradrenergic neurons innervate the gut. One population, which is also immunoreactive for neuropeptide Y, functions as vasoconstrictors and

projects to the spleen, mesenteric blood vessels and arterioles in the gut wall. A second population, which is immunoreactive for somatostatin, inhibits secretomotor neurons. This population terminates in the submucosal ganglia of the small intestine, cecum, and proximal colon. The third population inhibits motility and projects to the myenteric ganglia. Enteric sensory neurons project to the two populations of neurons that inhibit secretion and inhibit motility but not to the vasomotor neurons (Furness, 2003). Activation of postganglionic sympathetic fibers that course back to the myenteric plexus results in reflex sympathetic inhibition on regions of the GI wall. Studies of the colon indicate that this enteroenteric reflex is initiated by the activation of intestinofugal (enteric sensory) neurons by distention of the intestine. It appears that these neurons can be stimulated directly by the distention and by local neurons that synapse with them. Acidic chyme in the small intestine also activates an enteroenteric reflex, resulting in inhibition of gastric motility. Based on numerous experimental data, the reflex response produced by the sympathetic efferent fibers is thought to inhibit the motility of a more proximal (orally directed) region of the GI tract relative to the location of the initial stimulus. Therefore it appears that the enteroenteric reflex, via prevertebral ganglia, regulates the movement of luminal contents from a proximal to a distal direction (Furness, 2003).

The functional relationship between the sensory afferent fibers and sympathetic system becomes somewhat more complex when it is noted that sympathetic prevertebral ganglia receive additional input from the CNS via preganglionic sympathetic fibers (splanchnic nerves) and collateral branches of visceral afferent fibers that are conveying information to the spinal cord (see Fig. 10-19); therefore the sympathetic ganglia may serve a variety of functions related to GI activity. Sympathetic fibers controlling the vasculature may use these ganglia simply as a relay station in which preganglionic fibers cause the firing of postganglionic vasomotor fibers. However, and more importantly, the ganglia also may serve as an integrative center for collecting CNS input from preganglionic fibers, as well as peripheral input from sensory neurons in the GI wall. Neither of these inputs alone is capable of causing the postganglionic neurons to reach their firing threshold; therefore the continual activity of sensory neurons from the gut, in essence, determines the firing threshold of the postganglionic neurons. As long as this activity is at a high enough level, the spatial summation of these afferent fibers, together with the input from preganglionic sympathetic fibers, allows CNS information to reach the effectors. The necessity of summation to allow for proper GI function demonstrates the importance of sensory input to the prevertebral sympathetic ganglia. This input provides a means by which the prevertebral ganglia can regulate and adjust (modulate) incoming information from the CNS that is destined for the GI tract (Jänig, 1988).

Perhaps of equal importance is that the prevertebral ganglia are thought to be involved in the circuitry that protects the GI tract from potential or real injury. GI visceral afferents, the cell bodies of which are located in dorsal root ganglia, have been shown to transmit information from mechanoreceptors and receptors sensitive to molecules such as bradykinin and hydrogen chloride. As they course to the spinal cord, these afferent fibers send collateral branches into the prevertebral ganglia. This input to the prevertebral ganglia, which is only approximately 10% of all of the synapses at this location (Furness, 2003), and to the spinal cord provides the sensory limb for viscerovisceral, viscerosympathetic, and viscerosomatic reflexes (discussed later in this chapter), as well as for visceral sensation. The collateral branches synapsing in the ganglia are thought to cause a lowering of the firing threshold of the postganglionic fibers. This would allow spatial summation of the sensory afferent fibers and preganglionic fibers to occur more readily, thereby facilitating, for example, the motor limb of the intestino intestinal reflex (Jänig, 1988).

In summary, the enteric nervous system not only independently controls the GI tract, but also has an important functional relationship with extrinsic autonomic fibers. By modulating the enteric nervous system, parasympathetic preganglionic fibers stimulate gut motility and secretion and also relax the GI sphincters. The sympathetic postganglionic fibers not only synapse on cells of the enteric plexus, but also presynaptically inhibit preganglionic parasympathetic fibers (Gershon, 1981; Kiernan, 1998) and thus function to inhibit GI motility and secretion and also constrict the sphincters.

INNERVATION OF AUTONOMIC EFFECTORS
Innervation of the Immune System

Recent research indicates that the autonomic nervous system can influence the activity of the immune system. Evidence from animal studies (Jänig and Häbler, 2000) shows that sympathetic efferent fibers innervate primary and secondary lymphoid tissue. T lymphocytes and macrophages have been found close to the varicosities on the efferent fiber membranes. Panuncio et al. (1998) studied human lymph nodes and found sympathetic adrenergic fibers entering lymph nodes along blood vessels, primarily arteries. Other fibers were located in the parenchyma in T-cell regions. Postcapillary venules also were found to have nerve fibers associated with them, possibly for regulating the movement of lymphocytes into the lymph node. The spleen is another lymphatic organ that has been researched extensively and has been found to be innervated by sympathetic post-

ganglionic neurons (Jänig and Häbler, 2000). Studies of the feline spleen have shown that it is innervated by approximately 12,000 sympathetic fibers. Relative to the weight of the spleen compared with the weight of the kidney, the number of splenic sympathetic fibers is three times the number supplying the kidney. The fibers to the spleen appear to be different from sympathetic renal fibers, which function as vasoconstrictors. Some splenic fibers appear to function independently from arterial baroreceptor input and are activated reflexively to sensory input from the spleen, as well as the GI tract; therefore the sympathetic fibers may have other functions besides vasoconstriction and capsular contraction. Studies in rats show the alteration of various immune functions in the spleen with sympathetic nerve stimulation. These alterations include changes of cellular elements involved in immune responses after sympathectomy; decrease of immune responses after splenic nerve stimulation; and activation of certain other immune responses (e.g., stimulation of a specific hypothalamic region results in splenic nerve activity that correlates with the suppression of cytotoxic activity of splenic natural killer cells). Sato (1997) used anesthetized rats and looked at the effect of pinching the hind paws and brushing and pinching the skin on sympathetic activity in the spleen. The results showed a reflex response that included vasoconstriction and a decrease in cytotoxic activity of the natural killer cells.

In addition to the spleen, the immune system of the skin also may be influenced by the sympathetic nervous system. Effector tissues in the skin (i.e., sweat glands, arrector pili muscles, and vascular smooth muscle) are well supplied by sympathetic fibers. However, neurophysiologic studies have shown that some cutaneous sympathetic efferents are not associated with the innervation of those tissues. Although the function of these other fibers is unclear, they may be involved with the immune system (Jänig and Häbler, 2000). There is also an important relationship between the lymphatic tissue of the GI tract and the enteric division of the ANS. This division (see Enteric Nervous System), located in the wall of the gut, consists of the neuronal population that regulates GI motility and secretion. Receptors for neurotransmitters released from enteric neurons have been identified on lymphatic tissue cells located in the wall of the gut. During GI inflammation, toxins and inflammatory mediators can activate enteric neurons, which activate (bind to) the receptors on the lymphatic tissue cells. In addition, the enteric neurons inhibit sympathetic firing. Also, the chemical mediators can sensitize primary afferent nociceptors and recruit silent nociceptors, resulting in neurogenic inflammation. During this process, mast cells, which have a direct CNS innervation, release mediators such as serotonin, histamine, and nerve growth factor. These chemicals stimulate vagal afferent fibers and local enteric neurons. These neurons then initiate propulsive motor activity and secretion to rid the gut of the harmful agent. There also may be a link between the functional relationships of the cells of the immune system, the inflammatory process, and enteric neurons to irritable bowel syndrome (IBS). In some patients with this syndrome, there is an increase in the number of immune and inflammatory cells in the vicinity of nerve fiber terminals. This may indicate that enteric neurons are the target of an autoimmune response, which may be the cause of IBS symptoms (Hansen, 2003b).

Innervation of Peripheral Effectors

Cutaneous Effectors. Cutaneous autonomic effectors include blood vessels, sweat glands, adipose tissue, and arrector pili muscles. Similar to tissues of the immune system, but unlike most autonomic effectors, these cutaneous effectors are innervated by only the sympathetic division. Preganglionic fibers originate from cell bodies located in the intermediolateral cell column of the T1 to L2 or L3 cord segments, leave via ventral roots, and after traversing the white rami communicantes, synapse in the sympathetic chain ganglia. Postganglionic fibers, which include vasoconstrictor fibers, sudomotor fibers (to sweat glands), and pilomotor fibers, travel in gray rami to join the spinal nerve on its course to its dermatomal area of supply. (However, the area of skin innervated by sympathetic fibers has been found to be wider than the dermatomal distribution of the somatic fibers [Ogawa and Low, 1993].) More specifically, superior and middle cervical ganglia send postganglionic fibers to the head and neck; the stellate (cervicothoracic) ganglion (in conjunction with a small contribution from the middle ganglion) supplies the upper extremities; thoracic ganglia supply the trunk; and lower lumbar and upper sacral ganglia furnish postganglionic fibers for the skin of the lower extremities (Jänig, 1990; Williams et al., 1995). Because sympathetic efferents innervate cutaneous effectors covering the entire body, nearly all spinal nerves are likely to contain postganglionic sympathetic fibers. The sympathetic innervation of these cutaneous effectors is controlled primarily by the hypothalamus, and stimulation of these effectors is important for thermoregulation.

Blood Vessels Supplying Skeletal Muscles. During muscle activity, vasodilation (and subsequent increased blood flow) is primarily a result of local muscle tissue effects; for example, decreased oxygen in the contracting muscle causing the release of vasodilator substances. However, sympathetic fibers also innervate these blood vessels providing continuous vasomotor tone and when further activated, causing vasoconstric-

tion (sympathetic vasodilator fibers also exist in some lower animals) (Guyton, 1991). The adrenal medulla (innervated by preganglionic sympathetic fibers) is also involved in the regulation of blood flow to skeletal muscles by causing vasoconstriction (via the neurotransmitter norepinephrine, which binds to vasoconstrictor alpha receptors) and some vasodilation (via the neurotransmitter epinephrine, which binds to vasodilator beta receptors) (Guyton, 1991).

The origin of preganglionic neurons for the upper extremity blood vessels is the intermediolateral cell column of the T2 to T6 or T7 (primarily T2 and T3) cord segments. The axons enter the sympathetic chain ganglia through white rami communicantes and synapse predominantly in the stellate (cervicothoracic) ganglion. Postganglionic fibers leave the ganglion within gray rami to join spinal nerves and, subsequently, ventral rami destined to form the brachial plexus. The C8 and T1 ventral rami receive the greatest contribution of fibers; therefore the lower trunk of the brachial plexus conveys most of the peripheral sympathetic efferents. The lower trunk provides fibers to numerous terminal branches of the brachial plexus, including the median, ulnar, and radial nerves. As the postganglionic neurons travel with these nerves, they supply branches to the accompanying brachial, ulnar, and radial arteries, respectively. The lower extremity muscular arteries are supplied by sympathetic fibers originating in the T10 to L2 or L3 cord segments. These preganglionic fibers enter the sympathetic chain and synapse in the lumbar and sacral ganglia. Postganglionic neurons traverse the gray rami, join spinal nerves, and then enter ventral rami of the lumbosacral plexus. Some postganglionic efferents course with the femoral nerve to supply muscular branches of the femoral artery, whereas others travel with the tibial nerve to innervate the tibial vascular tree (Williams et al., 1995).

Surgical denervation of the peripheral vasculature can be accomplished by cutting the sympathetic chain or removing sympathetic ganglia (sympathectomy) or cutting preganglionic fibers at the appropriate location (Williams et al., 1995). This provides a treatment for relief of vasomotor spasms that occur in such disorders as Raynaud's disease and intermittent claudication. Sympathectomy also has been performed to influence vasomotor tone in hypertensive patients.

Innervation of the Heart and Lungs

Sympathetic Innervation. As with most autonomic effectors, the heart and lungs are innervated by both the sympathetic and parasympathetic divisions of the ANS. Sympathetic preganglionic neurons to both the heart and lungs originate in the T1 to T4 or T5 cord segments, enter the sympathetic chain, and synapse. The preganglionic sympathetic fibers associated with the innervation of the heart synapse in the thoracic ganglia that correspond to the spinal cord segments of origin. Many also ascend to synapse in all three cervical ganglia. Postganglionic fibers leave the ganglia as cardiac branches (nerves), which form part of the cardiac plexus (see Fig. 10-9, *B*). Sympathetic innervation of the heart results in cardiac acceleration and increased force of ventricular contraction. Coronary blood flow is primarily controlled by autoregulation of the coronary arteries in response to increased and decreased cardiac activity and subsequent metabolic needs of the muscle tissue. However, the coronary arteries are well innervated by sympathetic fibers and, although of minor importance functionally, these fibers on stimulation cause either vasoconstriction or vasodilation, depending on which receptor (alpha or beta, respectively) is activated (Guyton, 1991). Afferent information from the heart travels in all cardiac branches except the branch associated with the superior cervical ganglion (Williams et al., 1995).

Postganglionic sympathetic fibers to the lungs originate from the T2 to T5 sympathetic chain ganglia and pass through the cardiac plexus. However, they continue and course along the pulmonary arteries to form the pulmonary plexus. These postganglionic efferents provide bronchodilation and vasoconstriction to the lungs.

Parasympathetic Innervation. Parasympathetic innervation to the heart and lungs is provided by the vagus nerve (CN X). Cardiac preganglionic fibers originate in the brain stem medulla. Although most parasympathetic visceral efferents originate in the dorsal motor nucleus, some, possibly the majority, of efferents to the heart originate in or near the nucleus ambiguus (Loewy and Spyer, 1990; Noback, Strominger, and Demarest 1991; Williams et al., 1995; Kiernan, 1998; Nolte, 2002). Regardless of origin, the preganglionic fibers descend within the vagus nerve into the thoracic cavity as cardiac branches and become part of the cardiac plexus (see Fig. 10-9, *B*). They synapse in small cardiac ganglia located in the cardiac plexus and in the walls of the atria. Postganglionic parasympathetic fibers cause a decrease in ventricular contraction and cardiac deceleration. Although autoregulation of coronary arteries based on local metabolic needs is the primary mechanism of controlling coronary blood flow, a few parasympathetic fibers innervate these arteries and, on stimulation, result in a slight vasodilation (Guyton, 1991).

Vagal preganglionic fibers that innervate the lung aid the sympathetics in forming the pulmonary plexus. The preganglionic parasympathetic fibers synapse in small ganglia adjacent to the lung hilum. Postganglionic fibers continue into the lung to stimulate bronchoconstriction, vasodilation, and glandular secretion (Williams et al., 1995). These actions help to maintain the integrity of the epithelial lining of the bronchial tree.

Innervation to the Head

In general preganglionic sympathetic cell bodies for the head (and neck) are located in the T1 (primarily) to T3 (and some in T4 and T5) spinal cord segments. These fibers enter the sympathetic chain and ascend to the superior cervical ganglion, where they synapse. Postganglionic fibers leave the ganglion and travel with branches of the carotid arteries to gain access to autonomic effectors in the head (see Fig. 10-9, *A*). One large branch (the internal carotid nerve) leaves the ganglion branches to form the internal carotid plexus, which travels on the internal carotid artery into the cranial cavity. Some fibers (vasoconstrictors) of the plexus continue to the cerebral arteries, where they meet additional sympathetic fibers of the vertebral plexus. Other fibers leave the artery and travel to their destination by "hitching a ride" on cranial nerves in the region.

The perivascular plexus surrounding the external carotid artery and its branches contains fibers that are vasomotor, pilomotor, and secretomotor to all sweat glands of the face except for the sweat glands in the medial part of the forehead. These are supplied by branches of the internal carotid plexus (Watson and Vijayan, 1995; Salvesen, 2001).

Although sympathetic efferents employ arterial transportation, parasympathetic fibers to the head emerge from the brain stem as a part of the oculomotor, facial, and glossopharyngeal nerves. These nerves innervate glandular tissue and smooth muscle.

Although there is dual innervation to the lacrimal, mucosal, and salivary glands, the secretomotor fibers are parasympathetic (sympathetic fibers produce vasoconstriction). Parasympathetic fibers that innervate the lacrimal gland, nasal and palate mucosal glands, and major salivary glands (sublingual and submandibular) travel with the facial nerve. Preganglionic neurons originate in the superior salivatory nucleus located in the brain stem. Those en route to the lacrimal and mucosal glands synapse in the pterygopalatine ganglion, and those destined for the salivary glands synapse in the submandibular ganglion. Parasympathetic efferents innervating the parotid salivary gland course in the glossopharyngeal cranial nerve. These preganglionic fibers originate in the inferior salivatory nucleus of the brain stem and course to the otic ganglion. After synapsing, the postganglionic secretomotor fibers travel to the parotid gland (see Figs. 10-15 and 10-16, *A*).

The ANS is also intimately involved with the innervation of effectors located in the region of the orbit. These include the smooth muscle (Müller's muscle or superior tarsal muscle) of the eyelids, blood vessels of the eye, and the smooth muscle of the iris and ciliary body. This innervation is responsible for some of the functions that can be assessed during a neurologic examination. Regulation of blood flow to the eye is extremely important in maintaining an adequate nutrient supply to the retina. Retinal arterioles are autoregulated, but choroidal arterioles are autonomically innervated. Sympathetic activation causes vasoconstriction, whereas parasympathetic stimulation, via the facial nerve, is vasodilatory (Loewy, 1990b).

The upper eyelid contains skeletal muscle (levator palpebrae superioris), which is innervated by somatic efferents of the oculomotor nerve. It (and the lower eyelid to a lesser extent) also contains smooth muscle fibers (Müller's muscle or superior tarsal muscle) (Williams et al., 1995). The smooth muscle is innervated by sympathetic fibers. Because ptosis (drooping) of the upper eyelid is an important indicator of damage to the sympathetic nervous system, knowledge of the two innervations is necessary for differentiating a lesion involving the oculomotor nerve from a lesion of the sympathetic system.

Other smooth muscle fibers in this region are the intrinsic muscles of the eye (i.e., the sphincter and dilator pupillae muscles of the iris and the ciliary muscle of the ciliary body). The iris acts as a diaphragm and regulates the amount of light entering the eye. The dilator muscle is innervated by sympathetic postganglionic efferents that have left the internal carotid plexus to travel with the ophthalmic fibers of the trigeminal nerve. The parasympathetic innervation supplies the sphincter muscle fibers and is the motor arc of the pupillary light reflex. The origin of the parasympathetic preganglionic fibers is the Edinger-Westphal nucleus of the midbrain. The fibers emerge from the brain stem, lie superficially in the dorsomedial aspect of the oculomotor nerve, and travel to the ciliary ganglion located in the orbit (see Fig. 10-15). After synapsing, postganglionic fibers innervate the sphincter muscle fibers of the iris. When these fibers are activated to cause pupillary constriction, there is an accompanying inhibition of the innervation to the dilator muscle (Loewy, 1990b). During alert but resting periods, a constant sympathetic tone is sustained through hypothalamic input; parasympathetic fibers are inhibited at the same time (Cross, 1993b).

An additional smooth muscle, the ciliary muscle, also is involved in the normal function of the eye. This muscle controls the tension of the suspensory ligaments attached to the lens. Parasympathetic and some sympathetic fibers (the function of the latter is unclear) innervate the ciliary muscle. Controlling the regulation of the curvature and thus the refractive power of the lens via this muscle is essentially a parasympathetic function. This innervation allows focusing to occur when an object is close to the eye (accommodation). Of the total number of preganglionic fibers leaving the Edinger-Westphal nucleus, 94% travel to the ciliary muscle, whereas the remaining fibers supply the iris (Cross, 1993b). The accommodation-convergence reflex is necessary during near vision to correct for an unfocused image on the fovea (region of the retina associated with the most acute vision). The reflex response (mediated by CN III) results in an increase in lens curvature, pupillary constriction, and convergence of the eyes.

Knowledge of the innervation of the eye is important because pathologic conditions affecting the autonomic innervation can occur and because these eye functions can be tested in a neurologic examination. Pathologic conditions caused by disruption of parasympathetic fibers include the Argyll-Robertson pupil (associated with neurosyphilis), internal ophthalmoplegia, light-near dissociation, and Adie's pupil (Cross, 1993a). Horner's's syndrome is an example of a condition attributed to a lesion in the sympathetic system (see Clinical Applications).

Innervation of the Bladder

The bladder functions to store and evacuate urine. Control of bladder function occurs by a complex integration and coordination of bladder afferent fibers, sympathetic and parasympathetic efferent fibers, somatic efferent fibers (Fig. 10-20), pontine micturition centers, hypothalamic nuclei, and cortical areas (Carpenter and Sutin, 1983; de Groat and Steers, 1990; Abdel-Azim, Sullivan, and Yalla, 1991; Bradley, 1993; Blok and Holstege, 1998; Shefchyk, 2001, 2002). Sympathetic preganglionic neurons originate in cord segments T11 or T12 through L2 and synapse in corresponding ganglia and small ganglia in the superior and inferior hypogastric plexuses. Postganglionic fibers course in the vesical plexus (anterior fibers of the inferior hypogastric plexus) to the bladder. Some of these fibers inhibit the smooth muscle (detrusor) of the bladder wall, but many, and possibly the majority are also vasomotor, suggesting that sympathetic efferents may have no essential role in micturition. Other sympathetic fibers richly supply (especially in the male) and stimulate the nonstriated (smooth) muscle in the neck of the bladder (sphincter vesicae). Although this innervation may serve a minor function in maintaining urinary continence, its major role is to contract these muscle fibers during ejaculation (Carpenter and Sutin, 1983; Williams et al., 1995; Snell, 2001).

The parasympathetic innervation is the more important autonomic efferent supply to the detrusor muscle of the bladder. The parasympathetic fibers originate in the S2 to S4 spinal cord segments, pass into the cauda equina, emerge from the S2 to S4 pelvic (ventral) sacral foramina, and form pelvic splanchnic nerves (see Figs. 10-17 and 10-20). These nerves travel within the inferior hypogastric plexus and continue distally into the vesical plexus. These preganglionic fibers synapse with postganglionic neurons located in ganglia within the vesical plexus or within the bladder wall. The postganglionic fibers provide excitatory innervation to the detrusor

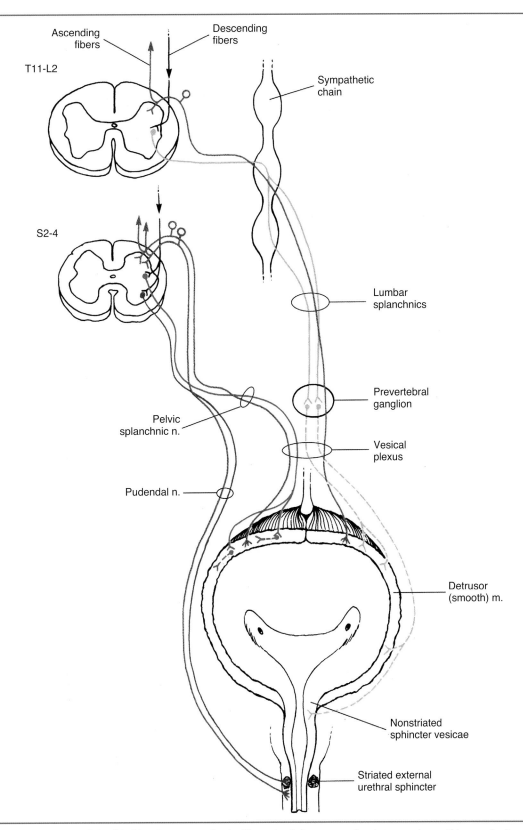

Ascending fibers

Descending fibers

T11-L2

Sympathetic chain

S2-4

Lumbar splanchnics

Prevertebral ganglion

Pelvic splanchnic n.

Vesical plexus

Pudendal n.

Detrusor (smooth) m.

Nonstriated sphincter vesicae

Striated external urethral sphincter

FIG. 10-20 Innervation of the bladder. Parasympathetic fibers (*red*) innervate the detrusor (smooth) muscle. Sympathetic fibers (*yellow*) are primarily vasomotor to the bladder wall but also supply the sphincter vesicae (nonstriated) muscle in the neck of the bladder, which functions to close the lumen of the neck during ejaculation. Somatic efferents (*blue*) coursing in the pudendal nerve also provide an important innervation to the external ventral sphincter (striated muscle). Afferent fibers (*green*) entering the cord may transmit information to higher centers, as well as provide the afferent arc for initiating the voiding response. Descending information from the hypothalamus and cerebral cortex also may modulate the spinal cord neurons.

muscle. (A few fibers supply and inhibit the nonstriated sphincter vesicae.)

Another important muscle involved with normal bladder function is the striated (voluntary) urethral sphincter muscle. The somatic motor neurons that innervate this muscle originate in Onuf's nucleus, which is located in the ventral horn of S2 to S4. These neurons course through the S2-4 ventral roots, spinal nerves, ventral rami, and travel in the pudendal nerve to reach the skeletal muscle fibers of the sphincter.

The bladder and lower urinary tract exist in two states: continence, which is bladder filling, and micturition, which is bladder voiding. During continence, sympathetic fibers facilitate bladder filling by causing relaxation of the detrusor muscle and contraction of the sphincter vesicae. In addition, somatic motor neurons fire and maintain the external urethral sphincter muscle in a tonically active state. Micturition is a reflex response and is initiated by sensory input from the bladder wall. Afferents course in the pudendal nerves, sympathetic nerves, and parasympathetic nerves. Sympathetic afferents include both nociceptive and nonnociceptive fibers. However, this information does not appear to be of major importance in the normal micturition reflex response initiated by distention (Shefchyk, 2002). The most important afferent fibers are those coursing with parasympathetic efferent fibers. These fibers are group A-delta fibers, which convey information concerning distention of the bladder wall, and C fibers, which are concerned with pain and temperature sense. The fibers travel in the pelvic splanchnic nerves and enter the sacral cord segments. Input via A-delta fibers is necessary to initiate the voiding response. Once this information has reached the cord, tract neurons ascend in the dorsal column, dorsolateral funiculus, and lateral funiculus to terminate in higher centers. One of these areas is the periaqueductal gray matter located in the midbrain, which projects to the micturition center located in the pons. This center acts as a switch and when bladder afferent activity reaches a specific threshold, the micturition response is turned on and continence is turned off. Descending fibers from the micturition center course through the lateral funiculus of the cord and, via interneurons, cause excitation of sacral preganglionic parasympathetic neurons, resulting in detrusor muscle contraction. The descending fibers from the micturition center also cause inhibition of somatic motor neurons, resulting in relaxation of the external urethral sphincter (Blok and Holstege, 1998; Shefchyk, 2001, 2002). Although the pontine center coordinates the micturition process, it in turn is modulated by the cerebral cortex (dorsolateral prefrontal cortex and anterior cingulate gyrus) and diencephalic (primarily the hypothalamus) structures, which also may project directly to the spinal cord. These areas may be involved with the attentiveness and response to micturition and determining the beginning

of micturition (de Groat and Steers, 1990; Bradley, 1993; Blok and Holstege, 1998). Descending cortical input allows voluntary control of voiding and allows one to start and stop micturition on demand. The connections between the spinal cord and brain stem form a spinobulbospinal reflex, which is instrumental for sustaining detrusor muscle contraction and relaxing the striated sphincter during micturition. Spinal cord lesions may disrupt the reflex, but spinal cord neurons can reorganize to allow group C afferent fibers to initiate a spinal reflex that produces an automatic reflex bladder (de Groat et al., 1990). This type of reflex results in voiding, whenever the bladder is full.

Innervation of Sexual Organs

The innervation of sexual organs, which is similar to that of the bladder, consists of sympathetic, parasympathetic, and somatic fibers (de Groat and Steers, 1990; Seftel, Oates, and Krane, 1991; Stewart, 1993). This section is primarily concerned with the innervation of male sexual organs, although innervation to homologous female organs is somewhat similar.

The sympathetic preganglionic fibers take origin from approximately the T10 to L2 cord segments (Fig. 10-21). The route of these fibers varies. Some preganglionic fibers synapse with postganglionic neurons in the sympathetic chain. The axons of these postganglionic neurons enter into the hypogastric nerves and continue into the inferior hypogastric (pelvic) plexus. Other preganglionic fibers travel in the superior hypogastric plexus and synapse in ganglia scattered in the inferior hypogastric plexus (Seftel, Oates, and Krane, 1991). In both cases the postganglionic fibers coursing within the inferior hypogastric plexus continue distally into the prostatic plexus (Williams et al., 1995). These fibers then leave the plexus as the cavernous nerve and innervate erectile tissue of the penis and smooth muscle in the seminal vesicles, prostate gland, vas deferens, and the nonstriated sphincter in the bladder neck. Parasympathetic preganglionic fibers originate from S2 to S4 and course in the pelvic splanchnic nerves (see Fig. 10-21). The pelvic splanchnic nerves synapse in ganglia in the inferior hypogastric (pelvic) plexus. Postganglionic fibers, in conjunction with postganglionic sympathetic fibers, continue to (and are the primary innervation of) erectile tissue, as well as glandular tissue in the seminal vesicles, prostate gland, and urethra.

The somatic nervous system is also involved with sexual function. The pudendal nerve contains sensory fibers that course from the penis to sacral cord segments. It also contains motor fibers that travel from the spinal cord to the bulbocavernosus and ischiocavernosus skeletal muscles. These motor neurons originate in Onuf's nucleus, which is located in the ventral horn of the S2 to S4 cord segments.

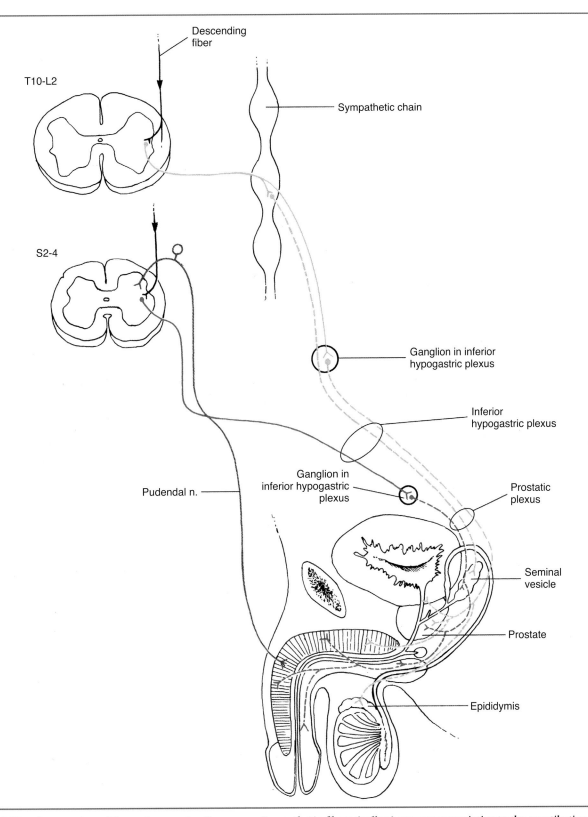

FIG. 10-21   Innervation of the male reproductive organs. Sympathetic fibers (*yellow*) are vasoconstrictive to the erectile tissue and also supply the glandular smooth muscle tissue. Parasympathetic fibers (*red*) are the major supply of the penile erectile tissue but also supply the glandular tissue. The pudendal nerve contains somatic efferent fibers (not pictured here) to the bulbocavernosus and ischiocavernosus muscles and afferent fibers (*green*) conveying sensory information from the penis. These afferent fibers form the sensory arc for reflexogenic erections. Descending fibers from the hypothalamus and limbic system structures send input to the spinal cord neurons, which initiate psychogenic erections.

The erection phase of sexual function can be initiated by stimuli such as visual, auditory, imaginative, and tactile. Evidence from spinal cord-injured patients indicates that there are two types of erection reflexes: psychogenic and reflexogenic. In healthy individuals, both types of reflexes probably act synergistically. Reflexogenic erections are sacral spinal reflexes consisting of afferent fibers in the pudendal nerve activating sacral parasympathetic efferent fibers (a small number of afferent fibers ascend in the dorsal columns to higher centers). Psychogenic erections begin in supraspinal centers, including the limbic system and the hypothalamus. The hypothalamus has been implicated as the integration center for the erection response (de Groat and Steers, 1990; Stewart, 1993).

Fibers from these supraspinal centers descend through the brain stem and the lateral white column (funiculus) of the spinal cord to synapse on lower thoracic and lumbar preganglionic sympathetic neurons and the sacral preganglionic parasympathetic neurons. The parasympathetic fibers initiate the erectile response by causing dilation of the arteries within the erectile tissue. However, the sympathetic fibers contribute to this reflex because they also can initiate a psychogenic erection (possibly through the use of different neurotransmitters) when the parasympathetic preganglionic neurons are lesioned (de Groat and Steers, 1990; Seftel, Oates, and Krane, 1991).

Emission and ejaculation are also a part of sexual function. Cortical modulation occurs, but the mechanism is complex and unclear. Emission is sympathetically controlled by neurons originating in the T10 to L2 or L3 cord segments (see previous discussion for the route of these sympathetic preganglionic and postganglionic fibers). This event includes the smooth muscle contraction of the vas deferens, seminal vesicles, prostate gland, and nonstriated sphincter vesicae (to prevent reflux of semen into the bladder during ejaculation) resulting in the deposition of semen into the prostatic urethra. The process of ejaculation consists of propelling the semen from the prostatic urethra through the membranous and penile parts of the urethra and out the urethral orifice. The bulbocavernosus and ischiocavernosus skeletal muscles, which are innervated by the pudendal nerve, contract during this event. The coordination of emission and ejaculation probably occurs by the integration of sensory afferent fibers, descending supraspinal input, and motor efferents in an ejaculation center located in the T12 to L2 cord segments (Seftel, Oates, and Krane, 1991).

VISCERAL AFFERENTS
General Considerations

Although the ANS is considered by some to consist primarily of an efferent limb, visceral afferent fibers have an important relationship with the efferent fibers.

Visceral afferent fibers, which since 1894 have been known to accompany autonomic efferents (Cervero and Foreman, 1990), provide information about changes in the body's internal environment. This input becomes integrated in the CNS and may participate in reflexes via autonomic and somatic efferents. These reflexes, such as the regulation of blood pressure and the chemical composition of the blood, aid the ANS in the control of homeostasis. However, visceral afferent fibers also mediate some conscious feelings, such as the visceral sensations of hunger, nausea, and distention. Although receptors of visceral afferent fibers do not respond to stimuli such as cutting or burning (as cutaneous receptors do), a pathologic condition or excessive distention produces visceral nociception. The continual barrage of impulses via visceral afferent fibers on the CNS is the probable cause of an individual's feeling of well-being or of discomfort.

Visceral afferent fibers convey information from peripheral receptors called interoceptors. These endings, which may be encapsulated or free nerve endings, are of variable shapes, such as knobs, loops, rings, tendrils, and complex encapsulated endings (Williams et al., 1995). They are found in the walls of the viscera, glands, blood vessels, epithelium, mesentery, and serosae. Some are described as mechanoreceptors and include numerous pacinian corpuscles. These are located in the abdominal mesenteries. Other mechanoreceptors are found in the serosal covering of the viscera and also in the blood vessels, and they may be stimulated by movement or distention. Still others, found in smooth muscle such as that of the bladder, monitor both contraction and distention (Willis and Coggeshall, 1991). Nociceptors of two types have been located in the heart and GI tract. Both respond to mechanical, thermal, and chemical stimuli. One group is comparable to the cutaneous A-delta fiber type, whereas the other group is similar to the cutaneous C-fiber type (Willis and Coggeshall, 1991). In addition, chemoreceptors and baroreceptors are special interoceptors that are located specifically in the aortic arch and the bifurcation of the left and right common carotid arteries.

The visceral afferent fibers are similar to somatic afferent fibers in that just one neuron extends from the receptor into the CNS. The visceral afferent fibers are found in both the sympathetic and parasympathetic divisions (the enteric nervous system afferent fibers have already been discussed) and travel with the autonomic efferents. The vast majority are unmyelinated; with the exception of those from the pacinian corpuscles located in the mesentery (see previous discussion). Although many of these afferent fibers are purely sensory, some fibers also have an efferent function. These fibers have the ability to release neurotransmitters such as substance P, CGRP, and ATP from their peripheral endings. The release of these chemicals results in neurogenic inflammation, which includes vasodilation, increased vascular permeability, altered smooth muscle contractility, and functional changes in cells typically involved with the inflammatory response. This event appears to be a widespread phenomenon that occurs in autonomic tissues within the cardiovascular, respiratory, and GI systems (Williams et al., 1995). The cell bodies of visceral afferent fibers that travel with parasympathetic efferents in the glossopharyngeal (CN IX) and vagus (CN X) nerves are located in the inferior (petrosal) ganglion of CN IX and the inferior (nodose) ganglion of CN X. The dorsal root ganglia of the second, third, and fourth sacral roots house visceral afferent cell bodies of fibers that travel with pelvic parasympathetic efferents. Cell bodies of afferent fibers associated with sympathetic fibers are located in the dorsal root ganglia of the thoracic and upper lumbar dorsal roots. These fibers course from the periphery along with sympathetic efferent fibers, pass through the prevertebral ganglia without synapsing, and enter the sympathetic trunk (Fig. 10-22). Then they pass through the white rami communicantes into the dorsal root and terminate in the cord segment from which the accompanying preganglionic fibers originate.

Electron microscopic and retrograde tracing methods show that a low density of fibers innervates the viscera in comparison to the innervation of the skin. Feline

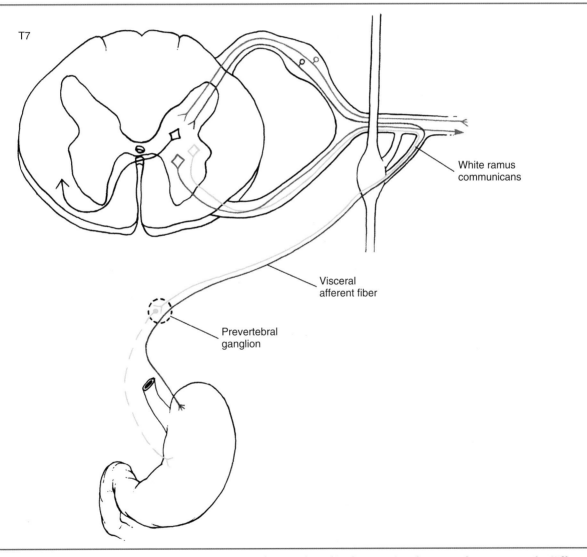

FIG. 10-22 The pathway of visceral afferent information into the spinal cord is shown using the stomach as an example. (Afferent fibers that travel in the vagus nerve and convey visceral information are not shown.) Note how the afferent fiber (*forest green*) travels with the sympathetic efferent fiber (*yellow*) but does not synapse in the prevertebral ganglion. Instead the afferent fiber synapses in the dorsal horn and has the capability of influencing numerous neurons, including preganglionic efferents, somatic efferents (*blue*), or tract neurons (*black*). In the case of visceral pain, viscerosomatic neurons also are receiving input from cutaneous sources (*purple fiber*), thus providing a mechanism for pain referral (see text for discussion).

studies demonstrate that approximately 16,000 sympathetic afferent fibers exist, and 6000 to 7000 of these are found in the greater splanchnic nerves (Cervero and Foreman, 1990). However, the total number of afferent fibers represents less than 20% of all sympathetic fibers and approximately 2% of the fibers located in dorsal roots of thoracic and lumbar spinal nerves. An obvious disparity is noticed when the parasympathetic afferent fibers are enumerated. Feline visceral afferent fibers in the vagus nerve number approximately 40,000 and pelvic afferent fibers approximately 7500. Of the total number of fibers in the vagus, 80% are afferent. In the pelvic nerves 50% of the fibers are afferent (Cervero and Foreman, 1990). The specific functional differences between the afferent fibers associated with the sympathetic division and those associated with the parasympathetic division are not clear. The parasympathetic division afferent fibers generally are thought to transmit input concerning activity of the viscera, such as GI motility and secretion. By monitoring the activity, these afferent fibers are able to mediate reflexes necessary for the proper regulation of visceral function. The sympathetic division afferent fibers appear to be concerned with sensations arising from the viscera, especially the sensation of pain (Cervero and Foreman, 1990).

Afferent Fibers Associated with the Parasympathetic Division

Afferent fibers coursing in the vagus nerve relay input from many sources (Williams et al., 1995). A partial list includes the following:

- Walls of the pharynx
- Thoracic structures
- Heart
- Walls of large vessels
- Mucosa and smooth muscle of the bronchial tree of the lung
- Connective tissue adjacent to the alveoli of the lung
- Abdominal structures
- Stomach and intestinal walls
- Digestive glands
- Kidneys

The glossopharyngeal nerve conveys visceral afferent information from the posterior region of the tongue, upper pharynx, tonsils, and the carotid sinus and carotid body.

The cell bodies of afferent fibers for both the vagus and glossopharyngeal nerves are located in their respective inferior ganglia. These ganglia are located adjacent to the jugular foramen of the skull. The afferent fibers of both CNs IX and X synapse in the nucleus of the tractus solitarius, which is located in the medulla oblongata of the brain stem. From here, axons project to numerous areas in the central autonomic network of the brain stem and diencephalon (see Control of Autonomic

Efferents and Figs. 10-28 and 10-29) and the cerebral cortex. The projections to the cerebral cortex travel by way of the thalamus. These cerebral projections allow for conscious awareness of sensations, such as hunger. When appropriate, reflexes also may be elicited. Examples include the swallowing, cough, cardiovascular, and respiratory reflexes.

Visceral afferent fibers from the pelvic viscera and distal colon enter the spinal cord via pelvic splanchnics. These fibers monitor stretch in the hollow viscera and possibly mediate nociception originating in the bladder and colon (Carpenter and Sutin, 1983; Cervero and Foreman, 1990).

Afferent Fibers Associated with the Sympathetic Division

As mentioned, input conveyed through sympathetic afferent fibers is concerned with visceral sensation, especially visceral nociception. The sensations that reach consciousness are poorly localized and, in the case of pain, may be referred and may produce hyperalgesia, as well. The cell bodies of these fibers are located in the dorsal root ganglia of the thoracic and upper lumbar dorsal roots. These visceral afferent fibers travel from the peripheral receptors in the cardiac, pulmonary, and splanchnic nerves and continue through the sympathetic trunk, white rami communicantes, dorsal roots, and finally terminate in the spinal cord.

Central Projections and the Referral of Pain

As mentioned, pain of visceral origin differs substantially from somatic pain, both in the clinical presentation to the painful stimuli and the neurologic mechanisms associated with the production of the pain. Numerous characteristics help to define visceral pain. Distention of the hollow muscular walled organs, ischemia, and inflammation of the viscera are stimuli that induce pain. However, the severity of the condition resulting in pain is not always a reflection of the severity of the pain experienced. For example, mild pain may be experienced with early appendicitis, whereas severe pain may be present with the fairly normal presence of gas in the GI tract. The least sensitive of the viscera tend to be the solid organs, whereas the serosae of the hollow organs appear to be the most sensitive. Also, a mildly painful or even nonpainful stimulus can result in severe pain (Al-Chaer and Traub, 2002) if an organ is already inflamed or altered pathologically (e.g., irritable bowel syndrome [IBS]). Visceral pain often is described as being either true or referred. True visceral pain is diffuse pain that is perceived as originating from deep, midline structures in the thorax or abdomen. It is often accompanied by the sense of nausea and ill-being. An example of this is during the early stage of appendicitis when the pain is initially felt in the midline. Referred pain also is diffuse and is localized to a distant cutaneous site or to muscles. Cervero and Laird (1999) have suggested that there are five important clinical characteristics associated with visceral pain:

1. Not all viscera (e.g., liver, kidney) are sensitive to painful stimuli. This is because of functional variances of the peripheral receptors and the phenomenon that some receptors of visceral afferents, when stimulated, do not evoke a conscious perception.

2. Visceral pain is not always linked to an injurious event. For example, distention of the bladder, although painful, does not damage the tissue, whereas cutting the gut wall is not painful.

3. Visceral pain is referred to distant locations based on the convergence of visceral afferent fibers and somatic afferent fibers on viscerosomatic neurons in the spinal cord.

4. Visceral pain is poorly localized and diffuse. This is a result of such factors as:
   a. The viscera are less densely innervated compared with somatic structures.
   b. The distribution of visceral afferent fibers terminating in cord segments is broader than somatic fibers, spanning as many as five segments (Chandler, Zhang, and Foreman, 1996; Jänig, 1996).
   c. A specific visceral sensory pathway is lacking.
   d. Viscerovisceral convergence occurs in the cord (Al-Chaer and Traub, 2002).

5. Visceral pain is accompanied by autonomic reflex and motor responses such as vomiting, changes in heart rate, or hypertonicity in skeletal muscles.

Neurotransmission of Visceral Pain. Peripheral receptors are located in the blood vessels, wall (of hollow organs), parenchyma of the visceral organs, and serosa (outer covering of certain organs). The receptors conveying nociception are sensitive to chemical, mechanical, and thermal stimuli and are classified physiologically as being either high or low threshold receptors. The high threshold receptors respond to noxious mechanical stimuli and are the lone receptors found in organs in which pain is the only conscious sensation (e.g., heart, ureter). There is a paucity of these in organs that respond to both innocuous and noxious sensations. Low threshold receptors respond primarily to both innocuous and noxious mechanical stimuli and are located, for example, in the colon and bladder (Cervero and Laird, 1999; Al-Chaer and Traub, 2002). The distribution of these receptors varies among the visceral organs. A third type of receptor, called the silent nociceptor, also is located in the viscera. The silent receptors are minimally responsive or unresponsive to normally occurring stimuli, but become activated by inflammation and various chemical insults.

Both high and low threshold afferent fibers are activated in brief acute visceral pain events. If the stimulation is prolonged or repetitive (e.g., in hypoxia or inflammation), the high and low threshold receptors become sensitized and the unresponsive silent nociceptors become activated, as well. The peripheral sensitization of these nociceptors is caused by the release of chemical mediators from the injured or inflamed tissue cells, which subsequently lower the firing threshold of the nociceptors. These events result in nociceptors being sensitive to and activated by normal innocuous stimuli. Activation of all of these afferent fibers produces a barrage of sensory input to dorsal horn viscerosomatic neurons, which results in hyperexcitability and hyperactivity of these neurons. All of this activity gives rise to visceral pain, which may be referred, and often is accompanied by hyperalgesia and allodynia. Hyperalgesia is an increase in sensitivity, resulting in enhanced pain perception. Allodynia is the perception of pain from a stimulus that is normally innocuous. The term *hyperalgesia* is used in this section to refer to both hyperalgesia and allodynia. This phenomenon also may be seen in the skin and other somatic tissues (e.g., muscle). (See Chapter 11 for a discussion of terms related to pain and pain referral and a discussion of peripheral and central hyperalgesia [sensitization] of nociception from somatic tissues related to the spine.) These dorsal horn neuronal changes are highly organized and specific, corresponding only to those neurons receiving input directly from the injured tissue (Cervero, 2000b). The dorsal horn neurons are described as forming an "irritable focus," and their collective alterations in excitability are called central sensitization (Cervero and Laird, 1999; Basbaum and Jessell, 2000; Cervero, 2000a,b; Al-Chaer and Traub, 2002). It is speculated that this event may be mediated by *N*-methyl-D-aspartate (NMDA) glutamate receptors and possibly neurokinin-1 substance P receptors (Basbaum and Jessell, 2000; Cervero, 2000b; Al-Chaer and Traub, 2002). Glutamate is a major excitatory neurotransmitter that is released from the sensory fibers and evokes a fast excitatory postsynaptic potential (EPSP). Neuropeptides such as substance P evoke slow EPSPs and appear to regulate the actions of glutamate. Glutamate and substance P are released together, coordinating the firing of the dorsal horn neurons. In addition, the neuronal hyperexcitability may be facilitated by positive feedback loops established between the dorsal horn neurons and higher centers. The presence of these feedback loops may explain the motor and autonomic reflex responses (e.g., nausea and hypertonicity in abdominal muscles) that accompany visceral pain experiences (Cervero and Laird, 1999). As long as peripheral sensitization of the nociceptors continues during the inflammatory process, normal physiologic (innocuous) stimuli activate afferent fibers and perpetuate the increased volley of sensory input to the "irritable focus" that was initiated by the acute injury. The increased excitability of these neurons in turn facilitates and sustains the effects of the sensory input from the viscera, resulting in an increase in pain intensity and duration. In addition, the normal function of the affected viscera may be altered because of the injury and inflammation, resulting in further activation of the sensitized nociceptors and even the recruitment of more distant nociceptors. Thus the presence of the central sensitization phenomenon in conjunction with normal physiologic visceral afferent activity results in the persistence of visceral pain even after the initial tissue injury is healing. Central sensitization may be the mechanism that produces hyperalgesia and allodynia both in sites to which pain is referred (referred hyperalgesia) (see section on pain referral) and in the same or nearby viscera (visceral hyperalgesia). Central sensitization also may be the mechanism underlying certain GI disorders such as IBS (Jänig, 1995; Cervero and Laird, 1999; Cervero, 2000a; Joshi and Gebhart, 2000). In IBS, pain is perceived by patients in the absence of any clear GI pathology. In this case, stimuli from normal GI activity results in the perception of pain or an increase in awareness of GI activity by the patient. This may result from peripheral sensitization or central sensitization and the activation of the hyperexcitable dorsal horn neurons (the "irritable focus") and increased activation of visceral nociceptive pathways. The condition also may be driven by output of the irritable focus and reflexive efferent activation of the GI tract, which increases abnormal gut contractions and stimulates further afferent input, establishing a positive feedback loop (Jänig, 1995). Treating this condition may include using agents that alter the receptors located in the periphery (i.e., the serotonin receptors) and dorsal horn (i.e., NMDA receptors), thus reducing peripheral and central sensitization (Cervero and Laird, 1999).

Visceral afferent fibers entering the spinal cord may initiate reflex responses or synapse on tract neurons. Neuron tracing techniques have shown that visceral afferent fibers synapse in numerous laminae, including I, V, VII, VIII, and X (Cervero and Foreman, 1990; Willis and Coggeshall, 1991). The more numerous unmyelinated fibers, such as those transmitting visceral nociception, enter the dorsolateral tract of Lissauer. They immediately enter the dorsal horn, as well as send collaterals up and down as many as five segments within Lissauer's tract before they enter the dorsal horn. These fibers synapse in laminae I and V on tract neurons that form the spinothalamic tract and also in laminae VII and VIII on the spinoreticular tract neurons (Cervero and Foreman, 1990). The spinoreticular tract projects to the reticular formation of the brain stem, which in turn projects to the intralaminar thalamic nucleus. From here, fibers

travel to the cerebral cortex and into the limbic system. The spinothalamic tract synapses in the ventral posterior and intralaminar thalamic nuclei, which project to the cerebral cortex. As the tract passes through the brain stem, it sends collateral fibers into the brain stem reticular formation (see Ascending Tracts in Chapter 9). Higher centers are activated through the interconnections and terminations of these two tracts. This allows a conscious perception of the nociception as pain and also allows the individual to respond to the pain. The spinothalamic tract helps to localize pain, although pain from the viscera is localized much less accurately than pain of somatic origin. Activating the reticular formation permits some localization and a conscious attentiveness to the pain. This is mediated not only by the reticular formation, but also by its connections with the thalamus and widespread areas of cerebral cortex, including the anterior cingulate cortex. Moreover, the accompanying discomfort and unpleasantness produce a particular affective mental state and subsequent behavioral patterns that are mediated through the phylogenetically older limbic system. Evidence gained from experimental studies and midline myelotomies (intentionally placed midline lesions of the spinal cord) performed to treat pain from pelvic cancer indicates that visceral information also ascends in the dorsal column of the cord (Cervero and Laird, 1999; Willis et al., 1999; Joshi and Gebhart, 2000; Nauta et al., 2000; Ness, 2000; Westlund, 2000; Al-Chaer and Traub, 2002; Palecek, Paleckova, and Willis, 2002). Postsynaptic dorsal column cells (PSDCs) are located around the central canal of the spinal cord. These cells are responsive to noxious and innocuous cutaneous stimuli, as well as mechanical and chemical visceral noxious stimuli. Axons from these cells in the sacral cord segments conveying pelvic visceral nociception ascend ipsilaterally in the midline of the dorsal column in an area distinct from mechanoreceptive ascending fibers. The fibers synapse in the gracile nucleus, and third-order neurons continue in the medial lemniscus. In addition to the fibers coursing in the medial lemniscus, some fibers synapse in the medullary reticular formation, periaqueductal gray, hypothalamus, amygdala, and medial areas of the thalamus. Fibers from thoracic PSDC cells carrying thoracic visceral nociception ascend at the lateral edge of the fasciculus gracilis and synapse in the gracile and cuneate nuclei. These dorsal column fibers may provide an alternate route, and possibly the major route, for transmitting visceral nociception to higher centers. Additional tracts that also have been associated with visceral nociception include the spino-(trigemino)parabrachial, spinohypothalamic, and spinosolitary tracts (Cervero and Laird, 1999; Al-Chaer and Traub, 2002).

The data that have demonstrated the termination of visceral afferent fibers in the spinal cord gray matter also lend credence to the convergence-projection theory of referred pain (Ruch, 1946). This theory maintains that referred pain occurs because of the convergence of visceral and somatic afferent fibers on the same pool of viscerosomatic neurons in the cord (see Fig. 10-22). Because somatic pain is more common than visceral pain, the higher centers misread the visceral input as originating from somatic afferent fibers. Therefore pain is referred to the area of skin and deep structures (e.g., muscle, bone) supplied by the somatic afferent fibers that have entered the same cord segments as the visceral afferent fibers. There is evidence suggesting there is viscerovisceral convergence among different organs as well (Al-Chaer and Traub, 2002; Giamberardino, 2003). The viscerosomatic neurons, located in laminae I, V, and X (Jänig, 1996) of the cord, are either tract neurons or local interneurons. The site of referral may be to the skin, muscles (or other deep somatic tissues), or both. In addition, referred pain often is accompanied by hyperalgesia. The hyperalgesia, which is an increased sensitivity to pain produced by noxious and innocuous (allodynia—see previous discussion) stimuli, is the result of peripheral sensitization of nociceptors and, more importantly, central sensitization. Although hyperalgesia is evident at the onset of the painful experience, it often persists longer than the pain associated with the initial visceral insult. This may occur for several reasons: (a) the persistence of the previously described plastic changes in the dorsal horn neurons make this area of the spinal cord function independently of peripheral nociceptive activation; (b) changes in the viscera persist longer than the initial focal lesion and send afferent input to the dorsal horn, maintaining the hyperactivity of the neurons; (c) viscerosomatic reflexes are activated back toward the peripheral sites, causing increased sensitivity of nociceptors (including muscle nociceptors) and therefore hyperalgesia; and (d) trophic changes occur in hyperalgesic somatic tissue. Studies in rat models of hyperalgesic muscle have shown morphofunctional changes (essentially characteristics associated with muscle atrophy) indicative of muscles undergoing sustained contractions, which often occur as a consequence of visceral referred pain. Examples of visceral pain referral to muscle is the referral to abdominal oblique and quadratus lumborum muscles seen in patients experiencing pain from renal calculus, referred pain to the rectus abdominis muscle as a result of biliary calculus, and referred pain to the inferior aspect of the rectus abdominis and pelvic muscles as a result of dysmenorrhea (Vecchiet, Vecchiet, and Giamberardino, 1999; Giamberardino, 2003).

A common example of pain referral to cutaneous sites occurs after a myocardial infarction or angina pectoris episode. The relationship between visceral afferent fibers and the spinothalamic tract for pain originating from the heart was determined from data obtained from experiments on primates. These investigations were designed to demonstrate that cardiac ischemia stimulates cardiac afferent fibers, which in turn synapse on spinothalamic tract cells. Bradykinin, a peptide released from ischemic cells, was injected into cardiac tissue and resulted in stimulation of afferent fibers. By measuring tract neuron discharge rates, it was shown that 15 seconds after bradykinin injection (the time needed for receptor activation), 75% of the spinothalamic tract cells increased their firing rate (Cervero and Foreman, 1990). These data support the theory that visceral afferent fibers converge on the same tract cells on which somatic afferent fibers terminate. The peripheral distribution of these same somatic afferent fibers becomes the general location of the pain referral. The afferent fibers subserving nociception from the heart course primarily in the middle and inferior cardiac nerves (to the middle and inferior cervical sympathetic ganglia) and left thoracic cardiac branches (Kiernan, 1998) and eventually enter the first five thoracic cord segments. Pain is most frequently referred superficially to the left side of the chest and left inner arm; however, pain often is referred to the neck and jaw also. It is speculated that the mechanism for this referral pattern is the convergence of cardiac afferent fibers with the upper cervical cord segments. Cardiac afferent fibers travel in sympathetic nerves and the vagus nerve. The vagal fibers enter the medulla and synapse in the nucleus of the tractus solitarius (NTS) and also send branches inferiorly into the C1-3 cord segments (see Relationship between the Dorsal Horn and the Trigeminal Nerve in Chapter 9). Fibers from the NTS also may send relay neurons to the C1-2 segments (Chandler, Zhang, and Foreman, 1996). These segments are the site of convergence of trigeminal afferent fibers serving the head, and somatic afferent fibers conveying sensory information from the area served by the C1-3 cord segments. This region of the dorsal horn provides the anatomic substrate for convergence of the trigeminal, somatic, and vagal afferent fibers on tract neurons (Chandler, Zhang, and Foreman, 1996; Chandler et al., 1999; Foreman, 1999) and subsequent misinterpretation of the origin by higher centers. Another theory explaining this referral pattern is that afferent information synapsing in thoracic spinal cord segments may ascend to upper cervical segments via propriospinal fibers. Also, visceral afferent fibers that enter the zone of Lissauer may ascend or descend as many as five cord segments before synapsing in the dorsal horn. These connections may provide a route for cardiac afferent fibers to directly terminate in the upper cervical segments (Chandler, Zhang, and Foreman, 1996), thus referring pain to the neck and even the head (via the connections to the spinal nucleus of the trigeminal nerve).

Another example of pain referral is that which occurs as a result of biliary calculus (gallstones). Sensory afferents from the gall bladder and bile ducts course in the right greater splanchnic nerve and into the T7 and T8 cord segments. The referral site is the right upper quadrant of the abdomen and right infrascapular region, corresponding to the T7 and T8 dermatomal patterns. As the disease progresses, inflammation of the peritoneum associated with the diaphragm occurs. (The involvement of the parietal serous membranes lining the inside wall of the abdominal and thoracic cavities has been described as viscerosomatic pain [FitzGerald and Folan-Curran, 2002].) The chemical mediators involved with the inflammatory process activate the peritoneal sensory fibers that travel in the phrenic nerve. These afferent fibers terminate in the C3-5 cord segments and thus can refer pain to the top of the shoulder.

Because pain is the most important clinical visceral sensation, knowledge of visceral pain referral patterns and the spinal cord segments to which visceral afferent fibers project (which is the same location as the sympathetic preganglionic cell bodies) is extremely important. This knowledge allows a clinician to more effectively diagnose pathologic conditions occurring in the viscera (Fig. 10-23 and Table 10-2).

Autonomic Reflexes

Reflexes are common events mediated by the nervous system. A reflex can be described simply as an involuntary action that occurs fairly quickly, regulates some effector function, and has no direct involvement with the cerebral cortex. The components of a reflex arc include a peripheral receptor and its afferent fiber, which form the sensory limb; an efferent fiber that forms the motor limb; and an effector. Depending on whether the reflex arc is monosynaptic or polysynaptic, there may or may not be interneurons connecting the afferent and efferent fibers. Both types of afferents (somatic and visceral) and efferents (somatic and visceral) may be involved, thus creating four major kinds of reflex arcs. These are somatosomatic, viscerosomatic, viscerovisceral, and somatovisceral.

Somatosomatic Reflexes. Somatosomatic reflexes consist of somatic afferent fibers that influence somatic effectors, that is, skeletal muscle. Chapter 9 discusses examples of this type of reflex, which included the muscle stretch reflex and superficial reflexes (cremasteric and abdominal). The flexor (withdrawal) reflex and the crossed extensor reflex also are examples of somatosomatic reflexes.

Viscerosomatic Reflexes. The existence of polysynaptic viscerovisceral and viscerosomatic reflexes implies that visceral afferent fibers are involved not only with the mediation of visceral functions, but also with the functions of somatic effectors (i.e., skeletal muscles). Physiologic activities that exemplify viscerosomatic reflex responses concern respiratory function and GI activity. Regulation of respiratory rhythmicity is under the control of respiratory centers located in the medulla.

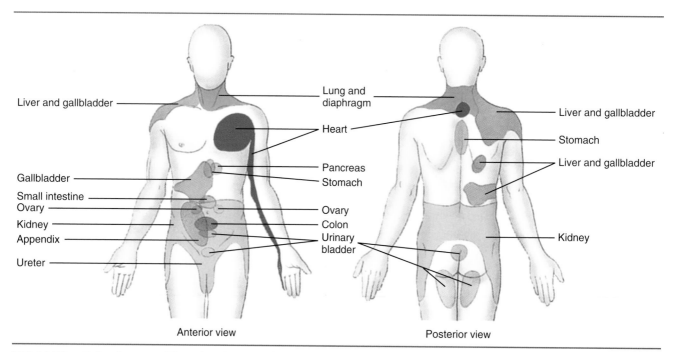

FIG. 10-23 Referral patterns. The colored regions show cutaneous areas to which visceral pain is referred (see text for discussion). (From Tortora GJ & Grabowski SR. [2003]. *Principles of anatomy and physiology* [10th ed.]. New York: John Wiley & Sons, Inc.)

Table 10-2   Origin of Preganglionic Autonomic Fibers

Structure	Sympathetic (Cord Segments)	Parasympathetic (Nuclei/Cord Segments)
Smooth muscle and glands of the head	T1-3 (T4 or T5)	Edinger-Westphal nucleus (CN III), superior salivatory (CN VII), and inferior salivatory nuclei (CN IX)
Cutaneous effectors	T1-L2 or L3	None
Blood vessels of upper extremity skeletal muscles	T2-6 or T7	None
Blood vessels of lower extremity skeletal muscles	T10-L2 or L3	None
Heart	T1-4 or T5	Dorsal motor nucleus of CN X and nucleus ambiguus
Lungs	T2-5	Dorsal motor nucleus of CN X
Stomach	T6-10	Dorsal motor nucleus of CN X
Small intestine	T9-10	Dorsal motor nucleus of CN X
Large intestine		
Ascending and transverse colon	T11-L1	Dorsal motor nucleus of CN X
Descending colon and rectum	L1-2	S2-4 cord segments
Liver and gallbladder	T7-9	Dorsal motor nucleus of CN X
Spleen	T6-10	Dorsal motor nucleus of CN X
Pancreas	T6-10	Dorsal motor nucleus of CN X
Adrenal gland (medulla)	T8-L1	None
Kidney	T10-L1	Dorsal motor nucleus of CN X
Bladder	T11-L2	S2-4 cord segments
Sex organs	T10-L2	S2-4 cord segments
Prostate	T11-L1	S2-4 cord segments
Uterus	T12-L1	S2-4 cord segments

These neurons receive input from lung receptors that inhibit inspiration and facilitate expiration. The Hering-Breuer reflex is activated to prevent overinflation of the lung in the hyperinflated state and when the tidal volume increases to greater than 1.5 L. Stretch receptors that lie in the bronchi and bronchioles of the lungs increase their firing rate as the lungs inflate. This information is conveyed via visceral afferent fibers in the vagus nerve to the nucleus of the tractus solitarius of the brain stem medulla. From this nucleus, neurons project into the respiratory center that inhibits inspiration. From here, descending fibers inhibit the motor neurons that innervate the skeletal muscles of respiration and subsequently terminate the inspiration phase. Other visceral afferent fibers that reflexively influence respiratory skeletal muscles course in the glossopharyngeal and vagus nerves from chemoreceptors located in the carotid and aortic bodies. A change in the carbon dioxide concentration causes a reflex change in the rate and depth of respiration. Abnormal stimuli such as visceral nociception also can produce skeletal muscle contractions. An example of this type of viscerosomatic reflex is the contraction of the abdominal skeletal musculature after excessive distention of a viscus or the inflammation of peritonitis (see section on referred pain).

Experiments on rabbits have shown that stimulation of organs such as the renal pelvis and small intestine cause reflex paravertebral muscle contractions. In addition, some pathologic conditions (e.g., coronary artery disease) cause stimulation of afferent fibers that produce not only skeletal muscle contractions, but also concurrent activation of autonomic effectors in somatic tissue that results in cutaneous vasomotor and sudomotor changes (Beal, 1985).

Viscerovisceral Reflexes. Visceral afferent fibers also mediate visceral reflex responses. Viscerovisceral reflex responses are common occurrences and are best exemplified in the functioning of the cardiovascular and GI systems. Changes in blood pressure are monitored by baroreceptors of the carotid sinus and aortic arch. For example, an increase in blood pressure stimulates the baroreceptors. The visceral afferent fibers from these course in the glossopharyngeal and vagus nerves to the brain stem, causing a reflex slowing of the heart rate via visceral efferent fibers in the vagus nerve and peripheral vasodilation via inhibition of sympathetic efferent fibers. Visceral afferent fibers from the GI tract and bladder convey information allowing for the normal functioning of digestion, elimination, and voiding. Sensory input such as distention produces reflex responses, including contraction of smooth muscle (in the wall and sphincters) and mucosal secretion.

The enteric nervous system is intimately involved with viscerovisceral reflex responses. For example, a toxic microbial organism may stimulate the intrinsic sensory neurons of the submucosal plexus that innervate the epithelium of the gut. Although the circuitry is not completely understood, these neurons cause reflex secretion of water and ions, a decrease in absorption, and, by means of the myenteric plexus, increased gut motility (Loewy, 1990a) (see section on Enteric Nervous System).

Somatovisceral Reflexes. The existence of somatovisceral reflexes indicates that visceral afferent fibers are not the sole initiators of visceral responses; somatic afferent fibers also can reflexively stimulate autonomic efferent fibers. This usually occurs when changes of skin temperature result in cutaneous vasomotor and sudomotor responses. Although evidence exists that stimulating the receptors of somatic afferent fibers produces changes in visceral activity, the exact neural circuitry for somatovisceral reflexes is not clearly understood.

Sato and colleagues (Sato, Sato, and Schmidt, 1984; Sato and Swenson, 1984; Sato, 1992a,b) have provided much evidence supporting the presence of somatovisceral reflexes. Using anesthetized rats, they stimulated the receptors of somatic afferent fibers from the skin, muscle, and knee joint and measured the reflex changes in heart rate, gut motility, bladder contractility, adrenal medullary nerve activity, and secretion of the adrenal medulla. Reflex responses to cutaneous stimuli produced the following varied responses depending on the type of stimuli and organ involved:

1. Noxious and innocuous mechanical stimuli and thermal stimuli produced an increase in heart rate.
2. Noxious pinching of the abdominal skin resulted in inhibited gastric motility, although motility sometimes was facilitated when the hind paw was pinched.
3. Stimulation of the perianal area caused increased efferent firing to and reflex contractions in a quiescent (slightly expanded) bladder, but this caused the inhibition of bladder contractions in an expanded bladder.
4. Noxious pinching of the skin and noxious thermal stimuli resulted in an increase in the secretory activity of and neural activity to (via the greater splanchnic nerve) the medulla of the adrenal gland, whereas innocuous stimuli had the opposite effect.

Type III and IV muscle afferent fibers, stimulated by intraarterial injections of potassium chloride (KCl) and bradykinin (both of which are algesic agents), produced the following effects on heart rate and smooth muscle of the bladder:

1. "Injection of KCl regularly accelerates heart rate. With bradykinin, both accelerations and decelerations can be observed" (Sato, 1992a).
2. Both substances had effects on the bladder similar to those initiated by cutaneous stimuli (i.e., excitation to the quiescent bladder and inhibition to the contractions of an expanded bladder).

Joint receptors from a normal and inflamed knee joint were stimulated by movements both within and beyond the joint's normal range of motion. Results showed that heart rate and secretory and nerve activity of the adrenal medulla increased when the normal knee joint was moved beyond its normal range and when the inflamed knee joint was moved within and beyond its normal range, with a greater increase occurring during the latter. These data indicated the variability that can occur in different effectors in response to various stimuli of somatic afferent fibers. These experiments showed that effectors could be mediated through both sympathetic or parasympathetic efferent fibers and that the response could be excitatory or inhibitory. Further, reflex responses may be integrated at the segmental level (spinal cord) or at the supraspinal level, and the data indicated that both paths were used. For example, segmental integration occurred for the cutaneovesical reflex of the quiescent bladder, cutaneoadrenal reflex, and cutaneogastric reflex, and supraspinal integration was necessary for the cutaneocardiac reflex and cutaneovesical reflex of the expanded bladder.

In other experiments exploring somatovisceral reflexes, different forces were applied to the lateral aspect of two regions of immobilized spines of anesthetized rats (Fig. 10-24) to study the effect on heart rate, blood pressure, and activity in the nerve to the adrenal medulla and renal nerve to the kidney (Sato and Swenson, 1984; Sato, 1992a). Lateral flexion resulting from applied mechanical force stimulated afferent fibers supplying the vertebral column and produced the following results:

1. A consistently large decrease in blood pressure that returned to normal after the stimulus was removed
2. An inconsistently small decrease in heart rate
3. A decrease in blood flow to the gastrocnemius and biceps femoris muscles, with a concomitant decrease in systemic arterial blood pressure
4. An initial decrease in activity in the renal nerve and subsequent recovery, both during the period of stimulation
5. An initial decrease in activity in the adrenal nerve with a gradual return to baseline activity, which was followed by an additional increase in activity (likely caused by a baroreceptor-mediated reflex response)

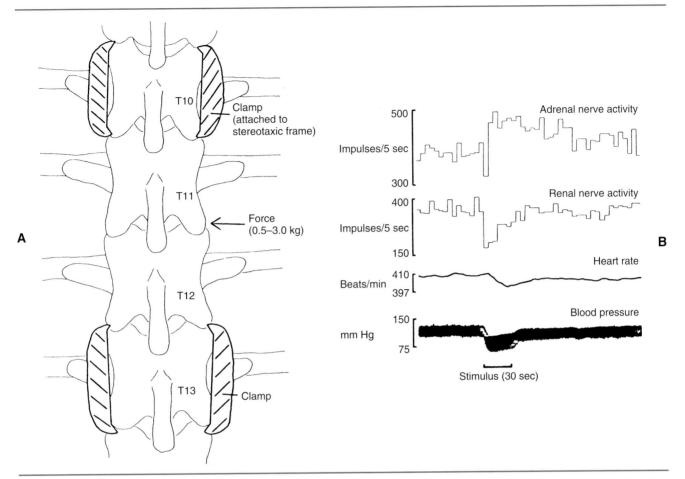

FIG. 10-24   **A,** Illustration of the stimulation procedure (thoracic spine shown). Segments isolated from skin and muscle, upper and lower segments fixed in a spinal stereotaxic device, and force exerted (0.5 to 3 kg) on mobile segments. **B,** Sample record from a central nervous system–intact animal with thoracic spine stimulation. Force (3 kg) delivered during the period marked by the dark bar below the blood pressure trace. (**A,** From Sato A & Swenson RS. [1984]. Sympathetic nervous system response to mechanical stress of the spinal column in rats. *J Manipulative Physiol Ther, 7(3),* 141-147.)

In summary, these experiments show that a stress applied to the spine initiates reflex arcs resulting in changes in heart rate, blood pressure, and activity in sympathetic efferents to the kidney and medulla of the adrenal gland. Based on this evidence, the neural components for this type of somatovisceral reflex do exist, and spinal manipulation may stimulate somatic afferent fibers to create similar somatovisceral reflex responses. Pathologic processes affecting the spine also may result in reflex changes in visceral activity (Sato, 1992a).

More recent studies have confirmed the fact that noxious and innocuous stimuli affect cardiovascular and other autonomic responses. Anatomic and experimental evidence has shown that numerous mechanoreptors are found in structures of the neck (e.g., skin, muscles, tendons, ligaments, periosteum, intervertebral discs, zygapophysial joints) that work in conjunction with the vestibular system to provide reflex responses to postural

changes (Bolton, 1998). Reflexes associated with postural adjustments include the cervicocollic reflex, tonic neck reflex, and cervico-ocular reflex. In addition, there is evidence that activation of neck receptors elicits reflexes that produce autonomic responses. Experimental studies on cats (Bolton et al., 1998) suggested that stimulation of afferents of cervical neck muscles produced cervicosympathetic and cervicorespiratory reflex responses. This was evident by changes seen in the splanchnic (sympathetic preganglionic neurons) and abdominal nerves (respiratory motoneurons), as well as the hypoglossal nerve. It has been established that input from neck afferents is relayed through brain stem vestibular nuclei to sympathetic and respiratory neurons. In addition, brain stem transections through the caudal medulla performed to separate the vestibular nuclei connections from the cord have shown that afferent fibers from the neck also stimulate sympathetic and respiratory nerves without relaying through the vestibular nuclei. However, transections through the middle of the medulla, which possibly interrupt descending fibers from the rostral ventrolateral (VL) medulla (part of the central autonomic control network), have been found to alter the activity of the sympathetic and respiratory neurons. Therefore based on the data from these experiments, a complex mechanism appears to exist to produce the physiologically normal cervicosympathetic and cervicorespiratory reflexes. This complex mechanism involves caudal brain stem and spinal cord structures that must be intact for these reflexes to take place.

In addition, numerous studies on anesthetized animals also indicate that autonomic reflex responses are seen in visceral organs in response to somatic stimuli. Some of the effector organs studied that demonstrated changes are the gastrointestinal tissues, heart, urinary bladder, vasculature of the peripheral nerves, vasculature of the cerebrum, medulla of the adrenal gland, and spleen (see overview article by Sato, 1997).

More recent animal studies also confirm that stimulation of somatic structures has an effect on autonomic responses. In one study, the effects of somatic stimuli were observed on the motility of the quiescent bladder. The results showed that there was an increase in bladder muscle tone in response to noxious chemical stimuli of the interspinous tissue but little change in bladder pressure in response to innocuous somatic stimuli (Budgell, Hotta, and Sato, 1998). Another animal study examined the effects of noxious chemical stimulation of interspinous tissues on gastric motility. The results showed that motility was strongly inhibited and that the reflex arc responsible for this action was segmentally located to the mid to lower thoracic region. Although both the vagus and sympathetic nerve supply to the stomach was found to be involved in the reflex, the sympathetic innervation appeared to be more important (Budgell and Suzuki, 2000).

It also has been demonstrated that cardiac function can be altered by the innocuous stimulation of mechanoreceptors through spinal manipulation. Budgell and Igarashi (2001) reported one case study of a young man with bradycardia and an arrhythmia. While being monitored continuously by electrocardiography, one cervical (C2) spinal manipulation was performed on the patient, which resulted in the coincidental disappearance of the arrhythmia. Although the result was clearly apparent, no distinct mechanism has yet to be proposed to explain the event. Another study investigated the effects of spinal manipulation (C1 and C2 levels) on healthy young adults on cardiac function. Results from this study, which used sham and authentic manipulations, demonstrated significant changes in heart rate and heart rate variability when only the authentic manipulations were performed (Budgell and Hirano, 2001).

NEUROTRANSMISSION OCCURRING AT THE AUTONOMIC GANGLIA AND NEUROEFFECTOR JUNCTIONS

The neurotransmission that occurs at the autonomic ganglion and neuroeffector junction is important physiologically and pharmacologically. The classical description of chemical transmission at these two locations was simply to explain the actions of the two major neurotransmitters: norepinephrine (also called noradrenaline) and acetylcholine. Fibers releasing those chemicals thus were called adrenergic and cholinergic, respectively. However, recent information has demonstrated that the autonomic ganglion and neuroeffector junction are regions of complex interactions involving not only acetylcholine and norepinephrine, but also cotransmitters and neuromodulators.

Ganglionic Transmission

As stated, the ganglion is the location of postganglionic cell bodies, and therefore the site in which preganglionic neurons synapse. Functionally it is the location in which information from the CNS, via preganglionic neurons, and the periphery, via collateral branches of afferent neurons (releasing substance P and CGRP [Iversen, Iversen, and Saper, 2000]), is integrated and then distributed to the peripheral effectors via postganglionic neurons. Each preganglionic neuron diverges onto many postganglionic neurons (divergence) and each postganglionic neuron in turn receives input from more than one preganglionic neuron (convergence) (see Fig. 10-4). The divergence occurring in the sympathetic system traditionally is thought to be greater compared with the divergence in the parasympathetic system so that the sympathetic system can produce widespread responses. This concept has been used to delineate the two systems. However, some authors suggest that the difference in divergence ratios should not be used to characterize the sympathetic and parasympathetic systems, but rather should be noted as the means by which small targets with distinct functions are regulated (limited divergence) and extensive effectors (targets) acting in unison are regulated (vast divergence) (Wang, Holst, and Powley, 1995; Jänig and Häbler, 2000). Each postganglionic cell is inhibited via dendrodendritic synapses with other postganglionic cells and interneurons, the latter being excited by preganglionic fibers (see Fig. 10-4) (Kiernan, 1998). The primary neurotransmitter released by preganglionic neurons at their synaptic boutons is ACh (Fig. 10-25). This binds to and activates nicotinic receptors (so-named because the effect can be reproduced using the drug nicotine) found on the postganglionic neurons. In addition to postganglionic neurons, nicotinic receptors also are found on skeletal

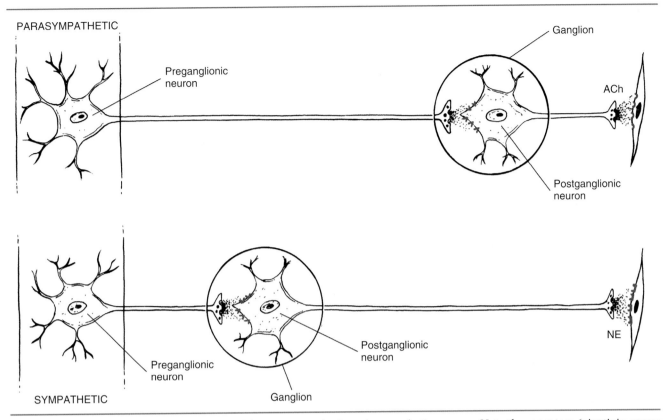

FIG. 10-25 Major neurotransmitters released by parasympathetic and sympathetic neurons. Note the receptors (nicotinic, *green;* muscarinic, *purple*; alpha, *blue*) to which the neurotransmitters bind. Preganglionic neurons of both systems and postganglionic parasympathetic neurons release acetylcholine (Ach). Postganglionic sympathetic neurons typically release norepinephrine. (Those two sweat glands release Ach.)

muscle cells and CNS neurons. The binding causes depolarization and the generation of a fast EPSP. Use of the nicotine receptors is regarded as the main mechanism for transmission in both sympathetic and parasympathetic divisions of the ANS (Iversen, Iversen, and Saper, 2000). However, if the preganglionic neuron is stimulated repeatedly, ganglionic ACh also binds to muscarinic receptors on postganglionic cells. These are G protein–coupled receptors that evoke slow EPSPs and inhibitory postsynaptic potentials (IPSPs). Neuropeptides such as enkephalins, neurotensin, somatostatin, substance P, VIP, and neuropeptide Y (Iversen, Iversen, and Saper, 2000; Bear, Conners, and Paradiso, 2001) are co-localized with (contained in) cholinergic preganglionic neurons. These molecules are important in helping to determine the overall activity of the postganglionic neuron. They act by modulating the postsynaptic membrane such that the membrane will reach threshold more easily when activated via a fast EPSP (Iversen, Iversen, and Saper, 2000; Bear, Conners, and Paradiso, 2001). Animal studies on sympathetic ganglia also show variability among postganglionic neurons in paravertebral (sympathetic chain) ganglia versus those in prevertebral ganglia. Paravertebral ganglia cells have consistent

properties (i.e., each preganglionic neuron evokes an EPSP via nicotinic receptor channels and an action potential always is produced). On the other hand, prevertebral ganglia cells do not have uniform properties, but instead can be divided into three groups based on their electrophysiologic, anatomic, and neurochemical differences (Jänig and Häbler, 2000). The transmission of information coursing through this site is complex and likely modulated and controlled based on the structure of the ganglion and the chemical diversity at the level of the preganglionic and postganglionic synapse and at the synapse of the interneuron pool.

Neuroeffector Transmission

Postganglionic neurons innervate the smooth muscle, cardiac muscle, and glands of the body. The axons are approximately 1 μm in diameter and typically are unmyelinated. Studies on the terminal endings of primarily sympathetic postganglionic axons show that they are different from somatic efferent fibers. The motor neurons that innervate skeletal muscle fibers do so at the neuromuscular junction at specialized regions on the postsynaptic membrane called the motor end plate. The neurotransmitter is released at this one site and binds to the receptors. On the other hand, postganglionic autonomic fibers branch extensively near the effector muscle cells, thus regulating the function of numerous muscle fibers. These fibers are arranged in bundles and some smooth muscle fibers are directly innervated, whereas the rest are electrically linked to the directly innervated cells by gap junctions. There are no well-defined presynaptic and postsynaptic specializations, nor just one transmission site. Instead the ends of the terminal branches of the postganglionic neurons are varicosed (i.e., they have a beaded appearance) (Fig. 10-26). Each of these beads or swellings (numbering from 10,000 to more than 2 million/mm^3) (Hamill, 1996) is called a varicosity, and it contains mitochondria and vesicles of stored neurotransmitters (100 to 1000 per varicosity in adrenergic fibers). Each varicosity is approximately 0.3 to 1 μm in diameter and is located approximately 4 μm from its neighboring varicosity (Hirst et al., 1996; Bennett, 1998). The membrane of each varicosity is devoid of its Schwann cell neurilemma. Because there are no postsynaptic specializations, the varicosities are dynamic and may move along the axons (Williams et al., 1995). Because these are strung out along the terminal

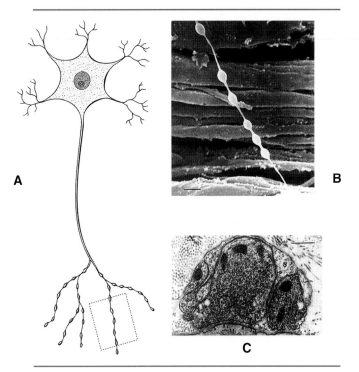

FIG. 10-26   A, Varicosities located on the distal portion of an autonomic neuron. **B,** Scanning electron micrograph of one terminal autonomic nerve fiber showing its varicosities (enlarged view of area outlined in **A**). This fiber is lying over the smooth muscle in the rat small intestine. **C,** Transmission electron micrograph of a section through a varicosity. (From Williams PL et al. [Eds.]. [1995]. *Gray's anatomy* [38th ed.]. Edinburgh: Churchill Livingstone.

fiber ending, the receptors are also spread over the surface of the effector cell membrane and each varicosity is a possible site for neurotransmission onto muscular (or glandular) tissue. The neurotransmitter, which is released typically en passage as the action potential travels along the axon, crosses the synaptic cleft and may diffuse a distance (as many as several hundred nanometers) before reaching its target receptors (Iversen, Iversen, and Saper, 2000). The synaptic cleft varies considerably in size from tissue to tissue, ranging from as little as 20 nm in densely innervated effector tissues (e.g., ductus deferens) to 1 to 2 μm in large elastic arteries (Williams et al., 1995).

The traditional description of chemical transmission at the neuroeffector junction has been based on the release of the "conventional" transmitters ACh, released by the parasympathetic postganglionic fibers, and NE, released by sympathetic postganglionic fibers (see Fig. 10-25). In general, these neurotransmitters are released and bind to and activate their specific receptors, which in turn release intracellular chemical messengers. In turn, these messengers initiate a cascade of cellular reactions; however, other chemical substances have been found to be involved with neurotransmission. For example, ATP is a co-transmitter with NE in adrenergic neurons, although its concentration relative to NE varies in different fibers. Neuropeptides are common substances that co-localize with both NE- and ACh-containing neurons and function to modulate neurotransmission. Neuropeptide Y is found in approximately 90% of postganglionic adrenergic fibers. It facilitates responses by acting postsynaptically on effector cells located more than 60 nm away. On densely innervated target cells that are 20 nm away, neuropeptide Y acts on the *presynaptic* membrane and dampens effector activity by inhibiting the release of ATP and NE. Neuropeptide Y often is associated with other neuropeptides such as galanin and dynorphin. The few sympathetic neurons that are cholinergic (e.g., to sweat glands) have been shown to often contain CGRP and VIP. Adenosine also modulates transmission of sympathetic neurons at both the presynaptic and postsynaptic junction (Iversen, Iversen, and Saper, 2000).

Parasympathetic postganglionic neurons have been found to co-localize VIP with ACh. VIP is a vasodilator that may function to assist effector activity by increasing blood flow, which is necessary in the process of glandular secretion (Iversen, Iversen, and Saper, 2000). Other populations of neurons use ATP or nitric oxide (or both) as co-transmitters (Williams et al., 1995). In addition, nitric oxide, which has been implicated in the mediation of smooth muscle relaxation, and ATP have been recognized as chemical substances associated with nonadrenergic, noncholinergic (NANC) fibers (Williams et al., 1995).

The actual physiologic response of effector tissues to postganglionic neuron activation is dependent on the neurotransmitter (and possible co-transmitters and co-modulators) released. More importantly, the response also is dependent on the presence and distribution of ligand receptors at the neuroeffector junction to which the neurotransmitter will bind. Depending on the physiologic status of the target cell, the concentration of receptors found on its postsynaptic membrane can be modified by the cell inserting or removing receptors into its cell membrane (up-regulation or down-regulation, respectively), thus affecting the binding capability of neurotransmitter and the resulting activity of the target cell.

NE is the primary neurotransmitter that sympathetic postganglionic fibers release, although fibers that innervate sweat glands release ACh. NE binds to adrenergic receptors, of which there are two major types, α (alpha) and β (beta). The α type is further subdivided into an α_1 type, which is subdivided into three subtypes (A, B, D), and an α_2 type, which is also subdivided into three subtypes (A, B, C) (Insel, 1996). The β receptor is divided into β_1, β_2, and β_3 types. Each type of adrenergic receptor is linked preferentially to specific subclasses of G proteins located in the cell membrane. Each G protein in turn is linked to specific effector molecules within the cell. For example, phospholipase C_β and adenylyl cyclase are examples of such effector molecules. Activation of the effector molecules in turn leads to changes in intracellular concentrations of second messengers (e.g., cyclic adenosine monophosphate [cAMP]), which results in the modulation of cellular activities (Insel, 1996).

The primary neurotransmitter that parasympathetic postganglionic fibers release is ACh. At the neuroeffector junction, ACh binds to muscarinic receptors. These receptors are so-named because administration of the alkaloid muscarine (derived from the *Amanita* mushroom) was found to mimic specific actions of the parasympathetic system. Muscarinic receptors are subdivided into three major classes: M_1, which is excitatory to ganglionic neurons and when activated modulates NE release; M_2, which decreases heart rate and contractility; and M_3, which causes smooth muscle contraction and increased glandular secretion (Hamill, 1996).

Adrenergic and muscarinic receptors are located on both presynaptic (postganglionic) and postsynaptic (target cell) membranes (Fig. 10-27). More specifically, M_1, M_2, and M_3 receptors are located on the postsynaptic membranes. Some muscarinic receptors are located on sympathetic neuron presynaptic membranes and these receptors inhibit the release of NE. Others are located on parasympathetic presynaptic membranes. When stimulated, these inhibit the further release of ACh. α_1 adrenergic receptors are located on postsynaptic membranes and when activated mediate smooth muscle

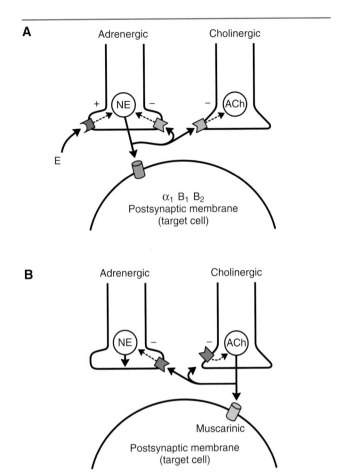

FIG. 10-27   Neuroeffector junction illustrating the multiple receptors on the presynaptic neuron and the postsynaptic (target) cell and their influence on the release of acetylcholine (ACh) and norepinephrine (NE). **A,** NE release is inhibited by presynaptic α_2 receptors (*blue*) which also inhibit the release of ACh from adjacent parasympathetic fibers. NE release is promoted by β_2 receptors (*red*) which bind epinephrine (E). α_1 (excitatory), β_1 (excitatory), and β_2 (excitatory and inhibitory) receptors (*green*) are located on the postsynaptic cell membrane. **B,** Presynaptic muscarinic receptors (*teal*) inhibit the release of excess ACh and inhibit neurotransmitter release from adjacent sympathetic fibers. Muscarinic receptors (*dark yellow*) are located on the postsynaptic cell membrane.

contraction in peripheral small arteries and large arterioles, dilator pupillae muscle, GI sphincters, bladder neck, and the vas deferens. α_2 receptors are located on sympathetic presynaptic membranes (as autoreceptors involved with an auto-feedback loop regulating NE release) and on neighboring parasympathetic presynaptic membranes. In both cases, when activated, neurotransmitter release is inhibited. β_1 receptors found on postsynaptic membranes cause increase in heart rate and force of contraction, and those found on cells in the kidney cause the secretion of renin. Renin is part of the pathway that forms the vasoconstrictor peptide, angiotensin II. β_2 receptors are activated by epinephrine (released from the medulla of the adrenal gland) and by locally released NE. These receptors are postsynaptic and cause relaxation of tracheal and bronchial smooth muscle and the ciliary muscle of the eye, and initiate glycogenolysis and gluconeogenesis in the hepatocytes of the liver. β_2 receptors also are found on presynaptic adrenergic fiber membranes acting as autoreceptors and causing the release of NE (FitzGerald and Folan-Curran, 2002). β_3 receptors are located in brown adipose tissue and the gallbladder. When activated, these receptors are thought to promote lipolysis and heat production in fat (Insel, 1996). Table 10-1 lists the effector tissues and their adrenergic receptor type.

In addition to the adrenergic and cholinergic receptor categories, there also are receptors for nitric oxide. These receptors function to relax vasculature smooth muscle. In addition, there are receptors that bind adenosine and ATP (called purinergic P_1 and purinergic P_2, respectively). Adenosine modulates sympathetic activity by activating presynaptic receptors that prevent further release of ATP and NE after intense sympathetic activation. It also inhibits cardiac and smooth muscle activity that is in direct opposition to NE-produced excitation. ATP is a cotransmitter with NE and is involved with the fast and slow responses observed in smooth muscle (Iversen, Iversen, and Saper, 2000).

Notice that controlling the activity of the target cell is dependent on the concentration and availability of neurotransmitter present in the synaptic cleft. This is linked to the release and removal of that neurotransmitter. The release is determined by the frequency of action potentials and influx of calcium ions, which in turn controls the release of neurotransmitter. In addition, noradrenergic presynaptic membranes include receptors that modulate the release of NE. These are the β_2 and α_2 adrenergic receptors (see the preceding) and receptors for histamine, prostaglandin E1, 5-hydroxytryptamine, ACh (all of which may decrease NE release), and angiotensin II (which promotes release of NE). The removal of NE at the synaptic cleft (and therefore the cessation of its action) occurs primarily by inactivation through either diffusion or uptake. Neuronal reuptake of NE results largely in the restorage of NE into vesicles, although some NE is degraded by monoamine oxidase (MAO). Uptake by the effector cell (extraneuronal) results in the degradation of NE, by MAO and catechol O-methyltransferase (COMT), into inactive metabolites. The inactive metabolites subsequently diffuse out of the cell and into the capillaries. Because of the large synaptic cleft, NE also is able to diffuse away from the junction and into capillaries. Removal by neuronal uptake occurs, the majority of the time (70%), in densely innervated tissues compared with removal by extraneuronal uptake (20%). However, diffusion and extraneuronal uptake may be more important in sparsely innervated tissues (Bray et al., 1994; Weisbrodt, 1998).

The control of ACh concentration is similar to that of NE in that action potentials trigger the release of ACh into the synaptic cleft. However, the removal of ACh is via degradation of ACh by acetylcholinesterase into choline and acetate. Subsequent reuptake returns choline to the nerve terminal. Also, ACh is removed by its diffusing away from the junction (Bray et al., 1994; Weisbrodt, 1998).

In summary, the mechanism of neurotransmission that occurs in the ANS is more complex than the simple traditional description of a sympathetic division, which uses NE, and a parasympathetic division, which uses ACh, to control the activities of visceral tissues of the body. Research has resulted in information that reveals concepts illustrating the complexity and versatility of ANS neurotransmission. Some of these advances, which have been discussed in the previous section, indicate that nerve fibers can release more than one neurotransmitter (co-transmission); that neuromodulation of neurotransmitter release and action can occur at either the presynaptic or postsynaptic membrane; and that the neuroeffector junction has structural and functional attributes that suit the overall functioning of the ANS and differ from the skeletal neuromuscular junction (Williams et al., 1995). Other factors contributing to the complexity of autonomic neuronal transmission are the presence of NANC fibers, which use peptides and modulate the function of the major neurotransmitters (FitzGerald and Folan-Curran, 2002); the presence of afferent neurons that release neurotransmitter from their peripheral endings (called sensorimotor nerves) and function in the autonomic control of the GI system, heart, lungs, ganglia, and vasculature; the discovery of integrative circuitry found not only in the enteric nervous system, but also in peripheral intrinsic ganglia associated with the heart, bladder, and respiratory structures; and plasticity (the ability to change) of autonomic neurons (demonstrated by variations in the expression of neurotransmitters, cotransmitters, and receptors) that occurs not only during normal development and aging processes, but also in response to hormones and nerve growth factors released as a result of injury, surgery, and disease states (Williams et al., 1995).

Pharmacologic Applications

The synapse between preganglionic and postganglionic neurons, and postganglionic fibers and effectors, is of interest pharmacologically. Various agents, some of which are produced synthetically, can produce numerous effects. Some mimic the actions of sympathetic (sympathomimetic) stimulation, and others mimic the actions of parasympathetic (parasympathomimetic) stimulation. Many agents block receptor sites or alter the deactivation mechanism of the neurotransmitter. Examples of blocking agents are high concentrations of nicotine, which act at the ganglion level and sustain postganglionic depolarization; atropine, which binds to muscarinic receptors (used to dilate the pupils and increase heart rate by blocking the effects of postganglionic parasympathetic stimulation); phenoxybenzamine, which blocks alpha-adrenergic receptors; propranolol, which blocks beta-adrenergic receptors (used to treat hypertension); and reserpine, which inhibits NE synthesis and storage (Snell, 2001).

Some pharmacologic agents also inhibit or inactivate acetylcholinesterase. Because ACh is not deactivated, it continues to stimulate cholinergic fibers. Examples of reversible anticholinesterase drugs are physostigmine and neostigmine, used in treating glaucoma and myasthenia gravis. Irreversible anticholinesterase drugs are also produced. Some of these are toxic, such as "nerve gas" (Carpenter and Sutin, 1983).

Pharmacologic agents can also mimic autonomic function by stimulating receptors. Phenylephrine (Neo-Synephrine; used to decrease nasal secretions) and isoproterenol (Isuprel; used as a bronchodilator during attacks of asthma) activate alpha and beta receptors, respectively. Pilocarpine can mimic parasympathetic activity and also is used in the treatment of glaucoma (constriction of the sphincter pupillae muscle allows drainage of the anterior chamber of the eye by opening the canals of Schlemm).

CONTROL OF AUTONOMIC EFFERENTS
Central Autonomic Network

The results of much investigation have clarified the components, neurotransmitters, and functions of the sympathetic and parasympathetic divisions of the ANS. However, not until relatively recently have the results of research begun to elucidate the complex neural circuitry that integrates and regulates autonomic efferents. This circuitry, called the central autonomic network, integrates the input it receives and subsequently activates numerous structures that are responsible for widespread autonomic, endocrine, and behavioral effects. For the visceral effectors to produce a response, the central autonomic network sends input to the preganglionic parasympathetic (primarily the vagal system) and sympathetic neurons. The central autonomic network is located in the brain stem and in more rostral structures. It includes many reciprocally connected nuclear areas such as the hypothalamus, NTS (the nucleus of the tractus solitarius), ventrolateral medulla (VLM), parabrachial nucleus, thalamus, and cerebral cortex (Fig. 10-28).

One integral component of this circuitry is the NTS (Loewy, 1990c; Barron and Chokroverty, 1993). This nucleus is bilateral and lies adjacent to the dorsal motor nucleus of the vagus in the dorsomedial aspect of the brain stem medulla rostral to the obex (Fig. 10-29 and see Fig. 9-12). Studies performed on rats show that the NTS is the major brain stem integrator of visceral afferent fibers, including those conveying cardiovascular, respiratory, GI, and taste information.

The NTS has been described as being divided into three parts. The rostral part receives input from the oral cavity, pharynx, and larynx. The intermediate portion receives input from the esophagus, stomach, and intestines. The caudal part receives cardiac and respiratory input (Benarroch, 2001; Gamboa-Esteves et al., 2001). Therefore the NTS is viscerotopically organized. Some afferent fibers terminate in organ-specific subnuclei, which in turn connect with appropriate preganglionic neurons and make reflex adjustments on effector organs. Other afferent fibers synapse on a common region of the caudal NTS called the commissural nucleus (Loewy, 1990c). This nucleus is reciprocally connected to many areas of the CNS, including the spinal cord. Evidence suggests that the NTS receives afferent input from the spinal cord via the spinosolitary tract (Gamboa-Esteves et al., 2001). Afferent fibers from superficial dorsal horn laminae (I to III) ascend in the dorsal column and synapse bilaterally in the caudal NTS. Ascending fibers from deeper laminae (IV to V) course in the dorsolateral white matter and synapse ipsilaterally in the lateral and caudal NTS. Thus somatic sensory input from spinal nerves may be integrated with visceral afferent input from cranial nerves and be used to initiate reflex responses in the cardiovascular system and respiratory system. In addition, trigeminal afferent fibers have been shown to terminate in the caudal NTS, which may explain cutaneous reflex responses occurring in the face in response to temperature changes (Amonoo-Kuofi, 1999). The connections of the cord and trigeminal system with the NTS provide the foundation for integration between somatic and autonomic components of the nervous system and possibly for somatovisceral and viscerovisceral reflex responses (Menetrey and Basbaum, 1987).

The NTS also has been implicated as being part of a descending pain control system. Electrical and chemical stimulation studies show that the NTS influences nociceptive transmission from the cord and that other known nuclei of the pain control system such as the periaqueductal gray (PAG) and raphe nuclei project to the NTS. In addition, data show that the NTS projects via the solitariospinal tract to the superficial and deep laminae of the dorsal horn (Amonoo-Kuofi, 1999; Gamboa-Esteves et al., 2001).

The NTS also has reciprocal connections with brain stem nuclei such as the VLM reticular formation and parabrachial nuclei, and forebrain nuclei such as the hypothalamus and amygdaloid complex.

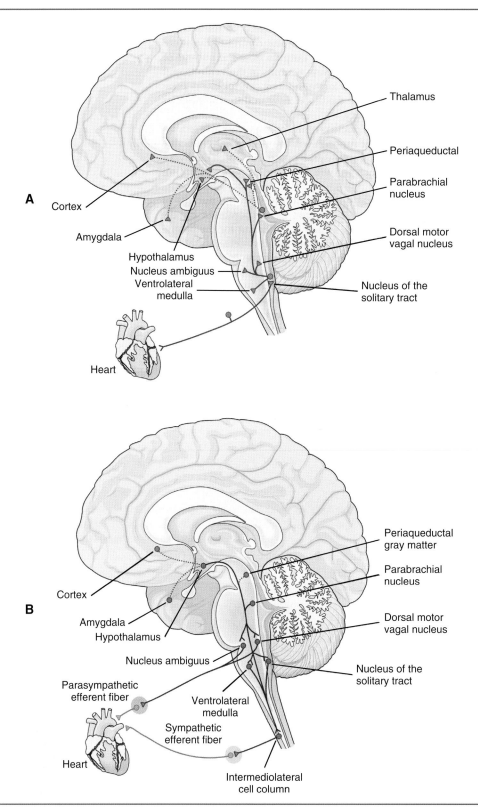

FIG. 10-28   Central autonomic connections. **A,** The distribution of visceral afferent information throughout the brain. The nucleus of the tractus solitarius (nucleus of the solitary tract) projects to preganglionic neurons, the ventrolateral medulla for reflex rsponses, and higher centers. The parabrachial nucleus also provides indirect input (*dotted lines*) to higher centers. **B,** The direct and indirect (*dotted lines*) output of the central autonomic network on parasympathetic and sympathetic preganglionic neurons. (From Kandel ER, Schwartz JH, & Jessell TM, [Eds.]. [2000]. *Principles of neural science* [4th ed.]. New York: McGraw-Hill.)

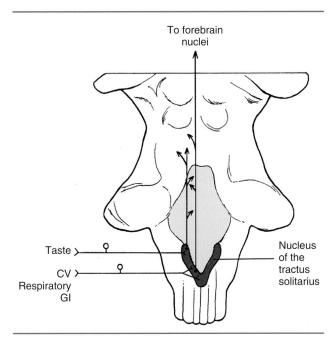

To forebrain
nuclei

Taste

CV
Respiratory
GI

Nucleus
of the
tractus
solitarius

FIG. 10-29 Nucleus of the tractus solitarius. This nucleus is an integrative center and a major component of the central autonomic network of the brain. The nucleus receives various afferent input, such as taste, cardiovascular, respiratory, and gastrointestinal. The output (*arrows*) is dispersed to numerous areas, including brain stem nuclei and forebrain nuclei (e.g., the thalamus and hypothalamus), resulting in reflex responses, as well as autonomic, endocrine, and behavioral responses.

The VLM reticular formation consists of a group of glutaminergic and catecholaminergic neurons located near the ventrolateral surface of the medulla. It functions as a relay center for sympathetic responses concerning blood pressure (Hamill, 1996; Amonoo-Kuofi, 1999). It receives input from the NTS concerning baroreceptor information. The VLM has reciprocal connections with the hypothalamus, central gray matter, and parabrachial nucleus, and it is divided into a rostral part (RVLM) and a caudal part (CVLM). A major projection of the RVLM is to the intermediolateral cell column of the spinal cord on neurons modulating vasomotor function. An increase in activation of the RVLM causes the release of vasopressin and catecholamines, resulting in an increase in blood pressure and heart rate. Decreasing the activity results in pronounced hypotension. The CVLM inhibits sympathetic activity indirectly via inhibitory neurons to the RVLM.

Another brain stem nucleus that is part of the central autonomic network is the parabrachial nucleus. This nucleus is located in the dorsolateral pons and is involved with the behavioral responses to visceral sensations, including taste. It receives the majority of its viscerotopically organized fibers from the NTS (Amonoo-Kuofi, 1999; Iversen, Iversen, and Saper, 2000; Benarroch, 2001) and is connected reciprocally to numerous regions.

These regions include the hypothalamus, PAG, amygdaloid complex, thalamus, and cerebral cortex. The parabrachial nucleus provides the major visceral afferent input to the thalamus.

The PAG is a nuclear region surrounding the cerebral aqueduct of the midbrain. It receives input from the NTS, parabrachial nucleus, hypothalamus, and dorsal horn of the spinal cord (nociception). It has a major role in integrating behavioral, somatic, autonomic, and antinociceptive responses to stress. Through its projections to pontine and medullary reticular formation neurons, the PAG also initiates typical "fight-or-flight" autonomic responses (Iversen, Iversen, and Saper, 2000; Benarroch, 2001).

The amygdaloid complex is a nuclear region located in the anterior temporal lobe of the cerebrum. It functions in the integration and regulation of autonomic responses associated with emotions, including conditioned behaviors such as fear. It receives input from the cerebral cortex, thalamus, and central autonomic network, and projects to the hypothalamus, PAG, NTS, VLM, and vagal nuclei (Iversen, Iversen, and Saper, 2000; Benarroch, 2001).

The viscerosensory thalamic nucleus, which receives information primarily from the parabrachial nucleus, is the ventroposterior parvocellular nucleus. This nucleus is located adjacent to the ventral posterior thalamic nucleus, which is the nucleus that receives nociceptive and thermoreceptive information via the spinothalamic tracts. This thalamic region is an area in which visceral information is integrated with somatic pain and temperature sensations providing a more comprehensive analysis of the integrity of the tissues of the body. The ventroposterior parvocellular nucleus projects viscerotopically to the anterior insular cortex (visceral sensory cortex), such that gustatory input terminates most anteriorly, cardiorespiratory input terminates most posteriorly, and GI input terminates in the middle. The insula is interconnected with the anterior tip of the cingulate cortex (the infralimbic area), which is considered to be a visceral motor region, and both areas send fibers to the amygdaloid complex, PAG, hypothalamus, parabrachial nucleus, NTS, and medullary reticular formation. The loss of conscious appreciation of visceral sensations, such as taste, can be the result of a lesion in the insular cortex. A loss of emotional responses to external stimuli (abulia) can be the result of a lesion in the anterior cingulate cortex (Iversen, Iversen, and Saper, 2000).

Hypothalamus

The hypothalamus has been considered to be heavily involved in the control of the ANS because data had shown that stimulating the anterior and posterior hypothalamic nuclei produced parasympathetic and sympathetic responses, respectively. Recent studies indicate that descending and ascending pathways of the cortex and basal forebrain that traverse hypothalamic neurons may be responsible for the autonomic responses. However, there is evidence that indicates that the paraventricular nucleus of the hypothalamus is involved with the autonomic regulation of blood volume. This occurs by input to the IML (intermediolateral) cell column of the cord, indirectly via the RVLM (which then projects to the IML cell column), and directly through fibers coursing to the IML cell column. These latter fibers also send collateral branches into the RVLM (Badoer, 2001).

Rather than functioning as the major controller of the autonomic nervous system, the hypothalamus is now considered to be an integrator of autonomic activity and endocrine function with behavior associated with the basic physiologic processes essential to homeostasis regulation (Iversen, Iversen, and Saper, 2000). The hypothalamus is able to maintain homeostasis by having access to sensory information from essentially all areas of the body. This occurs through neuronal input from numerous regions of the CNS and through information conveyed by the blood that is detected by hypothalamic neurons. Such information includes temperature, osmolarity, and glucose and hormone concentrations. The hypothalamus then compares this sensory input with the biologic set points for numerous physiologic processes and then initiates the necessary autonomic, endocrine, and behavioral responses to restore homeostasis. The hypothalamus is also intimately involved with the limbic system, which is a phylogenetically old system concerned with behaviors and visceral responses necessary for survival. Although important, the hypothalamus is just one part of the central autonomic network.

Descending Fibers and Other Autonomic Nervous System Influences

Preganglionic sympathetic neurons receive descending input from the hypothalamus (paraventricular nucleus), NTS, pontine noradrenergic cell group (A5), caudal raphe nuclei, and the RVLM. Interneuronal circuits in the intermediate gray matter of each sympathetic spinal cord level also can influence sympathetic output, although the exact mechanism is unclear (Loewy, 1990c). However, transneuronal studies of interneuronal input to preganglionic neurons suggest that the interneuronal circuits are located in laminae IV, V, VII, and X and are organized segmentally. There is no indication using transneuronal methods of any contralateral segmental or intersegmental projections of interneurons onto preganglionic neurons (Cabot, 1996).

In addition to the central autonomic network, the cerebellum and cerebral cortex have been implicated in playing a role in the production of autonomic responses. Data gathered from stimulation and ablation studies of

the cerebellum suggest that the cerebellum is involved at least with cardiovascular functions. On stimulation of the cerebral cortex (superior frontal gyrus, insula, and sensorimotor strip), changes in cardiovascular and respiratory functions, GI motility, and pupillary dilation are produced. These changes are caused by cortical projections that are likely channeled through the hypothalamus. However, the cerebellar and cerebral pathways mediating these autonomic responses are as yet unknown (Barron and Chokroverty, 1993).

Because the majority of this information was gathered from experiments performed on lower mammals, much research needs to be done to clarify the central autonomic circuitry of the human brain. Sympathetic and parasympathetic efferents are certainly under the control of numerous CNS structures that have formed a complex network. This network is linked in such a way that integration and modulation of the autonomic and endocrine systems are possible and behavioral responses can even be affected.

CLINICAL APPLICATIONS

A discussion of the vast number of lesions that can alter autonomic activity is beyond the scope of this chapter. Therefore the following are just a few examples of various pathologic processes that may cause autonomic dysfunction.

Denervation Hypersensitivity

Although total disruption of the innervation to skeletal muscles prohibits contraction from occurring, many viscera are autoregulated, and lesions of preganglionic and postganglionic fibers to these autonomic effectors may not cause total cessation of function. However, the autonomic effector may not function in the most efficient manner under these circumstances. Depending on its location, a lesion would likely eliminate the release of neurotransmitters either between the preganglionic and postganglionic neurons or between the postganglionic neuron and effector. When this occurs, the denervated structures show an increase in sensitivity to their neurotransmitters, which at times may be found in the circulation. This hypersensitivity is possibly caused by an increase in the number of cell membrane adrenergic receptor sites or by alterations in the reuptake mechanism of certain neurotransmitters (e.g., epinephrine) (Carpenter and Sutin, 1983; Snell, 2001). The effectors show greater sensitization as a result of sectioning postganglionic fibers rather than sectioning preganglionic fibers (Carpenter and Sutin, 1983).

An example of the effects of denervation hypersensitivity may be observed in the pupils of individuals who have Horner's's syndrome, which is caused by a disruption of sympathetic fibers (see the following discussion). If the individual's sympathetic nervous system is stimulated (e.g., overexcitement), epinephrine and NE are released from the medulla of the adrenal gland into the blood and cause the pupil to dilate (paradoxic pupillary response), even though the sympathetic innervation to the iris has been interrupted (Noback, Strominger, and Demarest, 1991). Administration of sympatheticomimetic agents to individuals with Horner's's syndrome also produces this same pupillary response (Cross, 1993a).

Horner's Syndrome

Horner's syndrome is primarily an acquired pathologic condition but rarely may occur as a congenital condition. This syndrome is caused by the interruption of the sympathetic innervation to effectors located in the head. Characteristic signs seen in Horner's syndrome are those associated with the ipsilateral loss of sympathetic innervation to the following structures: smooth muscle of the dilator pupillae muscle of the iris, producing pupillary constriction (miosis), which is more apparent in dim light; smooth muscle (Müller's or superior tarsal muscle) of the upper eyelid, producing ptosis; sweat glands of the face, causing anhidrosis; and smooth muscle of the blood vessels, resulting in vasodilation (this makes the skin flushed and warm to the touch). The patient also may appear to have enophthalmos ("sunken eye"). This feature actually is caused by the narrowed palpebral fissure after denervation of the upper eyelids. Because of its denervation, the dilator pupillae muscle also is hypersensitive to circulating adrenergic neurotransmitters (see previous discussion).

The neuronal pathway that supplies the effector tissues involved in Horner's syndrome includes a central pathway, preganglionic neurons, and postganglionic neurons. An interruption of any part of these components may result in Horner's syndrome. The central pathway is ipsilateral and polysynaptic and includes interconnected fibers from the insular cortex, amygdala, hypothalamus (hypothalamospinal fibers), and brain stem nuclei. Although the exact location is unclear, the hypothalamospinal fibers have been shown to descend in the lateral aspect of the brain stem and lateral funiculus of the cord and terminate in the region of the intermediolateral cell column (Fig. 10-30, *A*). Interruption of these fibers can be caused by tumors, multiple sclerosis, trauma, or vascular insufficiency, such as that seen in lateral medullary (Wallenberg's) syndrome. Preganglionic and postganglionic sympathetic fibers also can be disrupted, resulting in Horner's syndrome. Preganglionic fibers originating from the upper three thoracic segments enter the sympathetic chain, ascend, and synapse in the superior cervical ganglion. Postganglionic fibers to the effectors travel with the external and internal carotid arteries. Therefore an interruption of preganglionic fibers (along their pathway in the ventral roots or in the cervical sympathetic chain) or postganglionic fibers may also result in Horner's syndrome (see Fig. 10-30, *A*).

The preganglionic neuron axons are anatomically related to the spine, apex of the lung, cervical pleura, subclavian artery, common carotid artery, internal jugular vein, thyroid gland, and upper ribs. Lesions of any of these structures could affect the preganglionic fibers, resulting in Horner's syndrome (Amonoo-Kuofi, 1999). Examples of these lesions include an apical lung (Pancoast) tumor pressing on the stellate ganglion (Fig. 10-30, *B*), surgical trauma to the thorax or neck (e.g., during the anterior surgical approach to the lower cervical vertebrae [Ebraheim et al., 2000]), and a cervical spine fracture or dislocation (Cross, 1993a). Postganglionic fibers may be disrupted in the neck or within the cranium. A lesion distal to the superior cervical ganglion may produce variation in the clinical signs and symptoms presented by the patient, because the postganglionic fibers use several different arteries to travel to their effectors. Therefore the signs and symptoms depend on which postganglionic fibers have been damaged. The majority of sudomotor fibers to the face travel along the external carotid artery and its branches. The fibers to the eyelid, eyeball, and orbit course with the internal carotid artery and its plexus. Because this artery may be the site of an aneurysm or dissecting lesion, the postganglionic fibers become susceptible to disruption. Also, as the fibers pass by the trigeminal ganglion to enter the ophthalmic division of the trigeminal nerve, they may be lesioned as a result of irritation of the trigeminal nerve. This syndrome, known as Raeder's (paratrigeminal) syndrome, presents with ptosis, miosis, and enophthalmos. It can be differentiated from Horner's syndrome by the presence of ipsilateral facial pain (from irritation of the trigeminal ganglion), and the preservation of facial sweating. Raeder's syndrome also can be caused by aneurysms or dissections of the internal carotid artery, head trauma, parasellar masses, hypertension, vasculitis, and migraines (Amonoo-Kuofi, 1999).

Raynaud's Disease

Raynaud's disease is the result of vasospasms in the digital arteries and arterioles of the fingers (most frequently). Although rarely affected alone, the toes may become involved in conjunction with the fingers. Induced by cold, this painful episodic condition presents bilaterally as changes in skin color caused by vasoconstriction and later a reactive hyperemia. This phenomenon also may be present secondary to other disorders, such as thoracic outlet syndrome, carpal tunnel syndrome, connective tissue disorders, and occupational trauma (e.g., operating air hammers or chain saws).

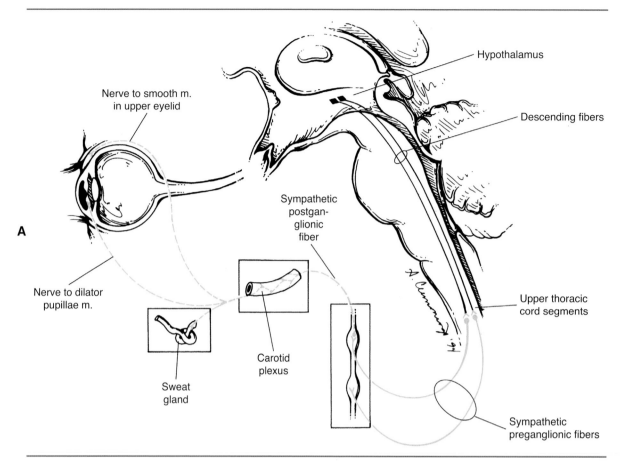

Nerve to smooth m.
in upper eyelid

Hypothalamus

Descending fibers

Sympathetic
postgan-
glionic
fiber

A

Nerve to dilator
pupillae m.

Upper thoracic
cord segments

Carotid
plexus

Sweat
gland

Sympathetic
preganglionic fibers

FIG. 10-30   Sites of lesions that may cause Horner's syndrome. **A,** An interruption of descending hypothalamic fibers within the brain stem of sympathetic preganglionic or sympathetic postganglionic fibers may produce the symptoms associated with Horner's syndrome.

Although conservative treatment should be attempted first, the administration of sympathetic pharmacologic blockers (e.g., reserpine) or even sympathectomy may be necessary to treat serious cases (Carpenter and Sutin, 1983; Khurana, 1993; Snell, 2001).

Hirschsprung's Disease

Hirschsprung's disease (megacolon) is a congenital condition affecting the enteric nervous system. It occurs as a result of neural and glial stem cells not migrating from the neural crest and therefore not developing into the myenteric plexus of a segment of the distal colon. This segment typically is a small area in the rectum, although it can be localized anywhere in the region between the midjejunum and anal canal. Because of the absence of the myenteric plexus, that segment of colon is left in a state of constriction. This subsequently blocks evacuation of the bowel and causes the region proximal to the constriction to become immensely dilated. If the affected area is large, the condition can be fatal during early development or childhood (Williams et al., 1995).

Complex Regional Pain Syndrome

Complex regional pain syndrome (CRPS) is a neurogenic pain condition (see Chapter 11) that most commonly occurs in either an upper or lower extremity, and that may be either localized or include the entire limb. This disorder is divided into two types: CRPS I, which was formerly known as reflex sympathetic dystrophy, and CRPS II, which was known as causalgia. CRPS I is the result of a minor injury (e.g., sprain, bruising), bone fracture, or surgery of the affected limb. In CRPS I there is typically no detectable nerve damage and the symptoms are not confined to any specific nerve distribution. CRPS II develops after a major peripheral nerve, or one of its branches, is damaged. The classic example for this type of injury is a bullet wound to a major nerve, but any similar trauma may produce CRPS II.

CRPS is characterized initially by signs and symptoms localized to the affected extremity. However, the signs and symptoms typically increase in severity and number over time, and the disease ultimately may spread to other ipsilateral areas or even to the contralateral limb. The

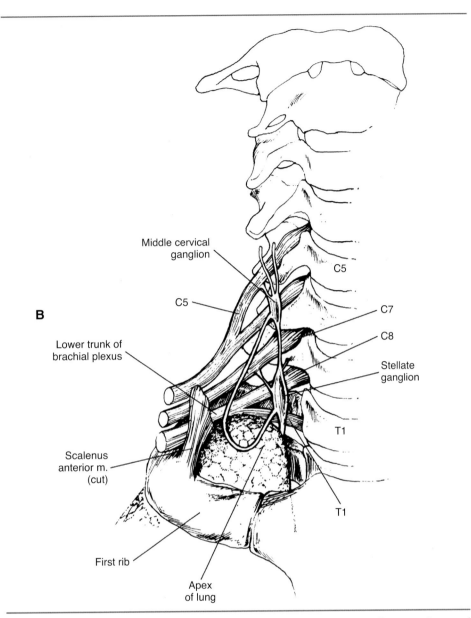

B

Middle cervical ganglion

C5

C5

C7

C8

Stellate ganglion

T1

Lower trunk of brachial plexus

Scalenus anterior m. (cut)

T1

First rib

Apex of lung

FIG. 10-30—cont'd   B, Because of the location of the lung apex, stellate ganglion, and lowest trunk of the brachial plexus, a tumor in the lung apex may result in Horner's syndrome and lesion signs in the upper extremity (as a result of pressure on the stellate ganglion and lowest trunk of the brachial plexus, respectively).

signs and symptoms, in order of general occurrence and progression are as follows:

1. Pain that is spontaneous, severe, and that may be associated with hyperalgesia and allodynia
2. Motor disturbances such as weakness, dystonia, increased physiologic tremors, and joint movement restrictions
3. Vasomotor and autonomic changes such as changes in skin color, temperature change in the affected limb, swelling, and sweating abnormalities
4. Trophic changes of the skin and subcutaneous tissues such as abnormal nail and hair growth

These clinical features of CRPS may be devastating. In addition to these signs and symptoms, a distinguishing feature of this condition is that its symptoms are disproportionate to the severity of the original insult (Walker and Cousins, 1997; Wasner, Backonja, and Baron, 1998; Schwartzman and Popescu, 2002; Turner-Stokes, 2002; Wasner et al., 2003). Because the clinical presentation includes disturbances in autonomic functions, a dysfunctional sympathetic nervous system has been implicated as causing or strongly influencing the condition. In fact, the involved pain often is called sympathetically maintained pain (SMP) because it can be relieved by sympatholytic procedures and it appears to be sustained by sympathetic efferent fibers. The most generally accepted model for the mechanism of the disease is that after acute tissue damage, polymodal nociceptors become sensitized because of both continuous stimulation by chemical mediators released during the inflammatory process and a lack of tissue healing. Under these pathologic conditions, the afferent fibers also become sensitive to catecholamines and upregulate adrenergic receptors. The release of NE from sympathetic fibers or circulating in the blood can activate these receptors located in the dorsal root ganglion, the periphery, and possibly the lesioned nerve. This event is called coupling of sympathetic efferent and afferent fibers. In addition, inflammatory chemical mediators such as bradykinin and nerve growth factor bind to sympathetic fiber varicosities, resulting in the release of prostaglandins and other mediators that can activate the primary afferent fibers and sustain nociceptive input (Jänig and Baron, 2003). Sympathetic afferent coupling occurs not only in cutaneous locations, but also in deep somatic tissues, resulting in patients experiencing painful bone, muscle, or joint tissues. The mechanism appears to be an indirect coupling involving the capillary bed and nonneuronal elements such as mast cells and macrophages (Jänig and Baron, 2003).

In the spinal cord, wide dynamic range dorsal horn neurons are sensitized by the activation of polymodal nociceptors. These sensitized neurons then can be activated by innocuous cutaneous mechanoreceptors, resulting in touch being perceived as pain (allodynia). The sympathetic neurons are activated locally, resulting in sympathetic efferent and afferent coupling. This is followed by the firing of the afferent neurons, which in turn activates the sensitized dorsal horn neurons (Gordon, 1996; Walker and Cousins, 1997; Wasner, Backonja, and Baron, 1998; Jänig and Baron, 2003). This positive feedback loop maintains hyperexcitability and allows the pain to persist.

Associated autonomic abnormalities in the regulation of temperature and sweating appear to be caused by changes in the autonomic circuitry within the central nervous system. Abnormal sympathetic reflex patterns in the affected limb may be related to CRPS (Wasner et al., 2003). In the acute stage, cutaneous vasodilation occurs as a result of functional inhibition of vasoconstrictor fibers (i.e., C fiber nociceptors release substance P and other neurochemicals that inhibit sympathetic activity or override it, resulting in vasodilation paradoxically in conjunction with increased sympathetic activity). In chronic cases, there is evidence that vasoconstrictor activity returns once the acute nociceptive response has faded, causing a decrease in skin temperature and blood flow. Another possible mechanism for autonomic disturbances is that changes in the neuronal circuitry

may prevent the descending fibers from higher centers from facilitating the activity of the cord circuits. These circuits normally control the activity of the preganglionic neurons that regulate cutaneous vasoconstriction and sudomotor secretion. Also, motor disturbances seem to be the result of a CNS mechanism in which there are changes of the cord circuitry involved with spinal reflexes. This may be the result of continuous nociceptive input and the plasticity of spinal synaptic circuitry. In addition, there may be a lack or abnormal integration of sensory and motor information at the cortical level, resulting in faulty planning and programming of autonomic motor activities. There is still no clear explanation for all of the mechanisms of the clinical features of edema and inflammation. Although the initial trauma initiates inflammatory processes, the continuation and amplification of these processes in CRPS are poorly understood. Sympathetic activity appears to be involved with maintaining the swelling, possibly through a coupling mechanism with peptidergic unmyelinated fibers. When activated, these fibers cause neurogenic inflammation by releasing peptides that vasodilate precapillary vessels and cause plasma extravasation from postcapillary vessels (Jänig and Baron, 2003). This inflammatory response may lead to increased efferent sympathetic activity and further irritation of the nociceptors. This positive feedback loop is thought to play a significant role in CRPS. Wasner et al. (2003) found that chemical mediators of neurogenic inflammation (e.g., CGRP, interleukin-6, nitric oxide, substance P) present in the plasma were elevated, thus supporting the premise that inflammation is involved in the early stages of CRPS and that sympathetic activation can influence the intensity of the inflammatory process.

CRPS is a complex disorder, and the exact mechanisms explaining its clinical characteristics are still not fully understood. However, CRPS appears to be a systemic disease that involves both PNS and CNS components.

Spinal Cord Injury

General Considerations. As mentioned in Chapter 9, an injury to the spinal cord may cause dysfunction in somatic motor activity and impair somatic sensory input. This same type of lesion also may have widespread and disastrous effects on the ANS. These effects may occur by destroying the preganglionic neuron cell bodies or removing the descending influence on preganglionic neurons from higher centers.

The latter scenario results in loss of input from the hypothalamus, medullary centers, and other centers on the preganglionic neurons below the level of the lesion.

The specific level of the lesion and the amount of neuronal loss determine which functions of the ANS are lost and which are retained. High lesions of upper thoracic or cervical segments are especially detrimental because they can eliminate all brain control on essential homeostatic mechanisms. These mechanisms are extremely important in permitting the body to respond to such events as environmental changes (e.g., temperature) or emotional stresses. For example, with complete lesions of the lower cervical spinal cord, all integration between segmental autonomic reflexes and descending influences is eliminated. This leaves any remaining control of bladder and bowel function, sexual function, cardiovascular regulation, and thermoregulation to the uninhibited reflex arcs formed by visceral afferent fibers and preganglionic sympathetic and sacral parasympathetic efferent fibers. This can be life threatening in the case of regulation of vasomotor tone and thermoregulation. The dysfunctions resulting from spinal cord injuries usually are most apparent in effectors that normally function automatically, usually are taken for granted (e.g., bladder and bowel function), but are an extremely important part of daily living.

Spinal Shock and Other Consequences. The initial reaction to a complete transection of the spinal cord is spinal shock, which affects somatic (see Chapter 9) and autonomic functions. Removing supraspinal input causes loss of all autonomic reflexes below the level of the lesion. This results in paralytic ileus and an areflexic, atonic bladder that is characterized by acute retention (Abdel-Azim, Sullivan, and Yalla, 1991) with overflow incontinence (Hanak and Scott, 1983; Adams and Victor, 1989; Snell, 2001). High thoracic or cervical transections also can result in profound hypotension from loss of vasomotor tone, loss of thermoregulation caused by impaired vasomotor tone, and possible loss of sweating and piloerection.

After the effects of spinal shock have worn off, autonomic functions and homeostatic control rely on the integrity of the afferent and efferent neurons below the level of the lesion, and a stage of heightened reflex activity ensues. This stage is characterized by hyperactivity in deep tendon reflexes, a spastic bladder (see Effects on Bladder Function), and heightened vasoconstrictor and sweating responses to epinephrine (see Denervation Hypersensitivity).

In addition to the disruption of bladder, bowel, and sexual functions, lesions causing quadriplegia continue to produce serious impairment of other ANS functions, because descending input to sympathetic efferents destined for the heart, peripheral blood vessels, sweat glands, and arrector pili muscles is severed. A specific example of a difficulty that arises from the loss of descending input to preganglionic sympathetic neurons is a marked decrease in the ability to regulate blood pressure. Normally a decrease in cerebral blood pressure, such

as would occur when sitting up from a supine position, is corrected easily. However, in patients with cervical cord injuries, the decrease in blood pressure stimulates baroreceptors, but the stimulation does not result in reflex sympathetic vasoconstriction. Therefore these patients are prone to orthostatic hypotension, and consciousness may be lost if the drop in blood pressure is severe enough. Also, the regulation of vasomotor tone in response to temperature changes or emotional stress (which usually acts as a sympathetic stimulus) is absent in dermatomes below the level of the lesion. For example, with an injury of the upper thoracic spinal cord (near T3) the face and neck may demonstrate flushing and sweating in response to a rise in temperature, but reflex vasodilation of the rest of the body does not occur (Appenzeller, 1986; Adams and Victor, 1989). These patients have difficulty controlling their body temperature.

Effects on Bladder Function. The normal functioning of the bladder is regulated by numerous areas in the CNS (see Fig. 10-20). The involvement of higher centers with sacral afferent and efferent neurons generates a sense of fullness and the need to void. These connections allow the suppression of voiding until an appropriate time, and provide the ability to start and stop voiding and evacuate the bladder completely. Lesions in the spinal cord disrupt this type of voluntary control. A disruption of the PNS or CNS components that control bladder function results in a neurogenic bladder (Benarroch et al., 1999). Neurogenic bladder is classified as reflex (upper motor neuron type) or nonreflex (lower motor neuron type). The reflex bladder consists of uninhibited and automatic (or spastic) types. A lesion in the medial frontal cortex results in an uninhibited bladder. Because the coordination between the detrusor muscle and the external urethral sphincter is preserved, there is urinary incontinence but not retention. Bladder volume and intravesical pressure are normal.

A complete lesion above the lumbosacral cord segments severs ascending sensory input to the brain and descending information from the brain and results in an automatic (spastic) bladder. The bladder is hyperreflexic, and stretch receptors initiate reflex contraction on filling. However, incomplete emptying occurs because of "detrusor-striated sphincter dyssynergia" (lack of coordination between the detrusor muscle and external urethral sphincter caused by the disruption of descending fibers) (de Groat et al., 1990; Abdel-Azim, Sullivan, and Yalla, 1991; Bradley, 1993). Bladder volume is decreased and intravesical pressure is increased. A lesion in sacral cord segments (conus medullaris) or the cauda equina destroys the innervation to the bladder and produces a nonreflex, flaccid (autonomous) bladder. The detrusor muscle is areflexic and atonic, and the bladder fills and overflows (overflow incontinence). Bladder volume is increased and intravesical pressure is decreased. Also, there is no perianal sensation or anal and bulbocavernosus reflexes, which are preserved in the uninhibited and spastic bladder conditions (Benarroch et al., 1999). Patients often can manage bladder function by learning and maintaining a routine of consistent fluid intake and by catheterization (preferably intermittent). In some instances, pharmacologic therapy may also be necessary. In patients with supraspinal lesions, surgical enlargement of the bladder (augmentation cystoplasty) also may become an option. In individuals with sacral cord lesions, micturition is possible by using the Credé (applying manual pressure to the suprapubic region) and Valsalva maneuvers (Abdel-Azim, Sullivan, and Yalla, 1991).

Effects on Bowel Function. Lesions that result in bladder dysfunction also affect bowel activity. The types of effectors involved with normal bowel function (i.e., smooth muscle and striated sphincters) are similar to those involved with bladder functions. The pattern of innervation of the bowel is similar to that of the bladder, as well. Thus similarities exist between the effects of spinal cord lesions on bowel function and the effects on bladder function. Loss of descending input from the brain eliminates the voluntary control of defecation, the awareness of the sensation to defecate, and the knowledge that defecation is occurring. Instead, the bowel is automatic, which means that it contracts in response to local reflexes. These reflexes are initiated by distention, irritation (e.g., suppositories), and in some instances digital anal stimulation. Management of bowel, as well as bladder, function is of great concern for the patient, and helping the patient become as independent as possible is a psychologic advantage. Setting aside a routine time for reflex bowel action is important for bowel training. Proper diet, fluid intake, positioning, and medication also can help to maximize the success of such training (Sutton, 1973).

Effects on Sexual Function. The extent to which their sexual functions are impaired is of great importance to many patients with spinal cord injuries. As with the urinary system, the genitalia receive parasympathetic, sympathetic, and somatic innervation (see Fig. 10-21). Male sexual dysfunction has been studied extensively, more so than female sexual dysfunction, most likely because fewer females experience spinal cord injuries and their functional loss is less detrimental. Similar to the effects seen in other organs, the degree of dysfunction depends on the completeness of the lesion and the level of the injury.

Erections can be psychogenic or reflexogenic (see previous discussion). The former are initiated by supraspinal input channeled through the hypothalamus and limbic systems to descend ultimately to parasympathetic

and sympathetic efferents (de Groat and Steers, 1990). Reflexogenic erections are elicited by exteroceptive stimuli and are mediated by a reflex arc that uses sacral cord segments. Both supraspinal and reflex connections probably work in concert in healthy individuals.

Patients with spinal cord injuries usually are still capable of having erections (Seftel, Oates, and Krane, 1991). Patients with complete lower motor neuron lesions in the sacral cord (conus medullaris) or cauda equina may still retain psychogenic erections via the sympathetic innervation of the penis, although reflexogenic erections are absent (de Groat and Steers, 1990; Seftel, Oates, and Krane, 1991). However, patients with complete upper motor neuron lesions above the T12 cord segment are incapable of psychogenic erections, although reflexogenic erections are usually present (Seftel, Oates, and Krane, 1991). Tactile stimulation of the genital area is the initiator of this reflex response. Incomplete lower or upper motor neuron lesions increase the chances of being able to have psychogenic erections.

Although erections occur frequently in spinal cord-injured patients, ejaculation is uncommon in patients with complete upper motor neuron lesions. The CNS mediation of ejaculation is highly complex, involving an ejaculatory center in the lower thoracolumbar spinal cord segments and in supraspinal areas, such as the cerebral cortex. Although the circuitry is not completely understood, these centers are thought to be vulnerable to injury. Infertility is a major problem among patients with spinal cord lesions because of the failure to ejaculate (Seftel, Oates, and Krane, 1991).

Conus Medullaris Syndrome. As mentioned previously, the pattern of innervation to the bladder, bowel, and genitalia is similar and involves sympathetic, parasympathetic, and somatic neurons. Lesions in the sacral segments produce a conus medullaris syndrome affecting the bladder, bowel, and genitalia in a manner described previously. Conus medullaris syndrome also results in anesthesia in the perianal region. Of diagnostic value is that this syndrome results in perianal sensory loss and autonomic disturbances, but the lower extremities retain their normal sensory and motor functions (Carpenter and Sutin, 1983).

Autonomic Dysreflexia. Spinal cord lesions of midthoracic and cervical segments also produce a condition called autonomic dysreflexia, also known as autonomic hyperreflexia. This syndrome is a widespread autonomic reflex reaction to afferent stimuli that is normally modulated by descending supraspinal input. The initiation of autonomic dysreflexia occurs when a noxious stimulus causes afferent fibers to fire and send input into the spinal cord below the level of the lesion.

Common stimuli are distention of the bladder, urinary tract infection, blockage or insertion of a catheter, rectal distention, and occasionally cutaneous stimulation and flexion contractures (Appenzeller, 1986; Benarroch, 1993). Without normal supraspinal inhibition, sympathetic efferents cause widespread reflex vasoconstriction in areas innervated by cord segments below the lesion, which results in hypertension. Baroreceptors monitoring the increase in blood pressure send information to vasomotor centers, which in turn attempt to correct this threatening situation. This results in bradycardia, and above the level of the lesion (usually in the face and neck), vasodilation, flushing, and profuse sweating occur.

However, because of the lesion, no corrective message reaches the sympathetic fibers below the spinal cord blockage; therefore vasoconstriction continues and is accompanied by piloerection and skin pallor (Naftchi et al., 1982b). Patients monitored during a hypertensive crisis exhibit an increase of their mean arterial pressure from 95 to 154 mmHg (Naftchi et al., 1982a). Others demonstrate a systolic pressure that may exceed 200 mm Hg (Ropper, 1993). This hypertension usually produces a throbbing headache and is extremely serious because it can result in seizures, localized neurologic deficits, myocardial infarction, visual defects, and cerebral hemorrhaging (Hanak and Scott, 1983; Adams and Victor, 1989; Benarroch, 1993). Immediate alleviation of this condition by identifying and removing the cause of the stimulus, which can produce a decrease in blood pressure within 2 to 10 minutes (Ropper, 1993), is imperative.

Conclusion. Lesions of the spinal cord producing dysfunction of normal sexual, bowel, and bladder activities cause not only considerable physical impairment, but also significant psychologic concern for the patient. Rehabilitation of the patient to as much independent control as possible with as little reliance on others as possible is extremely important. The location of the lesion determines the amount and type of function that remain, and the amount of remaining function determines the methods that may be used to achieve self-reliance.

As can be seen from the previous discussion, the effects of spinal cord injury to the somatic (see Chapter 9) and autonomic nervous systems can be considerable and in some cases life-threatening. The resulting loss of sensory and motor functions serves as a continual reminder of the importance of the intricate and complex neural circuitry that is necessary for the normal functioning of the human body.

REFERENCES

Abdel-Azim M, Sullivan M, & Yalla SV. (1991). Disorders of bladder function in spinal cord disease. *Neurol Clin, 9(3),* 727-740.

Adams RD & Victor M. (1989). *Principles of neurology* (4th ed.). St Louis: McGraw-Hill.

Al-Chaer ED & Traub RJ. (2002). Biological basis of visceral pain: Recent developments. *Pain, 96,* 221-225.

Amonoo-Kuofi HS. (1999). Horner's's syndrome revisited: With an update of the central pathway. *Clin Anat, 12,* 345-361.

Appenzeller O. (1986). *Clinical autonomic failure.* New York: Elsevier.

Badoer E. (2001). Hypothalamic paraventricular nucleus and cardiovascular regulation. *Clin Exp Pharm Physiol, 28,* 95-99.

Barron KD & Chokroverty S. (1993). Anatomy of the autonomic nervous system: Brain and brain stem. In PA Low (Ed.). *Clinical autonomic disorders.* Boston: Little, Brown.

Basbaum AI & Jessell TM. (2000). The perception of pain. In ER Kandel, JH Schwartz, & TM Jessell (Eds.). *Principles of neural science.* (4th ed.). New York: McGraw-Hill.

Beal MC. (1985). Viscerosomatic reflexes: A review. *J Am Osteopath Assoc, 85(12),* 53-68.

Bear MF, Conners BW, & Paradiso MA. (2001). *Neuroscience* (2nd ed.). Baltimore: Lippincott Williams & Wilkins.

Benarroch EE. (1993). Central autonomic disorders. In PA Low (Ed.). *Clinical autonomic disorders.* Boston: Little, Brown.

Benarroch EE. (2001). Pain-autonomic interactions: A selective review. *Clin Auto Res, 11,* 343-349.

Benarroch EE et al. (1999). *Medical neurosciences* (4th ed.). New York: Lippincott Williams & Wilkins.

Bennett MR. (1998). Transmission at sympathetic varicosities. *News Physiol Sci, 13,* 79-84.

Blok BFM & Holstege G. (1998). The central nervous system control of micturition in cats and humans. *Behav Brain Res, 92,* 119-125.

Bolton PS. (1998). The somatosensory system of the neck and its effects on the central nervous system. *JMPT, 21,* 553-563.

Bolton PS et al. (1998). Influences of neck afferents on sympathetic and respiratory nerve activity. *Brain Res Bull, 47,* 413-419.

Bradley WE. (1993). Autonomic regulation of the urinary bladder. In PA Low (Ed.). *Clinical autonomic disorders.* Boston: Little, Brown.

Bray JJ et al. (1994). *Lecture notes on human physiology* (3rd ed.). Cambridge, UK: Blackwell Science.

Budgell B & Hirano F. (2001). Innocuous mechanical stimulation of the neck and alterations in heart-rate variability in healthy young adults. *Autonom Neurosci Basic Clin, 91,* 96-99.

Budgell BS, Hotta J, & Sato A. (1998). Reflex responses of bladder motility after stimulation of interspinous tissues in the anesthetized rat. *JMPT, 21,* 593-599.

Budgell BS & Igarashi Y. (2001). Response of arrhythmia to spinal manipulation: Monitoring by ECG with analysis of heart-rate variability. *JNMS, 9,* 97-102.

Budgell B & Suzuki A. (2000). Inhibition of gastric motility by noxious chemical stimulation of interspinous tissues in the rat. *J ANS, 80,* 162-168.

Cabot JB. (1990). Sympathetic preganglionic neurons: Cytoarchitecture, ultrastructure, and biophysical properties. In AD Loewy & KM Spyer (Eds.). *Central regulation of autonomic functions.* New York: Oxford University Press.

Cabot JB. (1996). Some principles of the spinal organization of the sympathetic preganglionic outflow. *Prog Brain Res, 107,* 29-42.

Camilleri M. (1993). Autonomic regulation of gastrointestinal motility. In PA Low (Ed.). *Clinical autonomic disorders.* Boston: Little, Brown.

Carpenter MB & Sutin J. (1983). *Human neuroanatomy* (8th ed.). Baltimore: Williams & Wilkins.

Cervero F. (2000a). Visceral hyperalgesia revisited. *Lancet, 356,* 1127-1128.

Cervero F. (2000b). Visceral pain: Central sensitization. *Gut, 47(Suppl IV),* iv56-iv57.

Cervero F & Foreman RD. (1990). Sensory innervation of the viscera. In AD Loewy & KM Spyer (Eds.). *Central regulation of autonomic functions.* New York: Oxford University Press.

Cervero F & Laird JMA. (1999). Visceral pain. *Lancet, 353,* 2145-2148.

Chandler MJ et al. (1999). Convergence of trigeminal input with visceral and phrenic inputs on primate C1-C2 spinothalamic tract neurons. *Brain Res, 829,* 204-208.

Chandler MJ, Zhang J, & Foreman RD. (1996). Vagal, sympathetic and somatic sensory inputs to upper cervical (C1-C3) spinothalamic tract neurons in monkeys. *J Neurophysiol, 76(4),* 2555-2567.

Cross SA. (1993a). Autonomic disorders of the pupil, ciliary body, and lacrimal apparatus. In PA Low (Ed.). *Clinical autonomic disorders.* Boston: Little, Brown.

Cross SA. (1993b). Autonomic innervation of the eye. In PA Low (Ed.). *Clinical autonomic disorders*. Boston: Little, Brown.

de Groat WC & Steers WD. (1990). Autonomic regulation of the urinary bladder and sexual organs. In AD Loewy & KM Spyer (Eds.). *Central regulation of autonomic functions*. New York: Oxford University Press.

de Groat WC et al. (1990). Mechanisms underlying the recovery of urinary bladder function following spinal cord injury. *J Auton Nerv Syst, 30*, S71-S78.

Dodd J & Role LW. (1991). The autonomic nervous system. In ER Kandel, JH Schwartz, & TM Jessell (Eds.). *Principles of neural science* (3rd ed.). East Norwalk, Conn: Appleton & Lange.

Ebraheim NA et al. (2000). Vulnerability of the sympathetic trunk during the anterior approach to the lower cervical spine. *Spine, 25*, 1603-1606.

FitzGerald MJT & Folan-Curran J. (2002). *Clinical neuroanatomy and related neuroscience* (4th ed.). Edinburgh: WB Saunders.

Foreman RD. (1999). Mechanisms of cardiac pain. *Annu Rev Physiol, 61*, 143-167.

Furness JB. (2000). Types of neurons in the enteric nervous system. *J Auton Nerv Sys, 81*, 87-96.

Furness JB. (2003). Intestinofugal neurons and sympathetic reflexes that bypass the central nervous system. *J Comp Neurol, 455*, 281-284.

Gamboa-Esteves FO et al. (2001). Projection sites of superficial and deep spinal dorsal horn cells in the nucleus tractus solitarii of the rat. *Brain Res, 921*, 195-205.

Gershon MD. (1981). The enteric nervous system. *Annu Rev Neurosci, 4*, 227-272.

Giambernardino MA. (2003). Referred muscle pain/hyperalgesia and central sensitisation. *J Rehabil Med, 41*, 85-88.

Gordon N. (1996). Reflex sympathetic dystrophy. *Brain Dev, 18*, 257-262.

Grundy D. (2002). Neuroanatomy of visceral nociception: Vagal and splanchnic afferent. *Gut, 51*, i2-i5.

Guyton AC. (1991). *Textbook of medical physiology* (8th ed.). Philadelphia: WB Saunders.

Hamill RW. (1996). Peripheral autonomic nervous system. In D Robertson, PA Low, & RJ Polinsky (Eds.). *Primer on the autonomic nervous system*. New York: Academic Press.

Hanak M & Scott A. (1983). *Spinal cord injury*. New York: Springer.

Hansen MB. (2003a). The enteric nervous system I: Organization and classification. *Pharmacol Toxicol, 92*, 105-113.

Hansen MB. (2003b). The enteric nervous system II: Gastrointestinal functions. *Pharmacol Toxicol, 92*, 249-257.

Harati Y. (1993). Anatomy of the spinal and peripheral autonomic nervous system. In PA Low (Ed.). *Clinical autonomic disorders*. Boston: Little, Brown.

Hirst GDS et al. (1996). Transmission by post-ganglionic axons of the autonomic nervous system: The importance of the specialized neuroeffector junction. *Neuroscience, 73*, 7-23.

Insel PA. (1996). Adrenergic receptors: Evolving concepts and clinical implications. *N Engl J Med, 334*, 580-585.

Iversen S, Iversen L, & Saper CB. (2000). The autonomic nervous system and the hypothalamus. In ER Kandel, JH Schwartz, & TM Jessell (Eds.). *Principles of neural science* (4th ed.). New York: McGraw-Hill.

Jänig W. (1996). Neurobiology of visceral afferent neurons: Neuroanatomy, functions, organ regulations and sensations. *Biol Psychol, 42*, 29-51.

Jänig W. (1995). The sympathetic nervous system in pain. *Eur J Anaesthesiol, 12*, 53-60.

Jänig W. (1990). Functions of the sympathetic innervation of the skin. In AD Loewy & KM Spyer (Eds.). *Central regulation of autonomic functions*. New York: Oxford University Press.

Jänig W. (1988). Integration of gut function by sympathetic reflexes. *Baillieres Clin Gastroenterol, 2(1)*, 45-62.

Jänig W & Baron R. (2003). Complex regional pain syndrome: Mystery explained? *Lancet Neurol, 2*, 687-697.

Jänig W & Häbler H. (2000). Specificity in the organization of the autonomic nervous system: A basis for precise neural regulation of homeostatic and protective body functions. *Prog Brain Res, 122*, 351-367.

Joshi SK & Gebhart GF. (2000). Visceral pain. *Curr Rev Pain, 4*, 499-506.

Khurana RK. (1993). Acral sympathetic dysfunctions and hyperhidrosis. In PA Low (Ed.). *Clinical autonomic disorders*. Boston: Little, Brown.

Kiernan JA. (1998). *The human nervous system* (7th ed.). Philadelphia: JB Lippincott.

Loewy AD. (1990a). Anatomy of the autonomic nervous system: An overview. In AD Loewy & KM Spyer (Eds.). *Central regulation of autonomic functions*. New York: Oxford University Press.

Loewy AD. (1990b). Autonomic control of the eye. In AD Loewy & KM Spyer (Eds.). *Central regulation of autonomic functions*. New York: Oxford University Press.

Loewy AD. (1990c). Central autonomic pathways. In AD Loewy & KM Spyer (Eds.). *Central regulation of autonomic functions*. New York: Oxford University Press.

Loewy AD & Spyer KM. (1990). Vagal preganglionic neurons. In AD Loewy & KM Spyer (Eds.). *Central regulation of autonomic functions*. New York: Oxford University Press.

Menetrey D & Basbaum AI. (1987). Spinal and trigeminal projections to the nucleus of the solitary tract: A possible substrate for somatovisceral and viscerovisceral reflex activation. *J Comp Neurol, 255*, 439-450.

Mitchell GAG. (1953). *Anatomy of the autonomic nervous system*. Edinburgh: E&S Livingstone, 209-269.

Moore KL & Dalley AF. (1999). *Clinically oriented anatomy* (4th ed.). Baltimore: Williams & Wilkins.

Murata Y et al. (2000). Sensory innervation of the sacroiliac joint in rats. *Spine, 25*, 2015-2019.

Murata Y et al. (2003). Variations in the number and position of human lumbar sympathetic ganglia and rami communicantes. *Clin Anat, 16*, 108-113.

Naftchi NE et al. (1982a). Autonomic hyperreflexia: Hemodynamics, blood volume, serum dopamine-hydroxylase activity, and arterial prostaglandin PGE2. In NE Naftchi (Ed.). *Spinal cord injury*. New York: Spectrum.

Naftchi NE et al. (1982b). Relationship between serum dopamine-hydroxylase activity, catecholamine metabolism, and hemodynamic changes during paroxysmal hypertension in quadriplegia. In NE Naftchi (Ed.). *Spinal cord injury*. New York: Spectrum.

Nauta HJW et al. (2000). Punctate midline myelotomy for the relief of visceral cancer pain. *J Neurosurg: Spine, 92*, 125-130.

Ness TJ. (2000). Evidence for ascending visceral nociceptive information in the dorsal midline and lateral spinal cord. *Pain, 87*, 83-88.

Noback CR, Strominger NL, & Demarest RJ. (1991). *The human nervous system* (4th ed.). Philadelphia: Lea & Febiger.

Nolte J. (2002). *The human brain* (5th ed.). St Louis: Mosby.

Ogawa T & Low PA. (1993). Autonomic regulation of temperature and sweating. In PA Low (Ed.). *Clinical autonomic disorders*. Boston: Little, Brown.

Palecek J, Paleckova V, & Willis WD. (2002). The roles of pathways in the spinal cord lateral and dorsal funiculi in signaling nociceptive somatic and visceral stimuli in rats. *Pain, 96*, 297-307.

Panuncio AL et al. (1998). Adrenergic innervation in reactive human lymph nodes. *J Anat, 194*, 143-146.

Raybould HE. (1999). Nutrient tasting and signaling mechanisms in the gut. I. Sensing of lipid by the intestinal mucosa. *Am J Physiol, 277*, G751-G755.

Rocco AG, Palombi D, & Raeke D. (1995). Anatomy of the lumbar sympathetic chain. *Reg Anesth, 20*, 13-19.

Ropper AH. (1993). Acute autonomic emergencies in autonomic storm. In PA Low (Ed.). *Clinical autonomic disorders*. Boston: Little, Brown.

Ruch TC. (1946). Visceral sensation and referred pain. In JF Fulton (Ed.). *Howell's textbook of physiology* (15th ed.). Philadelphia: WB Saunders.

Salvesen R. (2001). Innervation of sweat glands in the forehead. A study in patients with Horner's's syndrome. *J Neurol Sci, 183*, 39-42.

Sato A. (1992a). The reflex effects of spinal somatic nerve stimulation on visceral function. *J Manipulative Physiol Ther, 15(1)*, 57-61.

Sato A. (1992b). Spinal reflex physiology. In S Haldeman (Ed.). *Principles and practice of chiropractic* (2nd ed.). East Norwalk, Conn: Appleton & Lange.

Sato A. (1997). Neural mechanisms of autonomic responses elicited by somatic sensory stimulation. *Neurosci Behav Physiol, 27*, 610-621.

Sato A, Sato Y, & Schmidt RF. (1984). Changes in blood pressure and heart rate induced by movements of normal and inflamed knee joints. *Neurosci Lett, 52*, 55-60.

Sato A & Swenson RS. (1984). Sympathetic nervous system response to mechanical stress of the spinal column in rats. *J Manipulative Physiol Ther, 7(3)*, 141-147.

Schwartzman RJ & Popescu A. (2002). *Curr Rheumatol Repts, 4*, 165-169.

Seftel AD, Oates RD, & Krane RJ. (1991). Disturbed sexual function in patients with spinal cord disease. *Neurol Clin, 9(3)*, 757-778.

Shefchyk S. (2001). Sacral spinal interneurons and the control of urinary bladder and urethral striated sphincter muscle function. *J Physiol, 533(1),* 57-63.

Shefchyk S. (2002). Spinal cord neural organization controlling the urinary bladder and striated sphincter. *Prog Brain Res, 137,* 71-82.

Snell RS. (2001). *Clinical neuroanatomy for medical students* (3rd ed.). Boston: Little, Brown.

Stewart JD. (1993). Autonomic regulation of sexual function. In PA Low (Ed.). *Clinical autonomic disorders.* Boston: Little, Brown.

Sutton NG. (1973). *Injuries of the spinal cord.* Toronto: Butterworth.

Taylor GS & Bywater RA. (1988). Intrinsic control of the gut. *Baillieres Clin Gastroenterol, 2(1),* 1-22.

Tortora GJ & Grabowski SR. (2003). *Principles of anatomy and physiology* (10th ed.). New York: John Wiley & Sons, Inc.

Turner-Stokes L. (2002). Reflex sympathetic dystrophy: A complex regional pain syndrome. *Disab Rehab, 24,* 939-947.

Vecchiet L, Vecchiet J, & Giamberardino MA. (1999). Referred muscle pain: Clinical and pathophysiologic aspects. *Curr Rev Pain, 3,* 489-498.

Walker SM & Cousins MJ. (1997), Complex regional pain syndromes: Including "reflex sympathetic dystrophy and causalgia." *Anaesth Int Care, 25,* 113- 125.

Wang FB, Holst M, & Powley TL. (1995). The ratio of pre- to postganglionic neurons and related issues in the autonomic nervous system. *Brain Res Rev, 21,* 93-115.

Wasner G, Backonja M, & Baron R. (1998). Complex regional pain syndromes (reflex sympathetic dystrophy and causalgia): Clinical characteristics, pathophysiologic mechanisms and therapy. *Neurol Clin, 16,* 851-868.

Wasner G et al. (2003). Complex regional pain syndrome: Diagnostic, mechanisms, CNS involvement and therapy. *Spinal Cord, 41,* 61-75.

Watson C & Vijayan N. (1995). The sympathetic innervation of the eyes and face: A clinicoanatomic review. *Clin Anat, 8,* 262-272.

Waxman SG. (2003). *Clinical neuroanatomy* (25th ed.). Chicago: McGraw-Hill.

Weisbrodt NW. (1998). Autonomic nervous system. In LR Johnson (Ed.). *Essential medical physiology* (2nd ed.). Philadelphia: Lippincott-Raven.

Westlund KN. (2000). Visceral nociception. *Curr Rev Pain, 4,* 478-487.

Williams PL et al. (1995). *Gray's anatomy* (38th ed.). Edinburgh: Churchill Livingstone.

Willis WD et al. (1999). A visceral pain pathway in the dorsal column of the spinal cord. *Proc Natl Acad Sci USA, 96(14),* 7675-7679.

Willis WD & Coggeshall RE. (1991). *Sensory mechanisms of the spinal cord* (2nd ed.). New York: Plenum Press.

CHAPTER 11

Pain of Spinal Origin

Gregory D. Cramer
Susan A. Darby
Robert J. Frysztak

The purpose of this chapter is to apply much of the information from previous chapters to the clinical setting. This is accomplished by discussing the case of a typical patient with low back pain. In addition, structural features of other regions of the spine particularly susceptible to injury or pathologic conditions also are mentioned briefly. The aspects of pain discussed in this chapter are meant to include the most common causes of discomfort. Exhaustive lists are beyond its scope. Fortunately, this subject has been reported thoroughly elsewhere (Kirkaldy-Willis, 1988a; Haldeman, 1992; Cavanaugh, 1995; Greenspan, 1995; Bogduk, 1997; Siddal and Cousins, 1997). This chapter discusses a challenging problem that faces clinicians continuously: their patients' pain.*

PATIENT BACKGROUND

On a bright Monday afternoon in January, Mr. S., a 40-year-old man, enters the waiting room. The receptionist recognizes Mr. S. as a previous patient. As she hands him a form inquiring about the details of his chief complaint, she notices his extremely slow gait and guarded stance. The receptionist retrieves his previous records while Mr. S. diligently fills out the form. At the earliest opportunity the receptionist hands the clinician the file previously compiled on Mr. S. and mentions that he appears to have "a nasty case of low back pain." As the practitioner (you) reviews the records, he or she immediately recalls Mr. S. as a patient from 3 years earlier. He had strained the muscles of his lower back while unloading bags of dry cement mix that he was planning to use for a home improvement project. The clinician suspects his complaint today may be related to this prior incident, and begins to analyze the perception of pain.

*Because of the clinical nature of the material in this chapter, no red rules to highlight information have been placed in the margins.

PERCEPTION OF PAIN

The general approach to patients complaining of pain is that it is real. It has both physical and psychologic components, one of which may predominate, and the pain always alters the personality of the individual (Kirkaldy-Willis, 1988b; Burton et al., 1995; Gillette, 1996; Kummel, 1996; Hildebrandt et al., 1997). This alteration of personality usually returns to the prepain state when the physical cause of the discomfort has sufficiently healed. In addition, pain always has a subjective component and is perceived by patients in relation to previous experiences with pain, usually from their early years (Weinstein, 1988).

Pain has been defined by the International Association for the Study of Pain as "an unpleasant sensory and emotional experience associated with actual or potential tissue damage, or described in terms of such damage" (Merskey, 1979). This group's committee on taxonomy goes on to state, "If a patient regards their experience as pain and if they report it in the same ways as pain caused by tissue damage, it should be accepted as pain" (Merskey, 1979). Therefore not all pain is the result of a nociceptive stimulus received and transmitted by a sensory receptor of a peripheral nerve (Weinstein, 1988).

Many other factors may influence the patient's perception of pain, including the following: the individual's general health, the nervous system's overall status, the pain's chronicity, and even the environment in which the patient lives (Haldeman, 1992). In addition, a person's work environment, work activities, and work satisfaction have all been found to affect the occurrence and outcome of back pain (Macfarlane et al., 1997; Pappageotgiou et al., 1997). Finally, the dorsal root ganglia, spinal cord, and higher centers are all capable of adjusting and regulating (modulating) painful stimuli. Therefore to continue with the example of Mr. S., the clinician may not fully appreciate and understand the severity of Mr. S.'s pain until he or she has had an opportunity to observe him on several different occasions (Kirkaldy-Willis, 1988b).

The characteristics and quality of pain, such as that experienced by Mr. S., can be important. For example, diffuse burning pain, which may or may not radiate into the lower extremity, can be of sympathetic origin. The afferent fibers of the recurrent meningeal nerve travel with sympathetic fibers. The peripheral (sensory) receptors of the nerves may be stimulated by arachnoiditis and postoperative fibrosis and could be a source of diffuse burning pain of sympathetic origin (Kirkaldy-Willis, 1988b). However, aching usually is the result of muscle tightness or soreness and frequently is relieved by stretching and short periods of rest. Other generalized lower extremity pain, excluding aching pain, often is associated with a vascular or neurogenic cause (Weinstein, 1988).

PAIN OF SOMATIC ORIGIN

The clinician now begins to consider the possible causes of Mr. S.'s current discomfort. Low back pain (LBP) can be defined as pain in the lumbar or sacral region that is "not more than a handbreadth" away from either side of the patient's vertebral column (Bogduk, 1992). Even though LBP is one of the most common complaints seen by physicians, it is one of the most difficult to understand (Weinstein, 1988). Recall that an anatomic structure must be supplied by nociceptive nerve endings (nerve endings sensitive to tissue damage; see Chapter 9) to be a cause of LBP, and Mr. S.'s perception of his LBP greatly depends on the factors described previously. Noncutaneous nociceptors are found in muscles, tendons, joint capsules, periosteum, perivenous tissues (vasa nervorum), and several visceral tissues (Greenspan, 1997). Therefore these are all potential sources of Mr. S.'s discomfort. Also recall that nociceptors may be stimulated by mechanical, thermal, or chemical means. Because the structures that receive nociceptive innervation are able to "generate pain," they are sometimes called pain generators. (Notice that the presence of the nociceptive endings in the damaged tissue is what actually allows the structure to function as a pain generator.) The nociceptive nerve endings respond to tissue damaging or potentially tissue damaging stimuli; that is, nociceptive nerve endings can fire before tissue damage actually occurs, thereby possibly preventing injury (Greenspan, 1997).

Once a nociceptor has depolarized, intrinsic and extrinsic physiologic changes can occur in its membrane properties that frequently allow it to become more sensitive to subsequent noxious stimuli. This increased sensitivity is known as hyperalgesia. The central nervous system (CNS) has several mechanisms by which it, too, may create hyperalgesia from an area of injury. Therefore after tissue is damaged, it is usually more sensitive to further nociception until healing has occurred. After pathologic conditions or injury, hyperalgesia also may be present in the healthy tissues surrounding the site of the lesion.

Frequently nociception of spinal origin is the result of damage to several structures, and the effects of hyperalgesia allow for nociception to be felt from tissues that, if injured to the same degree independently, might have gone unnoticed (Haldeman, 1992). (Hyperalgesia and other related concepts are discussed in further detail in the section Important Terms and General Concepts Related to Pain.)

Most pain has a physical cause, even though not all the structures supplied by nociceptors, and therefore capable of producing pain, are known (Haldeman, 1992). Those tissues that are supplied by nociceptive nerve endings usually can undergo a number of different pathologic processes that can lead to direct stimulation or sensitization of nociceptors (Haldeman, 1992).

One of the best ways to organize Mr. S.'s possible pain generators is to list them according to the four main sources of neural innervation to spinal structures: the anterior primary division (APD, ventral ramus), posterior primary division (PPD, dorsal ramus), recurrent meningeal nerve, and sensory fibers that course with the sympathetic nervous system (Fig. 11-1). All these afferent nerves have their cell bodies in the dorsal root ganglia (DRGs), which, with the exception of C1 and C2 (see Chapter 5), are located within the intervertebral foramina (IVFs) of the vertebral column. Note that the sensory fibers that are associated with the recurrent meningeal nerve and sympathetic nervous system provide a route for the transmission of nociception from somatic structures of the vertebral column's anterior aspect. Fibers arising from these sources pass through the APD for a short distance before reaching the spinal nerve. They then enter the dorsal root. Even though these nerves briefly pass through the ventral ramus,

they are best considered separately because they are important to nociception of spinal origin.

Anterior Primary Divisions (Ventral Rami)

To approach the cause of the discomfort experienced by Mr. S., first consider those structures innervated by the lumbar APDs (Box 11-1). The APDs of the lumbar region innervate much of the gluteal and inguinal regions, as well as the entire lower extremity. Although these regions may refer to the low back, they usually are accompanied by more localized pain from the structure that is either injured or affected by some form of pathologic process. More likely causes of back pain originating from structures innervated by APDs (ventral rami) are several muscles, including the psoas major, quadratus lumborum, and lateral intertransversarii. Strain or possibly increased tightness (what some would call "spasm") of these muscles can be a source of back pain. Abscess

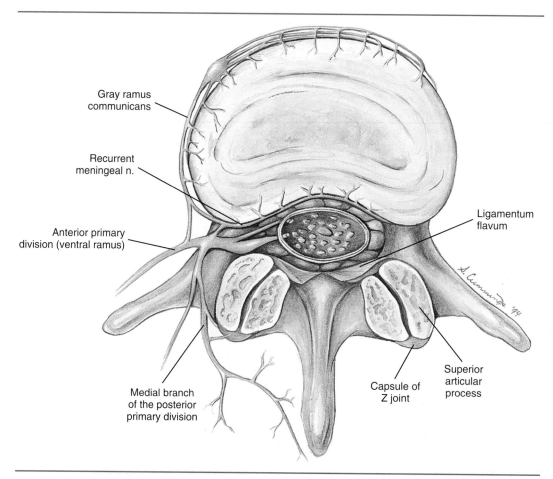

Gray ramus communicans

Recurrent meningeal n.

Anterior primary division (ventral ramus)

Ligamentum flavum

Medial branch of the posterior primary division

Capsule of Z joint

Superior articular process

FIG. 11-1   Horizontal view of a lumbar vertebra, the intervertebral foramina, the vertebral foramen, and the nerves associated with this region. Notice the innervation to the zygapophysial joint by the medial branch of the posterior primary division. Also notice the recurrent meningeal nerve innervating the posterior aspect of the intervertebral disc. The recurrent meningeal nerve also innervates the posterior longitudinal ligament and the anterior aspect of the spinal dura mater.

BOX 11-1
SPINE-RELATED STRUCTURES INNERVATED BY THE VENTRAL RAMUS

Possible Pain Generators

♦ Referred pain from structures innervated by nerves of the lumbar plexus
♦ Psoas muscle
♦ Quadratus lumborum muscle
♦ Intertransversarii muscles (lateral divisions)

within the psoas muscle also is a possible source of pain. The transverse processes (TPs) are innervated by the APD too, and a fracture of a TP or bruise to its periosteum may result in pain (Bogduk, 1983).

Posterior Primary Divisions (Dorsal Rami)

Discomfort such as that experienced by Mr. S. also may arise from structures innervated by the PPDs (dorsal rami) listed in Box 11-2. This list contains some of the most frequent causes of LBP, including the deep back muscles, which receive nociceptive innervation by means of nerves accompanying the vessels that supply these muscles; spinal ligaments (nociceptors are most numerous in the posterior longitudinal ligament, innervated by the recurrent meningeal nerve, and fewest in the interspinous ligament and ligamentum flavum); and the zygapophysial joints (Z joints). These are all high on the list of possible causes of pain similar to that

BOX 11-2
STRUCTURES INNERVATED BY THE DORSAL RAMUS

Possible Pain Generators

MEDIAL BRANCH OF THE DORSAL RAMUS INNERVATES

♦ Deepest back muscles (see Table 4-2)
♦ Zygapophysial joints
♦ Periosteum of posterior vertebral arch
♦ Interspinous, supraspinous, and intertransverse ligaments, ligamentum flavum
♦ Skin (in the case of upper cervical, middle cervical, and thoracic dorsal rami)

LATERAL BRANCH OF THE DORSAL RAMUS INNERVATES

♦ Erector spinae muscles
♦ Splenius capitis and cervicis muscles (cervical region)
♦ Skin

experienced by Mr. S. (Cavanaugh, 1995). Each of these groups of structures may be affected by a number of pathologic conditions or injuries. The muscles may be strained or affected by areas of myofascial tenderness ("trigger points") (Bogduk, 1983; Hubbard and Berkoff, 1993). The ligaments may be sprained. Pain from the Z joints may be difficult to localize because each Z joint receives innervation from the PPD of the same level and also from the PPD of the level above (Bogduk, 1976) and below (Jeffries, 1988). The Z joints may be fractured (fracture of an articular process) or inflamed as a result of arthritic changes. Discomfort also can arise from a Z joint articular capsule or synovial fold (Giles, 1987; Schwarzer et al., 1994) that has become entrapped within the Z joint or pinched between the articular surfaces (see Chapter 7). Degeneration of articular cartilage may produce inflammatory agents that may stimulate nociceptors of the Z joint articular capsules. Inactivity of the spinal joints, even if this inactivity is imposed on these joints by muscle guarding, may promote degeneration (Cramer et al., 2004) (Fig. 11-2) and pain (Kirkaldy-Willis, 1988b). In addition, the spinous processes may be fractured or may repeatedly collide with one another (Baastrup's syndrome). Finally, Sihvonen et al. (1995) found that the medial branch of the posterior primary division can become irritated or entrapped along its course, causing weakness of transversospinalis muscles (i.e., semispinalis, multifidus, and rotatores muscles) and low back pain. The LBP in this instance presumably results from irritation of the medial branch of the posterior primary division and also from abnormal stresses and loads being placed on pain generators of the spine as a result of the biomechanical changes caused by the muscle weakness.

Recurrent Meningeal Nerve

Structures innervated by the recurrent meningeal (sinuvertebral) nerve also may be a source of back pain (Raoul et al., 2002). The list in Box 11-3 identifies the structures supplied by these nerves. The periosteum of a vertebral body may be affected by fracture or neoplasm within the vertebral body. The basivertebral veins may be affected by intraosseous hypertension, crush fractures, or neoplasms of the vertebral body (Bogduk, 1983). The epidural veins may be affected by venous engorgement. The posterior aspect of the intervertebral disc (IVD) is also a pain generator (Schwarzer et al., 1994; Cavanaugh, 1995) that can be affected by internal disc disruption, protrusion of the nucleus pulposus through the outer layers of the anulus fibrosus, or tearing (sprain) of the outer layers of the anulus fibrosus (AF). Of related importance is that sensory innervation of degenerated IVDs extends into the deeper layers of the anulus fibrosus. That is, the process of IVD degeneration seems to

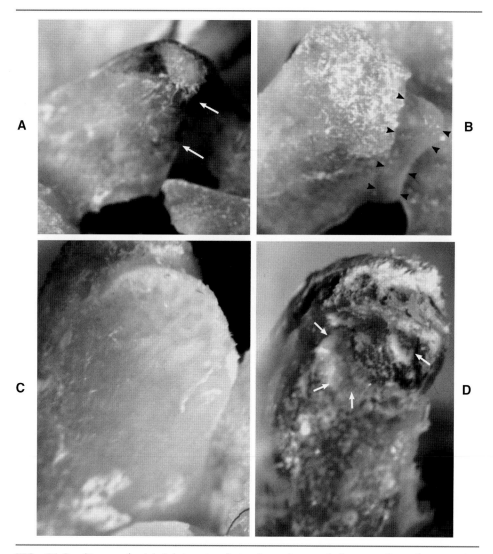

FIG. 11-2 Zygapophysial joint osteophyte formation and facet surface degeneration following induced hypomobility in an animal model (rat). The external surfaces of two L5 superior articular processes are shown in **A** (8-week control animal) and **B** (8-week fixation/hypomobility animal). **A,** Notice that the cephalad edge of the articular process is smooth in the control animal (*small white arrows*) with no signs of osteophytes, whereas in **B** a prominent osteophyte (*arrowheads*) is seen on the cephalad portion of the articular process of the 8-week fixation/hypomobility animal. The internal surfaces of two L5 superior articular facets are shown in **C** (1-week control animal) and **D** (4-week fixation/hypomobility animal). **C,** Notice that the articular facet of the control animal is smooth, whereas in **D** that of the 4-week fixation/hypomobility animal has marked roughening, pitting, and remodeling. The deep pitting is identified with white arrows. **D,** The remodeling is so marked that the ventral portion of the articular process (*bottom*) is out of the plane of maximum focus. (From Cramer GC et al. [2004]. Degenerative changes following spinal fixation in a small animal model. *J Manipulative Physiol Ther, 27,* 141-154.)

stimulate the nerves innervating the posterior, lateral, and anterior aspects of the IVD to grow deeper into the IVD, probably making them more capable of providing nociceptive sensation (Yoshizawa, O'Brien, and Thomas-Smith, 1980). Also innervated by the recurrent meningeal nerves is the posterior longitudinal ligament, which can

be torn (sprained) during severe hyperflexion injuries or may be pierced by an IVD protrusion. In addition, the anterior aspect of the dura mater may be compressed by an IVD protrusion or irritated by the release of chemical mediators associated with internal disc disruption (see Chapter 7).

Nerves Associated with the Sympathetic Nervous System

Finally, recall that several structures are innervated by nerves that arise directly from the sympathetic trunk and gray communicating rami (Box 11-4). The sensory fibers of these nerves follow the gray rami to the APD, where they enter the spinal nerve. They then reach the spinal cord by coursing through the dorsal roots. Pathologic conditions of the periosteum of the anterior and lateral aspects of the vertebral body, which are innervated by sensory fibers traveling with gray rami, may result in pain. Some of the most common causes of this type of pathologic condition include fracture, neoplasm, and osteomyelitis (Bogduk, 1983). Sprain of the anterior longitudinal ligament or outer layers of the anterior or lateral part of the anulus fibrosis also may result in nociception conducted by fibers that course with the gray communicating rami.

Under certain circumstances, the sympathetic nervous system can play a complex role with regard to pain (Jorgensen and Fossgreen, 1990; Budgell, Hotta, and Sato, 1995; Siddall and Cousins, 1997). Vascular changes, changes in perspiration (sudomotor), and changes in nail, hair, and bone structure can accompany chronic pain associated with the sympathetic nervous system

(Siddall and Cousins, 1997). This pain often is burning in nature and is associated with increased stimulation of sensory receptors. This is accompanied by an increased perception of pain in areas not associated with tissue damage (hyperalgesia), and also by an increased sensitivity to mechanical stimulation, including mechanical stimulation that previously would not be considered capable of producing pain (allodynia). The mechanism may be related to the finding that nociception from damaged or regrowing nerves and even nearby axons sometimes can be activated by norepinephrine from sympathetic stimulation. This activation is thought to result from alpha-adrenergic (norepinephrine) receptors developing on C (nociceptive) fibers after partial nerve injury (Greenspan, 1997). Once known as reflex sympathetic dystrophy, the term *complex regional pain syndrome* is now preferred (Plancarte and Calvillo, 1997). The pain of some patients with complex regional pain syndrome is related to the sympathetic nervous system (sympathetically maintained pain), although others' pain is not (sympathetically independent pain) (Greenspan, 1997). (See Sympathetically Maintained Pain later in this chapter and Complex Regional Pain Syndrome in Chapter 10).

Pain Generators Unique to the Cervical Region

If Mr. S. is also presenting with pain in the cervical region, other structures should be included on the list of possible pain generators. These include irritation of the nerves surrounding the vertebral artery and nociception arising from uncovertebral "joints."

Nociception arising from almost any structure innervated by the upper four cervical nerves may refer to the head, resulting in head pains and headaches (Campbell and Parsons, 1944; Edmeads, 1978; Bogduk, Lambert, and Duckworth, 1981; Bogduk, 1984; Aprill, Dwyer, and Bogduk, 1990; Dwyer, Aprill, and Bogduk, 1990; Darby and Cramer, 1994; Cramer, 1998). Pain originating from the region of the basiocciput and occipital condyles frequently refers to the orbital and frontal regions (Campbell and Parsons, 1944). A discussion of neck pain and its relationship to headache and head pain has been fully covered elsewhere (Vernon, 2001), and is beyond the scope of this chapter.

Autonomic reactions such as sweating, pallor, nausea, alterations of pulse, and other autonomic disturbances frequently have been observed in association with disturbances of the suboccipital and upper cervical spine. The intensity of these autonomic reactions seems to be proportional to the stimulus and proximity of the stimulus to the suboccipital region. The autonomic response ranges from mild subjective discomforts to measurable objective signs (Campbell and Parsons, 1944).

Pain Generators Unique to the Thoracic Region

If Mr. S. should present with discomfort of the thoracic region, the costocorporeal and costotransverse articulations should be added to the list of possible pain generators (see Chapter 6). Also a compression fracture of one or more of the thoracic vertebral bodies could be a realistic source of acute pain arising from the thoracic region.

Dorsal Root Ganglia

The neurons located in the dorsal root ganglia (DRG) serve as modulators of spinal nociception. They contain many neuropeptides (see Chapter 9) associated with the transmission of nociception (e.g., substance P, calcitonin gene-related peptide [CGRP], vasoactive intestinal peptide) (Weinstein, Claverie, and Gibson, 1988). These neuropeptides and other neuromodulators are secreted from the peripheral terminals of sensory nerves that transmit nociception. These substances are manufactured in the cell bodies of the DRG and reach the peripheral terminals (sensory endings) and the synaptic boutons found in the dorsal horn of the spinal cord by axonal transport mechanisms. The presence of neuropeptides and neuromodulators around the receptors may sensitize the receptors, making them more susceptible to depolarization (Weinstein, Claverie, and Gibson, 1988). (See the sections Important Terms and General Concepts Related to Pain, and Modulation of Nociception for more information on the modulation of nociception at the level of the peripheral nerve endings.)

SOMATIC REFERRED PAIN

Nociception arising from any of the somatic structures previously listed may be perceived by Mr. S. or a similar patient as being a considerable distance from the pain generator, even in an area innervated by different nerves than those innervating the pain generator. This is known as pain referral. The term *somatic referred pain* has been used to describe this type of back pain (Bogduk, 1992, 1997).

Several possible mechanisms of pain referral exist. Perhaps one of the most important mechanisms is the result of the internal organization of the spinal cord. The nociceptive information coming in from a pain generator is dispersed by either ascending or descending fibers that make up the dorsolateral tract of Lissauer (see Chapter 9). These fibers may ascend or descend several cord segments before synapsing. Thus nociceptive information, entering from several different spinal cord segments, converges on the same interneuronal pool; therefore this interneuronal pool receives primary sensory information from different somatic regions (Fig. 11-3). More specifically, the dorsal horn neurons in the extreme lateral aspect of the dorsal gray horn have been found to receive input from a wide variety of superficial and deep tissues. In fact, spinal tissues have been found to produce more convergence in the spinal cord than other tissues, a phenomenon termed *hyperconvergence* (Gillette, Kramis, and Roberts, 1993). Gillette, Kramis, and Roberts (1993) found that neurons within the skin, Z joint, spinal ligaments, and paraspinal muscles all caused firing of the same dorsal horn neurons. This dispersal of incoming afferents onto different-tract neurons, in combination with the convergence of several different afferents onto single tract neurons, most likely decreases the ability of the CNS to localize nociception (Haldeman, 1992; Darby and Cramer, 1994). In addition, excitatory and inhibitory interneurons found in laminae I and II in the spinal cord can be activated by nonnociceptive afferents, as well as by descending pathways, and also can modulate the output of second-order neurons, thus further altering the ability of the CNS to localize nociception. This type of dispersal and convergence also may be found at the second synapse along the nociceptive pathway. That synapse occurs in the ventral posterior lateral nucleus of the thalamus (see later discussion on pain pathway).

The ventral posterior lateral thalamic nucleus projects to the postcentral gyrus of the cerebral cortex. The region of the back is represented on a small area of the postcentral gyrus (sensory homunculus) of the cerebral cortex (see Fig. 9-5). The small size of the sensory cortex devoted to the back also may contribute to the poor localization of nociception of spinal origin (Haldeman, 1992). In addition, the tract neurons for ascending pain pathways most frequently carry nociceptive information from cutaneous areas. Therefore when the tract neurons are stimulated to fire, the cerebral cortex (where conscious awareness of nociception occurs) may interpret the impulse as originating from a cutaneous or other recently injured region. Either of these regions may be distant to the structure that is currently damaged or inflamed. This phenomenon sometimes is called pain memory (Carpenter and Sutin, 1983; Wyke, 1987; Nolte, 1988).

The existence of pain referral between somatic structures has been documented for some time (Kellgren, 1938; Inman and Saunders, 1944; Hockaday and Whitty, 1967; McCall, Park, and O'Brien, 1979). The term somatic referred pain is used currently when discussing pain of somatic origin that is felt distant to the structure generating the nociception (Box 11-5). This type of pain is characterized as dull and aching, difficult to localize, and fairly constant in nature (Bogduk, 1997). For future reference, these characteristics of somatic referred pain are highlighted in Box 11-6.

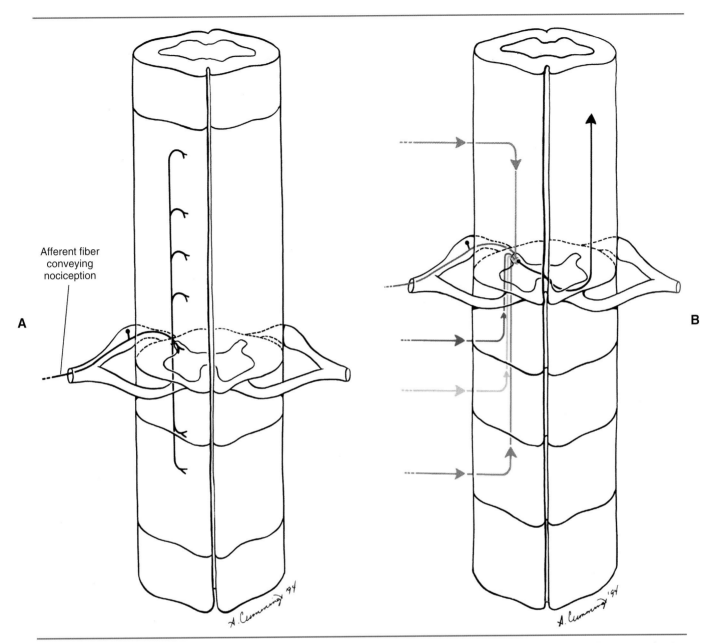

FIG. 11-3   A, Dispersion of afferents conducting nociception as they enter the spinal cord. **B,** Convergence of afferents conducting nociception onto a tract neuron.

Continued

Increased tenderness to deep palpation of the back muscles and hyperalgesia of innervated tissues may occur in areas of referred pain (Weinstein, 1988). An example of somatic referred pain is the pain arising from an inflamed Z joint, which may refer to the groin, buttock, greater trochanter of the femur, and posterior aspect of the thigh, extending to the knee and occasionally extending inferiorly to the leg's posterior and lateral calf (Weinstein, 1988; Yukawa et al., 1997).

Takebayashi et al. (2001) recently identified an additional explanation for pain referring to regions innervated by nerves originating at higher spinal levels than the nerves that typically supply a particular pain generator. These investigators found that, in rats, some of the nerve fibers innervating spinal tissues originate from dorsal root ganglia several segments above those at the same segmental levels as the damaged tissues. In other words, some of the nerves innervating Mr. S.'s L4-5 IVD may originate from his L1 or L2 DRG and refer pain into his inguinal region (innervated by L1 and L2). In rats the fibers that eventually reach the higher dorsal root ganglia course from the pain generator of origin to gray rami communicantes at the level of the pain generator, ascend in the sympathetic chain, and then course through

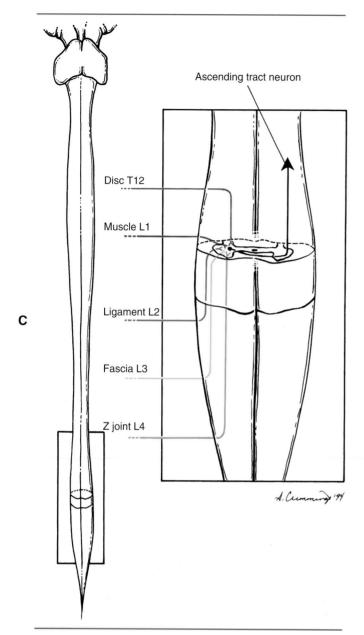

Ascending tract neuron

Disc T12

Muscle L1

Ligament L2

Fascia L3

Z joint L4

C

A. Cummings '94

FIG. 11-3—cont'd   C, Nociception from a variety of sources may influence the same pool of tract neurons.

the IVD at L4-5 or L5-S1 experience groin pain (Yukawa et al., 1997).

The threshold of nociceptors typically is lower than that of pain perception. This may result from the polysynaptic nature of the connections associated with most nociceptors. Many A-delta, and most C fibers synapse on one or more interneurons before reaching tract neurons of the ascending pathway that will transmit their information to the cortex, and each of these interneuronal connections is a site for possible modulation (inhibition). Another possible explanation of the difference in thresholds may result from central modulation of nociception via stimulation of mechanoreceptors (Greenspan, 1997). Consequently, activity of the muscles and the Z joints, as well as spinal manipulation of the Z joints, tends to decrease pain via a "gate control" type of mechanism (Melzack and Wall, 1965; Kirkaldy-Willis, 1988b). The work of Indahl et al. (1997) illustrates this point. In an elegant experiment using 29 adolescent pigs, these investigators stimulated the L3-4 IVD while recording muscle activity (by means of needle electromyography) from the multifidus and longissimus muscles. The stimulation of the IVD created an increased number of action potentials from the spinal muscles. The researchers then injected physiologic saline into the Z joint innervated by the same segmental level. The physiologic saline stretched the Z joint capsule. This resulted in significant decreased muscle activity. The authors concluded that stretching the Z joint capsule decreased multifidus muscle tightness (spasm) that was caused by pain arising from the IVDs (Indahl et al., 1997). Therefore if the pain was of somatic origin, Mr. S. might benefit most from treatment designed to promote activity and movement (Kirkaldy-Willis, 1988b). (See the section Modulation in the Spinal Cord for a more detailed explanation of the gate control theory.) Of related interest is that patients

another gray communicating ramus that connects to an anterior primary division at the higher segmental level. From here the fibers pass through the APD, spinal nerve, DRG, and dorsal root at the higher level before synapsing in the more superior spinal cord segment. This work has been supported by the animal research (also rats) of others (Ohtori et al., 1999, 2001). Therefore the anulus fibrosus of the IVD is supplied by nerves originating from several segments and from both the left and right sides (Nakamura, 1996). Although more work in humans is needed to verify these animal studies, the results are consistent with the findings of clinical research showing that approximately 4.1% of patients with protrusion of

with LBP have been found to have decreased proprioception, as measured by standing and then four-point kneeling 10 times in 30 seconds (Gill and Callaghan, 1998). Consequently, increased activity, joint movement, and rehabilitative and proprioceptive training exercises also may help to improve Mr. S.'s joint position sense. However, recall that under certain circumstances mechanoreceptors can be sensitized to cause pain once tissue damage is well established, probably by means of central sensitization at the dorsal horn of the spinal cord (mechanical hyperalgesia) (Greenspan, 1997). Therefore precautions also should be taken to avoid further compromising any damaged tissue.

All the discussed information was quickly recalled even before the clinician entered the examination room to see Mr. S. Just as the clinician steps into the room, he or she quickly remembers the pathways for the transmission of pain.

CENTRAL TRANSMISSION OF NOCICEPTION

Pain is the perception that results from the cerebral cortex's interpretation of nociceptive input by a variety of CNS structures (Basbaum and Jessell, 2000). Some of the CNS structures that have been implicated in contributing to this process include the dorsal horn of the spinal cord; excitatory and inhibitory interneurons in the spinal cord; ascending pathways; reticular formation of the brain stem; thalamus; and several areas of the cerebral cortex, including the primary sensory cortex, cingulate gyrus, and insular cortex (Craig and Bushnell, 1994; Craig et al., 1996). The interconnections of these areas and subsequent integration of the information result in the components associated with the sensation of pain. These components include discriminatory qualities, emotions, attentiveness to the painful area, and reflex responses involving both the autonomic and endocrine systems (Haldeman, 1992).

The afferent fibers that convey nociception are group A-delta and C fibers. These fibers enter the dorsolateral tract of Lissauer, located at the tip of the cord's dorsal horn. Some fibers continue directly into the gray matter of the dorsal horn, whereas their collateral branches ascend or descend numerous cord segments before entering the dorsal horn (see Fig. 11-3, A). The A-delta fibers convey nociception quickly and rapidly and terminate in lamina I and laminae V to VII. The group C fibers convey what is interpreted as a dull sensation of pain at a slow rate and terminate directly in lamina II and may indirectly (via interneurons) terminate in laminae V and VII. In addition, many of the neurons synapsing in lamina VII originate from both sides of the body, and may further contribute to the diffuse nature of many pain conditions (Basbaum and Jessell, 2000). The neurons that transmit the information to higher centers are located in various laminae of the gray matter (see Chapter 9). Surgical cordotomy procedures that relieve pain have shown that the most important fibers transmitting nociception to higher centers decussate in the ventral white commissure and then ascend in the anterolateral quadrant of the cord's white matter (Hoffert, 1989). Alternative pathways also may be involved, although their course and function in humans remain unclear (Besson, 1988; Hoffert, 1989) (see Chapter 9).

Spinothalamic Tract

The response of the brain to painful stimuli is intricate and complex, and there are several pathways associated with Mr. S.'s LBP. Nociceptive information is conveyed to higher centers by tracts in the anterolateral quadrant of the spinal cord. Two major tracts conduct this information in the cord's anterolateral quadrant, the spinothalamic tract (also called the neospinothalamic tract), and the spinoreticular tract. The spinothalamic tract conveys nociceptive information, which is perceived as sharp, pinpricklike pain, via fast conducting A-delta fibers. The integrity of this tract commonly is tested during a neurologic examination by asking the patient to differentiate the sensations of sharp versus dull. The cell bodies of the tract neurons are both nociceptive-specific and wide-dynamic-range neurons (sensitive to many types of stimuli) that are located in the dorsal horn primarily in laminae I and V to VII (Basbaum and Jessell, 2000). These axons decussate in the ventral white commissure within one or two segments of entry and ascend in the anterolateral white matter of the cord and through the brain stem. They synapse in the ventral posterior lateral nucleus and posterior nucleus, which comprise the lateral nuclear group of the thalamus (Fig. 11-4, A). From the thalamus, axons of the next order neurons course to the somesthetic region of the cortex, which is the postcentral gyrus and the posterior part of the paracentral lobule of the parietal lobe. As the axons of the spinothalamic tract ascend, body parts are represented in specific regions of the tract. This specific pattern is retained in the cerebral cortex, such that a specific area of cortex corresponds to the region of the body from which the sensory fibers originated. This cortical representation is called the sensory homunculus. The size of the body part represented on the homunculus reflects the amount of sensory innervation devoted to that body area. As mentioned, this unequal neuronal representation may be one reason that localization of sensations, such as pain, is more difficult in one region (e.g., back) than another (e.g., fingertips or lips). The information conveyed in the spinothalamic tract is processed in the region of the sensory homunculus. Here the nociception is perceived as pain that is acute, localized, and discriminatory.

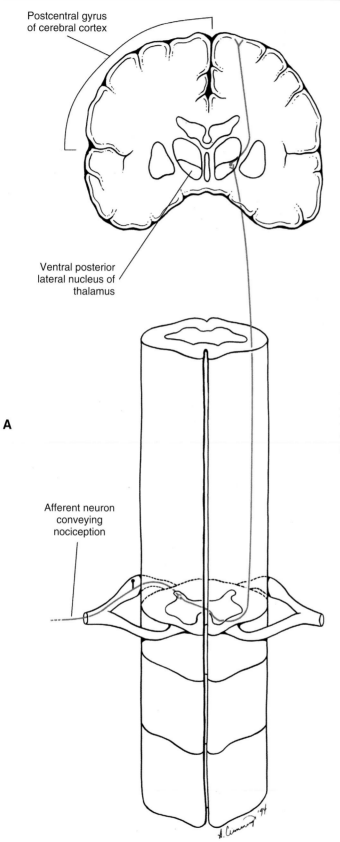

Postcentral gyrus
of cerebral cortex

Ventral posterior
lateral nucleus of
thalamus

A

Afferent neuron
conveying
nociception

FIG. 11-4 Ascending spinal cord tracts associated with nociception. **A,** The neospinothalamic tract is associated with localization of nociceptive stimulation. This pathway also is associated with the evaluation of the intensity of nociceptive stimulation.

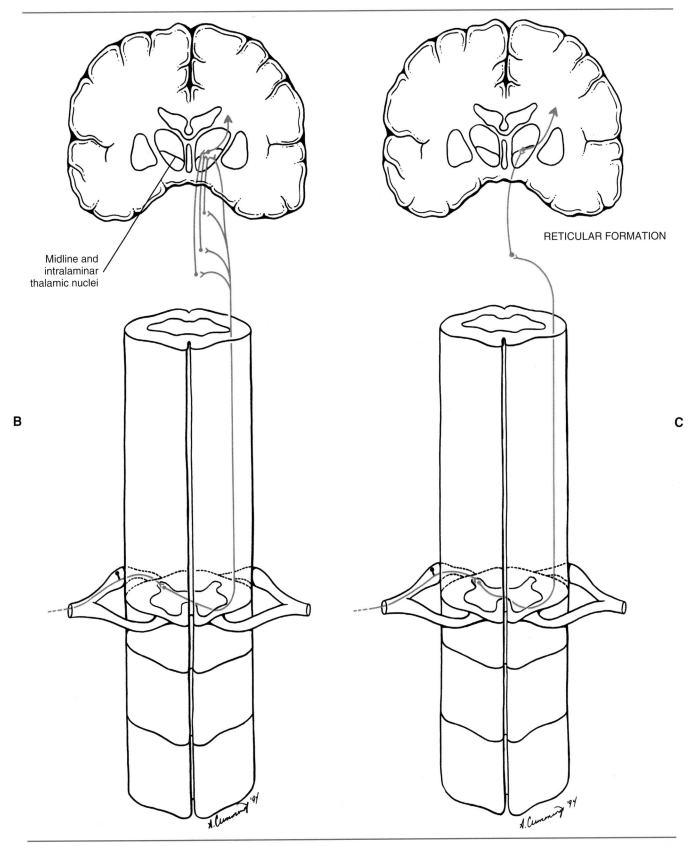

Midline and intralaminar thalamic nuclei

RETICULAR FORMATION

B

C

FIG. 11-4—cont'd   **B,** The paleospinothalamic tract, which sends collateral branches into the brain stem reticular formation, and, **C,** spinoreticular tract are most likely associated with the evaluation of nociceptive input as being unpleasant (painful). They both project to widespread areas of the cerebral cortex and are associated with the body's autonomic response to nociceptive stimuli (e.g., increased sympathetic stimulation).

Spinoreticular Tract

The other tract that ascends in the anterolateral quadrant is the spinoreticular tract (Fig. 11-4, *B* and *C*). The cell bodies of the spinoreticular tract are located in laminae VII and VIII. The nociceptive input to these neurons is polysynaptic; therefore these neurons are likely involved with more complex response properties of pain. The axons of these neurons ascend to the reticular formation of the brain stem and to the thalamus. The reticular formation is a complex network of neurons located throughout the core of the brain stem. It has numerous functions and is a major component of the ascending reticular activating system (ARAS), along with the thalamus and cerebral cortex. The ARAS provides the circuitry through which arousal and attentiveness are maintained. The tract neurons synapsing in the reticular formation form complex connections within this region and subsequently project to brain stem nuclei, the hypothalamus, and the midline and intralaminar nuclei of the thalamus. These latter nuclei are part of the medial nuclear group of the thalamus. Subsequent thalamic projections course to widespread, nonspecific areas of the cerebral cortex. In addition, the paleospinothalamic tract (also known as the spinoreticulothalamic tract) contributes collateral branches to the reticular formation as it ascends through the brain stem to the midline and intralaminar thalamic nuclei. The spinoreticular tract and spinoreticulothalamic fibers are not somatotopically organized. The nociceptive information conveyed in these fibers also may be involved with the generation of chronic pain and the qualities associated with that sensation. The focusing of the individual's attention on the painful area is most likely a function of the ARAS.

Dimensions of Pain

Pain appears to be of two dimensions. One is a sensory portion that is involved with identifying the location, intensity, quality, and other characteristics of the pain for an appropriate motor response. The other is the dimension of affect and motivation. This is the subjective awareness of the unpleasantness of the pain: the desire (motivation) to terminate, reduce, or escape the stimulus. It includes the emotions involved with present, short-term, or long-term implications of the pain (i.e., interference with one's life) and the cognitive processes of how to cope with the pain. Pain is a complex sensation, and multiple pathways that ascend both in series and in parallel terminate in numerous brain stem and cortical regions to participate in its processing. The pathway that serves the dimension of pain sensation is the (neo)spinothalamic pathway, sometimes called the lateral and more direct pathway. As discussed, this path-

way projects to the somatosensory cortex, which in turn projects to other cortical areas such as the posterior parietal lobe and insular cortex. From these two areas, projections continue to other areas (e.g., the amygdala and anterior cingulate cortex) that have reciprocal connections with the prefrontal cortex. This pathway may be involved not only with the rudimentary aspects of pain such as intensity, quality, and location; but also with integrating numerous somatosensory inputs. The integration of these inputs provides an overall feeling of the seriousness or threat of the pain stimulus to the body and self (Price, 2000). The aspect of affect and motivation to pain sensation is served by numerous pathways sometimes collectively called the medial pathway (Cross, 1994; Hudson, 2000; Sewards and Sewards, 2002). The spinoreticular and spinoreticulothalamic tracts (see previous section) and spinomesencephalic and spinohypothalamic tracts (see Chapter 9) terminate in brain stem nuclei, the thalamus, and hypothalamus (Price, 2000). Processing at these levels may produce elementary aspects of pain behavior by involving autonomic activation, escape responses, arousal, and fear. These attributes occur early in pain-processing stages when fear, defensive behavior, and visceral responses occur. The thalamic nuclei of this pathway (midline and intralaminar) project to the limbic system, which allows an individual to perceive a sensation as being uncomfortable, aching, or hurting (Haldeman, 1992). The component of the limbic system receiving this input is the anterior cingulate cortex (see Fig. 9-14). This region is considered to be a major cortical area for processing the emotional (motivational) component of pain (Hudson, 2000; Price, 2000; Raineville, 2002; Sewards and Sewards, 2002). The anterior cingulate cortex is indirectly and directly connected with many other areas including the posterior cingulate cortex, amygdala (which functions in the memory aspects of painful experiences), insular cortex (which functions in the autonomic component of the entire painful episode), parietal cortex, and prefrontal cortex. Because of these interactions, the anterior cingulate cortex may be a region that integrates pain information received from sensory cortices concerning recognition and threat of the painful experience with information received from the prefrontal cortex. This integration is considered important for individuals like Mr. S. to plan how to respond and cope with the painful experience.

IMPORTANT TERMS AND GENERAL CONCEPTS RELATED TO PAIN

The sensations that are generally thought of as painful are all perceptions by the cerebral cortex, and therefore subjective. These perceptions are based on previous experience and understanding that something injurious has occurred to the body. Most painful conditions experienced or described by patients have a physiologic basis, and understanding the mechanisms associated with the stimulation of nociceptors and the subsequent perception of pain is important to properly diagnose and treat any injury. The following section contains a list of many of the common terms used in further describing and differentiating diagnoses related to pain. Many of the terms used to describe, define, or classify pain for diagnostic purposes were developed specifically for use in clinical practice, hence the need here for additional physiologic descriptions to provide information related to the mechanisms associated with a particular term. Each term is followed immediately (in quotes) by the current definition as described by the International Association for the Study of Pain (Merskey and Bogduk, 1994), a physiologic or anatomic description for that term, and finally, a brief description, where appropriate, relating to Mr. S.

Terms Related to Pain

Nociceptor. "A receptor preferentially sensitive to a noxious stimulus or to a stimulus which would become noxious if prolonged." All nociceptors are specialized primary sensory neurons whose cell bodies are located in the dorsal root or trigeminal ganglia. The primary sensory endings are usually in the periphery, and they transmit their information into the CNS via central processes of either the dorsal root ganglia or trigeminal ganglia. There are three major classes of nociceptors: thermal, mechanical, and polymodal. Nociceptors transduce (convert) the mechanical, thermal, and chemical signals into action potentials that synapse in the dorsal horn (or spinal nucleus of the trigeminal nerve) onto second-order "pain" pathway neurons. The pain pathways eventually reach the cortex and are interpreted by the CNS as pain (see Central Transmission of Nociception for a detailed discussion of these pathways). Thermal nociceptors are activated by extreme temperatures ($>45°$ C or $<5°$ C) that could potentially damage the body. Mechanical nociceptors are activated by intense pressure or stretch. Polymodal nociceptors are activated by high-intensity mechanical, chemical, or thermal stimuli (Basbaum and Jessell, 2000). In addition, the viscera and many other tissues (including spinal tissues) contain "silent nociceptors" that normally are not activated by noxious stimuli. These receptors can be dramatically altered by inflammation or chemical insults, resulting in a significant lowering of their firing thresholds and a concomitant increase in their firing rate. Therefore these "silent nociceptors" may contribute to the development of secondary hyperalgesia or central sensitization (described later in this section).

Pain. "An unpleasant sensory and emotional experience associated with actual or potential tissue damage, or described in terms of such damage." Pain is always subjective, and based primarily on past experiences of noxious stimuli and their resulting effect on the body. Sensations such as burning, aching, pinching, stinging, and soreness all warn us that a certain activity or stimulus should be avoided. The greater the stimulus intensity, the greater is the urge for the individual to discontinue or avoid that stimulus in the future. Like the interpretation of all sensory stimuli, pain is a perception or elaboration created by the cerebral cortex based on both sensory and emotional experience associated with a particular set of stimuli. Perception of pain may or may not be directly related to nociception. For example, an injured athlete may not experience pain until after the game is ended. Pain can be classified as acute, persistent, or chronic. Acute and persistent pain motivate individuals to avoid the pain producing activity or seek help, whereas chronic pain appears to serve no useful purpose other than to make the patient miserable. Persistent pain can be further subdivided into either nociceptive or neuropathic pain (see definitions provided later in this section).

Allodynia. "Pain due to a stimulus which does not normally provoke pain." This term is used to describe conditions in which, because of some alteration in the CNS, a stimulus that is normally not painful is now considered painful. For example, light touch or moderate cold may evoke a painful response when applied to one area of the body (abnormal response), but be perceived as nonpainful (normal) elsewhere in the body. Most of the nociceptive afferent fibers entering the dorsal horn undergo a high degree of divergence before synapsing on their second-order pathways. The majority of these synapses are onto interneurons that influence the overall neural tone of the spinal cord associated with spinal reflexes, postural control, and the overall responsiveness of the system. In general, the responsiveness of these interneurons normally is suppressed by descending supraspinal pathways. After an injury, the increased afferent activity associated with nociceptive input may dramatically increase the overall output of the interneurons. Because of the large number of interneurons present in the dorsal horn and their subsequent activation by the increased nociceptive inputs, afferents of non-nociceptive fibers may subsequently activate nociceptive interneurons, thus triggering a painful response to a normally nonpainful stimulus. Allodynia also applies to conditions that may give rise to sensitization (described later in this section), such as sunburn, inflammation, or trauma. During the physical examination for Mr. S., the clinician should be sure to check for and note any nonpainful stimuli (e.g., light touch, wisp of cotton) that elicit a painful response.

Analgesia. "Absence of pain in response to stimulation which would normally be painful." Because pain is a perception controlled by the cerebral cortex, it can be modulated in many ways to alter the incoming nociceptive input and prevent the perception of the noxious stimulus. Every synapse of the nociceptive input is a potential site for modulation, and the CNS has a remarkable set of local (spinal cord) interneurons and descending modulatory pathways exclusively designed to interrupt the conveyance of the nociceptive input. If the input of the nociceptive signal can be attenuated or inhibited before reaching the cortex, then perception of the pain will be reduced or eliminated. (See the section Modulation of Nociception for a detailed analysis of the pathways involved.) In addition, exogenous agents such as aspirin or acetaminophen can alter the biochemical pathways responsible for production of inflammatory (nociceptive) agents, thereby reducing their effect on the nociceptors and thus their input into the CNS. Other agents, such as morphine, can mimic the effects of inhibitory neurotransmitters and dramatically reduce nociceptive input into the CNS.

Central Pain. "Pain initiated or caused by a primary lesion or dysfunction in the central nervous system." Any disease process, trauma, or space-occupying lesion affecting the CNS can alter normal functions of the tracts, nuclei, and cell bodies of the nervous system, including the somatosensory system. Remember that the CNS has no sensory afferents of its own, including nociceptors. Therefore normally it cannot detect the presence of these abnormalities, but alterations in normal functions indicate the presence of these pathologies. Both positive and negative signs can exist after lesions or dysfunctions occur within the CNS. Positive signs (paresthesias) are sensations that normally are not present, but can be experienced after the lesion, and include pain, dysesthesia, or tingling sensations. Negative signs are those that normally are present, but no longer are able to be perceived, such as loss of position sense, touch, or pain. Pressure on tracts can cause the axons to spontaneously fire. If those axons originated from nociceptors or their corresponding afferent pathways, then pain will be perceived coming from the area of the body normally innervated by those nociceptors, even though there is no noxious stimulus present. Nociceptive afferents, especially in the spinal cord and peripheral nerves, are most easily stimulated in this way, because of the limited (or completely absent) myelin present on those fibers. Lesions or dysfunction within the CNS also can cause swelling, edema, ischemia (because of compression of blood vessels), blockage of cerebrospinal fluid (CSF), and distention of the dura, all of which stimulate nociceptors outside of the CNS, thereby increasing the amount of pain associated with CNS lesions. In addition, these lesions can block normal signaling between the periphery and the cortex, or from the cortex to the spinal cord, thereby altering normal function and perception. Any lesion within the CNS that alters the normal processing of nociceptive information can be associated with central pain.

Hyperalgesia or Sensitization. "An increased response to a stimulus which is normally painful." Hyperalgesia differs from allodynia in that hyperalgesia is an increased sensitivity to pain because of a lowering of the nociceptor's threshold for pain by either peripheral or central mechanisms, whereas allodynia is a perception of pain from nonpainful stimuli. Hyperalgesia can be classified as primary (peripheral) and secondary (central).

Primary hyperalgesia. This occurs at the site of the injury when the nociceptive fiber is sensitized or directly stimulated by chemical agents released by the damaged tissue and nearby cells or the neuron itself (Fig. 11-5, *A* through *C*). Substances such as bradykinin, histamine, prostaglandins, leukotrienes, acetylcholine, serotonin, and substance P all directly affect nociceptors by lowering their threshold for activation. After tissue damage, a nociceptor responds with a greater number of action potentials to the same stimulus given before the injury occurred. In addition, some of the substances just listed can directly activate nociceptors, resulting in a further increase in nociceptive input into the CNS. Potassium, serotonin, bradykinin, and histamine all have been identified as activators of peripheral nociceptors (Fields, 1987). Activated nociceptors also can release chemical agents (e.g., substance P and CGRP) at the peripheral terminal that can either sensitize or activate other nearby nociceptors. These chemical agents are synthesized in the cell body (in the DRG) and transported down to the peripheral terminal.

Secondary hyperalgesia. Secondary hyperalgesia occurs during severe or persistent injury. In these situations C fibers fire repeatedly, thereby increasing the firing of neurons in the dorsal horn. This phenomenon is called "wind-up," and is dependent on the release of excitatory neurotransmitters (glutamate) from the C fibers, resulting in long-term changes in the sensitivity of the dorsal horn neurons. The resulting long-term changes in sensitivity are termed *central sensitization* (Fig. 11-5, *D* and *E*). According to Cavanaugh (1995):

"The sensitization of these dorsal horn neurons is characterized by reduced thresholds (allodynia), increased

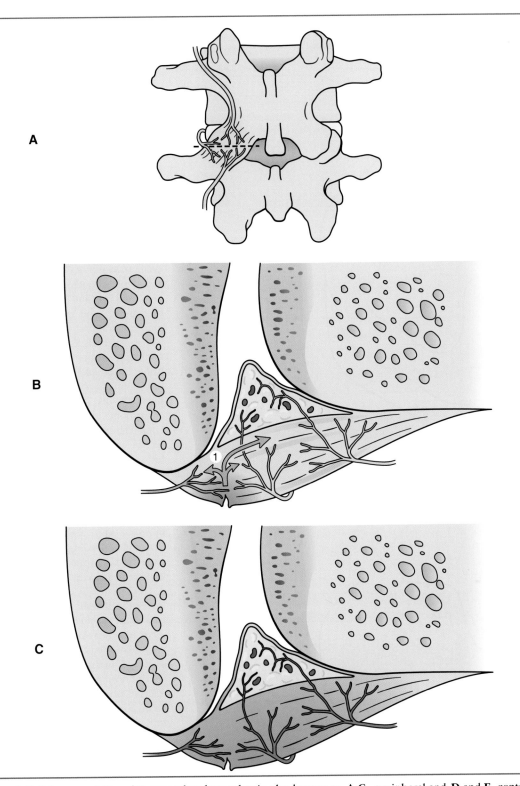

FIG. 11-5 **A-C,** Primary and, **D** and **E,** secondary hyperalgesia, also known as, **A-C,** peripheral and, **D** and **E,** central sensitization. **A,** Posterior view of a zygapophysial (Z) joint showing the innervation of the Z joint capsule from the posterior primary division (dorsal ramus) of the same level, the level above, and the level below. For example, if the vertebrae depicted are L3 and L4, the nerve that is the furthest lateral, *left,* in this figure would be the posterior primary division of the L3 spinal nerve, and the nerves coming from the level above and below would be the posterior primary divisions of the L2 and L4 spinal nerves, respectively. The dashed line through the joint shows the plane of section shown in **B** and **C. B,** Horizontal section of the same Z joint showing a torn area of the posterior aspect of the capsule. The orange color of the nerve to the left indicates that it is firing as a result of the chemokines, 1, that have been released in the area of tissue damage. **C,** Primary hyperalgesia (peripheral sensitization). The red color of the nerves has been used to indicate that they are firing at an increased rate. This means the nerves are responding to the same stimuli they previously experienced (e.g., movement) with a greater number of action potentials. In addition, the neurons are also firing spontaneously because of the chemokines (*1* in **B**) first released from the damaged tissue and subsequently also released from the nerve endings themselves.

Continued

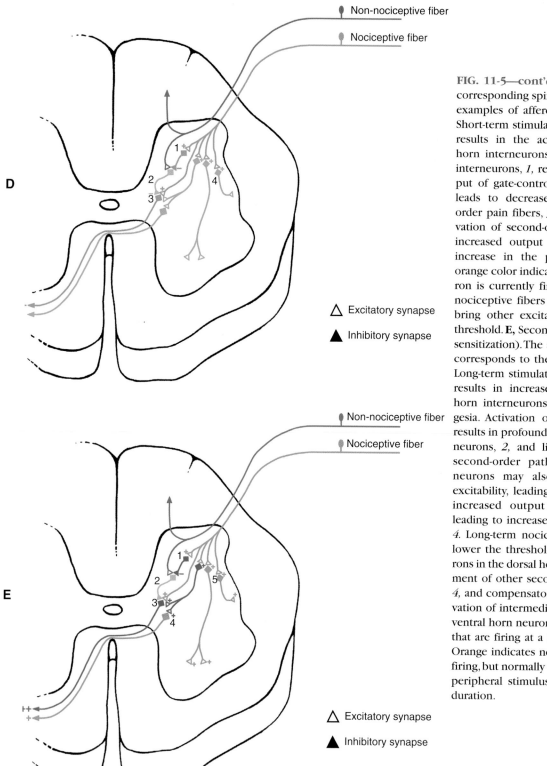

D

Non-nociceptive fiber

Nociceptive fiber

△ Excitatory synapse

▲ Inhibitory synapse

E

Non-nociceptive fiber

Nociceptive fiber

△ Excitatory synapse

▲ Inhibitory synapse

FIG. 11-5—cont'd   D, Cross section of a corresponding spinal cord segment showing examples of afferent neurons shown in **B.** Short-term stimulation of nociceptive fibers results in the activation of many dorsal horn interneurons. Activation of inhibitory interneurons, *1,* results in a decrease in output of gate-control interneurons, *2,* which leads to decreased inhibition of second-order pain fibers, *3.* In addition, direct activation of second-order fibers results in an increased output of these fibers and an increase in the perception of pain. The orange color indicates the second-order neuron is currently firing. Short stimulation of nociceptive fibers may not be sufficient to bring other excitatory interneurons, *4,* to threshold. **E,** Secondary hyperalgesia (central sensitization). The spinal cord segment now corresponds to the scenario depicted in **C.** Long-term stimulation of nociceptive fibers results in increased excitability of dorsal horn interneurons and secondary hyperalgesia. Activation of inhibitory neurons, *1,* results in profound decreases in gate-control neurons, *2,* and little or no inhibition of second-order pathways, *3.* Second-order neurons may also undergo changes in excitability, leading to spontaneous and/or increased output to nociceptive input, leading to increased output of these fibers, *4.* Long-term nociceptive activity may also lower the threshold of excitatory interneurons in the dorsal horn, leading to the recruitment of other second-order pain pathways, *4,* and compensatory effects, *5,* such as activation of intermediolateral (autonomic) and ventral horn neurons. Red indicates neurons that are firing at a higher rate than normal. Orange indicates neurons that are currently firing, but normally would not be firing if the peripheral stimulus was of relatively short duration.

spontaneous discharge, increased response to afferent input (hyperalgesia), increased response to repeated stimulation (wind-up), and the expansion of receptive fields. There is strong evidence that the release of excitatory amino acids and neuropeptides in the dorsal horn after noxious stimulation leads to central sensitization."

This long-term change in the excitability of dorsal horn neurons has been attributed to induction of immediate early genes, which results in upregulation in the expression of neuropeptides, neurotransmitters, and their receptors (Basbaum and Jessell, 2000). Alterations in the biochemical properties and overall excitability of dorsal horn neurons can lead to spontaneous pain, decrease the threshold for the production of pain, and constitute a "memory" for the C fiber input. Mr. S. could be experiencing both primary and secondary hyperalgesia (sensitization) associated with his current condition. Any damage to the vertebrae, IVDs, muscles, ligaments, and surrounding tissues could initiate primary hyperalgesia. In addition, because of his previous injury to this area, the CNS could very well have stored a "memory" for this type of pain in the form of lowered thresholds or increased excitability, and therefore central sensitization also may contribute to the severity of his pain.

Hypoalgesia. "Diminished pain in response to a normally painful stimulus." Hypoalgesia can be achieved by several mechanisms, all of which involve alteration of central synapses. These alterations in central synapses also help determine the overall level of tolerance for pain, or more specifically the threshold for perception of pain. Small to moderate increases in nociceptor activity essentially can be "ignored" by the CNS by increasing the level of inhibition via interneurons at any of the synaptic relays along the pathways to the cortex. Much of this "setting of the gain" of the pain systems occurs at the level of the spinal cord, specifically in the dorsal horn. Inhibitory interneurons found here can be activated by many systems, including nonnociceptive afferents, descending corticospinal tract axons, and other interneurons in the dorsal horn. Once perception of pain does occur, additional descending pathways can further inhibit nociceptive afferents (see Modulation of Nociception).

Neuralgia. "Pain in the distribution of a nerve or nerves." Pain associated with neuralgias is most often described as either lancinating or paroxysmal in quality. The pain can occur spontaneously or be triggered in response to minimal stimuli that normally would not elicit pain (allodynia). The most common example is *trigeminal neuralgia,* or *tic douloureux,* which consists of excruciating, paroxysmal, electric shock–like facial pain in the distribution of one branch of the trigeminal nerve (most often the maxillary division). Pain often is evoked by a tactile stimulus in a particular location,

called the trigger zone. Episodes of pain tend to become more frequent and present a progressively debilitating condition for the patient.

Neurogenic Pain. "Pain initiated or caused by a primary lesion, dysfunction, or transitory perturbation in the peripheral or central nervous system." Neurogenic pain normally involves sensitization of the nociceptors, dorsal root ganglia, and dorsal horn neurons. This includes both central sensitization and the wind-up phenomenon. Polymodal nociceptors normally have little or no spontaneous activity. However, after injury they become sensitized, resulting in increased spontaneous activity, decreased threshold, increased sensitivity to heat or cold, sensitivity to sympathetic stimulation, and antidromic release of neuropeptides (Benarroch et al., 1999). The clinical characteristics of neurogenic pain are spontaneous pain (burning, aching, or shocklike), hyperalgesia, and allodynia. Neurogenic pain includes deafferentation pain, sympathetically maintained pain, and neuropathic pain (see the following).

Deafferentation pain. This type of pain may be a complication of any injury anywhere along the course of the somatosensory pathway. For example, phantom limb pain is associated with peripheral nerves and spinal cord dysfunction after amputation, whereas multiple sclerosis can cause dysesthesia and pain resulting from demyelination in the spinal cord or brain stem. In addition, thalamic syndromes can lead to a severe burning sensation (dysesthesia) after a localized lesion within the thalamus.

Sympathetically maintained pain. This condition most often is characterized by the simultaneous occurrence of pain, local autonomic dysregulation (e.g., edema, vasomotor disturbances, abnormal sweating) and trophic changes of the skin, soft tissues, and bone. These changes most often are associated with lesions of peripheral nerves or nerve roots. Normally most nociceptive afferents have considerable divergence as they enter the dorsal horn, and many nociceptive afferents directly or indirectly activate multiple interneurons, reflex pathways, second-order neurons, and sympathetic neurons (Fig. 11-5, *D* and *E*). The activation of these sympathetic neurons in the intermediolateral cell column results in alterations in blood flow (vasoconstriction or vasodilation, as well as swelling, edema, and possibly trophic changes) that aid in healing injuries. However, this also contributes to sensitization and direct activation of nociceptors at and near the site of the injury (primary hyperalgesia) and typically an increased sensitivity to pain. When these normal physiologic responses continue past the time of healing, they then become pathologic in nature and contribute to sympathetically maintained pain. Two types have been recognized: reflex sympathetic dystrophy, or complex regional pain syndrome (CRPS) I, and causalgia, or CRPS II. CRPS I develops after an initiating noxious event, whereas CRPS II develops after a nerve injury. Although normally the CNS responds to both of these events with an appropriate physiologic response, any alteration or persistence of the sympathetically mediated response is considered abnormal (see also Complex Regional Pain Syndrome in Chapter 10). During the history and physical examination of Mr. S., the clinician should take care to note any of the preceding signs and symptoms to help determine the degree of sympathetic involvement in Mr. S.'s painful condition.

Neuropathic Pain. "Pain initiated or caused by a primary lesion or dysfunction in the nervous system." Neuropathic pain is a type of neurogenic pain. It is normally associated with painful nerve compression (e.g., IVD compression of a dorsal root or DRG) or after formation of posttraumatic neuromas following nerve lesion. This results in abnormal firing of the nerve in areas of demyelination, selective loss of large fiber–mediated segmental inhibition, and increased activity of small nociceptive fibers. The increased activity of the nociceptive fibers is thought to be mediated by local changes in extracellular ionic concentrations (increased Na^+ and decreased K^+ ions), which result in a depolarization of the unmyelinated and demyelinated fibers. Some confusion exists about the definition of neuropathic pain by using a "physiologic definition" of neuropathic pain that erroneously includes central sensitization processes associated with chronic pain (Portenoy, 1996). The use of the term or diagnosis of neuropathic pain should be avoided except in cases in which a clear anatomic lesion or physiologic dysfunction exists within the nervous system. Consequently, the physician should take care to note and substantiate any direct or indirect evidence that points to a lesion or dysfunction of the nervous system. If Mr. S. has an IVD compressing a dorsal root or DRG this could lead to neuropathic pain.

Nociceptive Pain. "Pain induced by direct stimulation of nociceptive afferents." Portenoy and Kanner (1996) defined nociceptive pain as "pain that is believed to be commensurate with the presumed degree of ongoing activation of peripheral nociceptors." Nociceptive pain is directly related to activation of normal pain mechanisms in response to tissue injury. Therefore any injury or condition that causes an increase in the normal activity of nociceptive afferents could be nociceptive pain *if* that increase in activity is recognized by the cortex. Indeed most nociceptive pain often is more severe than the perceived intensity of the stimulus because of the extensive network of inhibitory connec-

tions that exist to alter the threshold for perception of pain. The severity of the injury is not always directly related to the amount of pain perceived by the subject. Some overt injuries may produce an obvious painful condition. However, there are many stimuli (e.g., changes in local extracellular ion concentrations) that can activate nociceptors without obvious trauma or injury to the site of the painful condition. Acute pain is directly attributable most often to some trauma or altered condition that directly activates the nociceptors. However, chronic pain is much harder to define and treat, because the initial cause of the pain (activation of nociceptors) can be altered dramatically by central mechanisms. Stimulation of the nociceptors resulting from the initial injury may be dissociated from the ongoing perception of pain long after the injury has healed because of changes in second-order fibers, interneurons, and descending pathways. Therefore chronic pain may no longer be attributable to nociceptive pain.

Many of the structures in and around the lower back are possible pain generators that can initiate nociceptive pain and should be closely investigated in Mr. S. These structures include the muscles, tendons, joint capsules, periosteum, perivenous tissues (nervi vasorum), visceral tissues (Greenspan, 1997), transverse and spinous processes, spinal ligaments, Z joints, and the IVDs and the nerves themselves (nervi nervorum).

Pain Threshold. "The least experience of pain which a subject can recognize." Threshold was traditionally described as the least *stimulus intensity* at which a subject perceived pain. Because stimulus intensity is an external measure used to elicit a response from the subject, and cannot be a measure of pain, this term (stimulus intensity) was excluded from the current definition. However, pain is an experience defined by the subject, and consequently highly subjective. Therefore threshold is also highly subjective, and is directly related to the subject's current disposition. A subject who is energetic, feeling good, and in generally good health will most likely have a higher tolerance (higher threshold) to pain compared with a subject who is tired, injured, or suffering the effects of a cold, flu, or other seemingly unrelated illness.

General Concept Related to Pain

Physiologic and Pathophysiologic Pain. One method of categorizing pain is to divide it into two basic types, physiologic and pathophysiologic. The latter also is known as clinical pain. Physiologic pain is related to a stimulus (tissue damage) and the response to that stimulus by the nervous system (e.g., nociceptive pain). The response involves the spinal cord, as well as higher centers of the CNS. This type of pain is associated with the "hard-wiring" of the nervous system when responding to tissue damage. Pathophysiologic pain is the result of tissue (including nerve) inflammation and nerve injury inside or outside the CNS. The concept of pathophysiologic pain has developed as more knowledge has been acquired about the changes (some are long-term changes) that occur in the nervous system after tissue damage, and how these changes affect the response of the nervous system to nociceptive input (e.g., peripheral and central sensitization). The concept of pathophysiologic pain is particularly important when considering subacute and chronic pain syndromes (Siddall and Cousins, 1997).

MODULATION OF NOCICEPTION
Modulation at the Level of the Peripheral Nerves and Spinal Tissues (Pain Generators)

Damage to or section of a peripheral nerve results in biochemical and neurophysiologic changes in the nerve and surrounding tissues that lower the threshold of the affected nerve and the nerve endings of other nerves within the affected surrounding tissues (Fig. 11-5, *A* through *C*). These changes are mediated by the nerve endings themselves or by the DRG, and also can cause the nociceptive fibers to fire spontaneously (ectopically). In addition, a decrease in the blood supply anywhere along the course of myelinated nerves can cause a reduction of the myelination that also can lead to ectopic firing of the nerves. Ectopic firing of the afferent fibers is interpreted by the CNS as if a real stimulus onto a specific receptor had produced the event, and these impulses can be perceived as stabbing (sharp), radiating, or burning pain (Siddall and Cousins, 1997). Of related importance is that a much higher incidence of blocked lumbar segmental arteries and the middle sacral artery exists in patients with LBP compared with age-matched controls (Kauppila and Tallroth, 1993). Recall that these arteries supply the dorsal and ventral roots, spinal nerve, proximal portion of the anterior primary division, and a considerable portion of the posterior primary division and its medial and lateral branches. Therefore ischemia to any of these nerve fibers can lead to an increase in the amount of perceived pain through ectopic firing, even though no true peripheral nociceptive stimulus may be present.

Nerve fibers in the region become more sensitive to stimulation once tissue damage occurs, and motions or pressures that normally would not cause pain now may be perceived as quite painful (allodynia). The phenomenon of increased sensitivity of nociceptors after tissue damage is known as peripheral sensitization or primary hyperalgesia. Primary hyperalgesia (sensitization) has been verified experimentally in spinal tissues (Yamashita et al., 1990). This type of sensitization is caused by a combination of pain-mediating chemicals (e.g., substance P, bradykinin, histamine) released from tissue cells in the area of tissue damage, including inflammatory tissue cells (e.g., lymphocytes, mast cells), as well as neurotransmitters and related substances released from the nerve endings innervating the injured tissues. These events can lead to a prolonged sensation of pain to nociceptive stimuli. In addition, certain nociceptors, sometimes called "silent nociceptors," which normally have an extremely high threshold and do not fire even with mild to moderate tissue damage, begin to fire frequently once this "chemical soup" of pain mediators is found in the damaged tissues. Silent nociceptors have been well documented in muscle tissue and joint capsules and are thought to be present in the IVD. They are not found in skin (Cavanaugh, 1995; Greenspan, 1997). These silent nociceptors are also a component of peripheral sensitization. Conversely, endogenous opioids in the peripheral tissue may be released and activate opioid receptors found on the afferent fibers, thus modulating the membrane potential of the afferent fibers and resulting in a decrease of nociceptive input and ultimately in pain perception (Siddall and Cousins, 1997). Therefore the response of the peripheral nervous system to tissue damage is a complex one, and is the result of the competitive effects of pain mediators and endogenous opioids in the region surrounding the sensory nerve endings or a damaged nerve.

Modulation in the Spinal Cord

The neurotransmission of nociception can be modulated at the segmental level by the action of interneurons in the dorsal horn (Fig. 11-6). This mechanism has been known to exist since Melzack and Wall (1965) proposed the gate control theory. Since then the dorsal horn, and especially the superficial dorsal horn, has been extensively investigated. The data from this research have led to numerous questions concerning the details of the gate control theory, and subsequently the theory was revised. However, the general concept of the gate control theory appears to be accepted (McMahon, 1990; Willis and Coggeshall, 1991). Briefly this theory states that increased activity of large-diameter, low-threshold (nonnociceptive) afferents competitively inhibits the transmission of small-diameter (nociceptive) afferent fibers, thus decreasing nociceptive input by tract neurons to higher centers, resulting in a decrease in the perception of pain. This concept has led to effective therapies for relief of pain, such as transcutaneous nerve stimulation and dorsal column stimulation (McMahon, 1990).

The inhibition of the tract neurons conducting nociception most likely comes from a population of interneurons located in lamina II (substantia gelatinosa). Many

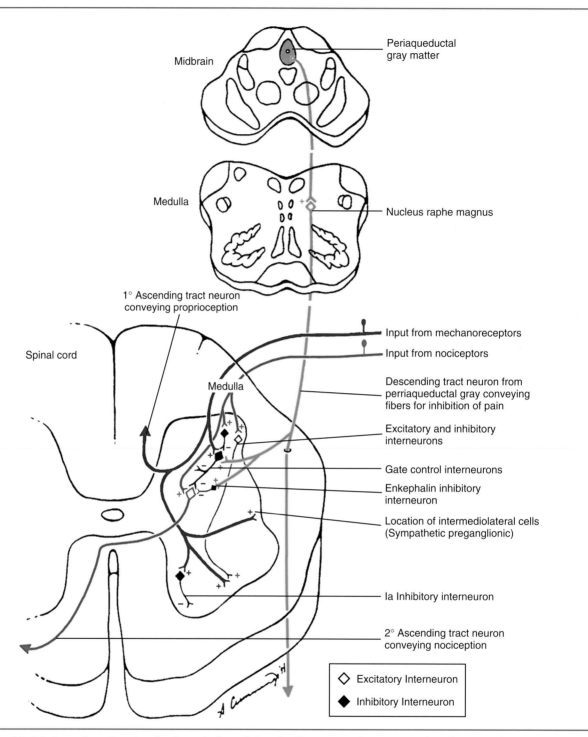

FIG. 11-6 Modulation of nociception in the spinal cord. Local afferents conducting impulses from mechanoreceptors and descending fibers from the nucleus raphe magnus are capable, via inhibitory interneurons, of inhibiting the second order tract neurons conducting nociception. Afferents conducting impulses from nociceptors also synapse onto interneurons in the dorsal horn. In addition, excitatory and inhibitory interneurons in the dorsal horn influence the gate control interneurons affecting nociception, as well as other spinal circuits to the ventral horn and sympathetic preganglionic cells in the intermediolateral cell column. Interneurons therefore play a key role in the modulation of nociception.

of these interneurons use enkephalins as neurotransmitters. These interneurons receive excitatory input (possibly indirectly) from large-diameter, low-threshold mechanoreceptive afferents. The interneurons, in turn, inhibit the neurons conducting nociception (Basbaum, 1984). Consequently a balance between the nonnociceptive inhibitory input and excitatory nociceptive input from small-diameter fibers is mediated by inhibitory interneurons, and is likely to be necessary for the normal processing of nociception (McMahon, 1990). This balance is probably the result of modulation originating from both the complex circuitry of the superficial dorsal horn and descending supraspinal pathways, and may explain, in part, the wide variability associated with tolerance to pain. In addition, stimulation of the nonnociceptive mechanoreceptors immediately after the activation of C fiber nociceptive afferents can reduce the output of the nociceptive neurons and possibly reduce the amount of central sensitization associated with activation of pain pathways. Further research is necessary to clarify this circuitry and its relationship to the descending input from regions in the brain stem (see following discussion).

Supraspinal Modulation

Evidence from studies in which electrical stimulation of regions of the brain stem produced analgesia (Basbaum and Fields, 1978) indicates that descending pathways can modulate nociceptive signals. One of the components of this endogenous pain control system is the periaqueductal gray (PAG) matter of the midbrain. This region has a major projection to the nucleus raphe magnus, which is located in the midline of the rostroventral medulla (see Fig. 11-6). This nucleus is rich in the neurotransmitter serotonin. Serotonergic fibers course into the dorsolateral funiculus of the spinal cord (raphe-spinal tract) from this region, and many fibers synapse on neurons in the superficial dorsal horn (laminae I and II). A second pathway stimulated by the PAG originates in the lateral tegmental nucleus of the brain stem and sends adrenergic neurons to stimulate interneurons that use enkephalin as a neurotransmitter. These interneurons also are found in the superficial dorsal horn of the spinal cord (Basbaum and Fields, 1984; Hendry, Hsiao, and Bushnell, 1999). The superficial dorsal horn receives input from afferent fibers conveying nociception. In addition, this is the location of the origin of the spinothalamic tracts (Basbaum and Fields, 1978; Jessell and Kelly, 1991) and the area involved with the segmental modulation of nociception (see previous section). The descending fibers synapse on several types of neurons. These include the inhibitory interneurons containing enkephalins (an opioid peptide) just discussed, and also the nociceptive projection (tract) neurons. The opioid-

containing (enkephalin) inhibitory interneurons are close to both primary nociceptive afferents and the tract neurons. In fact, the axonal afferent nociceptive endings and the dendrites of the tract neurons both contain opioid receptors (Jessell and Kelly, 1991). Pharmacologic studies have shown that the release of opioid peptides from the inhibitory interneurons block transmission of nociception by two mechanisms (see Fig. 11-6). One proposed mechanism is by binding to receptors on the presynaptic terminals of the primary afferent fibers and blocking their release of neurotransmitters, such as substance P. The enkephalins may bind to μ-opioid receptors by diffusing from their site of release to the presynaptic membrane of the primary afferent fibers (Basbaum, 1987; Besson, 1988; Jessell and Kelly, 1991; Basbaum and Jessell, 2000). The effect of these enkephalins on the presynaptic membrane is to hyperpolarize the membrane or shorten the duration of the incoming action potential (or both), which leads to a decrease in the amount of neurotransmitter released, and therefore a reduction of nociceptive information being transmitted to the CNS.

The second mechanism by which inhibitory interneurons can mediate spinal neurotransmission of nociception is by directly synapsing with the postsynaptic membrane of the tract neuron (see Fig. 11-6). This occurrence has been well documented (Basbaum, 1987; Besson, 1988; Jessell and Kelly, 1991). Through these connections, the tract neuron is made less excitable (by increasing K^+ conductance and thus hyperpolarizing the cell) and nociceptive transmission can be reduced substantially. Recall that the descending fibers from the PAG stimulated the enkephalin interneurons. Therefore analgesia can be produced by neural stimulation of the PAG. Analgesia also can be produced by the administration of opiates, such as morphine, into the CNS. The areas activated by the opiates are similar to those that produce analgesia when the PAG, rostroventral medulla, and enkephalin interneurons in the superficial dorsal horn are stimulated by normal neural transmission. This lends credence to the theory that endogenous opioid peptides, which have been found in the brain, can activate the descending control system to modulate pain perception (Jessell and Kelly, 1991).

In addition to the serotonergic descending pathway, other fibers descend from the pons (Basbaum, 1987; Hoffert, 1989) and appear to be involved with modulation of the nociceptive system. These descending fibers contain norepinephrine and also appear to inhibit nociception at the dorsal horn level. However, at the same time, collateral branches of these fibers synapse on the serotonergic neurons of the raphe nuclei. The subsequent release of norepinephrine at this level results in tonic inhibition of the raphe-spinal neurons (Basbaum, 1987), which tends to increase nociceptive transmission in the dorsal horn. Thus both systems provide a descending component to the mechanism for controlling pain. Feeding into these two systems is the nociceptive information transmitted through the ascending pathways (Basbaum and Fields, 1978). These ascending pathways possibly include the spinomesencephalic tract and input from the reticular formation (see Chapter 9). Also, possibly feeding into the two descending systems is stress-induced input channeled through the limbic system and hypothalamus (Jessell and Kelly, 1991). Therefore supraspinal modulation of pain is a complicated process that can be modulated at many levels by numerous different ascending and descending systems. This allows significant variability in the overall perception of pain based on the degree of tissue injury, physical activity of the individual, stimulation of other sensory systems, mental activity, psychologic factors (including stress), and other influences. Consequently, once the physical cause of Mr. S.'s problem is determined, many factors must be considered when developing a comprehensive treatment plan.

After a brief pause to review the nature of mechanical back pain, the clinician enters the room to greet Mr. S., and is now mentally prepared to consider the pain that is bothering Mr. S.

DIFFERENTIATION BETWEEN PAIN OF SOMATIC ORIGIN AND RADICULAR PAIN

On meeting Mr. S., the clinician notices that he is not seated in the consultation room but instead is standing and partially supporting himself on the edge of the desk located near the center of the room. Mr. S. appears to be in great pain. As the clinician approaches, Mr. S. lets go of the desk and slowly reaches to shake the clinician's hand. The clinician notices that in doing so, Mr. S. leans dramatically to the right and has his left hand placed along his left buttock. The clinician has read Mr. S.'s account of his chief complaint and has noted that he has been experiencing rather mild LBP on and off over the past 2 years. However, this morning while unloading his truck (Mr. S. drives a truck for a prominent soft drink manufacturer, and his job requires him to deliver the soda to grocery and convenience stores), he heard a "pop," and shortly thereafter felt extreme pain in his back that shot "like a lightning bolt" down his left leg (Fig. 11-7). During questioning, Mr. S. states the pain is a dull ache in his low back region (he moves his hand around a rather large area of his lower lumbar area and into his left buttock). He goes on to say that the lightning bolt pain is "on and off" and extends (he points) into his left posterior thigh and leg and the lateral aspect of the sole of his left foot. The clinician carefully questions Mr. S. about somatic and visceral symptoms of the head and neck, thorax, abdomen, and pelvis, and other possible injury to his lower extremity. The inquiries reveal that he has had no significant difficulties or symptoms arising from these regions.

The physical examination reveals Mr. S. to be an individual who, his present state excluded, is physically fit. His vital signs are normal. Chest and abdomen are normal to palpation, percussion, and auscultation, and he has no palpable inguinal hernia. Rectal examination is normal. Examination of his head, anterior neck, and cervical and upper thoracic regions are normal. Cranial nerves and upper extremity sensation, reflexes, and muscle strength are all normal.

Mr. S. has a great deal of muscle guarding of his lumbar region during the examination. The clinician notes marked tightness of his erector spinae muscles (possibly associated with hyperalgesia), and that he is particularly sensitive to percussion over the L5 spinous process. Reflexes, sensory findings (e.g., pinprick, ability to identify touch from a cotton swab, vibration sense), and motor strength of his right lower extremity are all normal. His left extremity reveals slight weakness of plantar flexion, slightly diminished Achilles reflex, and diminished sensation to pinprick and a wisp of cotton along the posterior leg and lateral aspect of the sole of the left foot. Nerve tension signs (straight leg raising and well leg raising) are positive (40 degrees on the left and 60 degrees on the right), reproducing the lightning bolt pain that extends down the left lower extremity into the sole of the left foot.

Because of his antalgic posture, description of a sharp stabbing pain, positive nerve tension signs, decreased sensation, and diminished Achilles reflex, the clinician strongly suspects that Mr. S. has a disc bulge or protrusion of the L5-S1 IVD. The clinician believes that the disc is compressing the S1 dorsal and ventral nerve roots (Figs. 11-7 through 11-9). Compression of this kind results in a type of pain frequently encountered in clinical practice, known as radicular pain. Radicular pain is caused by activation of sensory fibers at the level of the dorsal root or DRG. It is experienced as a thin band of sharp, shooting pain along the distribution of the nerve or nerves supplied by the affected dorsal root (Box 11-7).

Some of the causes of radicular pain include IVD protrusion, spinal (vertebral) canal stenosis (see Chapter 7), and other space-occupying lesions. The list in Box 11-8 shows several additional *causes* of radicular pain. Boxes 11-9 and 11-10 show the most likely *mechanisms* of radicular pain.

Roles of the Dorsal Root Ganglia and Nerve Roots in Pain of Radicular Origin

The results of compression on the DRG and nerve roots are myriad. Notice in Box 11-9 that mechanical deformation affects not only the nerve fibers within the dorsal

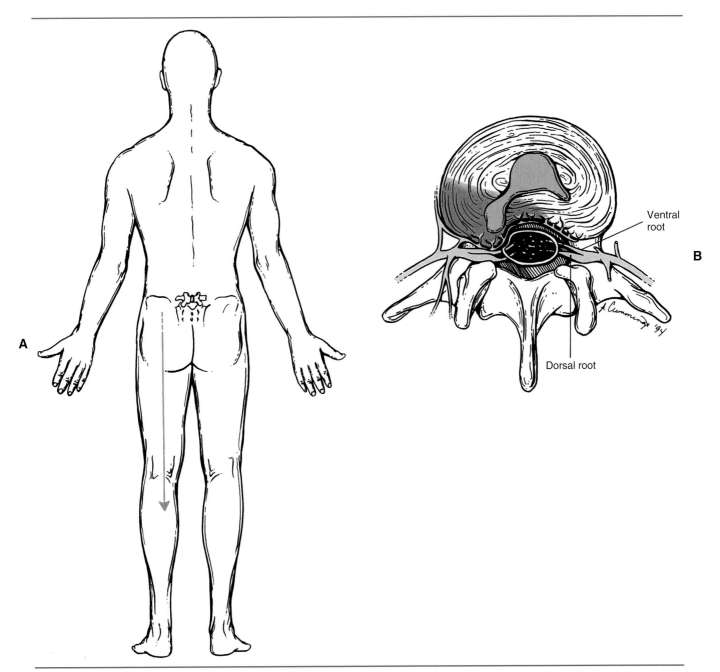

FIG. 11-7   A, Pain radiating into the lower extremity as a result of, **B,** an intervertebral disc protrusion. The disc protrusion is shown compressing the dorsal (and ventral) roots. This is one mechanism by which the sensation described as pain (and called radicular pain) may be felt radiating into the lower extremity. The sensation of pain also may be felt in the lower extremity after injury to or pathologic conditions of somatic structures (e.g., zygapophysial joints, ligaments, deep back muscles). The term *somatic referred pain* has been used to describe radiating discomfort produced by this latter mechanism (which is not demonstrated in this figure).

root, but also the blood vessels and connective tissue elements associated with the root (Dahlin et al., 1992). The spinal cord, nerve roots, and dorsal root ganglia (especially the dorsal root ganglia) are more susceptible to compression than peripheral nerves, and compression or inflammation anywhere along the cauda equina or DRGs can be associated with radiculopathy (Garfin et al.,

1995). Weinstein, (1988) has stated, "The intensity of the pain and its radicular nature are dependent on the strength of the stimulus" (i.e., amount of compression). As noted, the DRG is particularly sensitive to compression (Hanai, Matsui, and Hongo, 1996). Notice also in Box 11-9 that pressure on the DRG eventually results in decreased blood flow to sensory nerve cell bodies,

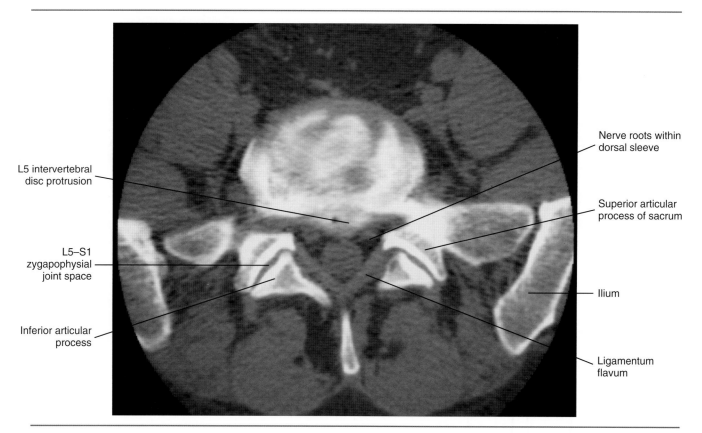

L5 intervertebral disc protrusion

L5–S1 zygapophysial joint space

Inferior articular process

Nerve roots within dorsal sleeve

Superior articular process of sacrum

Ilium

Ligamentum flavum

FIG. 11-8 Computed tomography discogram (radiopaque dye injected into the nucleus pulposus) of the L5-S1 region. Notice that a protrusion of the intervertebral disc can be seen on this horizontal image. The extension of the dye throughout the intervertebral disc (irregular radiopacity throughout intervertebral disc) is an indication of internal disc disruption. The circular structure contained within the "V" formed by the ligamenta flava is the cauda equina within the lumbar cistern and is surrounded by arachnoid and dura (thecal sac). (Computed tomography discogram courtesy Dr. Dennis Skogsbergh.)

which results in neural ischemia, and the neural ischemia is perceived as radicular pain (Rydevik, Myers, and Powell, 1989). In addition, histamine-like chemicals and membrane-bound substances (e.g., phospholipase A_2) within the nucleus pulposus (not in the anulus fibrosus) of a prolapsed or extruded IVD cause inflammation of the DRG, which also results in radicular pain, demyelination of nerve roots, and decreased nerve conduction velocities in the nerves affected by these chemical mediators (Rydevik, Brown, and Lundborg, 1984; Garfin, Rydevik, and Brown, 1991; Chen et al., 1997; Otani et al., 1997; Kayama et al., 1998; Özaktay, Kallakuri, and Cavanaugh, 1998). In addition, nucleus pulposus on nerve roots has been found to result in increased endoneurial fluid pressure, causing what has been called a "compartment syndrome of DRG." This compartment syndrome decreases blood flow in the DRG, augmenting radicular pain (Yabuki et al., 1998; Yabuki, Igarashi, and Kikuchi, 2000). Ectopic impulses (depolarization of neurons without extrinsic stimulation) are thought to occur from these changes and as a result to be one cause of radicular pain. These impulses normally occur during slight

mechanical pressure on the DRG, and may continue for up to 25 minutes after the removal of the compression. These continued ectopic impulses are known as "after-discharges." Such ectopic discharges may be related to the demyelination mentioned earlier in this paragraph. In addition, substance P (a neuromodulator) has been found in the DRGs of experimentally chronically compressed sensory roots in pigs (Cornefjord et al., 1995), and voltage-dependent ion channels are altered in DRGs associated with radiculopathy (Abe et al., 2002). These findings also may contribute to the ectopic discharges. Finally, the receptive fields of the neurons supplied by a compressed DRG are sensitized and expanded after the compression is removed (Cavanaugh, 1995; Hanai, Matsui, and Hongo, 1996).

Exposure of the DRG and nerve roots to both normal and degenerated nucleus pulposus also causes a decrease in the nerve conduction velocities of the axons passing through them (Otani et al., 1997; Iwabuchi et al., 2001; Ozawa, Atsuta, and Kato, 2001) that can take up to 8 weeks to resolve after exposure to nucleus pulposus tissue (Otani et al., 1997). Added to this are the findings

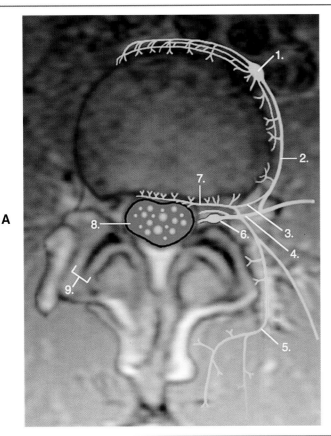

A

FIG. 11-9 The innervation of the intervertebral disc in horizontal section. **A,** Neural elements have been drawn onto a horizontal magnetic resonance imaging (MRI) scan. The top of the illustration is anterior and the bottom is posterior. Numbers indicate the following: *1,* sympathetic ganglion; *2,* gray ramus communicans; *3,* branch of the gray ramus coursing toward the intervertebral foramen to contribute to the recurrent meningeal (sinuvertebral) nerve; *4,* anterior primary division (ventral ramus); *5,* medial branch of posterior primary division (the lateral branch is seen coursing to the reader's right of the medial branch); *6,* dorsal root (spinal) ganglion and dural root sleeve (*red*) within the intervertebral foramen; *7,* recurrent meningeal (sinuvertebral) nerve; *8,* cauda equina (*yellow*) within the cerebrospinal fluid (*blue*) of the lumbar cistern of the subarachnoid space; *9,* zygapophysial joint. Notice that the intervertebral disc is receiving innervation from branches of the sympathetic ganglion (anteriorly), gray communicating ramus (laterally and posterolaterally), and recurrent meningeal nerve (posteriorly). Also notice that the zygapophysial joint is receiving innervation from the medial branch of the posterior primary division. (**A,** Photograph courtesy Ron Mensching and illustration courtesy Dino Juarez, The National University of Health Sciences.)

Continued

BOX 11-7
RADICULAR PAIN

Pain arising from the dorsal root or the dorsal root ganglion. Usually causes pain to be referred along a portion of the course of the nerve or nerves formed by the affected dorsal root. This is frequently along a dermatomal pattern.

BOX 11-8
STRUCTURES AND CONDITIONS THAT CAN IRRITATE THE DORSAL ROOTS (OR GANGLIA)

♦ Disc lesion
♦ Abscess (osteomyelitis and tuberculosis)
♦ Tumor of the spinal canal
♦ Spondylolisthesis
♦ Malformation of the vertebral canal
♦ Malformation of the spinal nerve root and its sheath
♦ Miscellaneous diseases of bone
♦ Histamine-like chemicals released from degenerating intervertebral disc

(Modified from Bogduk N. (1976). The anatomy of the lumbar intervertebral disc syndrome. *Med J Aust, 1,* 878-881.)

BOX 11-9
MECHANISM OF RADICULAR PAIN: 1

Pressure on dorsal root or dorsal root ganglion
↓
Edema within the nerves
↓
Further edema and hemorrhage within the dorsal root ganglion
↓
Decreased blood flow to sensory nerve cell bodies
↓
Ischemia of neural elements
Ischemia perceived as PAIN

(Modified from Rydevik BL, Myers RR, & Powell HC. (1989). Pressure increase in the dorsal root ganglion following mechanical compression. *Spine, 14(6),* 574-576.)

of Anzai et al. (2002), who in experiments using rats, found that nucleus pulposus placed on nerve roots caused wide-dynamic-range neurons of the dorsal horn of the spinal cord to have "enhanced responses to noxious stimuli for hours." Therefore nucleus pulposus placed on nerve roots resulted in the induction of hyperalgesia in rats.

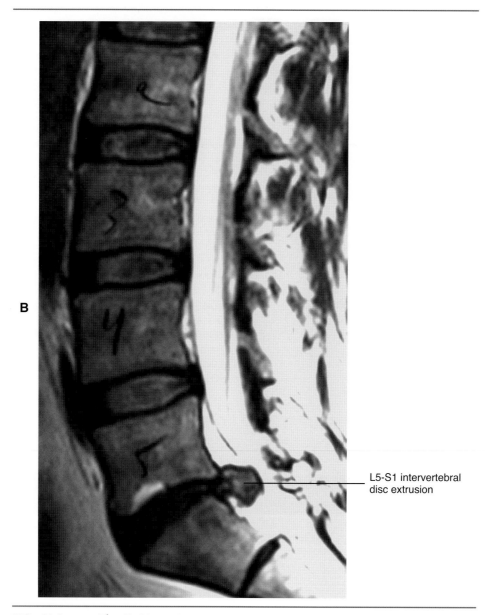

FIG. 11-9—cont'd **B,** Magnetic resonance imaging scan performed in a sagittal plane, showing extrusion of the L5-S1 intervertebral disc. (Magnetic resonance imaging courtesy Dr. Dennis Skogsbergh.)

The dorsal and ventral roots receive sensory innervation themselves via nervi nervorum. The nervi nervorum provide another mechanism by which pressure on the nerve roots can result in pain. The nervi nervorum are most sensitive to stretch, which may help to explain the effectiveness of orthopedic tests designed to stretch the spinal nerve and nerve roots (e.g., the straight leg raise test) (Cavanaugh, 1995). The dorsal and ventral roots originally were verified as a source of back pain by Smyth and Wright (1958), who tied nylon ligatures around nerve roots of patients during lumbar disc surgery and then pulled on the ligatures during the post-surgical recovery period. They found that nerve roots associated with IVD prolapse were much more sensitive to pulling (stretching) of the ligatures than adjacent nerve roots.

The nerve roots in the IVF may respond to pressure differently than those comprising the cauda equina within the spinal canal. The cauda equina may be more sensitive to compression than the distal aspects of the dorsal roots (Dahlin et al., 1992), and even a small amount of pressure (compression) may produce venous congestion of the intraneural microcirculation of nerve roots in the cauda equina (Olmarker et al., 1989). As

> **BOX 11-10**
> **MECHANISM OF RADICULAR PAIN: 2**
>
> Pressure on dorsal root or dorsal root ganglion by
> prolapsed intervertebral disc
> ↓
> Biochemical components of nucleus pulposus "spill" onto
> dural root sleeve of dorsal root ganglia
> ↓
> Inflammation of the dorsal root ganglia
> ↓
> Chemical radiculopathy
> Inflammation perceived as PAIN
>
> (Data from Rydevik B, Brown M, & Lundborg G. (1984).
> Pathoanatomy and pathophysiology of nerve root compression.
> *Spine, 9,* 7-15; and others.)

mentioned when discussing DRGs, the presence of
nucleus pulposus (NP) cells (not extracellular matrix) on
porcine cauda equina also results in decreased nerve
conduction velocities. The decreased conduction velocities result from Schwann cell damage (Olmarker,
Rydevik, and Nordborg, 1993; Olmarker et al., 1996,
1997). Kirkaldy-Willis (1988b) stated:

> Compromise of the cauda equina as a result of spinal
> stenosis may result in unusual sensations which may be
> "bizarre" in nature and may affect one or both limbs. . . .
> He may say that the legs feel as though they do not
> belong to him . . . or are made of rubber.

Other sensory and even motor modalities are also
influenced when a dorsal nerve root is affected (Box
11-11). Therefore radicular pain usually is accompanied
by paresthesia, hypesthesia, and decreased reflexes
(because the sensory limb of the deep tendon reflex is
affected). For the reason that the dorsal root and ventral
nerve root are adjacent to each other, compression of
the dorsal root usually is accompanied by compression

> **BOX 11-11**
> **DISTINGUISHING FEATURES OF RADICULAR PAIN**
>
> ◆ Sharp, shooting type of pain along the distribution of
>   the nerve(s) supplied by the affected dorsal root
> ◆ Long radiation into the upper or lower extremity
>   (although this does not necessarily have to be the case)
> ◆ Pain coursing along a fairly thin band
> ◆ Pain accompanied by paresthesia, hypesthesia, and
>   decreased reflexes
> ◆ Pain may be accompanied by motor weakness (as a
>   result of compromise of the ventral roots)

of the ventral nerve root as well. In addition to stimulation of the nervi nervorum of the root, which results
in pain, compression of the ventral (motor) root results
in motor weakness. Therefore radicular pain often may
be accompanied by motor weakness (see Box 11-11).
Because of the decreased motor function found with
compression of the ventral roots, needle electromyography of the paraspinal muscles can be useful in verifying the diagnosis of radiculopathy in difficult cases
(Haig, LeBreck, and Powley, 1995).

Chronic compression of nerve roots and DRGs results
in other unique physiologic responses. For example,
serotonin, a neurotransmitter previously discussed as
being involved in pain modulation, results in vasoconstriction in the blood vessels supplying nerve roots that
are chronically compressed but causes vasodilation of
vessels of healthy (uncompressed) nerve roots (Sekiguchi
et al., 2002). However, chronically compressed nerve
roots also seem to adapt to some extent. Kikuchi et al.
(1996) found that chronically compressed nerve roots
are less sensitive to acute compression than noncompressed nerve roots.

What may seem to some as an unrelated activity can
cause changes in the DRG in certain individuals. Whole
body vibration has been established as one cause of
LBP. Morphologic changes in the DRGs (i.e., increase in
number of mitochondria, lysosomes, and nuclear membrane clefts) have been found with whole body vibration
in rabbits. These changes are consistent with the formation of neuropeptides. This suggests the potential for
similar changes in humans with occupations attended by
whole body vibration. Such occupations include truck
driving, certain highway maintenance, and some construction occupations (McLain and Weinstein, 1991).
Because Mr. S. has this type of occupation (driving a
truck), his sensory neurons may be sensitized to additional stimulation.

Combined Somatic Referred and Radicular Pain

In addition to the radicular signs and symptoms just
discussed, Mr. S. also has diffuse LBP. This leads the
clinician to suspect that he may be experiencing two
different types of pain: somatic referred (nociceptive)
and radicular (neuropathic) pain.

Recall that pain of somatic origin displays certain
characteristics. Some of the generalized discomfort experienced by Mr. S. may be emanating from a lesion of a
somatic structure. A review of possible somatic pain
generators is useful, because only those structures innervated by nociceptive nerve endings are capable of
producing pain (see Boxes 11-1 through 11-4).

Mr. S. also appears to be experiencing pain and some
loss of function resulting from irritation of the left S1

nerve roots (dorsal and ventral). Therefore Mr. S. is simultaneously experiencing both radicular pain and pain arising from somatic structures. This is not unusual. Pain of spinal origin frequently arises from more than one pain generator. In addition, the referral zones of somatic referred pain and radicular pain frequently overlap. A patient with the symptoms and signs described for Mr. S. could be experiencing somatic referred pain originating from the posterior aspect of the anulus fibrosus, posterior longitudinal ligament, and anterior aspect of the dural root sleeve. The nociceptive input from these structures is carried by the recurrent meningeal nerve to the dorsal horn of the spinal cord and then follows the described pathways to higher centers.

The radicular pain and functional deficits (i.e., decreased Achilles reflex and loss of plantar flexion) of the left lower extremity described in this particular case are caused by compression of the S1 nerve roots between the bulging L5 IVD and the left superior articular process of S1. The mechanisms of nociception arising from compression of the dorsal root, as well as the mechanism of the loss of motor function from compression of the ventral root, are described earlier in this section.

Unique Role of the Intervertebral Discs in Low Back Pain

Like Mr. S., many patients experience low back and leg pain resulting from pathology of the IVD and from pressure on nerve roots or a DRG from a bulging IVD. A great deal of research related to the biology of the IVD and its role in back pain has been completed in resent years. This section summarizes some of the key findings of that research.

Common Pathologies of the Intervertebral Disc. Two of the most common problems associated with the IVD are IVD degeneration and IVD protrusion (herniation). The following sections discuss each of these pathologies separately; however, the two processes are not mutually exclusive. For example, extruded nucleus pulposus spontaneously produces increased amounts of matrix metalloproteinases, nitric oxide, interleukin-6, prostaglandin E_2, and other chemical mediators. These products may be intimately involved in both the biochemistry of disc degeneration and the pathophysiology of radiculopathy (Herzog, 1996; Kang et al., 1996).

Intervertebral disc degeneration. Intervertebral disc degeneration is difficult to define and is also difficult to separate from the normal aging process of the IVD. For these reasons, disc degeneration and normal aging of the disc frequently are discussed interchangeably. The IVD seems to age differently than other tissues of the body (probably as a result of its avascular nature), and many authors now conclude that the disc is unique in that it begins the degenerative process quite early in life (roughly the second decade). However, there is a wide variation in the aging and degenerative process of the disc, and some septuagenarians have the IVDs of 30-year-olds (and vice versa).

The hallmarks of disc degeneration are loss of fluid and fluid pressure, disruption or breakdown of collagen (including tearing of the anulus fibrosus) and proteoglycans, and sclerosis of the cartilaginous end plate (CEP) and adjacent subchondral bone.

There are several conditions that have been found to promote or even possibly initiate disc degeneration. Some of these conditions may not appear to have an obvious relationship. For example, advanced aortic atherosclerosis, presenting as calcium deposits in the posterior wall of the aorta, increases a person's risk of developing disc degeneration and is associated with the occurrence of back pain (Kauppila et al., 1997). Because of the histologic and biochemical nature of IVD degeneration, and the relationship of this condition to the aging process of the IVD, a more thorough discussion of the pathophysiology of IVD degeneration is presented in Chapter 14.

Protruded nucleus pulposus. A protruded or extruded nucleus pulposus frequently is considered to be the end stage of a rather long process. This process includes tearing of the inner layers of the AF with associated bulging outward of the remaining AF, followed by complete extrusion of part of the NP through the remaining layers of the AF (see Fig. 14-17, *E* and *F*). The terminology associated with this topic is confusing. When discussing IVD pathology with another clinician, agreeing upon a common set of terms is important. The following terminology was developed by a consensus process supported by the International Society for the Study of the Lumbar Spine (Andersson and Weinstein, 1996) (Fig. 11-10):

- *Disc bulge.* Expansion of disc material beyond its normal border (e.g., a normal disc during significant compression; or a degenerated, or aging, disc with decreased disc height.) The AF bulges in both cases.
- *Protrusion.* Discrete localized bulge in the AF; the disc material is displaced (i.e., the NP has protruded through the inner layers of the AF). Therefore a true herniation (through at least the inner fibers of the AF) is present.
- *Extrusion.* The NP has protruded through all layers of the AF, but remains attached to the disc of origin. Some authors subcategorize extrusion into subligamentous extrusion, which does not penetrate the posterior longitudinal ligament, and transligamentous extrusion, which does penetrate the posterior longitudinal ligament (Herzog, 1996).

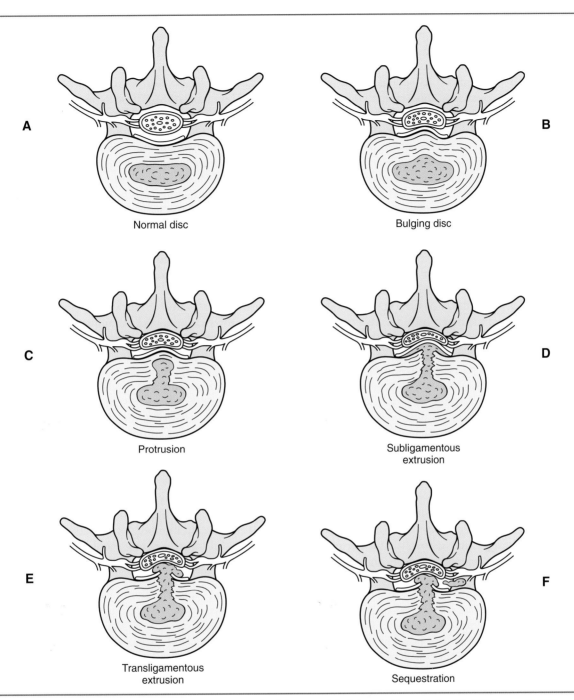

FIG. 11-10 Demonstration of terms related to intervertebral disc (IVD) bulging. **A**, Normal disc. **B**, IVD bulge. **C**, IVD protrusion. Notice the nucleus pulposus has herniated through several lamellae of the anulus fibrosus but has not passed through the most external lamella. **D** and **E**, IVD extrusion. The nucleus pulposus has passed through the most external lamella of the anulus fibrosus but remains attached to the host IVD. Extrusions can be further subdivided into, **D**, subligamentous or, **E**, transligamentous extrusions, depending upon whether or not the nucleus pulposus remains anterior to the posterior longitudinal ligament (subligamentous) or has pierced the ligament (transligamentous). **F**, Sequestration. Same as **D** and **E** except that a piece of the herniated fragment is no longer in contact with the remainder of the host nucleus pulposus. Note the sequestered fragment in **F** is to the reader's right (patient's left) of the transligamentous extrusion.

◆ *Sequestration*. A free disc fragment with no attachment to the host IVD is located in the epidural space. This free fragment can migrate superiorly, inferiorly, medially, or laterally. Sequestrations also can be subcategorized into subligamentous sequestration (*does not* penetrate the posterior longitudinal ligament), and transligamentous sequestration (*does* penetrate the posterior longitudinal ligament). On the rare occasions when the dura mater is adherent to the posterior longitudinal ligament, a transligamentous sequestration may penetrate the dura mater (Herzog, 1996).

Jönsson and Stromqvist (1996) found that a patient (such as Mr. S.) usually, but not always, exhibits more serious signs and symptoms with an increase in the severity of disc pathology from bulge, to prolapse and extrusion, to sequestration.

Although a significant number of people in their twenties suffer from painful, bulging IVDs (Salminen, 1995), protrusion and extrusion of the IVD occurs most commonly during the fourth and fifth decades of life. At this age the NP retains its relatively high fluid content and high hydrostatic pressure, but the AF may have acquired tears and fissures. In addition, during the fourth and fifth decades there is a relatively high level of activity, with exposure to external forces in jobs and sports. These factors combine to increase the likelihood of IVD protrusion and extrusion during this age period (Kraemer, 1995). Kraemer (1995) has called the increased incidence of IVD protrusion and extrusion during the fourth and fifth decades of life, "the midlife crisis of the disc."

Contrariwise, in the later decades, even though the AF has more fissures and ruptures, the NP is relatively dehydrated and does not move toward the periphery. In addition, external forces during sports and lifting on the job usually are reduced. The vertebral column has reduced motion (becomes "stiff"), but frequently becomes relatively pain free (Kraemer, 1995). This has been termed "the comfortable rigidity of the aging spine" (Kraemer, 1995). However, bony narrowing and stenosis of the spinal canal occurs more frequently in the elderly than earlier in life.

Once a disc fragment has extruded through the AF a complex series of events occurs (Fig. 11-11). This has been the topic of much recent research. First, the NP begins to absorb more fluid (i.e., swells) once it is extruded from the AF. This can result in increased pressure on the nearby DRG or dorsal and ventral nerve roots during the first several days after extrusion of the NP (Kraemer, 1995). In addition, an extruded, and even just a protruded, IVD initiates an inflammatory response. This inflammation has been found to be mediated by substances originating from the NP, as well as the response of the surrounding tissue to the NP-related substances. Such chemical mediators include nitric

oxide, Prostaglandin E_2, Phospholipase A_2, Interleukin-6, Interleukin-8, substance P, and mononuclear cells (Kang et al., 1996, 1997; O'Donnell and O'Donnell, 1996; Chen et al., 1997; Hashizume et al., 1997; Kawakami et al., 1997; Nygaard, Mellgren, and Østerud, 1997; Piperno et al., 1997; Ahn et al., 2002). These substances, and the inflammation associated with them, are probably significant in the production of the radicular pain associated with protruded, extruded, and sequestered nuclei pulposi (protruded nucleus pulposus [PNP]).* The pressure of a PNP on the DRG or dorsal root (which has recently been quantified in the lumbar region to be >53 mmHg) is also a cause of the radicular pain (Takahashi, Shima, and Porter, 1999). Experimentally, the combination of inflammatory substances and pressure on the DRG (or dorsal root) has been found to produce the most pronounced decrease in nerve conduction velocities. These changes in nerve conduction velocities may not be fully expressed until after 1 week of compression and exposure to the byproducts of inflammation (Takahashi et al., 2003). Therefore treatment often is directed at decreasing the inflammation, as well as decreasing the intradiscal pressure of the host disc (to "pull" the herniated NP back into the confines of the AF). Various nutritional and pharmaceutical approaches are used to treat the inflammation, and many manipulative procedures (such as flexion-distraction and other manipulative, or adjusting, techniques) and surgical procedures are used to treat the pressure on the neural elements caused by the PNP. In fact, Onel et al. (1989) found in a study using computed tomography (CT) to evaluate PNP in 30 subjects that traction resulted in "retraction" of extruded nuclear material in significant numbers of extruded IVDs. Decreasing the pressure on the neural elements also is thought to decrease inflammation as well.

Much recent research related to IVD protrusion in the cervical and lumbar regions (PNP in the thoracic region has not been studied as extensively) has found that PNP is a dynamic process, and that after approximately 1 to 3 weeks PNPs will usually begin a 2-month to 1-year process of resolution, resulting in significant resorption, and from a patient's standpoint (pain) often complete remission of signs and symptoms (Kraemer, 1995; Bush et al., 1997; Haro et al., 1997; Otani et al., 1997). In fact, Carreon et al. (1996) provided histologic evidence of resorption of sequestered NPs, and shrinkage of PNP has been seen on both CT and magnetic resonance imaging (MRI)) (Koike et al., 2003). The greatest reduction in size of a PNP (with or without extrusion) usually occurs between 6 months and 1 year after the initial protrusion occurs (Herzog, 1996). However, approximately 0.25%

---

*Throughout this section, PNP is used to refer to protrusion, extrusion, or sequestration of an IVD.

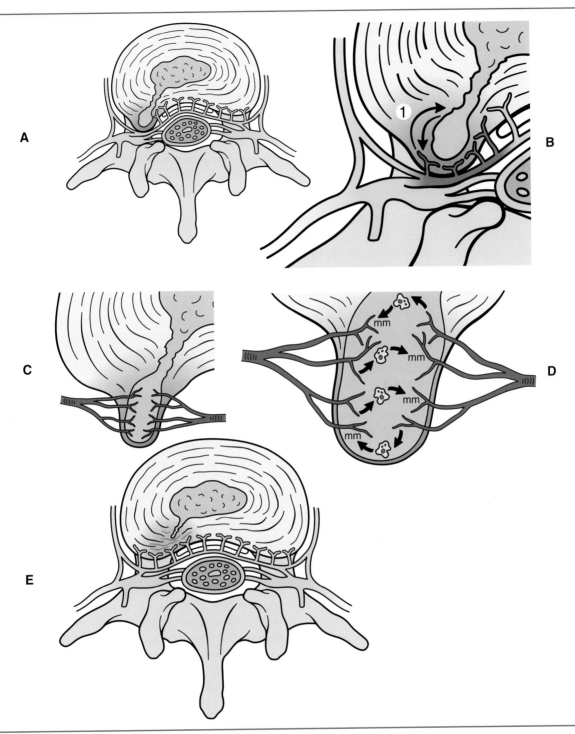

FIG. 11-11 Healing of an intervertebral disc (IVD) protrusion. **A,** A left posterolateral protrusion of the nucleus pulposus (NP, *blue*) through the majority of the lamellae of the anulus fibrosus (AF) has resulted in an inflammatory response (*red*). **B,** A close-up of the protruding IVD and the surrounding tissues shows that the inflammation has affected the nerves innervating the outer lamellae of the IVD. Both the IVD and nerves are shown releasing chemokines, *1,* including fibroblast growth factor, angiogenin, transforming growth factor-beta, platelet-derived endothelial cell growth factor, and vascular endothelial growth factor. **C,** An isolated view of the protruding IVD shows that in response to the chemokines just listed, new blood vessels grow (neovascularization) into the inflamed AF and NP. **D,** A close-up of the protruded NP and surrounding AF shows that macrophages (the cells in the NP) have made their way from the new blood vessels into the protruded NP. The macrophages in turn release matrix metalloproteinases (mm). The matrix metalloproteinases break down the extracellular matrix (primarily collagen and proteoglycans) within the protruded NP, and the absorption of the extracellular matrix into the vascular system results in shrinkage of the protrusion. **E,** Granulation (scar) tissue (gray) is laid down in the region of the AF surrounding the originally protruded and now retracting NP. The scar tissue eventually constricts, resulting in resolution of the IVD bulge. The greatest reduction in size of a protrusion (or extrusion or sequestration) usually occurs between 6 months and 1 year after the initial protrusion occurs (Herzog, 1996).

of LBP patients require surgery for PNP.* Cauda equina syndrome, severe acute motor weakness, and intolerable pain requiring permanent high-dose analgesics are among the strong indications for surgery (Kraemer, 1995; Andersson and Weinstein, 1996).

The process of PNP remission and resorption seems to begin with the ingrowth of new blood vessels onto the region of prolapse or into the extruded disc fragment (Fig. 11-11, C and D). Although the healthy adult IVD is avascular, the surrounding ligaments are supplied by blood vessels. In addition, the epidural space contains the relatively dense internal vertebral venous plexus. These vessels can allow a rather extensive system of branches to grow into the IVD after IVD protrusion, extrusion, and sequestration (Virri et al., 1996; Koike et al., 2003). This "neovascularization" probably results from the inflammatory process that was briefly described earlier, and the expression of chemokines, or cytokines, by the PNP. Some of the chemokines associated with the repair response also may be released from the nerve endings innervating the IVD (Ashton and Eisenstein, 1996; Palmgren et al., 1996) (Fig. 11-11, B). The release of cytokines by the nerve endings probably is related to the primary role of these nociceptive fibers to respond to noxious, including chemical, stimuli. These nerve endings are probably sensitive to the internal environment of the deeper layers of the AF as the chemicals seep toward the AF from the NP (McCarthy, 1993). The chemokines specifically associated with neovascularization include fibroblast growth factor, angiogenin, transforming growth factor-beta, platelet-derived endothelial cell growth factor, and vascular endothelial growth factor (Koike et al., 2003). Neovascularization seems to be closely associated with the resorption and scar formation (granulation tissue) associated with the healing process of PNP. In addition, chemokines are also expressed in the scar tissue of PNP, and inflammatory mediators are released from mononuclear cells found along the edge of the granulation tissue associated with PNP. These cytokines and inflammatory mediators are associated with the granulation tissue function to promote and continue the neovascularization and resorption process begun with the initial occurrence of the PNP (Doita et al., 1996; Haro et al., 1996; Minamide et al., 1999). In addition, chondrocytes within the IVD have been found to be chemotactic and they recruit monocytes (macrophages) that participate in IVD resorption (Kikuchi et al., 1998). The new vessels formed by the neovascularization process carry the macrophages into the PNP. The macrophages in turn secrete matrix metalloproteinases. These metalloproteinases further break down the extracellular matrix within the PNP, and the absorp-

tion of the extracellular matrix results in shrinkage of the PNP (Koike et al., 2003) (see Fig. 11-11, E).

Often portions of NP, AF, and CEP are found in varying concentrations in the extruded or sequestered IVD fragment. In such cases, NP undergoes resorption most rapidly, followed by AF, and then CEP (Kraemer, 1995; Carreon et al., 1996, 1997). In fact, a recent study showed that CEP inhibits the neovascularization associated with the resorption of the extruded disc fragment. Therefore higher concentrations of CEP in a given extruded fragment seem to slow the resorption process. This may help to explain the wide variation of healing rates seen clinically. In addition, cervical herniations often contain more CEP (Kokubun, Sakurai, Tanaka, 1996). This also may help to explain why cervical disc problems can be challenging clinically. However, sometimes a patient may, after several weeks, experience a decrease in pain even though the PNP remains the same size. This is thought to result from a change in the hydration of the extruded fragment and a complete or partial resolution of the inflammation and edema surrounding the affected nerve roots or DRG (Kraemer, 1995).

Clinicians often are amazed at the wide variation in pain patterns associated with disc problems. Recall that the AF of the IVD receives sensory innervation (Figs. 11-1 and 11-9, A). Consequently, damage to the AF can be a primary source of pain. In addition, degenerated and injured IVDs, as well as PNPs themselves, have been found to be more heavily innervated with sensory nerve endings than "healthy discs," and these more numerous nerve endings are accompanied with a higher concentration of the neuromodulator, substance P (Coppes et al., 1997). This ingrowth of nerves after IVD injury and the accompanying higher concentration of substance P in the region of the nerve endings make such an IVD more likely to be pain producing (a pain generator) if it is not allowed to heal properly, or if it is reinjured. In addition, the IVD also may contain silent nociceptors (see section Modulation at the Level of the Peripheral Nerves and Spinal Tissues [Pain Generators]), and the chemical mediators within the NP that were discussed earlier in this section may stimulate these silent nociceptors when the disc is injured, again resulting in pain (Cavanaugh, 1995). Recall that the specific nerves that supply the IVD are the recurrent meningeal nerve, to the posterior IVD; and fibers that course with the autonomic nervous system, to the anterior and lateral IVD. These nerves have a variable distribution pattern. Therefore discogenic pain (not including radicular pain) can present in a wide variety of patterns, including radiation into the groin or lower extremity. In addition, compression or inflammation of the DRG or the dorsal roots from a PNP or the inflammation associated with it, as described, results in the sharp stabbing pain, known as radicular pain, which radiates along the distribution of the nerves

---

*A large variation exists in the rates of surgery.

that are affected (see discussion of radicular pain in previous sections). Recall that radicular pain usually has a more distal radiation pattern than discogenic pain.

Animal studies have shown that an incision in the AF results in decreased nerve conduction velocities and morphologic changes in the dorsal roots. The cut AF allows "leakage of NP material," and the NP material (not a bulge or extrusion) close to the nerve roots is thought to be what causes the morphologic and physiologic changes in the nerve root (Kayama et al., 1996). Other studies also have shown that NP tissue simply placed near dorsal roots or DRGs results in decreased nerve conduction velocities (Otani et al., 1997), and phospholipase A_2, which is associated with PNP, has been found to cause demyelination of nerve roots (Chen et al., 1997). These findings help to explain the LBP (because of tearing of the AF) and radicular pain (from the DRG or dorsal roots) radiating into the lower extremity in patients with no evidence of PNP on MRI or even during surgery (Kayama et al., 1996). These findings are supported by those from human studies showing aching pain with radicular pain in patients with disc disruption but without compromise of the outer anular fibers (Ohnmeiss, Vanharanta, and Ekholm, 1997). Therefore even if Mr. S. has no evidence of PNP on MRI, he may still have an IVD injury. This makes a thorough history and physical examination important in all cases of LBP, and additional laboratory and neurophysiologic tests important in many cases of serious acute or chronic LBP.

Interaction between the Zygapophysial Joints and Intervertebral Discs

Even though the Z joints probably are not the primary source of back pain in the case of Mr. S., the structures of the posterior vertebral arch, and particularly the Z joints, also may contribute to radicular pain of discal origin. This is because Z joint facet arthrosis may further decrease the space available for the exiting nerve roots (Kirkaldy-Willis, 1988a) (Fig. 11-12). Chapter 7 discusses the role that may be played by facet arthrosis in the development of spinal (vertebral) canal stenosis and of IVF stenosis.

The reverse also is true. Disc degeneration may lead to increased stress on the Z joints. This can result in somatic pain, not originating from the articular cartilage but from pressure on the subchondral bone underlying the articular cartilage. The added pressure on the Z joints secondary to disc degeneration also may result in a small piece of soft tissue (articular capsule or Z joint synovial fold) being nipped between the facets (Hutton, 1990), which can also cause pain.

Recall that lumbar radiculopathy may be caused by chemical irritation. This also has been reproduced by selective nerve sheath injection with hypertonic saline (Rauschning, 1987). In addition, escape of radiopaque contrast medium into the nerve root canals (IVFs) has been repeatedly observed during facet joint arthrography. Because extraarticular synovial fluid is known to have strong tissue-irritating properties, Rauschning (1987) believes that "leakage of synovial fluid from ruptured intraspinal synovial cysts or weakened facet joint capsules may cause pain and possibly transient nerve root dysfunction." Therefore simultaneous radicular pain and somatic pain arising from the Z joints are a real possibility (see Fig. 11-12).

Other Considerations

Pain of Radicular Origin. Focus often is placed on the dermatomal pattern of radicular pain. Yet there is significant variation in dermatomal patterns from individual to individual, and the dermatomes themselves overlap. So the dermatomes are only a crude means to determine the origin of radicular pain. In addition, the peripheral portions of the nerves affected by compression or inflammation of a dorsal root or DRG also supply sensory innervation to structures of myotomal and sclerotomal origin (e.g., muscles, periosteum of bones, ligaments of the back and lower extremities). Therefore pain resulting from compression of a dorsal root or DRG sometimes is felt deeper than a dermatomal distribution, corresponding to the myotomal and sclerotomal distribution of the peripheral extension of these nerves (Weinstein, 1988). This deep pain can be felt superiorly, inferiorly, medially, or laterally (or any combination of these) from the corresponding dermatome.

Pain of Somatic Origin. Somatic referral of pain also is related to the embryologic origin of somatic pain generators. Recall that paraxial mesoderm, which surrounds the embryonic neural tube, condenses to form paired somites. Each somite subdivides into a dermomyotome (to form dermis and muscle) and sclerotome (to form the vertebrae, Z joints, the ligaments between the vertebrae, and the AF of the IVDs). Some embryologic myotomes migrate and fuse with one another. Therefore the dull aching somatic referred pain associated with myotomal patterns of pain referral, initiated by tissue damage of a somatic pain generator, may be large. Such myotomal patterns can occur with strain of the large erector spinae muscles. The deeper muscles (e.g., the transversospinalis group, interspinales, and intertransversarii muscles) remain more segmental in distribution and innervation. However, even the smaller muscles and the small joints of the spine frequently receive innervation from more than one spinal nerve. This overlap of segmental innervation also contributes to the broad referral patterns of somatic pain arising from the deep back structures (see the section Somatic Referred Pain for more details).

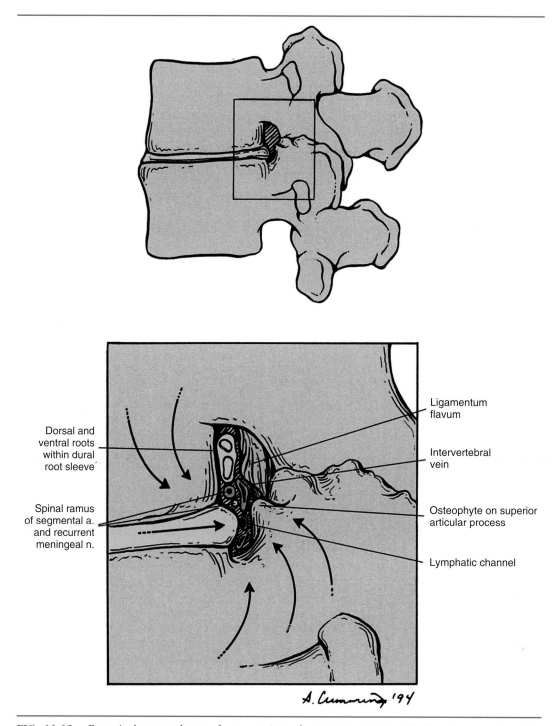

Dorsal and
ventral roots
within dural
root sleeve

Spinal ramus
of segmental a.
and recurrent
meningeal n.

Ligamentum
flavum

Intervertebral
vein

Osteophyte on superior
articular process

Lymphatic channel

A. Cumming '94

FIG. 11-12   Foraminal encroachment from a variety of sources (*arrows*), including intervertebral disc narrowing, intervertebral disc bulge, and zygapophysial joint arthrosis. Notice that as the two vertebrae approximate each other, the more superior body also shifts slightly posteriorly because of the disc narrowing.

The clinician turns to Mr. S. and notices that Mr. S.'s eyes are closed. The clinician's heart quickens, imagining that Mr. S. may have expired from old age during the time that the clinician has been considering the various ramifications of pain of spinal origin. However, the clinician is relieved as respiratory movements by Mr. S. are

noticed. Mr. S. is roused from his deep slumber so the examination can be finished. The clinician focuses the care of Mr. S. on his disc protrusion with radiculopathy, and during the next few weeks, Mr. S. responds well to the treatment. The investigation and treatment of Mr. S.'s pain have reignited the clinician's interest in the mechanism of back pain. Consequently, Mr. S. has provided a service to the clinician of almost equal value to the help that the clinician has given Mr. S.

Suggested Readings

The work of Bogduk (1997) provides a clear, well-organized, and well-referenced account of structures of the spine receiving nociceptive innervation. It also describes the mechanisms, as well as they are understood, of somatic referred and radicular pain. The books of Kirkaldy-Willis (1988) and Haldeman (1992), and the papers by Cavanaugh (1995), Greenspan (1995), and Siddall and Cousins (1997) provide excellent correlations between the basic science considerations of pain of spinal origin and clinical practice.

REFERENCES

Abe M et al. (2002). Changes in expression of voltage-dependent ion channel subunits in dorsal root ganglia of rats with radicular injury and pain. *Spine, 27*, 1517-1524.

Ahn SH et al. (2002). mRNA expression of cytokines and chemokines in herniated lumbar intervertebral discs. *Spine, 27*, 911-917.

Andersson GBJ & Weinstein JN. (1996). Disc herniation. *Spine, 21*, 1S.

Anzai H et al. (2002). Epidural application of nucleus pulposus enhances nociresponses of rat dorsal horn neurons. *Spine, 27*, E50-E55.

Aprill C, Dwyer A, & Bogduk N. (1990). Cervical zygapophyseal joint pain patterns II: A clinical evaluation. *Spine, 15*, 458-461.

Ashton IK & Eisenstein SM. (1996). The effect of substance P on the proliferation and proteoglycan deposition of cells derived from rabbit intervertebral disc. *Spine, 21*, 421-426.

Basbaum AI. (1984). Anatomical substrates of pain and pain modulation and their relationship to analgesic drug action. In M Kuhar & G Pasternak (Eds.). *Analgesics: Neurochemical, behavioral, and clinical perspectives*. New York: Raven Press.

Basbaum AI. (1987). Cytochemical studies of the neural circuitry underlying pain and pain control. *Acta Neurochir Suppl (Wien), 38*, 5-15.

Basbaum AI & Fields HL. (1978). Brain stem control of spinal pain-transmission neurons. *Annu Rev Physiol, 40*, 217-248.

Basbaum AI & Fields HL. (1984). Endogenous pain control systems: Brainstem spinal pathways and endorphin circuitry. *Annu Rev Neurosci, 7*, 309-338.

Basbaum AI & Jessell TM. (2000). The perception of pain. In ER Kandel, JH Schwartz, & TM Jessell (Eds.). *Principles of neural science* (4th ed.). New York: McGraw-Hill.

Benarroch EE et al. (1999). Leptin receptor immunoreactivity in sympathetic prevertebral ganglion neurons of mouse and rat. *Neurosci Lett, 265(2)*, 75-78.

Besson JM. (1988). The physiological basis of pain pathways and the segmental controls of pain. *Acta Anaesthesiol Belg, 39(3 Suppl 2)*, 47-51.

Bogduk N. (1976). The anatomy of the lumbar intervertebral disc syndrome. *Med J Aust, 1*, 878-881.

Bogduk N. (1983). The innervation of the lumbar spine. *Spine, 8*, 286-293.

Bogduk N. (1984). The rationale for patterns of neck and back pain. *Patient Management, 13*, 17-28.

Bogduk N. (1992). The causes of low back pain. *Med J Aust, 156*, 151-153.

Bogduk N, Lambert G, & Duckworth J. (1981). The anatomy and physiology of the vertebral nerve in relation to cervical migraine. *Cephalalgia, 1*, 11-24.

Bogduk N. (1997). *Clinical anatomy of the lumbar spine* (3rd ed.). London: Churchill Livingstone.

Budgell B, Hotta H, & Sato A. (1995). Spinovisceral reflexes evoked by noxious and innocuous stimulation of the lumbar spine. *J Neuromusculoskel Syst, 3*, 122-131.

Burton AK et al. (1995). Psychosocial predictors of outcome in acute and subchronic low back trouble. *Spine, 20*, 722-728.

Bush K et al. (1997). The pathomorphologic changes that accompany the resolution of cervical radiculopathy: A prospective study with repeat magnetic resonance imaging. *Spine, 22*, 183-186.

Campbell D & Parsons C. (1944). Referred head pain and its concomitants. *J Nerv Ment Dis, 99*, 544-551.

Carpenter MB & Sutin J. (1983). *Human neuroanatomy* (8th ed.). Baltimore: Williams & Wilkins.

Carreon LY et al. (1996). Histologic changes in the disc after cervical spine trauma: Evidence of disc absorption. *J Spinal Disord, 9*, 313-316.

Carreon LY et al. (1997). Neovascularization induced by anulus and its inhibition by cartilage end plate. Its role in disc absorption. *Spine, 22(13)*, 1429-1434.

Cavanaugh JM. (1995). Neural mechanisms of lumbar pain. *Spine, 20*, 1804-1809.

Chen C et al. (1997). Effects of phospholipase A2 on lumbar nerve root structure and function. *Spine, 22*, 1057-1064.

Coppes MH et al. (1997). Innervation of "painful" lumbar discs. *Spine, 22(20)*, 2342-2349.

Cornefjord M et al. (1995). Neuropeptide changes in compressed spinal nerve roots. *Spine, 20*, 670-673.

Cramer GC et al. (2004). Degenerative changes following spinal fixation in a small animal model. *J Manipulative Physiol Ther, 27*, 141-154.

Cramer LE. (1998). Preventing low back pain in industry. *JAMA, 280(23)*, 1993-1994.

Craig AD & Bushnell MC. (1994). The thermal grill illusion: Unmasking the burn of cold pain. *Science, 265(5169)*, 252-255.

Craig AD et al. (1996). Functional imaging of an illusion of pain. *Nature, 384(6606)*, 258-260.

Cross SA. (1994). Pathophysiology of pain. *Mayo Clin Proc, 69(4)*, 375-383.

Dahlin LB et al. (1992). Physiology of nerve compression. In S Haldeman (Ed.). *Principles and practice of chiropractic* (2nd ed.). East Norwalk, Conn: Appleton & Lange.

Darby S & Cramer G. (1994). Pain generators and pain pathways of the head and neck. In D Curl (Ed.). *Chiropractic approach to head pain*. Baltimore: Williams & Wilkins.

Doita M et al. (1996). Immunohistologic study of the ruptured intervertebral disc of the lumbar spine. *Spine, 21(2)*, 235-241.

Edmeads J. (1978). Headaches and head pains associated with diseases of the cervical spine. *Med Clin North Am, 62*, 533-544.

Fields HL. (1987). *Pain*. New York: McGraw-Hill.

Garfin SR, Rydevik BL, & Brown RA. (1991). Compression neuropathy of spinal nerve roots. *Spine, 16*, 162-166.

Garfin SR et al. (1995). Spinal nerve root compression. *Spine, 20*, 1810-1820.

Giles LGF. (1987). Lumbo-sacral zygapophysial joint tropism and its effect on hyaline cartilage. *Clin Biomechan, 2*, 2-6.

Gill KP & Callaghan MJ. (1998). The measurement of lumbar proprioception in individuals with and without low back pain. *Spine, 23*, 371-377.

Gillette RD. (1996). Behavioral factors in the management of back pain. *Am Fam Physician, 53*, 1313-1318.

Gillette RG, Kramis RC, & Roberts WJ. (1993). Characterization of spinal somatosensory neurons having receptive fields in lumbar tissues of cats. *Pain, 54*, 85-98.

Greenspan A. (1995). Bone island (enostosis): Current concept. A review. *Skeletal Radiol, 24(2)*, 111-115.

Greenspan JD. (1997). Nociceptors and the peripheral nervous system's role in pain. *J Hand Ther, April-June*, 78-85.

Haldeman S. (1992). The neurophysiology of spinal pain. In S Haldeman (Ed.). *Principles and practice of chiropractic* (2nd ed.). East Norwalk, Conn: Appleton & Lange.

Haig AJ, LeBreck DB, & Powley SG. (1995). Paraspinal mapping: Quantified needle electromyography of the paraspinal muscles in persons without low back pain. *Spine, 20*, 715-721.

Hanai F, Matsui N, & Hongo N. (1996). Changes in responses of wide dynamic range neurons in the spinal dorsal horn after dorsal root or dorsal root ganglion compression. *Spine, 21*, 1408-1415.

Haro H et al. (1997). Sequential dynamics of monocyte chemotactic protein-1 expression in herniated nucleus pulposus resorption. *J Orthop Res, 15(5)*, 734-741.

Hashizume H et al. (1997). Histochemical demonstration of nitric oxide in herniated lumbar discs: A clinical and animal model study. *Spine, 22*, 1080-1084.

Hendry SHC, Hsiao SS, & Bushnell MC. (1999). Somatic sensation. In MJ Zigmond et al. (Eds.). *Fundamental neuroscience*. San Diego: Academic Press.

Herzog RJ. (1996). The radiologic assessment for a lumbar disc herniation. *Spine, 21*, 19S-38S.

Hildebrandt J et al. (1997). Prediction of success from a multidisciplinary treatment program for chronic low back pain. *Spine, 22,* 990-1001.

Hockaday JM & Whitty CW. (1967). Patterns of referred pain in the normal subject. *Brain, 90(3),* 481-496.

Hoffert MJ. (1989). The neurophysiology of pain. *Neurol Clin, 7(2),* 183-203.

Hubbard DR & Berkoff GM. (1993). Myofascial trigger points show spontaneous needle EMG activity. *Spine, 18(13),* 1803-1807.

Hudson AJ. (2000). Pain perception and response: Central nervous system mechanisms. *Can J Neurol Sci, 27(1),* 2-16.

Hutton WC. (1990). The forces acting on a lumbar intervertebral joint. *J Manual Med, 5,* 66-67.

Indahl A et al. (1997). Interaction between the porcine lumbar intervertebral disc, zygapophysial joints, and paraspinal muscles. *Spine, 22,* 2834-2840.

Inman VT & Saunders JB. (1944). Referred pain from skeletal structures. *J Nerv Ment Dis, 996,* 660-667.

Iwabuchi M et al. (2001). Effects of anulus fibrosus and experimentally degenerated nucleus pulpous on nerve root conduction velocity. *Spine, 26,* 1651-1655.

Jessell TM & Kelly DD. (1991). Pain and analgesia. In ER Kandel, JH Schwartz, & TM Jessell (Eds.). *Principles of neural science* (3rd ed.). East Norwalk, Conn: Appleton & Lange.

Jönsson B & Stromqvist B. (1996). Neurologic signs in lumbar disc herniation. Preoperative affliction and postoperative recovery in 150 cases. *Acta Orthop Scand, 67(5),* 466-469.

Jorgensen LS & Fossgreen J. (1990). Back pain and spinal pathology in patients with functional upper abdominal pain. *Scand J Gastroenterol, 25(12),* 1235-1241.

Kang JD et al. (1996). Herniated lumbar intervertebral discs spontaneously produce matrix metalloproteinases, nitric oxide, interleukin-6, and prostaglandin E2. *Spine, 21,* 271-277.

Kang JD et al. (1997). Toward a biochemical understanding of human intervertebral disc degeneration and herniation: Contributions of nitric oxide, interleukins, prostaglandin E_2, and matrix metalloproteinases. *Spine, 22,* 1065-1073.

Kawakami M et al. (1997). The role of phospholipase A_2 and nitric oxide in pain-related behavior produced by an allograft of intervertebral disc material to the sciatic nerve of the rat. *Spine, 22,* 1074-1079.

Kauppila LI et al. (1997). Disc degeneration/back pain and calcification of the abdominal aorta: A 25-year follow-up study in Framingham. *Spine, 22,* 1642-1649.

Kauppila LI & Tallroth K. (1993). Postmortem angiographic findings for arteries supplying the lumbar spine: Their relationship to low-back symptoms. *J Spinal Disord, 6,* 124-129.

Kayama S et al. (1996). Incision of the annulus fibrosus induces nerve root morphologic, vascular, and functional changes: An experimental study. *Spine, 21,* 2539-2543.

Kayama S et al. (1998). Cultured autologous nucleus pulposus cells induce functional changes in spinal nerve roots. *Spine, 23,* 2155-2158.

Kellgren JH. (1938). Observations on referred pain arising from muscle, *Clin Sci, 3,* 175-190.

Kikuchi S et al. (1996). Increased resistance to acute compression injury in chronically compressed spinal nerve roots. *Spine, 21,* 2544-2550.

Kikuchi T et al. (1998). Monocyte chemoattractant protein-1 in the intervertebral disc. A histologic experimental model. *Spine, 23(10),* 1091-1099.

Kirkaldy-Willis WH. (1988a). The pathology and pathogenesis of LBP. In W Kirkaldy-Willis (Ed.). *Managing low back pain* (2nd ed.). New York: Churchill Livingstone.

Kirkaldy-Willis WH. (1988b). The mediation of pain. In W Kirkaldy-Willis (Ed.). *Managing low back pain* (2nd ed.). New York: Churchill Livingstone.

Koike Y et al. (2003). Angiogenesis and inflammatory cell infiltration in lumbar disc herniation. *Spine, 28(17),* 1928-1933.

Kokubun S, Sakurai M, & Tanaka Y. (1996). Cartilaginous end plate in cervical disc herniation. *Spine, 21(2),* 190-195.

Kraemer J. (1995). Natural course and prognosis of intervertebral disc diseases. International Society for the Study of the Lumbar Spine, Seattle, Washington, June 1994. *Spine, 20(6),* 635-639.

Kummel BM. (1996). Nonorganic signs of significance in low back pain. *Spine, 21,* 1077-1081.

Macfarlane GJ et al. (1997). Employment and physical work activities as predictors of future low back pain. *Spine, 22,* 1143-1149.

McCall IW, Park WM, & O'Brien JP. (1979). Induced pain referral from posterior lumbar elements in normal subjects. *Spine, 4(5),* 441-446.

McCarthy PW. (1993). Sparse substance P-like immunoreactivity in intervertebral discs. Nerve fibers and endings in the rat. *Acta Orthop Scand, 64(6),* 664-668.

McLain RF & Weinstein JN. (1991). Ultrastructural changes in the dorsal root ganglion associated with whole body vibration. *J Spinal Disord, 4,* 142-148.

McMahon S. (1990). The spinal modulation of pain. In JK Paterson & L Burn (Eds.). *Back pain: An international review.* Dordrecht, Netherlands: Kluwer.

Melzack R & Wall PD. (1965). Pain mechanisms: A new theory. *Science, 150(699),* 971-979.

Merskey H. (1979). Pain terms: A list with definitions and notes on usage. Recommended by the IASP subcommittee on taxonomy. *Pain, 6,* 249-252.

Merskey H & Bogduk N. (1994). *Classification of chronic pain: Descriptions of chronic pain syndromes and definitions of pain terms* (2nd ed.). Seattle: IASP Press.

Minamide A et al. (1999). Effects of basic fibroblast growth factor on spontaneous resorption of herniated intervertebral discs: An experimental study in the rabbit. *Spine, 24,* 940.

Nakamura S et al. (1996). Origin of nerves supplying the posterior portion of lumbar intervertebral discs in rats. *Spine, 21,* 917-924.

Nolte D. (1988). Bronchial hyperreactivity: Pingpong between cells, nerves and mediators. *Med Klin (Munich), 83(4),* 149-150.

Nygaard ØP, Mellgren SI, & Østerud B. (1997). The inflammatory properties of contained and noncontained lumbar disc herniation. *Spine, 22,* 2484-2488.

O'Donnell JL & O'Donnell AL. (1996). Prostaglandin E_2 content in herniated lumbar disc disease. *Spine, 21,* 1653-1656.

Ohnmeiss DD, Vanharanta H, & Ekholm J. (1997). Degree of disc disruption and lower extremity pain. *Spine, 22,* 1600-1605.

Ohtori S et al. (1999). Sensory innervation of the dorsal portion of the lumbar intervertebral disc in rats. *Spine, 24,* 2295.

Ohtori S et al. (2001). Neurones in the dorsal root ganglia of T13, L1 and L2 innervate the dorsal portion of lower lumbar discs in rats. A study using diI, an anterograde neurotracer. *J Bone Joint Surg Br, 83(8),* 1191-1194.

Olmarker K et al. (1989). Effects of experimental graded compression on blood flow in spinal nerve roots. A vital microscopic study on the porcine cauda equina. *J Orthop Res, 7(6),* 817-823.

Olmarker K et al. (1996). Ultrastructural changes in spinal nerve roots induced by autologous nucleus pulposus. *Spine, 21,* 411-414.

Olmarker K et al. (1997). The effects of normal, frozen, and hyaluronidase-digested nucleus pulposus on nerve root structure and function. *Spine, 22,* 471-476.

Olmarker K, Rydevik B, & Nordborg C. (1993). Autologous nucleus pulposus induces neurophysiologic and histologic changes in porcine cauda equina nerve roots. *Spine, 18,* 1425-1432.

Onel D et al. (1989). Computed tomographic investigation of the effect of traction on lumbar disc herniations. *Spine, 14(1),* 82-90.

Otani K et al. (1997). Experimental disc herniation. *Spine, 22,* 2894-2899.

Özaktay AC, Kallakuri S, & Cavanaugh JM. (1998). Phospholipase A2 sensitivity of the dorsal root ganglion. *Spine, 23,* 1297-1306.

Ozawa K, Atsuta Y, & Kato T. (2001). Chronic effects of the nucleus pulposus applied to nerve roots on ectopic firing and conduction velocity. *Spine, 26,* 2661-2665.

Palmgren T et al. (1996). Immunohistochemical demonstration of sensory and autonomic nerve terminals in herniated lumbar disc tissue. *Spine, 21(11),* 1301-1306.

Pappageotgiou AC et al. (1997). Psychosocial factors in the workplace: Do they predict new episodes of low back pain? *Spine, 22,* 1137-1142.

Pennie B & Agambar L. (1991). Patterns of injury and recovery in whiplash. *Injury, 22,* 57-59.

Piperno M et al. (1997). Phospholipase A_2 activity in herniated lumbar discs: Clinical correlations and inhibition by piroxicam. *Spine, 22,* 2061-2065.

Plancarte R & Calvillo O. (1997). Complex regional pain syndrome type 2 (Causalgia) after automated laser discectomy. *Spine, 22,* 459-462.

Portenoy R. (1996). Neuropathic pain. In R Portenoy & R Kanner (Eds.). *Pain management: Theory and practice.* Philadelphia: FA Davis.

Portenoy R & Kanner R. (1996). *Pain management: Theory and practice.* Philadelphia: FA Davis.

Price DD. (2000). Psychological and neural mechanisms of the affective dimension of pain. *Science, 288,* 1769-1772.

Raineville P. (2002). Brain mechanisms of pain affect and pain modulation. *Curr Opin Neurobiol, 12,* 195-204.

Raoul S et al. (2002). Role of the sinu-vertebral nerve in low back pain and anatomical basis of therapeutic implications. *Surg Radiol Anat, 24,* 366-371.

Rauschning W. (1987). Normal and pathologic anatomy of the lumbar root canals. *Spine, 12,* 1008-1019.

Rydevik B, Brown M, & Lundborg G. (1984). Pathoanatomy and pathophysiology of nerve root compression. *Spine, 9,* 7-15.

Rydevik BL, Myers RR, & Powell HC. (1989). Pressure increase in the dorsal root ganglion following mechanical compression. *Spine, 14(6),* 574-576.

Salminen JJ et al. (1995). Low back pain in the young. *Spine, 20,* 2101-2108.

Schwarzer AC et al. (1994b). The relative contributions of the disc and zygapophyseal joint in chronic low back pain. *Spine, 19,* 801-806.

Seaman DR & Cleveland C. (1999). Spinal pain syndromes: Nociceptive, neuropathic and psychologic mechanisms. *JMPT, 22,* 458-472.

Sekiguchi M et al. (2002). Nerve vasculature changes induced by serotonin under chronic cauda equine compression. *Spine, 27,* 1634-1639.

Sewards TV & Sewards MA. (2002). The medial pain system: Neural representations of the motivational aspect of pain. *Brain Res Bull, 59(3),* 163-180.

Siddal PJ & Cousins MJ. (1997). Spine update: Spinal pain mechanisms. *Spine, 22,* 98-104.

Sihvonen T et al. (1995). Dorsal ramus irritation associated with recurrent low back pain and its relief with local anesthetic or training therapy. *J Spinal Disord, 8,* 8-14.

Smyth MJ & Wright V. (1958). Sciatica and the intervertebral disc: An experimental study. *J Bone Joint Surg Am, 40-A (6),* 1401-1418.

Takahashi K, Shima I, & Porter RW. (1999). Nerve root pressure in lumbar disc herniation. *Spine, 24,* 2003.

Takahashi N et al. (2003). Pathomechanisms of nerve root injury caused by disc herniation: An experimental study of mechanical compression and chemical irritation. *Spine, 28,* 435-441.

Takebayashi T et al. (2001). Effect of nucleus pulposus on the neural activity of the dorsal root ganglion. *Spine, 26,* 940-945.

Vernon H. (Ed). (2001). *The cranio-cervical syndrome.* Oxford, UK: Butterworth Heinemann.

Virri J et al. (1996). Prevalence, morphology, and topography of blood vessels in herniated disc tissue. A comparative immunocytochemical study. *Spine, 21(16),* 1856-1863.

Weinstein J, Claverie W, & Gibson S. (1988). The pain of discography. *Spine, 13,* 1344-1348.

Weinstein WH. (1988). The perception of pain. In W Kirkaldy-Willis (Ed.). *Managing low back pain* (2nd ed.). New York: Churchill Livingstone.

Willis Jr WD & Coggeshall RE. (1991). *Sensory mechanisms of the spinal cord* (2nd ed.). New York: Plenum Press.

Wyke B. (1987). The neurology of back pain. In MIV Jayson (Ed). *The lumbar spine and back pain.* (3rd ed.). New York: Churchill Livingstone.

Yabuki S et al. (1998). Acute effects of nucleus pulposus on blood flow and endoneurial fluid pressure in rat dorsal root ganglia. *Spine, 23,* 2517-2523.

Yabuki S, Igarashi T, & Kikuchi S. (2000). Application of nucleus pulposus to the nerve root simultaneously reduces blood flow in dorsal root ganglion corresponding hindpaw in the rat. *Spine, 25,* 1471-1476.

Yamashita T et al. (1990). Mechanosensitive afferent units in the lumbar facet joint. *J Bone Joint Surg, 72-A,* 865-870.

Yoshizawa H, O'Brien J, & Thomas-Smith W. (1980). The neuropathology of the intervertebral discs removed for low back pain. *J Pathol, 132,* 95.

Yukawa Y et al. (1997). Groin pain associated with lower lumbar disc herniation. *Spine, 22,* 1736-1740.

PART III

Spinal Development, Pediatric Spine, and Microscopic Anatomy

CHAPTER 12

Development of the Spine and Spinal Cord

Barclay W. Bakkum
William E. Bachop

The human back can be identified as early as the end of the third week of development when the embryo consists of a disc of cells between the floor of the amnionic cavity and the roof of the yolk sac cavity (Fig. 12-1). Because the embryo is a flattened disc of cells, no complete body wall (i.e., no sides or front) exists, only the back (Brash, 1951b). Even at this early point, all the primordia that make up the definitive back are present: the surface ectoderm, neural tube, neural crest, notochord, and paraxial mesoderm. The posterior boundary of the back is the surface ectoderm flooring the amnionic cavity, and its anterior boundary is the endoderm roofing the yolk sac cavity.

BLASTOCYST

The human begins as the fertilized ovum, which cleaves itself into smaller and smaller embryonic cells known as blastomeres, each carrying all the genetic information needed to build any tissue or organ in the body (Williams et al., 1995). These cells at first form a solid sphere, but rearrangement and continued cell division produce a hollow sphere known as the blastocyst (Patten, 1964). The blastocyst is a single cell layer thick except at one pole, where the cells form into a disc that is two cell layers thick (Brash, 1951b) (Fig. 12-2, *A*). This disc is called the inner cell mass to distinguish it from all the other cells, which are referred to collectively as the trophoblast (Mossman, 1987). The hole in the center of the blastocyst is known as the blastocyst cavity.

The inner cell mass and the trophoblast have different fates. The former goes on to form the embryo proper. The latter can be likened to embryonic scaffolding that eventually is dismantled or discarded. Before that happens, trophoblast cells proliferate by mitosis until they are several cell layers thick. The innermost layer of the trophoblast still lines the blastocyst cavity. It remains cellular and is called the cytotrophoblast (Baxter, 1953). The cells in the outermost layer begin to lose their cell membranes, thus forming a syncytium known as the syncytiotrophoblast (Williams et al., 1995) (Fig. 12-2, *B*). This syncytium releases proteolytic enzymes that enable the blastocyst to digest its way into the lining of the uterus, called the endometrium. This process is known as implantation and usually is completed by the end of the second embryonic week. The implanted blastocyst does not leave the uterine wall until it bursts out in the form of a newborn (Beck et al., 1985).

Also during the second week of development, the inner cell mass has been changing (Williams et al., 1995). A space, the first sign of the amnionic (amniotic) cavity,

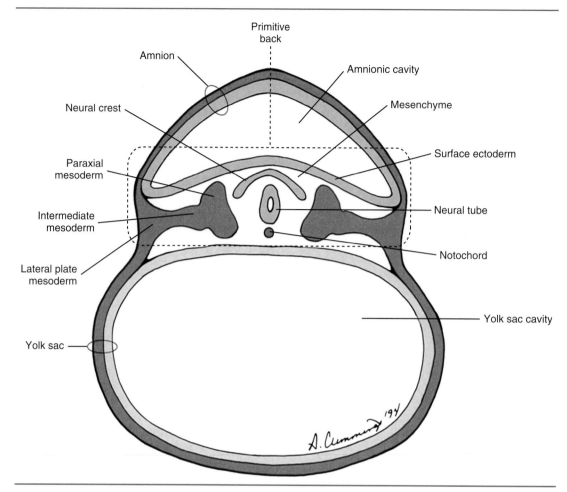

FIG. 12-1   Cross section of the primitive back at roughly the end of the third embryonic week.

has appeared within it (see Fig. 12-2, *B*). The amnionic cavity can be thought of as being enclosed by walls, a roof, and a floor (Langebartel, 1977). The roof and walls become the amnion. The floor becomes the dorsal surface of the embryo and later transforms into the outer layer of the skin on the newborn's back (Sadler, 2004). By this time the inner cell mass is attached to the cytotrophoblast by only a narrow bridge of cells that is called the connecting stalk (Fig. 12-3). The connecting stalk marks the tail or caudal end of the embryo just as the amnion marks its dorsal surface. A close observer would note that the cells in the inner cell mass have grouped themselves into two layers (see Fig. 12-2, *A*). One layer floors the amnionic cavity and is called the epiblast. The other layer roofs the blastocyst cavity and is called the hypoblast (Moore and Persaud, 2003). The hypoblast gives rise to a layer of cells that comes to line the blastocyst cavity. The blastocyst cavity then is known as the primitive yolk sac even though it contains a negligible amount of yolk (Scammon, 1953) (see Fig. 12-3).

The yolk sac cells next bud off other cells that deposit themselves on the outside of the yolk sac, where they make up a layer called extraembryonic mesoderm (Moore and Persaud, 2003) (Fig. 12-4). The triple layer, consisting of the cytotrophoblast sandwiched between the syncytiotrophoblast and extraembryonic mesoderm, is called the chorion and is the embryonic portion of the placenta (Goss, 1966). That means the cavity inside the chorion actually corresponds to the previous blastocyst cavity or primitive yolk sac (Sadler, 2004). To recognize the changes that have occurred (e.g., the imminent appearance of the secondary or definitive yolk sac and extraembryonic mesoderm), this cavity is renamed the extraembryonic coelom and is also called the chorionic cavity (Goss, 1966) (see Fig. 12-4).

GASTRULATION AND DEVELOPMENT OF THE NOTOCHORD

At the beginning of the third week of development, a narrow groove forms on the caudal portion of the dorsal surface of the epiblast known as the primitive streak (Hamilton and Mossman, 1972) (Fig. 12-5). Epiblast cells begin to migrate toward the primitive streak. Once there,

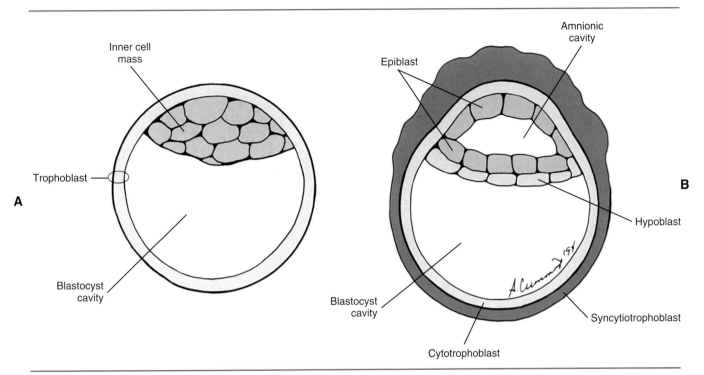

FIG. 12-2   Cross section of the blastocyst. **A,** At the beginning of the second embryonic week. **B,** In the middle of the second embryonic week.

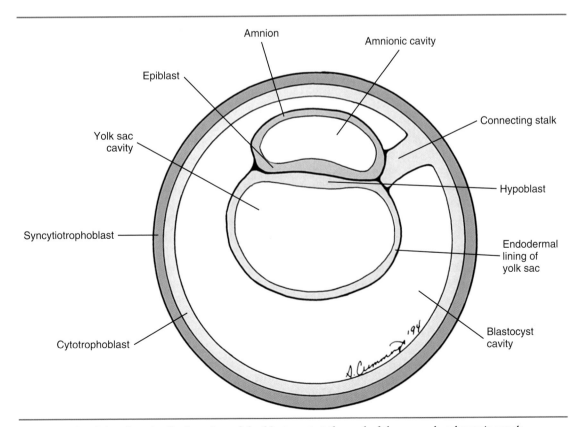

FIG. 12-3   Longitudinal section of the blastocyst at the end of the second embryonic week.

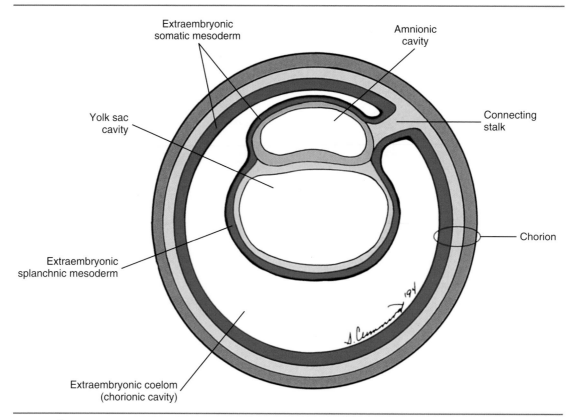

FIG. 12-4   Longitudinal section through bilaminar embryo at the end of the second embryonic week before appearance of mesoderm.

the cells detach from the epiblast and invaginate deep to it through the primitive streak. Once invaginated, the cells move in all directions. Some of these cells displace the hypoblast and form the endoderm (Sadler, 2004). The endoderm eventually will form the lining of the respiratory and gastrointestinal tracts. Other invaginating cells form a new layer of cells between the epiblast and the newly formed endoderm called the intraembryonic mesoderm. The cells remaining in the epiblast become the ectoderm. The ectoderm, mesoderm, and endoderm are the three germ layers from which the entire embryo will differentiate. The process of forming these germ layers and creating a trilaminar embryonic disc is known as gastrulation.

Some of the invaginated epiblast cells moving superiorly in the midline toward the future head turn into a structure known as the notochord (Fig. 12-6; see also Fig. 12-1). The notochord is a relatively rigid rod of cells that marks the longitudinal axis of the embryonic body and induces the nervous system to develop. The vertebral column later occupies this site, and by then the notochord has turned into the part of the intervertebral disc known as the nucleus pulposus.

NEURULATION

Also during the third week of development, the notochord induces the ectoderm to form a thickening along its length in the midline called the neural plate, which is the primordium of the entire nervous system (Arey, 1965). The cells of the neural plate are known as the neuroectoderm. A groove forms, which runs the length of the neural plate, with two folds flanking it. This neural groove deepens and sinks below the surface. The neural folds close over it, thus forming a hollow tube of neuroectoderm called the neural tube (Scothorne, 1976) (Fig. 12-7). The neural tube is the primordium of the brain and spinal cord, and the process of its formation is called neurulation. Other neuroectoderm cells invaginate along with the neural tube but remain apart from it (Romanes, 1972a,b). They are collectively known as the neural crest (see Fig. 12-7) and give rise, among other things, to many important components of the nervous system, including all sensory neurons, all postganglionic autonomic neurons, and all ganglia, both sensory and motor (Scothorne, 1976). The rest of the ectodermal cells, which are not part of the neural plate, are destined

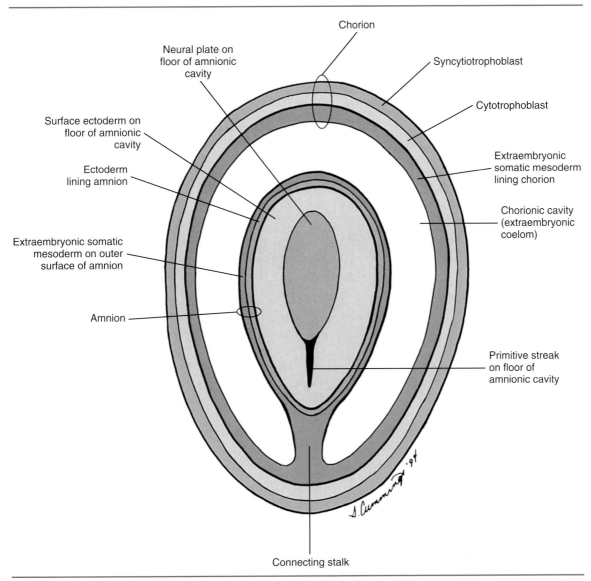

FIG. 12-5 Frontal section through chorion and amnion during third embryonic week revealing a view of the floor of the amnionic cavity as would be seen by an observer positioned on the roof of that cavity.

mostly to form the epidermis (the surface layer of the skin), and are appropriately named surface ectoderm.

SOMITE DEVELOPMENT

The mesoderm lying just lateral to the notochord parallels the long axis of the embryo and is called the paraxial mesoderm. Beginning during the third embryonic week, the paraxial mesoderm subdivides into blocks of cells known as somites, which are major contributors to the muscles, bones, and the dermis of the body. Just lateral to the somites on both sides of the embryo, other mesodermal cells have formed into a structure called intermediate mesoderm. The intermediate mesoderm eventually will develop into the majority of the genitourinary system (Fig. 12-8; see also Fig. 12-1). Lateral to the intermediate mesoderm is the lateral mesoderm, which will, along with the overlying ectoderm, form the lateral and ventral parts of the body wall.

The somites are staging areas from which mesoderm cells deploy to new locations (Sadler, 2004). The cells of the ventromedial portion of the somite will migrate toward the notochord and neural tube. These cells eventually produce hard tissues, such as bone, cartilage, and ligaments, so the part of the somite from which they are derived is appropriately called sclerotome (Harrison, 1972) (Fig. 12-9).

The rest of the somite is called the dermomyotome or epithelial plate of the somite. Traditionally, once myoblasts could be identified in the somite, termed

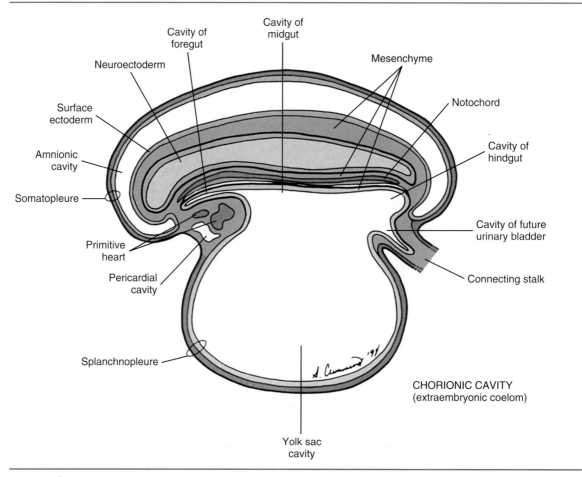

FIG. 12-6 Midsagittal section through embryo during the third embryonic week showing how folding has converted the proximal part of the yolk sac into a foregut (at the head end), a hindgut (at the tail end), and a midgut (which still lacks a floor and is confluent with the yolk sac cavity).

the myotome, the remainder of the somite was called the dermatome, which went on to form the dermis of the skin (Beck et al., 1985) (see Fig. 12-9). It is now believed that the superficial portion of the somite, the region of the traditionally defined dermatome, contributes a significant amount of muscle precursor cells as it elongates through the body wall (Williams et al., 1995). Also, the only dermis that appears to be derived exclusively from somites may be that covering the epaxial musculature, which is a much more restricted distribution than implied by the term dermatome. The remainder of the dermomyotome forms myoblasts that will eventually form skeletal muscles (Fischman, 1972) (see the following).

During the next several weeks, the amnion undergoes a series of folds creating the embryo's body wall and defining the lumen of the embryonic gut (Fig. 12-10). The embryo's body cut in cross section at this time appears as two concentric rings. The inner ring is the splanchnopleure; the outer is the somatopleure (Goss, 1966) (see

Fig. 12-8). The outer ring actually has the shape of a jeweler's signet ring. Tucked close together inside the signet part are the neural tube, neural crest, notochord, somites, intermediate mesoderm, and mesenchyme (see Fig. 12-8). The signet part corresponds to what is variously called the back, the posterior body wall, and the posterior abdominal or posterior thoracic wall (Callander, 1939; Grant, 1952; Davenport, 1966).

VERTEBRAL DEVELOPMENT

Typical Vertebrae

Vertebral development can be conveniently divided into four stages. The notochordal stage is first. The notochord not only forms the original basis for the development of the vertebrae by defining the axis of the embryo, it also forms some of the cells of the intervertebral disc. The second stage is the mesenchymal, or blastemal, stage. Mesenchyme is the connective tissue of the embryo that is, at least in the case of the vertebrae, derived from

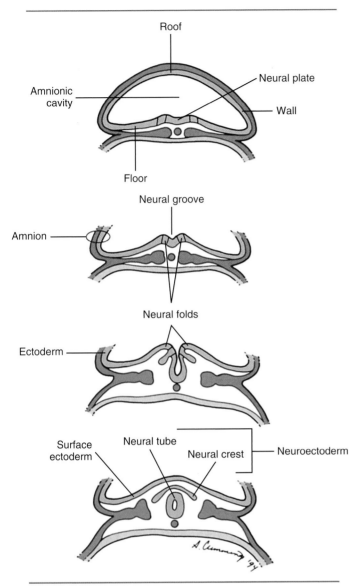

FIG. 12-7 Cross section through the amnionic (amniotic) cavity during the third embryonic week showing the formation of the neural tube and neural crest from its floor.

paraxial mesoderm. Each vertebra is formed from a mesenchymal model. The third stage is the cartilage stage, in which the vertebral mesenchyme is replaced by hyaline cartilage. The osseous stage is last, in which the hyaline cartilage is replaced by bone. Therefore each vertebra is formed by the process of endochondral ossification.

Cells of the sclerotome migrate medially from the somite to surround the neural tube and notochord (Breathnach, 1958). Instead of forming a continuous tunnel of cells, they form a series of discrete blocks of mesenchyme (Williams et al., 1995). Those cells ventral to the neural tube that specifically surround the notochord are known as the centrum. The cells dorsolateral

to the neural tube are called the neural arch (O'Rahilly, 1986) (Fig. 12-11). Each neural arch forms a pedicle, which projects ventromedially toward the centrum, and a lamina, which projects dorsomedially toward the corresponding lamina from the other side. The laminae eventually fuse and expand to form the spinous process. Cranial and caudal projections of the neural arch form articular processes, which will develop into the zygapophysial joints with adjacent vertebrae. A lateral projection of the neural arch forms the true transverse process. Projecting anterolaterally from the neural arch is the costal element, which expands to meet the tip of the transverse process. The patterning of the mesenchyme into presumptive vertebrae appears to be regulated by *HOX* genes (Sadler, 2004).

For years the accepted view has been that the sclerotome cells forming a centrum derived from two contiguous somites (Beck et al., 1985). This dual origin accounts for the staggered position of myotomes and centra (Sadler, 2004). This accepted view was challenged by Verbout (1985). However, experimental support for the accepted view also has been adduced (Bagnall et al., 1987). Most evidence still suggests that approximately the cranial half of a centrum is derived from the caudal portion of the somite above, whereas the caudal half of a centrum is derived from the cranial portion of the somite below (Williams, 1995) (Fig. 12-12).

Regardless of their origin, by the end of the second embryonic month, some of the mesenchymal cells of the vertebrae change into chondroblasts and begin laying down an extracellular cartilaginous matrix (Hall, 1978). There are typically two chondrification centers in each centrum, located on either side of the notochord. These rapidly replace the notochord in the region of the centrum with cartilage to form a single mass of cartilage (Williams et al., 1995) (see Fig. 12-11). Also, each side of the neural arch develops at least one chondrification center.

By the end of the embryonic period, primary ossification centers appear in the cartilaginous vertebra. These usually appear in a cranial to caudal pattern, beginning in the upper cervical region by approximately week 8 and reaching the sacral area by week 22 (Williams, 1995). Typically two primary ossifications centers form in the centrum (ventral and dorsal), which rapidly fuse into one center (Moore and Persaud, 2003). There is also a primary ossification center that develops in each side of the neural arch (O'Rahilly & Muller, 1992) (see Fig. 12-11). By birth, each vertebra consists of three bony segments connected by hyaline cartilage: the centrum and each half of the neural arch. The cartilages between the centrum and each neural arch actually are located within the region that will become the adult vertebral body. This region is known as the neurocentral synchondrosis (or junction) and usually fuses together into

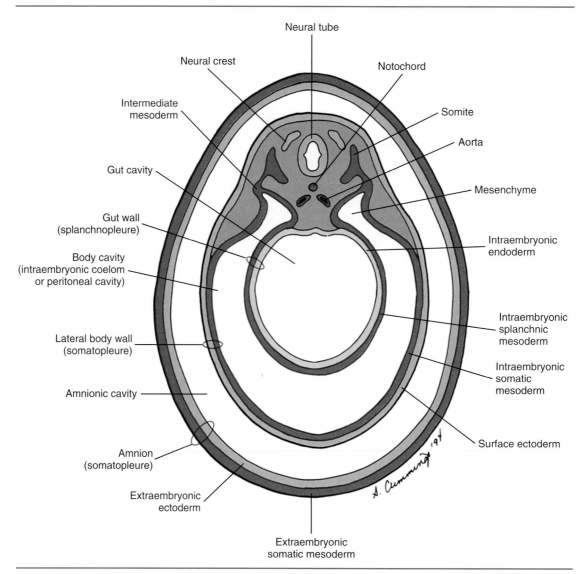

FIG. 12-8   Cross section through the two concentric tubes that run the length of the embryonic body at the end of the third embryonic week: the inner primitive gut tube (splanchnopleure) and the outer body wall tube (somatopleure). The space between them becomes the body cavity.

compact bone by age six (Maat et al., 1996). Therefore the terms vertebral body and centrum are not equivalent. Likewise the terms neural arch and vertebral arch are not synonymous. The vertebral body encompasses all of the centrum and a portion of each neural arch. The vertebral arch is only a portion of each neural arch (Trotter and Peterson, 1966).

At approximately the time of puberty, secondary ossification centers appear in the remaining cartilage (Sinclair, 1972) (see Fig. 12-11). Typically each vertebra develops five secondary ossification centers: one for the tip of each transverse process, one for the tip of the spinous process, and two anular apophyses (outdated

term: anular epophyses) one on the superior and one on the inferior rim of the vertebral body. A vertebra can increase in height and diameter before and after birth by employing intrinsic bone-depositing mechanisms around the circumference, or periosteum, and at the ends (Bogduk and Twomey, 1987). Also, there can be some variation in the distribution, and sometimes even number, of ossification centers from vertebra to vertebra, accounting for some of their individual variation (Inkster, 1951).

Although each vertebra has costal elements, the eventual fates of these elements vary by region of the spine. In the cervical spine, the costal elements eventually form most of the adult transverse process, including the

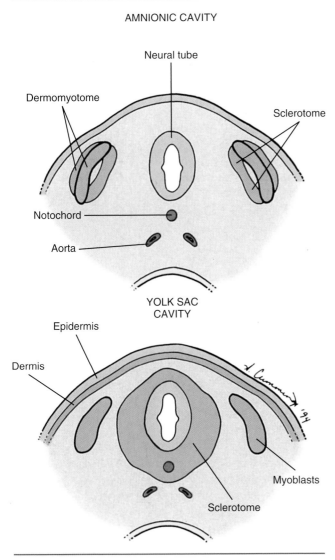

FIG. 12-9 Cross section through two stages in somite differentiation: before and after dermis and sclerotome cells have migrated to the destinations shown by the arrows.

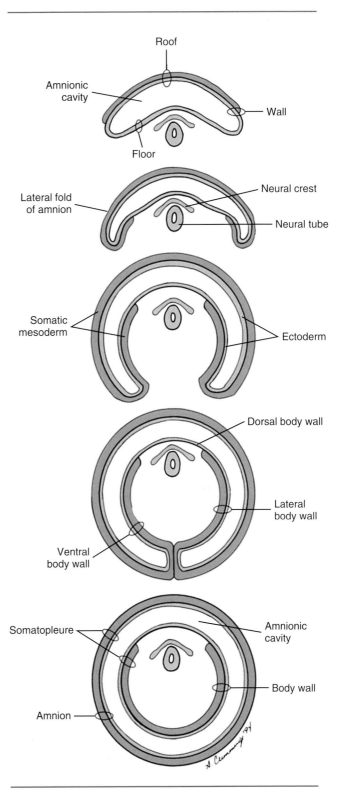

FIG. 12-10 Cross section through the amnionic cavity and neural tube showing how the original amnion transforms itself into two concentric tubes during the third embryonic week. The inner tube is the embryo's body wall; the outer is the definitive amnion.

portions that form the ventral and dorsolateral boundaries of the foramen of the transverse process. Only the portion of the adult transverse process that forms the dorsomedial border of the foramen of the transverse process develops from the embryonic transverse process. In the thoracic region, the costal elements reach their maximal length and form the ribs. In the lumbar spine, the costal elements form the anterior and lateral portions of the adult transverse processes. The embryonic transverse process forms only the dorsomedial portion of the adult lumbar transverse process, which includes the accessory process (Robertson, 1966).

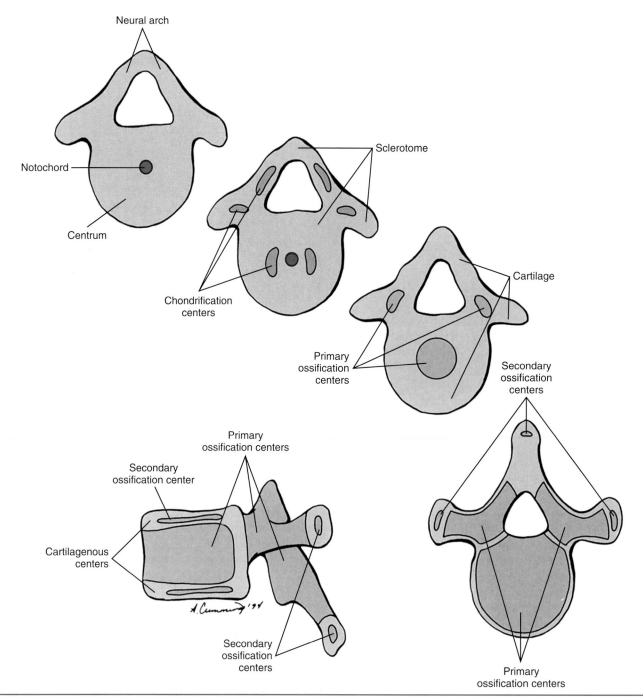

FIG. 12-11   Four cross-sectional views and a lateral view of a vertebra composed at first almost entirely of sclerotome cells (*tan*), which are gradually replaced by cartilage (*blue*), which is almost entirely replaced by bone (*purple*).

Atypical Vertebrae (Developmentally)

There are several vertebrae that have atypical patterns in their development. These include the atlas, axis, seventh cervical, lumbars, sacrum, and coccyx.

Atlas.   In the mesenchyme stage, most of the cells of the posterior aspect of the centrum of the first cervical vertebra actually become associated with the superior aspect of the cells of the centrum of the second cervical vertebra. This detachment of cells accounts for the lack of a vertebral body in the atlas and gives this bone its characteristic ring shape. These "extra" cells will become the odontoid process of the axis. The remaining cells of the anterior aspect of the centrum of the atlas will become the anterior arch of that bone. The atlas usually

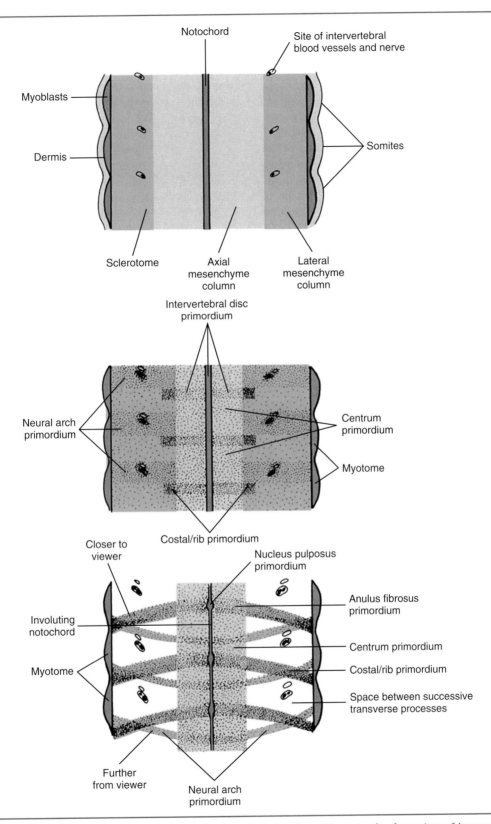

FIG. 12-12 Frontal section through notochord and somites depicting three stages in the formation of intervertebral discs and vertebrae. Cells migrate from the sclerotome to surround the notochord, but cell density is not the same everywhere along the notochordal length. Cell condensations mark the sites where intervertebral discs will appear. The vertebral centra will develop in the spaces between cell condensations. Other sclerotome cells located dorsolaterally form condensations that mark the sites where neural arches will appear. The spinal nerve and intervertebral blood vessels appear in the spaces between the developing neural arches. Other sclerotome cells located laterally condense next to the disc at the site where the costal element will appear.

is ossified from three ossification centers. There is one ossification center for each lateral mass. Also, a third ossification center forms for the anterior arch, but this center does not usually develop until after the time of birth (Pharaoh, 1956).

Axis. Most of the mesenchyme cells from the posterior aspect of the centrum of the atlas become associated with the superior aspect of the centrum of the axis. These cells will eventually become the odontoid process, although there is recent evidence that the odontoid process is not derived solely from the centrum of the atlas (David et al., 1998). The axis usually has five primary and two secondary ossification centers. The centrum and neural arches ossify in the typical manner (one center for each). At the beginning of the third trimester of pregnancy, two ossification centers appear laterally in the base of the cartilaginous odontoid process. A thin piece of cartilage may separate the base of the odontoid process and the body of the axis. This rudimentary disc ossifies slowly and may not completely disappear until the latter teenage years. A secondary ossification center forms in the apex of the odontoid process at approximately age 3 to 6 and unites with the rest of the odontoid process by approximately age 12. The last secondary ossification center is a typical anular apophysis associated with the inferior aspect of the body of the axis.

Seventh Cervical. The seventh cervical vertebra has the typical ossification centers with addition of separate secondary ossification centers for the costal processes. These appear at approximately the sixth fetal month and unite with the rest of the vertebra at approximately age 6. These may remain separate from the rest of the vertebra and form cervical ribs. Occasionally separate ossification centers for the costal processes can be found for the sixth, fifth, and even fourth cervical vertebrae (Williams et al., 1995).

Lumbars. Generally, the lumbar vertebrae ossify in the typical manner. In addition, there is usually a secondary ossification center that forms for each mamillary process.

Sacrum. The sacrum begins as five vertebral segments that eventually fuse into a single bone. Primary ossification centers for the centrum and neural arches of each sacral vertebra appear between the tenth and twelfth weeks of development. The neural arches and centra begin uniting during the second year. This process begins in the lower segments and is completed in the upper segments by the sixth year. The neural arches from both sides are usually fused by approximately the eighth year. Primary ossification centers also appear for the costal elements of the upper three (and sometimes more) segments superior and lateral to the pelvic sacral

foramina during the third trimester of pregnancy. The costal elements fuse with the corresponding neural arches during the second to fifth years and to the centra by approximately the eighth year. Laterally the conjoined neural arches and costal elements are separated from the segments above and below by epiphyseal cartilages. These epiphyseal cartilages are associated with the auricular surfaces. Around the time of puberty, various secondary ossification centers may form that are associated with the upper and lower aspects of the centra, spinous tubercles, transverse tubercles, and costal elements. The centers for the costal elements complete the ossification process for the auricular surfaces by age 20 (Pharaoh, 1956).

The bodies of the sacral vertebrae during early life are separated by intervertebral fibrocartilages. The margins of the bodies begin to fuse around age 18, beginning inferiorly. By the mid-twenties, the sacrum usually is a single, solid bone, although vestiges of the intervertebral fibrocartilages may persist (Williams et al., 1995).

Coccyx. Each segment of the coccyx ossifies from a single primary ossification center. The center for the first segment appears soon after the time of birth. Occasionally there are separate ossification centers that appear for the coccygeal cornua at approximately this same time (Williams et al., 1995). The ossification centers for the remaining coccygeal segments appear, from superior to inferior, variably during childhood and puberty, so that all of them have usually appeared by age 20. The segments gradually fuse with one another so that by age 30 the coccyx usually is a solid bone. The coccyx may variably fuse with the sacrum in later life.

Intervertebral Discs and Other Joints

Although the mesenchyme of the sclerotome replaces the notochordal tissue to form the centra of the vertebrae, the notochordal tissue located between the developing vertebrae actually expands to form the presumptive nucleus pulposus of the intervertebral discs (see Figs. 12-9 and 12-12). This expanded notochordal tissue is surrounded by sclerotomal mesenchyme called the perichordal disc. The perichordal disc will eventually form the anulus fibrosus and cartilaginous end plates. Around the sixth fetal month, the cells of the notochord begin to degenerate, being replaced by cells of the surrounding mesenchyme. This process continues so that all of the notochordal cells have disappeared by the end of the second decade of life (Williams et al., 1995). Therefore the only structures in the adult that are of notochordal origin are possibly some noncellular matrices of the nucleus pulposus.

The zygapophysial joints develop in a similar manner to other synovial joints from the mesenchyme of the sclerotome (Bogduk and Twomey, 1987). The mesenchyme between the presumptive articular processes condenses around the sixth fetal week. Around the periphery of this region, the mesenchyme differentiates into the capsular and flaval ligaments. Centrally the mesenchymal cells disappear to form the synovial cavity by a process of apoptosis. The mesenchyme lining the inside of the fibrous capsule eventually forms the synovial membrane.

The other ligaments associated with the spine (Walmsley, 1972), including the sacroiliac ligaments (Salsabili and Hogg, 1991), also develop as condensations of mesenchyme of the sclerotome. In the appropriate intervertebral regions, this mesenchyme condenses and forms dense regular collagenous connective tissue that becomes the various named ligaments.

Developmental Anomalies

Because the development of the vertebrae is a complicated process, it should not be surprising that developmental anomalies are common occurrences. Many of these do not pose any problems and are never detected or are incidental findings. On the other hand, some of these can have a profound impact on the health and lifestyle of the individual. Many of these conditions are discussed in further detail in other chapters. References to these chapters appear where appropriate.

Klippel-Feil Syndrome. Klippel-Feil Syndrome is a developmental anomaly of the cervical spine in which there is fusion or malformation of multiple vertebrae. There also may be absence of one or more cervical vertebrae. The head of a person with this problem appears low between the shoulders, and the neck usually appears too short. Commonly there is fusion of the lower cervical vertebrae into one large, misshapen bone, which reduces cervical ranges of motion.

Basilar Impression (Platybasia). Basilar impression is mainly a developmental defect in the occiput in which it appears to have been pushed superiorly by the cervical spine. Frequently there is an accompanying malformation of one or both of the upper cervical vertebrae. The atlas may be ankylosed to the occiput. Because the occipital condyles and the squama of the occiput are misshapen, the foramen magnum commonly is smaller in diameter and distorted. Also, the odontoid process can project unusually high into the area of the foramen magnum. These latter two malformations can lead to profound neurologic insult to the lower portion of the brain stem or upper region of the spinal cord. (See Chapter 5 for additional details.)

Occipital Vertebra. This is a condition in which there appears to be an occipital vertebra. There are two main forms of this anomaly. The first is a true occipital vertebra in which a rudimentary vertebra forms, almost always attached to the inferior aspect of the occiput. Usually a normal atlas is found below this malformation. This anomaly is thought to represent a vestige of the proatlas seen in primitive vertebrates and results from the improper incorporation of the occipital sclerotomes (Pharaoh, 1956).

The second form of this anomaly is an atlanto-occipital fusion; this is sometimes termed occipitalization. In this case, the articular processes of atlas and the occipital condyles are ankylosed. Other than this bony attachment of the two bones, both may be normal in appearance, although the atlas may be somewhat misshapen.

Detached Apex of Odontoid Process. This anomaly represents a nonunion of the apical region of the odontoid process with the rest of that process (see Figs. 13-10 and 13-13). There appears to be a small fragment of bone just above the odontoid process, which is commonly known as a terminal ossicle (ossiculum terminalis). The rest of the odontoid process appears somewhat shortened and blunted. This ossicle usually is embedded in the apical odontoid ligament. (See Chapter 13 for additional information.)

Os Odontoideum. Sometimes there is a nonunion of the odontoid process with the body of the axis (see Figs. 13-10 and 13-12). If this happens, the ununited ossicle is termed an os odontoideum. This can lead to a relatively unstable upper cervical region, although there usually is a soft tissue connection between the ossicle and the body of the axis. Trauma in the region that otherwise would not present much of a problem can lead to catastrophic consequences with this anomaly. (See Chapters 5 and 13 for additional information.)

Congenital Absence of the Odontoid Process. Obviously this rare anomaly can be dangerous. This condition represents a failure of mesenchymal or other (e.g., ossification) developmental centers of the odontoid process. Usually compensatory ankylosis in the region can be found, which may be the result of the increased mobility and instability in the region.

Accessory Ribs. Accessory ribs, usually rudimentary, are an overgrowth of the costal elements of either lumbar or cervical vertebrae (Fig. 12-13). Lumbar ribs are much more common than cervical ribs (Moore and Persaud, 2003), and usually cause no clinical problems. Cervical ribs may be involved in neurovascular insults in the region of the thoracic inlet, which are known commonly in clinical circles as a type of thoracic outlet syndrome. (See Cervicoaxillary Syndrome in Chapter 5.)

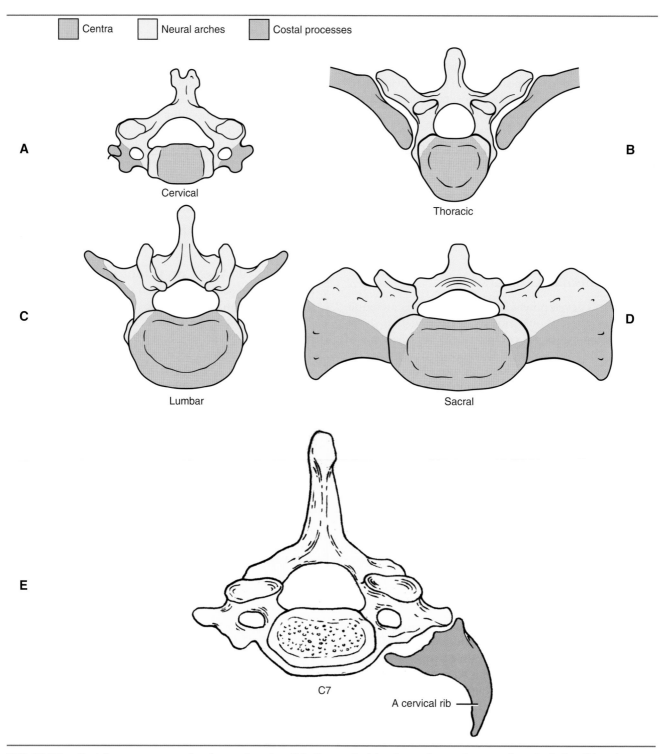

FIG. 12-13   Costal processes, neural arches, and centra of, **A,** the cervical (notice each costal process here includes all but the most proximal part of the posterior root of the transverse process); **B,** thoracic (which normally become ribs); **C,** lumbar; and, **D,** sacral regions of the vertebral column. **E,** Illustration showing a cervical rib. (**E,** Modified from Mathers LH. [1996]. *Clinical anatomy principles*, St Louis: Mosby.)

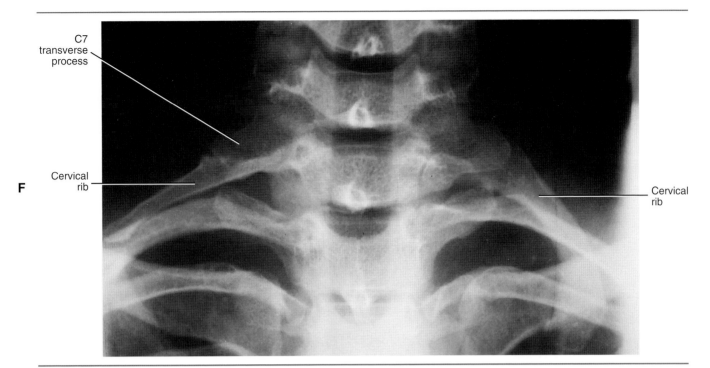

FIG. 12-13—cont'd   **F,** Anterior-posterior x-ray showing bilateral cervical ribs. Sizes of cervical ribs vary considerably. A cervical rib may, but does not always, articulate with the first thoracic rib or the sternum. When the cervical rib does not have an osseous anterior attachment, a fibrous band may extend from the anterior tip of the rib to the either the first thoracic rib or the sternum (see text for further details).

Hemivertebra. When only either the right or left half of a vertebral body develops, it results in the anomaly known as hemivertebra, or cuneiform vertebra, and usually occurs in the thoracic spine (Fig. 12-14, *A* and *B*). The problem presumably occurs in the cartilage stage of development or earlier. Because there are two chondrification centers for the centrum, right and left, it is hypothesized that one of these fails to develop (Rothman and Simeone, 1992). Usually the half of the vertebral body that is present becomes deformed because of weight bearing such that it is triangular in shape (when seen from in front, as in an AP plain film radiograph), with the apex directed medially. This deformation results in an obvious scoliosis that usually undergoes degenerative changes relatively early in life. Frequently two hemivertebrae can be found several segments away from each other. The two hemivertebrae are formed from opposite halves of the developmental centers. Thus they compensate for one another, decreasing the severity of the scoliosis.

Butterfly Vertebra. This is a deformity in which both halves of the vertebral body have formed but have not united properly in the midline (Fig. 12-14, *C* and *D*). Each half is usually wedge-shaped, such that each is not as tall in the midline as it is laterally. When viewed in

an AP plain film radiograph, the vertebral body has a shape that is reminiscent of a butterfly, hence the name of the deformity. The developmental problem presumably happens in the chondrification stage, or earlier, because of an imperfect union of the regions of the centrum formed by the side-by-side chondrification centers. This anomaly usually occurs in the thoracic spine and may cause spinal curvatures: kyphosis, scoliosis, or both.

Block Vertebra. This anomaly represents a nonsegmentation of the somites (Fig. 12-14, *E* and *F*). It results in the formation of a vertebra that is actually two adjacent vertebrae that are fused together into a single bone. The vertebral body is twice as high as normal. The vertebral arches usually are also fused together, although not always completely. This anomaly is most frequent in the lumbar spine, but can occur anywhere in the spine. It may result in a kyphotic deformity because of the tendency to overdevelopment of the posterior aspect of the vertebral body and underdevelopment of the anterior aspect.

Lumbosacral Transitional Segment. This is a general term for two types of developmental anomalies. One is when the L5 vertebra overdevelops, especially its

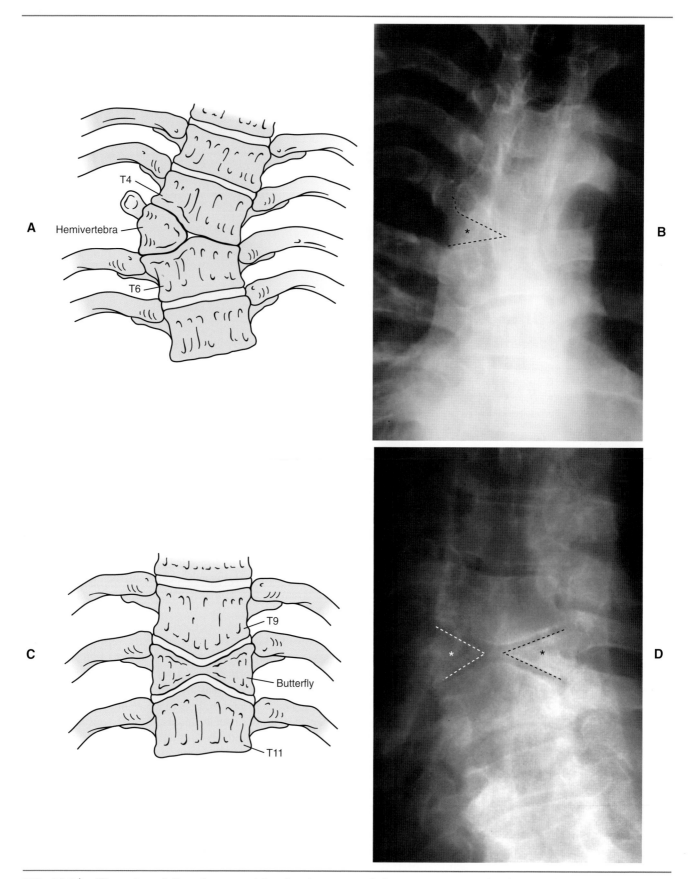

FIG. 12-14 Illustrations, *left,* and x-rays, *right,* showing many of the most common developmental anomalies. **A** and **B,** Hemivertebra (outline and asterisk on the anterior-posterior thoracic x-ray of **B**). **C** and **D,** Butterfly vertebra (outlines and asterisks on the anterior-posterior thoracic x-ray of **D** show that this butterfly vertebra is completely bisected in the midline). (X-rays courtesy Dr. Jeff Rich.)

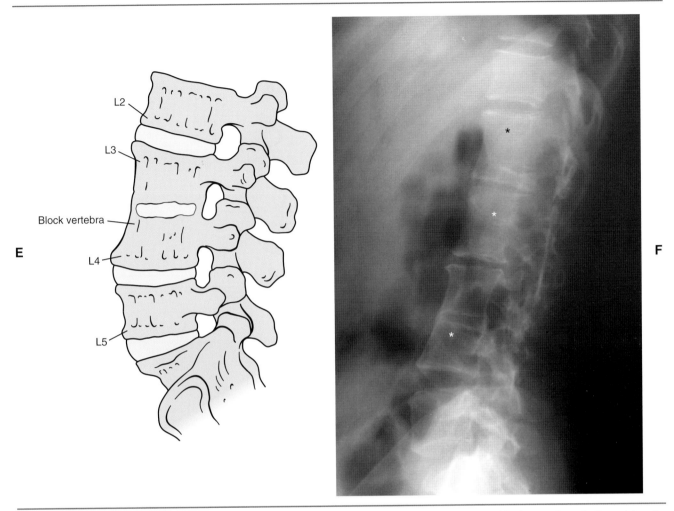

E   F

FIG. 12-14—cont'd   **E** and **F** Block vertebra (lumbar region, notice the three consecutive block vertebrae indicated by the asterisks in **F**).

Continued

transverse processes, and appears similar to the sacral segments. This specific anomaly is called a sacralization of L5 and is not too uncommon (Fig. 12-14, *G* and *H*). It may happen either unilaterally or, more often, bilaterally. This overdevelopment may go so far as to result in the actual fusion of L5 with S1. This fusion usually only involves one or, more often, both transverse processes. Sometimes L5 may completely fuse with S1 to form a sacrum that is truly composed of six segments. This type of anomaly, especially the types in which there is bilateral asymmetry, could cause altered biomechanics in the region. (See Chapter 7 for additional information.)

The other type of transitional segment in this region is when the S1 segment develops in such a way as to be more similar to a lumbar vertebra than a sacral segment. This usually is termed a lumbarization of S1. It is not as common as a sacralization of L5. This independence of S1 may go so far as to result in six true lumbar vertebrae.

This type of anomaly causes resultant changes in the structure of the sacroiliac joint.

Spina Bifida.   Spina bifida is the result of nonunion of the right and left halves of the neural arches (Fig. 12-15, *A* to *E*). Unfortunately it also may involve the underlying neural tissue, and if so, is one of the most serious vertebral anomalies. If no neural tissue is involved in the defect, it is termed spina bifida occulta, because there are rarely any clinical manifestations. This type of anomaly occurs most commonly in the lumbo-sacral region. In fact, the sacral hiatus may be considered a physiologic spina bifida. The second most common location is C1, in which case it is called agenesis of the atlas (see Chapter 13). Spina bifida occulta may be found in nearly 10% of the otherwise normal population (Sadler, 2004). In these cases, the separation between the halves of the vertebral arch usually is not wide, is filled

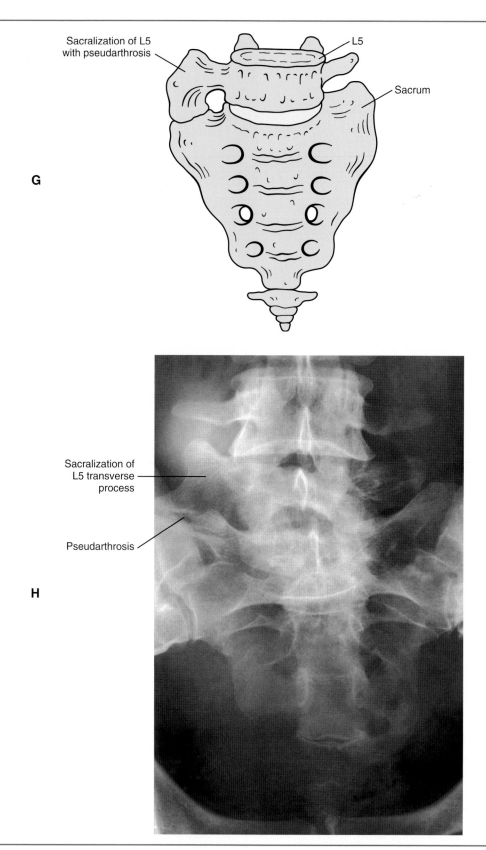

FIG. 12-14—cont'd **G** and **H** (anterior-posterior x-ray), Transitional segment between L5 and the sacrum (sacralization) forming an accessory joint (pseudarthrosis).

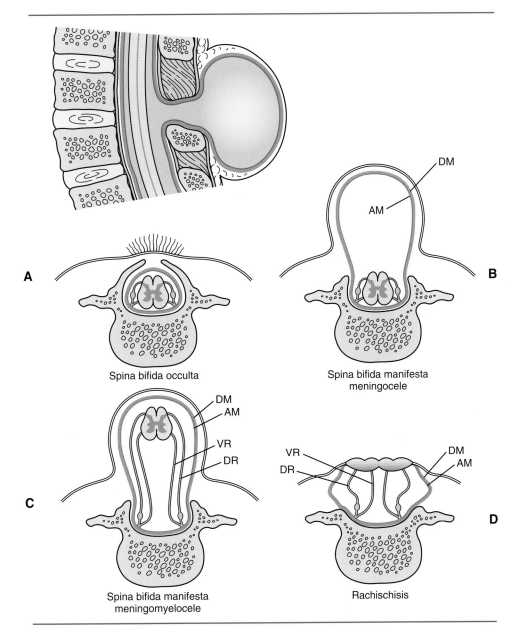

FIG. 12-15 Spina bifida. The orientation illustration in the upper left of the figure is of a midsagittal section through T11–L2 in a newborn with spina bifida manifesta (meningocele) at the level of T12. Parts **A** through **D** show the different types of spina bifida in horizontal sections through T12. **A,** Spina bifida occulta. **B** and **C,** Spina bifida manifesta showing, **B,** meningocele and, **C,** meningomyelocele. **D,** Rachischisis. Notice the neural tissue is completely exposed to the external environment in this latter condition. See text for further details on each of these types of spina bifida. *AM,* Arachnoid mater; *DM,* dura mater; *DR,* dorsal root; and, *VR,* ventral root.

Continued

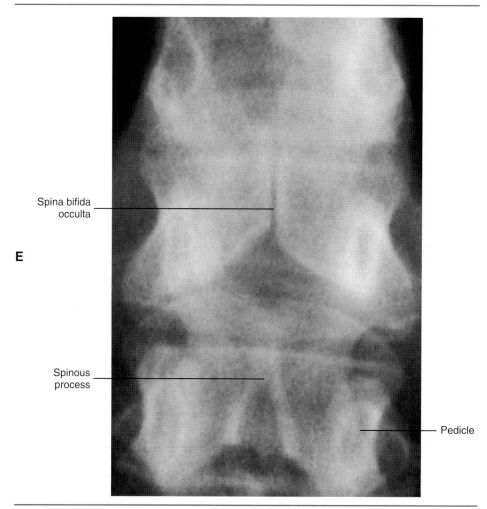

FIG. 12-15—cont'd   E, X-ray showing spina bifida occulta of a thoracic vertebra. (X-ray courtesy Dr. Jeffrey Rich.)

with connective tissue, and is covered with skin. Sometimes a tuft of hair may be found over the defect, especially in the lumbosacral region.

If the developmental defect involves not only osseous structures, but also the underlying neural tissue, it is termed spina bifida cystica or manifesta. These actually represent a form of neural tube defect and may occur in approximately 1/1000 births (Sadler, 2004). In these, neural tissue protrudes through the defect in the vertebral arch to form a cystlike sac. If only fluid-filled meninges protrude through the vertebral defect, it is termed meningocele. If true neural tissue also protrudes through the defect, it is known as meningomyelocele. Rarely the neural folds do not fuse properly with each other. Instead they fuse with the overlying surface ectoderm, resulting in a mass of flattened neural tissue. This is known as myeloschisis or rachischisis. Usually spina bifida cystica is found in the lumbosacral region,

but it may be associated with anencephaly when it is found in the cervical region. Spina bifida cystica usually results in severe neurologic deficits.

AXIAL MUSCLE DEVELOPMENT

Epaxial Muscles

While the sclerotome is starting to form the vertebrae, the dermomyotome is also continuing to develop. Cells along the craniomedial edge of the dermomyotome elongate in a cranial to caudal direction and are collectively called the myotome. These cells will form the epaxial muscles, which are dorsolateral to the vertebrae. The myotome of one somite soon encounters the myotomes cephalic and caudal to it. The cells of the myotome are postmitotic myoblasts that soon lose their individual identities and develop into the deep muscles of the back (Lockhart, 1951). The deep back muscles also are called the intrinsic or "true" muscles of the back and include the erector spinae and transversospinalis groups, two splenius muscles, and suboccipital muscles. Other deep back muscles that are epaxial in nature are the interspinales, levators costarum, and medial portions of the intertransversarii. These muscles are all innervated by the dorsal rami of spinal nerves (Joseph, 1976) (see Figs. 4-2 to 4-4).

Hypaxial Muscles

The cells of the ventrolateral edge of the dermomyotome at the levels of the limbs will migrate into the developing limb buds to form the limb musculature. The remainder of the cells of the dermomyotome will grow into the flank region of the trunk to form the hypaxial musculature (Langebartel, 1977). All of the hypaxial muscles, and also the limb muscles, are innervated by ventral rami of spinal nerves (Sadler, 2004).

The myoblasts from adjacent somites run into one another, lose their individual identities, and form the muscles of the thoracic and abdominal body wall (Williams et al., 1995). These include many muscles that can be seen from the back, such as the intercostal, lateral portions of the intertransversarii, subcostal, the two serratus posterior, and the external abdominal oblique muscles (Sinclair, 1972). Myoblasts move ventromedially toward the vertebral column, where they join with myoblasts from adjacent somites to form muscles located at the sides and front of the vertebral column (Lockhart, 1951). These muscles include the three scalenes, two longus (colli and capitis), two psoas, and quadratus lumborum (Snell, 1975). Other myoblasts form the two muscular sheets that roof and floor the abdominopelvic cavity, the thoracoabdominal and pelvic diaphragms (Arey, 1965; Moore and Persaud, 2003), both of which intersect the posterior body wall. Still other myoblasts move posteriorly to form the muscles that hold the scapula to the vertebral column or ribs (Corliss, 1976). These muscles include the rhomboids, levator scapulae, and serratus anterior, all of which are innervated by ventral rami that have been channeled through the brachial plexus (Leeson and Leeson, 1972) (see Fig. 4-1).

The scapula is somewhat of an intermediary between the bones visible from the back (spine and ribs) and the bone that extends from the elbow to the shoulder (humerus) (Breathnach, 1958). The shoulder muscles that connect the scapula to the humerus include the supraspinatus, infraspinatus, teres major, teres minor, subscapularis, and deltoid (Romanes, 1976). All but the subscapularis can be seen from behind (Crafts, 1966), but the gross anatomist does not regard them as back muscles, even though the average person might

(Hollinshead, 1982). These muscles develop from the ventrolateral edge of the dermomyotome and consequently are innervated by ventral rami of spinal nerves through the brachial plexus (Langebartel, 1977). However, one muscle connects the humerus directly to the posterior aspect of the trunk, largely bypassing the scapula (Sinclair, 1972). This muscle is the latissimus dorsi, and its origin can be traced back to this same region of the dermomyotome. It is also innervated by ventral rami through the brachial plexus (Lockhart, 1951).

The mentioned hypaxial muscles that migrated toward the back can be regarded as making up the extrinsic muscles of the back, just as the derivatives of true myotome make up the intrinsic musculature of the back (Mortenson and Pettersen, 1966). It is interesting to note that the muscles that began more dorsally in the somite, the epaxial muscles, eventually form the deep back muscles. The hypaxial muscles, even though they began more ventrally in the somite, migrate dorsally and eventually come to overlie the epaxial muscles, becoming the superficial back muscles (Scothorne, 1976). The extrinsic muscles, with one exception (trapezius), are innervated by ventral rami; the intrinsic muscles, with no exception, are innervated by dorsal rami (Lockhart, 1951).

Trapezius Muscle. One superficial, or extrinsic, back muscle may not be derived from the somites, but overlies those that do (Zuckerman, 1961). This muscle, the trapezius, may derive from the mesoderm located in the transition zone between the pharyngeal (branchial) arches and cervical somites (Lockhart, 1951). Its motor innervation comes from the same cranial nerve that innervates the most caudal branchial arches, the (spinal) accessory or eleventh, and its sensory innervation may come from cervical spinal nerves (Williams et al., 1995). However, some disagreement exists about how to interpret this dual innervation (Hollinshead, 1982).

NEURAL DEVELOPMENT IN THE BACK

Spinal Cord

The caudal portion of the neural tube will form the spinal cord or spinal medulla. Some neuroectodermal cells of the neural tube differentiate into macroglioblasts and others into neuroblasts (Clark, 1951). The latter soon take on the characteristics of a neuron-to-be (Williams et al., 1995). A blob of protoplasm, the future nerve cell body, contains the chromosomes. The cytoplasm streams out into fingerlike projections that become axons and dendrites (Sadler, 2004). Sometimes the cytoplasmic processes merely connect one side of the neural tube with the other, never leaving the tube (Noback and

Demarest, 1975). At other times, one cytoplasmic process travels down or up the spinal cord, or even to the brain stem itself, whereas other processes remain at the same level of the neural tube at which they originated (Williams et al., 1995).

A cytoplasmic process of one neuroblast usually travels with others having a common origin and destination (Williams et al., 1995). Such a bundle of cytoplasmic processes inside the neural tube is called a tract (Barr and Kiernan, 1993). The cytoplasmic processes traveling together originate from a group of nerve cell bodies in the primitive spinal cord and, for example, may terminate in the thalamus. These cytoplasmic processes form the spinothalamic tract (Goss, 1966). Sometimes the cytoplasmic process from a neuroblast leaves the spinal cord altogether (Durward, 1951) and, with many others, forms an aggregate known as the ventral root of the spinal nerve (Goss, 1966). An individual cytoplasmic process of this type finds its way to a particular region of a particular skeletal muscle. Along the way it has passed through a spinal nerve, the dorsal or ventral ramus of the spinal nerve, perhaps through a nerve plexus, and finally through a peripheral nerve (Larsell, 1953).

The derivatives of the neural tube (i.e., brain and spinal cord) are ensheathed in connective tissue layers termed the meninges. The innermost layer, which is intimately adhered to the surface of the central nervous system, is a thin layer of loose connective tissue called the pia mater. It is still uncertain as to whether the pia traces back to mesoderm or to neural crest (Williams et al., 1995). A similar uncertainty exists about the origin of the arachnoid mater, which faces the pia mater across the subarachnoid space (Carlson, 1981). It is generally agreed that the outermost meninx, the dura mater, derives from mesoderm (Williams et al., 1995). The spinal nerve roots also are ensheathed by meninges, mostly in the form of the dural root sleeves, which blend with the epineurium of the peripheral nerve.

Spinal Nerve Roots

Two cytoplasmic processes issue forth in opposite directions from most of the clusters of neural crest cells that are not destined to become autonomic neurons. One process travels dorsomedially into the neural tube, where as an axon (central process) it terminates in the region that becomes the dorsal horn of the gray matter (see Chapters 3 and 9). The central process synapses with neuroblasts derived from the neural tube in the dorsal horn. The central processes also can ascend the dorsal aspect of the spinal cord to form the dorsal columns (see Chapter 9). The second cytoplasmic process travels ventrolaterally, where it enters a spinal nerve as a dendrite (peripheral process). The cytoplasmic process going dorsomedially and the one traveling ventrolaterally, as well as the nerve cell body to

which they are both attached, are said to lie in the dorsal root of the spinal nerve. Such a dorsal root contains many other neuroblasts with the same shape and spatial configuration, and all their nerve cell bodies together form the spinal ganglion, also known as the dorsal root ganglion (Clark, 1951). This is a sensory ganglion, and no synapses occur within it. The dorsal root is called a sensory root because the current consensus holds that it contains only fibers of afferent neuroblasts derived from neural crest (Scothorne, 1976). The consensus also holds that the ventral root is a motor root and contains only axons of efferent neuroblasts derived from the neural tube (Cohen et al., 1992). That means that the spinal nerve formed by the intersection of the sensory and motor roots is a mixed nerve, and that the cell bodies of the nerve fibers are derived from both neural tube and neural crest (Clark, 1976) (see Fig. 3-12).

The dorsal and ventral roots are attached to the neural tube at one end and converge to form the spinal nerve at the other end (Clark, 1976). In the early embryo, the roots on one side are not much different in length from the roots on the opposite side and from one spinal level to another (Francis and Voneida, 1966). However, these relationships change with time (Sadler, 2004).

Each dorsal and corresponding ventral root grows laterally toward the paraxial mesoderm before the vertebrae have formed (Beck et al., 1985). Both eventually become trapped between the vertebra formed cephalic and the vertebra formed caudal to them (Hollinshead and Rosse, 1985) (see Fig. 12-12). When first formed, all these roots at all spinal levels have roughly the same length, and they all extend out laterally from the neural tube at approximately the same angle, nearly 90 degrees. However, when these roots become trapped they do not all remain the same length and do not all continue to make the same angle with the neural tube (Cohen et al., 1992). The dorsal and ventral roots that are trapped between a pair of vertebral primordia must elongate when the neural tube stays fixed in place because the vertebral primordia seem to be moving caudally. The vertebral primordia trapping cervical and thoracic roots move caudally the least, if at all, and thus their nerve roots elongate the least (Romanes, 1972a,b). By contrast, the vertebral primordia trapping lumbar and sacral roots move caudally the most, which means their nerve roots elongate the most (Snell, 1981) (see Fig. 3-8). The angle the elongated roots make with the neural tube also has been reduced less than 90 degrees to an acute angle, and the more elongated the root, the more acute the angle (Clark, 1976). The longest roots have had their angle reduced to 0 degrees, so they hang down vertically, paralleling the neural tube itself (Parke, 1992b). Early anatomists thought the dozens of nerve roots hanging down together caudal to the neural tube resembled a horse's tail, thus the name in Latin, cauda equina (Hollinshead, 1982) (see Fig. 3-11).

Autonomic Nervous System

Other neuroblasts are located elsewhere in the gray matter of the neural tube, in an area known as the lateral horn (Romanes, 1972a). Each neuroblast sends one of its cytoplasmic processes into the closest ventral root, not heading for skeletal muscle but rather toward non-skeletal muscle or glands (or both) (Sadler, 2004). Each process can change course, leave the spinal nerve it has entered, and travel to a nearby structure known as a sympathetic chain ganglion (Goss, 1966) (see Fig. 10-7). In so doing, the processes create a bridgelike structure called a white ramus communicans. It is known as white because this ramus is made up mostly of myelinated nerve fibers (Ellis, 1983).

These neuroblasts, stretching from the lateral horn (the future intermediolateral cell column) to a sympathetic chain ganglion, are myelinated and are called preganglionic neuroblasts (Romanes, 1972a,b). They function as motor neurons, which means the white ramus is made up of axons derived from the neural tube. As a rule, white rami are found attached only to the T1 through L2 spinal nerves (Crafts, 1966). The lateral horn corresponds to the nerve cell bodies, and the white ramus corresponds to the axons of the same neuroblasts, or preganglionic sympathetic neuroblasts (Durward, 1951). Above and below these spinal levels, there is no lateral horn, no white rami exist, and the ventral roots do not contain myelinated axons of preganglionic sympathetic neuroblasts (Bruce and Walmsley, 1939).

Some axons of preganglionic neuroblasts cross over a white ramus to a sympathetic chain ganglion but do not terminate within the ganglion (Francis and Voneida, 1966). Instead, they pass through the ganglion and continue up the sympathetic chain or down the chain to a sympathetic chain ganglion at a different spinal level, where they terminate (Langebartel, 1977). Inside they synapse with neuroblasts known as postganglionic sympathetics (Goss, 1966). Some axons of preganglionic neuroblasts reach sympathetic chain ganglia by way of white rami, but they do not terminate in any sympathetic chain ganglion (Goss, 1966). Instead, these preganglionic axons pass through the sympathetic chain ganglion without synapsing and continue on their way to a sympathetic ganglion in the abdominal cavity, where they terminate (Francis and Voneida, 1966). These are called splanchnic nerves (see Chapter 10). Some preganglionic neuroblasts have nerve cell bodies located in the gray matter of the sacral region of the neural tube and are classified as parasympathetic. Their axons travel long distances and terminate in parasympathetic ganglia located close to the pelvic organs they innervate (Scothorne, 1976). They synapse inside these parasympathetic ganglia with postganglionic parasympathetic neuroblasts located within or close to the organs (Romanes, 1972b).

All sympathetic and parasympathetic postganglionic neuroblasts, as well as the ganglia they help to form, derive from the neural crest (O'Rahilly and Muller, 1992). These motor ganglia are made up of the nerve cell bodies of postganglionic neuroblasts that migrated from the original site of the neural crest (i.e., dorsolateral to the neural tube) to the site of the ganglion. Most, if not all, postganglionic neuroblasts in a sympathetic chain ganglion send their cytoplasmic processes out of the ganglion to the closest spinal nerve and, in so doing, form a bridge called a gray ramus communicans. It is termed gray (as opposed to white) because this ramus is made up of unmyelinated nerve fibers (Romanes, 1972a). Once in the spinal nerve, the postganglionic axons twist their way through the branches of the spinal nerves. These include dorsal and ventral rami, nerve plexuses, when present, and peripheral nerves (Woodburne, 1983). The postganglionic axons terminate in the smooth muscle of blood vessels or in glands (Hollinshead and Rosse, 1985).

Although all spinal nerves have gray rami communicantes, sometimes the axons of postganglionic sympathetic neuroblasts shun the gray rami and are not distributed by a spinal nerve (Larsell, 1953). Instead, they travel directly to the organ they innervate (Durward, 1951). This is the case with the heart, in which the axons of postganglionic sympathetic neuroblasts make up the cardiac sympathetic nerves (Francis and Voneida, 1966). The nerve cell bodies for these postganglionic neuroblasts lie in cervical sympathetic chain ganglia (Durward, 1951).

VASCULAR DEVELOPMENT IN THE BACK

While all the mentioned embryonic and fetal events have been taking place, the ubiquitous mesoderm has been constructing the cardiovascular system (Brash, 1951a). On the surface of the yolk sac, reddish spots develop called blood islands. The redness is caused by hemoglobin in erythroblasts that appear inside these blood islands as they hollow out and become confluent with each other. Other vascular plexuses are formed in the same way throughout the embryo, but certain channels begin to predominate while others disappear (Yoffey, 1976). Two large channels located ventral to the foregut turn out to be the mesodermal rudiments of the heart. This primitive heart drains into vascular channels that have derived from the mesoderm that lies on either side of the nearby pharyngeal arches (Patten, 1953). These paired channels carry blood dorsally away from the heart to the left and right dorsal aortae, and they are called aortic arches (Yoffey, 1976) or aortic arch arteries (Moore and Persaud, 2003).

The blood entering the paired dorsal aortae moves into all the branches from this pair of arteries, which are the largest of the embryonic body. The paired branches going to the back have been called segmental arteries

(Hollinshead, 1982). The capillaries of the back return that blood to segmental veins that empty into paired anterior and posterior cardinal veins (Brash, 1951a). The anterior and posterior cardinals on each side empty into a common cardinal vein, and then two of these empty into the primitive heart (Sadler, 2004). The circulatory pathway is now complete, but restructuring of that vasculature commences almost at once (Hollinshead and Rosse, 1985).

Arteries

The aortic arches largely disappear, except for the third, fourth, and sixth pairs; those that remain are modified (Oelrich, 1966). The third pair is used to help build the carotid artery system (Walls, 1972). One component of that system, the external carotid artery, serves the back through two of its branches, the ascending pharyngeal and occipital (Williams et al., 1995).

The fourth pair of aortic arches also helps shunt blood toward the back by contributing to the formation of the subclavian artery and arch of the aorta. The subclavian artery sends blood through many of its branches to the back (Oelrich, 1966). A list of these branches includes the vertebral artery, branches of the costocervical trunk (the deep cervical and highest intercostal arteries), and branches of the thyrocervical trunk (the ascending cervical, transverse cervical, and suprascapular arteries) (Romanes, 1966).

As development proceeds, the two dorsal aortae fuse into a single aorta, located caudally, and the paired segmental arteries branching from this single aorta proceed to designations that vary, depending on the body region they serve. These segmental branches include intercostals, subcostals, and lumbars; all these send branches to the back (Williams et al., 1995). Those paired segmental arteries supplying paired organs embedded retroperitoneally in the embryo's posterior body wall are named after the organ they serve (i.e., renal, adrenal, and gonadal) (Brash, 1951a).

Before attenuation of the single dorsal aorta into an unpaired terminal artery known as the median sacral, the dorsal aorta gives off a pair of umbilical arteries that help to form the common iliac trunk on each side (Walls, 1972). The segmental arteries called the fifth lumbars also may help to form this trunk (Williams et al., 1995). One artery that branches from the common iliac trunk is the internal iliac artery, and it gives rise to two arteries that serve the back: the iliolumbar and lateral sacral (Parke, 1992a).

The aortic arches and dorsal aorta have been sending branches to the embryo's intervertebral foramina (IVFs) (Williams et al., 1995). By the time arterial differentiation is complete, the arteries supplying branches to the IVFs have undergone changes that vary according to the spinal level (Woodburne, 1983). In the cervical region, they branch from the ascending cervical, deep cervical, and primarily the vertebral arteries; in the thoracic region, they branch from the posterior intercostals and subcostal arteries; and in the abdominal region, they branch from the lumbar, iliolumbar, lateral sacral, and median sacral arteries (Oelrich, 1966). They rebranch once inside the IVF (Hollinshead, 1982), and in the process intersect three arteries that run the length of the spinal cord: the single anterior spinal and the two posterior spinal arteries (see Chapter 3).

The anterior spinal artery had formed near the juncture of the brain and spinal cord by the union of a branch from one vertebral artery with a branch from the other vertebral artery to form an artery that extends caudally on the cord's anterior aspect (Yoffey, 1976) (see Fig. 3-15). Each posterior spinal artery had branched from a vertebral and sometimes posterior inferior cerebellar artery. The posterior spinal artery extends caudally on the posterior aspect of the spinal cord (Walls, 1972). The posterior inferior cerebellar arteries were themselves branches from the vertebral arteries, which branch from the subclavian arteries (Goss, 1966). Thus the blood supply for the spinal cord and its adnexa (hard and soft tissues) originates from within the cranium by way of the vertebral arteries and, periodically all along the spine's length, by way of feeder arteries (i.e., tributaries of arteries that enter IVFs) (Parke, 1992a). Chapter 3 discusses the arterial supply of the spinal cord in further detail.

The previous account related how the embryo constructs mesodermal channels delivering blood to those back muscles that are called intrinsic, deep, or true. The embryo develops different channels to the other back muscles that have been designated extrinsic or superficial. These latter arteries branch from the subclavian or axillary and include the following: transverse cervical, suprascapular, scapular circumflex, posterior humeral circumflex, and thoracodorsal (Crafts, 1966). Their synonymy and variability is complex (Goss, 1966). Mesoderm also has formed channels returning blood from these superficial back muscles, and often these veins retrace the route of the arteries and also bear the same names (Hollinshead and Rosse, 1985). Their variability is even greater than that of the arteries (Brash, 1951a).

Veins

While all the arterial development has been happening, the mesoderm in the epidural space surrounding the spinal cord has been forming a network of veins (Romanes, 1966) (see Fig. 3-17). This plexus lies between the meninges and the vertebrae and is known as the internal (epidural) vertebral venous plexus. This plexus receives blood from the spinal cord and the vertebrae and channels it into the intervertebral veins (Walls, 1972). These veins exit the IVFs and ventral sacral foramina (Woodburne, 1983).

Outside the foramina, the intervertebral veins drain into veins called segmental by some (Hollinshead, 1982) and intersegmental by others (Brash, 1951a). These segmental/intersegmental veins receive specific names according to their spinal level (e.g., vertebrals, intercostals, lumbars, lateral sacrals) (Brash, 1951a). These veins carry the blood back to the heart by different routes. The vertebral veins drain into the brachiocephalic veins, which pass the blood to the superior vena cava (Romanes, 1966). The intercostal veins drain into the azygos system of veins (Gosling et al., 1990), and this variable system also drains the blood to the superior vena cava. The superior vena cava empties into the right atrium of the heart (Romanes, 1968).

The lumbar veins are even more variable in their drainage pattern (Brash, 1951a). The first and second lumbar veins drain into a vein called the ascending lumbar, which in turn drains into the subcostal vein or directly into the azygos (right side) veins or hemiazygos (left side). The subcostal vein drains into the azygos system, and the venous blood continues on to the heart by way of the superior vena cava (Oelrich, 1966). The third and fourth lumbar veins are tributaries to the inferior vena cava, which empties into the right atrium of the heart (Brash, 1951a). The fifth lumbar vein drains into the iliolumbar vein. The iliolumbar vein drains into the common iliac vein, itself a tributary of the inferior vena cava, which empties into the heart (Romanes, 1968). The intervertebral veins exiting from the ventral sacral foramina drain into the lateral sacral veins (Oelrich, 1966). From there the blood passes to the internal iliac vein, then to the common iliac vein, and finally into the inferior vena cava, which drains into the right atrium of the heart (Goss, 1966). These lower segmental veins frequently drain into the ascending lumbar vein as well.

The intervertebral veins draining into veins in the neck, thorax, and abdomen have a common pattern. In each case they intersect a vein running lengthwise. In the cervical region the intervertebral veins are linked vertically by the vertebral vein, because they are all tributaries to it (Brash, 1951a). In the thoracic region they are connected to the vertically running azygos system of veins (Goss, 1966). In the abdominal region they drain to the ascending lumbar vein (Romanes, 1968). In the pelvic region they are linked vertically by the lateral sacral vein (Brash, 1951a). At least one authority has regarded the azygos vein as a cephalic continuation of the ascending lumbar vein (Goss, 1966).

When the mesoderm constructed a venous plexus inside the vertebral canal, it also constructed one on the outside, the external vertebral venous plexus (Parke, 1992). This external plexus of veins drains the soft and hard tissues contiguous to it (Oelrich, 1966). This external plexus also anastomoses with the internal plexus of veins inside the vertebral canal (Hollinshead, 1982). Both venous plexuses drain into the segmental veins (Goss, 1966). (The latter includes the posterior intercostal, lumbar, and lateral sacral veins [Walls, 1972].) Thus the segmental veins receive blood from the vertebrae and the soft tissues that envelop them by way of the external venous plexus (O'Rahilly, 1986). All the blood from the two plexuses is added to the blood already in the segmental veins, blood that was returning from the deep muscles and skin of the back (Romanes, 1968). The blood next flows from these segmental veins into various definitive veins that the fetus has fashioned out of various precursor veins of the early embryo (Brash, 1951a).

The definitive vein that the blood from segmental veins in the cervical region ultimately drains into is known as the superior vena cava (Oelrich, 1966). It is derived from the right common cardinal vein and a part of the right anterior cardinal vein (Patten, 1953). Blood from segmental veins in the thoracic region drains into the azygos system of veins: the azygos, hemiazygos, and accessory hemiazygos veins (Walls, 1972). This azygos system forms from the embryo's posterior cardinal veins (Goss, 1966). According to Patten (1953), the embryo's supracardinal veins also may contribute. Blood from segmental veins in the lower lumbar and sacral regions drains into the ascending lumbar veins or the inferior vena cava, which forms from the posterior cardinal, subcardinal, and supracardinal veins of the embryo (Patten, 1953). Blood from the embryonic gonads, kidneys, and adrenal glands is delivered to the inferior vena cava by veins named after the organ they serve. They are all derived from the subcardinal veins of the embryo (Williams et al., 1995).

Virtually all the tissues making up the bulk of the posterior body wall are derived from mesoderm (e.g., the thoracic duct and its lymphatic tributaries and the various fasciae: superficial, deep, endothoracic, transversalis, and thoracolumbar) (Goss, 1966). However, the neural elements (e.g., the lumbosacral plexus) develop from ectoderm (Larsell, 1953).

Suggested Readings

Space limitations and other considerations do not allow discussion of investigative studies on the development of frog, chick, and mouse embryos as related to the human embryo (Ballard, 1964; Rugh, 1964). However, the reader has been provided a substantial amount of background information with which to continue the study of the enormous amount of information available in the field of human development (Rothman and Simeone, 1992). Readers requiring more depth and breadth than given in this chapter are recommended to consult the scholarly treatises of Parke (1992a,b) and O'Rahilly and Muller

(1992), both authorities in the field. They fill in the lacunae, sort through the controversies, and are reliable guides to primary sources in the literature. Also, some of the genetic control of development has been investigated recently (Moore and Persaud, 2003; Sadler, 2004). The reader also is encouraged to search the primary literature for the latest advances in this exciting field.

REFERENCES

Arey LB. (1965). *Developmental anatomy* (7th ed.). Philadelphia: WB Saunders.

Bagnall K et al. (1987). Some experimental data to support the theory of resegmentation in vertebral formations. *Anat Rec, 218,1* 12A.

Ballard WW. (1964). *Comparative embryology*. New York: Ronald Press.

Barr ML & Kiernan JA. (1993). *The human nervous system* (6th ed.). Philadelphia: JB Lippincott.

Baxter JS. (1953). *Frazer's manual of embryology*. London: Bailliere, Tindall & Cox.

Beck F et al. (1985). *Human embryology* (2nd ed.). Oxford, UK: Blackwell.

Bogduk N & Twomey LT. (1987). *Clinical anatomy of the lumbar spine*. Melbourne: Churchill Livingstone.

Brash JC. (1951a). Blood vascular and lymphatic systems. In JC Brash (Ed.). *Cunningham's textbook of anatomy* (9th ed.). London: Oxford University Press.

Brash JC. (1951b). Human embryology. In JC Brash (Ed.). *Cunningham's textbook of anatomy* (9th ed.). London: Oxford University Press.

Breathnach AS. (1958). *Frazer's anatomy of the human skeleton* (5th ed.). London: Churchill Livingstone.

Bruce J & Walmsley R. (1939). *Beesly and Johnston's manual of surgical anatomy*. London: Oxford University Press.

Callander CL. (1939). *Surgical anatomy* (2nd ed.). Philadelphia: WB Saunders.

Carlson BM. (1981). *Patten's foundations of embryology* (4th ed.). New York: McGraw-Hill.

Clark WE. (1951). Central nervous system. In JC Brash (Ed.). *Cunningham's textbook of anatomy* (9th ed.). London: Oxford University Press.

Clark WE. (1976). Central nervous system. In WJ Hamilton (Ed.). *Textbook of human anatomy* (2nd ed.). St Louis: Mosby.

Cohen MS et al. (1992). Anatomy of the spinal nerve roots in the lumbar and lower thoracic spine. In RR Rothman & FA Simeone (Eds.). *The spine* (3rd ed.). Philadelphia: WB Saunders.

Corliss CE. (1976). *Patten's human embryology*. New York: McGraw-Hill.

Crafts RC. (1966). *A textbook of human anatomy*. New York: Ronald Press.

Davenport HA. (1966). Introduction and topographic anatomy. In BJ Anson (Ed.). *Morris' human anatomy* (12th ed.). New York: McGraw-Hill.

David KM et al. (1998). Cartilaginous development of the human craniovertebral junction as visualized by a new three-dimensional computer reconstruction technique. *J Anat 192(Pt 2)*, 269-277.

Durward A. (1951). Peripheral nervous system. In JC Brash (Ed.). *Cunningham's textbook of anatomy* (9th ed.). London: Oxford University Press.

Ellis H. (1983). *Clinical anatomy* (7th ed.). Oxford: Blackwell.

Fischman DA. (1972). Development of striated muscle. In GH Bourne (Ed.). *The structure and function of muscle* (2nd ed.). New York: Academic Press.

Francis CC & Voneida JJ. (1966). The nervous system. In BJ Anson (Ed.). *Morris' human anatomy* (12th ed.). New York: McGraw-Hill.

Gosling JA et al. (1990). *Human anatomy* (2nd ed.). London: Gower Medical Publishing.

Goss CM. (1966). *Gray's anatomy of the human body* (28th ed.). Philadelphia: Lea & Febiger.

Grant JCB. (1952). *A method of anatomy* (5th ed.). Baltimore: Williams & Wilkins.

Hall BK. (1978). *Developmental and cellular skeletal biology*. New York: Academic Press.

Hamilton WJ & Mossman HW. (1972). *Human embryology* (4th ed.). Baltimore: Williams & Wilkins.

Harrison RG. (1972). Introduction to human embryology. In GJ Romanes (Ed.). *Cunningham's textbook of anatomy* (11th ed.). London: Oxford University Press.

Hollinshead WH. (1982). *The back and limbs. Anatomy for surgeons* (3rd ed.). Philadelphia: Harper & Row.

Hollinshead WH & Rosse C. (1985). *Textbook of anatomy* (4th ed.). Philadelphia: Harper & Row.

Inkster RG. (1951). Osteology. In JC Brash (Ed.). *Cunningham's textbook of anatomy* (9th ed.). London: Oxford University Press.

Joseph J. (1976). Locomotor system. In WJ Hamilton (Ed.). *Textbook of human anatomy* (2nd ed.). St Louis: Mosby.

Langebartel DA. (1977). *The anatomical primer*. Baltimore: University Park Press.

Larsell O. (1953). The nervous system. In JP Schaeffer (Ed.). *Morris' human anatomy* (11th ed.). New York: McGraw-Hill.

Leeson CR & Leeson TS. (1972). *Human structure*. Philadelphia: WB Saunders.

Lockhart RD. (1951). Myology. In JC Brash (Ed.). *Cunningham's textbook of anatomy* (9th ed.). London: Oxford University Press.

Maat GJR et al. (1996). Postnatal development and structure of the neurocentral junction. Its relevance for spinal surgery. *Spine 21(6)*, 661-666.

Moore KL & Persaud TVN. (2003). *The developing human* (7th ed.). Philadelphia: WB Saunders.

Mortenson O & Pettersen JC. (1966). The musculature. In BJ Anson (Ed.). *Morris' human anatomy* (12th ed.). New York: McGraw-Hill.

Mossman HW. (1987). *Vertebrate fetal membranes*. New Brunswick, NJ: Rutgers University Press.

Noback CR & Demarest RJ. (1975). *The human nervous system* (2nd ed.). New York: McGraw-Hill.

Oelrich TM. (1966). The cardiovascular system: Arteries and veins. In BJ Anson (Ed.). *Morris' human anatomy* (12th ed.). New York: McGraw-Hill.

O'Rahilly R. (1986). *Gardner-Gray-O'Rahilly anatomy: A regional study of human structure* (5th ed.). Philadelphia: WB Saunders.

O'Rahilly R & Muller F. (1992). *Human embryology and teratology*. New York: John Wiley & Sons.

Parke WW. (1992a). Applied anatomy of the spine. In RR Rothman & FA Simeone (Eds.). *The spine* (3rd ed.). Philadelphia: WB Saunders.

Parke WW. (1992b). Development of the spine. In RR Rothman & FA Simeone (Eds.). *The spine* (3rd ed.). Philadelphia: WB Saunders.

Patten BM. (1953). The cardiovascular system. In JP Schaeffer (Ed.). *Morris' human anatomy* (11th ed.). New York: McGraw-Hill.

Patten BM. (1964). *Foundations of embryology* (2nd ed.). New York: McGraw-Hill.

Pharaoh DO. (1956). *Chiropractic orthopedy*. Davenport, Iowa: Palmer School of Chiropractic.

Robertson GG. (1966). Developmental anatomy. In BJ Anson (Ed.). *Morris' human anatomy* (12th ed.). New York: McGraw-Hill.

Romanes GJ. (1966). *Cunningham's manual of practical anatomy* (13th ed.). London: Oxford University Press.

Romanes GJ. (1966). *Cunningham's manual of practical anatomy* (13th ed.). London: Oxford University Press.

Romanes GJ. (1972a). The central nervous system. In GJ Romanes (Ed.). *Cunningham's textbook of anatomy* (11th ed.). London: Oxford University Press.

Romanes GJ. (1972b). The peripheral nervous system. In GJ Romanes (Ed.), *Cunningham's textbook of anatomy* (11th ed.). London: Oxford University Press.

Romanes GJ. (1976). *Cunningham's manual of practical anatomy* (14th ed.). London: Oxford University Press.

Rothman RR & Simeone FA. (1992). *The spine* (3rd ed.). Philadelphia: WB Saunders.

Rugh R. (1964). *Vertebrate embryology*. New York: Harcourt, Brace, & World.

Sadler TW. (2004). *Langman's medical embryology* (9th ed.). Baltimore: Williams & Wilkins.

Salsabili N & Hogg DA. (1991). Development of the human sacroiliac joint. *Clin Anat, 4(2)*, 199-208.

Scammon RE. (1953). Developmental anatomy. In JP Schaeffer (Ed.). *Morris' human anatomy* (11th ed.). New York: McGraw-Hill.

Scothorne RJ. (1976). Peripheral nervous system. In WJ Hamilton (Ed.). *Textbook of human anatomy* (2nd ed.). St Louis: Mosby.

Sinclair DC. (1972). Muscles and fasciae. In GJ Romanes (Ed.). *Cunningham's textbook of anatomy* (11th ed.). London: Oxford University Press.

Snell RS. (1975). *Clinical embryology for medical students* (2nd ed.). Boston: Little, Brown.

Snell RS. (1981). *Clinical anatomy for medical students* (2nd ed.). Boston: Little, Brown.

Trotter M & Peterson RR. (1966). Osteology. In BJ Anson (Ed.). *Morris' human anatomy* (12th ed.). New York: McGraw-Hill.

Verbout AJ. (1985). The development of the vertebral column. *Adv Anat Embryo Cell Biol, 90,* 1-122.

Walls EW. (1972). The blood vascular and lymphatic systems. In GJ Romanes (Ed.). *Cunningham's textbook of anatomy* (11th ed.). London: Oxford University Press.

Walmsley R. (1972). Joints. In GJ Romanes (Ed.). *Cunningham's textbook of anatomy* (11th ed.). London: Oxford University Press.

Williams PL et al. (1995). *Gray's anatomy* (38th ed.). Edinburgh: Churchill Livingstone.

Woodburne RT. (1983). *Essentials of human anatomy* (7th ed.). New York: Oxford University Press.

Yoffey JM. (1976). Cardiovascular system. In WJ Hamilton (Ed.). *Textbook of human anatomy* (2nd ed.). St Louis: Mosby.

Zuckerman S. (1961). *A new system of anatomy*. London: Oxford University Press.

CHAPTER 13

Unique Anatomic Features of the Pediatric Spine

Gregory D. Cramer
Shi-Wei Yu

IMPORTANCE OF THE PEDIATRIC SPINE

Understanding the spines of children is important for a number of reasons. Contrary to common belief, a fairly high number of children, particularly adolescents, suffer from back pain, and the pain is recurrent in many (Burton et al., 1996). A study of children in Finland, conducted by Taimela et al. (1997), showed the following prevalence of back pain among children:
1% in 7-year-old children
6% in 10-year-old children

18% of 14- and 16-year-old children and approximately 8% of 15-year-old children have recurrent or continuous low back pain (Salminen et al., 1995).

No difference was found in the incidence of low back pain between males and females in the study. However, pain was identified as being chronic or recurrent in 26% of boys with low back pain and in 33% of girls with low back pain (Taimela et al., 1997). Perhaps surprisingly, intervertebral disc (IVD) degeneration has been identified in with magnetic resonance imaging (MRI) in 15-year-old children, and an unexpectedly high number of young people in their twenties have bulging IVDs that are thought to be the cause of their back pain (Kraemer, 1995; Salminen et al., 1995). IVD protrusion is more prevalent in taller adolescents who have less ability to forward flex than in those of average height with better mobility in forward flexion (Salminen, Erkintalo-Tertti, and Paajanen, 1993). As might be expected, the incidence of low back pain among children who are less physically active is higher than in children who engage in the average level of physical activity (Salminen et al., 1995). Fortunately low back pain in childhood and adolescence does not seem to be related to disabling back pain in adulthood (Burton et al., 1996).

The purpose of this chapter is to identify unique anatomic features related to the pediatric spine. A separate chapter on this topic is important because the spines of children are not just miniature versions of the spines of adults. For example, many of the differences related to the pediatric spine can be mistaken for fractures on the x-rays of children (Fesmire and Luten, 1989). Because normally children are not x-rayed unless the chief complaint is related to trauma, or suspected trauma or other serious pathology, the identification of fractures is a primary focus when viewing these x-ray films. Knowing the precise locations of the ossification centers and the locations of closure, or final union, of the primary and secondary centers of ossification is important because these sites are the regions that can be mistaken for fractures most easily.

Understanding pediatric spinal anatomy also is important for the proper planning of certain treatment procedures, such as spinal manipulation. For example, the zygapophysial (Z) joints are underdeveloped until approximately 10 years of age. Knowing the rate and stage of development of these structures allows a clinician to tailor the manipulation by significantly reducing the force in those individuals, and those age groups, when the joints of the spine are not yet fully developed.

This chapter begins with a discussion of the changes that occur with age in key anatomic structures of the spine. Next, clinically relevant developmental changes of the spine that are important to various diagnostic and treatment procedures are covered. The chapter ends with a brief discussion of common pediatric disorders related to the anatomy of the spine.

AGE-RELATED ANATOMIC CHANGES OF THE PEDIATRIC SPINE

The age-related changes to key anatomic structures of the spine are covered in several ways in this chapter. First, Table 13-1 describes the changes of key anatomic structures for several pediatric age groups. Notice that the key anatomic structures included in Table 13-1 are the curves of the spine, vertebral bodies, IVDs, intervertebral foramina (IVFs), Z joints, and neurologic elements in the vertebral canal. The age groups of Table 13-1 are newborn, 3 months, 2 years, and 10 years. Next, the following sections briefly summarize the most important anatomic changes for the age groups just listed. Finally, age-related changes of the Z joints and the IVFs are described. These two anatomic structures are featured because they undergo unique and clinically important changes with age.

The Newborn Spine

The primary curves (thoracic and sacral kyphoses) of the newborn spine are developed; however, the secondary curves are rudimentary. The vertebral bodies of the newborn spine are more or less ellipsoidal in shape. They are considerably ossified at birth (70%). The IVDs of the newborn are extremely large relative to their adult size, and the nucleus pulposus is more or less rounded in shape (Fig. 13-1).

At birth, the vertebral canal between L1-4 is 70% of its adult size; however, the L5 vertebral foramen and the L5-S1 vertebral canal are only 50% developed. The

remaining 30% of the L1-4 vertebral canal development is completed by the end of the first year of infancy, whereas the L5 vertebral foramen and canal continues to develop until approximately 5 years of age. Of clinical importance is that the vertebral canal does not undergo "catch-up growth;" that is, if development is incomplete in infancy the vertebral canal will remain smaller than normal throughout life (Ursu, Porter, and Navaratnam, 1996).

Newborn IVFs are relatively huge (Fig. 13-2). The term *capacious* is used sometimes to describe the size of the IVFs with respect to the relatively small foraminal contents of young children. Occasionally authors incorrectly apply the term capacious to the IVFs of adults (Crelin, 1973), whereas others have shown that this clearly is not the case (Hewitt, 1970; Giles, 1994). The main reason for the relatively large size of the IVFs in newborns is that the Z joints, which form the posterior border of the IVFs, are underdeveloped in young children (see Fig. 13-2). Both the superior and inferior articular processes are extremely small and the distal ends of both are primarily cartilaginous. The spines of newborns should be handled with extreme care for this reason.

The plane of articulation of the newborn Z joints is more horizontal in orientation than in the adult. This plane gradually becomes more vertically oriented until the age of 10 years, when the adult angle of approximately 45 degrees to the vertical plane is achieved (Kasai et al., 1996).

The 3-Month-Old Spine

The curves of the vertebral column at 3 months of age are already changing from those of the newborn. In addition to the primary curves of the thoracic and sacral regions (which have been present since birth), the cervical lordosis (which is a secondary curve) begins to develop at approximately 3 months of age. The formation of the cervical lordosis begins because the 3-month-old infant is beginning to lift up his or her head and look around.

The vertebral bodies are continuing to ossify at 3 months of age; they are now approximately 80% ossified, compared with the 70% ossification found in the newborn. The vertebral bodies also are becoming more rectangular in shape, rather than the ellipsoidal shape seen in newborns. The IVDs are narrowing from superior to inferior and the nucleus pulposus is taking on a more ellipsoidal shape, rather than the rounded shape of newborns (Fig. 13-3).

The IVFs of 3-month-old spines remain large, and the articular processes of the Z joints remain relatively underdeveloped (Fig. 13-4). The distal ends of the superior and inferior articular processes are still primarily composed of cartilage (see Fig. 13-4).

Table 13-1   Changes during Infancy and Childhood of Important Anatomic Structures

Age	Curves (Sagittal Plane)	Vertebral Body (Primary Ossification Center)	Intervertebral Disc	Intervertebral Foramen	Zygapophysial Joint
Newborn infant	Shallow primary curves; flexible	Ellipsoidal in shape; primary center >70% ossification	Nucleus pulposus is homogenous, gelatinous, translucent, and grayish in appearance; shape varies with level and development from ellipsoid to round; contains a thin band of primitive notochord	Elongated O shape; slightly larger superiorly than inferiorly; spinal nerve occupies the uppermost portion of the foramen, above the level of the disc; veins found in inferior portion of the foramen; fat makes up the majority of the foraminal contents	Wide joint space, tip of articular processes composed primarily of cartilage
3-month-old infant	Shallow primary curves, beginning of cervical curve; flexible	Rectangular in shape, but almost square; >80% ossification	Nucleus pulposus less spherical and more ellipsoid in shape; the thin band of primitive notochord disappears	Remains an elongated O shape; nerve slightly lower in position	Joint space is relatively narrower; articular cartilage is thick and uniform; tips of the articular processes remain cartilaginous
2-year-old child	All secondary and primary curves are present	Square in shape; >90% ossification	Nucleus pulposus is much thinner superior-inferior; no longer uniformly gelatinous; fibers have formed within the nucleus pulposus	Foramen remains capacious, but the superior part is distinctly wider than inferior part	Joint space remains unchanged, but articular cartilage is much thinner Tips of the articular processes remain cartilaginous
10-year-old child	Similar to adult	Rectangular in shape; almost complete ossification	Nucleus pulposus is compacted to a relatively small (compared with the newborn) rounded shape	Inverted pear shape in lumbar and thoracic regions, oval shape in cervical region; spinal nerve lies further superior than earlier; convex posterior disc border; posterior border of the foramen flattens by the enlarging ligamentum flavum*	Joint space and articular cartilage remain unchanged; meniscus, or infoldings of the inner layer of the capsules (synovial folds), are seen Tips of the articular processes are much less cartilaginous and have much more bone in them (more fully developed)

*The ligamenta flava begin as thin structures that are convex anteriorly. They thicken dramatically with age and are relatively thick by age 2. They continue to thicken until the age of 10, at which time their anterior border has flattened into the adult appearance.

The 2-Year-Old Spine

The primary thoracic and sacral curves are well defined at 2 years of age. In addition, both secondary curves have developed at this age. That is, the cervical lordosis developed at approximately 3 months of age, and the lumbar lordosis began between 9 and 12 months of age. Like the cervical lordosis, the lumbar lordosis is created by postural changes. Specifically the lumbar lordosis begins when the infant starts to pull himself or herself up to stand, and then begins to walk. The cervical lordosis is greater in infants less than 5 years of age than in children above this age and in adults. This is thought to be the result of holding up the comparatively heavy head with the relatively underdeveloped cervical vertebrae and cervical paraspinal musculature (Kasai et al., 1996).

The vertebral bodies of the 2-year-old child are almost 90% ossified, and are almost fully developed. They are more rectangular in shape than at 3 months, and the superior and inferior bony rims of the vertebral bodies are more "squared off" at this stage, rather than rounded, as in the 3-month-old infant. At 2 years the IVDs are narrowing from top to bottom, taking on more of an adult type of appearance, although significant further development remains to be completed (Fig. 13-5).

The IVFs of the 2-year-old spine remain capacious; however, they begin to slightly narrow at their inferior aspect, particularly in the lumbar region (Fig. 13-6). The superior and inferior articular processes, which form the Z joints, begin to grow into the posterior and inferior aspect of the IVFs and then become more fully ossified during this stage of development. Even with this added growth and ossification, the Z joints are still relatively underdeveloped, leaving the IVFs comparatively large (see Fig. 13-6).

The 10-Year-Old Spine

The neurocentral synchondrosis persists as a plate of growth cartilage until it completes its fusion and is completely replaced with bone at 3 to 6 years of age. This cartilage plate, and later bony plate, which is located within the posterolateral aspect of the fully developed vertebral body, extends from the superior to inferior anular apophyses. This bony plate persists throughout life (Maat, Matricali, and van Persijn van Meerten, 1996). These plates are thought to be the reason that burst fractures of the vertebral body usually do not enter the posterolateral aspect of the anatomic vertebral body, and why during such fractures a central segment of the vertebral body frequently protrudes directly posteriorly, between the "wedge shape" formed by the left and right bony plates found at the neurocentral junction (Maat, Matricali, and van Persijn van Meerten, 1996).

The primary and secondary curves are fully developed at 10 years of age. Although the cervical lordosis may be prominent in early childhood, it diminishes after the age of 5 and is absent in 14% of the late childhood and adolescent population until approximately 16 years of age. This is partially because the cervical vertebral bodies can be wedge shaped (shorter anteriorly) during this period of time. The anterior wedging of the vertebral bodies reduces the cervical lordosis and also can be mistaken for a compression fracture (Fesmire and Luten, 1989). However, the fact that the wedged vertebrae occur at multiple levels precludes fracture.

Ligamentous laxity typically exists in the cervical spines of children, especially those less than 8 years of age. Such laxity can create a pseudosubluxation (i.e., the appearance of dislocation) during forward flexion (Kasai et al., 1996) as seen on lateral x-rays. This phenomenon is found in 46% of children 1 to 8 years old. The pseudosubluxation usually is most marked between the second and third cervical vertebrae (Fesmire and Luten, 1989).

The vertebral bodies (VBs) of the spines of 10-year-old children are almost 100% ossified and begin to look like "little adult" vertebral bodies. The growth in vertical height of the VBs is similar to growth of the long bones with primary and secondary growth spurts. Growth in boys terminates approximately 2 years later than in girls (Kasai et al., 1996). The IVDs have more adultlike proportions as well, with further narrowing of the IVDs from superior to inferior and the nucleus pulposus more centrally located (Fig. 13-7).

Severe spinal injuries in children are relatively rare. For example, fracture dislocation in the cervical region of children less than 15 years of age accounts for only approximately 2% of all such injuries. Seventy-five percent of these injuries in children result from motor vehicle and diving accidents. In children less than 8 years of age almost all fractures in the cervical region occur at C1 or C2. This is probably because of the relatively heavy head and relatively lax ligaments of infants and young children (Fesmire and Luten, 1989). Spinal cord injuries also are rare in children less than 16 years of age, accounting for 1% to 3.3% of all spinal cord injuries, although some authors report a higher incidence in certain metropolitan areas. Approximately 20% (4% to 67%) of pediatric spinal cord injuries resulting from significant trauma show no radiographic abnormalities. This condition has been logically termed *spinal cord injury without radiographic abnormalities* (SCIWORA). Sometimes the neurologic deficits do not appear immediately; however, patients may report paresthesias after the trauma. For this reason all pediatric patients suffering from significant cervical spine trauma who describe feeling numbness and tingling after the trauma should be

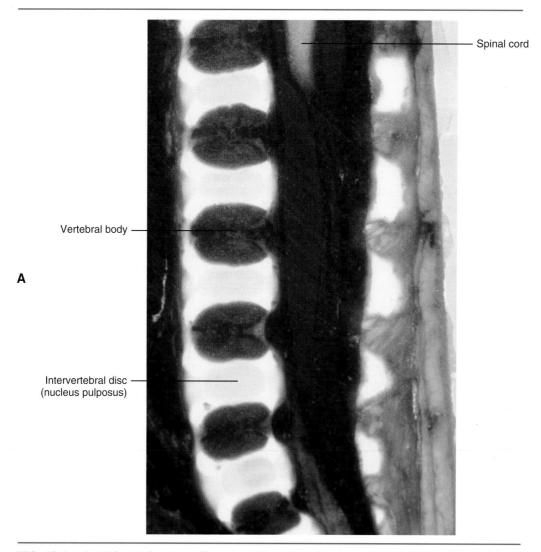

Spinal cord

Vertebral body

A

Intervertebral disc
(nucleus pulposus)

FIG. 13-1 **A,** Midsagittal section of a cadaveric newborn lumbar spine. Notice the large intervertebral discs and ellipsoidal vertebral bodies. (From Ho PS et al. [1988]. Progressive and regressive changes in the nucleus pulposus. Part I. The neonate. *Radiology, 169[1],* 87-91.)

examined carefully and considered to have cervical spinal cord injury until it is definitively ruled out over time (Fesmire and Luten, 1989).

The IVFs of 10-year-old children begin to take on a more adult type of appearance at approximately 6 to 10 years of age (notice the significant age range), having an inverted pear shape in the lumbar and thoracic regions, being much more narrow inferiorly than superiorly (Fig. 13-8), and an oval shape in the cervical region. This dramatic change in IVF shape at this age results from the significant development and full ossification of the superior and inferior articular processes that form the Z joints. As the superior articular process continues to grow and develop, it presses into the posterior and inferior aspects of the IVF. The anulus fibrosus also protrudes

slightly into the anterior and inferior aspect of the IVF. The result of these two structures moving into the inferior aspect of the IVF is a narrowing of that region. The ligamentum flavum continues to thicken since birth, and this ligament also helps narrow the posterior border of the IVF (see Fig. 13-8).

The IVF and articular process changes in this age range are important for a number of reasons. For example, once this age is reached, the Z joints are developed to the same proportions as adult Z joints. Therefore treatment procedures (e.g., spinal manipulation) can be employed in fashions more similar to those used with adults. Of course, the forces of manipulative procedures must be titrated to patients' size, body type, and weight.

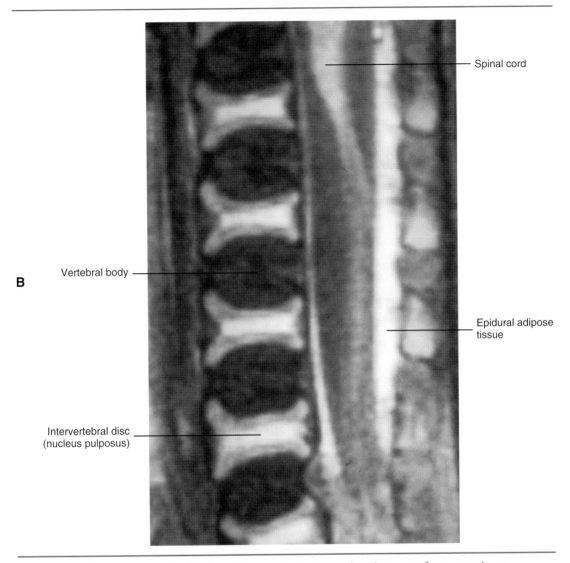

Spinal cord

Vertebral body

Epidural adipose tissue

Intervertebral disc (nucleus pulposus)

B

FIG. 13-1—cont'd   **B,** Midsagittal magnetic resonance imaging scan of same specimen.

Radicular pain from pathology within the IVF before this stage of development is rare and should be examined carefully. Space-occupying lesions large enough to cause radicular pain in the capacious IVFs of young children need to be large. Such large space-occupying lesions could be the result of neoplasia or a displaced bone fragment from a fracture, if trauma was associated with the event. Fortunately neoplasia (tumors) of the spine in children and adolescents less than 16 years of age is uncommon. Such tumors usually are accompanied by back pain and neurologic deficits, and usually can be identified on x-rays (Beer and Menezes, 1997). After the developmental period when the child is 6 to 10 years old (usually closer to the 10-year age group), and after the IVFs have reached their adult shape, the possibility exists (although rare) for an IVD to protrude far laterally into

the IVF, affecting the dorsal root ganglion or dorsal roots and causing radicular pain.

Key Anatomic Features of the Adult Spine Leading to Foraminal Stenosis

A better understanding of the process of spinal degeneration can be achieved by comparing and contrasting several of the key anatomic features of 10-year-old and adult spines. For example, the inverted pear shape of thoracic and lumbar IVFs and the oval shape of cervical IVFs is common to both healthy adult spines, as well as the spines of 10-year-old children. However, with advancing age the IVDs can narrow in some individuals, as a result of the breakdown of proteoglycans or secondary to trauma (see Chapter 14). As the IVD narrows, the

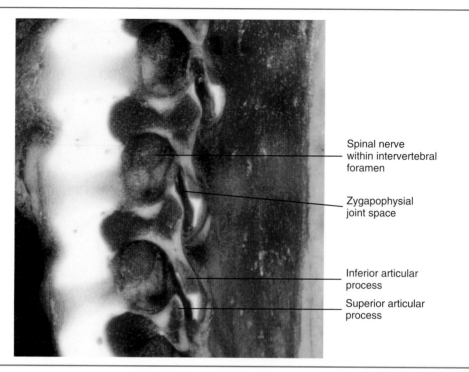

FIG. 13-2   Parasagittal section of a cadaveric newborn lumbar spine. Notice the large intervertebral foramina and underdeveloped articular processes forming the zygapophysial joints.

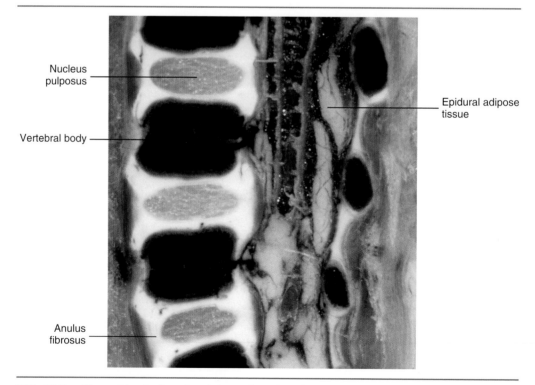

FIG. 13-3   Near midsagittal section (≈3 mm lateral to the midline; note medial aspects of laminae rather than spinous processes in section) of the lumbar region of a 3-month-old child. The vertebral bodies are now more rectangular in shape, and the intervertebral discs have narrowed from superior to inferior.

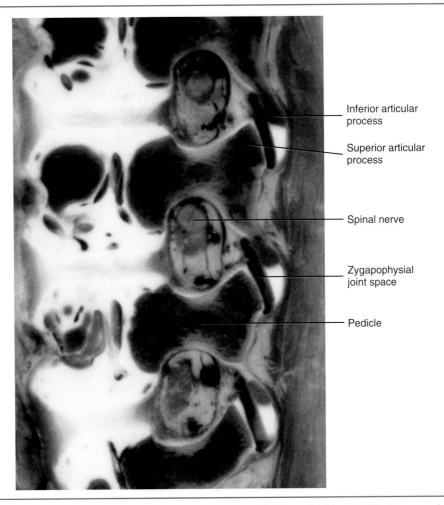

—— Inferior articular
process

—— Superior articular
process

—— Spinal nerve

—— Zygapophysial
joint space

—— Pedicle

FIG. 13-4   Parasagittal section of the lumbar region of a 3-month-old spine. The intervertebral foramina remain large and the articular processes remain underdeveloped. Notice the great amount of cartilage on the tips of the inferior articular processes. (From Yu S, Haughton VM & Rosenbaum AE. [1991]. Magnetic resonance imaging and anatomy of the spine. *Radiol Clin North Am, 29[4],* 691-710.)

anulus fibrosus can bulge into the region of the IVF. Narrowing of the IVD also causes the functional spinal unit (i.e., two vertebrae and the soft tissues between them) to narrow from top to bottom, causing the superior-to-inferior dimensions of the IVF to narrow. At the same time the bony vertebral end plates begin to widen as trabecula are laid down along the superior and inferior rims of the vertebral bodies. This bony change probably is secondary to the loss of fluid pressure in the nucleus pulposus; therefore more pressure is received by the anulus fibrosus and transferred along the rims of the vertebral bodies, causing the added trabeculae to be laid down in this region. This new bone frequently is dense and sclerotic and can appear more opaque on x-rays. The superior and inferior articular processes of the Z joint override one another as the two vertebrae surrounding the narrowing IVD come closer together and the IVF narrows. This overriding causes the superior

articular process of the vertebra below to fill the inferior aspect of the IVF, causing further stenosis. In addition, osteophytic bone changes (bone spurs) can occur on the articular processes. These bone spurs can protrude into the IVF, again resulting in additional IVF narrowing. Finally, as the two adjacent vertebrae continue to approximate each other, the ligamentum flavum thickens or in some cases can even buckle into the IVF, again resulting in further constriction of this region. These changes can result in foraminal stenosis. The changes associated with foraminal stenosis are summarized in Figure 11-12.

Summary of Clinically Relevant Changes of the Zygapophysial Joints

Recall that the articular processes have little bone in the newborn and are cartilaginous. They remain quite cartilaginous until approximately 6 to 10 years of age (closer

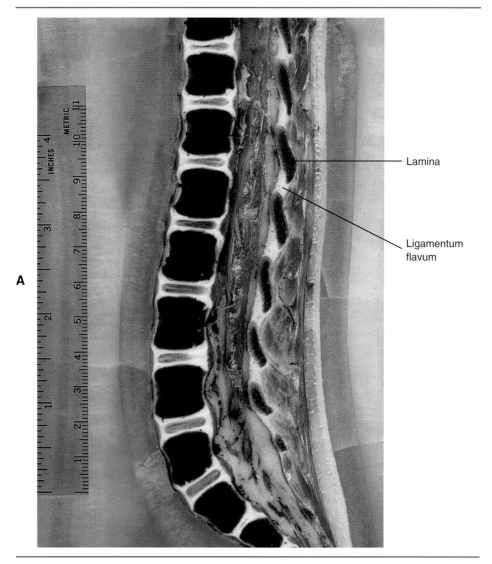

FIG. 13-5 **A,** Near midsagittal section (≈3 mm lateral to the midline; note laminae) of the lumbar region of a 2-year-old child. Note the square shape of the vertebral bodies.

to 10 years), when the cartilages of the tips of the superior and inferior articular processes gradually are replaced by bone. They then begin to attain the same proportions as articular processes of adult spines. The precise age of this maturation of the articular processes varies considerably from individual to individual.

The Z joint space in the newborn is wide, but it narrows fairly quickly and by 3 months of age the Z joint space already has narrowed considerably. The articular cartilage becomes thick at 3 months of age and then gradually begins to become thinner over the next 2 years. This cartilage remains relatively unchanged in thickness from 2 years of age until late puberty; then the articular cartilage begins to gradually thicken until the early twenties, eventually reaching up to 2 mm in thickness at 22 years of age.

Summary of Clinically Relevant Changes of the Intervertebral Foramina

As mentioned, the changes of the Z joints are related to the changes of the IVFs seen during infant and childhood development. Because the superior articular processes of infants and young children are relatively underdeveloped until approximately 6 to 10 years of age, they do not protrude into the IVFs as they do after this age period. Therefore the IVFs are rounded until approximately 6 to 10 years of age; after this age they gradually begin to take on their adult appearance (inverted pear-shaped in the thoracic and lumbar regions, oval in the cervical region). The thickening of the ligamenta flava also contributes to the development of the inverted pear-shaped adult lumbar and thoracic IVFs.

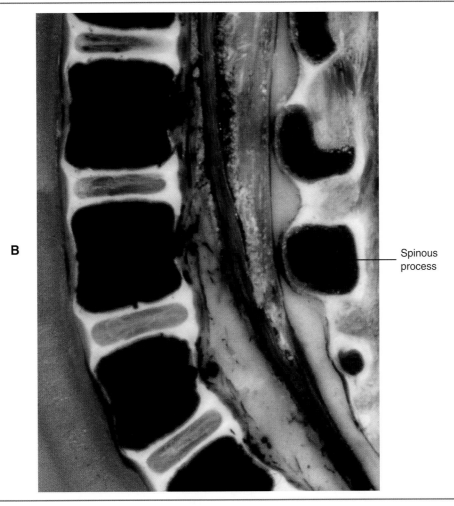

B

Spinous
process

FIG. 13-5—cont'd   B, Close-up of a midsagittal section (notice the spinous processes). The vertebral bodies are almost 90% ossified, and the intervertebral discs have narrowed considerably from 3 months of age.

CLINICALLY RELEVANT DEVELOPMENTAL ANATOMY IN CHILDREN

Developmental anomalies of the spine often are first noted during childhood. Also, many of the unique features of spinal development that can be confused as fractures on children's x-rays are related to spinal development or developmental anomalies of the vertebral column. Even though the topic of spinal development is fully covered in Chapter 12, the purpose of this section is to highlight the most clinically relevant aspects of spinal development that are most frequently encountered when evaluating the spines of children. Therefore this section begins with a brief review of some of the most common types of developmental anomalies. This is followed by a discussion of the normal development of the atypical vertebrae (C1 and C2), the relatively common developmental anomalies that occur in these vertebrae, and the potential consequences of these

anomalies. The last topic is a brief description of the development of the ring apophyses in typical vertebrae. These structures can be misinterpreted as fractures on x-rays if the normal time sequence of their development is not understood (Fesmire and Luten, 1989).

Developmental Anomalies of the Spine

There are many different types of developmental anomalies of the spine. However, the majority of the spinal anomalies seen on children's x-rays fall into the following categories:
1. Hemivertebra
2. Block vertebra
3. Multiple ossification centers
4. Asymmetric ossification centers
5. Fewer than normal ossification centers
   This section briefly discusses these anomalies.

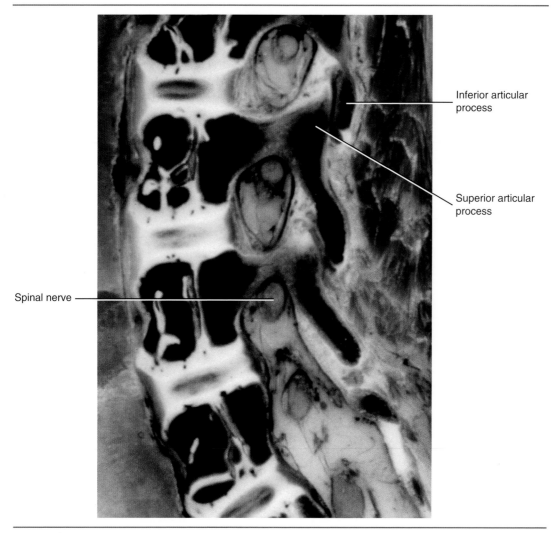

Inferior articular process

Superior articular process

Spinal nerve

FIG. 13-6 Parasagittal section of the lumbar region of a 2-year-old child. The intervertebral foramina remain capacious (although the inferior aspect has slightly narrowed), and the articular processes remain relatively underdeveloped.

Hemivertebra, or "half vertebrae," is a relatively common vertebral anomaly (see Fig. 12-14, *A* and *B*) in which the left or right half of the vertebral body, and possibly the posterior arch of the same vertebrae, fail to develop (see Chapter 12). If the sclerotomes migrate properly, the next step of development is for a portion of the migrated sclerotomes to develop into the "prototypes" of vertebra, while the remaining portions develop into the ligaments (including the anulus fibrosus) between adjacent vertebrae. This process of part of the sclerotomes becoming bony vertebrae and the other portions becoming ligamentous is known as segmentation; this process allows the development of moveable segments. If segmentation does not occur properly, then ossification continues along several bony segments without joints forming between the affected segments. The result is known as block vertebra (see Fig. 12-14, *E* and *F*).

In addition, variations of segmentation occur at the superior and inferior extremes of the vertebral column. These variations lead to anomalies of the occiput-C1 region and the L5-S1 region, and are discussed in Chapters 5 and 7, respectively, and also in Chapter 12.

Other developmental anomalies seen on pediatric spinal x-rays frequently are related to ossification centers: too many primary centers of ossification, too few primary centers of ossification, or asymmetry of the primary centers of ossification.

Unique Development of the Atypical Vertebrae

The first and second cervical vertebrae are atypical, even in the adult, and their development is atypical as well. The main, clinically relevant features of the development

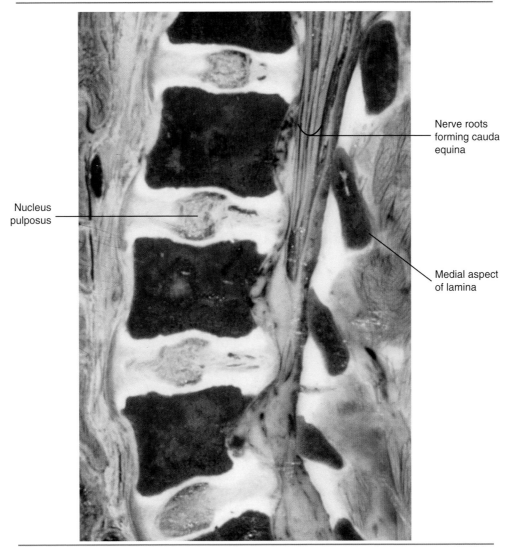

Nerve roots
forming cauda
equina

Nucleus
pulposus

Medial aspect
of lamina

FIG. 13-7 Near midsagittal section (≈3 mm lateral to the midline; note laminae) of the lumbar region of a 10-year-old child. The vertebral bodies are almost fully developed, and the intervertebral discs are fully developed.

of these two important vertebrae are discussed in the following text.

The Atlas. The first cervical vertebra (the atlas, or C1) develops from three primary centers of ossification: one in the anterior arch, and one in each lateral mass (Fig. 13-9). During development, these centers grow toward one another until the entire vertebra is ossified. The primary center of ossification in the anterior arch does not develop into a vertebral body, as is the case in other vertebra. In addition, this ossification center does not appear until the first postnatal year. It fuses with the two lateral masses at 7 to 9 years of age (Fesmire and Luten, 1989). Sometimes there is no primary center of ossification within the anterior arch. When this occurs, bone grows anteriorly from the ossification center in

each lateral mass. Fusion then may eventually occur at the center of the anterior arch. An anterior cleft remains in the anterior arch when the bone growth from the two lateral centers does not meet anteriorly (Fesmire and Luten, 1989).

Normally the primary centers of ossification for each lateral mass grow posteriorly and fuse in the center of the posterior arch at 4 to 7 years of age (Fesmire and Luten, 1989). A common anomaly of C1 is a lack of fusion of the posterior arch of the atlas. Such lack of fusion is termed agenesis of the atlas. Agenesis of the atlas has been statistically related to Arnold-Chiari malformation, or a descent of the cerebellar tonsils past the foramen magnum. For this reason a careful neurologic examination should be performed when an incidental finding of agenesis of the atlas is found on

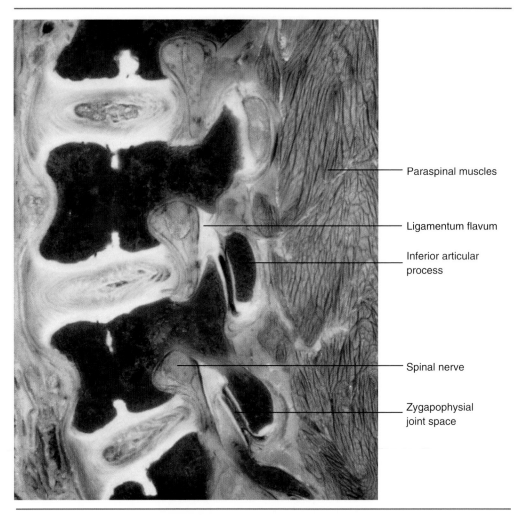

Paraspinal muscles

Ligamentum flavum

Inferior articular process

Spinal nerve

Zygapophysial joint space

FIG. 13-8 Parasagittal section of the lumbar region of a 10-year-old child. The intervertebral foramina (IVFs) have attained the "inverted pear" shape of a fully developed lumbar IVF. The articular processes also have significantly advanced in development. Notice the ligamenta flava forming the posterior border of the IVFs. Also notice Z joint synovial folds protruding into the labeled Z joint.

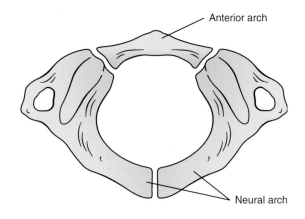

Anterior arch

Neural arch

FIG. 13-9 Development of the atlas (first cervical vertebra, C1). The atlas develops from three primary centers of ossification, one that will become the anterior arch, and one for each side of the neural arch. These latter centers will form the majority of the lateral masses and the posterior arch. The ossification center in the anterior arch appears during the first postnatal year and fuses with the centers in the lateral masses between 7 to 9 years of age. The left and right ossification centers of the neural arch will fuse posteriorly to complete the posterior arch of the atlas between the ages of 4 to 7 years. Failure of these latter two ossification centers to fuse posteriorly is termed *agenesis of the atlas*.

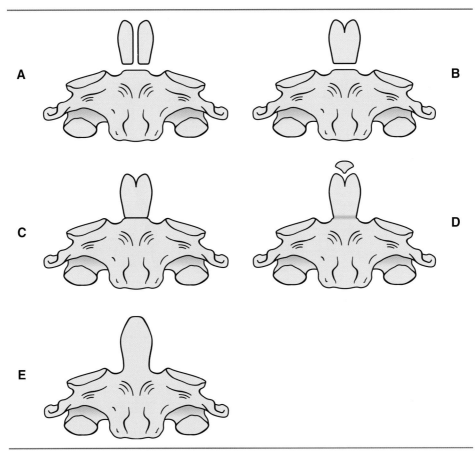

FIG. 13-10 Development of the odontoid process of the axis (second cervical vertebrae, C2). The odontoid process develops from two primary centers of ossification and one secondary center. The two primary centers are shown in **A,** before they have fused in the midline, which is depicted in **B.** The odontoid process has begun to fuse with the body of C2 in **C.** The secondary center of ossification, know as the ossiculum terminale is beginning to develop in **D.** This usually occurs between 3 and 6 years of age. The ossiculum terminale normally fuses with the remainder of the odontoid, **E,** by approximately 12 years of age. Notice that **E** also shows that the odontoid has completed its fusion with the body of C2. Lack of fusion of the odontoid with the body of C2 (persistence of what is shown in **B**) is termed os odontoideum, and lack of fusion of the secondary center of ossification is logically termed persistent ossiculum terminale (persistence of what is shown in **D**).

x-ray. Other anomalies related to C1 are too many primary centers of ossification or asymmetric primary centers of ossification.

Previously some investigators believed that because the nervous system is more fully developed than the skeletal system at birth, the spinal cord of newborns and young children might be more susceptible to compression at the C1-2 level than in adults. However, Jauregui et al. (1993), making measurements from MRI scans, found the midsagittal diameter of the vertebral canal at C1 in neonates to be 12.4 mm, leaving ample space for the spinal cord (13 mm is the accepted value in adults). They

also found that the vertebral foramen of the atlas, the atlanto-odontoid interspace, and the space available for the spinal cord underwent accelerated growth until the age of 5 years, allowing for Steele's rule of thirds for the vertebral foramen at C1 to be roughly maintained (i.e., one third of the foramen filled with spinal cord, one third with odontoid, and one third being "free space"). Recall from Chapter 5 that some ligamentous laxity in the upper cervical region is normal in children and the atlanto-odontoid interspace, which normally is less than 3 mm in adults, can be 3.5 to 5 mm in children 8 years old or younger (Fesmire and Luten, 1989).

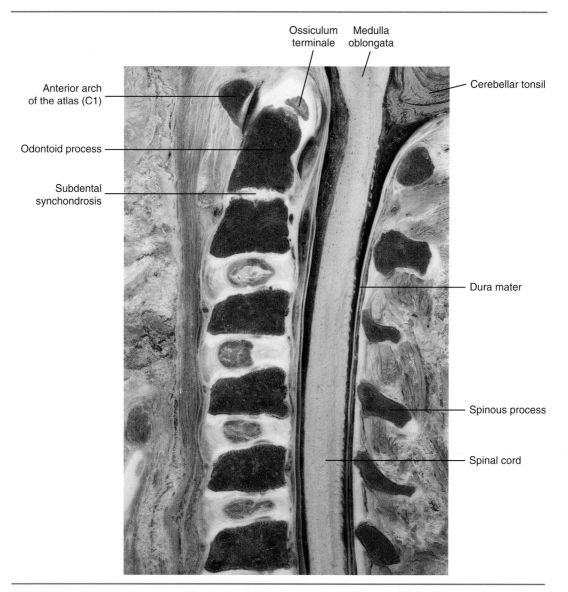

Ossiculum terminale

Medulla oblongata

Anterior arch of the atlas (C1)

Cerebellar tonsil

Odontoid process

Subdental synchondrosis

Dura mater

Spinous process

Spinal cord

FIG. 13-11 Midsagittal section of the cervical region in a 10-year-old spine. Notice the unfused subdental synchondrosis. Also notice that the ossiculum terminale has not yet fused with the remainder of the odontoid process. This is normal; the ossiculum terminale usually fuses by 11 to 12 years of age. (From Yu S et al. [1989]. Comparison of MR and diskography in detecting radial tears of the annulus: A postmortem study. *AJNR Am J Neuroradiol, 10[5],* 1077-1081.)

The Axis. The second cervical vertebra (the axis, or C2) has an atypical development (Fig. 13-10). The axis has the same three primary centers of ossification that correspond with the primary centers of typical vertebra (i.e., one in the vertebral body and one on each side of the posterior [vertebral] arch). The two ossification centers in the posterior arch normally fuse posteriorly in the midline at 2 to 3 years of age. The same two centers of ossification fuse anteriorly with the body of C2 at 3 to 6 years of age (Fesmire and Luten, 1989). However, in addition to the primary centers of ossification found in typical vertebrae, the odontoid process (dens) of the axis

(C2) has two primary centers of ossification of its own. These two ossification centers begin to fuse with one another by the eighth month of fetal development (Fesmire and Luten, 1989), but this newly united ossification center of the odontoid process does not begin to fuse with the body of C2 until 2 to 4 years of age. The region of fusion between the odontoid and the body of C2 is known as the dentocentral (subdental) synchondrosis (Fig. 13-11). Fusion usually occurs here along the outer rim of the odontoid process, leaving a cartilaginous remnant of an IVD within the confines of the rim of bone between the odontoid process and the body of C2. The

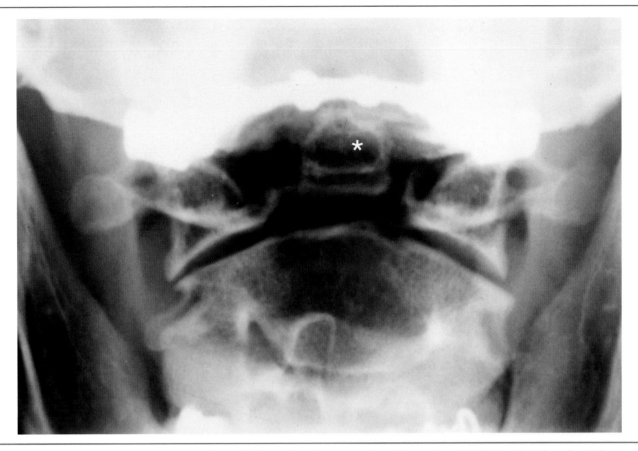

FIG. 13-12 Anterior-posterior open-mouth cervical x-ray showing an os odontoideum (*asterisk*). Notice that the odontoid process lacks a bony attachment to the body of C2.

rim of bony fusion around the subdental synchondrosis fuses by 4 years of age in 50% of individuals, and should be fused in all individuals by 6 years of age (Lefebvre et al., 1993); however, a remnant of nonunion may persist until late childhood, and can be seen on many anatomic specimens and x-rays until 11 to 12 years of age (Fesmire and Luten, 1989). This line of nonunion frequently is mistaken for a fracture, and it can be seen on x-ray throughout life in one third of the population. The centrally located subdental synchondrosis may never completely ossify and can be seen prominently on midsagittal cervical MRI scans of many individuals throughout their life (Fesmire and Luten, 1989).

There are times when the odontoid process never fuses with the body of C2, a condition known as os odontoideum (Figs. 13-10 through 13-12). However, some authors are convinced that most cases of os odontoideum are the result of a postnatal fracture (Lefebvre et al., 1993). This condition is discussed in detail in Chapters 5 (The Cervical Region) and 12 (Development of the Spine). Of particular clinical importance is that a

cartilage bridge can exist between the unfused odontoid and the body of C2. Such a bridge adds stability to the unfused odontoid. However, this cartilage bridge does not always remain firmly connected between the odontoid and the body of C2, and in other cases the cartilage bridge can fracture. A surgical attachment usually is indicated if no firm attachment exists.

A secondary center of ossification called the ossiculum terminale develops at the tip of the odontoid process (Fig. 13-13; see also Figs. 13-10 and 13-11). The ossiculum terminale first appears at 3 to 6 years of age and completes its fusion with the rest of the odontoid by approximately 12 years of age (Fesmire and Luten, 1989). Sometimes the ossiculum terminale does not fuse with the odontoid; this is termed persistent ossiculum terminale. This condition can be confused with a type I odontoid fracture (see Chapter 5). Careful examination of the margins between the free tip, or what on x-ray appears to be the free tip of the odontoid, and the remainder of the odontoid process usually reveals either roughened edges on the adjacent surfaces of the

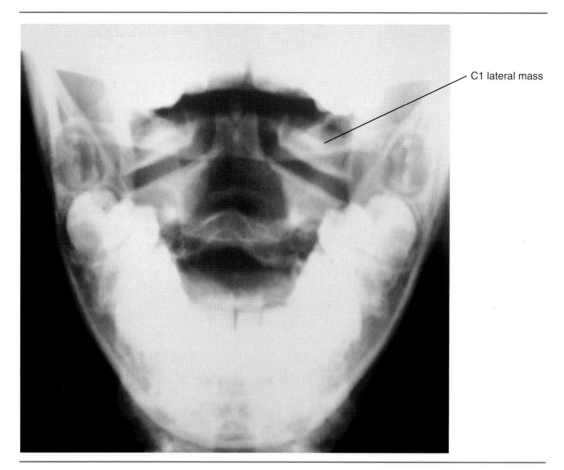

C1 lateral mass

FIG. 13-13   Anterior-posterior open-mouth cervical x-ray. Notice the odontoid process is apparent between the left and right lateral masses of the atlas (C1). The ossiculum terminale can be seen at the superior aspect of the odontoid.

odontoid and the ossiculum terminale, indicating a type I odontoid fracture, or smooth edges between these surfaces, indicating a true persistent ossiculum terminale.

Both the dentocentral synchondrosis and ossiculum terminale frequently can be seen on x-rays and MRI scans of the upper cervical region, and can be identified mistakenly as fractures or other pathology if the clinician does not remain aware of the patient's age and the normal development of this vertebra.

Key Feature in the Development of Typical Vertebrae

The anular (ring) apophyses appear on typical vertebrae just before puberty. The ring apophyses are secondary centers of ossification, located along the superior and inferior rims of the vertebral bodies (see Fig. 12-11). They do not extend all the way to the edge of the vertebral bodies; this can be seen on x-rays. They first appear on x-rays as early as 7 years of age in some children, and

their x-ray appearance can be mistaken for chip fractures (Fesmire and Luten, 1989). Although these structures do not fuse with the remainder of the vertebral body until approximately 25 years of age, they become difficult to see on x-rays after the late teenage years. Recall that further ossification and growth of the vertebral body do not occur once the ring apophyses fuse.

Location of the Conus Medullaris on Magnetic Resonance Imaging Scans of Children

MRI scans allow clear visualization of the spinal cord. Because of this, understanding the normal position of the spinal cord at different stages of childhood development becomes important. The conus medullaris (inferiormost part of the spinal cord) extends inferiorly to the second sacral segment in fetuses, but the rapid growth of the bony vertebral column during the fetal period causes the vertebral column to become longer

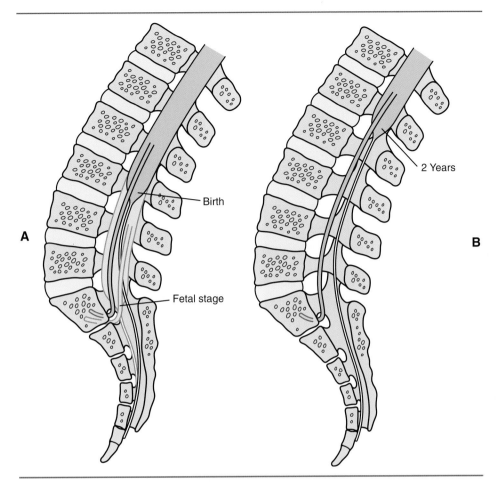

FIG. 13-14   Relative elevation of the conus medullaris during late fetal stage and early childhood development. **A,** The conus medullaris extends to the second sacral segment in fetuses, but the rapid growth of the bony vertebral column during the fetal period causes the vertebral column to become longer than the spinal cord. At birth the conus medullaris is at the level of the third lumbar vertebral body. **B,** Within the next several months to 2 years the spinal cord comes to lie approximately at the level of the first lumbar vertebral body.

than the spinal cord. Consequently, at birth the conus medullaris is at the level of the third lumbar vertebral body, and within the next several months to 2 years the spinal cord comes to lie at the level of the first lumbar vertebral body, where it remains throughout adulthood (Macdonald et al., 1999; Malas et al., 2000) (Fig. 13-14).

COMMON PEDIATRIC DISORDERS RELATED TO THE ANATOMY OF THE SPINE

Spondylolysis and Spondylolisthesis

Spondylolysis and spondylolisthesis are discussed in detail in Chapter 7. These clinical entities are mentioned here to highlight their occurrence in children. Spondylolysis, with or without spondylolisthesis, probably occurs with some frequency in children (Fig. 13-15). The youngest reported case of spondylolisthesis was that of a 4-month-old infant, and there have been several reported cases of this condition in infants less than 2 years of age (Fig. 13-16). However, pain from this condition is uncommon before the age of 9 (Lucey and Gross, 1995). As discussed in Chapter 7, the lack of pain in early cases of spondylolysis is probably because the nerves innervating the posterior vertebral arch do not extend to the pars interarticularis until after the age of 9 years. Consequently, in young children spondylolisthesis usually first manifests as variations of gait (wide-based, shuffling, or spastic), and then usually is identified on standard x-rays (Lucey and Gross, 1995). Because changes of gait also can be caused by neurologic and orthopedic disorders of the pelvis, hip, and lower extremities, neurologic and orthopedic conditions, along with

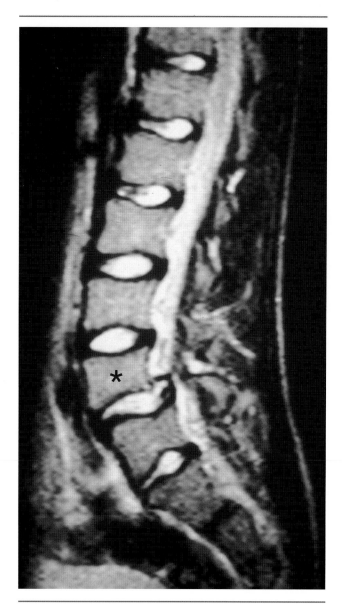

FIG. 13-15 Lumbar magnetic resonance imaging scan showing spondylolisthesis of L4 (asterisk on vertebral body of L4) in a 13-year-old boy.

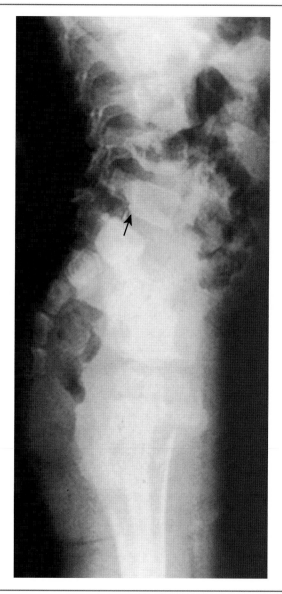

FIG. 13-16 X-ray showing a spondylolisthesis of L5 (*arrow*) in a 2-year-old girl. (From Lucey SD & Gross R. [1995]. Painful spondylolisthesis in a two-year-old child. *J Pediatr Orthop, 15,* 199-201.)

spondylolysis and spondylolisthesis, should be included in the differential diagnosis of infants with gait disorders with or without back pain.

Miyake et al. (1996) found that defects of the pars interarticularis in children resulted in retarded growth of the related articular processes and Z joint. When this occurred at L5, the result was more coronally facing L5-S1 articular facets that were more planar (i.e., the S1 superior articular facet was less concave and the L5 inferior articular facet was less convex) than normal.

The Normal Development of the Thoracic and Lumbar Curves and Scoliosis

A discussion of scoliosis can be found in Chapter 6. However, because idiopathic scoliosis is most commonly identified in the preteen or early teen years, the normal development of the thoracic and lumbar curves and scoliosis (Fig. 13-17) are briefly mentioned here.

Recall that the thoracic kyphosis normally increases during childhood, peaking at approximately 13 years of age. The lumbar lordosis decreases with age, becoming

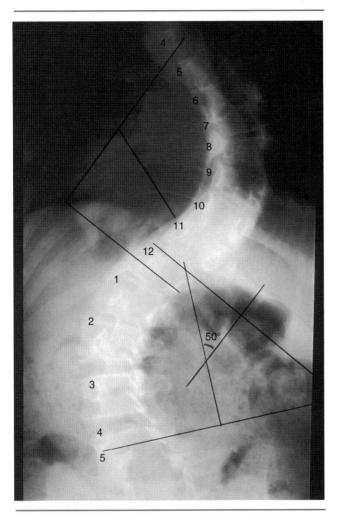

FIG. 13-17   X-ray of a 50-degree thoracolumbar scoliosis.

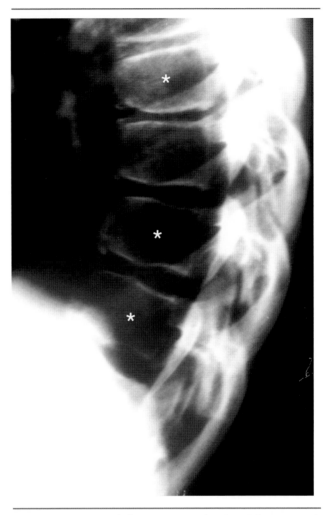

FIG. 13-18   Lateral thoracic x-ray showing Scheuermann's disease. Notice the roughened bony superior and inferior end plates, particularly of those vertebrae indicated by the asterisks.

the smallest at approximately 14 years of age (Nissinen et al., 1995). Much individual variation is seen in the development of these curves. Idiopathic scoliosis can develop during this time period, and lateral curves developing during the preteen and teenage years should be monitored closely.

Scheuermann's Disease

A more thorough discussion of Scheuermann's disease is also found in Chapter 6. This, too, is a condition of adolescence and should be considered when prolonged pain in the thoracic region, with or without pain in the upper lumbar region, is experienced in this age group. Recall that the hallmark of this condition is the irregular appearance of the bony end plates as seen on lateral x-rays (Fig. 13-18).

REFERENCES

Beer SJ & Menezes AH. (1997). Primary tumors of the spine in children. *Spine, 22,* 649-659.

Burton AK et al. (1996). The natural history of low back pain in adolescents. *Spine, 21,* 2323-2328.

Crelin ES. (1973). A scientific test of the chiropractic theory. *Amer Sci, 61,* 574-580.

Fesmire FM & Luten RC. (1989). The pediatric cervical spine: Developmental anatomy and clinical aspects. *J Emerg Med, 7,* 133-142.

Giles LGF. (1994). A histological investigation of human lower lumbar intervertebral canal (foramen) dimensions. *J Manipulative Physiol Ther, 17,* 4-14.

Hewitt W. (1970). The intervertebral foramen. *Physiotherapy, 56,* 332-336.

Jauregui N et al. (1993). Surgically related upper cervical spine canal anatomy in children. *Spine, 18,* 1939-1944.

Kraemer J. (1995). Presidential address: Natural course and prognosis of intervertebral disc diseases. *Spine, 20,* 635-539.

Kasai T et al. (1996). Growth of the cervical spine with special reference to its lordosis and mobility. *Spine, 21,* 2067-2073.

Krishna M & Upadhyay SS. (1996). Increased limb lengths in patients with shortened spine due to tuberculosis in early childhood. *Spine, 21,* 1045-1047.

Lafond G. (1962). Surgical treatment of spondylolisthesis. *Clin Orthop, 22,* 175.

Lefebvre S et al. (1993). Unstable os odontoideum in young children. *J CCA*, *37*, 141-144.

Lucey SD & Gross R. (1995). Painful spondylolisthesis in a two-year-old child. *J Pediatr Orthop*, *15*, 199-201.

Maat GJR, Matricali M, & van Persijn van Meerten EL. (1996). Postnatal development and structure of the neurocentral junction. *Spine*, *21*, 661-666.

Macdonald A et al. (1999). Level of termination of the spinal cord and the dural sac: A magnetic resonance study. *Clin Anat*, *12*, 149-152.

Malas MA et al. (2000). The relationship between the lumbosacral enlargement and the conus medullaris during the period of fetal development and adulthood. *Surg Radiol Anat*, *22*, 163-168.

Miyake R et al. (1996). Pathogenesis of sports-related spondylolisthesis in adolescents. Radiographic and magnetic resonance imaging study. *Am J Sports Med*, *24(1)*, 94-98.

Nissinen M et al. (1995). Left handedness and risk of thoracic hyperkyphosis in prepubertal schoolchildren. *Int J Epidemiol*, *24(6)*, 1178-1181.

Salminen JJ et al. (1995). Low back pain in the young. *Spine*, *20*, 2101-2108.

Salminen JJ, Erkintalo-Tertti MO, & Paajanen HEK. (1993). MRI findings of lumbar spine in the young: Correlation with leisure time physical activity, spinal mobility and trunk muscle strength in 15-year-old schoolchildren with or with out low back pain. *J Spinal Disord*, *6*, 386-391.

Taimela S et al. (1997). The prevalence of low back pain among children and adolescents. *Spine*, *22*, 1132-1136.

Ursu TRS, Porter RW, & Navaratnam V. (1996). Development of the lumbar and sacral vertebral canal *in utero*. *Spine*, *21*, 2705-2708.

CHAPTER 14

Microscopic Anatomy of the Zygapophysial Joints, Intervertebral Discs, and Other Major Tissues of the Back

Gregory D. Cramer
Barclay W. Bakkum
Peter C. Stathopoulos

Much of the current anatomic research related to the spine is concerned with the zygapophysial (Z) joints and the intervertebral discs (IVDs). The gross anatomy of these structures is covered in detail in Chapter 2. The characteristics of these structures unique to the cervical, thoracic, and lumbar regions are covered in Chapters 5, 6, and 7, respectively. Because much of the current investigation related to the Z joints and IVDs has been carried out in the lumbar region, Chapter 7 describes the Z joints and IVDs in significant detail. However, a considerable amount of the research on these two tissues is associated with their microscopic anatomy and molecular structure. The results of these investigations provide a greater understanding of normal, as well as pathologic, structure and function at the microscopic, ultrastructural (electron microscopic), and molecular levels.

As more information becomes available on the precise composition and arrangement of the tissues of normal and diseased Z joints, IVDs, and other tissues of the back, a better understanding of the biologic basis for current treatment develops. Continued investigation should lead to an increase in the understanding of spinal dysfunction. With changing concepts on the mechanisms of spinal dysfunction, new therapeutic approaches will undoubtedly emerge, and it will be necessary to keep abreast of these changing concepts to be able to effectively apply the new therapeutic approaches. Therefore an understanding of the microscopic anatomy of the tissues of the spine is extremely important to the clinician and researcher alike.

The purpose of this chapter is to provide the reader with comprehensive information on the microscopic anatomy of the Z joints and IVDs. A discussion of the normal composition of connective tissue in general and, more specifically, of hyaline cartilage and fibrocartilage in association with the Z joints and IVDs is also included.

Finishing out the chapter is a brief overview of the microscopic anatomy of the other major tissues in the region of the back.

MICROSCOPIC ANATOMY OF THE ZYGAPOPHYSIAL JOINTS

Bones in contact with one another are held together by connective tissue. This union forms a joint that, in some instances, is freely movable and lined by a synovial membrane. This type of joint is known as a synovial (diarthrodial) joint. The Z joints of the spine are of this type. The joints between contiguous vertebral bodies are formed by the IVDs and are classified as symphysis (symphyseal) joints. Symphysis joints are a type of cartilaginous joint or amphiarthrosis. The IVDs are tough, cushionlike pads consisting mainly of connective tissue, more specifically, specialized fibrocartilage. The IVDs are discussed later in this chapter.

As with all diarthrodial joints, the articular surfaces that form the Z joints are covered with shiny hyaline cartilage. This cartilage is lubricated by synovial fluid that allows the bones to glide smoothly over each other with minimal friction (Swann et al., 1974). A tough sleeve of dense connective tissue envelops the articular cartilages and joint cavity of the Z joints posteriorly. This connective tissue sleeve is known as the fibrous capsule. Anteriorly the ligamentum flavum takes the place of the articular capsule of the Z joint (Xu et al., 1991). A thin inner layer of highly vascularized connective tissue called the synovial membrane lines the joint capsule. Cells within the synovial membrane manufacture the synovial fluid.

This section discusses the microscopic anatomy of the articular cartilage, capsule, and synovial membrane of the Z joints. A working knowledge of connective tissue is important in treating pain of spinal origin because most tissues involved in the formation of the Z joints (and IVDs) are connective tissue, and pain arising from the Z joints is a significant cause of back pain (Mooney and Robertson, 1976; Kirkaldy-Willis, 1988). Therefore a section on connective tissue, including hyaline cartilage, immediately follows this section on Z joints.

Zygapophysial Joint Articular Cartilage

General Considerations. The articular cartilages lining the superior and inferior articular processes of each Z joint are similar in many respects to the articular cartilage associated with most synovial joints of the body. This means that the articular cartilage lining each of the articular processes of a Z joint is made up of a special variety of hyaline cartilage that is durable, lubricated by synovial fluid, compressible, and also able to withstand large compressive forces (Williams et al., 1995).

Recall that hyaline cartilage is not unique to the Z joints but is widely distributed in the body. In addition to lining the articular facets of Z joints, it also is found in a portion of the vertebral (cartilaginous) end plates of the IVDs, the nose, most of the laryngeal cartilages, C rings of the trachea, primary and secondary bronchi, costal cartilages of ribs, most articular cartilages of joints throughout the body, and the xiphoid process. It is also the type of cartilage present in the epiphyseal cartilage plates of growing long bones. Consequently, hyaline cartilage is essential for the growth and development of long bones before and after birth.

The purposes of Z joint articular cartilage is to protect the articular surfaces of the superior and inferior articular processes by acting as a shock absorber and to allow the articular surfaces to move across one another with little friction. Both functions are carried out efficiently. In fact, the coefficient of friction for typical articular surfaces is less than 0.002, which means that the two surfaces of a typical Z joint glide across each other with much greater ease than they would if they were both made of ice (the coefficient of friction for ice sliding on ice is <0.03) (Triano, 1992).

The articular cartilage of a single Z joint surface is small; in fact, the lumbar articular surfaces measure approximately 8 × 10 mm (Giles, 1992a,b). The Z joint articular cartilage also is approximately 1 to 2 mm thick (Figs. 14-1, 14-2, and 14-3). The concavity of the cartilage on lumbar superior articular facets is thicker than the periphery of the same surfaces. This is the opposite from that typically found in other joints of the body where the concavity of a joint surface usually is lined by thinner cartilage than that surrounding the concavity.

Z joint articular cartilage is made up of 75% water and 25% solids (Giles, 1992a,b) and consists of cells embedded in an abundant and firm matrix (Fig. 14-4). The cells that produce the cartilage matrix are chondroblasts, and in mature cartilage they are known as chondrocytes (Table 14-1). The matrix is made up of an intricate network of collagen fibers surrounded by proteoglycans and glycoproteins. The concentration of these constituents of articular cartilage differs from one part of the joint surface to another and also at different depths from the joint surface (Giles, 1992a,b).

Fresh hyaline cartilage is bluish white and translucent. In stained, fixed preparations, the matrix appears glassy, homogeneous, and smooth. Distributed throughout the matrix are spaces called lacunae, and within each lacuna is a chondrocyte. As with all articular cartilage, that of the Z joints has no nerve supply and no direct blood supply. Chondrocytes must receive nutrients by diffusion across the cartilage matrix from several sources. These sources include the blood vessels within the synovial membrane that is located along the peripheral margin of the nonarticular portion of the cartilage, the synovial fluid, and

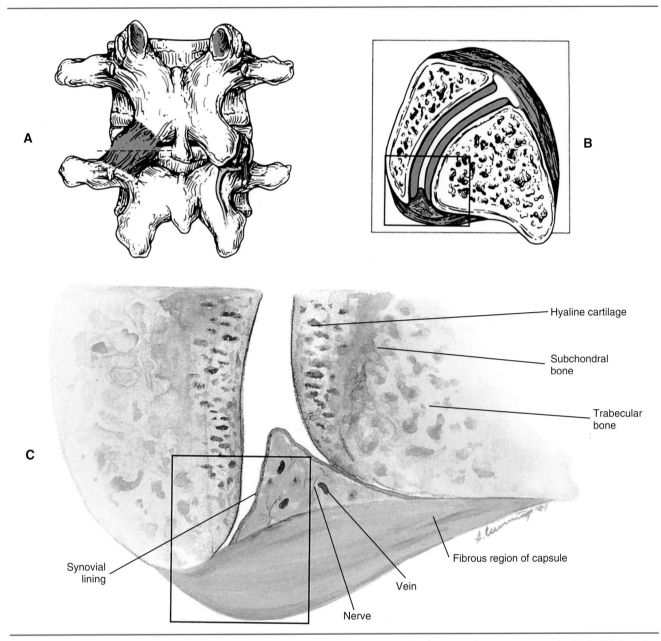

FIG. 14-1 Zygapophysial (Z) joint. **A** and **B,** Z joint from a posterior view and a horizontal section, respectively. **C,** Z joint after magnification by roughly a factor of 10. The articular cartilage, subchondral bone, and articular capsule are prominently displayed. In addition, a Z joint synovial fold is prominent. Notice that the articular capsule has an outer, tough fibrous region. The center of the synovial fold is more vascular and contains adipose tissue. A nerve can be seen passing through this latter region. A synovial lining can be seen on the deep surface of the articular capsule and the synovial fold. The box enclosing much of the synovial fold and a portion of the superior articular process is the region shown at higher magnification in Figure 14-7.

the blood vessels in the adjacent bone (Williams et al., 1995).

Chondrocytes are found singly in the lacunae. Commonly, especially in cartilage that is actively growing, the lacunae are grouped into clusters of two or more. These clusters are called cell nests or isogenous cell groups (Fig. 14-5). The cells within the nests have

arisen from the mitotic activity of a single chondrocyte; therefore the presence of isogenous cell groups signifies interstitial cartilage growth. This is supported by electron microscopy findings revealing that the chondrocytes within a cell nest exhibit a well-developed rough endoplasmic reticulum, a Golgi complex, and a large amount of glycogen and lipid.

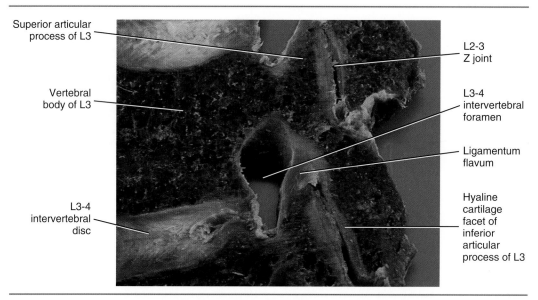

Superior articular process of L3

Vertebral body of L3

L3-4 intervertebral disc

L2-3 Z joint

L3-4 intervertebral foramen

Ligamentum flavum

Hyaline cartilage facet of inferior articular process of L3

FIG. 14-2   Parasagittal section through the L3 and L4 region of a cadaveric spine. Notice the ligamentum flavum covering the anterior (inner) aspect of the zygapophysial (Z) joint.

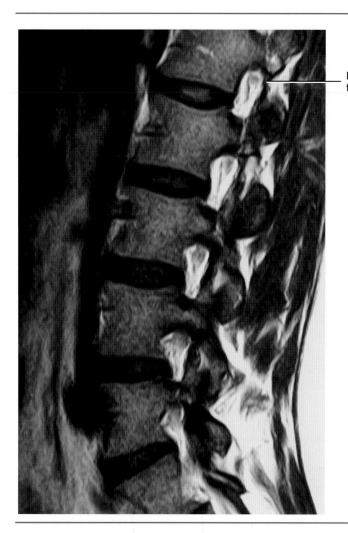

Ligamentum flavum

FIG. 14-3   Magnetic resonance imaging scan of the lumbar region performed in a parasagittal plane. The plane of section roughly corresponds to that of Figure 14-2. Notice the intervertebral discs, the intervertebral foramina, and their contents. (Magnetic resonance image courtesy Dr. Dennis Skogsbergh.)

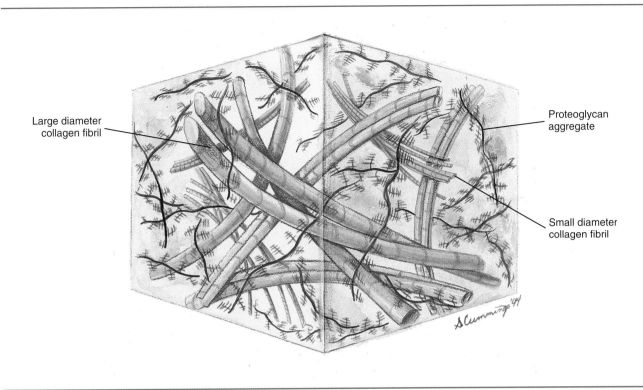

FIG. 14-4   Extracellular matrix of hyaline cartilage. Notice the abundance of collagen fibrils and proteoglycan aggregates.

Articular cartilage differs from typical hyaline cartilage in that the articular surface does not possess a covering of perichondrium (Giles, 1992b; Williams et al., 1995). Instead the cells of the articular surface appear flat and are closer together than they are farther within the cartilage matrix. In addition, the matrix of the articular surface becomes dense and fibrous. The collagen fibers, which course perpendicular to the articulating surface from deep within the cartilage matrix, curve as they reach the joint surface and become oriented parallel to the free edge of the articular cartilage.

Cartilage Matrix.   The cartilage matrix immediately surrounds the lacunae containing the chondrocytes. The matrix of hyaline cartilage consists of collagen (type II) fibers, a small number of elastic fibers, and an amorphous ground substance. The ground substance consists primarily of proteoglycans and glycoproteins. Each of these components of the cartilage matrix contributes to the strength, longevity, and resilience of this tissue.

Collagen.   The collagen component of hyaline cartilage consists of type II collagen fibers. These fibers are relatively thin and course in all directions within the cartilage. Usually they are not visible with the light microscope because they are masked by another compo-

nent of the cartilage matrix, the ground substance. The collagen fibers can be seen easily with an electron microscope.

Collagen functions to bind the cartilage together, protect the chondrocytes, allow for attachment of the articular cartilage to the subchondral bone, and help resist compressive loads (Giles, 1992a). Because collagen is an important constituent of all the connective tissue components of the Z joints and the IVDs, it is discussed in detail in Supporting Cells and Extracellular Matrix of Connective Tissue: Functional Components.

Ground substance.   Chemical analysis of the ground substance of the extracellular matrix of hyaline cartilage reveals that it contains a small amount of glycoproteins and a high concentration of three types of glycosaminoglycans: hyaluronic acid, chondroitin sulfate, and keratan sulfate. The chondroitin and keratan sulfates are joined to a core protein to form a proteoglycan monomer. These macromolecules interact with the collagen and elastic fibers of the hyaline cartilage matrix (Fig. 14-6).

The single core protein of the proteoglycan molecule has a molecular weight of 200,000 to 350,000 Da. The core proteins represent approximately 7% to 12% of the dry weight of cartilage. Bound to each core protein are 80 to 100 chondroitin 4-sulfate and chondroitin 6-sulfate

Table 14-1	The Cells of Connective Tissue			
Cell Type	**Function**	**Distribution**	**Characeristics**	**Miscellaneous**
Fibroblasts	Synthesize and secrete collagen, elastic fibers, reticular fibers, and proteoglycans (among other molecules) Support ligaments, tendons, bone, skin, blood vessels, and basement membranes	Throughout all loose and dense connective tissue	Flat, stellate cells with dark, ovoid, staining nuclei and one or two nucleoli Microscopically, may appear to be of different shapes because of the plane of sectioning	Most abundant cell type found in connective tissue proper
Chondroblasts	Synthesize and secrete extracelluar matrix of cartilage (collagen, elastic fibers, and glycosaminoglycans) Support articular cartilage	Present in hyaline cartilage of articulations (Z joints) and fibrocartilage of intervertebral discs; also found in elastic cartilage	Metabolically active with large vesicular nuclei and prominent nucleoli Cytoplasm pale and vacuolated because of high content of lipid and glycogen	Occupy artificial spaces, called lacunae, which are located in the matrix of cartilage Chondrocytes (mature chondroblasts) similar to chondroblasts except smaller with lower metabolic activity
Osteoblasts	Synthesize and secrete extracellular matrix of bone	In bone	Basophilic cytoplasm resulting from the presence of a large amount of rough endoplasmic reticulum that produces glycosaminoglycans and glycoproteins	Osteocytes (mature osteoblasts) similar to osteoblasts but less active in matrix secretion; occupy spaces in the matrix of bone known as lacunae
Myofibroblasts	Synthesize and secrete components of the extracellular matrix Capable of contractility	In blood vessels and skin throughout the body	Resemble fibroblasts with light microscopy, but ultrastructurally contain actin filaments for contraction	Develop during repair after tissue damage; produce collagen; contractile properties associated with retraction and shrinkage of fibrous (scar) tissue
Adipocytes	Synthesize and store lipids Provide a cushioning and padding function	Throughout body	Small nuclei with abundant lipid in cytoplasm	
Macrophages	Involved in phagocytosis	Throughout body	Derived from monocytes and assume several different forms	Highly motile cells that can move actively from one compartment of the body to another when stimulated by immunoglobulins and antigens
Mast cells	Functionally similar to basophils; granules of basophils and mast cells contain heparin (an anticoagulant), chondroitin sulfate, histamine, and leukotriene 3	In the lamina propria, especially of the digestive and respiratory systems; around blood vessels; and lining serous cavities	Cytoplasm stains basophilic and metrachromatic	

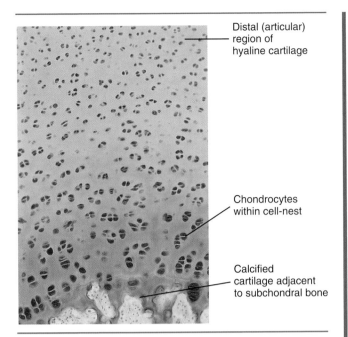

Distal (articular) region of hyaline cartilage

Chondrocytes within cell-nest

Calcified cartilage adjacent to subchondral bone

FIG. 14-5 Light micrograph of hyaline (articular) cartilage. The cartilage is from the distal tip of a fetal phalanx (magnification ×100). Developing articular cartilage of the zygapophysial joints is quite similar.

chains, each with a molecular weight of 20,000 Da. These two glycosaminoglycans make up 80% to 85% of the dry weight of hyaline cartilage. In addition, approximately 50 chains of keratan sulfate, each with a molecular weight of 5000 Da, are also attached to the core protein. Keratan sulfate contributes approximately 7% of the total dry weight of hyaline cartilage.

At one end of each core protein is a hyaluronic acid-binding region (see Fig. 14-6). At this site the proteoglycan units are joined to hyaluronic acid molecules to form long proteoglycan-hyaluronic acid (PG-HA) aggregates. The interaction of the proteoglycan monomer with hyaluronic acid is strengthened by the presence of a link protein (see Fig. 14-6). Proteoglycans and glycosaminoglycans are discussed in further detail later in this chapter with regard to the IVD.

Chondronectin is a glycoprotein found in cartilage. Glycoproteins differ from proteoglycans by their low carbohydrate content, different repeating disaccharide units, and the absence of sulfate esters. Chondronectin participates in the adhesion of chondrocytes to type II collagen. Common glycoproteins found in other body tissues include laminin and fibronectin. Laminin is found in basal laminae and is partially responsible for the adhesion of epithelial cells. Fibronectin is found in blood, plasma, fibroblasts, and some epithelial cells and helps to mediate normal cell adhesion and migration (Table 14-2).

Clinical and biomechanical considerations. Normally fluid moves out of articular cartilage when it is compressed and back into the cartilage when the Z joint is distracted. Such movement may help nutrients diffuse through the matrix to the chondrocytes. Articular cartilage can deform considerably when heavy compressive loads are applied to a joint. However, it returns to its previous state when the load is removed. If injured, articular cartilage heals rather slowly (a 1-mm defect heals in approximately 4 weeks). Passive movement of the joint may stimulate cartilage regeneration, whereas immobility results in the development of adhesions. Intermittent light weight-bearing activity does not stimulate cartilage regeneration but does stop the development of adhesions (Triano, 1992).

Articular cartilage becomes yellow, thinner, and more brittle with age, and undulations that may develop into ragged projections appear as a result of "wear and tear" of the joint surface (Williams et al., 1995). Also with age, fissures or cracks may develop in the articular cartilage. The development of such fissures is known as fibrillation of articular cartilage. The fissures may extend from the joint surface to the subchondral bone.

Zygapophysial Joint Articular Capsule

The Z joint capsules attach to the margins of the opposed superior and inferior articular facets of adjacent vertebrae throughout the vertebral column. The capsules are longer and looser in the cervical region than in the lumbar and thoracic regions. The articular capsule of a typical Z joint covers the joint's posterolateral surface. It consists of an outer layer of white and shining dense fibroelastic connective tissue with bundles of collagen fibers coursing parallel with one another. Deep to the outer fibrous layer is a vascular central layer that is softer and more extensible than the outer layer, and is made up of elastic fibers, similar to the ligamentum flavum, areolar tissue, and loose connective tissue. The third and deepest layer of the Z joint capsule is an inner smooth and shining layer consisting of a white synovial membrane (Giles and Taylor, 1987; Yamashita et al., 1996). The outer, connective tissue layer of the capsule is tough and is essentially made up of parallel bundles of collagen fibers that are primarily oriented in the horizontal plane. A few fibroblasts and fibrocytes and a small amount of ground substance also are found in this layer (see Supporting Cells and Extracellular Matrix of Connective Tissue: Functional Components). The collagen fibers of the capsule attach to the adjacent surfaces of the superior and inferior articular processes, just peripheral to the articular cartilage. In fact, a gradual transition occurs from the joint capsule to fibrocartilage and finally to the articular cartilage of the Z joint. The capsules have a rich sensory innervation, consisting of mechanoreceptors for proprioception and free nerve endings containing substance P for nociception (Giles and Taylor, 1987; Yamashita

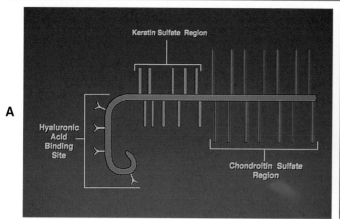

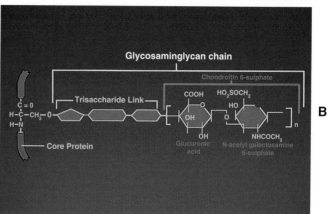

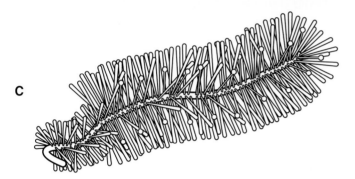

FIG. 14-6 **A,** Structure of a proteoglycan monomer. Notice several glycosaminoglycan chains (chondroitin sulfate and keratan sulfate) attached to a core protein. The protein molecule can attach to a long hyaluronic acid molecule to help to form a proteoglycan aggregate. **B,** An example of an individual glycosaminoglycan chain, in this case chondroitin 6-sulfate, and its attachment to the core protein. **C,** The "bottle-brush" appearance of a proteoglycan monomer. (**A** and **B,** Courtesy Dino Juarez, National University of Health Sciences.)

et al., 1996). However, they have a poor blood supply, which slows the healing of these structures once they are damaged (Giles, 1992b). The multifidus lumborum muscle attaches to the articular capsule, which lies just medial to the primary attachment of this muscle to the mamillary process. The multifidus lumborum muscle may put tension on the capsule and help keep it from being entrapped in the joint space (Taylor and Twomey, 1986).

The posterior and lateral aspect of each lumbar inferior articular process (IAP) has a "lip" that projects further posteriorly than the medial aspect of the IAP, which is more anteriorly located. Consequently, the articular capsule "wraps around" this posterior lip of the lateral aspect of the IAP before attaching to the more anteriorly positioned medial aspect of the IAP. The cervical and thoracic IAPs are oriented differently and do not have this posterior lip; consequently, their capsules do not have a wrap-around component. Boszczyk et al. (2001) found that this wrap-around region of the lumbar Z joint capsule was thicker and more fibrocartilaginous in nature (containing type II collagen, aggrecan, and link protein) than the thoracic Z joint capsules, which were found to be thinner and more purely fibrous (rather than fibrocartilaginous) in nature. The entheses (attachment sites) of the lumbar Z joint capsules to the lumbar infe-

rior and superior articular processes were found to have the same fibrocartilaginous make-up as the wrap-around portion, indicating that traction forces were placed on the entheses. The authors believed that the costovertebral (costocorporeal) and costotransverse articulations of the thoracic region, along with the spatial orientation of the thoracic articular processes, spared the thoracic capsules from the traction and compressive forces placed on the lumbar Z joint capsules (Boszczyk et al., 2001).

A detailed description of the fiber direction of the outer part of the lumbar Z joint capsules and the clinical significance of the fiber direction in the lumbar capsule is given in Chapter 7.

The articular capsules are thinner superiorly and inferiorly, where they form capsular recesses that cover fat-filled synovial pads. Defects exist within the superior and inferior aspects of the joint capsule and allow for the passage of small nerves and vessels. The synovial joint recesses and the development of synovial joint cysts are discussed in further detail with the lumbar region, where they have been studied the most extensively (see Chapter 7). Also, the specific innervation of the Z joint capsule by the medial branch of the posterior primary division (dorsal ramus) is discussed in Chapter 2.

Table 14-2   Fibers Found in Connective Tissue

Fiber Type	Function	Distribution	Miscellaneous
Collagen	Provides rigid support and tensile strength to tendons, ligaments, cartilage, bone, and intervertebral discs	Throughout body	Most abundant and most important of the extracellular fibrillar proteins in the human body
Fibrillin	Main component of extracellular microfibrils, which are one constituent of elastic fibers Microfibrils promote adhesion between different components of the extracellular matrix	Throughout body	Fibrillin is a glycoprotein that forms fibrils
Elastic fibers	Provide elasticity to tissues and allow them to recoil after stretching	Blood vessels, skin, and ligaments Large elastic fibers found in the ligamenta flava Also present in elastic cartilage of the ear, epiglottis, lungs, vocal cords, and pleura	Composed of glycoprotein microfilaments (fibrillin) surrounding a core region of elastin
Reticular fibers	Provide a fine scaffolding that supports the extracellular matrix in basal laminae (basement membranes)	Throughout body	Thin fibrils, identical to small collagen fibrils (about 20 nm in diameter); exhibit a 67-nm periodicity of type III collagen (see Table 14-3)
Fibronectin	Serves as an intermediate protein in the extracellular matrix, where it connects cells to other extracellular matrix components, especially collagen and certain glycosaminoglycans (e.g., heparin)	Throughout body	Dimer glycoprotein, synthesized by fibroblasts and some epithelial cells (molecular weight, 230 to 250 kilodaltons)

Ligamentum Flavum. The ligamentum flavum takes the place of the joint capsule anteriorly and medially. As discussed, this ligament passes from the anterior and inferior aspect of the lamina of the vertebra above to the posterior and superior aspect of the lamina of the vertebra below. However, the lateral fibers of this ligament course anterior to the Z joint, attach to its margins, and form its anterior capsule. Synovial extensions, or cysts, protrude out of the Z joint and along the attachment sites of the ligamentum flavum to the adjacent superior and inferior articular processes.

The ligamentum flavum is 80% elastic fibers and 20% collagen fibers. The elastic fibers within the ligamentum flavum prevent it from buckling into the intervertebral foramen (IVF) and vertebral canal, thus sparing the contents of these regions.

Synovial Membrane

The synovial membrane, synovium, or joint lining is a condensation of connective tissue that covers the inner surface of the fibrous capsule, thus forming a sac that encloses the joint cavity (Fig. 14-7). Therefore the region of a diarthrodial joint surrounded by a synovium is known as the synovial, or joint, cavity. The synovium covers the nonarticular bone enclosed within the joint capsule and courses to the margin of the articular cartilage, where a transition zone exists between the synovium and articular cartilage. The synovium does not cover the load-bearing surface of the cartilage. The joint cavity normally contains a small amount of a highly viscous, hyaluronic acid-rich fluid that lubricates the joint surfaces. This fluid is known as synovial fluid and is produced by the cells within the synovial membrane (see Synoviocytes). The major function of the synovial membrane is to produce synovial fluid. Another function is to absorb waste products of metabolism and cellular debris before they can accumulate in the Z joint cavity.

The innermost portion of the synovium is composed of one to three layers of specialized cells, known as synoviocytes or synovial lining cells. These cells form the intimal layer. Beneath this layer is a loose network of vascular areolar connective tissue that contains a rich blood supply. This layer is known as the synovial subintimal layer. It possesses many elastic fibers that probably serve to keep the synovium taut and prevent it from buckling into the joint cavity. The synovium is innervated by sensory nerve endings.

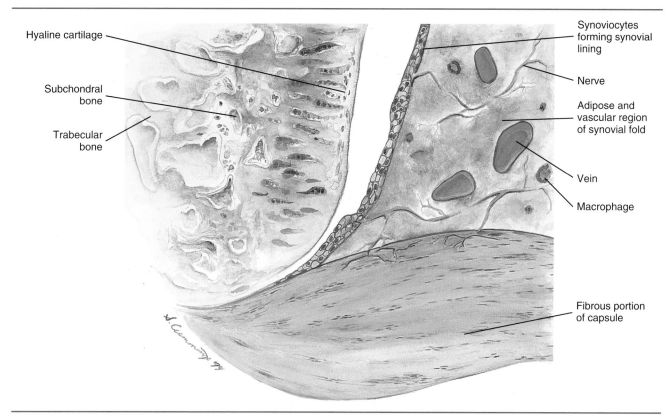

Hyaline cartilage

Subchondral bone

Trabecular bone

Synoviocytes forming synovial lining

Nerve

Adipose and vascular region of synovial fold

Vein

Macrophage

Fibrous portion of capsule

FIG. 14-7   Portion of the zygoapophysial (Z) joint at a magnification of approximately 40×. The region here is shown by the box in Figure 14-1. Portions of the articular cartilage, subchondral bone of the superior articular process and mamillary process, the articular capsule, and the Z joint synovial fold can be seen.

Typically projections of the synovial layer extend into the synovial cavity as Z joint synovial folds (Giles, 1992a). Their purpose is to fill in the small gaps along the periphery of the joint, where the articular cartilages of the opposing surfaces do not normally come in contact with one another. These folds also produce synovial fluid and provide an efficient mechanism for the distribution of this fluid directly into the joint cavity.

Z joint synovial folds contain a relatively large amount of adipose tissue at the region of their attachment to the fibrous layer of the articular capsule. They possess a nociceptive sensory nerve supply of free nerve endings containing substance P (Giles, 1987), and at times they may extend a considerable distance into the joint, in which case their central tips usually are fibrous. *Entrapment* of these folds between or *extrapment* of them peripheral to the articular surfaces of the Z joint have been implicated as possible causes of back pain (Mooney and Robertson, 1976; Giles and Taylor, 1987; Bogduk and Twomey, 1991). Giles (1992a) also states that traumatic synovitis of these folds may cause the release of pain-mediating agents and subsequent back pain.

Synoviocytes

Transmission electron microscopy studies reveal that a discontinuous layer of cells, known as synoviocytes, lines the free surface of the synovial membrane. Although synoviocytes resemble other connective tissue cells, they differ from ordinary fibroblasts (see Table 14-1) in their ultrastructural features and metabolic activities.

Synoviocytes have been classified into two types based on their cellular morphologic structure: fibroblast-like cells, or type A synoviocytes, and type B synoviocytes. Type A synoviocytes are somewhat numerous and are characterized by the presence of abundant cytoplasmic organelles such as endoplasmic reticulum. These cells are involved in secretion and are believed to synthesize hyaluronic acid and glycoproteins (see following discussion). Type B synoviocytes are similar to macrophages and are involved in phagocytosis. Types A and B synoviocytes are not connected by junctional complexes and do not rest on a basement membrane; therefore they do not constitute an epithelial lining of the joint cavity, although they do create a smooth secreting surface for the synovium. Small folds of synovium, or synovial villi, can be found periodically along the surface of the synovial membrane.

The synovial fluid produced by the type A synoviocytes is rich in hyaluronic acid and also contains protein, although its protein content is less than that of blood plasma (Triano, 1992; Williams et al., 1995). The hyaluronic acid imparts synovial fluid with great viscosity. Coiling of the hyaluronic acid molecules and interlocking between different molecules allow the synovial fluid to act as a shock absorber during compressive loads. However, during shear forces the coiled hyaluronic acid molecules straighten and the interlocking between molecules decreases, resulting in smooth, low-friction movement between the adjacent Z joint surfaces.

Supporting Cells and Extracellular Matrix of Connective Tissue: Functional Components

Because the Z joints are composed of connective tissue, a brief discussion of the normal characteristics of this type of tissue is essential for a complete understanding of the structure and function of the Z joints. Therefore this section discusses the cellular and extracellular components of connective tissue.

Early Connective Tissue (Mesenchyme). The connective tissue appearing in embryonic and early fetal development is called mesenchyme. When examined under the light microscope, this type of tissue is seen to be composed of large stellate or spindle-shaped cells that are separated by an abundant amount of intercellular substance. Early embryonic mesenchymal tissue does not contain fiber bundles. Instead, it is composed of fine reticular fibrils (type III collagen) embedded in a gelatinous, amorphous ground substance that is rich in glycosaminoglycans. Embryonic mesenchymal tissue is described as a multipotent or pluripotent tissue. This suggests that mesenchymal cells undergo extensive mitosis and are able to develop into many different types of connective tissue and related cells during fetal and adult life.

Mature Connective Tissue. Connective tissue is responsible for maintaining structural interrelationships between tissues and cells, including the tissues and cells of the spine. All connective tissue is composed of cells, extracellular fibers, an amorphous ground substance, and tissue fluid. The extracellular fibers and ground substance form the extracellular matrix. In contrast to other body tissues (e.g., epithelium, muscle), connective tissue contains fewer cells in proportion to the amount of extracellular matrix. Based on the composition of the extracellular matrix, adult connective tissue is classified into three main types: connective tissue proper, cartilage, and bone. The composition of the extracellular matrix varies among these three types. In connective tissue proper the extracellular matrix is soft; in cartilage it is much firmer, partially calcified, but flexible in nature; and in bone the matrix is rigid because of the presence of calcium salts, which are in the form of hydroxyapatite crystals.

Cartilage and bone are specialized types of connective tissue. Three histologic types of cartilage are encountered based on characteristics of the ground substance matrix:

◆ Hyaline cartilage
◆ Elastic cartilage
◆ Fibrocartilage

Hyaline cartilage is discussed in the previous section along with the Z joints, and fibrocartilage is discussed with the IVD. There is no elastic cartilage in spinal tissues; therefore this type of cartilage is not discussed in this chapter.

Cells of connective tissue. As mentioned, connective tissue consists of cells, fibers, and ground substance. The type of supportive resident cells found in connective tissue varies considerably and may include fibroblasts, chondroblasts and chondrocytes, and osteoblasts, osteoclasts, and osteocytes. These cells are important when considering the connective tissue of spinal structures. Adipocytes, mast cells, macrophages, and myofibroblasts are also found in connective tissue in various parts of the body. The functions and primary characteristics of these cells are listed in Table 14-1.

In addition to the fixed or resident cells of connective tissue described in Table 14-1, connective tissue also contains transient or immigrant cells. These include all the formed cellular elements found in blood with the exception of erythrocytes. The immigrant cells include the neutrophils, eosinophils, basophils, monocytes, lymphocytes, and plasma cells. When inflammation occurs, these immigrant cells leave the circulation and join fibroblasts and other connective tissue resident cells, such as macrophages. Once in the connective tissue, they fight microorganisms that cause inflammation and clean up (phagocytize) the debris that results from this process.

Fibers of connective tissue. The fiber component is another of the three elements of connective tissue. The types of fibers found in connective tissue are collagen, fibrillin, elastin, reticulum, and fibronectin. The functions of each of these are listed in Table 14-2.

Collagen Synthesis. Collagen is the most important fiber type of connective tissue. Collagen is a major component of connective tissue proper, cartilage, and bone. Collagen fibers are found in abundance throughout the articular capsule and hyaline cartilage of the Z joints and also throughout the IVDs. Collagen fibers are composed of collagen macromolecules, which are the most abundant protein in the human body. Collagen fibers are flexible and strong, and they are made up of a bundle of fine, threadlike subunits called collagen fibrils. Collagen is a stable protein under the physiologic conditions that exist in connective tissue; however, collagen is constantly being degraded and replenished by collagen-secreting cells.

It was believed for many years that collagen synthesis occurred primarily in fibroblasts, chondroblasts, osteoblasts, and odontoblasts; however, recent investigations in collagen biology indicate that many other cell types produce this unique protein. Collagen synthesis has been studied extensively in fibroblasts (Williams et al., 1995). Fibroblasts have the extensive rough endoplasmic reticulum and well-developed Golgi apparatus required of cells actively involved in protein synthesis. Labeled amino acids endocytosed by fibroblasts can be followed autoradiographically to the rough endoplasmic reticulum (rER), later to the Golgi complex, then to the outside of the fibroblast, and eventually to the newly formed collagen fibers. This evidence indicates that the collagen synthesis pathway is similar to that of other proteins. Fibroblasts synthesize collagen de novo and secrete it into the extracellular matrix. Fibroblasts also have the ability to break down collagen with specific degradative enzymes called collagenases.

Collagen is a ubiquitous substance that is extremely important in the integrity of both the Z joints and IVDs. Current research and possibly future treatments (nutritional and pharmacologic) related to these two regions of the spine may involve the individual steps of collagen synthesis. Because of the clinical importance of collagen synthesis, this pathway is discussed briefly here.

Collagen synthesis begins inside cells. However, the final processing and assembly into fibers takes place after collagen building blocks have been secreted outside the manufacturing cells. The intracellular events include synthesis of proalpha chains in the rER, hydroxylation and glycosylation of proalpha chains into triple helices in the Golgi apparatus, and formation of secretory granules (vesicles). The extracellular events include cleavage of extension peptides, fibrillogenesis and cross-linking, and assembly of fibrils into mature fibers (Fig. 14-8). Box 14-1 shows the events (steps) involved in collagen synthesis within the fibroblast (steps 1 through 9) and outside the fibroblast in the extracellular matrix (steps 10 through 12).

The amino acid composition of collagen is one of the features that makes collagen such a unique protein. Four amino acids compose most of the polypeptides in the collagen macromolecules. The principal amino acids that make up collagen are glycine (35%), proline (12%), hydroxyproline (10%), and alanine (11%). In the cytoplasm of the fibroblast, approximately 250 to 300 amino acids are combined by polyribosomes associated with rER to form a polypeptide with a molecular weight of 30,000 Da. This step of translation is performed under the control of messenger ribosomal ribonucleic acid (mRNA). Three polypeptide chains are combined into polypeptide alpha triple helices with a molecular weight of approximately 100,000 Da. These triple helices are released into the cisternae of rER (see Box 14-1, steps 1 through 3). Glycine is the third amino acid in each alpha chain of the newly formed triple helix. The amino acid after glycine frequently is proline, and the amino acid preceding the glycine frequently is hydroxyproline. Differences in the chemical structure of the alpha chains are responsible for at least 19 different types of collagen identified to date (Ross et al., 2003). Specifics of the 11 most common types of collagen can be found in Table 14-3.

Several modifications of the polypeptide chains occur within the cisternae of rER and the Golgi apparatus (see Box 14-1, steps 4 to 6 and Fig. 14-8). Disulfide bonds are formed within each polypeptide chain and between adjacent chains. Vitamin C is necessary for the formation of the disulfide bonds, and its absence results in certain types of collagen-related diseases such as scurvy. This bonding gives shape and stability to the triple-helix collagen macromolecule. The structure formed now constitutes a procollagen molecule. The procollagen molecule moves to the exterior of the cell via secretory granules (see Box 14-1, steps 7 to 9 and Fig. 14-8). Further modifications are made outside the cell. For example, enzymes cleave most of the uncoiled amino acids, thereby converting procollagen to tropocollagen molecules. These eventually aggregate to produce collagen fibrils (see Box 14-1, steps 10 to 12). Cross-links between lysine and hydroxylysine are then formed, giving the molecule its tensile strength. Changes in collagen cross-links have been seen in IVD degeneration (Duance et al., 1998).

The tropocollagen molecules are 300 nm long and 1.5 nm in diameter. They consist of three polypeptide chains that are twisted around one another to form a right-handed superhelix with a head and a tail end. Numerous tropocollagen molecules lie end-to-end and also in parallel chains or rows. All the molecules face the same direction, and approximately one fourth of the length of the tropocollagen molecule overlaps between the parallel rows. Therefore a tropocollagen molecule of one row ends approximately one fourth of the distance along the length of another tropocollagen molecule of an adjacent row. This configuration results in a regular 64- to 67-nm periodicity that is clearly visible on an

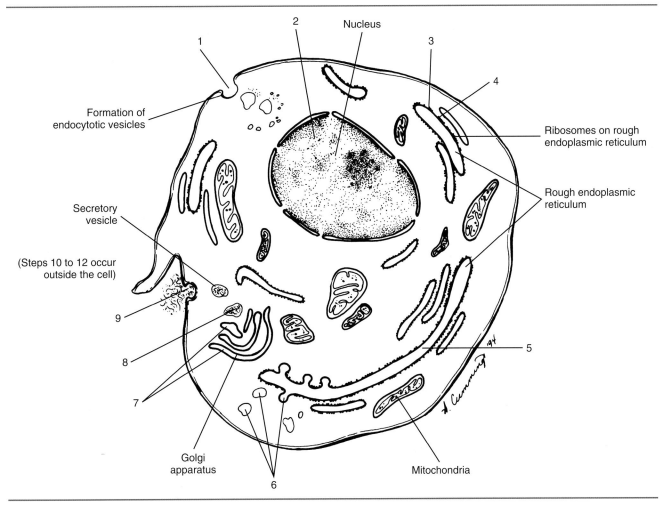

FIG. 14-8   Intracellular steps involved in collagen synthesis. The numbers refer to Box 14-1.

electron micrograph. Figure 14-9 shows collagen fibers within the IVD.

The finest strand of collagen that can be seen with the light microscope is the fibril, which is approximately 0.2 to 0.3 μm in diameter. A fibril is made up of still smaller units that have a diameter of 45 to 100 nm. These are called microfibrils. Newly formed microfibrils are only approximately 20 nm in diameter, and evidence shows that they increase in size with age. Most microfibrils are visible only with the electron microscope and demonstrate the characteristic cross-banding with a periodicity of 64 to 67 nm. The parallel assembly of microfibrils forms fibrils. The fibrils in turn aggregate in bundles to form the thicker collagen fibers. These fibers have a diameter ranging from 1 to 12 μm or more.

Types of Collagen. At present, 19 different types of collagen have been positively identified. They are designated as types I through XIX. Types I to V are the most abundant types of collagen. Types VI to XIX are considered less important because they occur in small quantities. Several of the minor types of collagen (types VI, IX, X, XI, XII, and XIV) are present in small amounts in the IVD (Duance et al., 1998). Table 14-3 lists the characteristics of the 11 most important types of collagen.

Types I, II, and III are arranged as ropelike fibrils and are the main forms of fibrillar collagen. Type I collagen consists of two alpha-1 chains and one alpha-2 chain and represents 90% of all collagen fibers distributed in connective tissue. Because type I fibers resist tensile stresses, their orientation and cross-linking vary according to the local environment. Type I collagen is found in bone, tendon, and the anulus fibrosus (AF) of the IVD. It is also found in the skin and cornea (see Table 14-3).

Type II collagen fibers are small, banded fibrils averaging 20 nm in diameter. They help to form the extracellular matrix of hyaline cartilage, including that of the Z joints and cartilaginous end plates (CEPs) of the IVDs. Type II collagen is the main type of collagen found in the nucleus pulposus (NP) of the IVD. It is also found

BOX 14-1
COLLAGEN SYNTHESIS

1. Uptake of amino acids via endocytosis
   ↓
2. Formation of messenger ribonucleic acid
   ↓
3. Synthesis, by ribosome, of alpha chains with peptides
   ↓
4. Hydroxylation of amino acids
   ↓
5. Glycosylation of specific hydroxyl-1 residues in rough endoplasmic reticulum (rER)
   ↓
6. Formation of procollagen in rER and movement into transfer vesicles
   ↓
7. Packaging of the procollagen by the Golgi complex into secretory vesicles
   ↓
8. Movement of vesicles to plasma membrane assisted by microfilaments and microtubules
   ↓
9. Exocytosis of procollagen
   ↓
10. Cleavage of procollagen to form tropocollagen
    ↓
11. Polymerization of tropocollagen into collagen microfibril
    ↓
12. Polymerization of collagen microfibrils into a complex, 1- to 12-μm collagen fiber

in elastic cartilage and the cornea and vitreous body of the eye. These fibers demonstrate a high electrostatic attraction for the chondroitin sulfate glycosaminoglycans. Type II collagen contains a higher degree of lysine hydroxylation than type I collagen.

Types III and IV collagen are well distributed throughout the body but are not found to any great extent in Z joints, IVDs, or other spinal tissues, although type III has been found in regions adjacent to spondylosis (Schollmeier, Lahr-Eigen, and Lewandrowski, 2000). The key features of these fibers and collagen types V through XI are listed in Table 14-3.

Ground Substance. The cells and fibers of connective tissue are surrounded by a translucent, fluidic, homogeneous, gel-like matrix called amorphous ground substance (Bloom and Fawcett, 1986). The ground substance exhibits no structural organization that is visible with light microscopy. Extracellular amorphous ground substance plays a vital role in the regulation of tissue nutrition, support, and maintenance of proper water content. Based on chemical analysis, the extracellular ground substance of connective tissue has the physical properties of a viscous solution or thin gel and consists of proteoglycans and glycosaminoglycans of various types. Proteoglycans and glycosaminoglycans are an important part of the hyaline cartilage of the Z joints and the cartilaginous (vertebral) end plates of the IVDs. They are also being studied with regard to the AF and NP of the IVD. Therefore glycosaminoglycans and proteoglycans are discussed in further detail with the articular cartilage of the Z joint (see previous discussion) and with the IVD (see following discussion).

MICROSCOPIC AND MOLECULAR STRUCTURE OF THE INTERVERTEBRAL DISCS

Symphyseal joints unite the vertebral bodies, and these joints are made up of the IVDs. The IVDs permit a limited amount of movement between the vertebral bodies while maintaining a union of great strength. The intrinsic stability of the motion segment (two adjacent vertebrae and the ligaments, including the disc, between them), and therefore of the whole spine, results mainly from the IVDs and the ligaments associated with them (Bogduk, 1997). The paraspinal and trunk muscles provide the spine's extrinsic stability.

IVDs (see Fig. 14-9) are important parts of the spinal column and play an active and important role in the spine's physiologic function. The physical properties, elasticity, and resiliency of the IVDs allow them to give support to the spine and allow motion to occur between adjacent vertebral segments, while also preventing too much motion from occurring between the same segments. The IVDs also allow the spine to return back to its original shape after being compressed or stretched (Chai Ben-Fu and Tang Xue-Ming, 1987).

The IVD consists of three main parts: the outer AF, which consists of a series of fibrocartilaginous rings (except in the cervical region, where it is a solid, crescent-shaped, fibrocartilaginous structure); the inner gelatinous NP; and the CEPs of hyaline-like cartilage. The end plates are located between the bony vertebrae and other parts of the IVD (Ghosh, 1990).

Each IVD is reinforced peripherally by circumferential ligaments (see Fig. 14-9, *A*). A thick anterior longitudinal ligament extends down the anterior aspect of the spinal column and is attached to the vertebral end plates. It provides additional anterior support to the AF. A thinner posterior longitudinal ligament spans across the posterior aspect of each disc and is firmly attached to the IVD's posterior aspect.

The IVD is specialized connective tissue designed to provide strength, mobility, and resistance to strain. All three parts of the IVD listed previously (Fig. 14-10; see also Fig. 14-9, *B*) consist of water, cells, proteoglycans

Table 14-3   Characteristics of Collagen Type I to XI

Collagen Type	Distribution	Light Microscopy	Ultrastructure	Produced By	Function
I	Outer anulus fibrosus, loose fibrous tissue, skin dermis, tendons, bones, ligaments, fascia, sclera, dentin, organ capsules, fibrocartilage	Large-banded collagen fiber, closely packed, thick, nonargyrophilic	Densely packed, thick fibrils with marked variation in diameter	Fibroblast, chondroblast, osteoblast, odontoblast	Resistance to tension
II	Z joint articular cartilage, intervertbral disc (anulus fibrosus, nucleus pulposus), cartilage end plate, hyaline and elastic cartilage, vitreous body of eye	Loose collagenous network visible only with picro-Sirius stain and polarized microscope	Very thin fibrils, embedded in abundant ground substance	Chondroblast	Resistant to intermittent pressure
III	Blood vessels, smooth muscle, endoneurium, bone marrow, uterus, lymphoid tissue, kidney, lung	Small-banded collagen fiber, forms reticular networks, weakly birefringent greenish fibers	Loosely packed, thin fibrils with more uniform diameter	Smooth muscle cells, fibroblast, reticulocyte, hepatocyte	Structural maintenance
IV	Epithelial and endothelial basement membranes, lens capsule	Sheetlike layers	Neither fibers nor fibrils	Endothelial and epithelial cells, muscle cells	Support and filtration
V	Basement membranes of placenta, smooth and skeletal muscle	Thin fibrils	*	Fibroblast	*
VI	Fine filaments of elastic tissue	Thin fibrils	*	Endothelial cells	*
VII	Anchoring fibrils in basement membrane of skin and amnion	Short, striated fibrils	*	Endothelial cells	*
VIII	Placental membranes, endothelium	*	*	Endothelial cells	*
IX	Cartilage	*	*	Chondrocytes	*
X	Mineralized cartilage	*	*	Hypertrophic chondrocytes	•
XI	Cartilage	*	*	Chondrocytes	*

*Insufficient data.

(PGs), and collagen. These components are found in varied concentrations in the three different regions of the disc. In fact, the varied concentrations of these basic components within the IVD make it a specialized type of connective tissue. For example, after an early age (≈2 years) the disc has no blood supply (except for the vessels within the vertebral bodies that are adjacent to the CEPs and remain until 11 to 12 years of age), and so receives its nutrition from the adjacent vertebral bodies. The PGs are essential in the process of attracting fluid and nutrition to the IVD from the adjacent vertebral bodies. The PGs are negatively charged and attract Na^+, which then attracts water and other nutrients by osmotic flow. The PGs have been found to actually regulate the amount and type of molecules entering the IVD. Breakdown of PG molecules in the IVD has been associated with the decreased fluid and tissue breakdown found in disc degeneration. Because chondroitin sulfate is a major component of the PGs, this substance and a related molecule, glucosamine sulfate, are frequently given as part of the conservative treatment of disc degeneration. Therefore PGs are important to the health and treatment of the IVD.

Collagen is another of the important components of the IVDs. As mentioned, the main type of collagen in the AF is type I, and is a ropelike molecule that is

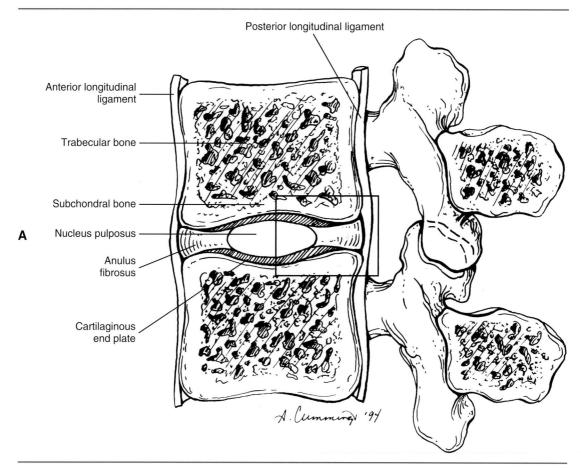

Posterior longitudinal ligament

Anterior longitudinal ligament

Trabecular bone

Subchondral bone

A

Nucleus pulposus

Anulus fibrosus

Cartilaginous end plate

A. Cummings '94

FIG. 14-9   **A,** Sagittal section of two adjacent vertebrae and the intervertebral disc between them.

tough and strong and gives the AF its ability to withstand the forces and loads placed on the IVD. The NP has a higher concentration of the less-well-organized type II collagen.

The cells make up the third important component of the IVD. The cells manufacture the collagen, as well as the PGs, of the disc. Because the CEP of the IVD has the greatest number of cells, this region may serve as the "manufacturing plant" for the important PGs and collagen of the IVD. The CEP also is permeable to fluids, thus allowing the fluids and metabolites from the adjacent vertebral bodies to diffuse into the NP and AF. The CEP has been found to be most permeable in its center, the part adjacent to the nucleus pulposus, and the NP has the greatest amount of fluid and hydrostatic pressure (fluid pressure) of the three parts of the IVD.

The hydrostatic pressure just mentioned is maintained by the fourth important constituent of the IVD: water. The water of the disc gives the disc the hydrostatic pressure needed to resist compression, while also allowing for adequate intersegmental movement. Remarkably the hydrostatic pressure of the IVD is also important in

resisting too much movement between vertebrae. Too much movement, of course, would damage the articular processes and possibly the neural elements housed within the vertebral canal.

Therefore each of the building blocks of the IVD is important and clinically relevant. In addition, each of the four constituents is closely related to the others. For example, the collagen fibers within the IVD become taut during movements of the spine and tend to restrain the PGs. The PGs in turn allow the IVD to deform. Because of its ability to absorb fluid (swell) and then to maintain its hydration (water), the PG gel of the NP is able to resist compression under large external loads (Weiss, 1988). The cells in turn maintain the proper levels of PGs and collagen fibers. Therefore the IVD is able to act as a lubricating cushion that prevents adjacent vertebrae from being eroded by abrasive forces during movement of the spinal column. The hydrated gelatinous NP serves to a certain extent as a shock absorber to reduce the impact between adjoining vertebrae (Junqueira and Carneiro, 2003), although the vertebral body helps in this function as well.

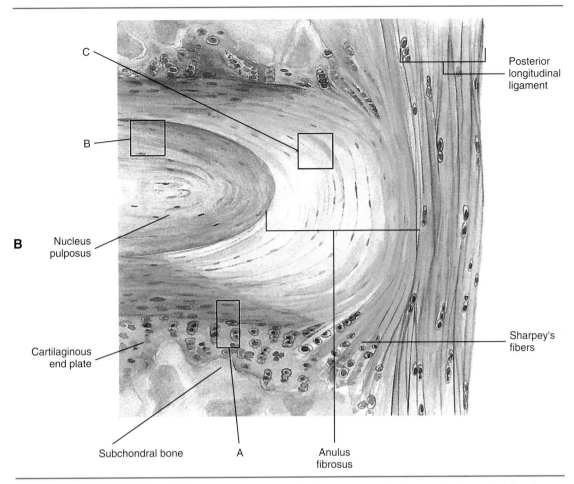

FIG. 14-9—cont'd   **B,** Shows the boxed region in **A** at higher magnification (magnification ≈ ×15). In addition to showing the anulus fibrosus (AF), nucleus pulposus, and cartilaginous end plate, the vertebral body and posterior longitudinal ligament are shown. Notice that the outer fibers of the AF attach to the cortical and subchondral bone of the vertebral body. These attachment sites are known as Sharpey's fibers. The collagen fibers of the inner layers of the AF enter the end plate and curve to run parallel to the discal surface of the vertebral body. (The boxes labeled **A, B,** and **C** refer to the regions shown in Figure 14-10.)

The histologic changes that take place in the IVD with advancing age have been described in postmortem studies by several investigators (Brown, 1971; Pritzker, 1977; Roberts et al., 1989, 1996; Boos et al., 2002). These changes include loss of distinction between the NP and AF, desiccation and fibrosis of the NP with fibrillation of the matrix, brown discoloration of the nucleus, fissuring of the nucleus and AF, fractures of the vertebral end plate, and osteophyte formation. Figure 14-11 demonstrates a series of events associated with degeneration of the IVD. Based on plain x-ray films, the fundamental diagnostic features of disc degeneration are reported to be disc space narrowing and osteophytosis. Decreased hydration as demonstrated by a decreased signal intensity of the IVD on T1- and T2-weighted magnetic resonance imaging (MRI) scans is also an indication of IVD degeneration. The section entitled Normal Aging of the Intervertebral

Discs and Intervertebral Disc Degeneration discusses the changes of IVD degeneration in further detail. In addition, Chapter 7 describes the consequences of these changes and the development of internal disc disruption. Chapter 2 describes the gross anatomic features of the IVD and the clinical relevance of these features, and Chapter 11 discusses IVD bulging, protrusion, and extrusion and their effects on the neural elements within the vertebral canal (i.e., cauda equina and dorsal root ganglia).

The next section of this chapter focuses on the typical microscopic anatomy and the composition of the AF, NP, and cartilaginous vertebral end plate. This section concludes with portions covering IVD aging and degeneration, PGs, and fibrocartilage. These last three portions have been included for readers interested in acquiring a deeper understanding of the biology of the IVD.

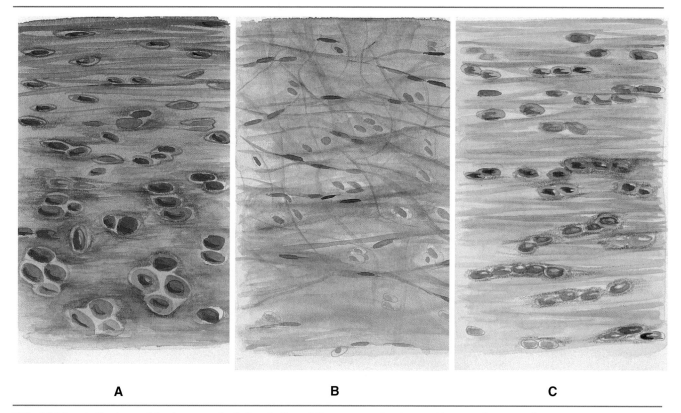

A   **B**   **C**

FIG. 14-10   **A,** Regions of the intervertebral disc. **A, B,** and **C** correspond to lettered boxes of Figure 14-9, *B.* **A,** Cartilaginous end plate. **B,** Nucleus pulposus. **C,** Anulus fibrosus. (**A, B,** and **C** represent a magnification ≈ ×100)

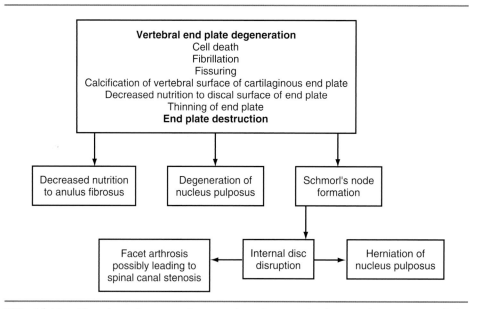

FIG. 14-11   Flowchart demonstrating a series of events leading to degeneration of the intervertebral disc.

Anulus Fibrosus

The AF is the rigid, outer series of rings (lamellae) that forms the peripheral portion of the IVD (Figs. 14-12 and 14-13). It functions to absorb pressure from the central well-hydrated (jellylike) NP. The tightly packed collagen fibers of the AF normally do not allow the large PG molecules of the NP to pass between them, even when the IVD is subjected to large compressive forces. The adult AF is not distinctly separated from the NP or cartilage of the vertebral end plates (Inerot and Axelsson, 1991).

The histologic features of the AF do not change much from childhood to maturity. The outer ring of the AF consists of an external tough layer of dense collagenous connective tissue, whereas the remainder of the AF is primarily composed of overlapping concentric layers of fibrocartilage. The outer part of the AF attaches to the margins of adjacent CEPs in infancy and childhood and to the outer rims of adjacent vertebral bodies in adolescence (see Fig. 14-9, *B,* Sharpey's fibers).

Light and electron microscopy indicate that a typical lumbar AF is composed of fibrocartilage and has a lamellar structure. Anteriorly the AF consists of more than 20 moderately thick lamellae. The outer lamellae are entirely fibrous and contain thick, tightly packed bundles of type I collagen fibers (Ghosh, 1990; Schollmeier, Lahr-Eigen, and Lewandrowski, 2000). Although the outer AF is composed of type I collagen (see Table 14-3), the fibers of the inner AF are composed of type II collagen (Bishop, 1992; Schollmeier, Lahr-Eigen, and Lewandrowski, 2000). The lamellae of the inner part of the AF also have a richer PG ground substance associated with them, which increases the capacity to resist compression (McDevitt, 1988). The collagen fibers in each lamella are orientated parallel to one another and form an angle of inclination (≈25 to 30 degrees) with the horizontal axis of the bony vertebral rims. The fibers of each consecutive layer form approximately a 120- to 130-degree angle with the fibers of adjacent lamellae. The lamellar structure and the angle of inclination of the collagen fibers enable the AF to sustain the normal forces of compression, torsion, and flexion that occur during movements of the IVD (Chai Ben-Fu and Tang Xue-Ming, 1987).

As mentioned, the anterior and lateral parts of the AF are composed of more than 20 moderately thick lamellae. The outer lamellae are loosely attached to the

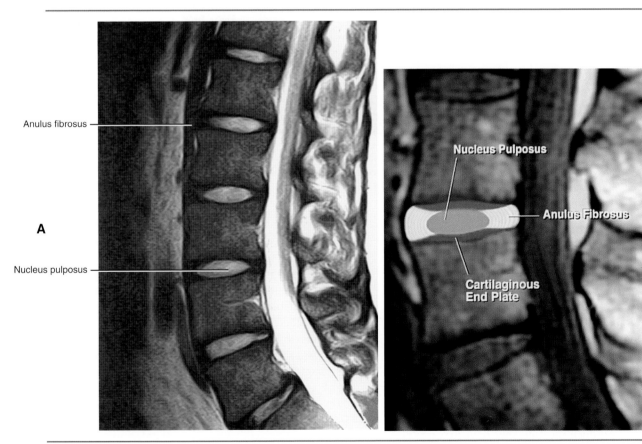

FIG. 14-12 **A,** Midsagittal magnetic resonance imaging scan of the lumbar region showing the intervertebral discs with adjacent vertebral bodies. **B,** Similar view with the parts of the intervertebral disc labeled. (Magnetic resonance image courtesy Dr. Dennis Skogsbergh.)

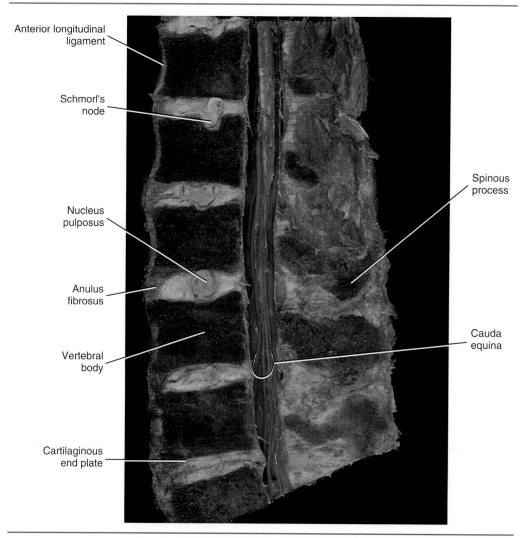

Anterior longitudinal
ligament

Schmorl's
node

Nucleus
pulposus

Anulus
fibrosus

Vertebral
body

Cartilaginous
end plate

Spinous
process

Cauda
equina

FIG. 14-13   Midsagittal section through a cadaveric lumbar spine. Notice that the cartilaginous end plates, the anuli fibrosi, and nuclei pulposi can be seen at several levels. Also notice the Schmorl's node, which has been labeled. (Compare with Figs. 14-15 and 14-16.)

strong anterior longitudinal ligament (Ghosh, 1990). The posterior and posterolateral parts of the AF are much thinner. They consist of 12 to 15 more closely arranged, thinner lamellae that follow the contour of the posterior parts of the adjacent vertebral bodies. The collagen fibers of the outer lamellae of the AF are fused with the lateral margin of the relatively thin posterior longitudinal ligament (Ghosh, 1990). As mentioned, the outer collagen fibers also attach to the posterior vertebral rims. The inner fibers of the AF are continuous with the CEPs (see following discussion and Fig. 14-9, *B*).

The cells of the AF are primarily chondrocytes. Although they produce cartilage, specific matrix proteins, the chondrocytes of the AF are of a different stage of differentiation than the chondrocytes of the growth plates of bones or of articular cartilage (Poiraudeau et al., 1999).

PG extraction from ground human lumbar AFs suggests that the PGs contain three regions: a chondroitin sulfate-rich region, a keratan sulfate-rich region, and a region that binds to hyaluronic acid (Table 14-4; see also Fig. 14-6). By binding to hyaluronic acid, the PGs are permitted to aggregate into PG macromolecules. Because of the immense clinical importance of PGs as they relate to the IVDs, a section devoted to this topic is found later in this chapter. However, characteristics of PGs specific to the AF are covered here.

Previous investigations of glycosaminoglycans and PGs of the IVDs have found that the PGs from the AF contain approximately 75% chondroitin sulfate and 25% keratan sulfate and hyaluronic acid (Antonopoulos et al., 1974; Stevens, Dondi, and Muir, 1979). These percentages are determined by analyzing the glucosamine/

Table 14-4   Glycosaminoglycans*

Name	Molecular Weight (Daltons)	Sulfation	Protein Linked	Disaccharide Composition	Distribution
Hyaluronic acid	10^6	No	No	D-Glucuronic acid + N-acetylglucosamine	Intervertebral disc, cartilage (including Z joint articular cartilage), synovial fluid, skin, vitreous body of eye, loose connective tissue, umbilical cord support fluid (Wharton's jelly)
Chondroitin sulfate	20,000	Yes	Yes	D-Glucuronic acid + N-acetygalactosamine	Intervertebral disc, cartilage (including Z joint articular cartilage), bone, skin, cornea, aorta, notochord
Dermatan sulfate	55,000	Yes	Yes	L-Iduronic acid or D-glucouronic acid + D-galactosamine	Skin, tendons, ligaments, fibrocartilage, blood vessels, heart
Heparan sulfate	15,000	Yes	Yes	D-Glucuronic acid or L-iduronic acid + D-galactosamine	Basement membranes, lung, liver, aorta
Keratan sulfate (I)	7000	Yes	Yes	D-Galactose + D-galactosamine	Cornea
Keratan sulfate (II)	7000	Yes	Yes	D-Galactose + D-galactosamine	Intervertebral disc (nucleus pulposus and anulus fibrosus), cartilage (including Z joint articular cartilage)

*Five main groups of glycosaminoglycans with different tissue distributions exist. Chondroitin sulfate exists as chondroitin sulfate-4 and chondroitin sulfate-6; both possess high levels of interaction with collagen type II. Dermatan sulfate demonstrates low levels of interaction, mainly with collagen type I. Heparan sulfate demonstrates intermediate levels of interaction with collagen types III and IV. Sulfation causes the molecules to be highly (−) charged and contributes to their ability to attract and bind Na+ and water.

galactosamine ratios (see Table 14-4) (Inerot and Axelsson, 1991). Both the hyaluronic acid and the keratan sulfate concentrations are higher in the AF than in hyaline cartilage (Antonopoulos et al., 1964; Hardingham and Adams, 1976). Also, the keratan sulfate region appears to be larger in AF PGs than in hyaline cartilage PGs. Fibrocartilage of human knee joint menisci has been shown also to contain dermatan sulfate. This molecule has not been detected in the human AF. Biochemically the absence of dermatan sulfate and the presence of types I and II collagen fibers suggest that the AF may be classified as an intermediate between hyaline cartilage and fibrocartilage (Inerot and Axelsson, 1991).

A study of the aging of IVD PG composition of canines and humans has shown that the keratan sulfate-rich region of the PG core protein (Fig. 14-6) is more resistant to proteolysis than the chondroitin sulfate-rich region. In addition, the number of keratan sulfate-rich fragments in human disc tissue increases with aging (Cole, Ghosh, and Taylor, 1986).

Clinical Considerations. Fluid moves in and out of the NP during the day, providing nutrients to the disc. During sleeping hours, the NP fills with fluid and presses against the AF. Therefore when an individual arises in the morning, the AF is tense and less flexible. This increase in AF tension after approximately 5 hours of rest may render it more vulnerable to injury after the rest.

Sudden movements of the lumbar spine, especially torsion coupled with flexion, can produce small tears in the AF. These tears usually occur in the posterior part of the AF, where the distribution of collagen fibers is less concentrated. Sometimes, tears in the AF may allow some of the soft jellylike NP to squeeze out into the vertebral canal. This latter condition is known as an extruded IVD (see Chapter 11). IVD extrusion is not as common a cause of back pain as once thought (see Chapter 7). However, the discs can be a source of pain without protrusion or extrusion (Bogduk, 1990). Contrary to previous reports (Malinsky, 1959; Wyke, 1987) that the IVD could not produce pain because it lacks nerve supply, several investigators (Yoshizawa, O'Brien, and Thomas-Smith, 1980; Bogduk et al., 1981) have confirmed that the lumbar discs do have a nerve supply and that nerve fibers and nerve endings have been demonstrated to exist in at least the outer third and possibly as far as the outer half of the AF. Most of these authors conclude that the lumbar disc is supplied with the necessary apparatus for the transmission of nociception and subsequent perception of pain. Chapters 2, 7, and 11 discuss the gross anatomy, including the innervation, and the clinical relevance of the IVD (including the AF) in further detail.

Nucleus Pulposus

Both fetal and infant discs have large notochordal NPs with abundant fluid mucoid matrices. The nucleus of a young disc is encapsulated along the periphery by the AF and on the superior and inferior surfaces by the CEPs (see following discussion). Perinatally the AF and CEPs are vascular, but their blood supply declines dramatically with childhood growth (Taylor, 1990); by 11 to 12 years of age, even the blood vessels that earlier supplied the IVD by entering the deepest parts of the CEPs from the vertebral bodies cannot be found. In fact, the adult NP is the largest avascular structure of the body. It receives nutrition primarily by means of diffusion from blood vessels within the subchondral bone of the adjacent vertebral bodies. This diffusion process by which the IVD receives its nutrients is known as imbibition.

The human NP is a highly hydrated tissue at birth, with a water content of 88% of its dry weight. This falls to 69% at 77 years of age. By comparison, the water content of the AF declines from 78% at birth to approximately 70% at 30 years, and thereafter it stays relatively constant (Gower and Pedrini, 1969). In adults, as the hydration declines with age, the tissues become firmer and lose their translucency, and the boundaries between the NP and AF become less distinguishable. Table 2-5 shows the relative concentrations of water, collagen, and PG (nonaggregated/aggregated ratio) of the NP and AF.

The higher water content of the NP, compared with that of the AF, is accompanied by a lower concentration of collagen in the NP. In addition, the collagen found in the NP is type II rather than type I, which is found in the AF. The individual fibrils of type II collagen are much smaller than those of type I (see Table 14-3). The fibers are also loosely arranged and are surrounded by a more abundant ground substance. In the NP, this ground substance contains a high percentage (65%) of hydrophilic, nonaggregated PGs.

Therefore the NP is a thick, jellylike region with a high concentration of fluid. It draws this fluid from the surrounding vertebral bodies. The fluid, a distillate of plasma, passes through the CEPs on its way to the NP. The NP also has relatively few cells. The cells are primarily notochordal cells in the young (see following discussion). These are then replaced by fibroblasts and chondrocytes. The adult NP makes up 35% to 50% of the IVD (Bishop, 1992). It normally lies slightly posterior to the IVD's center. Normal nuclear material moves backward and forward with flexion and extension movements of the spine, respectively.

The region of the adult NP that is adjacent to the CEPs contains a relative abundance of chondrocytes. The matrix surrounding the chondrocytes stain deeply with safranin and Alcian blue because of the presence of abundant PG macromolecules. Also in this region, vertically oriented collagen fibers extend from the end plate to the NP (Oda, Tamaka, and Tsukuki, 1988). These collagen fibers seem to be independent of the anchoring fibers of the AF. The attachment of these fibers to the end plate and the NP of the IVD may give stability to the IVD at times when the CEP is calcified or replaced by bone.

The Controversial Role of the Notochord in the Formation of the Nucleus Pulposus.
As mentioned, the NP is located in the center of the AF and occupies 35% to 50% of the IVD volume. In children the NP is large and is derived from the notochord (see Fig. 12-12). Gradually the transparent embryonic notochordal cells are replaced by a sparse population of chondrocytes and fibroblasts that originate in the CEP (Kim et al., 2003). In time these cells are partially replaced by fibrocartilage, which makes the NP more opaque and no longer transparent (Junqueira and Carneiro, 2003).

Several investigators have proposed that embryonic notochordal cells undergo degeneration and disappear soon after birth and that these cells have no further participation in the formation of the NP. Virchow (1857) wrote that the NP was formed from connective tissue. Luschka (1856, 1857) maintained that both the notochordal cells and the liquefaction of the inner layers of the surrounding connective tissue contributed to the formation of the NP. Peacock (1951) concluded that the NP was produced by mucoid degeneration of notochordal cells, which caused the disappearance of these cells and increased the mucoid matrix. However, Woelf et al. (1975) studied enzymes present in the NP and described the presence of enzymes that were associated with PG synthesis and oxidative activity. This indication of PG synthesis led them to conclude that human notochordal cells *do* contribute to the matrix of the NP in fetal and postnatal life.

Oda, Tamaka, and Tsukuki (1988) found that the NP was composed of tissue derived from the notochord in specimens collected from individuals ranging in age from 1 month to the midteens. They also found a fine fibrous tissue in the NP that was derived from the AF. No notochordal cells were demonstrated in the NP in the specimens that came from individuals 16 to 19 years of age. Also, the NP of the specimens had been replaced by fibrocartilage and dense collagenous fibrous tissue. These findings have been supported by those of Boos et al. (2002). Pritzker (1977) and Bishop (1992) suggested that the cells originating from the vertebral CEPs might be responsible for synthesizing the gelatinous matrix of the NP in mature IVDs. Kim et al. (2003) found in a rabbit model that the NP changes from having notochordal cells to chondrocyte-like cells. These cells were found to migrate from the adjacent CEP. The CEP chondrocytes began to migrate from the peripheral region of the CEP–NP interface, then the process progressed centrally, changing the notochordal NP into a fibrocartilaginous NP. Therefore notochordal cells probably contribute to the formation, development, and maintenance of the NP. However, this role declines as individuals reach their mid-teens. After this age, the vertebral end plate may continue to help the few cells left within the NP maintain the PG and collagen make-up of the NP.

Cartilaginous End Plate

As mentioned, the IVD is composed of a tougher, peripheral fibrocartilaginous AF and a central gelatinous NP, both of which are located between the superjacent and subjacent CEPs (Chai Ben-Fu and Tang Xue-Ming, 1987) (Figs. 14-12 and 14-13). The adult CEP is a thin strip ($\approx$0.6 to 3 mm thick) of hyaline-like cartilage (it transitions to fibrocartilage as it contacts the NP and AF) that contains many fine collagenous fibrils (similar to fibrocartilage) (Bishop, 1992; Roberts et al., 1996). The CEPs separate the NP and medial aspect of the AF from the subchondral bone of the adjacent vertebral bodies (see Figs. 14-9, 14-12, and 14-13). The subchondral bone of the vertebral bodies consists of a thin peripheral ring of compact bone that surrounds the CEP and a large central region that is cribriform in appearance, containing many small holes that pass to the cancellous bone of the vertebral body.

Developmentally each CEP is a part of the cartilage model of the vertebral body; however, the CEP does not have a firm attachment to the vertebral body. In fact, no fibrillar connections have been found between the CEP and adjacent vertebral body (Bishop, 1992), but the collagen fibers of the AF and NP enter the CEP and become enclosed in the CEP's ground substance (see Fig. 14-9, *B*). In addition, the CEP plays a vital role in the nutritional support of the IVD and may be the source of PG synthesis for the NP and AF (Bishop, 1992). Because the CEP is more closely related to the AF and NP than to the subchondral bone of the adjacent vertebral body, usually it is considered to be an integral part of the IVD.

Each CEP is composed of parallel lamellae of cells (primarily chondrocytes) and collagen fibers, arranged horizontally (Ghosh, 1990). As mentioned, the collagen fibers from the AF appear to continue into the CEP at the AF–CEP junction (Roberts et al., 1989). The CEP's ground substance consists of water within an amorphous matrix of PGs.

The CEPs have important mechanical functions. They contribute to the resilience of the motion segment. In addition, the CEPs participate in the hydrostatic distribution of the pressure absorbed by IVDs during loading (Broberg, 1983).

The CEPs are also thought to play an important role in the IVD's nutrition. Nutrients must diffuse from the blood vessels within the vertebral bodies, which contact the periphery of each CEP, through the cartilage matrix, eventually to reach the cells deep within the CEP. Only 10% of the adult bony end plate of the vertebral body is perforated by small vascular buds that make contact with the CEP (Maroudas, 1975). The vascular contacts are more plentiful in the central part of the CEP than in the peripheral regions (Roberts et al., 1989). The CEP and the NP have both a close anatomic and a close physiologic relationship with each other. The latter relationship is demonstrated by the fact that degeneration of a CEP may initiate the "degeneration" of the NP (see Chapter 7).

The ability to transport nutrients through cartilaginous tissues is known to depend on the make-up of the cartilage matrix, particularly the PG content of the matrix (Nachemson et al., 1970). The PG content (i.e., types of PGs present) and PG concentration controls the diffusion rate and distribution of charged solutes and macromolecules within the cartilage matrix. The CEP near the NP has a higher PG and water concentration than does the CEP adjacent to the AF. The CEP close to the AF (but not overlying it) also has a higher concentration of PGs, as well as a lower concentration of collagen, than the neighboring AF (Roberts et al., 1989). Therefore permeability is enhanced close to the NP and probably tapers off near the periphery of the CEP. If PGs in the CEP degrade (as has been found to occur with age and degeneration) or are lost, solutes can enter the IVD that normally would be excluded (e.g., chemokines or enzymes that could injure the IVD); also solutes (e.g., nutrients) that should remain in the IVD could escape (Roberts et al., 1996). This process also may initiate internal disc disruption (Crock, 1986; Chai Ben-Fu and Tang Xue-Ming, 1987).

Formation of bone inside the CEP, which occurs in some CEPs of certain individuals, also initiates a reduction of the nutritional route to the IVD as a whole. Bone formation may first cause the destruction of the discal surface of the CEP, which eventually contributes to the degeneration of the NP. Oda, Tamaka, and Tsukuki (1988) found that no adverse degenerative changes were observed in the NP when bone formation remained outside the CEP. This important finding might indicate the particular significance of the CEP in the maintenance of the NP.

Detailed histologic changes of the human cervical IVD from the neonate to the ninth decade, with special emphasis on the age changes of the NP and the CEP, were investigated by Oda, Tamaka, and Tsukuki (1988). They found that the CEP can be divided into two regions: the growth cartilage layer, which corresponds to the growth plate of a growing long bone, and the articular cartilage layer, which faces the NP (Fig. 14-14). The articular cartilage layer has been called the "zone of

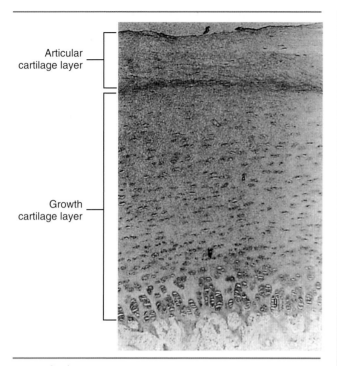

Articular cartilage layer

Growth cartilage layer

FIG. 14-14 Cartilaginous end plate of a newborn. Notice that it can be divided into two regions: the growth cartilage layer, which corresponds to the growth plate of a growing long bone, and the articular cartilage layer, which faces the nucleus pulposus. (From Oda J, Tamaka H, & Tsukuki N. (1988). Intervertebral disk changes with aging of human cervical vertebra: From the neonate to the eighties. *Spine, 13,* 1205-1211.)

resting cartilage" by other authors (Chandraraj, Briggs, and Opeskin, 1998). Oda, Tamaka, and Tsukuki (1988) also noted a fine fibrous tissue between the material derived from the notochordal cells in the NP and the articular cartilage layer of the CEP of the cervical discs of 1-month-old infants. The CEP of specimens collected from individuals 1 year old to the teenage years also contained the same two layers. The CEP of specimens from individuals over 20 years of age had lost the growth layer and was composed only of the articular layer. In people 20 to 30 years of age, the CEP began to calcify, and the calcified areas were invaded by blood vessels from the adjacent vertebral bodies. Calcification of the vertebral CEP has been related to degenerative change within the IVD as a whole (Bishop, 1992) (see Fig. 14-11).

End Plate Fracture (Schmorl's Nodes). Hydrostatic loading of the NP of the IVD causes bulges of the nucleus into the CEP. Fracture of the CEP can occur if the compressive force is great enough. CEP fractures, also known as traumatic Schmorl's nodes, have been noted in postmortem studies as features of disc degeneration (Vernon-Roberts and Pirie, 1977; Sachs et al., 1987) (see Fig. 14-13).

Schmorl's nodes are defined as herniations of the IVD through the CEP and bony end plate (Figs. 14-15 and 14-16; see also Fig. 14-13). They were first described in 1927 by a German pathologist, Christian G. Schmorl. These lesions are believed to be associated with trauma and occur most frequently in the lower thoracic and lumbar regions. Even though trauma is the most likely cause of Schmorl's node formation, a possible congenital origin, such as notochordal cell "rests" (i.e., pockets of notochordal cells that remain after they are normally displaced by chondrocytes or osteocytes) within the subchondral bone adjacent to the CEP, also has been suggested (Taylor, 1990; Pate, 1991). Such congenital defects could predispose one to a later CEP fracture.

Reported incidence of Schmorl's nodes ranges from 38% in radiologic studies to 76% in postmortem studies. Schmorl's nodes are thought to occur most commonly between the ages of 20 and 40, when the IVD has a relatively high fluid pressure (Chandraraj, Briggs, and Opeskin, 1998).

Schmorl's nodes probably predispose the IVD to early degenerative change, especially when observed in younger age groups. In fact, a dorsolumbar kyphosis, seen in adolescents, may be associated with Schmorl's nodes. Therefore CEP fractures should be considered a possible etiologic cause when an active adolescent patient has back pain of the thoracolumbar region.

Compression injury frequently results in an end plate fracture. This may completely resolve in some patients, or in others, inflammatory repair processes may extend into the NP and result in disc degradation (see Chapter 7). Such inflammatory disc degradation initiates internal disc disruption, which may become symptomatic. If the AF remains intact, isolated IVD resorption may follow, but if fissures and tears develop in the AF, the degraded nuclear material may extrude (Bogduk, 1990).

Normal Aging of the Intervertebral Discs and Intervertebral Disc Degeneration

The preceding sections on the three regions of the IVD have hinted at the fact that IVD degeneration is difficult to define and separate from the normal aging process of the IVD. The hallmarks of disc degeneration are loss of fluid pressure, disruption or breakdown of collagen and PGs, and sclerosis of the CEP and adjacent subchondral bone. All of these hallmark signs of IVD degeneration also can occur as part of the normal aging process of the IVD. For these reasons, disc degeneration and normal aging of the disc frequently are discussed interchangeably (Kraemer, 1995; Boos et al., 2002).

The IVD seems to age differently than other tissues of the body (probably as a result of its avascular nature), and many authors now conclude that the disc is unique in that it begins the degenerative process quite early in

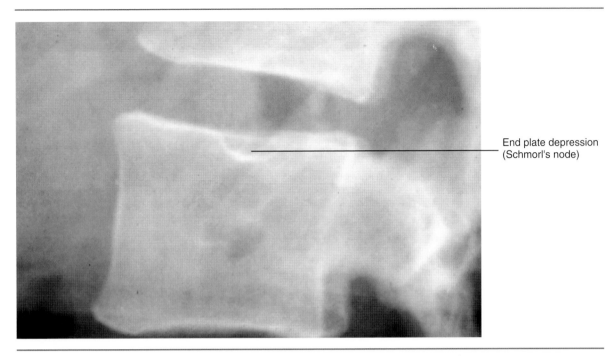

End plate depression
(Schmorl's node)

FIG. 14-15   X-ray demonstrating a Schmorl's node. (Compare with Figs. 14-13 and 14-16.) (Image courtesy Dr. Dennis Skogsbergh.)

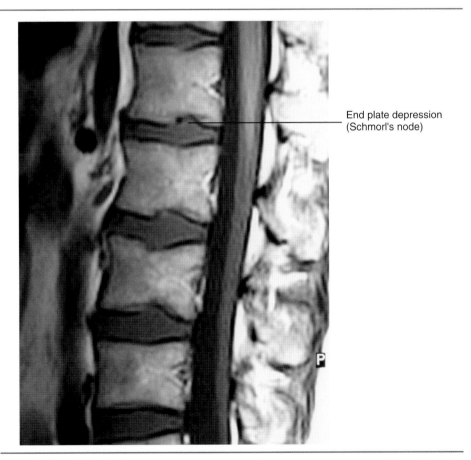

End plate depression
(Schmorl's node)

FIG. 14-16   Midsagittal magnetic resonance imaging scan demonstrating a Schmorl's node. (Compare with Figs. 14-13 and 14-15.) (Image courtesy Dr. Dennis Skogsbergh.)

life, roughly in the second decade or even earlier (Kraemer, 1995). However, there is a wide variation in the aging and degenerative process of the disc; some septuagenarians have the IVDs of 30-year-old people, and vice versa.

The first part of this section focuses on the normal aging process of the IVD and the relationship of this aging process to IVD degeneration. Figure 14-17 illustrates the changes that take place during aging and degeneration of the IVD. The second part of this section concentrates on unique characteristics of IVD degeneration and certain conditions that can promote or initiate IVD degeneration.

Summary of the Normal Aging of the Intervertebral Disc as a Whole.

The normal aging and degeneration of the IVD is closely related to the number of vessels that reach the IVD, especially the CEP. As the numbers of vessels decrease, and the nutrition provided and waste removed by these vessels decrease, the changes associated with IVD aging and degeneration increase (Brown et al., 1997; Chandraraj, Briggs, and Opeskin, 1998; Horner and Urban, 2001; Boos et al., 2002) (see Fig. 14-17).

Small vessels surround the IVD during fetal development. These vessels begin to decrease in number during the first 2 years of life, and the remaining vessels that course within the subchondral bone to enter the deepest layers of the CEP are almost completely obliterated by 11 to 12 years of age, leaving the IVD as the largest avascular structure of the body. The first significant degenerative changes in the IVD appear shortly thereafter, as early as 11 to 16 years of age. This is when the last blood vessels leave the CEP. As the vessels decrease in number in the CEP, a rather dramatic increase in cell death occurs in the remainder of the IVD. From this point on the NP and AF begin to show signs of degeneration (e.g., cell death, clefts, radial tears, degeneration of the extracellular matrix, and granular changes). Therefore even some teenagers may experience back pain as a result of IVD degeneration (Herzog, 1996). The increased cell death is replenished somewhat at this age by a marked increase in the proliferation of chondrocytes during this time (Boos et al., 2002).

The number of clefts and radial tears increases from 17 to 20 years of age, and the overall number of chondrocytes decreases as cell death, mucoid degeneration, and granular (scar tissue) changes begin to appear. These latter signs of degeneration increase throughout the second to the fourth decades of life. During the fifth and sixth decades of life the degenerative changes become the most severe; many clefts and tears filled with granular tissue become apparent throughout the IVD. Advanced tissue destruction and defects can be seen during this period of time. There is a high level of cell death (apoptosis) during these decades (Gruber and Hanley, 1998). Using a mouse model, Hutton et al. (1999) found that the rate of apoptosis in the CEP that occurs with aging and degeneration was also related to the rate of formation of osteophytes (spondylosis) along the superior and inferior margins of the vertebral bodies.

After 70 years of age the clefts and tears throughout the IVD have filled in with granular tissue, and the IVD takes on a homogenous "burnt out" appearance, making the NP, AF, and CEP difficult to distinguish from one another (Boos et al., 2002).

Normal Aging of the Nucleus Pulposus and Anulus Fibrosus.

The NP of fetal tissue contains many notochordal cells. The number of chondrocytes increases and the NP begins to take on slight mucoid characteristics during the first few months after birth. Subtle clefts develop in the NP during the next 2 years. The notochordal cells continue to die and the chondrocytes continue to increase in density between the ages of 3 and 10 years. There are virtually no notochordal cells left and there are significant clefts within the NP by 11 to 16 years of age. The number of clefts and radial fissures continue to increase until late in life (>70 years of age) when they have filled with granular (scar) tissue and are difficult to distinguish from the other tissue in the IVD. However, intranuclear clefts filled with fibrous (granular) tissue have been identified by means of T2-weighted MRI in patients just over 30 years of age (Herzog, 1996). The outer lamellae of the AF are the last to show signs of degeneration, and these signs in the AF appear in the seventh decade of life (Boos et al., 2002).

Normal Aging of the Cartilaginous End Plate.

The cartilaginous end plate (CEP) undergoes the earliest degenerative changes of the IVD. The CEP is well vascularized and slightly irregular in appearance during fetal development. Immediately after birth, the number of cells (primarily chondrocytes) increases dramatically and the cartilage takes on a disorganized appearance. During the next 16 years the number of blood vessels in the CEP steadily decreases, until there are no active vessels left by approximately 16 years of age (most are obliterated by 11 to 12 years of age) (Chandraraj, Briggs, and Opeskin, 1998; Boos et al., 2002). The decrease in active blood vessels is paralleled by the appearance of areas of obliterated vessels. These areas of obliterated vessels are already beginning to appear during the first 2 years of postnatal life. The number of regions of obliterated vessels dramatically increases until 16 years of age when these regions are the most pronounced. Between the ages of 11 to 16 years there is increased cell death in the CEP. The number of PGs also decreases and the extracellular matrix becomes more disorganized as cell death increases (Antoniou et al., 1996; Roberts et al., 1996; Gruber and Hanley, 2002). Because the PGs dictate the

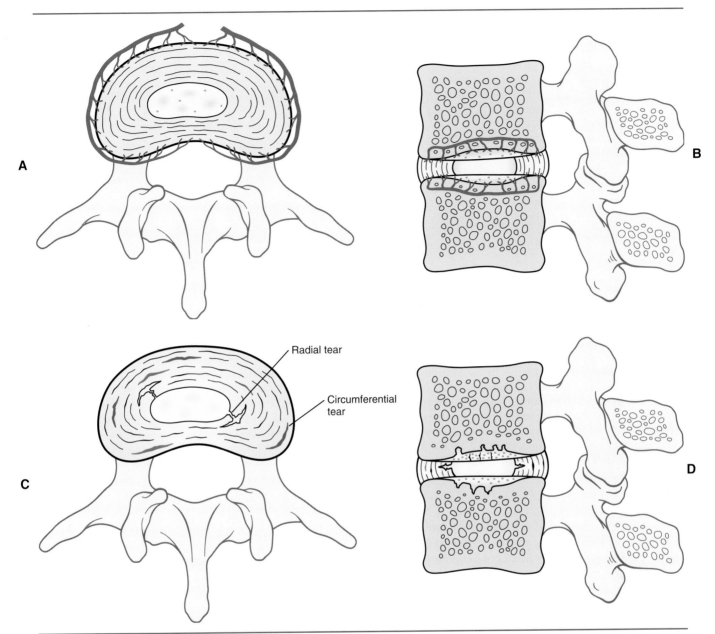

FIG. 14-17   Aging and degeneration of the intervertebral disc (IVD). Illustrations of superior views (left images, **A, C, E**) and midsagittal sections (right images, **B, D, F**) of the IVDs at the following three ages: **A** and **B,** Newborn; **C** and **D,** second decade of life; and, **E** and **F,** the sixth decade of life. Notice in the newborn that the IVD receives a blood supply. **A** shows the vessels that supply the periphery of the IVD and **B** shows those that supply the inner surfaces of the anulus fibrosus (AF), nucleus pulposus (NP), and cartilaginous end plates (CEP). The large horizontal vascular channels within the adjacent vertebral bodies in **B** are supplied by ascending and descending branches of the central arterial plexus of the vertebral bodies. This plexus and the ascending and descending branches are shown in Figure 2-4, *B.* The arteries shown here will regress and become obliterated in the next few years of life. Notice in **A** that the lamellae of the AF are tightly packed, the NP has a few cells within it (the nuclei are seen as dark blue dots), and the CEPs (above and below the NP and AF in **B**) are smooth and contain cells (primarily fibroblasts and chondrocytes). The changes shown in **C** and **D** can begin as early as the first decade of life, but usually do not become apparent until the second or third decades. The IVD is less well hydrated in **C** and **D** as the vessels shown in **A** and **B** regress. Some of the lamellae of the AF seen in **C** are separating to form circumferential tears, and two small radial tears have also begun to protrude through the innermost layers of the AF to connect to circumferential tears. There are virtually no cells remaining in the NP, and the superior CEP shows early signs of cracking (fissuring). Extensions of the cartilage of the superior and inferior CEPs can be seen plugging the vascular channels left by the obliterated vessels of the vertebral bodies that were shown in **B.** In spite of these changes, the CEPs in **D** have more cells at this stage than at any other time in their development.

Continued

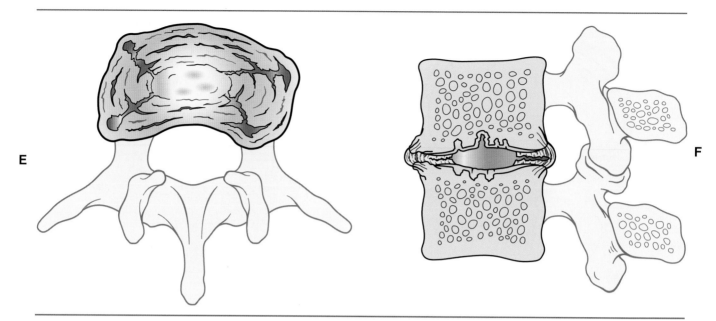

FIG. 14-17—cont'd   The IVDs in **E** and **F** show dramatic signs of aging and degeneration. Notice that the IVD in **E** has "spread out" as it dehydrates and is seen bulging in several locations. The IVD in **F** is shorter from superior to inferior, and the vertebral bodies have developed osteophytes (bone spurs) that are beginning to cover the AF above and below. **F** also shows Sharpey's fibers attaching the most peripheral layers of the AF to the adjacent bone of the osteophytes. The border between the AF and NP is indistinct in **E** and **F**, and many circumferential tears in the AF are connected by radial tears. This has allowed the NP to move through the radial tears (fissures) and fill the gaps in between the lamellae of the AF created by the circumferential tears. Some of the radial tears extend all the way to the periphery of the AF, and some of the circumferential tears show signs of scaring (i.e., the dark, narrow irregular tears). The CEPs in **F** are much thinner now and have begun to show more significant signs of aging as they become dry and brittle. Notice several regions where the NP has pushed well into the CEPs and is beginning to enter the vertebral body. (Please note: The ages at which the changes depicted in these illustrations occur are quite variable and may not progress to **E** and **F** in some individuals or may not be seen at all vertebral levels in others.)

solutes that are transported across the CEP and the rate of transport of these solutes, the decrease in the number of PGs may result in waste products building up in the IVD and nutrients being excluded from the IVD, both of which can lead to IVD degeneration.

Also between the ages of 11 to 16 years a significant numbers of cracks appear in the CEP. The CEP cracks are accompanied by corresponding microfractures of the adjacent subchondral bone. These findings often are associated with new bone formation in the subchondral bone. The CEP cracks and the microfractures in the subchondral bone continue to increase during the second through the sixth decades, when the subchondral bone becomes sclerotic and regions of the CEP calcify. This leads to an increased vulnerability of the CEP to Schmorl's node formation. In the seventh decade of life, the CEP stabilizes, and its appearance remains relatively the same throughout the remaining decades of life (Boos et al., 2002).

Normal Aging and Degeneration of the Bony End Plate.   Even though the bony end plate is not a part of the IVD, the fates of the bony and cartilaginous end plates are so closely linked that a brief discussion of the normal aging and degeneration of the bony end plate is warranted. The relationship between degeneration of the bony end plate and the formation of Schmorl's nodes is also of clinical importance.

During the first few years of life, vessels within the vertebral body course into the cartilage growth cap (not the CEP, but subjacent to it) of the superior and inferior ends of the vertebral body. Vessels course within "vascular canals" within this cartilage. Each vascular canal contains several vessels that extend into the CEP. As the cartilage of the growth cap is replaced by bone, the vessels recede, leaving "cartilage nodes," or areas of obliterated vessels, where the vascular canals once ended. These cartilage nodes fill with collagen from the CEP and NP and in some cases form what could be called "mini-Schmorl's nodes." Therefore the cartilage nodes represent weak spots in the vertebral bodies and allow with age nuclear material to extrude through the thinning CEP and into and through the cartilage nodes; with further increase in IVD pressures, true Schmorl's nodes are formed (Chandraraj, Briggs, and Opeskin, 1998). In addition, multiple Schmorl's nodes have been observed in individuals playing sports that create much axial loading (Hamanishi et al., 1994). Schmorl's nodes are also sometimes seen in conjunction with typical disc protrusions, suggesting that axial loading is causing the NP to protrude in many directions (Chandraraj, Briggs, and Opeskin, 1998).

Unique Features of Intervertebral Disc Degeneration. Recall from previous chapters that degeneration of the IVDs is accompanied by nerve and vascular ingrowths into the disc. Schwann cells of the nerves innervating the outer layers of the AF appear to play a role in this ingrowth (Johnson et al., 2001). The increased innervation is by free nerve endings containing increased substance P (nociceptors). Therefore injured or degenerated discs are more pain sensitive than noninjured or nondegenerated IVDs (Coppes et al., 1997). Also remember from previous chapters that the IVDs thrive on reasonable motion within normal physiologic limits. Consequently, frequent changes of postures improve and maintain the internal environment of the IVD, and an overly sedentary lifestyle is not good for the IVD and the entire spine (Kraemer, 1995). Also, spending prolonged periods of time in postures that produce increases in IVD hydrostatic pressure, such as prolonged standing while carrying loads and prolonged sitting (again, an overly sedentary lifestyle), can affect PG and collagen synthesis, inhibit disc nutrition, and also lead to IVD degeneration (Kraemer, 1995; Hutton et al., 1998, 1999, 2002). In fact, hydrostatic pressure within the IVD has been found to have significant influences on IVD cell metabolism. Normal pressure in the IVD is approximately 3 atm (atmospheres). Pressures at this level were found in experiments (in vitro) conducted by Handa et al. (1997) to stimulate the synthesis of PGs and inhibit the production of matrix metalloproteinases (which degrade the PGs and collagen of the IVD) in both the NP and inner AF. Pressures either above or below 1 to 3 atm were found to increase the rate of disc degeneration (decreased production of PGs and increased the production of matrix metalloproteinases). Lotz et al. (1998, 2000), using a mouse model, also found that prolonged graded compression resulted in graded IVD degeneration. They also noted that the IVDs showed signs of recuperation after having the increased pressures removed for 1 month.

Conditions that may promote or initiate intervertebral disc degeneration. Several conditions have been identified that promote or even possibly initiate disc degeneration. For example, traumatic Schmorl's node formation was previously mentioned as most likely being able to initiate IVD degeneration. In addition, extruded NP spontaneously produces increased amounts of matrix metalloproteinases, nitric oxide, interleukin-6, and prostaglandin E_2, and other chemokines (see Chapter 11). These products may be intimately involved in both the biochemistry of disc degeneration, as well as the pathophysiology of radiculopathy (Herzog, 1996; Kang et al., 1996, 1997; Crean et al., 1997; Duance et al., 1998).

Another condition that may promote or initiate IVD degeneration is advanced aortic atherosclerosis. This condition presents as calcium deposits in the posterior wall of the aorta and has been found to increase a person's risk of developing IVD degeneration, and is also associated with the occurrence of back pain (Kauppila et al., 1997).

Iwahashi et al. (2002) injected liquid nicotine into rabbits and then studied the IVDs. They found that nicotine reduced the vascular buds in the subchondral bone adjacent to the CEP and also decreased the lumen of the remaining vascular buds. In addition, nicotine administration resulted in necrosis in the NP and a "disturbance of the pattern of overlapping laminae" in the AF. These authors believe that a decrease in the vascular supply to the CEP led to a decrease in the oxygen tension in the CEP, which resulted in a decrease in the synthesis of PGs and collagen, both hallmarks of IVD degeneration (Iwahashi et al., 2002).

Potential treatments based on the basic science of the intervertebral disc. Adenovirus-mediated transfer of genes and the resultant production of therapeutic growth factors are being investigated as a means to further study the biology of the IVD and the potential for treatment for disc degeneration (Nishida et al., 1999); however, the low vascularity of the adult IVD may preclude the effective use of gene therapy in IVD disease (Boos et al., 2002).

As mentioned, decreased PG synthesis is related to IVD degeneration. Maeda and Kokubun (2000) also found an increased sensitivity of IVD cells to interleukin-1α with age and felt that this may be associated with IVD degeneration. Inner AF cells were found to be more sensitive to interleukin-1α than outer AF cells after normal aging. They believe this may explain why NP and the inner AF are the undergo degeneration before the outer lamellae of the AF. Maeda and Kokubun (2000) hypothesized that an interleukin-1α receptor antagonist protein introduced into the IVD may be beneficial in decreasing IVD degeneration by blocking the degenerative effects of interleukin-1α.

Glycosaminoglycans and Proteoglycans

The topic of glycosaminoglycans (GAGs) and PGs was introduced with connective tissue earlier in this chapter. GAGs and PGs are covered in further detail here because of their extreme importance in the IVD's proper functioning. Much of the relevant current research related to the IVD involves GAGs and PGs. In fact, "PGs are now thought to be the chief cellular indicators of disc functional capacity and appear to be the key to understanding the pathogenesis of disc degeneration" (Bishop, 1992).

The main function of GAGs and therefore PGs is structural; they interact with collagen fibers to provide support. In addition to providing support, GAGs, because of their ionic charge, are able to form electrostatic interactions with cationic molecules. This serves to transport electrolytes, water, and metabolites. The gel-like or viscous nature of the GAGs allows them to have a lubricating function in connective tissue and joints and also allows them to act as shock absorbers in the IVD.

Proteoglycan Monomers and Proteoglycan Aggregates. PG monomers are complex macromolecules composed of many GAGs covalently bonded to a core protein of varying length. Three dimensionally, the side chains attached to the core protein form the shape of a "bottle brush" (see Fig. 14-6). The short branches of the bottle brush represent keratan sulfate, and the long ones represent chondroitin sulfate. PG monomers group together to form PG aggregates. The backbone of a PG aggregate is hyaluronic acid. Hyaluronic acid is a long coil-like chain composed of alternating molecules of glucuronic acid and glucosamine. The PG monomers are attached to hyaluronic acid by a link protein.

Glycosaminoglycans. GAGs refer to long-chain, unbranched carbohydrate polymers composed of repeating disaccharide units of glucosamine (or galactosamine) and glucuronic acid attached to a protein core. The hexosamine (glucosamine and galactosamine) usually is sulfated (see Table 14-4). However, an exception among the GAGs to this general pattern is hyaluronic acid, which is the longest GAG and has no sulfated hexosamines. Most of the sugar molecules of GAG chains are negatively charged and repel each other. This negative charge attracts numerous Na^+ ions, which are osmotically active. This causes a large amount of water to rush into the matrix and creates a swelling hydrostatic pressure. This hydrostatic pressure enables the matrix of cartilage and the IVD to withstand compressive forces.

GAGs are synthesized within the cells of the connective tissue in which they are found. For instance, the fibroblast is the primary cell type of connective tissue proper, and it produces and maintains the ground substance of this tissue, which primarily consists of GAGs. Chondroblasts are cells that produce the ground substance of cartilage, and osteoblasts produce the ground substance of bone. The GAGs for the entire IVD are probably primarily produced by the cells within the CEP. The time it takes to replace the PGs in the human IVD is considerable (approximately 3 years) and is longer than the replacement time of other species (Table 14-5). Therefore much time is needed before complete repair

Table 14-5 Comparison of Turnover Time (Days) for Proteoglycan Molecules from Various Regions of the Intervertebral Discs of Dogs, Pigs, and Humans

Region of Disc	Dog (3 Years of Age)	Pig (3 Years of Age)	Human* (30 Years of Age)
Nucleus pulposus	750	900	1350
Outer anulus (anterior)	350	500	900
Inner anulus (anterior)	420	700	1050
Outer anulus (posterior)	510	630	990
Inner anulus (posterior)	630	800	1170

*Note that for a 30-year-old human, it takes more than 3 years to replace proteoglycan molecules.

of pathologic conditions or damage to the IVD can take place, and in some cases (especially if the CEP is damaged) repair may not be possible (Moore et al., 1996).

The principal GAGs of the extracellular matrix include the following:

◆ Hyaluronic acid
◆ Chondroitin sulfate
◆ Dermatan sulfate
◆ Heparan sulfate
◆ Keratan sulfate

These five types of GAGs differ in the following important ways: molecular weight, length of the chain, and type of disaccharide units. Table 14-4 summarizes the major characteristics of the principal GAGs. GAGs tend to exist in various configurations, which results in a variety of electrostatic charges among GAGs and allows them to participate in various degrees of interactions with adjoining chains. This variety of configurations and interactions of GAGs contributes to the formation of additional physical and chemical characteristics of the extracellular matrix.

Hyaluronic acid is by far the largest GAG, consisting of an estimated 2500 disaccharide units. Its molecular weight is approximately 10^6 Da. Hyaluronic acid is the major GAG of synovial fluid and many tissues (see Table 14-4). It is partially responsible for swelling within the extracellular matrix and also for attracting cells to the site of an injury. As mentioned previously, PG monomers also bind to hyaluronic acid to form PG aggregates.

Chondroitin 4-sulfate and chondroitin 6-sulfate consist of glucuronic acid and N-acetylgalactosamine. These two GAGs are similar in structure and function (see Table 14-4). Chondroitin 4-sulfate is the most abundant GAG found in the body and is present in immature cartilage. Chondroitin 6-sulfate is distributed in mature cartilage and other tissues. Decreased sulfation of the chondroitin sulfates has been related to IVD degeneration (Hutton et al., 1997).

Dermatan sulfate is the major GAG of skin, from which it derives its name. It is also distributed in tendons, ligaments, fibrocartilage, and other tissues. However, it is not found in the IVD or Z joints. Dermatan sulfate has a high affinity to associate closely with collagen type I fibers (see Tables 14-3 and 14-4).

Keratan sulfate is the shortest of the GAGs (see Table 14-4). It is found in skeletal tissue, as well as the cornea (keratan sulfate type I). Along with hyaluronic acid and chondroitin sulfate, keratan sulfate is a main contributor of cartilage PGs. It is also found in abundance in the NP of the IVD.

Heparan sulfate is associated with collagen type III reticular fibers, which are found in large amounts in basal laminae. Heparan sulfate is also distributed in the lungs, liver, and aorta. However, it is not found to any great extent in the Z joints or IVDs.

Fibrocartilage

Because the AF and NP of the IVDs are considered to be specialized fibrocartilage, a brief discussion of the general characteristics of this type of cartilage is included here.

Light microscopy reveals that fibrocartilage appears similar to dense connective tissue and hyaline cartilage (Fig. 14-18). Its matrix contains obvious thick bundles of type I collagen fibers (see Table 14-3). The collagen bundles are distributed in parallel beams among rows of chondrocytes. The chondrocytes are smaller than those of hyaline or elastic cartilage and are easily distinguished from the fibroblasts, also present in fibrocartilage, because chondrocytes lie within round or oval lacunae. Because of the presence of the collagen fibers and a lesser amount of GAGs, the matrix of fibrocartilage stains more eosinophilic than hyaline or elastic cartilage. Also, fibrocartilage, unlike nonarticular hyaline and elastic cartilage, is not enveloped by a perichondrium. Fibrocartilage is distributed in the IVD (see the previous discussions) and articular cartilages. It is also found in the pubic symphysis, ligamentum teres femoris capitis, glenoid ligament, and the intraarticular cartilages of some joints.

MICROSCOPIC ANATOMY OF OTHER MAJOR TISSUES IN THE BACK

The other tissues of the spine are similar in make-up to these same tissues in other regions of the body. However, an understanding of these tissues is essential to a comprehension of the structure and function of the spine. Therefore the remainder of the chapter gives a cursory overview of the microscopic anatomy of the other major tissues in the region of the back. These include connective tissues other than those previously discussed, skeletal muscle, and neural tissue. The reader is encouraged to consult histology texts for more in-depth information concerning these tissues.

Connective Tissue

As stated, connective tissue is the tissue that binds together and is the support for the various structures of the body. All connective tissues have three components: cells, fibers, and ground substance (including water). It is the relative amounts and structures of these components that determine the types of connective tissues found in the body. There are various classifications of connective tissues, but in general there are embryonic connective tissue, connective tissue proper, and specialized connective tissue (Ross et al., 2003). Each of these can be further subdivided:

- Embryonic connective tissue
    - Mesenchyme
    - Mucous connective tissue
- Connective tissue proper
    - Loose
    - Dense
        - Irregular
        - Regular
- Specialized connective tissue
    - Adipose tissue
    - Blood
    - Hemopoietic tissue
    - Lymphatic tissue
    - Bone
    - Cartilage

Of the embryonic connective tissues, mesenchyme has been discussed. Mucous connective tissue is found only in the umbilical cord and is beyond the scope of this text. Also, blood, lymphatic, and hemopoietic tissues are not discussed here. Cartilage has been thoroughly discussed, but connective tissue proper, adipose tissue, and bone are briefly covered.

Connective Tissue Proper. Connective tissue proper is tissue that, rather intuitively, seems to fall into the category of tissue that holds things together. It can be subdivided into two types: loose and dense (Junqueira and Carneiro, 2003). This is based mostly on the relative amounts of fibers that can be found in the extracellular matrix. Further, dense connective tissue can be thought of as having two varieties, based mostly on the arrangement of the fibers in the extracellular matrix: irregular and regular.

Loose or areolar connective tissue is characterized by a large amount of fluid ground substance (Fig. 14-19). There are moderate amounts of cells and fibers that

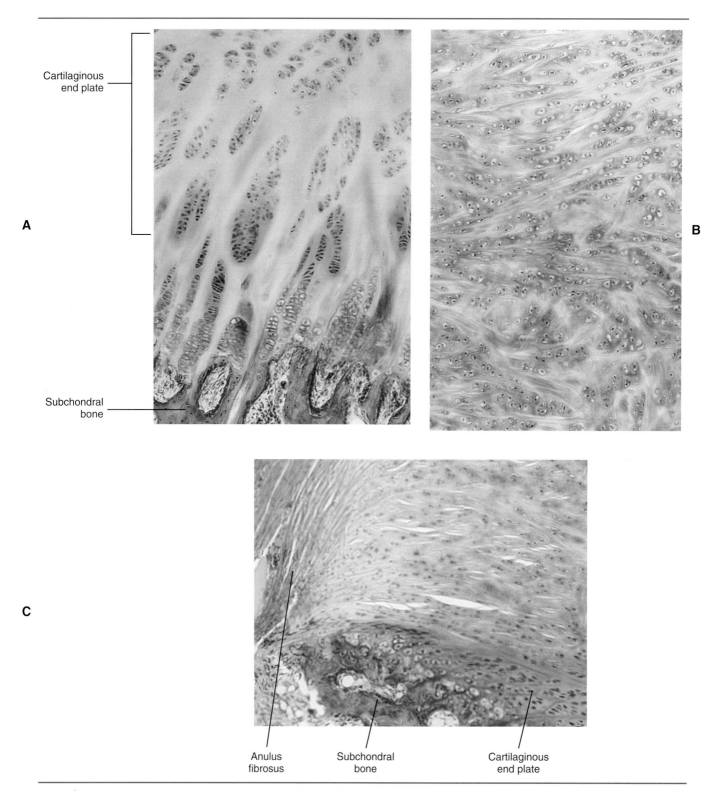

FIG. 14-18   Light micrographs demonstrating the fibrocartilaginous make-up and distinguishing features of the three component parts of the intervertebral disc. This specimen is from a mammalian fetus. **A,** Cartilaginous end plate (magnification ×100). **B,** Developing nucleus pulposus (magnification ×100). Notice the haphazard arrangement of the cells and fibrous elements in this region. **C,** Portion of the anulus fibrosus.

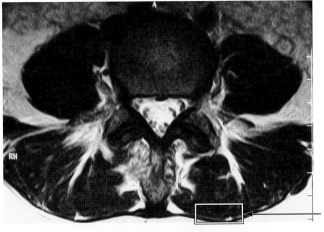

A

B

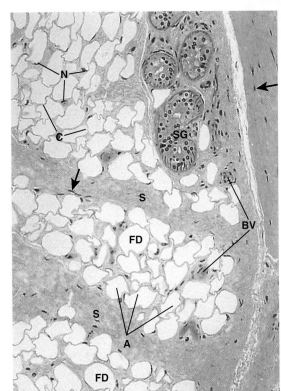

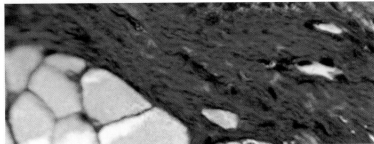

FIG. 14-19 Fascia and ligaments. **A,** Horizontal MRI scan through the lower lumbar region. Box labeled *B* indicates an area containing superficial and deep fascia, the focus of *B*. **B,** *left,* Superficial fascia (132× magnification). Notice the adipose cells and loose arrangement of collagen fibers. *A,* Adipocytes; *BV,* blood vessels; *C,* cytoplasm of adipocytes; *FD,* fat droplets; *N,* nuclei; *S,* connective tissue septa; *SG,* sweat gland; and, *arrows,* fibroblast nuclei. **B,** *right,* Deep fascia (132× magnification). Notice the regularly dense arrangement of cells and collagen fibers.

Continued

are loosely, or not closely, arranged in this matrix. The cells are predominantly fibroblasts and macrophages, but other cell types common to connective tissue also can be found, especially lymphoid cells and mast cells. All three connective tissue fiber types (elastic, collagen [mostly type I], and reticular) are represented. In general, connective tissues do not have as rich of a blood supply as other, more metabolically active tissues (e.g., neural tissue), but for a connective tissue, loose connective tissue is quite vascular. The functional characteristics of this type of tissue are that it is rather flexible but not

strong. It is commonly found in the body. In the region of the back, it mainly supports epithelia (e.g., papillary layer of the dermis) surrounds bundles of muscle cells (perimysium), and ensheaths lymphatic and blood vessels. Loose connective tissue, along with adipose tissue (see the following), also forms the superficial fascia.

Dense irregular connective tissue has large numbers of fibers that are arranged in bundles that are oriented in various directions (see Fig. 14-19). These fibers are mostly collagen fibers composed of type I collagen. There are relatively few cells, which are mostly fibroblasts,

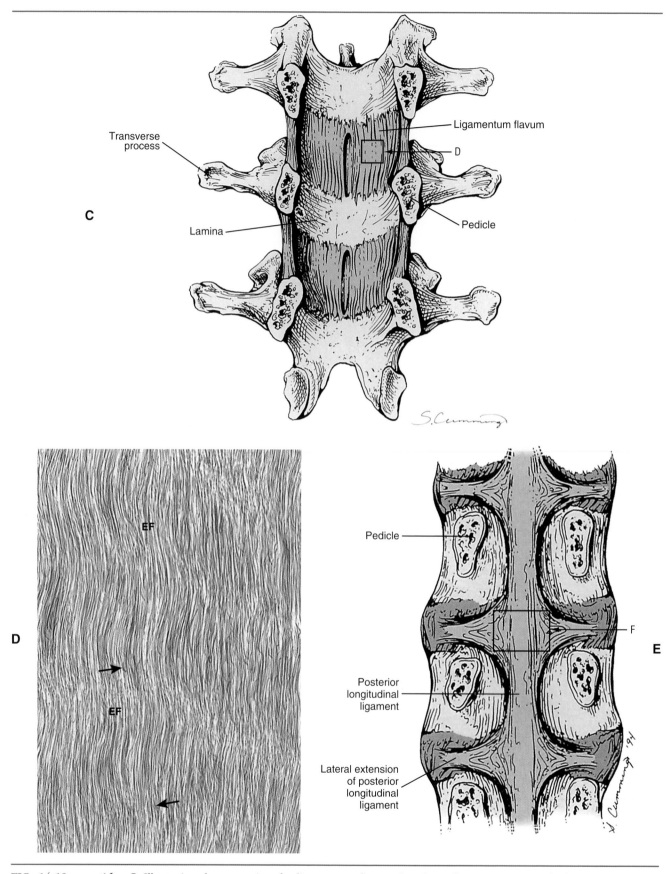

FIG. 14-19—cont'd   **C,** Illustration demonstrating the ligamentum flavum (an elastic ligament). Notice the box indicating the region depicted in *D*. **D,** Ligamentum flavum (132× magnification). Notice the regular arrangement of, *EF,* the elastic fibers in this ligament. *Arrows,* Fibroblasts. **E,** Illustration demonstrating, *F,* the posterior longitudinal ligament, a typical spinal ligament from a histologic perspective. Notice the box indicating the region depicted in *F*.

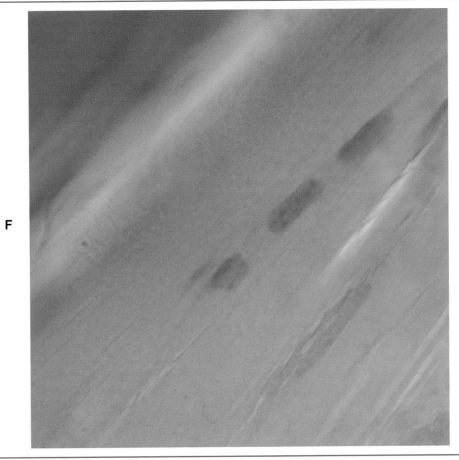

FIG. 14-19—cont'd   **F,** A typical ligament (approximately 100x magnification). Notice the elongated fibroblast nuclei between tightly packed bundles of regularly arranged collagen fibers. (**B,** *left,* From Gartner LP & Hiatt JL. [2000]. *Color atlas of histology* [3rd ed.]. Philadelphia: Lippincott Williams and Wilkins. **B,** *right,* From Junqueira LC & Carneiro L. [2002]. *Basic histology text and atlas* [10th ed.]. Chicago: McGraw Hill. D, From Gartner LP & Hiatt JL. [2000]. *Color atlas of histology* (3rd ed.). Philadelphia: Lippincott Williams and Wilkins.)

and little ground substance, when compared with loose connective tissue. Therefore it is less flexible but much stronger than loose connective tissue. The three-dimensional arrangement of the fibers gives this tissue good strength in all directions. In the region of the back, dense irregular connective tissue may be found mostly in the reticular or deep layer of the dermis.

The components of dense regular connective tissue are similar to those of dense irregular connective tissue, but their arrangement is different. In this case, the bundles of fibers are arranged linearly, with rows of cells, mostly fibroblasts, and a minimal amount of ground substance located between the bundles. This arrangement gives a tremendous amount of resistance to traction stresses in one direction (parallel to the fibers). In the back region, three main types of structures are composed of this tissue: tendons, ligaments, and deep fascia.

Tendons, the structures that connect muscles to bone, are composed of closely packed bundles of collagen fibers (see Fig. 14-21). These fibers are almost exclusively type I collagen. Between the bundles of fibers are rows of tendinocytes, which resemble fibroblasts. The bundles of collagen fibers are grouped together into fascicles, which are continuous with the corresponding fascicles of the muscle to which they attach (see the following). Each fascicle is invested or surrounded by a thin layer of loose connective tissue called the endotendineum. The endotendineum contains blood vessels and nerves. Surrounding the entire tendon is a thin layer of dense irregular connective tissue called the epitendineum. The endotendineum septa are continuous with the epitendineum.

Ligaments connect bones or cartilages and serve to support and strengthen joints. Like tendons, the bundles of fibers are linearly arranged in ligaments, although not quite as uniformly (Ross, 2003). Also, unlike tendons, there is no fascicular arrangement of the bundles of fibers, making ligaments less vascular than tendons. In most ligaments of the body, the fibers are predominantly type I collagen fibers, giving a great amount of tensile strength, but no elasticity (see Fig. 14-19). Because of the high amount of collagen, these ligaments appear white to the naked eye, and sometimes this dense regular collagenous tissue is called white connective tissue. One exception to this is the ligamentum flavum. It is composed of dense regular connective tissue, but most of the fibers in its extracellular matrix are elastic fibers, not collagen fibers. Under the microscope, longitudinal sections of these bundles of elastic fibers have a distinctive wavy appearance (see Fig. 14-19). This type of fiber gives the ligamentum flavum not only good tensile strength but also elasticity. Masses of elastic fibers have a distinct yellow-orange color when viewed by the naked eye. Therefore dense regular elastic connective tissue sometimes is known as yellow connective tissue. This coloration is also responsible for the name flaval ligament, because *flavus* means yellow in Latin.

The deep fascia also is composed of dense regular collagenous connective tissue. Its structure is similar to tendons, but instead of having the bundles of collagenous fibers arranged in fasciculi, the fibers are arranged into multiple layers. The fibers of each layer are parallel to each other, but the fibers of the various layers usually have a different orientation to the fibers of adjacent layers. This arrangement gives the deep fascia excellent tensile strength in many different directions in the same plane.

Adipose tissue. Fat-storing cells, or adipocytes, can be found throughout most of the loose connective tissue of the body. In the regions where these adipocytes are the predominant cell type, the tissue is called adipose tissue. The triglycerides in adipose tissue represent the main store of excess caloric energy in the body. Lipids are an efficient form of energy storage, because more than 9 kcal of energy are in 1 gram of lipid, as opposed to around 4 kcal/g of either carbohydrate or protein. Also, this tissue also acts as insulation for the body because fat is a poor conductor of heat and much of the adipose tissue is located subcutaneously. There are two types of adipose tissue found in the body: white and brown.

White adipose tissue, which actually looks yellow in humans, is characterized by having adipocytes with a single droplet of neutral fat. These cells are described as unilocular. White adipose tissue makes up the vast majority of adipose tissue in the body. Most of the superficial fascia of the body is basically white adipose tissue. When closely packed together, the adipocytes are mostly round or polyhedral. The fat droplet takes up the majority of the volume of each cell, so much so that the cytoplasm forms only a thin rim on the periphery of the cell. Also, the nucleus is flattened and eccentrically located; therefore adipocytes are sometimes known as signet ring cells. Each adipocyte is surrounded by a meshwork of reticular

fibers that are composed of type III collagen. Adipose tissue is incompletely subdivided into lobules by connective tissue septa, which contain a rich vascular supply and network of nerves. Adipose tissue is highly vascularized, so much so that the ratio of blood volume to cytoplasm volume is greater in adipose tissue than in skeletal muscle (Junqueria and Carneiro, 2003). The storage and mobilization of fat are regulated by a complex interplay of hormonal and neurologic mechanisms. Besides being an energy storage tissue, adipose tissue also has a secretory function. It produces a hormone known as leptin, which appears to be a circulating satiety factor involved in the regulation of food intake.

In brown adipose tissue, the adipocytes store fat in multiple droplets and are known as multilocular. The fat looks distinctly brown in color when seen by the naked eye. Brown adipose tissue is important in thermoregulation. The oxidation of fatty acids in the mitochondria of brown fat cells is uncoupled from the production of adenosine triphosphate (ATP); therefore the energy produced by these mitochondria is dissipated as heat. Brown fat is found abundantly in animals that hibernate. In humans, it can be found in late-term fetuses and newborns and may be important in heat regulation for the first few months of life. By the end of the first decade of life, the amount of brown adipose tissue is greatly diminished, such that there are negligible amounts of it in the adult.

Bone.   Bone is a specialized connective tissue in which the extracellular matrix is mineralized mostly by calcium phosphate in the form of hydroxyapatite crystals. This makes bone tissue hard, such that it forms the rigid support of the body as the skeleton. Bone also plays a vital role in the regulation of blood calcium levels by acting as a reservoir for both calcium and phosphate. Therefore unlike the dried skeletons that are studied in school, bone is a living, highly vascular, constantly changing tissue.

The organic portions of the extracellular matrix are composed of fibers and ground substance. The vast majority of the fibers are type I collagen fibers. These make up the main structural component of the extracellular matrix of bone (Ross et al., 2003). The ground substance is composed of mostly GAGs that are similar to those of other connective tissues (see the preceding). Several special glycoproteins found only in the ground substance of bone tissue appear to be involved with the promotion of mineralization of the matrix. During the mineralization process, the mineral salts become associated not only with the ground substance but also with the collagen fibers.

Within the extracellular matrix are physical holes known as lacunae (singular, lacuna). Each contains a cell known as an osteocyte. Because there is little to no diffusion through the hardened extracellular matrix, there are tunnels in the matrix known as canaliculi, which contain cytoplasmic processes of osteocytes. At the point where the process of one osteocyte encounters the process of a different osteocyte in the canaliculus is a gap junction. This allows communication and diffusion of materials between the osteocytes.

Three other types of cells are associated with bone tissue:

- Osteoprogenitor cells
- Osteoblasts
- Osteoclasts

Osteoprogenitor cells are found primarily on the outer and inner surfaces of bone tissue. They are pluripotential cells of mesenchymal origin that undergo a continual process of mitosis. They mostly give rise to osteoblasts, although during bone repair (e.g., after fracture) they may give rise to other types of cells involved in that process.

Osteoblasts are the differentiated bone cells that give rise to bone matrix. They secrete both collagen and ground substance in an unmineralized form known as osteoid. This addition of new osteoid on the existing surface of bone tissue is known as appositional growth. Active osteoblasts exhibit the same cytoplasmic architecture as other cells that secrete large amounts of protein (e.g., abundant rough endoplasmic reticulum and a well-developed Golgi apparatus). In actively growing bones, osteoblasts are found alongside each other exclusively on the surfaces of bone tissue in a way reminiscent of simple cuboidal epithelium, but without any basal lamina. Although osteoblasts appear to be polar in nature and secrete osteoid on only one side, occasionally an osteoblast become completely surrounded by osteoid. When this happens, a new lacuna is formed, and the cell becomes known as an osteocyte.

Osteoclasts are the bone cells responsible for resorption of bone matrix. They are large, multinucleated cells that are in physical contact with the surface of bone tissue. At this contact point the cytoplasm of these cells forms many folds that look like microvilli, giving it the appearance of a ruffled border. Lysosomal hydrolases are released from this ruffled border that digest the bone matrix outside the cell, creating shallow indentations in the bone matrix known as resorption bays or Howship's lacunae. Osteoclasts appear to endocytose the digested bone matrix, because large numbers of coated vesicles can be found in the region of the ruffled border. Osteoclasts, unlike osteoprogenitor cells, appear to originate from the same mononuclear hemopoietic progenitor cells that give rise to neutrophilic granulocyte and monocyte lineages. This makes osteoclasts closely related to macrophages, in both origin and function.

There are two main arrangements of bone tissue seen in mature bone (e.g., the vertebrae) (Fig. 14-20). A dense layer of compact bone forms the outer portion of bones.

Spongy, or cancellous, bone, which consists of a network of bony trabeculae (from the Latin, beam) and spicules, forms the interior of the vertebrae. The spaces between the trabeculae are known as the marrow cavities and are occupied by blood vessels and bone marrow, which is the main hemopoietic tissue of the body.

Compact bone consists of collections of cylindrical units of concentric lamellae (singular, lamella) or layers of mineralized extracellular matrix surrounding a centrally located canal. These units are known as osteons or haversian systems. The collagen fibers within a single lamella are arranged parallel with each other, but in different directions when compared with adjacent lamellae. This arrangement, reminiscent of plywood, gives compact bone tissue great strength. The centrally located canal is known as the osteonal or haversian canal and contains blood vessels, nerves, and some loose connective tissue. The haversian canals usually run parallel to the long axis of the bone. Lacunae, containing osteocytes, are located mostly between the concentric lamellae, although some may be located within the lamellae. Canaliculi, containing osteocyte processes, generally are arranged in a radial pattern with respect to the haversian canals. Perforating or Volkmann's canals are channels carrying blood vessels and nerves that travel from the superficial surface of the bone to the marrow cavities. They usually run perpendicular or oblique to the haversian canals, such that the Volkmann's canals also connect haversian canals with each other.

Spongy bone is similar in structure to compact bone, except that the matrix is arranged in trabeculae and spicules. If the trabeculae are relatively thick, they may contain true osteons, otherwise the trabeculae are composed of irregularly arranged lamellae of matrix and lacunae. There are numerous interconnecting marrow cavities of various sizes between the portions of bony matrix. This honeycomb arrangement of the mineralized matrix gives cancellous bone great strength with relatively little weight.

The bones of the skeleton can be called organs because they are composed of several tissues. Not only are they composed of bone tissue, they also have other connective tissues (e.g., hemopoietic and adipose tissues, blood vessels, nerves) and usually some sort of specialized articular regions (e.g., in the vertebrae; see the preceding). A layer of dense connective tissue called periosteum covers the outer surface of bones, except where there are specializations for the formation of a joint. The periosteum has a more fibrous outer layer with fibroblasts and type I collagen fibers. The inner layer is more cellular and consists mostly of osteoprogenitor cells. There are special bundles of periosteal collagen fibers called Sharpey's fibers that penetrate into the bone matrix and attach the periosteum to the bone. Periosteum contains a rich vascular supply and network of nerves. Endosteum is the

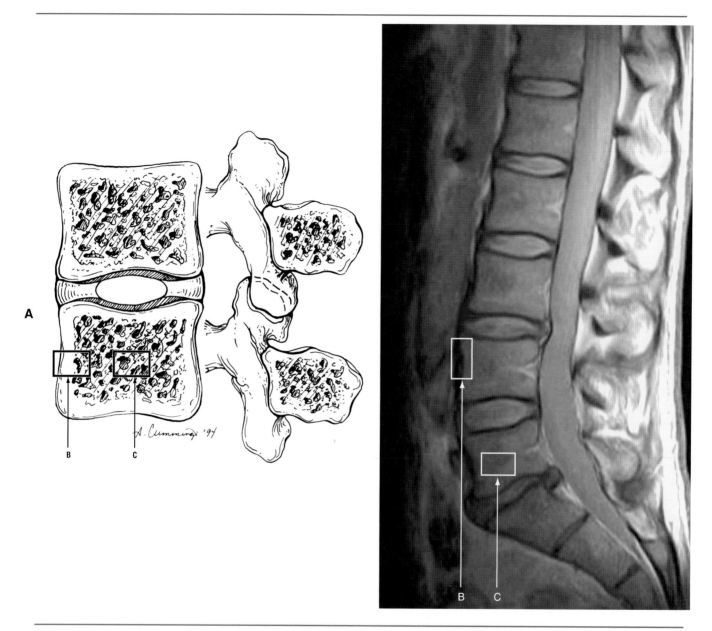

FIG. 14-20   Bone. **A,** Boxes indicate, *B,* cortical bone and, *C,* cancellous bone that are demonstrated in the corresponding parts of this figure.

connective tissue layer that lines the inner surface of bones and surrounds the marrow cavity. It is thinner than the periosteum, being mostly a single layer of osteoprogenitor cells with a minimal amount of extracellular matrix.

Skeletal Muscle

Muscle tissue is responsible for motion of the body as a whole and for the movements of various parts of the body in relation to each other. It is characterized by having elongated cells that are arranged parallel to one another. The primary physiologic property of muscle

tissue is the ability to contract or forcefully shorten the length of its cells. There are three types of muscle tissue that can be recognized in the body. Skeletal muscle has cylindrical, multinucleated cells that exhibit cross striations. It is found in the named muscles of the body and is under voluntary control. Cardiac muscle also has cross striations, but the cells are branched and each has only one nucleus. It is found exclusively in the myocardium of the heart and is involuntary. Smooth muscle has spindle-shaped cells with no cross striations. It is mostly found in the walls of viscera and the vascular system, in the arrector pili muscles of the skin, and in the intrinsic muscles of the eye. It is under autonomic and

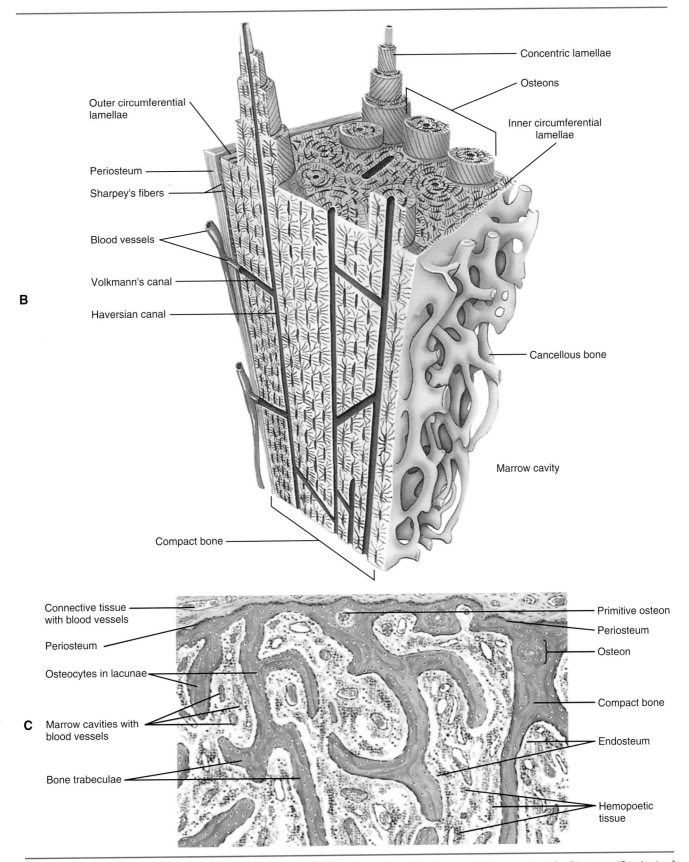

FIG. 14-20—cont'd   **B,** Illustration of cortical bone (compact bone). **C,** Light micrograph (approximately 40× magnification) of cancellous bone (spongy bone, trabecular bone). See text for details. (**B,** From Gartner LP & Hiatt JL. [2000.] *Color atlas of histology* [3rd ed.]. Philadelphia: Lippincott Williams & Wilkins. C, From Eroschenko VP. [2005]. *diFiore's atlas of histology with functional correlations* [10th ed.]. Philadelphia: Lippincott Williams & Wilkins.)

hormonal control. Although there is smooth muscle in the walls of the blood vessels in the back, and the skin of the back has arrector pili muscles, neither smooth nor cardiac muscle is discussed here.

Skeletal muscle cells are known as muscle fibers (Fig. 14-21). Do not confuse this use of the term fiber with connective tissue fibers. In muscle, the term fiber refers to a cell, but in connective tissue, fibers are extracellular structures that are produced by fibroblasts. Each skeletal muscle fiber is enveloped by endomysium, which is a thin layer of reticular fibers. Skeletal muscle fibers are found grouped into fascicles or bundles by thicker connective tissue layers. Each of these connective tissue layers is called a perimysium. There are various sizes and hierarchies of fascicles and their corresponding perimysia. These fascicles are continuous with the fascicles of the corresponding tendons of attachment for the muscle. An entire muscle is made up of a variable number of muscle fascicles that is entirely surrounded by a dense connective tissue layer called epimysium. The rich blood, lymphatic, and nerve supply of a muscle enters through and ramifies within these connective tissue layers. Also, these connective tissue layers, especially the endomysium, isolate each skeletal muscle fiber from its neighbors. This means that, unlike in cardiac and smooth muscle, each skeletal muscle fiber must be specifically stimulated to contract by the nervous system. This allows a great amount of control of the force produced by a muscle.

Each skeletal muscle fiber is multinucleated because it developed from the fusion of multiple cells known as myoblasts. Myoblasts forming the muscles in the region of the back are of mesenchymal origin (see Chapter 12). The nuclei of muscle fibers are elongated and characteristically found in the periphery of the cytoplasm, just below the sarcolemma or plasma membrane of the cell. The majority of the cytoplasm is filled with contractile elements known as myofibrils that extend the entire length of the muscle fiber (Ross et al., 2003). Myofibrils are composed of bundles of thick and thin myofilaments that are organized in a specific pattern. Each myofilament is composed of specific protein molecules (see the following). Surrounding each myofibril is a well-developed smooth endoplasmic reticulum known as the sarcoplasmic reticulum. Numerous mitochondria and glycogen deposits are in the regions between the myofibrils. The sarcolemma has numerous invaginations known as T (transverse) tubules that penetrate the cytoplasm to encircle each myofibril at regular intervals. Flanking the T tubules are expanded regions of the sarcoplasmic reticulum known as terminal cisternae. These function as Ca^{++} sinks. The sarcolemma can be depolarized by the neural stimulation at a special synapse known as the neuromuscular (myoneural) junction or motor end plate. A single axon may synapse with only one muscle fiber in muscles that need fine motor control (e.g., in some laryngeal muscles) or up to a couple hundred fibers in muscles that have more mass actions (e.g., quadriceps femoris muscles) (Junqueira and Carneiro, 2003).

When viewed in longitudinal section, skeletal muscle fibers exhibit cross striations of alternating light and dark bands (see Fig. 14-21). The dark bands are known as A bands because they are anisotropic to polarized light. The light bands are known as I bands because they are isotropic to polarized light. Sometimes visible at the light microscopic level, but more commonly seen at the ultrastructural level, are Z bands (discs or lines) (German, *zwischen,* between), which bisect the I bands. A sarcomere is the functional unit of organization of the myofilaments within the myofibril. A sarcomere runs from Z band to Z band. It is linear repetitions of these sarcomere units that form the myofibrils. The cross striations seen at the light microscopic level are the result of the sarcomeres being arranged in register between adjacent myofibrils.

At the electron microscopic level, each sarcomere can be seen to consist of several bands that are created by the relationships that the thin and thick myofilaments have with each other (see Fig. 14-21). The I band is made up of thin myofilaments whose ends are anchored in the Z band. The A band is composed of thick myofilaments. The A band is bisected by a lighter area known as the H band (German, *helle,* light). In the middle of the H band is a narrow, dense region known as the M band (disc or line) (German, *mitte,* middle). The M band represents the anchored region of the middle of the thick myofilaments and is the center of the sarcomere. The thick and thin myofilaments partially overlap each other; therefore the dark portion of the A band actually is the region of overlap and consists of both thick and thin myofilaments. The H band is the region of the sarcomere that contains only thick myofilaments.

Thin myofilaments are composed of three proteins: F actin, tropomyosin, and troponin. G (globular) actin monomers polymerize into double-stranded, helically arranged F (filamentous) actin. In the groove between the two strands is a myosin-binding site on each G actin. Tropomyosin is a filamentous protein that lies in the groove of F actin and sterically inhibits the myosin-binding sites of the actin. Troponin is a globular protein that attaches to tropomyosin and also has a Ca^{++}-binding site.

Thick myofilaments are composed of myosin that has a filamentous ("tail") portion and a globular ("head") portion. The tail portion is the part that is anchored at the M line. The head portion is located in the region of overlap of the thick and thin myofilaments and projects at nearly a right angle with respect to the tail portion of the molecule. The head has a binding site for actin and a binding site for ATP, which also acts as an ATPase.

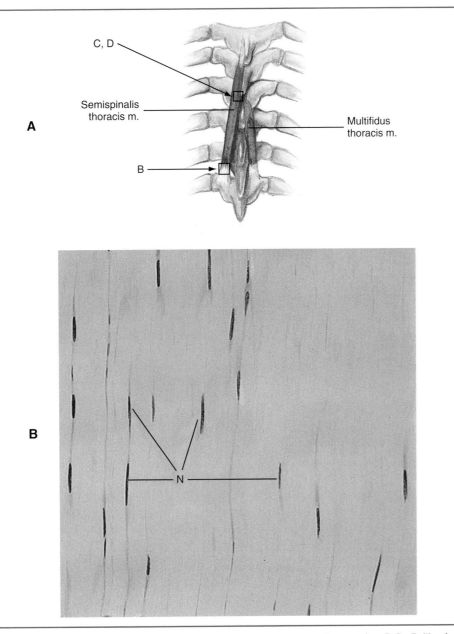

FIG. 14-21   Muscle and tendon. **A,** Boxes indicate the regions illustrated in **B-D. B,** Tendon (270× magnification). Notice the rows of elongated fibroblast nuclei (N) between tightly packed bundles of very regularly arranged collagen fibers.

Continued

Briefly the mechanism that explains how skeletal muscles contract that has received the most acceptance is the sliding filament hypothesis (Pollard and Earnshaw, 2002). The process is initiated when the sarcolemma is depolarized by neural activation of the neuromuscular junction. This depolarization is carried to the sarcoplasmic reticulum by the T tubules, which causes Ca^{++} release from the terminal cisternae. The Ca^{++} binds to troponin and causes a conformational change in that molecule. This conformational change in troponin causes the attached tropomyosin to shift position such that the myosin-binding site of actin is made available. Myosin and actin then bind to each other. Although there are many myosin heads projecting off a single thick myofilament, at any given time only a few are aligned in such a way that they can bind to actin. This binding of myosin and actin causes an ATP molecule (that is already bound to myosin) to be split into adenosine diphosphate (ADP) and Pi. The resultant release of energy causes a conformational change in the myosin head in relation to the

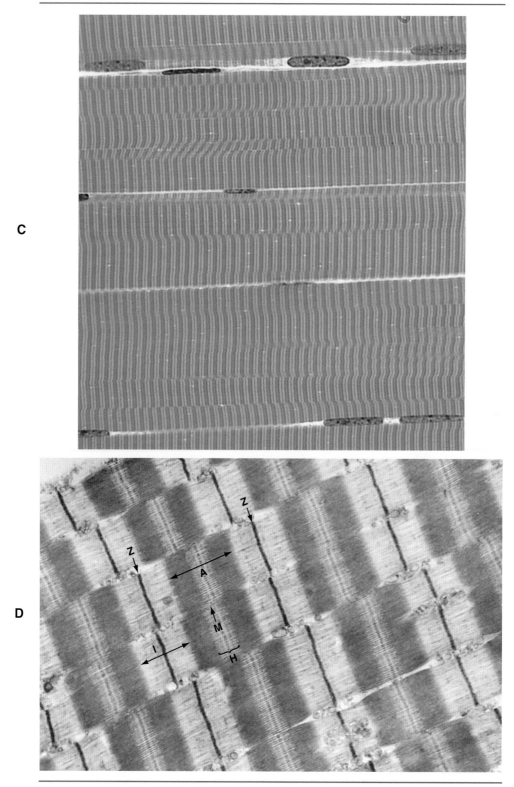

FIG. 14-21—cont'd **C,** Skeletal muscle (540× magnification). **D,** Ultrastructure of a sarcomere from skeletal muscle (approximately 130,000× magnification). The lines and bands have been labeled. See text for further details. (**B,** From Gartner LP & Hiatt JL. [2001]. *Color textbook of histology* [2nd ed.]. Philadelphia: Saunders. **D,** From Leeson TS & Leeson CR. [1981]. Histology [4th ed]. Philadelphia: W.B. Saunders.)

tail. This pulls the attached actin toward the center of the sarcomere, and creates contraction. The conformational change in the myosin head causes release of the ADP, and a new ATP molecule binds to the site. The binding of the new ATP molecule causes the release of actin and the myosin head to return to its original conformation. Therefore with contraction, the thin myofilaments are pulled and slide along the thick myofilaments toward the center of the sarcomere, hence the name of the hypothesis. This explains why the I and H bands get narrower and the Z bands get closer together during contraction. It must be remembered that a single muscle contraction ("twitch") is the result of hundreds of these binding and unbinding cycles.

Not only do muscles receive motor innervation, which stimulates contraction, but they also have sensory innervation. The specialized proprioceptive element in muscle is called a muscle spindle, from its fusiform shape. A muscle spindle consists of a connective tissue capsule that is filled with fluid. In the fluid-filled space are some specialized muscle fibers known as intrafusal fibers. The regular muscle fibers that make up the majority of the muscle sometimes are known as extrafusal fibers. There are two types of intrafusal fibers, based on the arrangement of their nuclei. In the nuclear bag cells, the nuclei are clumped in the center of the cell. In the other type of cell, known as nuclear chain cells, the nuclei form a row. Each intrafusal fiber has a sensory neuron terminal associated with the center of the cell. In addition, the ends of the intrafusal fibers, which have contractile capability, receive motor innervation in the form of a gamma motor neuron. Muscle spindles are stretch receptors (see Chapter 9).

Tendons also have sensory innervation that plays a role in proprioception. This is in the form of encapsulated receptors known as Golgi tendon organs. These receptors are typically found in the tendon near the tendon–muscle interface. Golgi tendon organs appear to signal tension on a tendon (see Chapter 9).

Neural Tissue

The nervous system is the chief organ system that correlates the adjustments and reactions of the body to internal and external environmental conditions. Anatomically it is divided into the central and peripheral nervous systems. The central nervous system (CNS) consists of the encephalon or brain and spinal medulla or cord. The peripheral nervous system (PNS) is the rest of the mass of neural tissue, which includes peripheral nerves, collections of nerve cell bodies known as ganglia, and specialized nerve endings. The nervous system also can be divided into functional units known as the somatic and autonomic nervous systems. The somatic nervous system supplies all of the parts of the body except viscera, smooth muscle, and glands. The autonomic nervous system supplies the targets that the somatic nervous system does not. It can be divided into a generally energy-mobilizing portion known as the sympathetic nervous system and a generally energy-sparing portion called the parasympathetic nervous system (see Chapter 10).

Nerve tissue is made up of two principal types of cells: neurons or nerve cells and neuroglia or supporting cells. Neurons are the functional units of the nervous system that can conduct electrochemical impulses known as action potentials. Action potentials are transient depolarizations of the cell membrane of the neuron. Neurons are arranged into networks in which the impulses travel from one part of the system to another. There are specialized contacts between neurons that allow the transmission of signals from one neuron to the next that are called synapses.

Neuroglia cells are the nonconducting cells of the nervous system. They serve to support the neurons in various ways that include physical protection, trophic functions, participation in impulse conduction, and, in the CNS, defense.

Neurons. The human nervous system contains more than 10 billion neurons (Ross et al., 2003). Functionally, there are three general categories of neurons: afferent, efferent, and interneurons. Afferent neurons carry information, generally sensory in nature, from the periphery into the CNS. Efferent neurons carry information, much of which is motor, from the CNS to targets in the periphery. Interneurons, which make up the vast majority of the neurons in the nervous system, communicate between neurons within the CNS.

Each neuron consists of a cell body and processes, known as axons and dendrites (Fig. 14-22). The cell body (soma or perikaryon) contains the nucleus of the cell. Unfortunately, a couple of terms can be confusing. The term nucleus can refer not only to the organelle of the neuron that contains the genetic material, but also it is the term used to denote a collection of nerve cell bodies within the CNS. The term neuron not only is used for the conductive cells of the nervous system, but also it is sometimes used to refer only to the nerve cell body. This latter definition of the term neuron is used more often when referring to the nerve cell bodies that are found in the nuclei of the CNS or in peripheral ganglia. Besides the nucleus of the cell, the cell body contains the usual cytoplasmic organelles present that maintain the cell. Prominent in the cytoplasm are stacks of rough endoplasmic reticulum called Nissl substance or bodies. These are necessary because neurons synthesize a large amount of proteins. Mitochondria also are represented in large numbers because of the high metabolic activity associated with neurons.

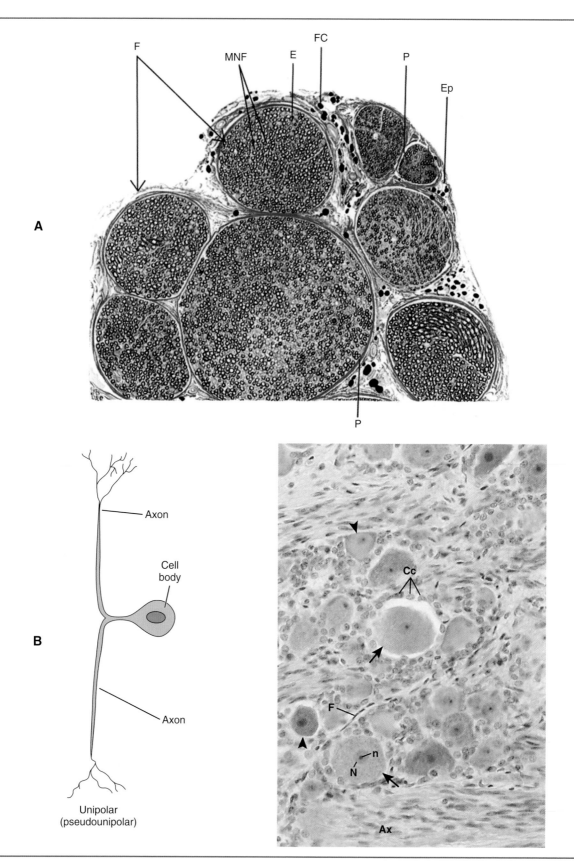

FIG. 14-22 Nervous tissue. **A,** Cross section of a peripheral nerve. *E,* Endoneurium; *Ep,* epineurium; *F,* fasciculi; *FC,* fat cells; *MNF,* myelinated nerve fibers; and, *P,* perineurium. **B,** Illustration, *left,* of a pseudounipolar neuron and a light micrograph (*right,* 270× magnification) of a dorsal root ganglion showing large (*arrows*) and small (*arrowheads*) cell bodies and cell processes (axons, Ax) of many such neurons. *F,* Fibroblasts; *Cc,* cell bodies of satellite cells; *N,* nucleus; and, *n,* nucleolus.

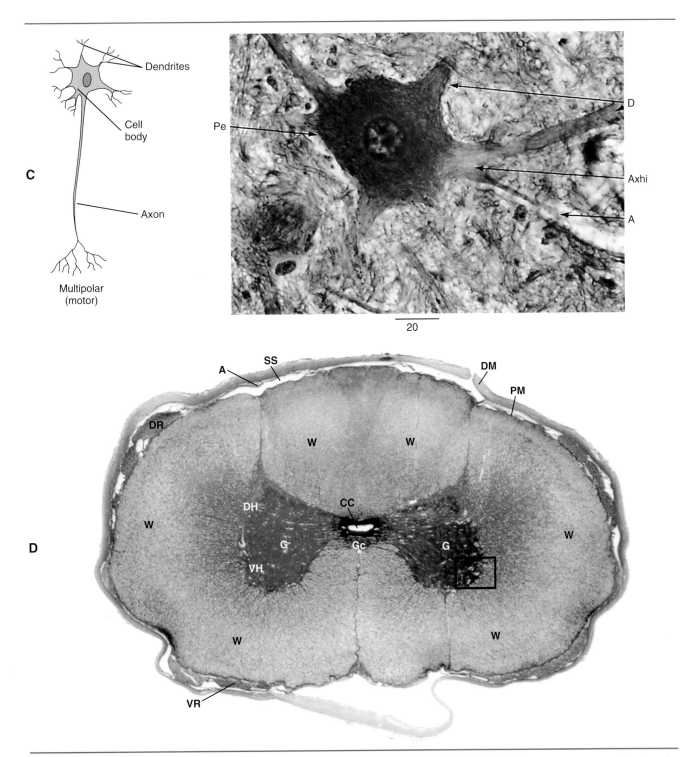

FIG. 14-22—cont'd   C, Illustration, *left,* of a multipolar neuron and a light micrograph (*right,* 612× magnification) showing the cell body (notice the axon hillock) and the proximal aspect of the cell processes (dendrites and axon) of a multipolar neuron. *A,* Axon; *Axhi,* axon hillock; *D,* dendrite; and, *Pe,* perikaryon. **D,** Cross section of the spinal cord (21× magnification) with inset (for **E**) demonstrating the interface between the ventral gray horn and the adjacent white matter (132× magnification). *A,* Arachnoid mater; *CC,* central canal; *DH,* dorsal horn; *DM,* dura mater; *DR,* dorsal root; *G,* gray matter; *Gc,* anterior gray commissure; *PM,* pia mater; *SS,* subarachnoid space; *VH,* ventral horn; *VR,* ventral root; and, *W,* white matter (approximately 10× magnification).

Continued

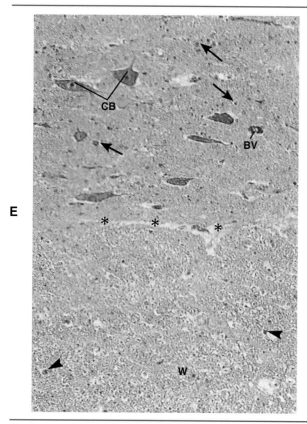

E

FIG. 14-22—cont'd   **E,** Region identified in the inset of **D.** This region includes both gray matter of the ventral horn of the spinal cord and the adjacent white matter, *W. BV,* Blood vessel; *CB,* cell bodies of multipolar neurons; *****, interface between gray and white matter; *arrowheads,* nuclei of glial cells within the white mater; and, *full arrows,* nuclei of glial cells within the gray matter (approximately 40 x magnification). (**A,** From Williams PL et al. [Eds.]. [1995]. *Gray's anatomy* [38th ed.]. Edinburgh: Churchill Livingstone. **B,** *left,* and, **C,** *left,* From Gartner LP & Hiatt JL. [2001]. *Color textbook of histology* [2nd ed.]. Philadelphia: Saunders. **B,** *right;* **D;** and **E;** From Gartner LP & Hiatt JL. [2000]. *Color atlas of histology* [3rd ed.]. Philadelphia; Lippincott Williams and Wilkins. C, right, From Bergmann RA & Afifi AK. [1974]. Atlas of microscopic anatomy: A companion to histology and neuroanatomy. Philadelphia: W.B. Saunders Company.

Besides a cell body, each neuron has a variable number of processes. Each neuron has a single axon that carries impulses away from the soma and forms a synapse (or synapses) where it contacts another neuron or other effector target. Most axons ramify distally such that a typical neuron in the CNS forms more than 1000 synapses (Kandel and Siegelbaum, 2000). The specific portion of the axon that helps form a synapse is known as the axon terminal or terminal bouton. The region of the cell body from which the axon arises is known as the axon hillock. There is a characteristic lack of Nissl substance in this region. Just distal to the axon hillock is the initial segment of the axon. It is in this location that action potentials are generated. Most axons are relatively long, as compared with dendrites, and many are myelinated. Neurons almost always have dendrites that carry impulses toward the soma. Typically dendrites are short, thicker in diameter than axons, and unmyelinated. In most neurons the dendrites ramify extensively into what is known as the dendritic tree. Neurons may be classified by the number of processes they have. Multipolar neurons have one axon and two or more dendrites. Motor neurons and interneurons typically have this morphology. Bipolar neurons have one axon and one dendrite. They are only found associated with the neural circuitry of the special senses. Pseudounipolar or unipolar neurons have a single process that is axonal in structure. Actually during development these cells had a separate dendrite and axon that fused together to make a single process attaching to the soma. This single process splits into a central process that enters the CNS and a peripheral process that terminates peripherally as a sensory receptor. Only primary afferent neurons have this arrangement.

Because most synthetic activity is restricted to the soma of the neurons, it is necessary to have an axonal transport system to move materials along the processes of the neuron, including dendrites. This transport system uses mostly microtubules and intermediate filaments to move materials. Axonal transport is a bidirectional system. Anterograde transport carries material from the soma to the periphery of the cell, whereas retrograde transport moves molecules from the periphery to the cell body. It has been shown that various types of materials in the cell are transported at different speeds such that both slow and fast axonal transport systems are recognized in neurons.

A synapse is the site of functional apposition between neurons, at which an impulse is transmitted from one neuron (the presynaptic neuron) to another (the postsynaptic neuron). Synapses are also found between neurons and their nonneural effector (target) cells (e.g., muscle or gland cells). Synapses may be formed between various parts of neurons. Most commonly they are axodendritic, in which a presynaptic axon forms a synapse with a postsynaptic dendrite. Many times in the CNS, the postsynaptic dendrite has a special structure for the synapse known as a dendritic spine that may help modify synaptic activity. Synapses may also form between axons and cell bodies of neurons (axosomatic) and between axons of two neurons (axoaxonic). In vertebrates, almost all synapses are chemical synapses in which the conduction of impulses from one neuron to the next is achieved by the release of a chemical neurotransmitter (e.g., acetylcholine, norepinephrine, and glycine) by the presynaptic terminal. The neurotransmitter diffuses across the synaptic cleft, which is the 20- to 30-nm space that separates the two neurons involved in the synapse. The neurotransmitter then may either excite (depolarize) or inhibit (hyperpolarize) the cell membrane of the postsynaptic neuron. This is achieved by interaction of the neurotransmitter with ion channels that are located in the postsynaptic membrane. These ion channels appear to be organized by an electron-dense structure known as the postsynaptic density. There are a few electrical synapses known as nexuses that can be found in certain places of the vertebrate CNS. These allow action potentials to spread directly from one neuron to the next and are structurally and functionally identical to the gap junctions that occur between cardiac muscle cells and between smooth muscle cells.

A typical neuron in the CNS is postsynaptic to or receives thousands of synapses (Kandel and Siegelbaum, 2000). Ultimately whether an action potential is generated in the postsynaptic neuron depends on the summation of all of the synaptic activity on the neuron. If the synaptic activity sufficiently depolarizes the cell membrane to reach threshold, an action potential is generated in the initial segment of the axon and carried by the axon to the synapse(s) for which it is presynaptic. If threshold is not reached, the cell does not generate an action potential, and the impulse from the presynaptic neurons is not passed along the neural circuit.

Neuroglia. There are approximately 10 times more neuroglia or glial cells than neurons in the mammalian nervous system (Junqueira and Carneiro, 2003). These supporting cells surround the nerve cell bodies and processes and furnish the microenvironment for the neurons. Sometimes only the supporting cells of the CNS are termed neuroglia, whereas the ones in the PNS are referred to only as supporting cells or peripheral neuroglia (Ross et al., 2003). The various types of neuroglia include the following:

◆ Schwann cells
◆ Oligodendrocytes
◆ Astrocytes
◆ Satellite cells
◆ Ependymal cells
◆ Microglia

Schwann cells are associated with axons in the PNS. These axons are called either myelinated or unmyelinated. If the axon is unmyelinated, it is embedded within a simple cleft in the Schwann cell (Ross et al., 2003). This helps maintain the microenvironment of the unmyelinated axon. Unlike with myelinated axons, a single Schwann cell may be associated with multiple unmyelinated axons. A lipid-rich layer known as the myelin sheath surrounds myelinated axons and acts as an insulator (or more correctly, a capacitor) for the axon, allowing saltatory proliferation of the action potentials

carried by the axon. The myelin sheath is composed of layers of the plasmalemma of the Schwann cells. Each Schwann cell wraps tightly around a single axon multiple times in a spiral fashion reminiscent of a cinnamon roll. The Schwann cell cytoplasm of each layer is removed such that the layers of the Schwann cell membrane fuse with each other to form the lipoprotein complex known as myelin. A thin cytoplasmic rim remains and surrounds the myelin. This rim is known as the neurilemma. Islands of cytoplasm found in the myelin sheath are known as clefts of Schmidt-Lanterman and appear to be necessary for Schwann cell maintenance. The myelin sheath is interrupted at intervals by the nodes of Ranvier. These gaps between adjacent Schwann cells are necessary for saltatory conduction of action potentials. Saltatory conduction causes the axon cell membrane in the gap between two Schwann cells to depolarize; the depolarization then "skips" from one gap to the next along the axon. Saltatory conduction dramatically increases the conduction velocity of axons.

Oligodendrocytes or oligodendroglia are associated with axons in the CNS. They provide the myelination for these axons in a way similar to that of Schwann cells in the PNS. Unlike Schwann cells, which surround a single axon, oligodendrocytes surround more than one axon. Oligodendrocytes have several dendritelike processes, hence the name of the cell, each of which surrounds an axon. There are other biochemical differences in the myelination of CNS versus PNS axons that may be involved in the lack of regenerative ability of CNS axons.

Astrocytes are support cells of the CNS. These are by far the most numerous type of glial cell. Each has a cell body with numerous processes giving it a starlike shape, hence the name. Cells with fewer, longer processes are known as fibrous astrocytes and are located in the white matter. Cells with more numerous, shorter processes are called protoplasmic astrocytes and are found in the gray matter. Astrocytes completely surround the neurons of the CNS, except where they are myelinated by the oligodendrocytes. Astrocytes have a unique type of intermediate filament made of glial fibrillar acidic protein that helps these cells provide strong structural support to the neurons. Astrocytes also help relate neurons to capillaries. In fact, some astrocytes have processes with expanded end-feet that attach to capillaries. These appear to have a role in maintaining the blood–brain barrier. Astrocytes appear to help regulate the movement of metabolites and wastes into and out of neurons along with controlling the ionic concentration of the extracellular compartment. Therefore astrocytes appear to play a major role in maintaining the microenvironment of the CNS neurons and their synapses.

Satellite cells surround the soma of neurons in peripheral ganglia. Ganglia or peripheral ganglia are collections of nerve cell bodies in the PNS. Satellite cells appear to have a similar function to Schwann cells associated with unmyelinated axons in the PNS or astrocytes in the CNS. They help establish and maintain the microenvironment of the cell bodies of neurons in the ganglia.

Ependymal cells form the simple cuboidal to columnar epithelial lining of the ventricles of the brain and the central canal of the spinal cord, which are the remnants of the lumen of the neural tube. The basal surfaces of the ependymal cells interdigitate with astrocyte processes. The apical surfaces of ependymal cells have cilia that may help move cerebrospinal fluid. Microvilli also can be found on the apical surface of these cells. These may be involved with absorption of cerebrospinal fluid.

Microglia are elongated cells that are relatively small and possess several irregular processes. They are actively phagocytic in regions of injury or disease. They represent the mononuclear phagocytic system in the CNS. As such they are derived from the bone marrow and migrate to the CNS by way of blood vessels.

Organization of the Central Nervous System.

As stated, the CNS consists of the brain and spinal cord. All of the cells of the CNS, with the exception of microglia, are derived from the neural tube (see Chapter 12). When sectioned and viewed with the naked eye, there are regions that look lighter in color (white matter) and darker in color (gray matter). White matter consists mostly of myelinated and unmyelinated nerve fibers along with their associated oligodendrocytes and astrocytes. The presence of large amounts of the fatty myelin is responsible for the lighter color. There are no neuron cell bodies in white matter. Gray matter is composed of nerve cell bodies, dendrites, axons (myelinated and unmyelinated), and associated glial cells. Sometimes the term neuropil is used to describe the mass of neuronal processes in the gray matter. Synapses are located in the regions of gray matter. The relative lack of myelin in these regions is responsible for their darker color. In much of the brain, the gray matter is located peripherally, whereas the white matter is more internal, although the regions of gray and white matter are not separated as simply in the brain stem. Discrete groups of functionally related nerve cell bodies in the gray matter in the CNS sometimes are called nuclei.

The relationship of the gray and white matter in the spinal cord is reversed when compared with that of most of the brain. The gray matter of the spinal cord is internal and forms the general shape of a capital H. The ventral cornua or horns contain neurons that are involved in motor function. Very large, multipolar neurons are located here that innervate skeletal muscles. The axons of these neurons form the ventral roots of the spinal nerves. The dorsal horns have neurons, most of which are relatively smaller in size, which are concerned with sensory functions. Sensory input into the dorsal horns enters by way of the dorsal roots of the spinal nerves. Several discrete nuclei are recognized in the gray matter of the spinal cord. In the center of the spinal cord is the central canal that is the remnant of the caudal portion of the neural tube lumen and is lined with ependymal cells.

The white matter surrounds the gray matter of the spinal cord. This tissue consists of various functionally related columns of fibers called tracts or fasciculi that mostly run in a vertical fashion to carry information to and from the brain. Other groups of fibers called commissures also connect structures on opposite sides of the spinal cord. Many other intersegmental fibers can be found in the white matter of the spinal cord.

Few connective tissues are associated within the brain and spinal cord, so they are soft and watery in nature; however, three layers of connective tissue, known as meninges (singular, meninx) surround the CNS. These layers are of mesenchymal origin. They are, from superficial to deep: dura mater, arachnoid, and pia mater. The dura mater or pachymeninx is the thickest and toughest. It consists of dense irregular collagenous connective tissue. Unlike around the brain, where it fuses with the inner periosteum of the skull, the dura mater surrounding the spinal cord is separated from the vertebrae by a fat-filled epidural space. The inner surface of the dura and also the outer surface in the region of the spinal canal are covered with a simple squamous epithelium. The dura mater has a rich blood supply and is innervated.

The other two layers of the meninges are thin compared with the dura mater and are sometimes collectively known as the leptomeninges. The arachnoid is a thin avascular layer of connective tissue that is loosely adherent to the dura and separated from the dura mater by a potential space. The arachnoid also has delicate trabeculae composed of loose connective tissue that connect it with the pia mater. These trabeculae give the arachnoid a spider-web appearance, hence the name. The regions between the trabeculae are collectively called the subarachnoid space. The subarachnoid space is filled with cerebrospinal fluid. Both inner and outer surfaces of the arachnoid, including the trabeculae, are lined with a simple squamous epithelium. The pia mater is a very thin layer of loose connective tissue that is intimately attached to the entire surface of the CNS. It also surrounds the perivascular connective tissue of the arteries and veins, but not capillaries, of the brain and spinal cord. The outer surface of the pia mater (facing the arachnoid) is lined with a simple squamous epithelium.

The capillaries of the CNS are less permeable to certain substances than in other parts of the body. This decreased permeability of these capillaries is termed the blood–brain barrier. It is mostly the result of occluding junctions between the endothelial cells, making these continuous-type capillaries. These occluding junctions are morphologically similar to tight junctions of other types of epithelia. The end-feet of astrocytes that are associated with these capillaries also seem to be involved in this blood–brain barrier, especially in maintaining water homeostasis in the CNS (Ross et al., 2003).

Organization of the Peripheral Nervous System. The main components of the PNS are nerves, ganglia, and nerve endings. Other than the nerve endings described previously (i.e., muscle spindles and Golgi tendon organs), the structure of the other types of nerve endings, which are mostly cutaneous in nature, is beyond the scope of this discussion. See Peripheral Receptors in Chapter 9 for a discussion of this topic.

Nerves, or peripheral nerves, are bundles of nerve fibers, usually both myelinated and unmyelinated, held together by connective tissue. Nerve fiber is a confusing term, because it can be defined in different ways. Most commonly the term nerve fiber refers to an axon with its associated coverings (e.g., myelin or Schwann cell). It also can be used to describe an axon only, whereas alternatively sometimes it is used to denote any process of a neuron, including both dendrites and axons. In the spinal nerves, the cell bodies for the motor axons are located in the anterior horn of the spinal cord. The cell bodies for the sensory nerve fibers are located in the dorsal root ganglion (see the following).

Surrounding each Schwann-cell ensheathed axon is a thin layer of reticular fibers called the endoneurium. These fibers appear to be produced by the Schwann cells, because there is a lack of fibroblasts in the vicinity. The fibers run both parallel to and around the axons, functionally binding them into fascicles. Around each fascicle of axons is the perineurium. It is made up of one or more layers of flattened epithelial-like cells. When there is more than one layer of perineurial cells (e.g., in the larger-caliber nerve fascicles) these cells appear to produce collagen fibers. They may even be contractile, given the large amount of actin found in their cytoplasm (Ross et al., 2003). Tight junctions connect the perineurial cells. Therefore perineurium acts as a metabolic diffusion barrier for the nerve fibers and establishes a blood–nerve barrier similar to the blood–brain barrier of the CNS. This protective function of the perineurium seems important to the normal functioning of peripheral nerves. In fact, there is a dearth of classic connective tissue cells, including most immune system cells, within peripheral nerves. About the only cells other than Schwann cells that can be found within a peripheral nerve are the occasional fibroblast and some mast cells. Surrounding the entire nerve is a relatively thick, dense, irregular collagenous connective tissue layer known as the epineurium. In larger nerves adipose tissue may be associated with the epineurium. Blood vessels (vasi nervorum) and nerves (nervi nervorum) supplying the nerve penetrate into the epineurium and travel in the perineurium. The tissue at the level of the endoneurium is poorly vascularized, and metabolic exchange must happen through diffusion from the perineurium. In the region of the intervertebral foramen, the epineurium of the spinal nerves becomes continuous with the dural root sleeve surrounding the spinal nerve roots (see Chapter 3).

Ganglia are collections of nerve cell bodies in the PNS that have a connective tissue framework and capsule for support. There are two varieties of ganglia. The first is sensory ganglia. The neuronal cells in these ganglia are pseudounipolar. Each cell body is surrounded by cuboidal-shaped satellite cells. The fibers associated with sensory ganglia are the peripheral and central processes of the pseudounipolar neurons. These fibers only travel through the ganglion and do not synapse. Dorsal root ganglia are the example of this type of ganglion in the region of the back. The second type of ganglion is the autonomic ganglion. The cell bodies of the multipolar postganglionic autonomic neurons reside in these ganglia. Usually there is a layer of relatively flattened satellite cells surrounding the cell bodies of these neurons. Unlike the sensory ganglia, in which no synapses occur, there is an abundance of synapses in autonomic ganglia. These are where the axons of preganglionic autonomic neurons synapse with the dendrites of the postganglionic autonomic neurons. The ganglia of the sympathetic gangliated chains are examples of this type of ganglion in the region of the back.

REFERENCES

Antoniou J et al. (1996). The human lumbar end plate. *Spine, 21,* 1153-1161.

Antonopoulos CA et al. (1964). Determination of glycosaminoglycans from tissue on the microgram scale. *Biochem Biophys Acta, 83,* 1-19.

Antonopoulos CA et al. (1974). Extraction and purification of proteoglycans from various types of connective tissue. *Biochem Biophys Acta, 338,* 108-119.

Bishop P. (1992). Pathophysiology of the intervertebral disc. In S Haldeman (Ed.). *Principles and practice of chiropractic* (2nd ed.). East Norwalk, Conn: Appleton & Lange.

Bloom W & Fawcett D. (1986). *Textbook of histology* (3rd ed.). Philadelphia: WB Saunders.

Bogduk N. (1990). Pathology of lumbar disc pain. *Manual Med, 5,* 72-79.

Bogduk N. (1997). *Clinical anatomy of the lumbar spine.* London: Churchill Livingstone.

Bogduk N et al. (1981). The nerve supply to the human lumbar intervertebral discs. *J Anat, 132,* 39-56.

Boos N et al. (2002). Classification of age-related changes in lumbar intervertebral discs: 2002 Volvo award in basic science. *Spine, 27,* 2631-2644.

Boszczyk BM et al. (2001). An immunohistochemical study of the dorsal capsule of the lumbar and thoracic facet joints. *Spine, 26,* E338-E343.

Broberg KB. (1983). On the mechanical behavior of intervertebral disc. *Spine, 8,* 151-161.

Brown MD. (1971). The pathophysiology of disc disease. *Orthop Clin North Am, 2,* 359-370.

Chai Ben-Fu & Tang Xue-Ming. (1987). Electron microscopic observation of normal, protruding and ruptured lumbar intervertebral discs. *Chin Med J, 100(9),* 723-730.

Chandraraj S, Briggs CA, & Opeskin K. (1998). Disc herniations in the young and end-plate vascularity. *Clin Anat, 11(3),* 171-176.

Cole TC, Ghosh P, & Taylor TK. (1986). Variations of the proteoglycans of the canine intervertebral disk with aging. *Biochem Biophys Acta, 19,* 209-219.

Coppes MH et al. (1997). Innervation of 'painful' lumbar discs. *Spine, 22,* 2342-2349.

Crean JKG et al. (1997). Matrix metalloproteinases in the human intervertebral disc: Role in disc degeneration and scoliosis. *Spine, 22,* 2877-2884.

Crock HV. (1986). Internal disc disruption: A challenge to disc prolapse fifty years on. *Spine, 1,* 650-653.

Duance VC et al. (1998). Changes in collagen cross-linking in degenerative disc disease and scoliosis. *Spine, 23,* 2545-2551.

Ghosh P. (1990). Basic biochemistry of the intervertebral disc and its variation with ageing and degeneration. *J Man Med, 5,* 48-51.

Giles LG. (1992a). The pathophysiology of the zygapophysial joints. In S Haldeman (Ed.). *Principles and practice of chiropractic* (2nd ed.). East Norwalk, Conn: Appleton & Lange.

Giles LG. (1992b). The surface lamina of the articular cartilage of human zygapophyseal joints. *Anat Rec, 233,* 350-356.

Giles LG & Taylor JR. (1987). Human zygapophyseal joint capsule and synovial fold innervation. *Br J Rheumatol, 26,* 93-98.

Gower WE & Pedrini V. (1969). Age related variations in protein polysaccharides from human nucleus pulposus, anulus fibrosus, and costal cartilage. *J Bone Joint Surg, 51,* 1154-1162.

Gruber H & Hanley EJ. (1998). Analysis of aging and degeneration of the human intervertebral disc: Comparison of surgical specimens with normal controls. *Spine, 23,* 751-757.

Gruber HE & Hanley Jr. EN (2002). Ultrastructure of the human intervertebral disc during aging and degeneration: Comparison of surgical and control specimens. *Spine, 27,* 798-805.

Hamanishi C et al. (1994). Schmorl's nodes on magnetic resonance imaging. Their incidence and clinical relevance. *Spine, 19(4),* 450-453.

Handa T et al. (1997). Effects of hydrostatic pressure on matrix synthesis and matrix metalloproteinase production in the human lumbar intervertebral disc. *Spine, 22,* 1085-1091.

Hardingham TE & Adams PA. (1976). A method for the determination of hyaluronate in the presence of glycosaminoglycans and its application to human intervertebral disc. *Biochem J, 159,* 143-147.

Herzog RJ. (1996). The radiologic assessment for a lumbar disc herniation. *Spine, 21,* 19S-38S.

Horner HA & Urban JP. (2001). 2001 Volvo Award Winner in Basic Science Studies: Effect of nutrient supply on the viability of cells from the nucleus pulposus of the intervertebral disc. *Spine, 26(23),* 2543-2549.

Hutton WC et al. (1997). Analysis of chondroitin sulfate in lumbar intervertebral discs at two different stages of degeneration as assessed by discogram. *J Spinal Disord, 10,* 47-54.

Hutton WC et al. (1998). The effect of compressive force applied to the intervertebral disc in vivo: A study of proteoglycans and collagen. *Spine, 23,* 2524-2537.

Hutton WC et al. (1999). The effect of hydrostatic pressure on intervertebral disc metabolism. *Spine, 24(15),* 1507-1515.

Hutton WC et al. (2002). Effect of tail suspension (or simulated weightlessness) on the lumbar intervertebral disc: Study of proteoglycans and collagen. *Spine, 27(12),* 1286-1290.

Inerot S & Axelsson I. (1991). Structure and composition of proteoglycans from human anulus fibrosus. *Connect Tissue Res, 26,* 47-63.

Iwahashi M. (2002). Mechanism of intervertebral disc degeneration caused by nicotine in rabbits to explicate intervertebral disc disorders caused by smoking. *Spine, 27(13),* 1396-1401.

Johnson WEB et al. (2001). Immunohistochemical detection of Schwann cells in innervated and vascularized human intervertebral discs. *Spine, 26,* 2550-2557.

Junqueira LC & Carneiro JCL. (2003). *Basic histology* (10th ed.). New York: Lange Medical Books McGraw-Hill.

Kandel ER & Siegelbaum SA. (2000). Overview of synaptic transmission. In ER Kandel et al. (Eds.). *Principles of neural science* (4th ed.). New York: McGraw-Hill.

Kang JD et al. (1996). Herniated lumbar intervertebral discs spontaneously produce matrix metalloproteinases, nitric oxide, interleukin-6, and prostaglandin E2. *Spine, 21,* 271-277.

Kang JD et al. (1997). Toward a biochemical understanding of human intervertebral disc degeneration and herniation: Contributions of nitric oxide, interleukins, prostaglandin E$_2$, and matrix metalloproteinases. *Spine, 22,* 1065-1073.

Kauppila LI et al. (1997). Disc degeneration/back pain and calcification of the abdominal aorta: A 25-year follow-up study in Framingham. *Spine, 22,* 1642-1649.

Kim KW et al. (2003). The origin of chondrocytes in the nucleus pulposus and histologic findings associated with the transition of a notochordal nucleus pulposus to a fibrocartilaginous nucleus pulposus in intact rabbit intervertebral discs. *Spine, 28(10),* 982-990.

Kirkaldy-Willis WH. (1988). The pathology and pathogenesis of low back pain. In W Kirkaldy-Willis (Ed.). *Managing low back pain* (2nd ed.). New York: Churchill Livingstone.

Kraemer J. (1995). Natural course and prognosis of intervertebral disc diseases. International Society for the Study of the Lumbar Spine Seattle, Washington, June 1994. *Spine, 20(6),* 635-639.

Lotz JC et al. (1998). Compression-induced degeneration of the intervertebral disc: An in vivo mouse model and finite-element study. *Spine, 23,* 2493-2506.

Lotz JC, Chin BA, & Urban JP. (2000). Intervertebral disc cell death is dependent on the magnitude and duration of spinal loading. *Spine, 25,* 1477-1483.

Luschka H. (1856). Die altersveranderungen der zwischenwirbellnorpel. *Virchows Arch, 11,* 8.

Luschka H. (1857). Uber gallertartige auswuchse am clivus blumenbachii. *Virchows Arch, 11,* 8.

Maeda S & Kokubun S. (2000). Changes with age in proteoglycan synthesis in cells cultured in vitro from the inner and outer rabbit annulus fibrosus. Responses to interleukin-1 and interleukin-1 receptor antagonist protein. *Spine, 25(2),* 166-169.

Malinsky J. (1959). The ontogenetic development of nerve terminations in the intervertebral discs of man. *Acta Anat, 38,* 96-113.

Maroudas A et al. (1975). Factors involved in the nutrition of the human intervertebral disc. *J Anat, 120,* 13-130.

McDevitt CA. (1988). Proteoglycans of the intervertebral disc. In P Ghosh (Ed.). *Biology of the intervertebral disc.* Boca Raton, Fla: CRC Press.

Mooney V & Robertson J. (1976). The facet syndrome. *Clin Orthop Res, 115,* 149-156.

Moore RJ et al. (1996). The origin and fate of herniated lumbar intervertebral disc tissue. *Spine, 21,* 2149-2155.

Nachemson A et al. (1970). In vitro diffusion of dye through the end plates and the annulus fibrosus of human lumbar intervertebral disks. *Acta Orthop Scand, 41,* 589-607.

Nishida K et al. (1999). Modulation of the biologic activity of the rabbit intervertebral disc by gene therapy: An in vivo study of adenovirus-mediated transfer of the human transforming growth factor β1 encoding gene. *Spine, 24,* 2419.

Oda J, Tamaka H, & Tsukuki N. (1988). Intervertebral disk changes with aging of human cervical vertebra: From the neonate to the eighties. *Spine, 13,* 1205-1211.

Pate D. (1991). Roentgen report: Schmorl's nodes. *MPI's Dynam Chiro,* Sept. 13.

Peacock A. (1951). Observation on the prenatal development of the intervertebral disc in man. *J Anat, 185,* 260-274.

Pollard TD & Earnshaw WC. (2002). *Cell biology.* Philadelphia: WB Saunders.

Poiraudeau S et al. (1999). Phenotypic characteristics of rabbit intervertebral disc cells. Comparison with cartilage cells from the same animals. *Spine, 24,* 837-844.

Pritzker PH. (1977). Aging and degeneration in the lumbar intervertebral disc. *Orthop Clin, 8,* 65-77.

Roberts S et al. (1989). Biochemical and structural properties of the vertebral end plate and its relation to the intervertebral disc. *Spine, 14,* 166-174.

Roberts S et al. (1996). Transport properties of the human cartilage end plate in relation to its composition and calcification. *Spine, 21(4),* 415-420.

Ross MH et al. (2003). *Histology* (4th ed.). Baltimore: Lippincott Williams & Wilkins.

Sachs BL et al. (1987). Dallas discogram description: A new classification of CT/discography in low-back disorders. *Spine, 12,* 287-294.

Schollmeier G, Lahr-Eigen R, & Lewandrowski KU. (2000). Observations on fiber-forming collagens in the anulus fibrosus. *Spine, 25(21),* 2736-2741.

Stevens RL, Dondi PG, & Muir H. (1979). Proteoglycans of the intervertebral disk: Absence of degradation during the isolation of proteoglycans from the intervertebral disk. *Biochem J, 179,* 573-578.

Swann DA et al. (1974). Role of hyaluronic acid in joint lubrication. *Annu Rev Dis, 33,* 318-326.

Taylor JR & Twomey LT. (1986). Age changes in lumbar zygapophyseal joints: Observations on structure and function. *Spine, 11,* 739-745.

Taylor JR. (1990). The development and adult structure of lumbar intervertebral discs. *J Man Med, 5,* 43-47.

Triano J. (1992). Interaction of spinal biomechanics and physiology. In S Haldeman (Ed.). *Principles and practice of chiropractic* (2nd ed.). East Norwalk, Conn: Appleton & Lange.

Trout JJ et al. (1982). Ultrastructure of the human intervertebral disc. I. Changes in notochordal cells with age. *Tissue Cell, 14(2),* 359-369.

Vernon-Roberts B & Pirie CJ. (1977). Degenerative changes in the intervertebral disks of the lumbar spine and their sequelae. *Rheumatol Rehabil, 16,* 13-21.

Virchow RL. (1857). *Untersuchung uber die entwickelung des schadel grindes in gesunden und krankhaften zustande und uber den eintfuss derselben auf schadelform, gesichsbildun und gehirnbau.* Berlin: G. Reimer.

Weiss L. (1988). *Histology* (6th ed.). New York: McGraw-Hill.

Williams PL et al. (1995). *Gray's anatomy* (38th ed.). Edinburgh: Churchill Livingstone.

Woelf HJ et al. (1975). Role of the notochord in human intervertebral disc. I. Fetus and infant. *Clin Orthop Rel Res, 39,* 205-212.

Wyke B. (1987). The neurology of back pain. In MIV Jayson (Ed.). *The lumbar spine and back pain* (3rd ed.). New York: Churchill Livingstone.

Xu GL et al. (1991). Normal variations of the lumbar facet joint capsules. *Clin Anat, 4,* 117-122.

Yamashita T et al. (1996). A morphological study of the fibrous capsule of the human lumbar facet joint. *Spine, 21,* 538-543.

Yoshizawa H, O'Brien J, & Thomas-Smith W. (1980). The neuropathology of the intervertebral discs removed for low back pain. *J Pathol, 132,* 95.

Index

Page numbers with "t" denote tables, those with "f" denote figures, and those with "b" denote boxes.